Quick Reference to Standard Protocols for All Nursing Interventions

All nursing skills must include certain basic steps for the safety and well-being of the client and the nurse. To prevent repetition, these steps are referred to at the beginning and end of each skill as standard protocols. The complete Standard Protocols include the essential steps that must be done consistently with each client contact in order to deliver responsible and safe nursing care.

BEFORE THE SKILL

1. **Verify physician's orders if skill is a dependent or collaborative nursing intervention.** Independent nursing interventions are verified with the nursing care plan or primary nurse. *Dependent and collaborative interventions include the most invasive procedures, such as medication administration and urinary catheterization.*

2. **Gather equipment/supplies and complete necessary charges according to agency policy.** Some equipment is reusable and is kept at the bedside. Some equipment is disposable and charged to the client as used. *Check agency policy.*

   SUPPLIES for all nursing interventions:
   - Armband (or picture) for client identification.
   - Consent Form if required by agency policy.
   - Clean gloves if contact with mucous membranes, nonintact skin, or moist body substances is anticipated. (Prior to selecting gloves, determine if client/nurse has a latex allergy and select nonlatex gloves).

3. **Perform hand hygiene for at least 10-15 seconds before each client contact.** (See Hand Hygiene, Chapter 4). *Check manufacturer's label for recommended duration for specific products.*

4. **Identify the client by checking identification bracelet and having the client state name (if able to do so).** Use at least two client identifiers (neither to be the client's room number). In many long-term care settings, identification bracelets are not used; however, pictures are available for identification. *Clients with difficulty hearing or altered level of consciousness may answer to a name other than their own. Additional bracelets may also be used to indicate safety concerns, such as allergies.*

5. **Introduce yourself to client (and family), including your name and title or role.** In this text "family" is used in an expanded sense to include husband/wife, domestic partner, or significant others. *Clients have the right to know the credentials of the persons providing their care.*

6. **Explain what you plan to do.** *Understanding what is being done reduces clients' level of anxiety and enhances their ability to cooperate.*

7. **Identify tea... e client can expect i...**

8. **Assess client ... h the intervention is still appropriate.** *Eac... ncludes assessment to indicate specific assessment indicated. Check for allergies as appropriate.*

9. **Adjust the bed to appropriate height and lower side rail on the side nearest you.** *Check locks on the bed wheel. Minimizes caregiver's muscle strain and prevents injury. Prevents bed from moving.*

10. **Provide adequate lighting for procedure.** *Ensures adequate illumination of client's body and equipment.*

11. **Provide privacy for client. Position and drape client as needed.**

DURING THE SKILL

12. **Promote client independence and involvement if possible.** *Participation enhances client motivation and cooperation.*

13. **Assess client tolerance. Be alert for signs of discomfort and fatigue.** *Ability to tolerate interventions varies depending on severity of illness or pain. Use nursing judgment to provide rest and comfort measures.*

COMPLETION PROTOCOL (END OF SKILL)

14. **Assist client to a position of comfort, and organize needed toiletry or personal items within reach.**

15. **Be certain client has a way to call for help and knows how to use it.** *Minimizes risk of falls.*

16. **Raise the appropriate number of side rails and lower the bed to the lowest position.** Nursing judgment may allow alert, cooperative clients to have side rails down.

17. **Dispose of used supplies and equipment.** Leave client room tidy. (*See CDC Guidelines, Chapter 4.*)

18. **Remove and dispose of gloves, if used. Perform hand hygiene for at least 10 to 15 seconds.** *Wearing gloves does not eliminate the need for hand hygiene.*

19. **Document and report client's response and expected or unexpected outcomes.** *Enhances continuity of nursing care.*

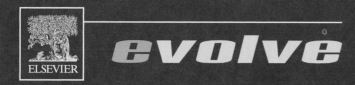

ELSEVIER *evolve*

Nursing Interventions & Clinical Skills

Thanks to my family, especially Mary Ann, Jess, and Kim
who are always ready to give guidance and support
in the challenges and changes that life brings
and
to the Associate Degree Nursing Faculty
who provide inspiration and motivation for student nurses
as they make the challenging transition toward competency in nursing practice.

MARTHA KEENE ELKIN

To the clinical nurses at the bedside, the nurse educators,
and the nurse researchers who work together to maintain excellence in nursing.

ANNE GRIFFIN PERRY

To my new professional colleagues, the nurses of Siteman Cancer Center.
They are a unique group of professionals who spend each day
pursuing excellence in patient and family care.

PATRICIA A. POTTER

NURSING INTERVENTIONS & CLINICAL SKILLS

4th EDITION

Martha Keene Elkin, RN, MSN, IBCLC

Nursing Educator for Associate Degree Nursing
Private Practice Lactation Consultant
Mother Care of Maine, Comprehensive Breastfeeding Services
Sumner, Maine

Anne Griffin Perry, RN, MSN, EdD, FAAN

Professor and Chairperson, Department of Primary Care and Health Systems Nursing
Southern Illinois University
Edwardsville, Illinois

Patricia A. Potter, RN, PhD, FAAN, CMAC

Research Scientist
Siteman Cancer Center
Barnes-Jewish Hospital
St. Louis, Missouri

with over 900 illustrations

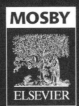

MOSBY

ELSEVIER

MOSBY
ELSEVIER

11830 Westline Industrial Drive
St. Louis, Missouri 63146

NURSING INTERVENTIONS & CLINICAL SKILLS

ISBN 978-0-323-04458-5

Notice

Knowledge and best practice in this field are constantly changing. As new research and experience broaden our knowledge, changes in practice, treatment and drug therapy may become necessary or appropriate. Readers are advised to check the most current information provided (i) on procedures featured or (ii) by the manufacturer of each product to be administered, to verify the recommended dose or formula, the method and duration of administration, and contraindications. It is the responsibility of the practitioner, relying on their own experience and knowledge of the patient, to make diagnoses, to determine dosages and the best treatment for each individual patient, and to take all appropriate safety precautions. To the fullest extent of the law, neither the Publisher nor the Authors assumes any liability for any injury and/or damage to persons or property arising out or related to any use of the material contained in this book.

Previous editions copyrighted 2004, 2000, 1996.

International Standard Book Number 978-0-323-04458-5

Executive Editor: Susan R. Epstein
Senior Developmental Editors: Robyn L. Brinks, Jean Sims Fornango
Editorial Assistant: Mary Jo Adams
Publishing Services Manager: John Rogers
Senior Project Manager: Cheryl A. Abbott
Senior Designer: Julia Dummitt

Printed in Canada

Last digit is the print number: 9 8 7 6 5 4 3 2

Barbara J. Berger, RN, MSN
Clinical Nurse Specialist
Southwest General Health Center Partnering with
    University Hospitals Health System
Middleburg Heights, Ohio

Janice C. Colwell, RN, MS, CWOCN
Clinical Nurse Specialist/Wound, Ostomy, and Skin Care
University of Chicago
Chicago, Illinois

Kelly Jo Cone, RN, BSN, MS, PhD, CNE
Associate Professor, Graduate Program
Saint Francis Medical Center College of Nursing
Peoria, Illinois

Karen S. Conners, RNC, MSN
Nurse Practitioner
Wildwood, Missouri

Wanda Cleveland Dubuisson, RN, PhD(c)
Associate Professor and Director of Graduate Program
Joseph and Nancy Fail School of Nursing at William Carey
    University
Hattiesburg, Mississippi

Susan Fetzer, BA, BSN, MSN, MBA, PhD
Associate Professor
University of New Hampshire
Durham, New Hampshire

Amy Hall, RN, PhD
Associate Professor and Chair, Department of Nursing and
    Health Sciences
University of Evansville
Evansville, Indiana

Maureen B. Huhmann, MS, RD
Assistant Professor
University of Medicine and Dentistry of New Jersey
New Brunswick, New Jersey;
Clinical Dietician
The Cancer Institute of New Jersey
New Brunswick, New Jersey

Kristine M. L'Ecuyer, RN, MSN, CCNS
Associate Professor
Saint Louis University School of Nursing
St. Louis, Missouri

Constance C. Maxey, RN-BC, MSN
Practice Consultant
Barnes-Jewish Hospital
St. Louis, Missouri

Peter R. Miller, RN, MSN, ONC
Instructor
Central Maine Medical Center School of Nursing
Lewiston, Maine

Karen Montalto, RN, DNSc
Coordinator, Non-Traditional Nursing Programs School/
    Hospital
Neumann College
Aston, Pennsylvania

Kim Campbell Oliveri, RN, MS, CS
Clinical Nurse Specialist
Beth Israel Deaconess Medical Center
Boston, Massachusetts

Wendy R. Ostendorf, RN, EdD
Associate Professor of Nursing
Neumann College
Aston, Pennsylvania

Shirley E. Otto, MSN, CRNI, OCN, AOCN
Oncology Practice Development Specialist
Via Christi Regional Medical Center
Wichita, Kansas

Jacqueline Raybuck Saleeby, RN, PhD, BCCS
Associate Professor
Barnes-Jewish College of Nursing
St. Louis, Missouri

Lynn Schallom, RN, MSN, CCRN, CCNS
Surgical Critical Care Clinical Nurse Specialist
Barnes-Jewish Hospital
St. Louis, Missouri

Kelly Schwartz, RN, BSN
Practice Consultant
Barnes-Jewish Hospital
St. Louis, Missouri

Julie Snyder, RN, MSN, BC
Adjunct Instructor
Old Dominion University School of Nursing
Norfolk, Virginia

Patricia A. Stockert, RN, PhD
Associate Dean Undergraduate Program
Saint Francis Medical Center College of Nursing
Peoria, Illinois

Donna L. Thompson, MSN, CRNP, BC, CCCN
Assistant Professor
Neumann College
Aston, Pennsylvania;
Continence Specialist
FairAcres Geriatric Center
Lima, Pennsylvania

Paula Vehlow, RN, MS
Professor
Lincoln Land Community College
Springfield, Illinois

Terry Wood, RN, PhD
Assistant Professor
Barnes-Jewish College of Nursing
St. Louis, Missouri

Rita Wunderlich, RN, MSN, PhD
Assistant Professor
Saint Louis University School of Nursing
St. Louis, Missouri

Rhonda Yancey, RN, BSN
Practice Consultant
Barnes-Jewish Hospital
St. Louis, Missouri

Valerie J. Yancey, RN, PhD, CHPN, HNC
Associate Professor
Southern Illinois University Edwardsville
Edwardsville, Illinois

Reviewers

JoAnn Acierno, RN, BSN
Assistant Professor, BSN Program
Clarkson College
Omaha, Nebraska

Joni Adams, RN, ADN, BSN, MSN
Assistant Professor
Ivy Tech Community College of Indiana
Evansville, Indiana

Colleen Andreoni, APRN, BC-NP
Nurse Practitioner
Rife & Associates Family Medicine
Orland Park, Illinois

Sylvia Baird, RN, BSN, MM
Manager Patient Safety
Spectrum Health
Grand Rapids, Michigan

Andrea Baptiste, MA, CIE
Biomechanist/Ergonomist
James A Haley VA Hospital
Tampa, Florida

Doris Bartlett, BSN, MS
Assistant Professor
Bethel College
Mishawaka, Indiana

M. J. Basti, RN, MSN
Instructor, Health Education
Cuesta Community College
San Luis Obispo, California

Julie Baylor, RN, PhD
Assistant Professor
Bradley University
Peoria, Illinois

Joanne Bonesteel, RN, MS
Nursing Faculty
Associate Degree Program
Excelsior College School of Nursing
Albany, New York

Greg Brooks, MS, ARNP
Instructor
Nurse Practitioner Program
University of Oklahoma College of Nursing
Oklahoma City, Oklahoma

Sheryl Kathleen Buckner, RN, MS
Academic and Staff Developer and Clinical Instructor
University of Oklahoma College of Nursing
Oklahoma City, Oklahoma

Jeanie Burt, RN, MSN, MA
Assistant Professor
Harding University College of Nursing
Searcy, Arkansas

Shari Clarke, APRN, MSN
Clinical Faculty
Kennesaw State University
Kennesaw, Georgia;
Adjunct Faculty
Georgia State University
Atlanta, Georgia

Susan S. Erue, RN, BSN, MS, PhD
Professor and Chair
Division of Nursing
Iowa Wesleyan College
Mt. Pleasant, Iowa

Sharon Lyon Garcia, RN, BSN
Nursing Program Director, PNE
McDowell Technical Community College
Marion, North Carolina

Yvette Conerly Glenn, MSN, FNP-C, CWS, APRN
Wound Care Specialist
VA Illiana HealthCare System
Danville, Illinois

Stephanie C. Greer, RN, MSN
Associate Degree Nursing Instructor
Southwest Mississippi Community College
Summit, Mississippi

Adrienne Hentemann, RN, BSN, MS
Administrative Care Services Manager
Spectrum Health
Grand Rapids, Michigan

Monica M. Hentemann, BSN, OCN
Registered Nurse
Spectrum Health
Grand Rapids, Michigan

Patricia J. Hutchison, RN, MSN, CDE
Education Coordinator
Grove City Medical Center
Grove City, Pennsylvania

Susie Huyer, RN, MSN
Faculty
University of Phoenix Online;
Administrator
Heartland Hospice
Fairfax, Virginia

Linda Kerby, BSN, MA, BA, RNC
Educational Consultant
Mastery Educational Consultants
Leawood, Kansas

Patricia T. Ketcham, RN, MSN
Adjunct Assistant Professor
Nursing Laboratory Manager
Oakland University School of Nursing
Rochester, Michigan

Joyce Kunzelman, RN, BScN, GNC(c)
Clinical Nurse Educator
Interior Health Authority
Vernon, B.C., Canada

Ronnette C. Langhorne, RN, MS
Assistant Professor
Thomas Nelson Community College
Hampton, Virginia

Sue Engman Lazear, RN, MN
Director
Specialists in Medical Education
Woodinville, Washington

Robin Lockhart, RN, MSN
Assistant Professor
Midwestern State University
Wichita Falls, Texas

Laura Logan, RN, CNS, MSN
School of Nursing Faculty
Stephen F. Austin State University
Nacogdoches, Texas

Barbara Maxwell, BSN, MS, MSN, CNS
Program Coordinator, Associate Professor
SUNY Ulster
Stone Ridge, New York

Lesia McBride, RN, BSN
Clinical Research Manager
Community Hospital Anderson
Anderson, Indiana

Lora J. McIntyre, RN, MSN
Assistant Professor of Nursing
Kent State University
Ashtabula, Ohio

Elaine Princevalli, RN, BSN, MS
Instructor, Practical Nurse Education
State of Connecticut Department of Education
Hamden, Connecticut

Anita Reed, RN, MSN
Clinical Nursing Faculty
St. Elizabeth School of Nursing
Lafayette, Indiana

Katie Frommelt Selle, RN(c), MA
Associate Professor of Nursing
Clarke College
Dubuque, Iowa

Gale Sewell, RN, MSN
Assistant Professor
Kent State University
Ashtabula, Ohio

Susan Parnell Scholtz, RN, DNS(c)
Associate Professor of Nursing
Moravian College
Bethlehem, Pennsylvania

Tamara Shields, RN, MS, CFNP
Nursing Faculty
St. Elizabeth School of Nursing
Lafayette, Indiana

Mary Surman, RN, BSN, CWOCN
Certified Wound, Ostomy, Continence Nurse
Our Lady of the Lake Regional Medical Center
Baton Rouge, Louisiana

Marianne Swihart, RN, BSN, MEd, MSN, CRNI, CWON, PCCN
Assistant Director of Nursing
Pasco Hernando Community College
New Port Richey, Florida

Mary Tedesco-Schneck, MSN, CPNP
Assistant Professor
Husson College
Bangor, Maine

Scott C. Thigpen RN, MSN, CCRN, CEN
Assistant Professor of Nursing
South Georgia College
Douglas, Georgia

Lynne Tier, RN, MSN, LNC
Associate Professor of Nursing
Learning Center Coordinator
Florida Hospital College of Health Sciences
Orlando, Florida

Anne Vaughan, MSN, BSN
Clinical Instructor
Bellarmine University
Louisville, Kentucky

Michelle H. Villegas, RN, MSN
Assistant Professor
Midwestern State University
Wichita Falls, Texas

Katherine West, BSN, MSEd, CIC
Infection Control Consultant
Infection Control/Emerging Concepts, Inc.
Manassas, Virginia

Toni Wortham, RN, BSN, MSN
Professor
Madisonville Community College
Madisonville, Kentucky

Janice Womack, RN
Associate Nurse Executive
Northwest Georgia Regional Hospital
Rome, Georgia

Contributors to Previous Editions

Elizabeth A. Ayello, RN, BSN, MS, PhD, CS, CETN
Clinical Assistant Professor of Nursing
New York University
New York, New York

Margaret R. Benz, RN, MSN(R), BC, APN
Adjunct Assistant Professor
Saint Louis University School of Nursing
St. Louis, Missouri

V. Christine Champagne, APRN, BC
Adult Nurse Practitioner
Midwest Chest Consultants
St. Charles, Missouri

Eileen Costantinou, RN, MSN
Practice Consultant
Barnes-Jewish Hospital
St. Louis, Missouri

Deborah Crump, RN, MS, CHPN
Hospice/Palliative Care Nurse
Androscoggin Home Care and Hospice
Oxford, Maine

Sheila A. Cunningham, BSN, MSN
Assistant Professor
Neumann College
Aston, Pennsylvania

Julie Eddins, RN, BSN, MSN, CRNI
Staff Nurse, IV Therapy
Barnes Hospital—Christian Health Services
Faculty
The Jewish College of Nursing and Allied Health
St. Louis, Missouri

Deborah Oldenburg Erickson, RN, BSN, MSN
Instructor, School of Nursing
Methodist Medical Center of Illinois
Peoria, Illinois

Joan O. Ervin, RN, BSN, MN, CCRN
Adjunct Faculty
Florence Darlington Technical College
Florence, South Carolina

Melba J. Figgins, MSN, BSN
Associate Professor
The University of Tennessee at Martin
Martin, Tennessee

Janet B. Fox-Moatz, RN, BSN, MSN
Assistant Professor
Neumann College
Aston, Pennsylvania

Lynn C. Hadaway, MEd, RNC, CRNI
Principal
Hadaway and Associates
Milner, Georgia

Susan A. Hauser, RN, BSN, BA, MS
Instructor
Mansfield General Hospital School of Nursing
Mansfield, Ohio

Mimi Hirshberg, RN, MSN
Barnes College of Nursing and Health Studies
University of Missouri—St. Louis;
    IV Therapist
Vascular Access Service
Barnes-Jewish Hospital
St. Louis, Missouri

Carolyn Chaney Hoskins, RN, BSN, MSN
Clinical Instructor
Rockingham Community College
Wentworth, North Carolina

Meredith Hunt, MSN, RNC, NP
Nurse Practitioner
TriCounty Health Services
Norway, Maine

Nancy Jackson, RN, BSn, MSN(R), CCRN
Pulmonary Clinical Nurse Specialist
St. Mary's Health Center
St. Louis, Missouri

Linda Kerby, BSN, MA, BA, RNC
Educational Consultant
Mastery Educational Consultants
Leawood, Kansas

Marilee Kuhrik, BSN, MSN, PhD
Associate Professor
Colorado Mountain College
Glenwood Springs, Colorado

Nancy Kuhrik, BSN, MSN, PhD
Associate Professor
Colorado Mountain College
Glenwood Springs, Colorado

Amy Lawn, BSN, MS, CIC
Infection Control Coordinator
Spectrum Health
Grand Rapids, Michigan

Antoinette Kanne Ledbetter, RN, BSN, MS, TNS
Clinical Education Coordinator
Missouri Baptist Medical Center
St. Louis, Missouri

Mary MacDonald, RN, MSN
Staff Educator
Spectrum Health
Grand Rapids, Michigan

Mary Kay Knight Macheca, RN, MSN(R), CS, ANP, CDE
Adult Nurse Practitioner/Certified Diabetes Educator
The Bortz Diabetes Control Center
Richmond Heights, Missouri

Cynthia L. Maskey, RN, MS
Professor, Associate Degree Nursing
Lincoln Land Community College
Springfield, Illinois

Barbara McGeever, RN, RSM, BSN, MSN, DNS(c)
Assistant Professor
Neumann College
Aston, Pennsylvania

Mary "Dee" Miller, RN, BSN, MS, CIC
Clinical Nursing Specialist/Infection Control and Epidemiology
St. Joseph's Hospital and Medical Center;
Faculty, BSN and MSN Nursing and Business
University of Phoenix
Phoenix, Arizona

Rose M. Miller, RN, BSN, MSN, MPA, ACLS
Instructor
Wallace College
Dothan, Alabama

Kathleen Mulryan, RN, BSN, MSN
Professor
LaGuardia Community College
Long Island, New York

Elaine K. Neel, RN, BSN, MSN
Instructor, School of Nursing
Methodist Medical Center of Illinois
Peoria, Illinois

Marsha Evans Orr, RN, MS
Owner
CreativEnergy, LLC Healthcare Consultants
Mesa, Arizona

Deborah Paul-Cheadle, RN
Registered Nurse, Infection Control
Spectrum Health
Grand Rapids, Michigan

Roberta J. Richmond, RN, MSN, CCRN
Cardiac Case Manager
Central Maine Medical Center
Lewiston, Maine

Paulette D. Rollant, RN, BSN, MSN, PhD, CCRN
Consultant and President
Adult Health Clinical Specialist
Multi-Resources, Inc.
Grantville, Georgia

Linette M. Sarti, RN, BSN, CNOR
Senior Coordinator
University Community Hospital
Tampa, Florida

Phyllis G. Stallard, BSN, MSN, ACCE
Assistant Professor
Neumann College
Aston, Pennsylvania

Victoria Steelman, RN, PhD, CNOR
Advanced Practice Nurse, Intensive and Surgical Services
University of Iowa Hospitals and Clinics
Iowa City, Iowa

Sue G. Thacker, RNC, BSN, MS, PhD
Professor
Wytheville Community College
Wytheville, Virginia

Nancy Tomaselli, RN, MSN, CS, CRNP, CWOCN, CLNC
President and CEO
Premier Health Solutions, LLC
Cherry Hill, New Jersey

Stephanie Trinkl, BSN, MSN
Instructor, Department of Nursing
Immaculata College
Immaculata, Pennsylvania

Kathryn Tripp, BSN
Nursing Instructor
Southeastern Community College
Keokuk, Iowa

Pamela Becker Weilitz, RN, MSN(R), CN, ANP
Board Certified Adult Nurse Practitioner
    and Medical-Surgical Clinical Nurse Specialist
Private Practice
St. Louis, Missouri;
Assistant Clinical Professor
Saint Louis University School of Nursing
St. Louis, Missouri

Jana L. Weindel-Dees, RN, BSN, MSN
Registered Nurse
Barnes-Jewish Hospital
St. Louis, Missouri

Joan Domigan Wentz, RN, MSN
Assistant Professor
Barnes-Jewish Hospital
College of Nursing and Allied Health
St. Louis, Missouri

Trudie Wierda, RN, MSN
Staff Educator
Spectrum Health
Grand Rapids, Michigan

Laurel A. Wiersema-Bryant, RN, MSN, CS
Clinical Nurse Specialist, Adult Nurse Practitioner
Barnes-Jewish Hospital
St. Louis, Missouri

Elizabeth R. Dunaway, RN, BSN, MA, CIC
Infection Control Consultant for Special Projects
Kitsap County Health District
Bremerton, Washington

Preface to the Student

This text is designed to be clear and easy to follow. The five-step nursing process provides the overall framework that is also used in most nursing textbooks. Each section and every feature is developed to describe how to perform the skills and how to effectively provide nursing care. Corresponding checklists enable self-evaluation of your performance for each of the skills in the text. These checklists can be purchased separately (ISBN 978-0-323-04736-4) or packaged with the text (ISBN 978-0-323-04898-9).

Quick Reference to Standard Protocols for all Nursing Skills highlights basic essential steps required for every nursing skill. Placing this information inside the front cover of the text and including a reminder at the beginning of each skill reduces repetition and quickly directs you to the essential steps of the individual skill.

Evidence in Practice sections provide you with information about current research and new evidence to influence nursing practice.

 A special **Glove Logo** reminds you when to apply clean gloves.

Chapter Format: Chapters open with a list of skills and pages for ease in location. Introductory information relating to these skills includes purposes, influencing factors, and principles.

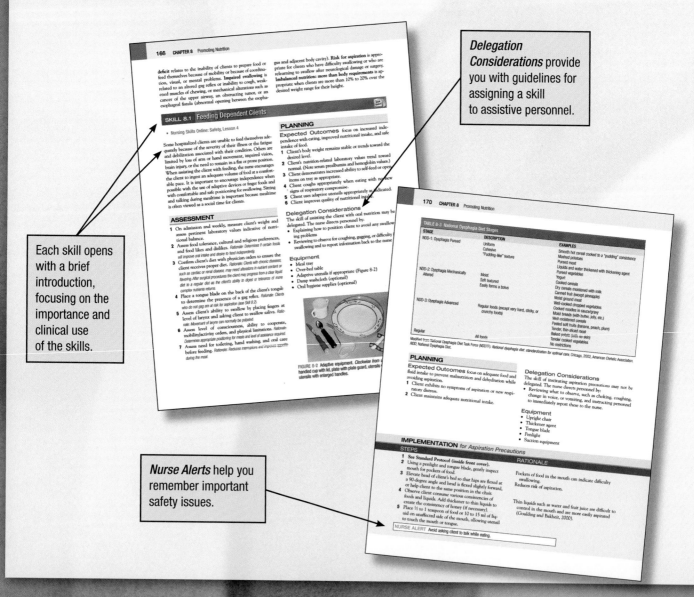

Delegation Considerations provide you with guidelines for assigning a skill to assistive personnel.

Each skill opens with a brief introduction, focusing on the importance and clinical use of the skills.

Nurse Alerts help you remember important safety issues.

Each skill is presented in an easy-to-follow two-column format with *Rationale for key steps* that explain why specific techniques are used.

A special *Glove Logo* reminds you when to apply clean gloves.

More than 900 *full-color photographs and drawings* with legends clearly show how steps are performed.

Communication Tips guide you in preparing clients for what they will experience (see, hear, or feel) as the skill is performed.

Unexpected Outcomes and Related Interventions describe how to assess for complications related to each skill and take the appropriate action.

Sample Documentation shows you how to record a narrative note with proper terminology and phrasing.

Special Considerations highlight specific needs for children and older adults and help you to work in home care and long-term care settings.

SKILL 8.1 Feeding Dependent Clients **167**

IMPLEMENTATION for Feeding Dependent Clients

STEPS	RATIONALE
1 See Standard Protocol (inside front cover).	
2 Offer toileting and hand washing before meal.	Increases level of comfort.
3 Offer toothbrush or mouthwash before meal.	May improve appetite in client with stomatitis or other oral hygiene problems.
4 Check the environment for distractions. Reduce the noise level if possible.	
5 Position client appropriately for safe eating within limitations of ability.	Positioning helps improve swallowing and digestion and avoids aspiration.
a. Up in chair	
b. High-Fowler's position if flat in bed	
c. Side-lying position if flat in bed (see illustration)	
6 Assess tray for completeness and correct diet.	Prevents intake of incomplete or incorrect diet.
7 Assist client with setting up meal tray if client is unable to do so: Open packages, cut up food, apply seasonings/condiments, butter bread, and place napkin.	Reduces effort needed to self-feed.
8 Place adaptive utensils on tray if indicated, and instruct in their use.	
9 If client is visually impaired, identify food location on plate as if it were a clock (e.g., the chicken is at 12 o'clock) (see illustration).	Visually impaired client may feed self when given adequate information about tray.
10 Pace feeding to avoid client fatigue. Ask client the order in which he or she wishes to eat food. Interact with client during mealtime. Verbally encourage self-feeding attempts.	Gives client some control of situation and avoids embarrassment about limitations. Social interaction may improve appetite.

COMMUNICATION TIP Use simple verbal prompts and touch, for example, "Here is your bread" (place bread in the client's hand). Pantomime desired behaviors, such as drinking a beverage.

11 Assist client with washing hands and repositioning as desired.	
12 Monitor intake and output (I&O) (see Skill 9.1) and calorie count.	Physician's orders may require identifying the specific number of calories consumed. The dietitian usually completes this; however, the nurse is vital in the recording of percentages of menu items consumed.
13 See Completion Protocol (inside front cover).	

STEP 5b. High-Fowler's position.

12

9   3

6

STEP 9 Location of food using clock.

---

168 CHAPTER 8 Promoting Nutrition

EVALUATION

1 Monitor body weight daily or weekly.
2 Monitor laboratory values as ordered.
3 Observe client's technique for self-feeding; certain items, part or all of meal.
4 Observe client for choking, coughing, gagging, or food left in the mouth during eating.
5 Observe use of adaptive utensils.
6 Observe amount of food on tray after meal.

Unexpected Outcomes and Related Interventions

1 Client refuses to eat food offered.
  a. Determine if client has other food preferences, cultural influences, or religious restrictions.
  b. Determine if client's ability and desire to eat is better at other times of the day.
2 Client chokes on food.
  a. Use suction equipment if necessary to clear food from airway.
  b. If choking occurs repeatedly, stop feeding and notify physician.
3 Food sits on side or back of mouth (see Skill 8.2).
  a. Initiate interventions to assist dysphagic clients with eating (see Skill 8.2).

Recording and Reporting

• Record the food and fluids actually consumed (for calorie count and I&O) and the degree of participation/independence. Describe client's ability to swallow and any choking that occurs.
• Report any choking or food tolerance/intolerance and significant changes to the dietitian.

Sample Documentation

0800 Able to feed self 5 bites with encouragement. Reported, "That is all I can do." Remaining breakfast fed to client. No difficulty swallowing or coughing noted. Consumed 70% of meal.

Special Considerations

Pediatric Considerations
• Food allergies are common in infancy because the immature intestinal tract is more permeable to proteins. Food allergies may be prevented by avoiding cow's milk for the first 6 months.
• Age affects the requirements for essential nutrients. Periods of rapid growth increase the need for calories, protein, vitamins, and minerals. A child requires more calories per kilogram of body weight than an adult.

Geriatric Considerations
• Changes in taste perception, oral mucus and saliva production, and dentition with aging may affect the client's food choices and ability to chew or swallow. Assess the client's food patterns for nutrient, calorie, and fluid adequacy.
• Older adults may have difficulty eating because of physical symptoms or lack of teeth or dentures.
• Thirst sensation may diminish in older adults, leading to inadequate fluid intake or dehydration.

Home Care Considerations
• Homebound older adults may benefit from Meals on Wheels, which can provide as many as three meals per day depending on the client's community (Meals on Wheels, 2006).
• Clients who are unable to feed themselves independently may eat better if other family members participate at mealtimes to avoid social isolation.

Long-Term Care Considerations
• Institutionalized older adults often have nutrition issues related to poor appetite, infections, weight loss, pressure ulcers, and polypharmacy. In 2005 the American Dietetic Association (ADA) published a position statement endorsing liberalized diets for older adults in long-term care (Niedert, 2005).

SKILL 8.2 Aspiration Precautions

Aspiration in the adult client usually occurs as a result of difficulties in swallowing (dysphagia). Swallowing dysfunction, better known as dysphagia, is associated with multiple myogenic, neurogenic, and obstructive causes (Box 8-5). Dysphagia is a decreased ability to voluntarily pass fluids and/or solids from the mouth to the stomach. Swallowing is a complex event, requiring both voluntary and involuntary movements. It requires the coordination of cranial nerves and the muscles of the tongue, pharynx, larynx, and jaw. Clients with neuromuscular diseases involving the brain, brain stem, cranial nerves, or muscles of swallowing should

be assessed for swallowing difficulties before feeding. Notify the care provider immediately if a client complains of difficulty swallowing or displays the following characteristics:
• Cough and/or voice change (hoarseness) after swallowing
• Weak involuntary cough or delayed cough (as long as 2 minutes after swallowing)
• Abnormal lip closure and slowed tongue movement; tongue weakness
• Slow, weak, or uncoordinated speech
• Regurgitation and pocketing of food

Preface to the Instructor

We are grateful for the enthusiastic responses to *Nursing Interventions & Clinical Skills* and have carefully preserved the features that made it unique: its streamlined and concise approach, language, and format easily understood by beginning and advanced nursing students. Generous use of color photographs illustrates skills and the way they are best learned and performed.

This 4th edition builds on the basic organization and format of the previous editions. Early chapters include basic skills typically introduced before or during initial clinical experiences, such as infection control, safety, hygiene, and vital signs. Later chapters focus on more complex skills often encountered in medical-surgical nursing, such as gastric intubation and enteral nutrition. All chapters include a brief introduction including evidence in practice and a unique segment that describes related nursing diagnoses in a way that helps students identify their potential application. Skills are presented in the nursing process format. Steps of the skills include parallel rationales to explain underlying scientific principles and research-based best practice techniques. Hundreds of close-up, full-color photographs facilitate learning. Delegation considerations; communication tips; and pediatric, geriatric, home care, and long-term care considerations help students adapt skills into the context of clinical care.

We have enlisted contributors and clinical consultants throughout the country who have provided their expertise in revising and updating each chapter. We carefully reviewed and refined the contributors' material ourselves to maintain a consistent organization and writing level to help beginning nursing students effectively grasp essential information.

KEY FEATURES

- Comprehensive coverage of nursing skills from the beginning basic skills to the complex advanced skills of central lines, parenteral nutrition, mechanical ventilation, and dialysis.
- Over 900 full-color photographs are conveniently placed near the accompanying text.
- Standard Protocols for beginning and completion of each skill emphasize safety and infection control practices.
- CDC hand hygiene guidelines are incorporated.
- A Glove Logo is used to visually highlight the circumstances when the use of clean gloves is recommended.
- Sterile Gloving is visually highlighted in skills to emphasize the importance of this essential action.

- Delegation Considerations are included in the planning section for each skill to help the learner identify when delegation to assistive personnel is appropriate and what to include to clarify expectations regarding performance of the task.
- Communication Tips provide guidelines on how to prepare, support, and instruct clients during a skill. In addition, there are tips that help students know when to offer valuable instruction.
- Recording and Reporting provides a concise, bulleted list of information to be documented and reported.
- Sample Documentation provides examples of clear, concise variance notes or narrative documentation.
- Special Considerations include guidelines for adaptation of skills in various settings, including home care and long-term care, and highlight specific needs for children and older adults.
- Legends for illustrations allow for quick identification of figures and skill steps.

NEW FEATURES

- Revised and streamlined quick reference for Standard Protocols.
- Evidence in Practice section to highlight current research and evidence related to the skills within the chapter.
- Cross referencing to corresponding skill in the skills online lessons as appropriate.
- Streamlined Delegation Considerations to guide the student in using "The Five Rights of Delegation" to safely delegate appropriate skills.
- Incorporation of the "Do Not Use" listing of abbreviations.
- Expanded Client Teaching incorporated into Communication Tips to assist students to more effectively prepare clients for self-care.

NEW CONTENT

- The **Evidence-Based Practice** section in each chapter summarizes a related nursing research study and its findings and explains its application to nursing practice.
- **New Skills and Procedural Guidelines** prepare students for practice.
  - Musculoskeletal and Neurological Assessment
  - Obtaining Blood Pressure from Lower Extremity by Auscultation
  - Breast and Testicular Self-Examinations

- **NCLEX® Style Review Questions** for each chapter include the new alternate-item format questions to help students begin to prepare for NCLEX exams.
- Cross references to **Nursing Skills Online** are provided at the beginning of skills that are included in the course to direct students to the appropriate lesson.
- Over 80 **video clips** from Mosby's Nursing Skills Videos are provided on the Evolve site for both students and faculty. Related skills in the book are flagged with a reminder to "View Video."

TEACHING-LEARNING PACKAGE

The comprehensive teaching and learning package includes the following:

- *Instructor's Resource with Test Bank* (available online or as a CD-ROM) includes a list of skills and procedural guidelines, teaching strategies, clinical activities, and answers to critical thinking and NCLEX exercises. The expanded ExamView Test Bank includes nearly 1000 NCLEX-style multiple choice questions.
- *Skills Performance Checklists for Nursing Interventions and Clinical Skills*, 4th edition, is sold separately or packaged with the text.
- *Mosby's Nursing Skills Video Series* provides valuable visual reinforcement for learning and is also available in CD-ROM format.
- *Skills Exercises* accompany the innovative series of engaging, action-packed videos that provide clear demonstrations of how to perform key nursing procedures in real-life clinical situations. Actual nurses perform each skill, incorporating contemporary concepts such as delegation, critical thinking, standard CDC precautions, and communication techniques.

- The *EVOLVE* site includes Weblinks and skills video clips.
- *Nursing Skills Online* consists of 17 modules, with each module comprising several lessons. Each lesson provides a content overview, a variety of interactive exercises, self-check activities, and an exam. The program features an abundance of visual aids such as photographs, drawings, boxes and tables, graphics, and video and animation clips to engage and hold the learner's interest. Students can easily navigate through manageable segments, with frequent interactive experiences that test comprehension and ask them to apply concepts. Students can also view the video for each skill from start to finish, pausing and repeating segments as desired. Each module concludes with a test that covers content from all lessons within the module. Scoring the final test interacts with the grade book function for group courses.

We hope that each chapter will help students develop a solid base on which to build the knowledge and ability to use critical thinking and the nursing process to provide nursing care for clients safely, effectively, and with an awareness of why, as well as how, the steps of each skill are performed.

Acknowledgments

We wish to acknowledge clinical nurses, educators, and students who provided valuable feedback and input into the revision of this text. Clinical nurses and educators offer their comments, recommendation, and suggestions. Students provide valuable insight into the needs of the students. Our contributors lend their clinical wisdom and expertise to assist in creating a state-of-the-art textbook. Our reviewers take their clinical expertise and offer insight and constructive feedback.

Thanks to the talented and dedicated professionals at Elsevier: Suzi Epstein, Executive Editor, who provided support, leadership, enthusiasm, and a healthy sense of humor during the revision process. Robyn L. Brinks and Jean Sims Fornango, Senior Developmental Editors, who spent countless hours tracking the progress of this text. Their organizational skills, commitment to accuracy, and dedication to quality kept the project on target. Mary Jo Adams, Editorial Assistant, who cheerfully assisted with countless details. John Rogers, Publishing Services Manager, and Cheryl Abbott, Senior Project Manager, whose organization, careful editing, and guidance of the project through the production process helped to ensure an accurate, consistent book. Julia Dummitt whose creativity provides an attractive and unique visual appeal to the text. These contributions significantly enhance the learning process.

Finally, thanks to our friends, families, and colleagues for their understanding, patience, and encouragement.

Martha "Marty" Keene Elkin
Anne Griffin Perry
Patricia A. Potter

Contents

Professional Nursing Practice

MEDIA RESOURCES

- **evolve** http://evolve.elsevier.com/Elkin

Nursing practice is an art and a science. Nurses apply critical thinking while performing a variety of nursing skills in accordance with the standards established by their state's Nurse Practice Act, national nursing organizations, and the community of practitioners with whom they work. Nurses are members of a *profession*, a group of people with specialized education, knowledge, and skills that serve a specific need. Professional nurses have autonomy in decision making and practice and function within a code of ethics for nursing practice. Nurses who act "professionally" are knowledgeable, conscientious, and responsible to themselves and others.

DEFINITION OF NURSING

In 1955 the American Nurses Association (ANA) defined the practice of professional nursing to include "the performance of skills requiring substantial critical thinking and specialized judgment with knowledge of biological, physical, and social sciences." Virginia Henderson wrote the following definition of nursing, which was adopted by the International Council of Nurses (ICN) in 1973:

> The unique function of the nurse is to assist the individual, sick or well, in the performance of those activities contributing to health, its recovery, or to a peaceful death that he would perform unaided if he had the necessary strength, will, or knowledge. And to do this in such a way as to help the client gain independence as rapidly as possible.

According to the ANA *Nursing's Social Policy Statement* (2003), definitions of professional nursing have evolved to acknowledge six essential features:

1. Provision of a caring relationship that facilitates health and healing
2. Attention to the range of human experiences and responses to health and illness within the physical and social environments
3. Integration of objective data with knowledge gained from an appreciation of the patient or group's subjective experience
4. Application of scientific knowledge to the processes of diagnosis and treatment through the use of judgment and critical thinking
5. Advancement of professional nursing knowledge through scholarly inquiry
6. Influence on social and public policy to promote social justice

Nurses assume many roles when caring for clients. Nurses are caregivers who display sensitivity and compassion when attending to clients' complex needs. Nurses are teachers who facilitate learning as an interactive process that results in knowledge to improve, maintain, and promote health.

**Leavell and Clark's
Three Levels of Prevention**

Primary Prevention

Health Promotion
Health education
Good standard of nutrition adjusted to
   developmental phases of life
Attention to personality development
Provision of adequate housing and recreation,
   as well as agreeable working conditions
Marriage counseling and sex education
Genetic screening
Periodic selective examinations

Specific Protection
Use of specific immunizations
Attention to personal hygiene
Use of environmental sanitation
Protection against occupational hazards
Protection from accidents
Use of specific nutrients
Protection from carcinogens
Avoidance of allergens

Secondary Prevention

Early Diagnosis and Prompt Treatment
Case-finding measures: individual and mass
   screening surveys
Selective examinations to
   Cure and prevent disease process
   Prevent spread of communicable disease
   Prevent complications and sequelae
   Shorten period of disability

Disability Limitations
Adequate treatment to arrest disease process and
   prevent further complications and sequelae
Provision of facilities to limit disability and
   prevent death

Tertiary Prevention

Restoration and Rehabilitation
Provision of hospital and community facilities for
   retraining and education to maximize use of
   remaining capacities
Education of public and industry to use rehabilitated
   persons to fullest possible extent
Selective placement
Work therapy in hospitals
Use of sheltered colony

Figure 1-1 The three levels of prevention developed by Leavell and Clark. (Data from Leavell H, Clark AE: *Preventive medicine for doctors in the community,* ed 3, New York, 1965, McGraw-Hill; modified from Edelman CL, Mandle CL: *Health promotion throughout the lifespan,* ed 6, St Louis, 2005, Mosby.)

Nurses are counselors who help individuals to recognize and cope with problems and improve relationships. Nurses are client advocates who defend client rights and encourage caregivers to provide the best possible care. Nurses are leaders who influence others to improve the health status of individuals and groups and improve the systems of delivery of health care in a variety of settings. Nurses are managers who plan and provide adequate staffing patterns, coordinate and supervise the delivery of nursing care, and ensure that high standards of nursing care are delivered.

As clinicians, nurses may be generalists who are able to function in a variety of medical-surgical settings. Others are specialists in areas such as gerontological nursing (care of older adults), pediatric nursing (care of children and adolescents), perinatal nursing (care of families before, during, or after childbirth), community health nursing, or psychiatric and mental health nursing. Nurses who obtain advanced graduate education assume roles as educators, clinical nurse specialists, and nurse practitioners.

NURSING PRACTICE

Nursing practice involves the delivery of client care with nurses integrating cognitive, interpersonal, and psychomotor skills. With each client encounter, nurses learn to practice nursing in the most safe, effective, and appropriate manner possible.

Cognitive Skills

The cognitive skills of critical thinking and clinical decision making are interrelated. Nurses assist clients in solving problems and finding solutions to their health problems to maintain, regain, or improve their health. Nurses apply knowledge from nursing, biological, physical, and social sciences to make the decisions necessary to promote clients' well-being. Selecting nursing interventions requires knowledge of the rationale for each intervention and recognition of normal and abnormal physiological and psychological responses. Expert nursing practice involves developing a sound knowledge base and applying what you learn from experiences in caring for clients.

Interpersonal Skills

Caring is the essence of nursing practice. Caring means being connected. Because caring determines what matters to a person, it describes a wide range of involvements, from parental love to friendship, from caring for one's work to caring for one's clients. Caring is specific and relational for each client you meet. Caring is essential to your ability to work with people in a respectful and therapeutic way. Caring is more than "taking care of"; it is also "caring for" and "caring about" each client. An important aspect of caring is the use of interpersonal skills including clear, open, and honest communication and teaching and counseling at the client's level of understanding. Effective communication improves your ability to know your client and helps you to recognize your client's problems, find solutions, and then implement those solutions. Effective education helps clients become healthier and more self-sufficient.

Psychomotor Skills

This text features a vast array of psychomotor skills and procedures typically used in client care. No skill should be performed without adequate knowledge and application of astute critical thinking. Advances in technology have required nurses to be able to operate complex equipment while remaining focused on clients' needs. Psychomotor skills involve providing direct care to clients, such as changing a dressing, giving an injection, or bathing. With the application of knowledge and caring interpersonal skills, psychomotor skills are performed smoothly, confidently, and efficiently.

SPECTRUM OF HEALTH CARE

Health care occurs at the primary, secondary, and tertiary levels of prevention (Figure 1-1). Prevention includes all activities that limit either the onset or the progression of a disease (Edelman and Mandle, 2005). Primary prevention is true prevention with the focus on health. Health is a positive, dynamic state that is more than merely the absence of disease. Primary prevention precedes disease or dysfunction and is applied to clients considered physically and emotionally healthy (Edelman and Mandle, 2005). It is not a therapeutic level of care. Primary prevention can be delivered to an individual or to a general population, for example, well baby care taught to a mother, management of a city's water system, and control of mosquito populations. The U.S. Department of Health and Human Services (USDHHS) has a national strategy to promote health called *Healthy People 2010* (USDHHS, 2000). The objectives of this program include continuing the objectives identified for *Healthy People 2000* to increase the span of healthy life by risk reduction, health services and protection, and research.

Secondary prevention focuses on persons who are experiencing health problems or illnesses and who are at risk for developing complications or worsening conditions. Activities are directed at diagnosis and prompt intervention, reducing the severity of disease, and enabling a client to return to a normal level of health as soon as possible (Edelman and Mandle, 2005). Secondary prevention includes screening techniques and treating early stages of disease to limit disability.

Tertiary prevention occurs when a defect or disability is permanent and irreversible. It involves minimizing the effects of long-term disease or disability by interventions directed at preventing complications or deterioration (Edelman and Mandle, 2005). Activities are directed at rehabilitation rather than diagnosis or treatment.

The health care system provides six levels of care: preventive, primary, secondary, tertiary, restorative, and continuing (Figure 1-2). Levels of care describe the scope of services and settings where health care is offered to clients in all stages of health and illness. For example, preventive care settings focus on education and prevention (e.g., care activities in the physician's office or the home), whereas tertiary care settings focus on highly technical care (e.g., care delivered in the intensive care unit [ICU] setting). Levels of care are not the same as levels of prevention. Levels of prevention describe the focus of health-related activities. At any level of care, nurses and other health care providers offer a variety of levels of prevention. The nurse working in an acute care, tertiary setting, for example, monitors the recovery of a postoperative

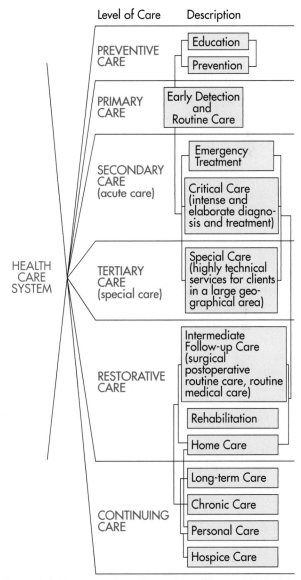

Figure 1-2 Spectrum of health services delivery. (Modified from Cambridge Research Institute: Trends affecting the US health care system, 262, Health Planning Information Series, Human Resources Administration, Public Health Service, Department of Health, Education, and Welfare, Washington, DC, 1976, revised and updated 1992, US Government Printing Office.)

open heart surgery client while also providing health promotion information to the client and family concerning healthy diet and exercise.

LEGAL CONCEPTS

Client Rights and Responsibilities

In 2003, the American Hospital Association (AHA) adopted *The Patient Care Partnership: Understanding Expectations, Rights, and Responsibilities* (Box 1-1). Health care institutions are encouraged to adapt and simplify the language to promote client and family understanding within their institution. Hospitals distribute informational brochures that offer simple and clear explanations of patient rights and responsibilities. Effective health care requires collaboration between clients and physicians and other health care professionals. Open and honest communication, respect for personal and professional values, and sensitivity to differences are integral to optimal client care. Health care settings must provide a foundation for understanding and respecting the rights and responsibilities of clients, their families, physicians, and other caregivers. Hospitals must ensure a health care ethic that respects the role of clients in decision making about treatment choices and other aspects of their care. In addition, hospitals must be sensitive to cultural, racial, linguistical, religious, age, gender, and other differences, as well as the needs of persons with disabilities.

The collaborative nature of health care requires that clients, or their families, participate in their care and recognizes that "family is defined by the client" (Dudley, 2001). The effectiveness of care and client satisfaction with the course of treatment depend to a large extent on the client fulfilling certain responsibilities. Clients are responsible for providing information about past illnesses, hospitalizations, medications, and other matters related to health status. To participate effectively in decision making, clients are encouraged to take responsibility for requesting additional information or clarifying their health status or treatment when they do not fully understand information and instructions. Clients must inform their physicians and other caregivers if they anticipate problems in following prescribed treatment.

A client may have an advance directive, which documents the client's wishes in the event that the client becomes incapacitated and unable to speak for himself or herself. This requires that the client, family, and health care providers face issues related to quality of life and end-of-life care. Clients are also responsible for ensuring that the health care institution has a copy of their written advance directive if they have one.

Clients should also be aware of the hospital's obligation to be reasonably efficient and equitable in providing care to other clients and the community. The hospital's rules and regulations are designed to help the hospital meet this obligation. Clients and their families are responsible for making reasonable accommodations to the needs of the hospital, other clients, medical staff, and hospital employees. Clients are responsible for providing necessary information for insurance claims and for working with the hospital to make payment arrangements, when necessary.

Informed Consent

The law requires that the person who performs an invasive procedure discuss it with the client in understandable terms. Informed consent involves a clear explanation of the treatments or procedure, names and qualifications of the persons involved, potential risks, and alternatives. The person obtaining consent must invite and answer all questions. Nurses are responsible for assessing clients' understanding and ability to make informed decisions. This includes protecting a client's rights, identifying related fears, determining the client's level of understanding, and obtaining approval of the procedure. The nurse is an advocate for the client and serves as a witness to the client's signature on the agency form. Ask the client to state in his or her own words what information was conveyed by the physician or provider. If there is any doubt about understanding or the client's decision, notify the care provider.

Nurse Practice Acts

Nurse Practice Acts define the scope of nursing practice and expanded nursing roles, set educational requirements for nurses, and distinguish between nursing and medical practice *for each state*. The authorization to practice nursing requires licensure by the State Board of Nursing. Each board sets rules and regulations that define the practice of nursing more specifically (e.g., which professional group can start intravenous [IV] therapy or prescribe medications). Professional nurses must understand the legal limits influencing their practice. This, coupled with good judgment and sound decision making, ensures safe and appropriate nursing care.

Most Nurse Practice Acts are purposefully broad so as not to limit the professional responsibilities of the nurse. Institutions and agencies may interpret specific actions allowed under the acts, but they cannot modify, expand, or restrict the act's intent. The primary intent of the state Nurse Practice Acts is to protect the public from unskilled, undereducated, and unlicensed personnel.

Standards of Care

Nursing standards of care are the legal guidelines for minimally safe and adequate nursing practice. Standards are defined in the Nurse Practice Acts of the State Board of Nursing of each state, the state and federal hospital licensing laws, professional and specialty organization standards, and the written policies and procedures of the employing institution (Mikos, 2004). Standards of care offer guidelines that establish expectations for the provision of safe and appropriate nursing care.

The ANA has established standards of nursing practice and policy statements that delineate the scope, function, and role of the nurse and establish clinical practice

BOX 1-1 The Patient Care Partnership: Understanding Expectations, Rights, and Responsibilities

When you need hospital care, your doctor and the nurses and other professionals at our hospital are committed to working with you and your family to meet your health care needs. Our dedicated doctors and staff serve the community in all its ethnic, religious, and economic diversity. Our goal is for you and your family to have the same care and attention we would want for our families and ourselves.

The sections explain some of the basics of how you can expect to be treated during your hospital stay. They also cover what we will need from you to care for you better. If you have questions at any time, please ask them. Unasked or unanswered questions can add to the stress of being in the hospital. Your comfort and confidence in your care are very important to us.

What to Expect During Your Hospital Stay

- **High quality hospital care.** Our first priority is to provide you the care you need, when you need it, with skill, compassion, and respect. Tell your caregivers if you have concerns about your care or if you have pain. You have the right to know the identity of doctors, nurses, and others involved in your care, as well as when they are students, residents, or other trainees.

- **A clean and safe environment.** Our hospital works hard to keep you safe. We use special policies and procedures to avoid mistakes in your care and keep you free from abuse or neglect. If anything unexpected and significant happens during your hospital stay, you will be told what happened, and any resulting changes in your care will be discussed with you.

- **Involvement in your care.** You and your doctor often make decisions about your care before you go to the hospital. Other times, especially in emergencies, those decisions are made during your hospital stay. When decision making takes place, it should include:

  Discussing your medical condition and information about medically appropriate treatment choices. To make informed decisions with your doctor, you need to understand:
  - The benefits and risks of each treatment.
  - Whether your treatment is experimental or part of a research study.
  - What you can reasonably expect from your treatment and any long-term effects it might have on your quality of life.
  - What you and your family will need to do after you leave the hospital.
  - The financial consequences of using uncovered services or out-of-network providers.

  Please tell your caregivers if you need more information about treatment choices.

  Discussing your treatment plan. When you enter the hospital, you sign a general consent to treatment. In some cases, such as surgery or experimental treatment, you may be asked to confirm in writing that you understand what is planned and agree to it. This process protects your right to consent to or refuse a treatment. Your doctor will explain the medical consequences of refusing recommended treatment. It also protects your right to decide if you want to participate in a research study.

  Getting information from you. Your caregivers need complete and correct information about your health and coverage so that they can make good decisions about your care. That includes:
  - Past illnesses, surgeries, or hospital stays.

- Past allergic reactions.
- Any medications or dietary supplements (such as vitamins and herbs) that you are taking.
- Any network or admission requirements under your health plan.

Understanding your health care goals and values. You may have health care goals and values or spiritual beliefs that are important to your well-being. They will be taken into account as much as possible throughout your hospital stay. Make sure your doctor, your family, and your care team know your wishes.

Understanding who should make decisions when you cannot. If you have signed a health care power of attorney stating who should speak for you if you become unable to make health care decisions for yourself, or a "living will" or "advance directive" that states your wishes about end-of-life care, give copies to your doctor, your family, and your care team. If you or your family need help making difficult decisions, counselors, chaplains, and others are available to help.

- **Protection of your privacy.** We respect the confidentiality of your relationship with your doctor and other caregivers, and the sensitive information about your health and health care that are part of that relationship. State and federal laws and hospital operating policies protect the privacy of your medical information. You will receive a Notice of Privacy Practices that describes the ways that we use, disclose, and safeguard patient information and that explains how you can obtain a copy of information from our records about your care.

- **Preparing you and your family for when you leave the hospital.** Your doctor works with hospital staff and professionals in your community. You and your family also play an important role in your care. The success of your treatment often depends on your efforts to follow medication, diet, and therapy plans. Your family may need to help care for you at home. You can expect us to help you identify sources of follow-up care and to let you know if our hospital has a financial interest in any referrals. As long as you agree we can share information about your care with them, we will coordinate our activities with your caregivers outside the hospital. You can also expect to receive information and, where possible, training about the self-care you will need when you go home.

- **Help with your bill and filing insurance claims.** Our staff will file claims for you with health care insurers or other programs such as Medicare and Medicaid. They will also help your doctor with needed documentation. Hospital bills and insurance coverage are often confusing. If you have questions about your bill, contact our business office. If you need help understanding your insurance coverage or health plan, start with your insurance company or health benefits manager. If you do not have health coverage, we will try to help you and your family find financial help or make other arrangements. We need your help with collecting needed information and other requirements to obtain coverage or assistance.

- While you are here, you will receive more detailed notices about some of the rights you have as a hospital patient and how to exercise them. We are always interested in improving. If you have questions, comments, or concerns, please contact: _____ _____.

Adapted from American Hospital Association: *The patient care partnership: understanding expectations, rights, and responsibilities,* Chicago, 2003, AHA. Reprinted with permission from the American Hospital Association, copyright 2003.

BOX 1-2 Standards of Practice

1 The registered nurse *collects comprehensive data* pertinent to the client's health or the situation in a systematic and ongoing process.
2 The registered nurse *analyzes* the assessment data to determine the diagnoses or issues.
3 The registered nurse *identifies* expected outcomes for a plan individualized to the client or the situation and validates the diagnoses or issue with the client, family, and other health care providers.
4 The registered nurse *develops* a plan that prescribes strategies and alternatives to attain expected outcomes and provides for continuity.
5 The registered nurse *implements* the plan in a safe and timely manner using evidence-based interventions and coordinates the care.
6 The registered nurse *evaluates* progress toward attainment of outcomes.

Reprinted from American Nurses Association: *Nursing: scope and standards of practice*, Silver Spring, MD © 2004, Nursesbooks.org.

BOX 1-3 The Five Rights of Delegation

Right Task: One that can safely be delegated for a specific client, such as repetitive tasks that require little supervision and that are relatively noninvasive.
Right Circumstances: Appropriate client, setting, and resources.
Right Person: Right person delegates the right task to the most appropriate person, to be performed on the right client.
Right Direction/Communication: Clear, concise description of the task, including its objective, limits, and expectations.
Right Supervision: Appropriate monitoring, evaluation, intervention (as needed), and feedback.

Reproduced from National Council of State Boards of Nursing: *The five rights of delegation*, http://www.ncsbn.org, accessed May 2006.

---

standards. These standards serve as guidelines and correlate to the nursing process (Box 1-2). It is important for professional nurses to be involved in establishing and maintaining standards of practice, because these standards define the responsibility and accountability for the profession. In addition, professional and government organizations have developed clinical practice guidelines for management of certain symptoms of diseases. These guidelines reflect current research that supports changes in practice. For example, the Agency for Healthcare Research and Quality (AHRQ) has evidence-based guidelines in the areas of pain management and pressure ulcer prevention and treatment.

Delegation

As a result of the changing demands in health care systems and increasing need for accessible, affordable, quality health care, there has been a trend toward using a variety of health care workers with different levels of education and training. Professional nurses find themselves in situations that require more support to perform the daily, routine tasks of care. A registered nurse (RN) needs time to coordinate care delivery for groups of clients, to conduct individual assessments, and to make judgments about a client's therapeutic needs. One solution is the addition of more ancillary personnel who can perform basic nursing care for more stable clients.

Delegation is the transfer of responsibility for the performance of a task from one individual to another while retaining accountability for the outcome (ANA, 2006). An RN may choose to delegate client care to ancillary staff, including licensed practical/vocational nurses (LPNs/LVNs) and assistive personnel (AP, e.g., certified nursing assistants [CNAs] and nursing technicians). Many LPNs/LVNs cannot actually delegate tasks to CNAs and nursing technicians. Nurses must be familiar with their state's Nurse Practice Act. One purpose of delegation is to improve efficiency, but the RN retains the accountability for the total nursing care of a client. In delegation, there is a decision-making process that takes into ac-

count which tasks can be delegated and in what type of situation. An RN may delegate components of care but not the nursing process itself (ANA, 2006).

It is important to recognize that nurses delegate tasks, not clients. Furthermore, a nurse should not automatically delegate a task because it is a task but because it is appropriate for someone else to perform the task. For example, the nurse is always responsible for assessing a client's ongoing status, but if the client is stable, the nurse can delegate vital sign monitoring to AP. These personnel work as the nurse's assistants or partners and perform tasks that the nurse determines are safe and appropriate for them to provide.

When delegating, the nurse must know the ancillary caregiver's education, skills, and experience, as well as the caregiver's demonstrated and documented evidence of current competency. Always provide clear expectations regarding performance of the task and evaluate the effectiveness of the performance in relation to established standards. AP are important members of the health care team and can be effective and productive when their contributions are effectively utilized, recognized, and valued. Box 1-3 lists the Five Rights of Delegation recommended by the National Council of State Boards of Nursing (2006).

Each skill within this text describes delegation considerations that should be taken into account as RNs, and in many cases LPNs/LVNs, perform the skill. The considerations highlight the types of precautions and directives that RNs and LPNs/LVNs provide when delegating. Part of delegation includes specific directives regarding how tasks are adapted to meet client needs and under what circumstances the caregiver should communicate with the licensed nurse. Appropriate delegation requires the nurse to (Keeling and others, 2000):

- Assess the knowledge and skills of the delegate
- Match tasks to the delegate's skills
- Communicate clearly, offering specific directions and a time period in which to complete a task
- Listen attentively to whether the delegate understands his or her responsibilities
- Provide feedback regarding the delegate's performance, regardless of outcome

BOX 1-4 Role of the LPN/LVN in the Nursing Process

Assessment: Observe and report significant cues (e.g., signs, symptoms) to RN or physician.
Diagnosis: Assist in validating current nursing diagnoses.
Planning: Assist with goal identification and priority setting; suggest nursing interventions.
Implementation: Carry out physician and nursing orders.
Evaluation: Assist with evaluation of progress toward goals and suggest alternative nursing interventions when necessary.

Modified from Christensen B, Kockrow E: *Foundations of nursing,* ed 5, St Louis, 2005, Mosby.

Nurse Professions and Roles

Registered nurses (RNs) are professionals who have completed a course of study at a state-approved school of nursing and passed the National Council Licensure Examination for Registered Nurses (NCLEX-RN). An RN uses the nursing process to assess, diagnose, plan, intervene, and evaluate client needs and responses to care; coordinates care delivery for groups of clients; makes the professional judgments necessary to adjust therapies and deliver care; delivers complex therapies; and provides client education and counseling. To achieve their complex role, RNs direct and coordinate other personnel in the timely delivery of client care.

Licensed practical nurses/licensed vocational nurses (LPNs/LVNs) receive 12 to 18 months of education in basic nursing techniques. LPNs/LVNs work under the supervision of a professional RN or physician. Although the LPN/LVN uses the nursing process under the direction of the RN, there are some limitations based on the scope of practice determined by the Nurse Practice Act in each state (Box 1-4). In many states the LPN administers medications and with additional education may initiate IV therapy.

Certified nurse assistants (CNAs) have 2 to 3 months of basic nursing care training with a focus on basic skills administered in hospitals and long-term care facilities. They may be trained to perform basic skills such as vital signs, hygiene, mobility, and care of the environment without gaining knowledge of the underlying scientific principles. In some states they may take a training course for nonparenteral medication administration to enable them to pass oral medications to stable clients in long-term care settings. This training emphasizes the "how to" with extremely limited awareness of the pharmacology and depends on the skillful abilities of RNs to assess and evaluate the medications given by someone else.

Assistive personnel (AP) include nursing technicians. They typically have on-the-job training of specific, repetitive, noninvasive tasks limited to a particular health care setting. In most settings many tasks are beyond the scope of a nursing technician, including irrigating catheters or wounds, inserting gastrointestinal (GI) tubes, administering tube feedings, and managing intravascular catheters. Each health care agency defines the type of nursing procedures AP can perform.

CLINICAL NURSING PRACTICE

When caring for clients, nurses are responsible for making accurate and appropriate clinical decisions. Clinical decision making is what separates professional nurses from unlicensed personnel. Critical thinking and application of the nursing process enable nurses to make the type of decisions needed to provide excellent nursing care.

Critical Thinking

Critical thinking allows nurses to make high-quality judgments about client care. For example, when your client's condition begins to change with a slowed response to questions, a grimace when turning to the side, reluctance to move, and sweating, critical thinking lets you make clinical inferences; in this situation you determine that the client might be in pain. You would then assess the situation more thoroughly and act to relieve the client's discomfort. Critical thinking is a reasoning process. It requires a commitment and a desire to grow intellectually. A critical thinker identifies and challenges assumptions, considers what is important in a situation, explores alternatives, sets priorities, draws conclusions, and thus makes informed decisions.

A useful critical thinking model for nursing practice includes five components: knowledge, experience, attitudes, and standards, all integrated and applied through the fifth component, the nursing process. This model is useful in making clinical decisions and judgments. The nurse's knowledge base includes information and theory from the basic sciences, humanities, behavioral sciences, and nursing. Experience includes your clinical learning experiences, as well as personal experiences. Clinical experience is the laboratory for testing nursing knowledge. A critical thinker has 11 central critical thinking attitudes: confidence, independence, fairness, responsibility, risk taking, discipline, perseverance, creativity, curiosity, integrity, and humility (Paul, 1993). Each time a nurse cares for a client, these attitudes provide guidelines for how to approach the client's health care problem and make the appropriate care decisions. Standards refer to the use of intellectual and professional standards. Intellectual standards are guidelines for rational thought. For example, you must use the standards of being clear, precise, specific, accurate, and relevant when you interview a client to learn about his or her health history. Professional standards include standards of ethics and evidence-based criteria in making decisions. The process of critical thinking comes together with the nursing process to allow nurses to use knowledge and experience in becoming competent professionals.

The Nursing Process

The nursing process includes five steps: assessment, nursing diagnosis, planning, implementation, and evaluation (Table 1-1). The purpose of the process is to diagnose and treat human responses to actual or potential health problems (ANA, 2003). The format for the nursing process offers a common language and way for nurses to "think through" clients' clinical problems (Kataoka-Yahiro and Saylor, 1994).

Assessment

The nursing process begins with assessment, the deliberate and systematic collection of data. The nurse collects data about clients to determine clients' current and past health status, functional status, and coping patterns. Assessment data includes information from interviewing the client and others significant to a situation, conducting a physical assessment, conferring with health care team members, and reviewing information in the client record. Both subjective and objective data come together to form a clinical picture of each client. Assessment is an ongoing process of data collection beginning with the first contact with a client and continuing with each additional contact. During assessment the nurse gathers data, analyzes and interprets the information, and organizes information into meaningful clusters to make nursing diagnoses.

Nursing Diagnosis

A nursing diagnosis is a clinical judgment about individual, family, or community responses to actual or potential health problems or life processes (NANDA-I, 2005). It is a statement that describes the client's response to a health problem that the nurse is licensed and competent to treat. A nursing diagnosis provides the basis for selection of nursing interventions.

The diagnostic process flows from the nurse's assessment and includes decision-making steps. After assessing a client's database and interpreting the patterns of clustered data from an assessment, the nurse forms diagnostic conclusions. Some of the conclusions lead to nursing diagnoses, but others do not. It is important to recognize that the outcome of the nursing diagnostic process includes problems treated by nurses (nursing diagnoses) and problems treated by several disciplines (collaborative problems). Together, these problems represent the range of conditions nurses manage.

Box 1-5 outlines the steps for forming a nursing diagnosis. North American Nursing Diagnosis Association International (NANDA-I)–approved nursing diagnoses have identified sets of defining characteristics that support identification of each nursing diagnosis (NANDA-I, 2005). After analyzing clusters of data, the nurse begins to consider diagnoses that might apply to the client. Carefully examine defining characteristics that either support or eliminate a nursing diagnosis. The absence of certain defining characteristics suggests that you reject a diagnosis. To be accurate, review all characteristics, eliminate irrelevant ones, and confirm relevant ones.

While focusing on patterns of defining characteristics, compare a client's pattern of data with data that is consistent with normal, healthful patterns. Use accepted norms as a basis for comparison. Judge whether the grouped signs and symptoms are normal for the client and whether they are within the range of healthful responses. Isolate defining characteristics not within healthy norms to identify the

TABLE 1-1 Summary of the Nursing Process		
COMPONENT	**PURPOSE**	**STEPS**
Assessment	To gather, verify, and communicate data about client to establish database	1. Collect nursing health history 2. Perform physical examination 3. Collect laboratory data 4. Validate data 5. Cluster data 6. Document data
Nursing diagnosis	To identify client's health care needs and formulate nursing diagnoses	1. Analyze and interpret data 2. Identify client problems 3. Formulate nursing diagnoses 4. Document nursing diagnoses
Planning	To identify client's goals, determine priorities of care, determine expected outcomes, and select nursing interventions to achieve goals of care	1. Identify client goals 2. Establish expected outcomes 3. Select nursing interventions 4. Delegate interventions 5. Write nursing care plan 6. Consults with client and health care team
Implementation	To administer nursing interventions necessary for accomplishing care plan	1. Reassess client's status 2. Review and modifying existing care plan 3. Perform nursing interventions
Evaluation	To determine extent to which goals of care have been achieved	1. Compare client response to criteria 2. Analyze reasons for results and conclusions 3. Modify care plan

client's diagnosis (Table 1-2). Before finalizing a nursing diagnosis, identify the client's general health care needs or problems. Considering all assessment data and focusing on the more relevant data help the nurse individualize nursing diagnoses. For example, a client may present with a general exercise tolerance problem. However, NANDA-I has a variety of diagnoses that apply to activity (e.g., activity intolerance, risk for activity intolerance, fatigue, impaired walking). Carefully review the selection of defining characteristics for the client, then select the correct diagnostic label.

Components of a Nursing Diagnosis. A nursing diagnosis consists of a two-part format that gives meaning and relevance to a client's health problems. The two-part format includes the NANDA-I diagnostic label followed by a statement of a related factor.

- The diagnostic label is a problem statement describing a physiological or psychological response to a health problem (e.g., **impaired skin integrity**).
- The etiology statement describes related or contributing factors that influence development of the response (e.g., **immobility**).

The diagnostic label may be an actual nursing diagnosis, a risk nursing diagnosis, or a wellness nursing diagnosis. An actual nursing diagnosis describes human response to health conditions or life processes that exist in an individual, family, or community. For example, **acute pain, diarrhea,** and **anxiety** are actual nursing diagnoses. A risk nursing diagnosis describes human responses to health conditions or life processes that have a chance of developing. For example, an overweight client with a spinal cord injury might have a diagnosis of **risk for impaired skin integrity.** The key assessment for risk diagnoses is the data that supports the client's vulnerability or risk. A wellness diagnosis describes human responses to level of wellness in an individual, group, or community that have a readiness for improvement (NANDA-I, 2005). Examples include **readiness for enhanced family coping** and **readiness for enhanced spiritual well-being.**

The related factor is a condition or etiology identified from the client's assessment data. It is associated with the client's actual or potential response to a health problem (e.g., **activity intolerance related to generalized weakness**). Related factors include four categories: patho-physiological, treatment-related, situational, and maturational. The "related to" phrase is not a cause-and-effect statement; rather it indicates that the etiology is associated with the problem. The inclusion of the "related to" phrase requires the nurse to use critical thinking to individualize the diagnosis and subsequent interventions. Remember, it is essential that the related factor communicate something that nurses can address within the domain of nursing practice. Interventions are selected based primarily on the "related factor" of the nursing diagnosis. Validate the related factor with the client when possible. For example, the diagnosis of **impaired physical mobility** could be related to **pain, weakness,** or **lack of balance.** Interventions for pain are obviously different from those for weakness or lack of balance.

Errors can occur in the diagnostic process. Collect data in an organized way to avoid inaccurate or missing data. Reduce errors in the diagnostic statement by identifying the client's response rather than the medical diagnosis, identifying a NANDA-I diagnostic statement rather than a symptom, identifying a treatable etiology rather than a clinical sign or chronic problem, and identifying the client's problem rather than the nursing intervention.

This text includes information in each chapter that identifies examples of nursing diagnoses related to the interventions and skills for that chapter. This information includes a description of the diagnostic statement, related factors that may be pertinent, and the focus for related nursing care.

Planning

After assessing a client's condition and identifying nursing diagnoses, the nurse develops a plan of care. This step includes setting client-centered goals and expected outcomes and prescribing nursing interventions. Another part of planning is to set priorities for a client. Remember that a single client often has multiple diagnoses and collaborative problems. Also being able to wisely set priorities ensures more timely and effective care when the nurse must care for groups of clients.

A client-centered goal is a specific and measurable behavior or response that reflects a client's highest level of

---

BOX 1-5 Creating a Nursing Diagnosis

1. Start with information from a client assessment. From the assessment, make a complete list of all significant cues, such as signs and symptoms, laboratory data, subjective data (client's report of symptoms), and data from medical history. Group cues according to clusters or patterns of significant cues in ways that make sense (e.g., recent weight loss, sore mouth, and reduced appetite indicate a nutrition problem). Each group of cues forms the defining characteristics for a nursing diagnosis label (e.g., body weight 20% or more under ideal, sore inflamed buccal cavity, lack of interest in food).
2. Identify the client problem or response from the NANDA-I list. This becomes the stem or label and the first part of the diagnostic statement. Use the exact NANDA-I words (e.g., imbalanced nutrition, less than body requirements).
3. Determine the etiology or contributing factors for the diagnosis. This becomes the "related to" part of the statement. From the assessment, ask, "What makes or maintains the client's unhealthy response?" What is associated with the defining characteristics? The related factor should be a condition or situation that nurses can independently treat or alleviate (e.g., inability to ingest food). Compare the client's contributing factors to those listed by NANDA-I.

TABLE 1-2 Example of the Diagnostic Process

ASSESSMENT	DATA CLUSTERS	ANALYSIS	NURSING DIAGNOSIS
Inspection of skin	Open lesion on sacrum 1 × 1 cm Red area 3 cm around coccyx	Pressure on coccyx	Impaired skin integrity related to immobility secondary to traction
Palpation of skin	Skin moist from diaphoresis Tenderness noted around lesion	Skin moisture promotes breakdown	
Historical data	Fractured left leg on 5/3 Positioned on back for traction to leg for 2 weeks; anticipate 4 more weeks minimum	Immobility	

wellness, for example, "Client performs insulin self-injection techniques for diabetes within 1 month." A goal is realistic and based on client needs and resources. It offers the predicted resolution of a problem, evidence of progress toward problem resolution, or continued maintenance of good health or function (Carpenito-Moyet, 2005).

An expected outcome is a specific measurable change in a client's status that is expected to occur in response to nursing care, for example, "Client will demonstrate syringe preparation with insulin by 3/20." At the time specified, the nurse evaluates the client's progress toward achievement, and the plan of care continues or is revised. An outcome is an objective measure of goal achievement. Meeting outcomes resolves the etiology for the nursing diagnosis. Expected outcomes provide a focus or direction for nursing care. Several expected outcomes are usually developed for each nursing diagnosis and goal. Often one nursing action is not enough to resolve a client problem.

There are seven guidelines for writing goals and expected outcomes:

1 Client centered—State what the client will do
2 Singular goal or outcome—Address one behavior or response
3 Observable—Determine through observation whether change has taken place
4 Measurable—Set standards against which to measure client's response, for example, "Apical pulse will be between 60 and 100 beats per minute"
5 Time limited—Time frame for each goal and outcome indicates when response is expected to occur
6 Mutual factors—Client agrees on direction and time limits of care
7 Realistic—Set goals and outcomes the client is able to reach

Priority setting involves ranking nursing diagnoses in order of importance. Priorities help the nurse anticipate and sequence nursing interventions. Classify priorities as high, intermediate, or low. Nursing diagnoses that, if untreated, result in harm to the client have the highest priorities. For example, **risk for other-directed violence, acute pain,** and **impaired gas exchange** are high-priority diagnoses that deal with the client's safety, comfort, and adequate oxygenation. Maslow's hierarchy of needs can act as a useful guide in setting priorities. These needs include, in the order of priority, physiological safety, love and belonging, esteem, and self-actualization. Priorities

can be psychological. Avoid classifying only physiological nursing diagnoses as high priority. Intermediate priorities involve the nonemergent, non–life threatening needs of the client. Low-priority diagnoses are client needs that are usually not directly related to a specific illness but may affect the client's future well-being.

Always determine priorities by involving the client. When the client is not aware of the significance of a particular intervention, explanations and teaching can help the client understand why one aspect of care is more important than another. Often it is appropriate to address the client's priorities before focusing on other areas of concern.

Implementation

Implementation involves the provision of care to clients. It describes the performance of nursing interventions necessary for achieving the goals and expected outcomes in the plan of care. Interventions include both direct and indirect care individualized to the client's needs. An intervention includes what, when, how much, how far, how long, how often, where, by whom, and with what. For example, in the case of a client with a nursing diagnosis of **impaired physical mobility,** the intervention "Encourage ambulation" is not adequate. Acceptable nursing interventions may include "Assist with walking to bathroom two times on 5/9" and "Assist with ambulating in hall at least 20 feet three times on 5/10."

Direct care interventions are treatments performed through interaction with the client. Examples include physical care techniques (e.g., urinary catheter insertion, administration of injections), activities of daily living (ADLs, e.g., bathing, dressing), education or counseling, and preventive nursing measures. Indirect care interventions are treatments performed away from the client but on behalf of the client or group of clients (Dochterman and Bulechek, 2004). Examples include management of the client's environment (e.g., safety and infection control), documentation, and interdisciplinary collaboration.

Evaluation

Evaluation involves examination of a condition or situation and then a judgment as to whether change has occurred. If exercise is a selected nursing intervention, the nurse evaluates the client's vital signs after ambulation to determine activity tolerance. When removing a surgical dressing, the nurse evaluates the wound to see whether healing has occurred since the last dressing change. The nursing process is dynamic and continuous, and evaluation is an ongoing process. The evaluation process includes five elements: (1) identifying evaluative criteria (these are the expected outcomes to measure); (2) collecting data to determine whether criteria are met; (3) interpreting and summarizing findings; (4) documenting findings; and (5) stopping, continuing, or revising the plan of care. Proper evaluation lets the nurse answer the following questions: What is the client's response to nursing care? Was the therapy effective?

Sometimes expected outcomes are not met, and evaluation of a client's progress reveals the need to revise approaches to care, introduce different interventions, or continue current interventions for a longer time. When expected outcomes are achieved, the nursing diagnosis can be documented as "resolved." Keeping focus on evaluation of the client's progress lessens the chance of the nurse becoming distracted by the tasks of care.

EVIDENCE-BASED PRACTICE

Evidence-based practice is the conscientious use of current best knowledge coupled with a clinician's expertise and clients' values and preferences when making clinical decisions (Melnyk and Fineout-Overholt, 2005). It uses the best scientific information available and applies this information to bedside client care. Although acquired in many ways, knowledge is information; discovery is the creative process of obtaining new knowledge. Historically nurses acquired new knowledge by tradition as one generation of nurses passed knowledge to the next. Because of many rapid changes in today's world, nurses need to seek relevant information from the scientific literature in addition to the experience of experts. The use of best evidence has been shown to improve client outcomes. Nurses must pursue, critique, and analyze best evidence and the possible implications for practice. During client care, ask yourself, "Are we using the best approach available in care of this client? What is the level of knowledge about the client's problem? How does the knowledge relate to my situation or the client's situation? How can this knowledge be applied?" It is essential for nurses to use a systematic approach, evidence-based information, and critical thinking to achieve the goal of the best possible client outcomes.

COMMUNICATION WITHIN THE HEALTH CARE TEAM

Client care requires effective communication among all members of the health care team. The two most common communication sources the nurse relies on are a client's record and reports. A client's record or chart is a confidential, permanent legal documentation of information relevant to the client's health care. It is a continuing account of the client's health status and the treatment provided by the health care team. Reports are oral, written, or audiotaped exchanges of information between members of the health care team. Common reports include change-of-shift reports, telephone and transfer reports, and incident reports. Nurses give verbal or taped reports when responsibility for care is being transferred to another health professional. A physician may call a nursing unit to receive a verbal report on a client's progress. The laboratory provides written reports or results of diagnostic tests.

Confidentiality

Do not disclose information about clients' status to other clients, family members (unless the client grants permission), or health care staff not involved in clients' care. Legal and ethical obligations require that nurses keep information about clients strictly confidential. In 1996, legislation to protect patient privacy for health information in the form of the Health Insurance Portability and Accountability Act (HIPAA) was proposed; the Act was finalized in 2003 with specific guidelines for communication of clients' personal health information (USDHHS, 2003). Under this legislation clients have access to their medical records and consent must be received from the client before information is released for health-related purposes. These standards require the USDHHS to establish national standards for electronic health care transactions and national identifiers for providers, health plans, and employers. HIPAA also addresses the security and privacy of health data. Adopting these standards will improve the efficiency and effectiveness of the nation's health care system by encouraging the widespread use of electronic data interchange in health care.

When health care professionals use records for data gathering, research, or education, records may be used only with permission and according to established agency, state, and federal guidelines. Many states require reporting of certain infectious or communicable diseases through the public health department, which must be done through proper channels.

Nurses may not disclose a client's status, including diagnosis, laboratory results, and prognosis, to other clients or staff not involved in the client's care. Nurses must be aware of confidentiality issues in elevators, waiting areas, and during lunch and coffee breaks. It is essential that protection be provided for the privacy and rights of clients who do not want information about their health information shared with others. For example, a nurse is responsible for respecting a client's wishes with regard to informing family members of a terminal illness. Further, a nurse cannot assume that a client's family members know all of the client's history, particularly with respect to private issues such as mental illness, medications, pregnancy, abortion, birth control, or sexually transmitted diseases (STDs).

The Medical Record

The medical record is a legal document. Through accurate documentation the record serves as a description of exactly what happens to a client in the health care system. The purpose of the record is to provide information for communication, education, assessment, research, financial billing, auditing, and legal accountability. Nursing care actually provided may have been excellent; however, in a court of law, "care not documented is care not done." The nursing process shapes a nurse's approach and direction of care, and good reporting and documentation reflect the nursing process.

- Assessments are recorded to offer a database from which health care team members can draw conclusions about the client's problems.
- Information about the client's concerns or condition assists caregivers in problem identification, planning, and setting priorities.
- Description of detailed care activities reflects the implementation of the plan.
- Evaluation of client responses to nursing care determines the client's success in achieving expected outcomes of care.

Nurses involved in the direct care of clients are responsible for documenting thorough assessments of a client's condition, descriptions of changes in a client's condition, a detailed accounting of nursing interventions, and an evaluation of the client's response to care.

Guidelines for Effective Documentation and Reporting

Nurses use various methods for recording and reporting. Regardless of the method, certain basic guidelines must be followed.

Factual

A factual record or report contains descriptive and objective information about what a nurse sees, hears, feels, or smells. An example of an objective description is "pulse 54, strong, and irregular." Avoid words such as *good*, *adequate*, *fair*, or *poor* that are subject to interpretation. Inferences are conclusions based on factual data. An example of an inference is "The client has a poor appetite." The factual data is "The client ate only two bites of toast for breakfast." Suppose that in one case the client was nauseated, whereas in another case the client was hungry but did not like the food on the tray. If nurses document inferences or conclusions without supportive factual data, misinterpretations about the client's health status occur.

Subjective data includes clients' perceptions about their health problems. Document subjective information using the client's words in quotes, for example, the client states she is "nauseated" or the client states she "does not like the food choices." In both cases, it would be helpful to document the actual food intake, as well as the subjective data.

Accurate

Accurate documentation uses clear, precise, accurate, and relevant measurements as a means to make comparisons and to determine when a client's condition has changed. Charting that an "abdominal wound is 5 cm in length, without redness or edema" is more accurate and descriptive than the statement "large abdominal wound is healing well." Accurate charting requires you to use only approved Joint Commission on Accreditation of Healthcare Organizations (JCAHO) or agency abbreviations and write out all terms that may be confusing. JCAHO has published an official "Do Not Use" list because of potential errors particularly in the area of medication administration (see Chapter 15). Correct spelling is essential, because terms can easily be misinterpreted (e.g., *accept* or *except*, *dysphagia* or *dysphasia*).

When observations are reported to another caregiver and interventions are performed by someone else, clearly indicate that fact (e.g., "Surgical dressings removed by Dr. Kline. Pulse of 104 reported to J. Kemp, RN"). End each entry with first name or first initial, last name, and title. For nursing students, include the approved abbreviation for the school and their program level.

Complete

Complete and concise information is essential to describe a client's clinical progress. Consider the following example of what may occur when a note has not been recorded completely.

A nurse explains and demonstrates a teaching session about giving insulin injections. The client eagerly expresses a desire to give the next injection when it is due. Documentation is as follows: "Discussed learning about insulin injection technique." During the next shift, another nurse spends time demonstrating the injection technique and assessing the client's readiness to give the injection because the previous teaching was not communicated. As a result, time is wasted, with the nurse repeating information the client previously learned instead of coaching the client through a self-injection.

Concise

Concise documentation facilitates efficient retrieval of pertinent information. When you learn to write concisely, less time is needed for documentation. A comparison of a concise and lengthy note follows:

Concise, Factual Entry	Lengthy Entry Using Vague Terms
0900 Left toes cool and pale, without inflammation, capillary return >5 sec; left pedal pulse 1+; right pedal pulse 4+. Describes pain in left foot as dull, aching 4 (scale 0-10).	0900 The client's left toes are cool, with pale color. There is no inflammation. There is slow capillary return present greater than 5 seconds. Dorsalis pedis pulse in left foot is weak, and the client complains of some discomfort. The pain in left foot is described as aching at a level of 4 on a scale of 0-10.

Current

Making prompt entries is essential in effective documentation (JCAHO, 2005). Delays in documentation result in serious omissions and untimely client care delays. Communicate the following at the time of occurrence:

1 Critical changes in vital signs
2 Pain assessment
3 Administration of medications and treatments
4 Preparation for diagnostic tests or surgery
5 Change in client status and who was notified
6 Client response to an intervention
7 Admission, transfer, discharge, or death of a client

Writing scratch notes on a work pad at the time of an event helps ensure accuracy when completing formal documentation. Many agencies use military time, a 24-hour time cycle. The military clock ends with midnight at 2400 and begins at 1 minute after midnight at 0001. The following examples compare standard with military time: 10:22 am is 1022 military time; 3:15 pm is 1515 military time (Figure 1-3).

Organized

Organized notes are written in a logical order. For example, an organized note follows the nursing process as the nurse describes the assessment, interventions, and client's response in a sequence. An organized note is also more effective when it is concise, clear, and to the point. When making a record entry, make a list of what to include before beginning to write in the permanent legal record. Identifying pertinent content is helpful in deleting unnecessary words.

The following compares a well-organized note with a disorganized note:

Organized Note	Disorganized Note
7/17 0630 Client reports sharp pain 9 (scale 0-10) in left lower quadrant of abdomen, worsened by turning onto right side. Positioning on left side decreases pain to 8 (scale 0-10). Abdomen is tender to touch and rigid. Bowel sounds are absent. Dr. Phillips notified. To x-ray for CT scan of abdomen. T. Reis, RN	7/17 0630 Client experiencing sharp pain in lower quadrant of abdomen. MD notified. Abdomen tender to touch, rigid, with bowel sounds absent. Positioning on left side offers minimal relief of pain. CT scan ordered of the abdomen. J. Adams, RN

Methods of Recording

The method of recording selected by a nursing service reflects the philosophy of the department. Staff use the same method throughout an agency. There are several acceptable methods: problem-oriented medical records (POMRs), source records, and charting by exception (CBE). The POMR organizes written information in a way to correspond to the nursing process. Organization of data is by problem or diagnosis. Ideally each member of the health care team contributes to a single list of client problems. Each recording includes a database, problem list, care plan, and progress notes. A source record is a way to organize chart information by each discipline. This format does not organize information by client problems. The advantage of a source record is that caregivers can easily locate the section of the chart to make entries. A disadvantage of the source record is fragmented data. CBE is an approach that defines criteria for normal nursing assessments and standards of practice for interventions. CBE simply involves completing a flow sheet that incorporates those standards, thus minimizing the need for lengthy narrative notes. However, the CBE system can be used inappropriately when nurses fail to enter notes that describe abnormal findings or unexpected changes in a client's condition.

Computerized Documentation

The majority of health care facilities have some type of electronic health record and documentation system. Computerized documentation can minimize repetitive clerical and monitoring tasks. Systems improve accuracy, timeliness, completeness, and communication across health disciplines. Data is more quickly retrievable. There is an increased risk of unauthorized individuals gaining access to computerized information. Do not share your password to enter and sign off computer files. Avoid leaving a computer terminal unattended when logged on. Follow agency protocol for correcting errors. Follow agency policy if you accidentally delete backup files. Avoid leaving information about a client displayed on a monitor where others see it. Follow confidentiality procedures for documenting sensitive client information.

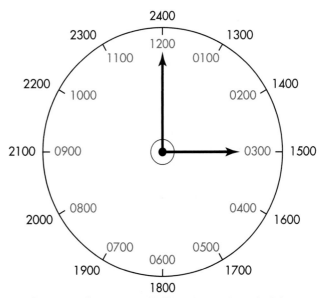

Figure 1-3 Comparison of military time and standard time.

SKILL 1.1   Documenting Nurses' Progress Notes

Nurses practice in a variety of settings and use a variety of forms and formats to communicate specific information about a client's health care. Documentation is a major indicator of quality and an important means of communication of the nursing care provided. Ideally, forms are designed to make data easy to find and interpret and to avoid unnecessary duplication. Most nursing forms have a place for client identification, date and times, and a key to indicate the meaning of abbreviations or entries used and the type of information required. Because of legal requirements, certain documentation rules must be followed.

BOX 1-6   Nursing Documentation Forms and Worksheets

Nursing History Forms
Completed when a client is admitted to a nursing unit. A nursing assessment must be completed for each client at the time of admission to a health care agency. The history includes basic biographical data (e.g., age, method of admission, physician), admitting medical diagnosis or chief complaint, and a brief medical-surgical history (e.g., previous surgeries or illnesses, allergies, medication history, client's perceptions about illness or hospitalization, physical assessment of all body systems). Encourages a systematic complete assessment and identification of relevant nursing diagnoses. Provides baseline data to compare with changes in the client's condition.

Graphic Sheets and Flow Sheets
Forms include routine observations made on a repeated basis using a check mark (e.g., when bath is given, client is turned). When completing a flow sheet, the nurse should review previous entries to identify changes.

Computerized Client Care Summary
Includes pertinent information about clients and their ongoing care plans, such as basic demographic data (e.g., age, religion), physician's name, primary medical diagnosis, current physician's orders, nursing orders or interventions, scheduled tests or procedures, safety precautions to use in the client's care, and factors related to ADLs.

Nursing Kardex (Worksheet)
Includes information needed for daily care on a flip card or in a notebook. Usually kept at the nurses' station. Information can be used for change-of-shift report and facilitates access to information without referring to the client record. Includes demographical data, tests ordered, therapies, and information related to ADLs. May include standardized or individualized nursing care plans.

BOX 1-7   Formats for Documentation

SOAP: Subjective data, Objective data, Assessment or Analysis, and Plan. Usually based on a numbered list of problems or nursing diagnoses.

   1 Anxiety related to preparation for surgery.
   S: Subjective data—The client's statements regarding the problem (e.g., Client stated, "I am dreading this surgery because last time I had a terrible reaction to the anesthesia and had such terrible pain when they made me get out of bed.").
   O: Objective data—Observations that support or are related to subjective data (e.g., frequent turning in bed and loud, agitated voice).
   A: Assessment/Analysis—Conclusions reached based on data (e.g., fear related to pain/anesthesia).
   P: Plan—The plan for dealing with the situation (e.g., "Notified anesthesiologist, Dr. Moore, of experience. Discussed alternatives for anesthesia and pain-control options. Stressed importance of activity for circulation and healing. Encouraged to keep nurses informed of pain level and need for medication and told client that pain usually is present, but manageable.").

PIE: Problem, Intervention, and Evaluation. Problem-oriented system in which progress notes are written based on a list of numbered or labeled client problems.

   P: Problem—Preoperative anxiety: Client stated, "I am dreading this surgery because last time I had a terrible reaction to the anesthesia and had such terrible pain when they made me get out of bed." Observed frequent turning in bed and loud, agitated voice.
   I: Intervention—Notified anesthesiologist, Dr. Moore, of experience. Discussed with client alternatives for anesthesia and pain-control options. Stressed importance of activity for circulation and healing.

   Told to keep nurses informed of pain level and need for medication. Told client that pain usually is present, but manageable.
   E: Evaluation—Client stated she was "very relieved." Stated she would tell the nurses about pain.

DAR: Data, Action, and client Response. Used in focus charting; a way to organize progress notes to make them more clear and organized.

   D: Data—Client states, "I am dreading this surgery because last time I had a terrible reaction to the anesthesia and had such terrible pain when they made me get out of bed." Observed frequent turning in bed and loud, agitated voice.
   A: Action—Notified anesthesiologist, Dr. Moore, of experience. Discussed alternatives for anesthesia and pain-control options. Stressed importance of activity for circulation and healing. Encouraged to keep nurses informed of pain level and need for medication and told client that pain usually is present, but manageable.
   R: Response—Client stated she was "very relieved." Stated she would tell the nurses about pain.

Narrative Note. Describes client data in a narrative paragraph. For example:

   Client states, "I am dreading this surgery because last time I had a terrible reaction to the anesthesia and had such terrible pain when they made me get out of bed." Observed frequent turning in bed and loud, agitated voice. Notified anesthesiologist, Dr. Moore, of experience. Discussed alternatives for anesthesia and pain-control options. Stressed importance of activity for circulation and healing. Encouraged to keep nurses informed of pain level and need for medication and told client that pain usually is present, but manageable.

Medical record forms that nurses have traditionally used for documentation include nursing admission history, physical assessment and vital signs graphic, medication administration records, nurses' notes, and nursing care flow sheets (Box 1-6). Many agencies have a variety of worksheets that are useful for routine client care and that are not a permanent part of the record. One example is a computerized care summary printed and updated each shift that includes current orders for ADLs, diagnostic tests ordered, and in some cases standard or individualized nursing care plans. In some long-term care agencies where information is not computerized a "Kardex" is handwritten in pencil to serve this purpose.

Because the nursing process shapes a nurse's approach to client care, good documentation reflects the nursing process. Nurses record assessment data to provide all health care team members a database from which to make decisions about clients' needs and problems. After developing a plan of care, with goals and expected outcomes, document a description of nursing care provided. Evaluation of care communicates the client's degree of progress toward wellness and success in meeting expected outcomes of care. One of the major challenges of effective documentation is to complete it in a timely fashion. Prompt documentation increases accuracy and promotes effective communication to other members of the health care team.

Progress notes are a format for documenting a record of a client's progress. A variety of formats may be used for progress notes, including SOAP (Subjective data, Objective data, Assessment or Analysis, and Plan); SOAPE (SOAP plus Evaluation); PIE (Problem, Intervention, and Evaluation); APIE (Assessment, Plan, Intervention, and Evaluation); and DAR (Data, Action, and client Response), used in focus charting (Box 1-7). Any caregiver needs to be able to read a progress note and understand what type of problem a client has, the level of care provided, and the results of the interventions. The nurse who is responsible for the client care provided signs each entry. The signature includes the full name and title.

ASSESSMENT

1 Review assessments, goals and expected outcomes, interventions, and client responses as soon as possible after contact with each client. *Rationale: Facilitates identifying the type of information to communicate in a progress note.*

PLANNING

Expected Outcomes focus on documentation that reflects appropriate information to describe the client's changing clinical status and response to nursing interventions.

Delegation Considerations

Some routine documentation may be delegated to AP, including vital signs, intake and output (I&O), and routine care related to ADLs. Documentation is best done by the individual who provides the care, to the extent possible.

Equipment

- Worksheets, nursing Kardex or client care profile, nursing care plan, critical pathway, or multidisciplinary treatment plan

IMPLEMENTATION *for Documenting Nurses' Progress Notes*

STEPS	RATIONALE
1 Identify the forms you are expected to maintain and where they are located.	
2 After each client contact, identify information that needs to be documented. Consider:	Improves quality and accuracy of documentation and promotes effective communication to other members of the health care team.
a. Abnormal findings	
b. Changes in status	
c. New problems identified	
3 Document in a timely fashion, without leaving open spaces between notes, and include date and time.	Increases accuracy and helps prevent omission of significant information.
4 Using agency format, document the following:	Ensures relevant information about client's clinical progress is available in written form.
a. Pertinent, factual, objective data	
b. Selected subjective data that validates or clarifies	
c. Nursing actions taken	
d. Client responses to actions taken	
e. Additional plans that should be implemented	

STEPS	RATIONALE
f. To whom the information has been reported, including name and status	When follow-up is needed, documenting to whom information was reported shares responsibility with that individual.
5 Sign progress note with full name or first initial and last name and status according to agency policy. Students are usually required to indicate their level of education and school affiliation.	Identifies person legally responsible for client care provided.

EVALUATION

1 Review previously documented entries with those you are about to enter, noting if there is significant change in the client's status.

Special Considerations

Home Care Considerations

• Documentation provides evidence of achieving nursing standards and is the basis for reimbursement for home health care services.
• Both quality of care and justification for financial reimbursement depend on effective documentation.
• Because Medicare has specific guidelines for eligibility for reimbursement, documentation that fulfills these guidelines is essential.

• Some parts of the record are needed in the home, whereas other parts are needed in the agency office; modems and laptop computers are helping address these varied needs.

Long-Term Care Considerations

• For stable long-term care residents, certain documentation entries may be made weekly or monthly.
• Outside agencies such as the state department of health determine the standards and policies for long-term care documentation.
• The RN is responsible for identifying and documenting episodic changes that may require more intensive nursing intervention and pertinent data for residents who become ill.

SKILL 1.2 Giving a Change-of-Shift Report

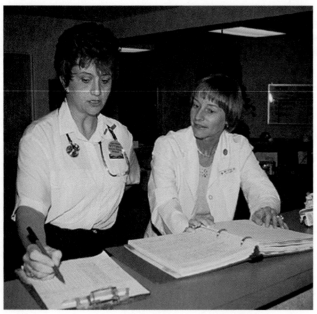

Figure 1-4 Giving a change-of-shift report.

In addition to written documentation, nurses report information about their assigned clients to the nurses working on the next shift. The purpose of the report is to provide continuity of care for the client. Recently, the JCAHO (2006) developed the *National Patient Safety Goals* for institutions to standardize an approach to "hand off" communication that includes an opportunity to ask and respond to questions. In the past, a change-of-shift report has often been given in a report room by audiotape. However, if audiotape is used, the outgoing staff must now remain available to answer questions from staff who are about to work the next shift (Figure 1-4). Oral reports are given either in a conference room or during walking rounds with nurses from both shifts participating. Regardless of the reporting method, it is beneficial to allow time for clarification or updates before the previous nurses leave the unit. Reports given in person or on rounds allow immediate feedback when questions are raised. Confidentiality must be maintained.

ASSESSMENT

1 Review information on worksheets, get report from co-workers to whom care has been delegated, and gather other relevant information (e.g., pertinent assessment data, laboratory reports, physicians' orders). *Rationale: Data reported needs to be relevant and timely, reflecting changes during the shift. Preparation enhances a clear, well-organized report.*

PLANNING

Expected Outcomes focus on identifying appropriate information to report to the nurses on the next shift.

Delegation Considerations

The skill of change-of-shift report may not be delegated.
- LPNs/LVNs may report on clients they care for directly.
- AP report to a nurse (e.g., apparent change in client's level of pain, reduction in level of consciousness, change in vital signs) so that the nurse may include any pertinent information (after validation) in the report.

Equipment

- Worksheets, nursing Kardex or client care profile, nursing care plan, critical pathway, or multidisciplinary treatment plan
- Tape recorder (according to agency policy)

IMPLEMENTATION *for Giving a Change-of-Shift Report*

STEPS	RATIONALE
1 Develop an organized format for delivering report that provides a description of client's needs and concerns.	Organizes data based on priorities and is individualized by the reporting nurse.
2 For each client, include:	
a. Background information—Client's name, gender, age, and current primary reason for hospitalization. Also include any known allergies, emergency code status (i.e., "do not resuscitate" [DNR]), and special needs as related to any physical challenges (e.g., blind, hearing deficit, amputee).	A more in-depth background report may be needed if a nurse new to a unit or an inexperienced nurse will be working the next shift.
b. Assessment data—Provide objective observations and measurements made by the nurse during the shift. Describe client's condition, and emphasize any recent changes. Include any relevant information reported by client, family, or health care team members, such as laboratory data and diagnostic test results.	Oncoming nurse will use data as a baseline for comparison during next shift.
c. Nursing diagnoses—If appropriate, state the nursing diagnoses appropriate for client. (Some agencies do not use nursing diagnosis in report.)	Clarifies the type of problems client is experiencing.
d. Interventions and evaluation (steps can be combined in a report).	Clarifies client's current responses to health problems.
(1) Describe therapies or treatments administered during shift and expected outcomes (e.g., medication changes, laboratory results, consultation visits). Specify how interventions are uniquely given for this client. Explain client's response and whether outcomes are met. Do not explain basic steps of procedure.	Staff learn the effect interventions are having on client's recovery and progress.
(2) Describe instructions given in teaching plan and client's ability to demonstrate learning.	Ensures continuity of teaching, minimizing repetition, but communicating any needs for reinforcement.
e. Family information—Report on family visitation or involvement, specifically as it influenced client. Explain if family members were included in care procedures or instruction.	Informs staff of level of involvement family members have assumed in client's care.

STEPS	RATIONALE
f. Discharge plan—Client's progress in reaching discharge is reviewed on an ongoing basis during each change-of-shift report. Discuss status of educational progress, communication with referral agencies, and preparation of family members for clients being discharged. This plan also identifies the roles and responsibilities of the multidisciplinary team and their follow-up visits.	All team members need to collaborate to follow the plan of care that promotes discharge each day to facilitate a smooth transition from hospital or health care facility to home.
g. Current priorities—Explain clearly the priorities to which oncoming nurse must attend.	Allows nurse to organize, make assignments, and plan by identification of which clients will need to be monitored most closely.
(1) Report on status of client undergoing significant clinical changes.	
(2) Report on immediate treatment planned for newly admitted client.	
(3) Explain status of specific preparatory activities for clients undergoing diagnostic or treatment procedures.	Ensures preparatory procedures will be completed on time to avoid treatment or diagnostic delay.
(4) Describe current physical status of clients returning from diagnostic or operative procedures.	Directs type of observations and treatments needed post procedure.

EVALUATION

1 Ask staff from the oncoming shift if they have questions regarding information reported.

2 When using a tape recorder, periodically self-evaluate for clarity, organization, rate of speaking, and volume level.

Special Considerations
Home Care Considerations

- Often a nurse is able to provide continuity of care for clients by having an assigned caseload for visits, making reporting on a daily basis unnecessary.

Long-Term Care Considerations

- Report in long-term care settings is similar to report in acute care settings with the exception that many clients are stable, or changes are often not apparent on a daily basis. In long-term care, periodic assessment and evaluation are done and reported according to established standards.

NCLEX® Style Questions

1 Mrs. Elvin is admitted to the hospital for the first time at 52 years of age. She is scheduled for surgery. Her neighbor and best friend are with her, and she tells the admitting nurse that this is her only "family." She also tells you that she has a question about the scheduled surgery. Legally and ethically the first priority of the nurse before asking the client to sign the surgery consent form is:
1. Notify the care provider that the client has a question about the surgery.
2. Identify the client's level of understanding and approval of the surgical procedure.
3. Inform the client of her right to implement an advance directive.
4. Inform the neighbor of her responsibility for informing the physician of anticipated problems in following prescribed treatment.

2 Mr. Joplin has been hospitalized in an acute care setting for pain control and treatment of cancer. Following assessment the nurse identifies a diagnosis of acute pain. The plan of care includes vital signs every 4 hours, I&O, medication for pain control, and bed rest. What can be delegated to assistive personnel?
1. Assessment of the pain
2. Obtaining pertinent factual objective data
3. Evaluation of client responses to interventions
4. Vital signs and measuring I&O

3 Special considerations for documentation of client care in the long-term care setting include:
1. Identifying and documenting episodic changes when clients become ill and more intensive nursing interventions are required
2. Daily documentation of subjective data that confirms that the client is well cared for
3. Weekly documentation of safety precautions utilized
4. Frequency of family interactions and support

4 The nurse checks on Mr. Rawls, a 62-year-old man who was admitted to the hospital with pneumonia. Mr. Rawls has been coughing profusely and has required suctioning. He also has an IV infusion of antibiotics. Mr. Rawls is febrile with a temperature of 101° F (38.3° C). Mr. Rawls asks the nurse if he can perhaps have a bed bath because he has been perspiring profusely. The most appropriate task for the nurse to delegate to the LPN/LVN working with her today is:
1. Vital signs
2. Administering IV antibiotics
3. Suctioning
4. Administering a bed bath

5 Anne Jenkins is caring for Mr. Niles, a 64-year-old client who had surgery for a benign tumor of the prostate. She enters the client's room to conduct an assessment and explains, "I want to ask you a few questions and check you carefully to see how you are doing this morning." While Anne inspects Mr. Niles' IV site, she notices redness. When she palpates over the site, Mr. Niles has a grimace on his face. Anne asks, "Is that area tender?" When the client admits to discomfort, Anne explains that Mr. Niles might be developing phlebitis, inflammation of the vein. In this situation, Anne has demonstrated which of the following skills?
1. Psychomotor
2. Cognitive
3. Interpersonal
4. Ethical

References for all chapters appear in Appendix D.

2

Facilitating Communication

MEDIA RESOURCES

- **evolve** http://evolve.elsevier.com/Elkin

- **View Video!** Video Clips

Communication is a basic human need and the foundation for establishing a caring relationship between the nurse and the client. Communication involves the expression of emotions, ideas, and thoughts through verbal (words or written language) and nonverbal (e.g., behaviors) exchanges. Verbal communication includes both the spoken and written word. Nonverbal communication includes body movement, physical appearance, personal space, touch, and facial expression. The interaction between the skilled nurse and the client progresses to a therapeutic level in which the nurse offers goal-directed activities to help the client share thoughts and feelings. With time and practice, nurses develop skills that limit social interactions and maintain a congenial and warm style that helps clients feel comfortable in sharing ideas and feelings.

Multiple essential interpersonal skills are necessary to communicate therapeutically with clients. These skills include having empathy and a nonjudgmental attitude, being aware of both verbal and nonverbal communication, using appropriate body language, being patient and sensitive to clients' cues, and giving feedback appropriately.

The basic elements of communication include a message, a sender, a receiver, and feedback (Figure 2-1). The message is the information expressed, which can be motivated by experience, emotions, ideas, or actions. The message may be sent through channels including visual, auditory, and tactile senses. Generally, the more channels used, the better the message is understood.

For communication to be effective, the receiver must be aware of the sender's message. The message received is understood as filtered through perceptions shaped from previous experiences. People tend to interpret life experiences through general assumptions and values they hold; in essence, this is the concept of filtering. The more aware people are of how these assumptions influence how they perceive the world and others, the more open they can be when interacting with others.

Feedback, verbal or nonverbal, is a response to the sender that can indicate if the meaning of the message sent was received. Because communication is a two-way process, the nurse gives feedback to clients and seeks feedback from clients to validate clients' understanding of the messages sent.

Communication is a complex process that is influenced by many factors (Box 2-1). Each person is unique and associates different ideas with a message and interprets it differently than any other person. For example, a facial expression may convey anger to one person and pain to another. It is essential for nurses to clarify messages so that incorrect inferences and miscommunication with the client are avoided.

Silence can be therapeutic. It gives the nurse and client time to think. It is important for the nurse to notice the client's inner feelings. It is also important to pay attention to a client's nonverbal behavior for cues that suggest what the client is feeling. Reflecting the nurse's impressions can validate what the client is experiencing. If silence lasts too long or becomes uncomfortable for the client, it can be helpful to say, "You seem very quiet," or "Could you tell me what you need right now?" or "How are you feeling?"

Barriers to effective therapeutic communication techniques exist in the form of ineffective responses and behaviors (Box 2-2). The use of these nontherapeutic techniques can hinder the therapeutic relationship between the client and the nurse.

Effective communication can be learned and requires practice, as does any other skill. An attitude of acceptance is helpful to promote open communication. To listen effectively, it helps to face clients, maintain eye contact, pay attention to what is being conveyed, and give feedback to verify accurate understanding. Even though the nurse may not agree with clients, the nurse can accept clients' rights to their opinions. It is best to avoid arguing with clients. Instead simply reflect understanding of what clients are communicating without agreeing or disagreeing.

Preoccupation with the techniques of communication can interfere with rather than enhance the communication process. Ineffective communication may not halt conversation, but it often tends to inhibit clients' willingness to express concerns openly. The nurse needs to find an appropriate place, allow sufficient time, and facilitate communication according to clients' circumstances and needs. Table 2-1 summarizes techniques that facilitate and inhibit communication.

CULTURAL CONSIDERATIONS RELATING TO COMMUNICATION

It is important to recognize cultural diversity and to demonstrate respect for people as unique individuals. Culture is just one factor that influences communication between two persons. Awareness of cultural norms or values enhances understanding of nonverbal cues. Consider any potential communication differences to effectively communicate with persons from other cultures, including cultural perspective, heritage, and health traditions of both the client and the nurse. Questions to consider include the following: Who is the nurse from a cultural perspective? Who is the client from a cultural perspective? What is the nurse's heritage? What is the client's heritage? What are the health traditions of the nurse's heritage? What are the health traditions of the client's heritage? Transcultural communication is most effective when each person attempts to understand the other's point of view from that person's cultural heritage.

Use of language, gestures, and vocal emphasis of words: Take care to determine if understanding was achieved. Avoid overly technical jargon, or terms unique to a culture.

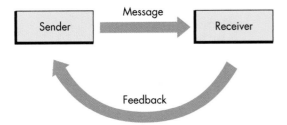

FIGURE 2-1 Communication is a two-way process.

BOX 2-1 Factors that Influence Communication

Perceptions: Personal views based on past experiences.
Values: Beliefs a person considers important in life.
Emotions: Subjective feelings about a situation (e.g., anger, fear, frustration, pain, anxiety, personal appearance).
Sociocultural background: Language, gestures, and attitudes common for a specific group of people relating to family origin, occupation, or lifestyle.
Knowledge level: Level of education and experience influences a person's knowledge base.
Roles and relationships: Conversation between two nurses differs from that between nurse and client.
Environment: Noise, lack of privacy, and distractions influence effectiveness.
Space and territoriality: Distance of 18 inches to 4 feet is ideal for sitting with a client for an interaction. Clients from different cultures may have different needs for personal space.

BOX 2-2 Ineffective Responses and Behaviors

- Not listening
- Talking too much
- Looking too busy
- Using clichés
- Seeming uncomfortable with silence
- Laughing nervously
- Not paying attention
- Smiling inappropriately
- Being opinionated
- Showing disapproval
- Avoiding sensitive topics
- Belittling feelings
- Arguing
- Minimizing problems
- Being superficial
- Being defensive
- Changing the subject
- Focusing on personal problems of the nurse
- Having a closed posture
- Making flippant remarks
- Ignoring the client
- Lying/being insincere
- Making false promises
- Making sarcastic remarks

From Keltner N, Schwecke L, Bostrom C: *Psychiatric nursing: a psychotherapeutic management approach,* ed 4, St Louis, 2003, Mosby.

TABLE 2-1 Facilitating and Inhibiting Communication

TECHNIQUE	EXAMPLES	RATIONALE
Initiating and Encouraging Interaction		
Giving information	"It is time for me to…" "I will be here until…"	Informs client of facts needed to understand situation. Provides a means to build trust and develop a knowledge base for clients to make decisions.
Stating observations	"You are smiling." "I see you are up already."	By calling client's attention to what is observed, nurse encourages client to be aware of behavior.
Open questions/comments	"What is your biggest concern?" "Tell me about your health."	Allows client to choose the topic of discussion according to circumstances and needs.
General leads	"And then?" "Go on…" "Say more…"	Encourages client to continue talking.
Focused questions/comments	"Tell me about your pain or comfort." "What did your doctor say?" "How has your family reacted?" "What is your biggest fear?"	Encourages client to give more information about specific topic of concern.
Helping Client Identify and Express Feelings		
Sharing observations	"You look tense." "You seem uncomfortable when…"	Promotes client's awareness of nonverbal behavior and feelings underlying the behavior. Helps clarify meaning of the behavior.
Paraphrasing	Client: "I could not sleep last night." Nurse: "You've had trouble sleeping?"	Encourages client to describe the situation more fully. Demonstrates that nurse is listening and concerned.
Reflecting feelings	"You were angry when that happened?" "You seem upset…"	Focuses client on identified feelings based on verbal or non-verbal cues.
Focused comments	"That seems worth talking about more." "Tell me more about…"	Encourages client to think about and describe a particular concern in more detail.
Ensuring Mutual Understanding		
Seeking clarification	"I don't quite follow you…" "Do you mean…?" "Are you saying that…?"	Encourages client to expand on a topic that is not yet clear or that seems contradictory.
Summarizing	"So there are three things you are upset about, your family being too busy, your diet, and being in the hospital so long."	Reduces the interaction to three or four points identified by nurse as significant. Allows client to agree or add other concerns.
Validation	"Did I understand you correctly that…?" "What made you decide to eat that when you know it gives you stomach pain?"	Allows clarification of ideas that nurse may have interpreted differently than intended by client.
Inhibiting Communication		
"Why" questions	"Why did you go back to bed?"	Asks client to justify reasons. Implies criticism and makes client feel defensive. Better to state what happened and encourage telling the whole story, e.g., "I noticed you went back to bed."
Sidestepping or changing subject	Client: "I'm having a hard time with my family." Nurse: "Do you have any grandchildren?"	Eases nurse's own discomfort and avoids exploring topic identified by client.
False reassurance	"Everything will be okay." "Surgery is no big deal."	This is vague and simplistic and tends to belittle client's concerns. It does not invite a response.
Giving advice	"You really should exercise more." "You shouldn't eat fast food every day."	This keeps client from actively engaging in finding a solution. Often client knows what should/should not be done and needs to explore alternative ways of dealing with issue.
Stereotyped responses	"You have the best doctor in town." "All clients with cancer worry about that."	This does not invite client to respond.
Defensiveness	"The nurses here work very hard." "Your doctor is extremely busy."	Moves focus away from client's feelings without acknowledging concerns.

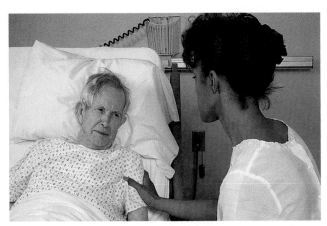

FIGURE 2-2 Therapeutic use of touch needs to take cultural factors into consideration.

Eye contact: Direct eye contact is valued in some cultures, whereas other cultures find it improper and intrusive; for example, it may be improper to make eye contact with authority figure.

Use of touch/personal space: Some cultures are "noncontact" cultures and have needs for clear boundaries; other cultures value close contact, handshakes, and embracing (Figure 2-2).

Time orientation: Many cultures are oriented to the present; some cultures value planning for the future.

Nonverbal behaviors: Use gestures with shared meaning.

Nurses need to adopt an attitude of flexibility, respect, and interest to bridge any communication barriers imposed by cultural differences.

The United States has become more culturally and ethnically diverse, reflecting a mixture of health care beliefs and practices. As society has become more diverse, it is essential for health care providers, including nurses, to learn about cultural and ethnic differences. This process begins with self-awareness; this involves getting to know oneself: one's personality, values, beliefs, and ethics when caring for clients who are different from oneself (Purnell and Paulanka, 2003).

Clients with limited English proficiency may not possess adequate vocabulary skills to communicate effectively. If a client does not speak the nurse's language, a translator or interpreter is needed (Dysart-Gale, 2005; Martin and others, 2005). Interpreters serve to decode the client's words and provide meaning behind the message, whereas translators just restate the words from one language to another. Often, the client speaks the nurse's language with limited ability or uses language with meaning different from the nurse's meaning. For example, the client may know customary greetings such as "How are you?" and not understand "pain" or "nausea." When communication fails, avoid the tendency to speak louder, stop talking, concentrate on the tasks, or begin doing things for, rather than with, the client. Inappropriate responses may result in painful isolation, anger, or misunderstanding for the client and inability of the client to cooperate. Trained interpreters and translators can positively affect persons with limited English proficiency by improving client

satisfaction, quality of care, and outcomes (Flores, 2005). Special approaches to communicate to clients who speak different languages are described in Box 2-3.

Helpful communication skills with clients of a different culture include tact, consideration, and respect. The nurse can convey empathy and genuine interest to facilitate complete information sharing. In addition, personal space needs to be respected when interviewing multicultural clients. The use of nonverbal communication, such as eye contact, gestures, and body language, varies among cultures (Purnell and Paulanka, 2003). Nurses need to take appropriate steps to preserve cultural differences while helping clients to change only the health care patterns that are not helpful.

SENSORY AND MOTOR ALTERATIONS

Clients with sensory losses require communication techniques that maximize existing sensory and motor functions. Some clients are unable to speak because of physical or neurological alterations, such as paralysis; a tube in the trachea to facilitate breathing (Figure 2-3); or a stroke resulting in aphasia, difficulty understanding or verbalizing. When a client experiences receptive aphasia, there is impaired comprehension of both written and spoken language. Expressive aphasia affects the motor function of speech so that the client has difficulty speaking and writing; however, the client can hear and understand. For clients with speech difficulties, speech pathologists are helpful. Body actions such as the use of touch and reading the client's body language facilitate a better understanding of the client's attitude and needs (Sundin and Jansson, 2003).

Hearing impairment affects one's quality of life and may be easily overlooked by health care providers. Communication is impaired when a message is lost or misinterpreted because the message is not heard due to the client's hearing alterations. Nurses have used aids such as pictures, electronic communication, two-way text messaging, and communica-

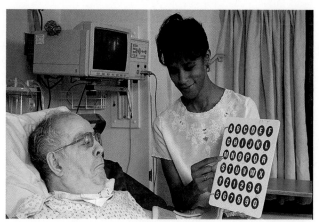

FIGURE 2-3 Communication tools for client who cannot speak because of tracheostomy.

> **BOX 2-4 Communication Aids**
>
> - Pad and felt-tipped pen or magic slate
> - Board with words, letters, or pictures denoting basic needs (e.g., water, bedpan, pain medication)
> - Call bells or alarms
> - Sign language
> - Use of eye blinks or movement of fingers for simple responses (e.g., "yes" or "no")
> - Flash cards with pictures rather than words
> - Computer/electronic devices

tion software to communicate with clients successfully (Akamatsu, Mayer, and Farelly, 2005; Beck and others, 2005; Houts and others, 2005). American Sign Language (ASL) interpreters have been used with hearing-impaired clients via telemedicine (Lopez and others, 2004). Communication aids can facilitate communication (Box 2-4).

EVIDENCE IN PRACTICE

Sundin K, Jansson L: 'Understanding and being understood' as a creative caring phenomenon—in care of patients with stroke and aphasia, *J Clin Nurs* 12(1):107-116, 2003.

Researchers examined the meaning of understanding and being understood in the care of clients with aphasia after stroke. This study was conducted because communication with these clients is often difficult because of their communication impairments. Also, these impairments may affect the quality of nurse-client interactions. The researchers videotaped nurses interacting with clients with aphasia while helping them with their activities of daily living (ADLs). A narrative and reflective interview was conducted with the nurses after the videotaping. The data was analyzed for themes related to understanding and being under-

stood within the context of the therapeutic nurse-client relationship. Several themes emerged, including silent dialogue, comprehending and mediating through body actions, striving for cooperation, and supporting attitude and permissive atmosphere. Through the use of touch, a sense of calm and comfort is conveyed to clients. Touch may also mediate acceptance of the client. Nonverbal communication is important to convey feelings and attitudes between the nurse and the client. The nurse encourages the client to manage his or her own care and will intervene if necessary. The nurse who listens in a nondemanding way facilitates open communication. This research suggests that the quality of the nurse-client interaction is enhanced when nurses encounter the client in a caring way, which includes understanding and being understood.

NURSING DIAGNOSES

Impaired verbal communication is an appropriate diagnosis when the focus is to enhance effective communication for a client with decreased or absent ability to use or understand language. **Anxiety** may be appropriate when the focus is to help the client deal with symptoms of anxiety, including muscle tension, shakiness, or restlessness. **Situational low self-esteem** may be appropriate when a person has a predominantly negative self-appraisal, including inability to handle situations and difficulty making decisions.

| SKILL 2.1 | Establishing the Nurse-Client Relationship | |

A therapeutic nurse-client relationship is the foundation of nursing care and involves client-centered, goal-directed interactions using therapeutic communication skills (Hagerty and Patusky, 2003). Therapeutic communication empowers clients to make decisions. Factors that influence communication include the client's perceptions, values, sociocultural background, and knowledge level. Therapeutic communication differs from social communication in

that it is client centered and goal directed with limited disclosure from the professional. However, an important aspect of therapeutic communication is the nurse's ability to show caring for the client. Caring establishes trust and creates an openness on the part of the client to communicate.

Usually nurses avoid sharing details of their personal lives with clients. Personal self-disclosure by the nurse may occur when it may be of help to the client, such as helping the client focus on key issues. This may assist the nurse in establishing a professional relationship with the client. Social communication that involves equal opportunity for personal disclosure and in which both participants seek to have personal needs met is not appropriate between nurses and clients (Keltner, Schwecke, and Bostrom, 2003).

The nurse-client relationship is characterized by three overlapping phases: orientation, working, and termination (Hagerty and Patusky, 2003). The orientation phase involves learning about the client and any initial concerns and needs. In the orientation phase, roles of the nurse or other health care professional are clarified, information is collected, goals are established, misunderstandings are clarified, and rapport is established between the nurse and the client. It is quite common for a nurse to encounter a client who needs comfort and support while experiencing threatening situations. A newly diagnosed illness, separation from family, the discomfort of surgery or diagnostic and treatment procedures, grief, and loss are just a few examples of health-related situations that may require the skill of comforting.

After orientation, the working phase begins. Examples of a variety of communication techniques that may facilitate or inhibit communication during the working phase are presented in Table 2-1. Active listening and empathy are two of the most effective ways to facilitate communication. Active listening conveys interest in the client's needs, concerns, and problems, and requires complete attention to understand the entire verbal and nonverbal message. Empathy is the act of effectively communicating to other persons that their feelings are understood. After people know their feelings have been accepted, they do not have to struggle to explain or justify their reactions (Fortinash and Holoday-Worret, 2004). Listening techniques are learned behaviors. At first they seem awkward and time consuming, but, as with any skill, they become more comfortable with practice. It is essential that the nurse appear natural, relaxed, and at ease while listening.

A nurse prepares for termination generally at the beginning of the relationship by indicating the purpose of the communication session and the amount of time available. The termination phase consists of evaluation and summary of progress toward identified goals.

ASSESSMENT

1 Determine client's need to communicate (e.g., client who constantly uses call light, is crying, does not understand an illness, has just been admitted to the hospital or nursing home).

2 Assess reason client needs health care.

3 Assess factors about self and client that normally influence communication: perceptions, values and beliefs, emotions, sociocultural background, severity of illness, knowledge, age level, verbal ability, roles and relationships, environmental setting, physical comfort, and discomfort. *Rationale: Facilitates accurate assessment of the experiences of the client.*

4 Assess client's language and ability to speak. Does the client have difficulty finding words or associating ideas with accurate word symbols? Does the client have difficulty with expression of language and/or reception of messages? *Rationale: Identifies the appropriate communication aids to be used (e.g., use of an interpreter, use of communication board).*

5 Observe client's pattern of communication and verbal or nonverbal behavior (e.g., gestures, tone of voice, eye contact). *Rationale: Patterns of communication may influence the type and manner of communication used by the nurse.*

6 Encourage the client to ask for clarification at any time during the communication. *Rationale: Gives the client a sense of control and keeps the channels of communication open.*

7 Identify cultural influences that affect communication. What language does the client predominantly use in thinking? Does the client need an interpreter or translator? Is the client able to read and/or write in English? What verbal or nonverbal communication shows respect (e.g., tempo, eye/body contact, topic restrictions)? *Rationale: Knowledge of cultural factors facilitates communication (Flores, 2005).*

PLANNING

Expected Outcomes focus on using therapeutic communication skills to obtain information about the client's ideas, needs, and concerns.

1 Client expresses ability to communicate with the nurse without feeling threatened or defensive.

2 Client expresses thoughts and feelings to the nurse through verbal and nonverbal communication.

3 Client identifies factors that provide support and comfort.

4 Client verbalizes feeling understood.

Delegation Considerations

The skill of establishing a therapeutic nurse-client relationship is a professional nursing skill and may not be delegated. Assistive personnel (AP) may observe and receive a lot of important information because of the length of time they are with the client. It is essential for AP to be aware of the following guidelines:

• All information discussed must be considered confidential.

• Client concerns, including anger and anxiety, should be communicated to the nurse to determine if additional nursing interventions are needed.

• All interactions need to be respectful and kind, including special considerations for clients who have cognitive or sensory impairment.

• Be aware of nonverbal behaviors, both of self and client.

IMPLEMENTATION *for Establishing the Nurse-Client Relationship*

STEPS	RATIONALE
Orientation Phase	
1 Create a climate of warmth and acceptance. Consider the need to alter the environment by lowering noise level and providing privacy and comfort. Also consider timing in relation to visitors or personal routines.	Environmental factors can promote open communication.
2 Be aware of cultural and gender differences. Plan for identified difficulties associated with culture, language, age, and gender. Consider inability to read or write English.	These factors can influence expression of discomfort, anxiety, or confusion.
3 Acknowledge and respond to physical discomforts, if any, by positioning, medication, or other comfort measures. Consider individual preferences and expressed needs.	Physical discomfort, difficulty breathing, and pain interfere with communication.
4 Provide an introduction by addressing the client by name and introducing self and role. For example, "Hello, my name is Jane Jones, and I am the student nurse who will take care of you today."	
5 Be aware of nonverbal cues that are both sent and received (e.g., eye contact, facial expression, posture, body language). Be particularly alert to behaviors that are incongruent with the client's verbal message.	Incongruence is an indication that something may be interfering with open communication. Behaviors are often more accurate than words, and clarification may be indicated before proceeding.
6 Explain purpose of the interaction when information is to be shared.	Confidentiality is maintained when client information is shared only with members of the health care team.
7 Encourage the client to ask for clarification at any time during the communication.	
Working Phase	
8 Ask one question at a time, and allow sufficient time to answer. Use direct and open-ended questions. Avoid asking questions about information that may not have yet been disclosed to the client (e.g., medical diagnosis).	Encourages client to tell a more complete story.
9 Use clear and concise statements with a client who experiences altered levels of consciousness and cognition; repeat information.	Helps client receive your message correctly.
10 Focus on understanding the client, providing feedback, encouraging problem solving, and providing an atmosphere of warmth and acceptance.	Need to clarify clients' misinterpretations because clients experiencing emotionally charged situations may not comprehend the message (Keltner, Schwecke, and Bostrom, 2003).
11 Adjust the amount and quality of time for communicating depending on client's needs.	Flexibility and adaptation of techniques may be necessary to encourage client's self-expression.
12 Provide empathy, which involves a sensitive and accurate awareness of client's feelings.	Empathy helps clients explain and explore their feelings so that problem solving may occur.
13 Remain centered on any current client concern. Avoid introducing new information.	Clients may be overwhelmed by additional information. Talking about self or other people or events shifts the focus away from clients (Fortinash and Holoday-Worret, 2004).
14 Communicate understanding by repeating what you understand the message to be (e.g., "I understand you...," "I hear you saying...," "I sense that..."). Offer feedback to clarify message.	Communicating understanding tends to decrease the intensity of feelings and conveys empathy (Keltner, Schwecke, and Bostrom, 2003).

STEPS	RATIONALE
15 Offer honest reassurance to the extent possible (e.g., that someone cares, that there is hope, that client is not alone).	Shows interest and concern for client (Keltner, Schwecke, and Bostrom, 2003).
16 Allow silence, which can be an effective means of allowing organization of thoughts and processing of information. When client becomes emotionally upset or cries, a quiet period can be helpful.	Provides acceptance and willingness to wait for client to be ready to continue.
17 Avoid communication barriers (see Table 2-1).	Barriers may not halt interaction, but tend to divert conversation to less meaningful topics.
Termination Phase	
18 Explore support services available and what services the client has previously used. Refer to other health professionals as appropriate.	
19 Summarize with clients what was discussed during the interaction. Ask clients to state their understanding of the information shared or conclusion reached.	Encourages the client to compare perceptions with the nurse and to determine if clarifications need to be made.

EVALUATION

1 Observe client's verbal and nonverbal responses (e.g., body language, verbal statements) after discussion of feelings and circumstances that have been identified.

2 Ask client for feedback regarding message communicated. Was communication accurately interpreted by caregivers?

3 Verify if information obtained from client is accurate regarding client's thoughts, needs, and concerns.

Unexpected Outcomes and Related Interventions

1 Client continues to verbally and nonverbally express feelings of anxiety, fear, anger, confusion, distrust, and helplessness.
a. Assess client's level of anxiety, fear, and distrust.
b. Come back at another time to repeat the message.
c. Determine influences affecting clear communication (e.g., cultural issues, literacy issues, physical limits).
2 Feedback between nurse and client reveals a lack of understanding.
a. Assess for and remove barriers to communication.
b. Repeat the message using another approach if possible.
3 Nurse is unable to acquire information about client's ideas, fears, and concerns.
a. Try alternative communication techniques to promote the client's willingness to communicate openly.
b. Rephrase question after time for understanding and response.
c. Offer another professional for the client to talk with to obtain the necessary information.

Recording and Reporting
- Record information-related interventions and client responses.
- Report pertinent information, subjective data, and nonverbal cues, including response to illness, response to therapy, and questions or concerns.

Sample Documentation
1345 Expresses anxiety about current hospitalization. Is fidgeting in the bed, wringing his hands. Expressed much concern about fears of cancer with recent diagnostic tests. Encouraged to talk with his wife and the physician about concerns and questions.

Special Considerations
Pediatric Considerations
- Use vocabulary that is familiar to the child, based on the child's level of understanding.
- Evaluate the child's usual patterns of communication.
- Consider the child's developmental level to select the most appropriate communication techniques (e.g., storytelling and drawing). Be sure to include parent and child (Hockenberry, 2005).

Geriatric Considerations
- Be aware of any cognitive or sensory impairment.
- Each client needs to be assessed individually. Avoid stereotyping older adults as having cognitive or sensory impairments.
- Speak face-to-face with the hard-of-hearing client, articulate clearly in a moderate tone of voice, and assess whether the client hears and understands the words.

- Nurses should make sure older clients with visual impairments use assistive devices such as eyeglasses and large-print reading material to aid in communication.

Home Care Considerations
- Identify a primary caregiver for the client. This individual may be a family member, friend, or neighbor.
- Assess the client's and primary caregiver's level of understanding regarding the client's condition.

- Incorporate the client's usual daily habits and routines into the communication event (e.g., bathing and dressing client).

Long-Term Care Considerations
- Incorporate the client's usual daily habits and routines into the communication event (e.g., bathing and dressing client).

SKILL 2.2   Interviewing

The interview involves communication initiated for a specific purpose and focused on a specific content area, such as the initial assessment of newly admitted clients or obtaining a health history in a health care provider's office. In nursing, the interviewer obtains information about the client's health state, lifestyle, support systems, patterns of illness, patterns of adaptation, strengths and limitations, and resources. This information can be used for an admission database or health history and provides data for identifying the client's expectations and for responding appropriately to individualized client needs.

The interview can facilitate a positive nurse-client relationship, which makes it easier for clients to ask questions about the health care environment and expectations regarding daily routines and procedures. It is important to encourage clients to ask questions at any time. They also have the right not to answer questions. Indicating the purpose of the interview helps to establish trust and to put the client at ease.

The interview is best scheduled at a time when interruptions will be minimal and visitors are not present. In some cases it is beneficial to include family members in the interview while the focus is clearly kept with identifying the client's needs. Before beginning, the nurse tells the client the purpose of the interview and the types of data to be obtained. Then time is spent becoming acquainted with the client. Establish a time frame for the interview, and honor this commitment to the client. Ask questions to form a database from which a care plan can be developed (Box 2-5). Carefully observe for evidence of discomfort and be willing to stop the interview when appropriate.

A direct-question technique is a structured format requiring one- or two-word answers and is frequently used to clarify previous information or obtain basic routine information (e.g., allergies, marital status). The open-ended question technique is used to promote a more complete description of identified areas of concern. Examples of open-ended questions/comments include "What are your health concerns?" "How have you been feeling?" and "Tell me about your problem."

ASSESSMENT

1   Review available information, which may include admission information such as name, address, age, marital status, employment, and reason for admission or reason for office visit.
2   Consider factors that may influence ability or willingness of client or significant other to respond to questions, such as physical pain, nausea, or anxiety. *Rationale: These factors may need to be alleviated before the interview.*
3   Determine if client is alert and oriented. Assess for hearing and speech difficulties. *Rationale: These factors may interfere with the interview, and another source of information will be needed.*
4   Consider factors that may influence ability of client to communicate, such as cultural or language barriers.

PLANNING

Expected Outcomes focus on gathering information through the interview process for a database to develop an appropriate plan of care.
1   Client (or significant other) is able to describe health concerns.
2   Verbal and nonverbal messages are congruent.

Delegation Considerations
The skill of interviewing cannot be delegated.

BOX 2-5   Interview Database

- Health-related concerns
- Perception of health status
- Past health problems and therapies
- Effect of health status on role; influence on relationship with members of household
- Influence on occupation
- Ability to complete ADLs

IMPLEMENTATION *for Interviewing*

STEPS	RATIONALE
1 Greet client and significant others and introduce yourself by name and job title. Tell client the reason for the interview and how long you expect it to last. Assure client that this information will be kept confidential.	Allays anxiety about divulging information to a stranger and encourages participation. The nurse may need to modify communication approaches, as needed, to accommodate the client's culture and practices.
2 Provide privacy and eliminate distractions, unnecessary noise, and interruptions by going to a quiet unoccupied room and/or closing the door. If others are present, ask client if they should stay.	Distractions and interruptions may interfere with therapeutic interactions between nurse and client.
3 Sit facing client at approximately the same eye level (see illustration).	This facilitates active listening and places client more at ease. It may be necessary to avoid direct eye contact with a client whose culture views it as inappropriate.
4 If client is alert enough to state name, where he or she is, and what day it is, proceed with the interview. Confirm information obtained from client with other caregivers or family members if client is disoriented or confused or does not seem reliable.	Alert and oriented client is a reliable source of information.
5 If client is talkative, refocus the interview when client strays from the topic.	
6 Ask what led client to seek health care. Attempt to obtain a descriptive account of all the events in the order in which they occurred. Ask open-ended questions and listen to client's story.	Active listening encourages the exchange of information. Conducting an interview by only asking questions may make client feel like a subject of interrogation.
7 Observe and clarify nonverbal behaviors. Validate with client the emotions or messages conveyed. Use validation as a communication tool.	Provides a focus for collecting more specific and accurate data related to the primary areas of concern.
8 For each symptom client reports, determine when, where, and under what circumstances it occurred. Also determine location; quality; quantity; duration; and aggravating, alleviating, and associated factors (Table 2-2).	
9 For each symptom, also clarify the absence of other related symptoms.	
10 Identify past hospitalizations, past surgical procedures and complications, and previous major health problems.	

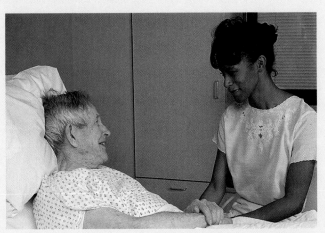

STEP 3 Sitting facing the client may facilitate communication.

STEPS	RATIONALE
11 Determine whether client regularly takes medications and, if so, for what period of time. Ask the name, reason for taking, dosage, and frequency. Specifically ask about dietary supplements or over-the-counter (OTC) medications such as aspirin, acetaminophen, ibuprofen, laxatives, sleeping pills, diet pills, herbal supplements/remedies, or other types of alternative therapies.	Clients may not think of dietary supplements or OTC medications, because these do not require prescriptions. However, both of these classifications of medications may have interactive effects with current or future prescribed medications.
12 Clarify if client takes narcotics, insulin, digitalis, contraceptives, steroids, or hormone replacements.	Clients may not mention these if such drugs seem unrelated to the reason for admission or when they think that the physician would have previously conveyed this information.
13 Identify risk factors related to lifestyle that influence the client's health, knowledge level, and awareness of the risk.	Risk factors include smoking, alcohol use, drug abuse, lack of exercise, stress, nutritional factors (e.g., fluids, cholesterol, carbohydrates, fiber, salt), exposure to violence, and unprotected sexual activity.
14 Continue with additional areas of interest or concern according to the focus of the interview.	
15 Give information that tells clients you are nearly finished.	This offers client a chance to ask final questions.
16 Summarize your understanding of client's health concerns.	

TABLE 2-2 Dimensions of a Symptom

DIMENSIONS	QUESTIONS TO ASK
Location	"Where do you feel it?"
	"Does it move around?"
	"Show me where."
Quality or character	"What is it like? Sharp, dull, stabbing, aching?"
Severity	"On a scale of 0 to 10, with 10 the worst, how would you rate what you feel right now?"
	"What is the worst it has been?"
	"In what ways does this interfere with your usual activities?"
Timing	"When did you first notice it?"
	"How long does it last?"
	"How often does it happen?"
Setting	"Does it occur in a particular place or under certain circumstances?"
Aggravating or alleviating factors	"What makes it better?"
	"What makes it worse?"
	"When does it change?"
	"Have you noticed other changes associated with this?"

EVALUATION

1 Ask if client or significant other has had an adequate opportunity to describe health concerns.

2 Observe client's nonverbal expressions during interview. Do they match verbal statements?

Unexpected Outcomes and Related Interventions

1 Family or significant other answers for client, even when client is capable of answering.

a. Direct the question to client, using client's name.

b. Avoid eye contact with family member.

c. Acknowledge the answer given by a family member, then state you are interested specifically in what client has to say about it.

d. Conclude the interview, and resume again after the family members are gone. If necessary, you may suggest that family take a break for a while, get coffee or a meal, or walk outside briefly for some fresh air.

2 Client is unable to communicate, and family members are present.

a. Interview family member as you would client.

b. Explore the needs of family and client.

Recording and Reporting

- List what is to be included in the admission profile:
  - Reason for admission
  - Medical-surgical history, family history
  - Allergies
  - Health habits, including cultural beliefs about health
  - Current prescribed therapies (include all OTC medications and supplements)
  - Current unprescribed therapies/alternative treatments

Sample Documentation

Documentation involves use of a standard assessment form for a database.

Special Considerations

Pediatric Considerations

- Evaluate the child's usual pattern of communication, including use of age-appropriate language.
- Consider the child's developmental level when interviewing the child.

- Include parents in the interviewing process when appropriate.

Geriatric Considerations

- Be aware of any cognitive or sensory impairment.
- Encourage clients with auditory and/or visual impairments to use assistive devices to aid in communication.

Home Care Considerations

- Assess for the presence of any cognitive or physical impairments that may hinder communication.
- Identify the client's primary caregiver and include in interviewing process.
- Assess client's and caregiver's level of understanding regarding client's condition.

Long-Term Care Considerations

- Assess for cognitive impairment or physical difficulties that may impair the client's communication.
- Identify who constitutes the client's support system, and include in interviewing process when appropriate.
- Assess client's level of understanding regarding health condition.

SKILL 2.3 Communicating with an Anxious Client

Anxiety can result from many factors. A newly diagnosed illness, separation from loved ones, the threat of pending diagnostic tests or surgical procedures, a language barrier, and expectations of life changes are just a few factors that can cause anxiety. How successfully a client copes with anxiety depends in part on previous experiences, the presence of other stressors, the significance of the event causing anxiety, and the availability of supportive resources. The nurse can help to decrease anxiety through effective communication. Communication methods reviewed in this skill may help an anxious client clarify factors causing anxiety and cope more effectively. There are stages of anxiety with corresponding behavioral manifestations: mild, moderate, severe, and panic (Box 2-6).

ASSESSMENT

1 Observe for physical, behavioral, and verbal cues such as dry mouth, sweaty palms, tone of voice, frequent use of call light, difficulty concentrating, wringing of hands, and statements such as "I am scared." *Rationale: Behaviors are indicative of anxiety.*

2 Assess for possible factors causing client anxiety (e.g., hospitalization, fatigue, fear, pain).

3 Assess factors influencing communication with the client (e.g., environment, timing, presence of others,

---

BOX 2-6 Behavioral Manifestations of Anxiety: Stages of Anxiety

Mild Anxiety
- Increased auditory and visual perception
- Increased awareness of relationships
- Increased alertness
- Able to problem solve

Moderate Anxiety
- Selective inattention
- Decreased perceptual field
- Focus only on relevant information
- Muscle tension; diaphoresis

Severe Anxiety
- Focus on fragmented details
- Headache, nausea, dizziness
- Unable to see connections between details
- Inability to recall events

Panic State of Anxiety
- Does not notice surroundings
- Feeling of terror
- Unable to cope with any problem

values, experiences, need for personal space because of heightened anxiety).

4 Assess own level of anxiety as nurse, and make a conscious effort to remain calm. *Rationale: Anxiety is highly contagious, and one's own anxiety can worsen the client's anxiety.*

PLANNING

Expected Outcomes focus on reducing the client's anxiety through the use of effective communication techniques.

1 Client establishes rapport, achieves a sense of calm, and discusses coping and decision making about current situation.
2 Client's physical and emotional discomforts are acknowledged.
3. Client discusses factors causing anxiety.

Delegation Considerations

Communicating for the purpose of reducing anxiety cannot be delegated. AP may have the occasion to interact with anxious clients and must know what to observe and report to the nurse.

IMPLEMENTATION *for Communicating with an Anxious Client*

STEPS	RATIONALE
1 Provide brief, simple introduction; introduce yourself and explain purpose of interaction.	Anxiety may limit amount of information client understands.
2 Use appropriate nonverbal behaviors (e.g., relaxed posture, eye contact). Stay with the client at the bedside.	Clients experiencing emotionally charged situations may not comprehend the verbally delivered message. Focus on understanding the client, providing feedback, assisting in problem solving, and providing an atmosphere of warmth and acceptance.
3 Use appropriate responses that are clear and concise.	Promotes effective communication so that the client can explore causes of anxiety and steps to alleviate anxious feelings.
4 Help client acquire alternative coping strategies, such as progressive relaxation, slow deep-breathing exercises, and visual imagery (see Chapter 10).	Stress-reduction techniques are nonpharmacological strategies that client can use to reduce anxiety.
5 Minimize noise in physical setting.	Decreasing environmental stimuli may reduce client's anxiety.
6 Adjust the amount and quality of time for communicating depending on client's needs.	Flexibility and adaptation of techniques may be necessary based on client's ability to communicate, level of anxiety, and need for more time to establish trust.

EVALUATION

1 Have client discuss ways to cope with anxiety in the future and make decisions about current situation.
2 Observe for continuing presence of physical signs and symptoms or behaviors reflecting anxiety.
3 Ask client to discuss factors causing anxiety.

Unexpected Outcomes and Related Interventions

1 Physical signs and symptoms of anxiety continue.
a. Utilize refocusing or distraction skills, such as relaxation and imagery, to reduce anxiety (see Skill 10.2).
b. Be direct and clear when communicating with client, to avoid misunderstanding.
c. Touch, when used appropriately, may help control feelings of panic.

d. Administering an antianxiety medication as prescribed may be necessary.

Recording and Reporting

- Cause of anxiety
- Nonverbal behaviors
- Methods used to relieve anxiety (pharmacological and nonpharmacological methods)
- Client response (verbal and nonverbal)

Sample Documentation

1130 Complains of headaches and dizziness. Does not recall that the doctor is coming to see him to discuss the upcoming surgery. Able to follow directions for using progressive relaxation techniques. Will periodically check in on client in his room and will evaluate level of anxiety in 1 hr.

Special Considerations
Pediatric Considerations
- Evaluate the child's usual pattern of communication, including use of age-appropriate language.
- Anxiety may be expressed through restless behavior, physical complaints, or behavioral regression.

Geriatric Considerations
- Be aware of any cognitive or sensory impairment.
- Anxiety is often the result of change in usual patterns and environment.

Home Care Considerations
- Determine community resources to assist client and caregiver with coping strategies.

Long-Term Care Considerations
- Assess for cognitive impairment or physical difficulties that may impair client's communication and cause social isolation.

SKILL 2.4 Communicating with an Angry Client

The degree and frequency of anger range from everyday mild annoyance to anger related to feelings of helplessness and powerlessness. There are positive functions of anger, including anger as an energizing behavior, anger to protect positive image, and anger to give a person greater control over a situation. Anger may be directly related to a client's experience with illness, or it can be associated with problems that existed before the client entered the health care system.

It is important for the nurse to understand that in many cases the client's ability to express anger is important to recovery. When a client has experienced a significant loss, anger becomes a means to help cope with grief. A client may express anger toward the nurse, but the anger often hides a specific problem or concern. A client diagnosed as having cancer may voice anger with the nurse's care instead of expressing a fear of dying.

It can be stressful for a nurse to deal with an angry client. Anger can represent rejection or disapproval of the nurse's care. A nurse's efforts at satisfying the needs of one angry client can result in a failure to meet the priorities of other clients. The nurse needs to allow the client to express anger openly and not feel threatened by the client's words.

Ultimately rage may develop when usual coping methods are no longer effective to manage the situation. Anger is the common underlying factor associated with a potential for violence. In the health care setting, the nurse may become the target of the client's anger when the client cannot express it toward a significant other. Deescalation skills are useful techniques for managing the potentially violent client. These skills range from using nonthreatening verbal and nonverbal messages to safely disengaging and controlling the aggressor physically (Fortinash and Holoday-Worret, 2004).

The client's anger cannot be allowed to compromise care. Skills for communicating with an angry client or a potentially violent client will allow a nurse to assist the client in dealing with anger constructively and in refocusing emotional energy toward effective problem solving.

ASSESSMENT

1. Observe for behaviors that indicate the client is angry (e.g., pacing, clenched fists, loud voice, throwing objects) and/or client expression that indicates anger (e.g., repeated questioning of the nurse, irrational complaints about care, no adherence to requests, belligerent outbursts, threats).
2. Assess factors that influence communication of the angry client, such as refusal to comply with treatment goals, use of sarcasm or hostile behavior, having a low frustration level, or being emotionally immature.
3. Consider resources available to assist in communicating with the potentially violent client, such as other members of the health care team and family members.

PLANNING

Expected Outcomes focus on promoting effective and socially appropriate verbal and nonverbal expressions of anger.
1. Client's feelings of anger subside without harm to self or others.
2. Client's anger is diffused, and problem solving is initiated.

Delegation Considerations
Therapeutic communication is a goal of all client interactions. All AP who may have contact with angry clients (e.g., security personnel, AP on psychiatric units) must be able to effectively communicate with those clients.

IMPLEMENTATION *for Communicating with an Angry Client*

STEPS	RATIONALE
1 Create a climate of client acceptance. Maintain a nonthreatening verbal approach using a calm tone of voice. Try to determine the source of the anger. Use an open body language with a concerned nonthreatening facial expression, open arms (not folded), hands not in pockets, relaxed posture, and a safe distance (e.g., not invading the client's personal space).	A relaxed atmosphere may prevent further escalation.
2 Respond to the potentially violent client with therapeutic silence, and allow client to ventilate feelings. Use active listening for understanding. Do not argue with client. Avoid defensiveness with client.	These techniques often deescalate anger, because anger expends emotional and physical energy; client runs out of momentum and energy to maintain anger at a high level. Arguing will escalate anger.
3 Answer questions calmly and honestly. If client presents a power-struggle type of question (e.g., "Who said you were in charge; I don't have to listen to you"), set limits using clear, concise language. Inform client of potential consequences, and follow through with consequences if behaviors are not altered.	By setting limits on power-struggle questions, structure is provided and anger is diffused (Fortinash and Holoday-Worret, 2004).
4 Maintain personal space. It may be necessary to have someone with you and to keep the door open. Position self between the client and the exit.	Steps promote nurses' safety when client becomes violent.
5 If the client is making verbal threats to harm others, remain calm yet professional and continue to set limits with inappropriate behavior. If a distinct likelihood of imminent harm to others is present, notify the proper authorities (e.g., nurse manager, security).	Angry clients lose the ability to process information rationally and therefore may impulsively express themselves through intimidation.
6 Focus on understanding the client, providing feedback, assisting in problem solving, and providing an atmosphere of warmth and acceptance nonverbally.	Clients experiencing emotionally charged situations may not comprehend the nurses' verbal message.

> **NURSE ALERT** The potentially violent client can be impulsive and explosive, and therefore it is imperative the nurse keep personal safety skills in mind. In this case, avoid touch.

STEPS	RATIONALE
7 Adjust the amount and quality of time for communicating depending on the client's needs. Try to listen and reflect understanding of the client's anger first, then return later to deliver the message.	It is futile to try to communicate a complicated message to a client in the height of anger.
8 If the client appears to be calm and anger is diffused, explore alternatives to the situation or feelings of anger.	May prevent future explosive outbursts and teach the client effective ways of dealing with anger.
9 Encourage safe coping behaviors (e.g., physical exercise as a means of directing energy in an acceptable way, writing about negative thoughts).	

EVALUATION

1 Ask client if feelings of anger have subsided.
2 Determine client's ability to answer questions and solve problems.

Unexpected Outcomes and Related Interventions

1 Client continues to demonstrate behaviors or verbal expression of anger or violence. Nurse is unable to assist the client in relieving source of anger or in expressing anger openly without violent acts.
   a. If anger continues to escalate, reassess factors contributing to anger.
   b. Remove or alter factors contributing to anger.
   c. Provide security measures (see agency protocol).

Recording and Reporting

- Observations related to factors precipitating anger, using exact quotes
- Threats of violence made and who was notified
- Nursing action for deescalation and limit setting
- Client response

Sample Documentation

1800 Client expressed extreme anger toward staff related to food served cold and no-smoking policy. Stated, "I just can't take this abuse any more. I have to get out of here now." Threatened to leave the hospital against medical advice. The nurse manager and the client's doctor were notified. Encouraged to write about his feelings; family plans to stay with client until he is more calm.

Special Considerations
Pediatric Considerations

- Children tend to have less internal control over their behaviors; immediately setting limits for inappropriate behaviors exhibited by child is effective (Hockenberry, 2005).

Geriatric Considerations

- Clients who have cognitive impairments may exhibit tantrumlike behaviors in response to real or perceived frustration. The nurse can use distraction techniques to remove the cognitively impaired adult client from the disturbing stimuli, or the nurse can use redirection to an activity that is pleasurable to the client.

Home Care Considerations

- Personal safety for the nurse against potentially violent clients or family members extends to all health care settings, including the client's home. The nurse may be in a potentially dangerous situation while giving care to the client at home; the nurse may give care to the client without support from other staff members.
- Be aware of physical surroundings, including possible exits. Maintain nonthreatening position, including body language, position, and rate of speech, when interacting with an angry or potentially violent client. The nurse should attempt to deescalate the client. If deescalation does not occur and the nurse feels safety may be threatened, the nurse should call for assistance or remove staff from situation.
- Have numbers for emergency use posted near phone (e.g., mental health provider, emergency response units, neighbors).

Long-Term Care Considerations

- The nurse should not enter an unsafe environment. In all settings, the nurse needs to be aware of both verbal and nonverbal cues that indicate escalating anger. In settings in which additional support is not readily available, it is also important to be aware of physical surroundings, possible exits, and communication systems to call for assistance (e.g., telephone, emergency call system). A quick exit is appropriate if efforts to deescalate are not successful.

SKILL 2.5   Communicating with a Depressed Client

Depression is a mood disorder that may have many causes. Persons with mild depression describe themselves as feeling sad, blue, downcast, and tearful. They commonly feel apathetic, hopeless, helpless, worthless, guilty, and angry. Other symptoms include difficulty sleeping or sleeping too much, irritability, weight loss or gain, headaches, and feelings of fatigue regardless of the amount of sleep. In some cases there is a high level of anxiety, physical complaints, and social isolation. Thoughts of death and decreased libido may also occur (Keltner, Schwecke, and Bostrom, 2003). Many clients in acute care settings who suffer from either acute or chronic health conditions have symptoms of depression. Some clients have been formally diagnosed and are treated with medications and/or psychotherapy; others may not have been diagnosed and therefore have not been treated.

ASSESSMENT

1   Assess for physical, behavioral, and verbal cues that indicate client is depressed, such as feelings of sadness, tearfulness, difficulty concentrating, increase in reports of physical complaints, and statements such as "I am sad/depressed."
2   Assess for possible factors causing client's depression (e.g., acute or chronic illness, personal vulnerability, past history).
3   Assess factors influencing communication with client (e.g., environment, timing, presence of others, values, experiences, poor concentration).
4   Nurse may need to confer with family members about possible causes of client's depression, including past history of the illness.

PLANNING

Expected Outcomes focus on recognizing symptoms of depression within the client and reducing client's depression through the use of effective therapeutic communication techniques.

1   Client talks about factors that increase sadness and anxiety.
2   Client states coping strategies that improve well-being.

Delegation Considerations

Therapeutic communication with a depressed client cannot be delegated. The nurse directs personnel on the behaviors (e.g., tearfulness, sadness) to report to the nurse.

IMPLEMENTATION *for Communicating with a Depressed Client*

STEPS	RATIONALE
1 Provide brief, simple introduction; introduce yourself, and explain purpose of interaction.	Symptoms associated with depression may limit amount of information client can understand.
2 Accept client as he or she is and focus on positive aspects of client. Provide positive feedback.	Depressed clients often have low self-esteem, and this approach helps to focus on their strengths.
3 Be honest and empathetic.	Facilitates the development of trust.
4 Use appropriate nonverbal behaviors and active listening skills.	Nonverbal messages to client convey the nurse's interest and help to alleviate depressive symptoms.
5 Use appropriate verbal techniques that are clear and concise. Use brief statements that both acknowledge current feeling state and provide direction.	Conveys empathy.
6 Use open-ended questions, such as "Tell me about how you are feeling."	Encourages the client to continue talking, facilitating a discussion of symptoms and circumstances.
7 Encourage small decisions and independent actions. Or when necessary, make decisions that clients are not ready to make.	Depressed clients may be overly dependent and indecisive.
8 Listen to symptoms and provide comfort measures such as back massage, relaxation, and guided imagery.	Depressed clients often have multiple somatic complaints.
9 Spend time and provide honest affirmation with client who is withdrawn.	Communicates the client's worth.
10 Ask, "Are you having thoughts of suicide?" If the answer is yes, ask, "Have you thought about how you would do it?" (*plan*); "Do you have what you need?" (*means*); "Have you thought about when you would do it?" (*time set*).	Depressed clients are at increased risk for suicide. Ninety-five percent of all suicide hotline callers will answer no at some point in this series of questions or indicate that the time is set for some date in the future. The more developed the plan, the greater the risk of suicide (Keltner, Schwecke, and Bostrom, 2003).
11 Simply talking about their problems for a length of time will give suicidal people relief from loneliness and pent-up feelings.	Awareness that another person cares and a feeling of being understood can decrease client's agitated state and help client get through a difficult time. Client also gets tired, and body chemistry changes.
12 Avoid arguments, problem solving, advice giving, quick referrals, belittling, or making the client feel that he or she has to justify suicidal feelings.	The reality is not how bad the client's problem is, but how badly the problem is hurting the client.
13 Refer to a trained mental health professional.	A person who feels suicidal needs treatment and follow-up.

EVALUATION

1 Observe for continuing presence of physical signs and symptoms or behaviors reflecting depression.
2 Have client discuss ways to cope with depression in the future and make decisions about own care.
3 Evaluate client's ability to discuss factors contributing to depression.

Unexpected Outcomes and Related Interventions

1 Client continues to have physical complaints and anxiety that seem to be related to unrelieved depression.
a. Evaluate support system.
b. Refer client to mental health professional for consultation.

Recording and Reporting

- Record subjective and objective behaviors (associated with depression) and interventions and client's response to ensure continuity of care between nurses.

Sample Documentation

1200 Sitting slumped over in room alone; still in nightclothes, hair uncombed, and with no makeup. Client states, "I feel so alone; my husband recently died and my kids made me sell my home and move to assisted living." Complains of fatigue and reports trouble sleeping. Has lost 25 lbs in 6 months. Encouraged to talk about her feelings. Tearful. Will encourage family to visit more often and talk openly about her losses.

Special Considerations

Pediatric Considerations

- Children manifest depression through physical (increased somatic complaints) and behavioral (difficulty in school, social isolation) signs, restless behavior, or behavioral regression and may be unable to express depression verbally (Hockenberry, 2005).

Geriatric Considerations

- Depression among older adults is a major health concern.
- It is important to differentiate depression and any underlying medical illness in this population because the symptoms may overlap.
- Suicide risk is increased in older adults (Keltner, Schwecke, and Bostrom, 2003).

Home Care Considerations

- Depression may be seen in home care settings and should be managed based on client's presenting behaviors with a consideration of any cognitive or physical impairments.

NCLEX® Style Questions

1 When observing and interpreting a client's nonverbal communication, the nurse should know that:
   1. Clients are usually very aware of their nonverbal cues.
   2. Verbal responses are more important than nonverbal cues.
   3. Nonverbal cues have obvious meaning and are easily interpreted.
   4. Nonverbal cues provide significant information and need to be validated.

2 A client has been withdrawn, suspicious, and explosive since admission. He is wary of staff and other clients. Which approach by the nurse is most appropriate?
   1. Refraining from touch
   2. Patting his arm when he seems frightened
   3. Reaching out to shake his hand as an initial greeting
   4. Placing an arm around his shoulders while walking down the hall

3 The nurse tells a client, "I notice you seem to become irritated when we discuss your relationship with your husband." Which communication technique is the nurse using?
   1. Interpreting
   2. Clarifying
   3. Giving information
   4. Making observations

4 Which of the following approaches creates a barrier to communication?
   1. Using too many different skills during a single interaction
   2. Giving advice rather than encouraging the client to problem solve
   3. Allowing the client to become too anxious before changing the subject
   4. Focusing on what the client is saying rather than on the skill used

5 The client states, "I get pretty discouraged when I realize I have been struggling with these issues for over a year." The nurse responds, "Yes you have, but lots of other people take even longer to resolve their problems; don't be so hard on yourself." What does this interaction represent?
   1. The client is expressing a lack of willingness to collaborate with the nurse.
   2. The client is offering the opportunity for the nurse to revise the plan of care.
   3. The nurse has responded ineffectively to the client's concerns.
   4. The nurse is using techniques consistent with the evaluation phase of the nurse-client relationship.

References for all chapters appear in Appendix D.

3

Promoting a Safe Environment

MEDIA RESOURCES

- **evolve** http://evolve.elsevier.com/Elkin
- **View Video!** Video Clips
- Nursing Skills Online

Client safety is one of the most important issues in health care. It is often defined as freedom from physical and psychological injury. Nurses in every health care setting are responsible for identifying and eliminating safety hazards. Following agency policy and procedures and providing ongoing communication with clients and families are two of many ways to maintain the safety and security of clients.

The Joint Commission on Accreditation of Healthcare Organizations (JCAHO) has released the *National Patient Safety Goals* since 2003 (JCAHO, 2005b). An expert multidisciplinary panel conducts a systematic review of national databases to identify relevant new goals for health care organizations. A sentinel event is defined by the JCAHO as an unexpected occurrence involving death, serious physical or psychological injury, or risk thereof. Sentinel events include any process variation (e.g., medication administration, restraint application procedures) for which a recurrence would carry a significant chance of a serious adverse outcome (JCAHO, 2006).

Sentinel events that occur across the country trigger the identification of client safety goals. Each client safety goal has a set of evidence-based recommendations on which health care agencies must focus their attention. Box 3-1 cites the JCAHO 2006 *National Patient Safety Goals* for hospitals and critical access hospitals.

Clients within health care settings are at risk for injury from falls, as well as client-inherent, procedure-related, and equipment-related accidents. Falls account for up to 90% of all reported incidents in hospitals. Client-inherent accidents include events such as self-inflicted cuts, burns, and ingestion or injection of foreign substances. Procedure-related accidents include medication and fluid administration errors and improper performance of procedures. Equipment-related accidents result from the electrical malfunction, disrepair, or misuse of equipment.

EVIDENCE IN PRACTICE

Riefkohl E and others: Medications and falls in the elderly: a review of the evidence and practical considerations, *P&T* 28(11):724, 2003.

Falls are a common health problem in the elderly population. The use of medications is one of the factors contributing to balance problems and the risk of falls. The research literature suggests that psychotropic drugs (e.g., Haldol, Thorazine), anticonvulsants, and certain cardiac drugs increase the risk of falling (Riefkohl and others, 2003). In addition, clients using three or more medications appear to be at increased risk for recurrent falls, particularly if doses of the individual medications are high. A thorough assessment of each client's medications should be made periodically. This involves an accurate listing of all medications a client takes, including over-the-counter (OTC) and herbal products. Ambulatory clients are encouraged to bring their medications with them to clinic visits to facilitate accuracy in the assessment.

NURSING DIAGNOSES

Risk for injury (trauma) is appropriate for clients who face external (e.g., chemical agent, health care provider, environmental design) and internal (e.g., malnutrition, developmental alterations) conditions that interfere with their defenses to avoid injury. **Risk for falls** is appropriate for clients susceptible to falling because of previous history, mobility limitations, medication use, disease, and environmental conditions. **Risk for impaired skin integrity** and **impaired physical mobility** apply to clients who require temporary physical restraint. **Deficient knowledge** related to a lack of knowledge of safety precautions is appropriate when teaching the client and family about safety issues.

BOX 3-1 2006 *National Patient Safety Goals* for Hospitals and Critical Access Hospitals

- Improve the accuracy of client identification; use at least two client identifiers (neither to be the client's room number) when administering medications, blood products, or treatments and when taking specimens.
- For verbal or telephone orders or telephone reporting, verify the complete order or test result by having person receiving the order/report "read back" the complete order/result.
- Standardize a list of abbreviations, acronyms, and symbols that are not to be used throughout an organization.
- Measure, assess, and, if appropriate, take action to improve timeliness of reporting, as well as timeliness of receipt by the responsible licensed caregiver of critical test results and values.
- Implement a standardized approach to "hand off" communications (e.g., change-of-shift report) and include an opportunity to ask and respond to questions.
- Improve the safety of using medications.
- Reduce the risk of health care–associated infections (HAIs).
- Accurately and completely reconcile medications across the continuum of care. Implement a process for obtaining and documenting a complete list of client's current medications upon the client's admission to the organization and with the client's involvement. Compare medications the organization provides to those on list. Communicate a complete list of the client's medications to the next provider of service when referring or transferring a client to another setting, provider, or level of care within or outside the organization.
- Reduce the risk of client harm resulting from falls. Implement a fall-reduction program and evaluate the effectiveness of the program.

© Joint Commission on Accreditation of Healthcare Organizations: 2006. Reprinted with permission.

PROCEDURAL GUIDELINE 3-1

Fire, Electrical, and Radiation Safety

Fire and Electrical Safety

Health care agency engineering departments routinely check and maintain all electrical devices. Each biomedical device (e.g., suction machine, intravenous [IV] pump) must have a current safety inspection sticker. All devices must be properly grounded, using a three-prong electrical plug. Generally clients are discouraged from bringing electrical devices to health care agencies. If a client brings a device, it must be inspected for safe wiring and function before use. Although smoking is usually not allowed in facilities, smoking-related fires continue to pose a significant risk because of unauthorized smoking in beds and bathrooms.

All health care agencies routinely have employees participate in fire safety training. The best intervention is prevention of fires. Health care personnel report the exact location of the fire, contain it, and extinguish it if possible. All personnel are then mobilized to evacuate clients if necessary. Nursing measures also include complying with the agency's smoking policies and keeping combustible materials away from heat sources. Some agencies have fire doors that are held open by magnets and close automatically when a fire alarm sounds. Always keep equipment away from fire doors.

Radiation Safety

Radioactive materials are significant health hazards. Hospitals have strict guidelines for the care of clients who receive radiation therapy or have radioactive implants. The safe handling, use, and disposal of radioactive materials is under the management of the Nuclear Regulatory Commission (NRC). Staff must strictly limit time of exposure and distance to the source of radiation. Clients are often restricted to specific floors of a hospital when radioactive materials are used.

PROCEDURAL GUIDELINE 3-1—cont'd

Chemical Safety

Chemicals found in some medications (e.g., chemotherapeutic agents), anesthetic gases, cleaning solutions, and disinfectants can be potentially toxic. Some chemicals can cause damage or irritation to the body after skin contact, if ingested, or when vapors are inhaled. Health care facilities must provide their employees access to a Material Safety Data Sheet (MSDS) for each hazardous chemical used. An MSDS offers detailed information about the chemical, any health hazards imposed, precautions for safe handling and use, and steps to take in case the material is released or spilled.

Fire, Electrical, and Radiation Safety
Delegation Considerations

The skill of fire, electrical, and radiation safety can be delegated. In the event of a fire or electrical or radioactive event, a nurse leads the health care team in an emergency response.

Equipment
Fire
- Appropriate fire extinguisher for fire: Type A, B, C, or ABC.

Radiation
- Protective radiation shield (lead apron)
- Lead-shielded container if required
- Radiation exposure badge or dosimeter
- Clean gloves
- Radioactive materials caution sign for client's door

Procedural Steps

1 Review agency guidelines for fire, electrical, and radiation safety.
2 Familiarize yourself with location of emergency equipment (e.g., fire alarms, fire extinguisher, emergency cart).
3 Know your clients' medical conditions, particularly mobility and level of cognition and responsiveness in case there is a need for evacuation.
4 For clients receiving radioactive implants, assess their knowledge of risks of radiation exposure, purpose of safety precautions, and whether they are pregnant or may have visitors who are pregnant.

5 **Fire Safety** (a helpful acronym is **RACE**)
a. **R**escue the client from immediate injury by removing from area or shielding from fire to avoid burns.
b. **A**ctivate the fire alarm immediately. Follow agency policy for alerting staff to respond. (In many situations, perform Steps a and b simultaneously by using the call system to alert staff while you help clients at risk.)
c. **C**ontain the fire.
   (1) Close all doors and windows.
   (2) Turn off oxygen and electrical equipment.
   (3) Place wet towels along base of doors.
d. **E**vacuate clients.
   (1) Direct ambulatory clients to walk by themselves to a safe area. Know the fire exits and emergency evacuation route.
   (2) Move bedridden clients by stretcher, bed, or wheelchair.
   (3) If client is on life support, maintain client's respiratory status manually until client is removed from fire area.
   (4) Use appropriate carrying method.
      (a) Place on blanket and drag client out of area.
      (b) Use two-person swing: Place client in sitting position and have two staff members form a seat by clasping forearms together (see illustration). Lift client into "seat" and carry out of area of danger (see illustration).
      (c) Use a "back-strap" method: Stand in front of client and place client's arms around your neck. Grasp client's wrists firmly against your chest. Pull client onto your back, and carry out of danger.

> **NURSE ALERT** Consider the client's weight and size when choosing evacuation carry. Have a staff member assist to avoid injury.

   (5) Extinguish fire using appropriate fire extinguisher: Type A for ordinary combustibles (e.g., wood, cloth, paper, most plastics); Type B for flammable liquids (e.g., gasoline, grease, anesthetic gas); Type C for electrical equipment; Type ABC for any type of fire.

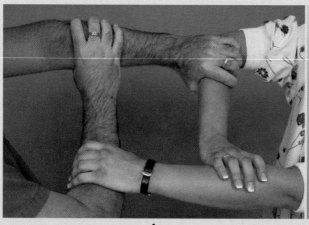
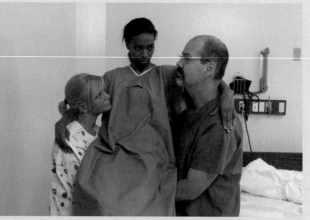

| A | B |

STEP 5d.(4)(b) A, Hands positioned to form two-person evacuation swing. **B,** Client is seated firmly on swing and holds nurses by shoulders for emergency evacuation.

PROCEDURAL GUIDELINE 3-1—cont'd

(6) To use extinguisher (see illustrations):
  (a) Pull the pin.
  (b) Aim the nozzle at base of fire and squeeze extinguisher handles, sweeping from side to side to coat area evenly.

6 **Electrical Safety**
  a. If client receives electrical shock, immediately disengage electrical source, then assess for presence of a pulse.
  b. If client is pulseless, institute emergency resuscitation (see Skill 35.1).
  c. Notify emergency personnel and client's physician.
  d. If client has a pulse and remains alert and oriented, obtain vital signs and assess the skin for signs of thermal injury.

7 **Radiation Safety**
  a. Place client in a private room with private bath, and place sign "Caution: Radioactive Material" on door.
  b. Wear a radiation exposure dosimeter when caring for client receiving radiation or radioactive implant.
  c. Explain treatment plan to client and family, including activity limitations, safety regulations, and time and distance limits (e.g., visitors are usually limited to 30 minutes a day and must stay at least 6 feet away from radiation source).
  d. Provide activities and distractions for client.
  e. Rotate care providers during client's stay on unit. (NOTE: Pregnant care providers cannot be assigned to client.)
  f. When entering client's room, wear a protective lead apron and gloves. Have family wear protective garments also.
  g. Follow agency policy for removal of laboratory specimens, dietary tray, dressings, linens, trash, and body fluids.

h. After caring for client, wash gloves before removing, and dispose of them in designated waste container. Perform thorough hand hygiene.
i. When client is discharged from facility, request a radiation safety officer to conduct a survey of sources of radiation.

Recording and Reporting
- Follow agency policy for reporting a sentinel event. Documentation will likely be made as sentinel event report and not in nurses' notes.
- Document in nurses' notes any education provided to client and family.

Special Considerations
Geriatric Considerations
- Physiological changes that accompany aging, such as a slower reaction time, muscular weakness, reduced pain and temperature perception, vision changes, confusion, and memory loss, place older adults at increased risk for injury.

Home Care Considerations
- The client is the final decision maker in the types of safety alterations made in the home. Financial resources must be considered. (See Chapter 38.)

Long-Term Care Considerations
- In a long-term care or assisted living setting, personnel protocols should address staff members' specific duties and posts, including notification procedure for fire department and management of exit maneuvers (Ebersole and others, 2004).

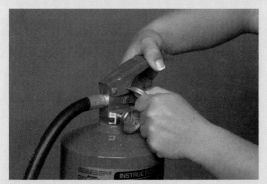

STEP 5d.(6)(a) Remove safety pin from fire extinguisher.

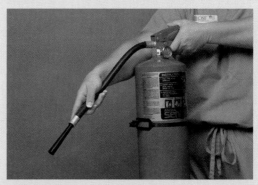

STEP 5d.(6)(b) Aim hose at base of fire and squeeze handles, sweeping from side to side.

SKILL 3.1 Fall Prevention

- Nursing Skills Online: Safety, Lesson 1

In 2001 more than 1.6 million older adults were treated in emergency departments for fall-related injuries, and nearly 388,000 were hospitalized (CDC, 2003). During 2002, nearly 13,000 adults age 65 and older died of fall-related injuries (CDC, 2006). Frail older adults are at particular risk because of impaired strength, mobility, balance, and endurance. How-ever, clients of all ages are at risk for falling when they receive care within a health care facility. The effects of medications, use of sedation, environmental barriers, and signs and symptoms of disease become contributing factors for falls. It is important to inform all clients, young and old, when they may be at risk for falling and instruct them to ask for assistance.

The JCAHO (2005a) recommends that all health care organizations have a formal fall-prevention program. There

---

BOX 3-2 RISK* Assessment Tools for Falls

TOOL 1: Risk Assessment Tool for Falls

Directions: Place a check mark in front of elements that apply to your client. The decision of whether a client is at risk for falls is based on your nursing judgment. *Guideline:* A client who has a check mark in front of an element with an asterisk (*) or four or more of the other elements would be identified as at risk for falls.

General Data
___ Age over 60
___ History of falls before admission*
___ Postoperative/admitted for surgery
___ Smoker

Physical Condition
___ Dizziness/imbalance
___ Unsteady gait
___ Diseases/other problems affecting weight-bearing joints
___ Weakness
___ Paresis
___ Seizure disorder
___ Impairment of vision
___ Impairment of hearing
___ Diarrhea
___ Urinary frequency

Mental Status
___ Confusion/disorientation*
___ Impaired memory or judgment
___ Inability to understand or follow directions

Medications
___ Diuretics or diuretic effects
___ Hypotensive or central nervous system (CNS) suppressants (e.g., narcotic, sedative, psychotropic, hypnotic, tranquilizer, antihypertensive, antidepressant)
___ Medication that increases gastrointestinal (GI) motility (e.g., laxative, enema)

Ambulatory Devices Used
___ Cane
___ Crutches
___ Walker
___ Wheelchair
___ Geriatric (Geri) chair
___ Braces

TOOL 2: Reassessment Is Safe "Kare" (Risk) Tool

Directions: Place a check mark in front of any element that applies to your client. A client who has a check mark in front of any of the first four elements would be identified as at risk for falls. In addition, when a high-risk client has a check mark in front of the element "Use of a wheelchair," the client is considered to be at greater risk for falls.
___ Unsteady gait/dizziness/imbalance
___ Impaired memory or judgment
___ Weakness
___ History of falls
___ Use of a wheelchair

*RISK, Reassessment Is Safe "Kare."

From *Rehabilitation Nursing,* 16(2), 68. Reprinted with permission of Association of Rehabilitation Nurses, 4700 W. Lake Avenue, Glenview, IL 60025-1485. Copyright © Association of Rehabilitation Nurses 1991.

---

is evidence to show that hospital-based fall-prevention programs, which focus on a multidimensional approach for reducing falls, can reduce fall rates (RNAO, 2002; CDC, 2006). Effective fall-prevention programs include a risk assessment, medication reviews with modification, use of assistive devices, exercise and strength training, and education for home safety (CDC, 2006).

Accurately assess clients and their environment for fall risk factors. Although there is little evidence that modifying the home environment alone will reduce fall risk (CDC, 2006), measures to reduce or eliminate hazards can minimize client injury. In the home setting, older adults are more likely to fall in the bedroom, bathroom, and kitchen. These falls most often occur while transferring from beds, chairs, and toilets; getting into or out of bathtubs; tripping over carpet edges or doorway thresholds; slipping on wet surfaces; and descending stairs (Tideiksaar, 1989). Therefore, carefully assess a client's home environment and inform the client or family member of potential hazards. Chapter 38 covers home safety assessment in-depth.

In the hospital setting, there are a variety of fall risk factor screening tools. A risk factor screening is conducted on all clients. The Joanna Briggs Institute (2001) notes that if a history of falls is detected, a fall-related assessment and subsequent proper interventions are likely to reduce future probability of falls. Because there are multiple known risk factors for falls, no one assessment tool has been shown to be most sensitive and specific to analyze fall risk (RNAO, 2002). The Reassessment Is Safe "Kare" (RISK) assessment tools (Box 3-2) include a client's physical and mental status, medications, and devices used to ambulate to determine the degree of fall risk. Nursing measures are chosen based on an individual client's fall risk score, medical condition, and the environment.

Nurses institute a number of environmental interventions for client safety. The call light/intercom system (Figure 3-1) allows clients to signal caregivers when they need assistance. Explain how to operate the call system to the client and family and place the call device within a client's reach.

A full set of raised side rails (two to a bed or four to a bed) may be considered a physical restraint. There is much debate within health care as to whether side rails are protective or whether they contribute to client injury, especially when a client cannot voluntarily lower a side rail (Gallinagh and others, 2002). Capezuti and others (2002) found that bilateral side rail use among older nursing home residents does

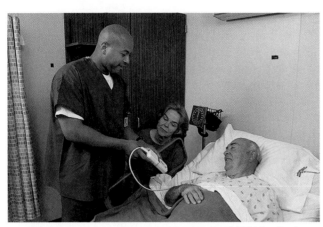

FIGURE 3-1 Nurse demonstrates use of call light to client.

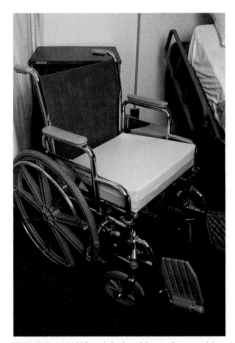

FIGURE 3-2 Wheelchair with wedge cushion in place.

not appear to significantly reduce the likelihood of falls and may actually become a serious hazard. Some clients attempt to climb over side rails to get out of bed. In addition, there have been cases of client entrapment with the use of side rails (Powell-Cope and others, 2005). Entrapment occurs when a client is caught, trapped, or entangled in hospital-bed components. Depending on a bed's design, there is a space or gap left between a side rail and the mattress edge. As a result clients may have their head, neck, or chest entrapped when they attempt to exit the bed, often leading to fatal injuries (Powell-Cope and others, 2005). Raising only one of two, or three of four, side rails gives clients room to exit a bed safely and to maneuver within the bed.

Wheels on beds and wheelchairs must be locked when stationary. Keep beds in the low position after providing client care. Place clients in a Geri chair or in a wheelchair

with a wedge cushion (Figure 3-2). These devices are designed to keep clients from getting up unassisted. Use a wheelchair only to transport clients rather than leaving a client in a wheelchair for an extended time. Visual cues, such as color-coded arm bands or signs on the door, are found to effectively identify risk-prone clients within an institution.

Electronic bed and chair alarms are available to warn nursing staff when a client who needs assistances tries to leave the bed or chair on his or her own. An Ambularm is worn on the leg and signals when the leg is in a dependent position, such as over a side rail or on the floor (see Skill 3.2). Additional devices include pressure-sensitive strips placed beneath the client and under the buttocks on either a bed or chair and a tether alarm clipped to the client's garment. These devices alert staff that a client is at risk of falling. Staff can then respond in a timely manner.

ASSESSMENT

1 Assess the client's motor, sensory, balance, and cognitive status, including ability to follow directions and cooperate. For the older adult, pay attention to risk factors, including impaired memory and cognition, fatigue, osteoporosis, osteoarthritis, urinary tract infection (UTI), dehydration, decreased hearing, decreased night vision, cataracts or glaucoma, orthostatic hypotension, decreased balance, slowed nervous system response, history of stroke, incontinence, or Parkinson's disease. *Rationale: Physiological alterations predispose client to falls.*

2 Assess client's medication history (including OTC medications and herbal products) for use of antidepressants, antipsychotics, benzodiazepines, antihypertensives, antihistamines, anticonvulsants, nonsteroidal antiinflammatory drugs (NSAIDs), corticosteroids, diuretics, muscle relaxants, antiarrhythmics, digoxin, nitrates, hypoglycemics, antiparkinson drugs, and histamine (H2) receptors. *Rationale: These medications may increase risk for falls (Elsaris and others, 2003).*

3 Assess client for history of previous fall (Cwikel and others, 2001). Be specific in your assessment, following the SPLATT acronym (Meiner and Lueckenotte, 2006):
   Symptoms at time of fall
   Previous fall
   Location of fall
   Activity at time of fall
   Time of fall
   Trauma post fall
   Rationale: Previous history of fall increases risk of repeated fall.

4 Assess risk factors in health care facility or home that pose a threat to client's safety (e.g., improperly lighted room, clutter in walking path). *Rationale: Reveals client's environmental risk factors for falls.*

5 Perform the timed "Get Up and Go" test, which measures the time it takes to rise from a standard chair, walk 3 meters, turn, walk back to the chair, and sit down. *Ra-*

tionale: Measures physical mobility in older adult. Useful in screening for altered balance and gait (Tinetti, 2003).

6 Determine what client knows about risks for falling and steps he or she takes to prevent falls.

PLANNING

Expected Outcomes focus on preventing client injury and on appropriate use of safety equipment.

1 Client's environment is free of hazards.

2 Client or family member is able to identify safety risks.

3 Client does not fall or suffer injury while in the health care agency or home.

Delegation Considerations

The skill of assessing a client's risk for falling cannot be delegated. Skills used to prevent falls can be delegated. The nurse directs personnel by:

- Explaining client's mobility limitations and any specific measures to minimize risks.
- Teaching specific environmental safety precautions to use (e.g., bed locked in low position, call bell within reach, nonskid footwear).

Equipment

- RISK assessment tool for falls
- Hospital bed with side rails
- Call light/intercom system
- Safety belt

IMPLEMENTATION *for Fall Prevention*

STEPS	RATIONALE
1 See Standard Protocol (inside front cover).	

> **NURSE ALERT** Before using any equipment for the first time, know the safety features and proper method of operation.

STEPS	RATIONALE
2 Adjust bed to proper height, and lower side rail on side of client contact.	Allows for proper body mechanics to reduce risk of injury. Height of bed allows ambulatory client to get in and out of bed safely.
3 Orient client to call light/intercom system.	
a. Provide client with hearing aid and glasses if used.	
b. Demonstrate to both client and family how to turn call bell on and off at bedside and in bathroom (see Figure 3-1).	Ensures client is able to activate call system correctly and quickly.
c. Have client/family return demonstration.	Reinforces understanding and evaluates ability to manipulate controls.
d. Explain best times for client/family to use call bell/intercom (e.g., to use bathroom, to get out of bed, to report pain).	Will increase likelihood of nurse being able to respond before client tries to get out of bed unassisted.
e. Secure call bell in an accessible location, such as on side rails or clipped to bedding. Make sure client can reach device easily and is aware of its location.	Prevents client from searching for device, overreaching, and possibly falling out of bed.
4 Use of hospital bed and side rails:	
a. Explain to client/family the two reasons for using side rails: preventing falls and turning self in bed.	Promotes client and family cooperation.
b. Check agency policies regarding side rail use.	Side rails are considered a restraint device when used to prevent the ambulatory client from getting out of bed voluntarily (CMS, 2000).
c. In a four side rail bed, keep the top two side rails up, lower two rails down, and bed in low position with bed wheels locked (see illustration). Check agency policy.	Minimizes risk of client falling out of bed. With bed in low position, if client climbs out of bed and falls, trauma may be reduced.
d. Leave one upper side rail up and one down. Follow this guideline when client is oriented and able to get out of bed independently.	Side rail can be used to enhance transfer and repositioning ability.

> **NURSE ALERT** Side rails may cause entrapment of the head and body. Assess for excessive gaps and openings between bed frame and mattress. Use side rail netting or protective padding to prevent mattress from being pushed to one side.

STEPS	RATIONALE
5 Arrange necessary items (e.g., water pitcher, telephone, reading materials, dentures) within client's easy reach and in a logical way, placing them consistently in same location.	Facilitates independence and self-care and prevents falls from attempts to reach too far.
6 Provide clear instructions to client/family regarding mobility restrictions, ambulation assistance, and transfer techniques.	Clients/family members need to know when to call caregivers for assistance.
7 Explain to client specific safety measures to prevent falls (e.g., wear well-fitting flat footwear with nonskid soles, dangle feet for a few minutes before standing, walk slowly, ask for help if dizzy or weak).	Safety precautions prevent slipping and loss of balance from orthostatic hypotension.
8 Make sure ambulatory client's pathway to bathroom facilities is clear. Remove unnecessary objects from rooms (e.g., extra IV poles).	
9 Provide adequate glare-free lighting throughout room.	Reduces likelihood of falling over objects. Glare may be a problem for older adults because of vision changes.
10 Confer with physical therapy on feasibility of gait training and muscle-strengthening exercise.	Single intervention strategies shown to reduce risk of falls among older adults include gait and exercise training (Tinetti, 2003).
11 Confer with physician on possibility of reducing or adjusting number of medications client receives.	Number of medications can be reduced safely if a balance is achieved between benefits of medications and risk of adverse events (Tinetti, 2003).
12 Safe transport using a wheelchair:	
a. During transfer, position wheelchair on same side of bed as client's strong or unaffected side (see Skill 6.2).	Facilitates client's ability to assist in transfer to chair.
b. Securely lock brakes on both wheels when transferring client into or out of wheelchair.	Keeps chair steady and secure.
c. Raise footplates before transfer; lower footplates, placing client's feet on them, after client is seated.	Promotes client's stability during transfer.
d. Have client sit with buttocks well back in seat. Use a seat belt or wedge cushion if available.	Protects client from sliding out of chair.
e. Back wheelchair into and out of elevator, rear large wheels first.	Makes a smoother ride and prevents smaller wheels from catching in the crack between elevator and floor.

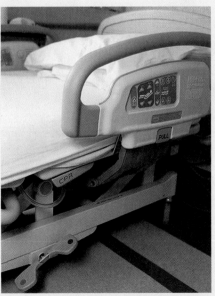

STEP 4c. Hospital bed should be kept in low position with wheels locked and upper side rails up (as appropriate).

STEPS	RATIONALE
f. When navigating on a ramp or incline, turn so that the chair pushes against your body, which is between the chair and the bottom of the ramp.	Prevents a runaway wheelchair that can pull away and roll faster down ramp than intended.

13 Safe transport using a stretcher:

> **COMMUNICATION TIP** Clients are not to be left on a stretcher unattended, especially when medicated or confused.

a. Lock wheels during transfer from bed to stretcher or stretcher to bed.	Prevents bed and stretcher from moving apart.
b. Use a safety belt across client's upper thighs, or raise side rails (see illustration).	Reduces risk of falling from stretcher.
c. Push stretcher from end where client's head rests. For stretchers with stationary wheels on one end and swivel wheels on other end, head of stretcher has stationary wheels.	Protects client's head in case of a collision.
d. Move stretcher into elevator head first.	Facilitates entry without bumping the sides.

14 Assisting the client with ambulation:

a. Depending on client's strength and ability to ambulate, use safety measures to protect against falls (see Skill 6.3).

> **COMMUNICATION TIP** When ambulating clients, talk about the risks for falls: "Your medications may make you feel dizzy or weak. Always ask for help before trying to walk until this passes." Also let the client who has a fear of falling know that confidence can be regained with continued practice.

15 See Completion Protocol (inside front cover).

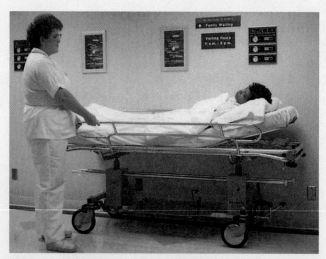

STEP 13b. Side rails are raised to prevent client from rolling off stretcher.

EVALUATION

1 Observe client's immediate environment for presence of hazards.

2 Evaluate need for assistive devices such as walker or bedside commode.

3 Ask client/family to identify safety risks.

4 Determine client's response to safety modifications and that no falls or injuries have occurred.

Unexpected Outcomes and Related Interventions

1 Client starts to fall while ambulating with a caregiver.

a. Put both arms around client's waist or grasp gait belt.

b. Stand with feet apart to provide broad base of support.

c. Extend one leg and let client slide against it to the floor (Figure 3-3, A).

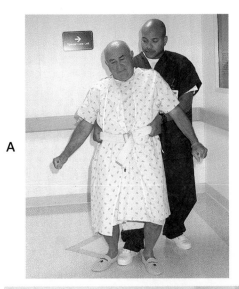

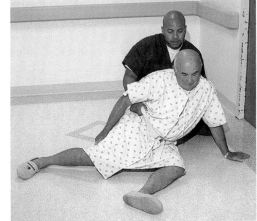

FIGURE 3-3 A, Stand with feet apart to provide broad base of support; extend one leg for client to slide against to the floor. **B,** Bend knees to lower body as client slides to floor.

d. Bend knees to lower body as client slides to floor (Figure 3-3, *B*).
2 Client suffers a fall.
a. Call for assistance.
b. Assess client for injury and stay with the client until assistance arrives to help lift client to bed or to a wheelchair.
c. Notify physician.
d. Note pertinent events related to fall and treatment provided in medical record.
e. Follow institution's sentinel event reporting policy.
f. Evaluate client and environment to determine whether fall could have been prevented.
g. Reinforce identified risks with client, and review safety measures needed to prevent a fall.

Recording and Reporting

- Record in progress notes specific interventions to prevent falls and promote safety.
- Report client's fall risks and measures taken to reduce risks to all health care personnel.
- Report immediately if the client sustains a fall or an injury.

Sample Documentation

0900 Fall risk assessment completed. Client placed on fall precautions due to history of falls, weakness, and urinary frequency. Call bell within reach, side rails up ×2, hourly room checks, night-light on at all times, bedside commode in place. Instructed to call for help when ambulating. Client voiced understanding.

1615 Found client on floor in bathroom after responding to emergency call light. Client stated, "I slipped on the wet floor." Alert and oriented ×3. No apparent injury from fall. BP 110/74, P 82 and regular, R 20. Assisted to bed and instructed to call for help before getting out of bed. Voiced understanding. Call bell placed within client's reach. Side rails up ×2. Dr. Justine and family notified of fall.

Special Considerations

Pediatric Considerations

- Never leave a child of any age unattended on a raised surface (Hockenberry and Wilson, 2007).
- Place hoods or tents over an infant's or child's crib to prevent accidental falls.
- Place gates at both ends of stairs to prevent toddlers from falling.
- Toddlers and children should wear helmets to protect the head from risk of injury while bicycling, skateboarding, or riding a scooter.

Geriatric Considerations

- Older clients with short-term memory loss or cognitive dysfunction may be unable to follow directions and may attempt to climb out of bed or get up from a chair unassisted.
- Older adults, especially postmenopausal women, are at risk for fractured hips. Fractures can cause independent clients to become more dependent or immobilized (Meiner and Lueckenotte, 2006).

Home Care Considerations

- Assess home environment and institute safety measures as appropriate (see Chapter 38).
- Items should be kept in their familiar positions and within easy reach.
- If client has a history of falls and lives alone, recommend he or she wear an electronic safety alert device. The device is turned on by the wearer to alert a monitoring site to call emergency services for help.

Long-Term Care Considerations

- Clients who wander from a nursing facility are at risk for injury. Specific interventions such as electronic wandering devices can be used to reduce this risk.
- Make sure assistive devices (e.g., canes, hand rails, walkers) are in proper working order.

SKILL 3.2 Designing a Restraint-Free Environment

Restraints, both chemical and physical (see Skill 3.3), restrict a client's physical activity or normal access to the body and are not a usual part of treatment indicated by a client's condition or symptoms (CMS, 2000). Serious and sometimes fatal complications can develop from the use of restraints. Because of the risks associated with restraint use, current legislation emphasizes reducing the use of restraints. A restraint-free environment is the first goal of care for all clients.

Clients at risk for falling or wandering present special safety challenges when trying to create a restraint-free environment. Wandering is defined as meandering, aimless, or repetitive locomotion that exposes a client to harm and is frequently in conflict with boundaries, limits, or obstacles (NANDA, 2005). This is a common problem in clients who are confused or disoriented. The interruption of wandering may cause more distress for a client. It is more helpful to identify the stimulus for wandering and modify the environment so that wandering is not likely to be hazardous (Ebersole and Hess, 2001).

Modifications of the environment are effective alternatives to restraints. More frequent observation of clients, involvement of family during visitation, and frequent reorientation are also helpful measures. Introduction of meaningful and familiar stimuli within a client's environment can reduce the types of behaviors (e.g., wandering, restlessness, confusion) that in the past led to restraint use.

ASSESSMENT

1 Assess client's physical and mental status, such as orientation; level of consciousness; ability to understand, remember, and follow directions; balance; gait; vision; hearing; bowel/bladder routine; level of pain; laboratory values; and presence of orthostatic hypotension. *Rationale: Identifies safety risks and physiological cause for behavior.*

2 Review prescribed medications (e.g., sedatives, hypnotics, diuretics [see Skill 3.1]) for interactions and untoward effects. *Rationale: Medication interactions or side effects often contribute to risk for falls or altered mental status.*

> **NURSE ALERT** Client's inability to understand or follow directions indicates client needs constant supervision.

3 For clients at risk for wandering, assess for cognitive decline (Mini-Mental State Examination [MMSE]) and wandering patterns (Algase Wandering Scale) (Algase and others, 2001). Also determine reasons for wandering (e.g., discomfort, boredom, looking for something that is "lost," overstimulation). *Rationale: Determines cause and nature of wandering and helps in selection of interventions.*

PLANNING

Expected Outcomes focus on maintaining client safety while avoiding the need for physical restraints.

1 Client will be injury free and/or will not inflict injury on others.

2 Client will display cooperative behavior toward staff, visitors, and other clients.

Delegation Considerations

The skill of assessing client behaviors and making decisions about less restrictive interventions cannot be delegated. Actions for promoting a safe environment may be delegated. The nurse directs personnel to:

- Report specific client behaviors and actions (e.g., client confusion, getting out of bed unassisted, combativeness).

Equipment

- Visual or auditory stimuli (e.g., calendar, clock, radio, television)
- Diversional activities (e.g., puzzles, games, audio books, music, videotapes)
- Wedge pillow
- Ambularm or pressure-sensitive bed or chair alarm

IMPLEMENTATION *for Designing a Restraint-Free Environment*

STEPS	RATIONALE
1 See Standard Protocol (inside front cover).	
2 Orient client and family to surroundings, introduce to staff, and explain all treatments and procedures.	Promotes client understanding and cooperation.

> **COMMUNICATION TIP** When orienting client, approach client in a calm, nonthreatening, professional manner. Repeat orientation information often, especially when the environment has changed from what the client is accustomed to.

STEPS	RATIONALE
3 Provide the same caregivers to the extent possible. Encourage family and friends to stay with the client. Companions can be helpful. In some institutions, volunteers can be good companions.	Reduces anxiety and increases safety when one person provides care and supervision is constant.
4 Place client in a room that is easily accessible to caregivers.	Facilitates close observation. Watching the unit's activities distracts client (Rogers and Bocchino, 1999).
5 Be sure client has glasses, hearing aid, or other sensory-aid devices on and functioning. Then, provide visual and auditory stimuli meaningful to specific client (e.g., calendar, radio [client's choice of music], family pictures) (see illustration).	Sensory deficit increases risk of confusion and disorientation. Meaningful stimuli orients client to day, time, and physical surroundings.

> **NURSE ALERT** Getting out of bed for toileting is one of the most common events leading to a client's fall, especially during evening or night hours when room is darkened.

6 Meet client's basic needs (e.g., toileting, relief of pain or hunger) as soon as possible.	Meeting basic needs in a timely fashion decreases client discomfort and anxiety.
7 Provide scheduled ambulation, chair activity, and toileting (e.g., ask client every 2 hours if needing to void). Organize treatments so client has long uninterrupted periods throughout the day.	Regular opportunity to void avoids risk of client trying to reach bathroom alone. Provides for sleep and rest periods. Constant activity may result in overstimulation.
8 Position IV catheters, urinary catheters, and tubes/drains out of client view, or use camouflage by wrapping IV site with bandage or stockinet, placing undergarments on client with urinary catheter, or covering abdominal feeding tubes/drains with loose abdominal binder.	Maintains medical treatment and reduces client access to tubes/lines.
9 Use stress reduction techniques such as back rub, massage, and imagery (see Chapter 10).	Reduced stress offers client energy to be channeled more appropriately.
10 Use diversional activities such as puzzles, games, books, folding towels, drawing/coloring, or an object to hold. Be sure it is an activity in which client expresses interest.	Meaningful diversional activities provide distraction, help to reduce boredom, and provide tactile stimulation. Minimizes wandering.
11 Use a pressure-sensitive bed or chair pad with alarms. To use Ambularm monitoring device:	Alerts staff to an unsteady client who is standing or rising up without help.
a. Explain use of device to client and family.	
b. Measure client's thigh circumference just above knee to determine appropriate size. For leg circumference less than 18 inches, use regular size; use large size for 18 inches or greater.	Band that is too loose may slip off; band that is too tight may interfere with circulation or cause skin irritation.

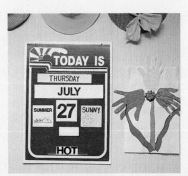

STEP 5 Calendar with large print orients client to physical surroundings. (From Sorrentino SA: *Assisting with patient care,* St Louis, 1999, Mosby.)

STEPS	RATIONALE

> **NURSE ALERT** Use of Ambularm is contraindicated in the presence of impaired circulation, swelling, skin irritation, or breaks in the skin.

   c. Test battery and alarm by touching snaps to corresponding snaps on leg band.

   d. Apply leg band just above knee and snap battery securely in place (see illustration).

   e. Instruct client that alarm will sound unless leg is kept in horizontal position (see illustration).

   f. To assist client to ambulate, deactivate alarm by unsnapping device from leg band.

12 Consult with physical therapy, speech therapy, and occupational therapy for appropriate activities to provide stimulation and exercise.

13 Eliminate invasive treatments as soon as possible (e.g. tube feedings, blood sampling).

                                                 Stimuli increase client's restlessness.

14 **See Completion Protocol (inside front cover).**

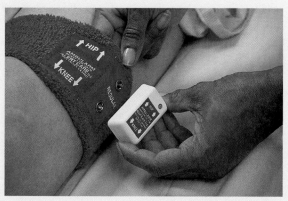

STEP 11d. Snap battery in place to activate alarm. (Courtesy AlertCare, Mill Valley, Calif.)

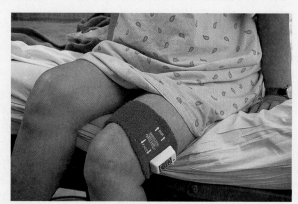

STEP 11e. Audio alarm will sound when client approaches near-vertical position. (Courtesy AlertCare, Mill Valley, Calif.)

EVALUATION

1 Observe client for any injuries.

2 Observe client's behavior toward staff, visitors, and other clients.

Unexpected Outcomes and Related Interventions

1 Client displays behaviors that increase risk for injury to self or others.

   a. Review episodes for a pattern (e.g., activity, time of day) that indicates alternatives that could eliminate the behavior.

   b. Discuss with all caregivers and support service personnel alternative interventions to promote safe, consistent care.

2 Client sustains an injury or is out of control, placing others at risk for injury.

   a. Notify physician, and complete a sentinel event report according to agency policy.

   b. Identify alternative measures to promote safety without a restraint.

   c. As a last resort, identify appropriate restraint to use (see Skill 3.3).

Recording and Reporting

• Document all behaviors that relate to cognitive status and ability to maintain safety: orientation to time, place, and person; ability to follow directions; mood and emotional status; understanding of condition and treatment plan; medication effects related to behaviors; interventions used; and client response.

Sample Documentation

   0900 Up and dressed; oriented to person, but not time or place. Upset and crying when unable to call wife on the telephone. Pacing in room. Reoriented to place. Explained to client wife is due to visit later in afternoon. Set radio to favorite talk show.

1000 Participated for 15 minutes with ball toss to music at O.T.; then resting in rocking chair, smiling, and interacting socially with roommate.

Special Considerations

Pediatric Considerations

- Distraction techniques can decrease the need for restraints. Examples include having a child hold a stuffed animal while an IV is being inserted, or blowing bubbles while a drain is being removed.

Geriatric Considerations

- A sudden onset of confusion, weakness, and functional decline in a previously oriented client may indicate the presence of an underlying illness in the older adult.
- Assess for physical causes of behavior changes such as urinary or respiratory infection, hypoxia, fever, fluid and electrolyte imbalance, side effects of multiple drug administration, depression, anemia, hypothyroidism, or fecal impaction (Ebersole and Hess, 2001).

Home Care Considerations

- Clients at risk for self-injury or violence toward others need intensive supervision. Family and/or caregiver must recognize this need and be willing and able to provide it.

Long-Term Care Considerations

- Allow the client to reminisce about past events to cultivate a sense of security, to enhance the client's identity, and to help maintain orientation.
- For wanderers, provide environmental modifications, for example, offer secure place for clients to wander (large safe, walking area); increase visual appeal of environment with tactile boards or three-dimensional wall art; place gridlines in front of doors to decrease exit seeking; make exits less accessible by covering panic bar with cloth and allow walking where doors are not in the path; use large-print signs and portrait-like photos to aid in finding way; use multiple and different kinds of locks on doors (Futrell, Melillo, and Titler, 2002).

SKILL 3.3 Applying Physical Restraints

- Nursing Skills Online: Safety, Lesson 2

Physical or chemical restraints should be the last resort and used only when all other reasonable alternatives have failed. Restraints are a temporary means to maintain client safety. A physician's order is required and must be based on a face-to-face assessment of the client (Figure 3-4). The order must be current and specify the duration and circumstances under which the restraint is to be used. Orders should be renewed according to agency policy (usually every 24 hours) and based on reassessment and reevaluation of the restrained client. Regulatory agencies such as the JCAHO (2005a) and the Centers for Medicare & Medicaid Services (CMS, 2004) outline standards regarding safe use of restraints. It is a requirement in long-term care settings to obtain informed consent from family members before using restraints on clients.

Clients needing temporary restraints include those at risk for falls and confused or combative clients at risk for self-injury or violence to self or others. In addition, health care providers apply restraints to prevent interruption of therapy such as an IV catheter, urinary or surgical drains, or life support equipment.

Restraints are either physical or chemical. A physical restraint is any manual method or physical or mechanical device that the client is unable to remove. Chemical restraints are medications, such as antianxiety agents and sedatives, used to control the client's behavior. The use of restraints is associated with serious complications, including pressure ulcers, constipation, urinary and fecal incontinence, and urinary retention. In some cases restricted breathing or circulation has resulted in death. Loss of self-esteem, humiliation, fear, and anger are additional serious concerns. The Food and Drug Administration (FDA), which regulates restraints as medical devices, requires manufacturers to label restraints as "prescription only." Many clients do not easily accept use of restraints. Cultural values affect how clients and family members perceive use of restraints. Before using restraints, assess the meaning of restraints to both the client and family. Culturally sensitive care may include removing restraints when family members are present.

ASSESSMENT

1 Assess client's behavior, such as confusion, disorientation, agitation, restlessness, combativeness, or inability to follow directions. *Rationale: If client's behavior continues despite treatment, use of physical restraint may be needed.*
2 Review agency policies regarding restraints. Check physician's order for purpose, type, location, and time or duration of restraint. Determine if a signed consent for use of restraint is needed. *Rationale: Physician's order for the least restrictive type of restraint is required.*
3 Review manufacturer's instructions for restraint application and determine the most appropriate size restraint. *Rationale: Correct application of appropriately sized restraint reduces risk of injury.*

Barnes-Jewish Hospital Physical Restraint and Seclusion Order Form

Date: _____ Patient Name _____ Registration Number _____

Medical-Surgical Restraint* Medical Reason: _____ Describe the specific behavior the patient exhibits that supports the need for restraint: _____ Time: From_____ to_____ (not to exceed 24°) *Renewal of orders and assessment for continued need required every 24 hours **Behavior Management Restraint or Seclusion**** Medical Reason: ☐ Disruptive/dangerous behavior or _____ Describe the specific behavior the patient exhibits that supports the need for restraint: _____ Time: From_____ to_____ (not to exceed 4°) Face to Face assessment evaluation required with in 1 hour **Renewal of orders and assessment for continued need required: Every 4 hours if patient ≥ 18 years of age Every 2 hours for ages 9 - 17; Every 1 hour for children under 8 years of age	**Restraint Type** (List less to most restrictive) ☐ Mittens ☐ Elbow Immobilizer ☐ 4 Bed rails up ☐ Vail Bed ☐ Soft limb ☐ Other: _____ For ED and Psychiatry ONLY (List least to most restrictive) ☐ Seclusion ☐ Locked Limb	**Restraint Location** ☐ LUE ☐ RUE ☐ LLE ☐ RLE	**RESTRAINT ORDER NEEDED** Remove this section when the order is written and signed.

_____ SIGNATURE _____   _____ PRINTED NAME _____   _____ PAGER OR PHONE _____
BJ 3343-354 V9 (09/03)

FIGURE 3-4 Restraint order form. (Courtesy Barnes-Jewish Hospital, BJC Health Care, St Louis, Mo.)

4 Inspect the area where the restraint is to be placed. Note any nearby tubing or devices. Assess condition of the skin, sensation, adequacy of circulation, and range of joint motion. *Rationale: Provides baseline assessment.*

> **NURSE ALERT** Restraints should not interfere with equipment such as IV tubes. They are not placed over access devices, such as an arteriovenous (AV) dialysis shunt.

PLANNING

Expected Outcomes focus on protecting the client from injury and maintaining prescribed therapy.
1 Client will maintain intact skin integrity, pulses, temperature, color, and sensation of restrained body part.
2 Client will be free of injury.
3 Client's therapies will be uninterrupted.
4 Restraint will be discontinued as soon as possible.
5 Client's self-esteem and dignity will be maintained.

Delegation Considerations

The skill of assessing client's behavior, orientation to the environment, need for restraints, and appropriate use cannot be delegated. The nurse may delegate the application of a restraint. The nurse directs personnel regarding:
• The appropriate type of restraint to use.
• How to routinely check the client's circulation, skin integrity, and breathing.
• When and how to change the client's position and provide range-of-motion (ROM) exercises, toileting, and skin care.
• When to report signs and symptoms of client not tolerating restraint (e.g., increased agitation, constricted circulation, change in skin integrity, changes in breathing).

Equipment

• Proper restraint
• Padding (if needed)

IMPLEMENTATION *for Applying Physical Restraints*

STEPS	RATIONALE
1 See Standard Protocol (inside front cover).	

> **COMMUNICATION TIP** Explain reason for restraint to both client and family, and stress that restraint is temporary and protective. Discuss other measures taken to avoid restraint and explain that they were inadequate.

STEPS	RATIONALE
2 Approach client in a calm, confident manner and explain what you are going to do.	Reduces anxiety and promotes cooperation.
3 Be sure client is comfortable and in proper body alignment.	Promotes comfort, prevents contractures, and prevents neurovascular injury.
4 If necessary, pad skin and bony prominences that will be under restraint.	Protects skin from irritation.

STEPS	RATIONALE

5 Apply proper-size restraint; *follow manufacturer's directions.*

a. **Belt restraint:**

Have client in a sitting position. Apply over clothes, gown, or pajamas. Make sure it is placed at the waist, not the chest or abdomen. Remove wrinkles or creases while placing around the waist, and avoid excessive tightness. Bring ties through slots in belt. Help client lie down if in bed (see illustrations).

Restrains center of gravity and prevents client from rolling off stretcher or falling out of bed. Tight application or misplacement can interfere with breathing.

b. **Extremity (ankle or wrist) restraint:**

Commercially available limb restraints are made of sheepskin with foam padding. Wrap limb restraint around wrist or ankle with soft part toward skin and secured snugly (but not tightly) in place by Velcro strap. Insert two fingers under secured restraint (see illustration).

Maintains immobilization of extremity to protect client from fall or accidental removal of device (e.g., IV tube, Foley catheter). Tight restraints may constrict circulation or ventilation and cause neurovascular injury or cause therapeutic devices to become occluded. Checking for constriction prevents neurovascular injury.

> **NURSE ALERT** Client with extremity restraint is at risk for aspiration if positioned supine. Place client in lateral position or with head of bed elevated, rather than supine.

c. **Mitten restraint:**

A thumbless mitten device restrains client's hands. Place hand in mitten, being sure Velcro strap(s) are around wrist rather than forearm (see illustration).

Prevents client from dislodging invasive equipment, removing dressings, or scratching, yet allows greater movement than a wrist restraint.

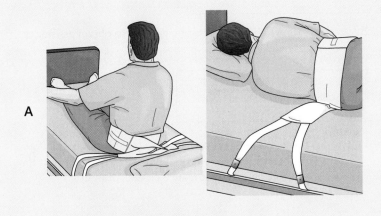

A

B

STEP 5 A, Apply belt restraint with client sitting. (From Sorrentino SA: *Mosby's textbook for nursing assistants,* ed 6, St Louis, 2000, Mosby.) **B,** A properly applied belt restraint allows client to turn in bed.

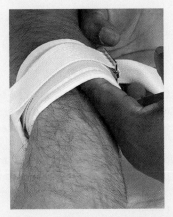

STEP 5b. Securing an extremity restraint. Check restraint for constriction by inserting two fingers under restraint. (From Sorrentino SA: *Mosby's textbook for nursing assistants,* ed 6, St Louis, 2000, Mosby.)

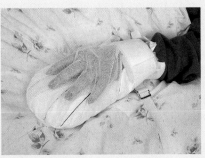

STEP 5c. Mitten restraint. (Courtesy JT Posey, Arcadia, Calif.)

STEPS	RATIONALE

d. **Elbow restraint (Freedom splint):**
Restraint consists of piece of fabric with slots in which tongue blades are placed. Insert client's arm so that elbow joint rests against padded area with tongue blades, keeping joint rigid.

Commonly used with infants and children to prevent elbow flexion. May also be used for adults.

> **NURSE ALERT** This text does not address application of vest restraints. Many health care agencies have banned the use of the jacket (vest) restraint because of the fatal injuries associated with its use.

6 Attach restraint straps to portion of bed frame that moves when head of bed is raised or lowered. ***Do not attach to side rails.*** Can also attach restraint to chair frame for client in chair or wheelchair.

When bed is raised or lowered, strap will not tighten and restrict circulation. Attaching to side rail could cause serious injury when lowered.

7 Secure restraint with a quick-release tie. ***Do not tie in a knot.***

Allows for quick release in an emergency.

8 Assess proper placement of restraint, including skin integrity, pulses, temperature, color, and sensation of the restrained body part. Remove restraints at least every 2 hours (JCAHO, 2005a) and evaluate client each time. Perform ROM exercises. If client is violent or noncompliant, remove one restraint at a time and/or have staff assistance while removing restraints.

Provides opportunity to change client's position, perform full ROM, toileting, and exercise and to provide food or fluids.

> **NURSE ALERT** Violent or aggressive client must never be left unattended while restraints are off.

9 Secure call light or intercom system within reach.

Allows client, family, or caregiver to obtain assistance quickly.

> **NURSE ALERT** Restraints restrict movement, making clients unable to perform activities of daily living (ADLs) without assistance. Providing food/fluids and assisting with toileting and other activities is essential.

10 Leave bed or chair with wheels locked. Keep bed in lowest position.

Locked wheels prevent bed or chair from moving if client attempts to get out. If client falls when bed is in lowest position, this will reduce chance of injury.

11 See Completion Protocol (inside front cover).

EVALUATION

1 Evaluate for proper placement of restraint, skin integrity, pulses, temperature, color, and sensation of restrained body part *at least every 2 hours* or sooner according to client need and agency policy (JCAHO, 2005a).

2 Inspect client for any injury resulting from immobility.

3 Observe IV catheters, urinary catheters, and drainage tubes to determine that they are positioned correctly and that therapy remains uninterrupted.

4 Evaluate client's need for restraint at least every 24 hours or more often depending on purpose of restraint (e.g., behavioral use requires review every 2 to 4 hours). Face-to-face evaluation by physician is required and new order obtained if restraint is to be continued (JCAHO, 2005a).

5 Observe client's behavior and reaction to the presence of restraints.

Unexpected Outcomes and Related Interventions

1 Skin underlying restraint becomes reddened or damaged.

a. Provide appropriate skin therapy (see Chapter 22).

b. Notify the physician, and reassess the need for continued use of restraint. Use a different type of restraint or use additional padding.

c. Consider whether alternatives to restraint can be used.

d. Remove restraints more frequently. Change wet or soiled restraints.

2 Client has altered neurovascular status to an extremity (cyanosis; pallor; coldness of the skin; or complaints of tingling, pain, or numbness).

a. Remove restraint immediately; stay with the client.

b. Notify the physician.

3 Client becomes confused, disoriented, or agitated.

a. Identify reason for change in behavior, and attempt to eliminate cause.

b. Use restraint alternatives, such as companionship or supervision, pain relief, other comfort measures, changing or eliminating bothersome treatments, reality orientation, music therapy, therapeutic touch, reminiscence, behavior modification, companionship, crafts, or active listening (Ledford and Mentes, 1997).

c. Determine need for more or less sensory stimulation.

Recording and Reporting

- Record nursing interventions tried to ensure client's safety before use of restraints.
- Record client's behavior before restraints applied, level of orientation, and client or family member's statement of understanding of the purpose of restraint and consent for application.
- Record type and location of restraint applied, time restraint was applied, and specific assessments related to breathing, circulation, skin integrity, and musculoskeletal system integrity.
- Record client's behavior after restraint application, times client was assessed, attempts to use alternatives to restraint and client's response, times restraint was released (temporarily and permanently), and client's response when restraints removed.

Sample Documentation

2020 Client has repeatedly attempted to get out of bed. Remains disoriented to name, date, and location. Provided sitter and attempted to reorient repeatedly without success. Conferred with Dr. Lynch. Client must remain on bed rest postoperatively following spinal surgery. Dr. Lynch here to assess client, ordered belt restraint for next 24 hours.

2030 Belt restraint applied around waist, able to breathe deeply without restriction. Skin under restraint is intact, without redness. Client able to move extremities. Initiating hourly observations of client. Family at bedside.

Special Considerations
Pediatric Considerations

- When a child needs to be restrained for a procedure, it is best that the person applying the restraint not be the child's parent or guardian.
- When an infant or child requires short-term restraint for treatment or examination that involves the head and neck, a mummy wrap can be effective (Figure 3-5) (Hockenberry and Wilson, 2007).
- Remain with the infant while restrained, and remove the restraint immediately after treatment is complete. If restraint is required for an extended period of time, remove it at least every 2 hours.

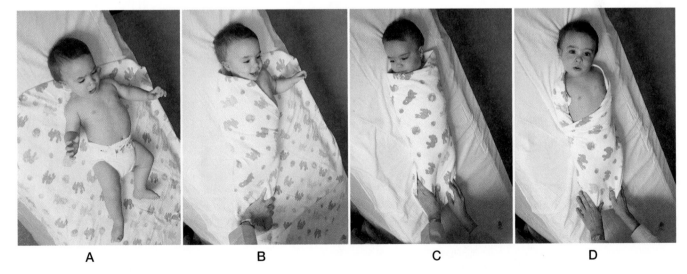

A   B   C   D

FIGURE 3-5 Application of mummy restraint. **A,** Infant placed on folded corner of blanket. **B,** One corner of blanket brought across body and secured beneath body. **C,** Second corner brought across body and secured, and lower corner folded and tucked or pinned in place. **D,** Modified mummy restraint with chest uncovered. (From Wong DL and others: *Whaley and Wong's nursing care of infants and children,* ed 6, St Louis, 1999, Mosby.)

Geriatric Considerations
- Restrained older adults respond to restraints with anger, fear, humiliation, demoralization, discomfort, and resignation (Strumpf and others, 1998).

Home Care Considerations
- If a restraint is needed for use at home, a physician's order is required and clear instructions should be given to the caregiver regarding proper application, care needed while in restraint, and potential complications.

Long-Term Care Considerations
- The need for restraints and the risk of injury can be reduced by individual assessment of risk factors, creative planning, modifying the environment, and promoting functional restoration (Ebersole and Hess, 2001).

PROCEDURAL GUIDELINE 3-2
Documenting Sentinel Events

An incident is defined as any unusual occurrence or situation that is likely to lead to undesirable effects or that varies from established policies and procedures or practices. A factual account of an adverse event, including action taken and outcome, must be documented on the medical record. In addition, the person who reports the incident must complete a confidential incident report to help identify circumstances or system problems that may be correctable. The first priority is always the safety of the individual involved in the incident. After that person is safe, it is important to document the incident completely.

If an incident involves serious physical or psychological injury or death, or the risk thereof, it will be reported as a sentinel event. Examples of sentinel events include a client fall, needlestick injury, medication administration error, and surgery on the wrong body part. The phrase "or the risk thereof" includes any process variation for which a recurrence would carry a significant chance of a serious adverse outcome. Note that the definition does include "near misses." Such events are called "sentinel" because they signal the need for immediate investigation and response.

Because any incident can result in a lawsuit, accuracy in reporting is essential. The incident report establishes a factual basis for what happened and the condition of the person involved. Incident reports provide a means for keeping all appropriate persons informed and offer a factual comparison for later developments. Clients' medical records are legally recoverable and can be used in court through a subpoena if information in the medical record validates that a report was completed. Therefore, do not make reference to an incident report in the client's medical record. A comparison of a correct and incorrect incident report entry follows:

Correct Entry	Incorrect Entry
1800 Client found on floor at foot of bed; able to respond to name when called. 2-cm abrasion noted across left forehead. Complains of pain in left arm; client states, "I used my arm to break the fall." No apparent injury to arm; ROM within normal limits. Vital signs stable. Instructed to use call light when attempting to ambulate. Dr. Smith notified, arrived on floor, examined client at 1825; ordered x-ray of left arm and placed client on fall-prevention protocol.	Client found on floor at foot of bed; probably fell on way to bathroom. Small abrasion over left forehead. Reports he also fell on left arm. Dr. Smith notified, saw client. Client instructed to use call light when needing to go to bathroom. X-ray completed as ordered.

Writing an Incident Report
Delegation Considerations
The completion of an incident report cannot be delegated.
- Any staff member who witnesses the event or first finds the client/visitor must report the incident to the staff nurse in charge.
- A registered nurse (RN) completes the incident report.
- The nurse informs personnel of the immediate actions and observations to make after an incident.

Equipment
- Incident report form

Procedural Steps
1. When first finding the client/visitor or learning of the incident, observe the client/visitor carefully and note the condition of the immediate surroundings. Systematically and carefully determine exactly what was involved and factors that may have contributed to the incident.
2. Assess the client/visitor for injury. Determine if there is any potential risk to the client and whether there is need to notify the physician.
3. Ask clients/visitors to describe what occurred, in their own words.
4. Complete the incident report form as promptly as possible, completely, and accurately, within the time dictated by agency policy (e.g., 8 to 24 hours).
5. Describe objectively what was observed when the incident was discovered, taking care to avoid personal opinions and feelings. Include time of event, witnesses (name and status), condition of individual, and who was notified.
6. Describe measures taken by any caregivers at the time of the incident, including assessment of body systems.
7. Sign the report and obtain additional signatures (e.g., physician, nursing supervisor) as required by agency policy.
8. Document factual data on the client's medical record, including the incident and related assessments and interventions. Do not include details contrary to agency policy. Do not include reference to completed incident report.
9. Seek to identify actions that could help prevent similar occurrences. Implement precautions to minimize client's risk for repeat incident.

SKILL 3.4 **Seizure Precautions**

A seizure involves a sudden, violent, involuntary series of muscle contractions that occur rhythmically, such as during acute or chronic seizure disorders, febrile episodes (especially in children), and after a head injury. Status epilepticus, characterized by prolonged seizures lasting more than 10 minutes or a series of seizures that occur in rapid succession over 30 minutes, is a medical emergency (Ignatavicius and Workman, 2002). Observation during a seizure is critical. Observe a client carefully before, during, and after the seizure, so that the episode can be documented accurately. Careful observation may help determine the type of seizure.

Oral airways for the purpose of maintaining the client's airway during a seizure are no longer recommended. Forcing something into the client's mouth could result in injury to the jaw, tongue, or teeth and cause stimulation of the gag reflex, thus causing vomiting, aspiration, and respiratory distress (National Institute of Neurological Disorder and Stroke, 2001). An airway is inserted only when there is clear access for insertion. Padded tongue blades do not belong at the bedside.

ASSESSMENT

1 Assess seizure history and knowledge of precipitating factors, noting frequency of seizures, presence of aura, and sequence of events, if known. Confer with family. *Rationale: Provides a baseline to evaluate onset of seizure activity.*
2 Assess for medical and surgical conditions that may lead to seizures or worsen existing seizure condition (e.g., electrolyte disturbance, heart disease, excessive fatigue, alcohol or caffeine use). *Rationale: These factors are common conditions that precipitate seizures.*

3 Assess medication history and client's adherence. Note therapeutic drug levels of anticonvulsants if available. *Rationale: Seizure medications must be taken as prescribed and not stopped suddenly. This may precipitate a seizure.*

PLANNING

Expected Outcomes focus on maintenance of self-esteem and prevention of injury, airway obstruction, and aspiration.
1 Client does not suffer traumatic physical injury during a seizure.
2 Client's airway is patent during seizure activity.
3 Client verbalizes positive self-feelings after a seizure episode.

Delegation Considerations
Assessment of client's risk for seizures cannot be delegated. Care of client on seizure precautions can be delegated. The nurse directs personnel by:
- Informing personnel of client's seizure pattern.
- Instructing personnel to react quickly in event of seizure by protecting client from a fall, not to attempt to restrain client, and not to place anything in client's mouth.

Equipment
- Padding for side rails and headboard
- Suction machine and Yankauer suction catheter
- Oral airway
- Oxygen via nasal cannula or face mask
- IV insertion equipment: 0.9% normal saline (NS) infusion
- Emergency medications: IV diazepam, lorazepam, valproate, phenytoin
- Clean gloves

IMPLEMENTATION *for Seizure Precautions*

STEPS	RATIONALE
1 **See Standard Protocol (inside front cover).**	
2 For clients with known risk, keep bed in lowest position with side rails up. Have oral suction equipment ready at bedside.	Modifications to environment minimize risks associated with seizure activity. Oral suctioning may be required after a seizure to prevent aspiration of secretions.
3 Provide or encourage use of bracelet or identification card noting existing seizure disorder and medications taken.	Communicates client's risk for seizure activity to emergency health care providers.

COMMUNICATION TIP Explain to the client and family what to expect during a seizure and the safety measures that are in place to protect the client from injury.

STEPS	RATIONALE

4 Seizure Response:

a. Position client safely. (1) If standing or sitting, guide client to floor and protect head by cradling in nurse's lap or placing pillow under head. Turn client onto side. (2) If client is in bed, turn client to side and raise side rails.

Position protects client from traumatic injury, especially head injury.

b. Stay with client.

c. Clear surrounding area of furniture.

Ensures emergency response staff can access client.

d. Keep client in side-lying position, supporting head flexed slightly forward (see illustration).

Position prevents tongue from blocking airway and promotes drainage of secretions, reducing risk of aspiration.

e. Do not restrain. Loosen restrictive clothing/gown.

Prevents musculoskeletal injury and airway obstruction.

f. Do not force any objects into client's mouth, such as fingers, medicine, tongue depressor, or airway when teeth are clenched.

Prevents injury to mouth and to nurse's hands.

g. Maintain client's airway, suction as needed, and provide oxygen if ordered. *Use oral airway only if easy access to oral cavity is possible.*

Prevents hypoxia during seizure activity.

h. Observe sequence and timing of seizure activity. Note type of seizure activity (tonic, clonic, staring, blinking), whether more than one type of seizure occurs, sequence of seizure progression, level of consciousness, nature of breathing, presence of incontinence.

Assists in accurate documentation, diagnosis, and eventual treatment of seizure.

i. Provide client privacy if possible. Have staff control flow of visitors in area.

Embarrassment is common after a seizure.

5 Status epilepticus is a medical emergency; call physician and response team immediately.

Airway occlusion and aspiration are potential complications of this medical emergency.

a. 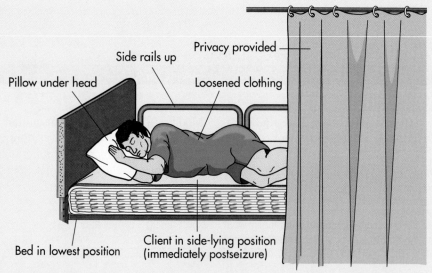 Insert an oral airway (see Chapter 35) when jaw is relaxed between seizure activity. Hold airway with curved side up, insert downward until airway reaches back of throat, then rotate downward and follow natural curve of tongue.

NURSE ALERT Do not place fingers in client's mouth. Client may accidentally bite nurse's fingers during seizure. Do not force airway into client's mouth.

Side rails up

Privacy provided

Pillow under head

Loosened clothing

Bed in lowest position

Client in side-lying position (immediately postseizure)

STEP 4d. Position of client following seizure and when on seizure precautions.

STEPS	RATIONALE
b. Access oxygen and suction equipment, keeping airway patent.	Intensive monitoring and treatment are required for this medical emergency.
c. Prepare for IV insertion, if saline lock or catheter not in place. Client usually will receive 0.9% sodium chloride.	
6 After seizure, assist client to position of comfort in bed with side rails up and bed in lowest position.	Provides for continued safety.
7 Explain what happened, and provide a quiet, nonstimulating environment. Client may be confused and experiencing postictal drowsiness. Foster an atmosphere of acceptance and give time for client to express feelings.	Clients who accept the reality of a disease and integrate this into their own self-concept have higher levels of self-esteem.
8 Pad side rails and headboard if indicated.	Reduces risk for traumatic injury from future seizures. Do not use pillows to pad side rails as they pose a suffocation risk.
9 See Completion Protocol (inside front cover).	

EVALUATION

1 Examine client to determine presence of any traumatic injuries resulting from seizure.

2 Evaluate airway and oxygenation status, mental status, and orientation after seizure.

3 Ask client to verbalize feelings after the seizure.

Unexpected Outcomes and Related Interventions

1 Client suffers traumatic injury.

a. Continue to protect client from further injury.

b. Notify the physician immediately.

c. Ensure environment is free of safety hazards.

2 Client verbalizes feelings of embarrassment and humiliation.

a. Offer support and allow client to verbalize feelings.

b. Encourage client and family to participate in decision making and planning care.

Recording and Reporting

• Record timing of seizure activity and sequence of events.

• Record presence of aura (if any), level of consciousness, posture, color, movements of extremities, incontinence, and client's status (physical and emotional) immediately following seizure.

• Report to physician immediately as seizure begins. Status epilepticus is an emergency.

Sample Documentation

1000 Observed client sitting in chair in room. Cry heard; client observed sliding to floor, not responding to verbal stimuli. Client assisted to floor with head supported. Pillow placed under head. Tonic and clonic movements of all four extremities noted, lasting 2 minutes. Color remained good; respiratory pattern slightly irregular. No incontinence noted. At conclusion of tonic and clonic movements, client slept for 20 minutes; respirations 16 per minute and regular.

1020 Client awake and alert. Requested nurse describe sequence of events. Stated that this was his "usual type of seizure."

Special Considerations
Pediatric Considerations

• Teach parents what to observe for in seizures, because many times they are present at onset.

• Children with severe atonic seizures may be encouraged to wear helmets.

Geriatric Considerations

• Older adults may have symptoms that block the recognition of a seizure disorder such as confusion lasting several days, unusual behaviors, or receptive and expressive language problems (Lannon, 1995).

• Older adults metabolize anticonvulsants more slowly; therefore drugs accumulate and cause toxicity. Monitor therapeutic blood levels of drugs closely.

• Do not try to remove dentures during a seizure. If they loosen, tilt head slightly forward and remove after seizure.

Home Care Considerations

• Discuss with family precipitating factors and care of the client experiencing a seizure.

• Unless seizure activity is well controlled, instruct client to not take tub baths or engage in activities such as swimming unless a knowledgeable family member is present. Driving may also be restricted until seizures are controlled for at least 1 year.

NCLEX® Style Questions

1 You enter the nurses' lounge and find a fire in the waste can. The receptacle is filled with paper and plastic cups. Which of the following types of fire extinguishers would you use to extinguish this type of fire?
1. Type A
2. Type B
3. Type C
4. Type ABC

2 When a client has a wrist restraint in place, the restraint should be removed for assessment of the client's extremity at least every:
1. 1 hour
2. 2 hours
3. 4 to 6 hours
4. Shift

3 Place the following steps for applying a wrist restraint in the correct order:
1. Insert two fingers under restraint to check for tightness.
2. Adjust bed to proper height; lower side rail on side of client contact.
3. Perform ROM exercises on involved extremity.
4. Secure restraint with a quick-release tie.
5. If necessary, pad bony prominences where restraints will be placed.
6. Secure call light.
7. Apply the proper-size restraint.
8. Remove restraint at least every 2 hours.
9. Attach restraint straps to bed frame.

4 Mr. Kyle is a 72-year-old retired professor who has been hospitalized since yesterday for a fractured ankle that was surgically repaired. He has an IV infusing D5NS with 20 mEq KCl at 100 ml/hr. The doctors have been trying to treat his low potassium level. Mr. Kyle is also receiving an antihypertensive, diuretic, and antibiotic. His wife reports, "He seems confused at times and not sure where he is." You enter the client's room and find him trying to remove his IV by pulling at the dressing. He is alert but not sure of the date or year. He has been hospitalized in the past. Mr. Kyle's risk for falls includes which of the following:
1. Impaired memory
2. Previous hospitalization
3. Age
4. Four medications
5. Use of diuretic
6. Surgery

References for all chapters appear in Appendix D.

Medical Aseptic Techniques

4

MEDIA RESOURCES

- **evolve** http://evolve.elsevier.com/Elkin

- **View Video!** Video Clips

- Nursing Skills Online

Infection control is one of the nurse's most important responsibilities. Clients in all health care settings are at risk for acquiring infections because of lower resistance to infection, exposure within health care facilities to an increased number of and more types of disease-causing organisms, and the performance of invasive procedures. Infection-control practices reduce or eliminate sources and transmission of infection to protect clients and health care providers from disease. Knowledge of communicable disease, the chain of infection, and critical thinking associated with how and when to use infection-control practices cannot be overemphasized. The nurse's role is vital in the prevention and control of infection.

Nosocomial or health care–associated infections (HAIs) are those that develop as a result of a stay or visit in a health care facility and that were not present or incubating at the time of admission (Bobo, 1994). In hospitals alone, HAIs account for an estimated 2 million infections, 90,000 deaths, and $4.5 billion in excess health care costs annually (CDC, 2006a). Such infections are more likely to develop in persons with chronic illnesses or compromised immunity and in older adults who are poorly nourished. Invasive diagnostic procedures such as bronchoscopy or gastroscopy and treatment with broad-spectrum antibiotics have also been shown to increase the risk for such infection (Arnold and McDonald, 2005; Stricof, 2005). There are two types of HAIs: exogenous and endogenous. Exogenous infection comes from microorganisms outside the client, such as *Salmonella* and *Aspergillus* organisms, which do not exist as normal flora. Endogenous infection occurs when part of the client's flora becomes altered and overgrowth results (e.g., infection from staphylococci, enterococci, and yeasts). Such an infection occurs when clients receive broad-spectrum antibiotics that alter normal flora. The number of microorganisms (dose) needed to cause an HAI depends on the virulence of the organism, the client's susceptibility, and the body site affected. Nurses are responsible for teaching clients and their families about the source and transmission of infections, reason for susceptibility, and infection-control principles.

The mere presence of a pathogen does not mean that an infection will begin. Development of an infection occurs in a cyclical process. This is described as the chain of infection, which depends on the presence of six elements: (1) an infectious agent or pathogen, (2) a reservoir or source for pathogen growth, (3) a portal of exit from the reservoir, (4) a method or mode of transmission, (5) a portal of entrance into the host, and (6) a susceptible host. An infection develops if the chain remains intact (Figure 4-1). However, a nurse who uses infection-control practices can break an element of the chain so that infection is not transmitted (Table 4-1). For example, cleansing contaminated objects, changing soiled dressings, wearing gloves when handling blood or body fluids, and performing hand hygiene after glove removal are just a few ways to break the infection chain. Asepsis is defined as the absence of disease-producing (pathogenic) organisms that involves the purposeful prevention of transfer of microorganisms (DeCastro, 2002). The two types of aseptic technique a nurse practices are medical and surgical asepsis (see Chapter 5).

Medical asepsis, or clean technique, includes procedures used to reduce the number of and prevent the spread of microorganisms. Hand hygiene, barrier techniques (e.g., use of gloves and gown), and routine environmental cleaning are examples of medical asepsis. Surgical asepsis, or sterile technique, includes procedures used to eliminate all microorganisms from an area. Sterilization destroys all microorganisms and their spores (Rutala, 1996). Nurses in the operating room (OR), labor and delivery (L&D), and procedural areas practice sterile technique. Surgical aseptic techniques are more rigid than those performed under medical asepsis.

In 1996 the Centers for Disease Control and Prevention (CDC) published guidelines for the set of precautions known as *standard precautions* (Garner, 1996). Part of the rationale for the development of standard precautions is the fact that any client may be a source for infection. Most microorganisms causing infections or disease are in colonized body substances of clients, regardless of whether a culture confirmed an infection and a diagnosis was made.

Body substances such as feces, urine, mucus, and wound drainage can contain potentially infectious organisms.

The risk all clients have for carrying an infection thus requires health care workers to use standard precautions to prevent exposure. Fundamental to standard precautions is the use of barrier protection. Barrier protection includes the appropriate use of personal protective equipment (PPE) such as gloves, masks or respirators, eyewear, and gowns to protect from exposure to blood and body fluids.

Barrier protection protects the health care worker from the client's blood and body fluids and helps prevent the transfer of organisms to other clients, health care workers, and the environment. It is also an important technique for protecting those clients who are immunosuppressed (e.g., clients with cancer who are receiving chemotherapy). Some form of PPE is indicated for all clients who potentially have an infection that can be transmitted to others. Because of the increased attention to the prevention of certain diseases, such as hepatitis B, acquired immunodeficiency syndrome (AIDS), and tuberculosis (TB), the CDC (1988; 1994) and the Occupational Safety and Health Administration (OSHA) (1994; 2001) have stressed the importance of barrier protection.

As advocates, nurses help to ensure that all health care providers (e.g., respiratory therapists, physicians, other nurses) working with clients and support staff (e.g., housekeepers) maintain infection-control practices at all times. This applies also to family members. When a hospitalized client has an infection, the nurse decides on the optimal room placement to minimize the chances of infection spreading to other clients. In addition, two clients with "like" infections can be placed in the same room. This is called *cohorting*. The knowledgeable and judicious use of infection-control practices can make a difference as to whether a client recovers from an illness or develops serious or even fatal complications.

EVIDENCE IN PRACTICE

Hilburn J and others: Use of alcohol hand sanitizer as an infection control strategy in an acute care facility, *Am J Infect Control* 31(2):109-116, 2003.

Hand washing is still believed to be the most important and effective infection-control measure. However, compliance among health care workers was found to be unacceptably low. Deterrents to hand-washing compliance include the amount of time required for soap-and-water hand washing with heavy workloads, skin irritation and dryness from frequent hand washing, inconvenient access to sinks, and inadequate knowledge of hand-hygiene protocols (CDC, 2002). An alternative to hand washing shown to improve asepsis compliance is alcohol hand rubs. Hilburn and others (2003) conducted a study on an acute care orthopedic unit for 16 months. Baseline data on infection rates were collected for 6 months, and then an alcohol gel hand sanitizer was made available for use by caregivers, clients, and visitors on the unit. The sanitizer was placed on wall-mounted dispensers outside client rooms,

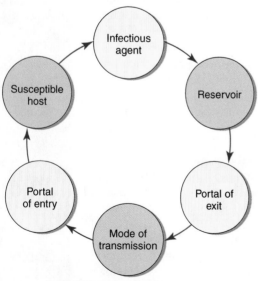

FIGURE 4-1 Chain of infection.

TABLE 4-1 Breaking the Chain of Infection

ELEMENT OF INFECTION CHAIN	MEDICAL ASEPTIC PRACTICES
1. Infectious agent (pathogenic organism capable of causing disease)	*Cleanse contaminated objects:* Perform cleaning, disinfection, and sterilization.
2. Reservoir (site or source of microorganism growth)	*Control sources of body fluids and drainage:* Perform hand hygiene. Bathe client with soap and water. Change soiled dressings. Dispose of soiled tissues, dressings, or linen in moisture-resistant bags. Place syringes, uncapped hypodermic needles, and intravenous (IV) needles in designated puncture-proof containers. Keep table surfaces clean and dry. Do not leave bottled solutions open for prolonged periods. Keep solutions tightly capped. Keep surgical wound drainage tubes and collection bags patent. Empty and dispose of drainage suction bottles according to agency policy.
3. Portal of exit (means by which microorganisms leave a site)	*Respiratory:* Avoid talking, sneezing, or coughing directly over wound or sterile dressing field. Cover nose and mouth when sneezing or coughing. Wear mask if suffering from respiratory tract infection. *Urine, feces, emesis, and blood:* Wear clean gloves when handling blood and body fluids. Wear gowns and eyewear if there is a chance of splashing fluids. Handle all laboratory specimens as if infectious.
4. Transmission (means of spread)	*Reduce microorganism spread:* Perform hand hygiene. Use personal set of care items for each client. Avoid shaking bed linen or clothes; dust with damp cloth. Avoid contact of soiled item with uniform. Discard any item that touches the floor. Follow standard precautions or select transmission-based isolation precautions.
5. Portal of entry (site through which microorganism enters a host)	*Skin and mucosa:* Maintain skin and mucous membrane integrity; lubricate skin; offer frequent hygiene; turn and position. Cover wounds as needed. Clean wound sites thoroughly. Dispose of used needles in puncture-proof container. *Urinary:* Keep all drainage systems closed and intact, maintaining downward flow.
6. Host (client)	*Reduce susceptibility to infection:* Provide adequate nutrition. Ensure adequate rest. Promote body defenses against infection. Provide immunization.

in bottles on medication and treatment carts, and in dispensers at the nurses' stations. Nurses were also given 4-oz bottles to carry in their pockets. The unit experienced a 36.1% decline in infection rates during the 10-month period when the hand sanitizer was used. Alcohol hand sanitizers improve compliance with hand hygiene because they are convenient, quick to use, and gentle on the skin.

NURSING DIAGNOSES

Risk for infection relates to clients who have specific risk factors that increase their potential for acquiring an infection, such as pathological conditions (immunosuppression, chronic disease, or obesity), treatments (surgery, invasive procedures, or steroids), situational factors (inadequate immunizations, or lack of hand washing by caregiver), or maturation (the very young and very old). A diagnosis of **deficient knowledge** regarding infection prevention is appropriate when clients are in need of information about infection-control measures. Clients can experience **anxiety, fear,** or a feeling of **powerlessness** when restricted to their rooms for isolation precautions or when they are required to use protective barriers. **Social isolation** may also be appropriate when use of protective barriers and environmental restrictions are required.

SKILL 4.1   Hand Hygiene

• Nursing Skills Online: Infection Control, Lesson 2

Hand hygiene is a general term that applies to hand washing, antiseptic hand wash, antiseptic hand rub, or surgical hand antisepsis. Hand washing refers to washing hands thoroughly with plain soap and water. An antiseptic hand wash is defined as washing hands with water and soap containing an antiseptic agent. The use of antimicrobial soap (antiseptic) is encouraged in health care settings. Antimicrobials effectively reduce bacterial counts on the hands and often have residual antimicrobial effects for several hours. There are a number of effective antimicrobial soaps that contain alcohols, chlorhexidine gluconate (CHG), triclosan, and iodophors. Certain antimicrobial soaps can irritate the skin, and their use must be weighed against the potential for skin irritation. Using an antiseptic hand rub means to apply an antiseptic alcohol-based waterless product to all surfaces of the hands to reduce the number of microorganisms present. These alcohol-based foams or gels contain cosmetic emollients to prevent skin dryness. Surgical hand antisepsis is an antiseptic hand wash or antiseptic hand rub performed preoperatively by surgical personnel (see Chapter 19). Antiseptic detergent preparations often have persistent antimicrobial activity after use (CDC, 2002).

Contaminated hands cause the transmission of infection. For example, a nurse caring for a client who has excessive pulmonary secretions assists the client in expectorating mucus and disposes of the tissues in a bedside trash container. The client's roommate asks the nurse to open a carton of milk on the meal tray. The nurse then leaves the room to prepare a dose of medication due in 5 minutes. If the nurse does not perform hand hygiene before each of these actions, organisms from the first client's mucus could easily transfer to the roommate's food and to the medication container. Health care workers function in a fast-paced environment when good client care demands attention to detail. With an increased workload, frequent interruptions in care activity, and multiple nursing tasks, compliance with hand hygiene can be a challenge. *Hand hygiene is not an option.* It is a critical responsibility of all health care workers.

The CDC Healthcare Infection Control Practices Advisory Committee (HICPAC) released new guidelines for hand hygiene in health care settings (CDC, 2002). The development of alcohol-based hand antiseptics for reducing bacterial counts on the hands offers an alternative to traditional hand washing that is highly effective (Hilburn and others, 2003; Girou and others, 2002). Hand hygiene effectively reduces HAIs when performed correctly. The decision to perform hand hygiene depends on four factors: (1) the intensity or degree of contact with clients or contaminated objects, (2) the amount of contamination that may occur with the contact, (3) the client's or health care worker's susceptibility to infection, and (4) the procedure or activity to be performed (Larson, 2000). The CDC recommends the following guidelines for hand hygiene:

1 When hands are visibly dirty or contaminated with proteinaceous material or are visibly soiled with blood or other body fluids, wash hands with either plain soap and water or an antimicrobial soap and water. The recommended duration for lathering hands is *at least 15 seconds* and preferably 30 seconds.
2 Wash hands with soap and water before and after eating.
3 Wash hands with soap and water after using the restroom.
4 Wash hands if exposed to spore-forming organisms such as *Clostridium difficile* or *Bacillus anthracis*.
5 If hands are not visibly soiled, use an alcohol-based hand rub for routinely decontaminating the hands in all of the following clinical situations:
a. Before having direct contact with clients.
b. Before applying sterile gloves.
c. Before inserting indwelling urinary catheters, peripheral vascular catheters, or other invasive devices that do not require a surgical procedure.
d. After contact with a client's intact skin (e.g., after taking a pulse or blood pressure, after lifting a client).
e. After contact with body fluids or excretions, mucous membranes, nonintact skin, and wound dressings *if hands are not visibly soiled*.
f. When moving from a contaminated body site to a clean body site during client care.
g. After contact with inanimate objects (e.g., medical equipment) in the immediate vicinity of the client.
h. After removing gloves.

Note that an antiseptic hand wash may be performed in all situations when an alcohol-based hand rub is indicated.

ASSESSMENT

1 Inspect surface of hands for breaks or cuts in skin or cuticles. Cover any skin lesions with a dressing before providing client care. If lesions are too large to cover, you may be restricted from direct client care. *Rationale: Open cuts or wounds can harbor high concentrations of microorganisms. Agency policy often prevents nurses from caring for high-risk clients if open lesions are present on hands.*
2 Inspect hands for visible soiling. *Rationale: Visible soiling requires hand washing with soap and water.*
3 Note condition of nails. Avoid artificial nails, extenders, and long or unkempt nails. Natural nail tips should be less than ¼ inch long. Do not wear artificial nails or extenders when caring for high-risk clients (e.g., intensive care unit [ICU], OR). See agency policy. *Rationale: Subungual areas of hand harbor high concentrations of bacteria. Long nails and chipped or old polish increase number of bacteria re-*

siding on nails, requiring more vigorous hand hygiene. Artificial nails increase the microbial load on hands (CDC, 2002).

4 Consider the type of nursing activity being performed. *Rationale: Determines hand hygiene technique to use.*

PLANNING

Expected Outcomes focus on preventing the transmission of infection.

1 Hands and areas under fingernails are clean and free of debris.

Delegation Considerations

All health care providers perform meticulous hand hygiene. If you observe other nurses, physicians, or therapists incor-rectly performing hand hygiene, reinforce the importance of the technique and the correct procedural steps.

Equipment
Hand Washing
- Easy-to-reach sink with warm running water
- Antimicrobial soap
- Paper towels or air dryer
- Clean orangewood stick (optional)

Antiseptic Hand Rub
- Alcohol-based waterless antiseptic containing emollient

IMPLEMENTATION *for Hand Hygiene*

STEPS	RATIONALE
1 Push wristwatch and long uniform sleeves above wrists. Avoid wearing rings; however, there is no definitive evidence that rings increase microbial load on the hands (CDC, 2002).	Provides complete access to fingers, hands, and wrists. There have been studies showing that skin underneath rings can be more heavily colonized than comparable areas of skin on fingers without rings. Gram-negative bacilli and *Staphylococcus aureus* are commonly found under rings (Boyce and Pittet, 2001).
2 Antiseptic hand rub:	
a. Dispense ample amount of product into palm of one hand (see illustration).	Use enough product to thoroughly cover hands.
b. Rub hands together, covering all surfaces of hands and fingers with antiseptic (see illustration).	Provides enough time for antimicrobial solution to work.
c. Rub hands together until the alcohol is dry. Allow hands to completely dry before applying gloves.	Removes transient organisms. Ensures complete antimicrobial action.
3 Hand washing using antiseptic soap:	
a. Be sure fingernails are short, filed, and smooth.	Many microorganisms on hands come from the subungual region (beneath the fingernails).

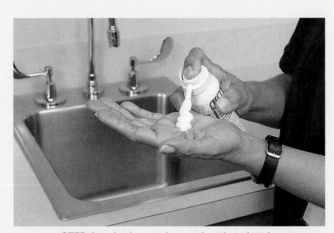

STEP 2a. Apply waterless antiseptic to hands.

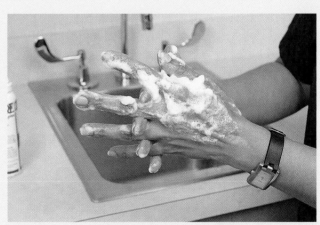

STEP 2b. Rub hands thoroughly.

STEPS	RATIONALE
b. Stand in front of sink, keeping hands and uniform away from sink surface. (If hands touch sink during hand washing, repeat steps.)	Inside of sink is a contaminated area. Reaching over sink increases risk of touching edge, which is contaminated.
c. Turn on water. Turn faucet on or push knee pedals laterally to regulate flow and temperature.	Knee pedals within the OR and treatment areas are preferred to prevent hand contact with faucet. Faucet handles have been found to likely be contaminated with organic debris and microorganisms (Griffith and others, 2003).
d. Avoid splashing water against uniform.	Microorganisms travel and grow in moisture.
e. Regulate flow of water so that temperature is warm.	
f. Wet hands and wrists thoroughly under running water. Keep hands and forearms lower than elbows during washing.	Hands are the most contaminated parts to be washed. Water flows from least to most contaminated area, rinsing microorganisms into sink.
g. Apply 3 to 5 ml of antiseptic soap (see product recommendation) and rub hands together vigorously, lathering thoroughly (see illustration). Soap granules and leaflet preparations may be used instead.	Necessary to ensure that all surfaces of hands and fingers are covered and cleansed.

> **NURSE ALERT** The decision whether to use an antiseptic or not is dependent on the procedure you will perform and the client's immune status. However, acute care hospitals usually have only antiseptic soap.

h. Perform hand hygiene using plenty of lather and friction *for at least 15 seconds.* Interlace fingers and rub palms and backs of hands with circular motion at least 5 times each. Keep fingertips down to facilitate removal of microorganisms.	Soap cleanses by emulsifying fat and oil and lowering surface tension. Friction and rubbing mechanically loosen and remove dirt and transient bacteria. Interlacing fingers and thumbs ensures that you cleanse all surfaces. Adequate time is needed to expose skin surfaces to antimicrobial agent.
i. Areas underlying fingernails are often soiled. Clean with fingernails of other hand and additional soap or clean with an orangewood stick *(optional).*	Area under nails can be highly contaminated, which increases risk for transmission of infection from nurse to client.

> **NURSE ALERT** Do not tear or cut skin under or around nail.

j. Rinse hands and wrists thoroughly, keeping hands down and elbows up (see illustration).	Rinsing mechanically washes away dirt and microorganisms.

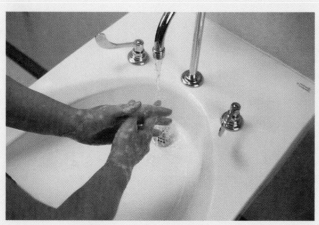

STEP 3g. Lathering hands thoroughly.

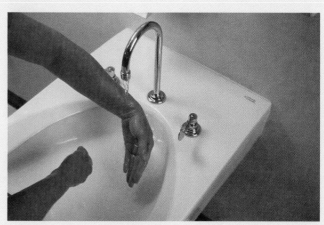

STEP 3j. Rinsing hands.

STEPS	RATIONALE
k. Dry hands thoroughly from fingers to wrists and forearms with paper towel or warm air dryer.	Drying from cleanest (fingertips) to least clean (forearms) area avoids contamination. Drying prevents chapping and roughened skin.

> **NURSE ALERT** Paper towels should dispense cleanly without hand or paper-towel contact with other surfaces. Reaching into the dispenser cabinet and touching the paper slot increases the risk of contamination (Harrison and others, 2003).

STEPS	RATIONALE
l. If used, discard paper towel in proper container.	Prevents transfer of microorganisms.
m. Use clean dry paper towel to turn off hand faucet. Avoiding touching handles with hands (see illustration). Turn off water with knee pedals (if applicable).	Prevents transfer of pathogens from faucet to hands. Faucet handles have been found to likely be contaminated with organic debris and microorganisms (Griffith and others, 2003).
n. If hands are dry or chapped at end of shift, use a small amount of lotion or barrier cream dispensed from an individual-use container.	There is a risk of organism growth in lotion, so it should not be applied during client care activities. Large, refillable containers of lotion have been associated with nosocomial or HAIs.

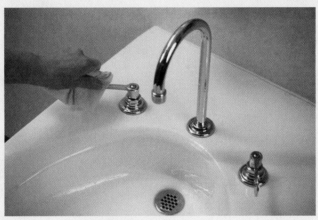

STEP 3m. Turning off faucet.

EVALUATION

1 Inspect surfaces of hands for obvious signs of soil or other contaminants.

2 Inspect hands for dermatitis or cracked skin.

Unexpected Outcomes and Related Interventions

1 Hands or areas under fingernails remain soiled.

a. Repeat hand hygiene.

2 Repeated use of soaps or antiseptics cause dermatitis or cracked skin.

a. Rinse and dry hands thoroughly; avoid excessive amounts of soap and antiseptic; try various products; use hand lotions or barrier creams. Use alcohol-based hand antiseptic rub whenever hands are not visibly soiled.

Recording and Reporting

• It is unnecessary to document hand washing.

• Report dermatitis, psoriasis, and cuts to agency's employee health and/or infection-control department.

PROCEDURAL GUIDELINE 4-1

Using Clean Gloves

- Nursing Skills Online: Infection Control, Lessons 1 and 2

Standard precautions require nurses to wear clean gloves before coming in contact with mucous membranes, nonintact skin, blood, body fluids, or other infectious material. Nurses wear gloves routinely when performing a variety of procedures (e.g., nasogastric tube insertion, enema administration, perineal hygiene, removal of soiled dressings). In addition, nurses with cuts; abrasions; or oozing, draining wounds on the hands must wear gloves (Larson, 1996). Always inspect gloves before use for cuts, tears, or holes. Gloves found with any of these deficiencies will not provide proper barrier protection. Clean gloves are easy to apply. Remove gloves and perform hand hygiene after caring for a client. Also, change gloves during client care if moving from a contaminated site to a clean body site. (For example, after administering an enema, dispose of gloves and perform hand hygiene before providing a bed bath.)

Latex allergies are occurring with more frequency in the health care field, not only in health care workers but also in clients. For this reason, latex-free gloves are more commonly used in health care settings Chapter 5 describes in detail the approach for assessing clients for latex allergies. If redness, inflammation, extreme dryness, or vesicles appear on the hands, an evaluation by a physician is indicated. When latex gloves are not available, synthetic vinyl gloves offer an excellent alternative.

Before performing a procedure that requires gloves, ask the client about latex allergies. The Food and Drug Administration (FDA) requires all clients to be asked about latex and requires caregivers to document the presence of a latex allergy. A latex allergy can bring on respiratory arrest, which is a life-threatening event. The nurse cannot use any latex when caring for clients with latex allergies.

Hand lotion is most beneficial just after washing and lightly drying the hands. Avoid using lotions that contain mineral oil or petroleum as their main ingredients, because these impair the integrity of latex and the effectiveness of gloves. Use the facility-provided lotion at the end of a work shift. Lotion is a culture media for organisms. Do not share a lotion bottle or buy large economy jugs to refill a small portable container.

Using Clean Gloves
Delegation Considerations
All health care providers use clean gloves. If you observe caregivers failing to use gloves when necessary, reinforce the importance of the procedure.

Equipment
- 1 pair of clean gloves (latex or latex-free)

Procedural Steps
1 **Glove Application:**
a. Inspect surface of hands for breaks or cuts in skin or cuticles. Cover any skin lesions with a dressing before providing client care. If lesions are too large to cover, you may be restricted from direct client care.
b. Inspect skin for redness, inflammation, extreme dryness, or vesicles that may indicate latex allergy.
c. Apply gloves (no special technique required). If wearing an isolation gown, pull cuffs of gloves over cuffs of gown. If not wearing a gown, pull up the gloves to cover the wrist (see illustration).
d. Interlink fingers to adjust glove fit.

2 **Glove Removal:**
a. Remove first glove by grasping outer surface of lower cuff, taking care to touch only glove to glove (see illustration).
b. Pull glove inside out over hand, taking care to touch only inside of glove with hand.
c. Grasp soiled glove in remaining gloved hand.
d. With ungloved hand, tuck finger inside cuff of remaining glove and pull it off, inside out, enclosing both soiled gloves. Discard in container (see illustration).
3 Perform hand hygiene.

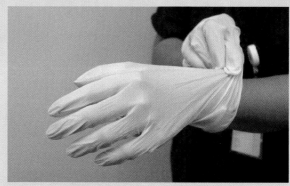

STEP 1c. Pull glove cuff up over wrist.

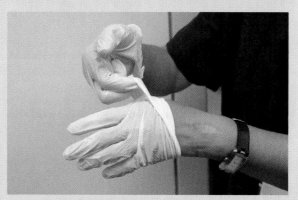

STEP 2a. Remove first glove.

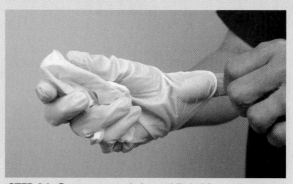

STEP 2d. Remove second glove while holding soiled glove.

SKILL 4.2   Caring for Clients Under Isolation Precautions

Nurses must follow standard precautions in the care of all clients. Table 4-2 describes CDC standard precautions, the primary strategies for reducing the risk of transmission of blood-borne and other pathogens. In 2004, the CDC added respiratory hygiene/cough etiquette to standard precautions as a measure to contain respiratory secretions in those clients with signs and symptoms. A health care agency must provide clients with tissues and no-touch containers for tissue disposal and provide dispensers of alcohol-based hand rub and masks (Siegel, 2005). Adherence to standard precautions has been associated with decreased skin and mucous membrane exposures and percutaneous injuries (e.g., needlestick injuries) (McCoy and others, 2001).

In cases in which clients are infected or colonized with specific microorganisms, the CDC recommends isolation precautions in addition to standard precautions (HICPAC,

1996). HICPAC published revised guidelines for isolation precautions in 1996. Health care facilities modify these guidelines, according to need and as dictated by state or local regulations. Isolation precautions are based on the assumption that microorganisms transmit by several routes; the five main routes are contact, droplet, air, common vehicle, and vector. The guidelines recommend the use of barrier precautions to interrupt the mode of transmission (see Procedural Guideline 4-1). Isolation or barrier precautions prescribe the specific use of PPE when a client is infected or colonized with specific organisms.

The CDC has also published guidelines for prevention of transmission of certain drug-resistant organisms (Garner, 1996). These guidelines, primarily for microorganisms such as vancomycin-resistant enterococci (VRE), vancomycin-resistant S. *aureus* (VRSA), and methicillin-resistant

---

TABLE 4-2   Centers for Disease Control and Prevention Isolation Guidelines

Standard Precautions (Tier One)

Standard precautions apply to blood, all body fluids, secretions, excretions (except sweat), nonintact skin, and mucous membranes.

Hand hygiene is performed between client contacts; after contact with blood, body fluids, secretions, and excretions and after contact with equipment or articles contaminated by them; and immediately after gloves are removed.

Gloves are worn when touching blood, body fluids, secretions, excretions, nonintact skin, mucous membranes, or contaminated items. Gloves should be removed and hand hygiene performed between client care encounters.

Masks, eye protection, or face shields are worn if client care activities generate splashes or sprays of blood or body fluids.

Gowns are worn if soiling of clothing is likely from blood or body fluids. Perform hand hygiene after removing gown.

Client care equipment is properly cleaned and reprocessed, and single-use items are discarded.

Contaminated linen is placed in leak-proof bag and handled so as to prevent skin and mucous membrane exposure.

All sharp instruments and needles are discarded in a puncture-resistant container (OSHA, 2001). Health care institutions should make available needleless devices. Any needles should be disposed of uncapped, or a mechanical device should be used for recapping.

A private room is unnecessary unless the client's hygiene is unacceptable. Check with an infection-control professional.

Respiratory hygiene/cough etiquette: Have clients cover the nose/mouth when coughing or sneezing; use tissues to contain respiratory secretions and dispose in nearest waste container; perform hand hygiene after contacting respiratory secretions and contaminated objects/materials; contain respiratory secretions with procedure or surgical mask; sit at least 3 feet away from others if coughing.

Transmission-Based Precautions (Tier Two)

CATEGORY	DISEASE	BARRIER PROTECTION
Airborne precautions	Droplet nuclei smaller than 5 μm; measles; chickenpox (varicella); disseminated varicella zoster; pulmonary or laryngeal TB	Private room; negative-pressure airflow of at least 6 to 12 exchanges per hour; mask or respiratory protection device (Siegel, 2005)
Droplet precautions	Droplets larger than 5 μm; diphtheria (pharyngeal); rubella; streptococcal pharyngitis, pneumonia, or scarlet fever in infants and young children; pertussis; mumps; mycoplasm pneumonia; meningococcal pneumonia or sepsis; pneumonic plague	Private room or cohort clients; mask
Contact precautions	Direct client or environmental contact; colonization or infection with multidrug-resistant organism; respiratory syncytial virus (RSV); shigella and other enteric pathogens; major wound infections; herpes simplex; scabies, varicella zoster (disseminated)	Private room or cohort clients; gloves, gowns
Protective environment	Allogeneic hematopoietic stem cell transplants	Private room; positive airflow with 12 or more air exchanges per hour; gloves, gowns

Modified from Garner JS: Guidelines for isolation precautions in hospitals, *Am J Infect Control* 24:24, 1996; and Siegel J: Isolation systems. In Carrico R, editor: *APIC text of infection control and epidemiology,* Washington, DC, 2005, Association for Professionals in Infection Control and Epidemiology.

S. aureus (MRSA), are stricter than other published recommendations.

The three types of transmission-based precautions may be combined for diseases that have multiple routes of transmission. When used singularly or in combination, they are to be used in addition to standard precautions when required by the specific infection. When a client requires isolation, determine the reason and the mode of transmission. Evaluate the tasks to be performed to identify the barrier equipment needed. For example, a client in respiratory isolation for measles has an organism that can be carried airborne. A mask is necessary when entering the room for any reason. To hold and feed an infant, it would be appropriate to wear both a mask and gown, to protect clothing from secretions from the infant's nose or mouth. It would be appropriate to add gloves to assist in intubating the infant. When a client is in contact isolation for a resistant organism in sputum and has been coughing, wear a gown, gloves, and mask within 3 feet of the client. It is acceptable to enter the room without any protective equipment to initially meet the client.

One important aspect of care for a client in isolation is appropriate compliance with hand hygiene and the changing of gloves between exposures to body sites and client equipment. Inadequate glove changes and hand hygiene between exposures to body sites can potentially lead to contamination of previously uncolonized sites (Kim and others, 2003). For example, do not allow microorganisms in a client's respiratory secretions to spread to the hub of a central line catheter on your gloved hands. Change gloves after the client expectorates, perform hand hygiene, and reapply gloves in such a situation. Noncompliance with glove changing and hand hygiene increases the risk of nosocomial or HAIs. Remember the guidelines for hand hygiene (see Skill 4.1) and apply them whenever you care for a client in isolation.

Taking care of a client requires understanding the chain of infection and how organisms travel to a receptive host. The most common mode of transmission is the hands. *Wash or decontaminate hands after every client contact*, or more often if exposed to body substances, even when gloves have been worn. Be aware of unconscious actions such as rubbing the eyes or nose, picking teeth, or biting fingernails. For respiratory or droplet-spread organisms, assume a safe zone beyond 3 to 5 feet from a client, unless the client is on airborne precautions. It is appropriate to walk into the room of a client in isolation, without barrier equipment, to introduce yourself and be seen without your face covered. This is a good opportunity to inform the client why it is necessary to wear masks, gowns, or gloves while performing certain tasks.

When a client requires isolation in a private room, remember that loneliness can easily develop. Isolation disrupts normal social relationships with visitors and caregivers. A client who suffers from an infectious disease may also experience self-concept or body image changes. When a client from another culture requires isolation, extra caution must be used to be sure the client and family understand the purpose of isolation. For example, the isolation of a loved one is considered disrespectful and uncaring in many collectivistic cultures (Hispanics, Africans, and Asians) (Mashaba, 2002). Unless the nurse acts to minimize the client's feelings of psychological and physical isolation, the client's emotional state can interfere with recovery.

ASSESSMENT

1 Assess client's medical history and possible indications for isolation (e.g., purulent productive cough, major draining wound). Review the precautions necessary for the specific isolation system.
2 Review laboratory test results (e.g., wound culture, acid-fast bacillus [AFB] smears, changes in white blood cell [WBC] count). *Rationale: Reveals type of organism infecting a client.*
3 Consider types of care measures to be performed while in client's room. *Rationale: Allows nurse to organize all equipment needed in room.*
4 Determine from nursing care plan, nursing colleagues, or family members the client's emotional state and reaction to isolation. Also assess client's understanding of purpose of isolation.
5 Assess whether the client has a known latex allergy. If an allergy is present, use latex-free gloves and refer to agency policy and resources available to provide full latex-free care. *Rationale: Protects client from serious allergic response.*

PLANNING

Expected Outcomes focus on preventing transmission of infection to nurse and other clients and improving client's knowledge of the purpose of isolation.
1 Client and/or family verbalizes purpose of isolation and treatment plan.
2 Infection does not develop in neighboring clients.

Delegation Considerations
Assessment of a client's status and type of care measures to perform cannot be delegated. Basic care procedures performed under isolation can be delegated. The nurse directs personnel by:
- Clarifying for personnel the type of isolation system implemented.
- Instructing personnel on the type of clinical changes to report.

Equipment
- Clean gloves
- Mask
- Eyewear, protective goggles or glasses, face shield

- Isolation gown
- Disinfectant swab (e.g., isopropyl alcohol with or without chlorhexidine)
- Medication

- Hygiene items
- Linen bag
- Sharps container
- Biohazard waste bag

IMPLEMENTATION *for Caring for Clients Under Isolation Precautions*

STEPS	RATIONALE
1 See Standard Protocol (inside front cover).	
2 Prepare all equipment to be taken into client's room. In many cases dedicated equipment, such as stethoscopes, blood pressure equipment, and thermometers, should remain in the room until client is discharged. If client is infected or colonized with resistant organism (e.g., VRE, MRSA), equipment remains in room and is thoroughly disinfected prior to removal from room (see agency policy).	The CDC recommends use of dedicated noncritical client care equipment (Garner, 1996).
3 Enter the client's room, and remain by the door. Introduce yourself, and explain the care you are to provide and the purpose of isolation precautions before applying PPE.	Allows client to sense the nurse's caring without exposing nurse to risk of infection transmission.
4 Prepare for entrance into isolation room.	
a. Apply gown, being sure it covers all outer garments; pull sleeves down to wrist. Tie securely at neck and waist.	Prevents transmission of infection when client has excessive drainage or discharge. Also reduces contamination of clothing from splashes or splatters.
b. Apply either surgical mask or respirator around mouth and nose (type depends on type of organism and facility policy). Tie or attach a mask securely to make sure it fits snugly.	Prevents exposure to airborne microorganisms or exposure to microorganisms from splashing of fluids.
c. Apply eyewear or goggles snugly around face and eyes (when needed) (see illustration).	Protects nurse from exposure to microorganisms that may occur during splashing of contaminated fluids.

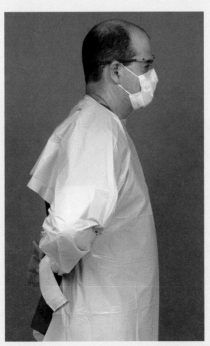

STEP 4c. Nurse with protective gown, mask, and goggles.

STEPS	RATIONALE

d. 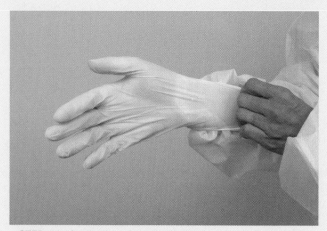 **Apply clean gloves.** (NOTE: Unpowdered latex-free gloves must be worn if client or health care worker has a latex allergy.) If you wear gloves with the gown, bring glove cuffs over edge of gown sleeves (see illustration).

Gloves are applied last so that they can be placed over the cuffs of the gown.

> **COMMUNICATION TIP** Reassure clients and families that isolation is used for diseases that are easily spread. It protects other clients in the facility from exposure to the microorganism. Be positive, and focus on what they can do (e.g., receive/send mail, watch TV, use the phone, receive visitors). Assure them that the goal is for isolation to be as short and pleasant as possible.

5 Enter client's room. Arrange supplies and equipment. (If equipment will be removed from room for reuse, place on clean paper towel.)

Minimizes contamination of care items.

6 Assess vital signs.
a. Follow routine procedures.
b. Avoid contact of stethoscope or blood pressure cuff with infective material. Wipe off with disinfectant after use.

If stethoscope is used later on other clients, there is a risk of transmitting infection unless it is disinfected.

c. If stethoscope is to be reused, clean diaphragm or bell and ear tips with disinfectant swab. Set aside on clean surface.

Cleaning with disinfectant before reuse reduces bacterial colonies (Guinto and others, 2002). Earpieces of stethoscopes have been found to be easily contaminated with *S. aureus*.

d. Use an individual electronic or disposable thermometer.

Prevents cross contamination.

> **NURSE ALERT** If disposable thermometer reveals presence of a fever, assess for other signs and symptoms and then confirm with an electronic thermometer (Potter and others, 2003).

7 Administer medications (see Chapters 16 and 17).
a. Give oral medication in wrapper or cup.
b. Dispose of wrapper or cup in plastic-lined container.
c. Administer injection, being sure to wear gloves.

Reduces risk of exposure to blood.

d. Discard needleless syringe or safety sheathed needle into designated sharps container (see illustration).

Needleless devices should be used to reduce the risk of needle sticks and sharps injuries to health care workers (OSHA, 2001).

> **NURSE ALERT** Hepatitis B virus (HBV) and hepatitis C virus (HCV) are the most prevalent blood-borne pathogens. Spread occurs mainly through direct parenteral or percutaneous exposure to tainted blood (Sattar and others, 2001).

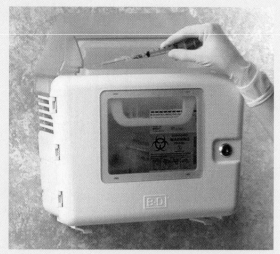

STEP 4d. Application of clean glove over edge of gown sleeve.

STEP 7d. Dispose of needle and syringe in sharps receptacle. *(Courtesy and copyright Becton, Dickinson and Company.)*

STEPS	RATIONALE

8 Administer hygiene, encouraging client to discuss questions or concerns about isolation.

COMMUNICATION TIP This is an excellent time to provide informal teaching.

a. Avoid allowing isolation gown to become wet. Carry washbasin outward away from gown; avoid leaning against wet tabletop.

Moisture allows organisms to travel through gown to uniform.

b. Remove linen from bed; avoid contact with isolation gown. Place in leak-proof linen bag.

Linen soiled by client's body fluids is handled so as to prevent contact with clean gown.

c. Provide clean bed linen and set of towels.

d. Change gloves and perform hand hygiene if hands become excessively soiled and further care is necessary.

9 Collect specimens (see Chapter 13).

a. Place specimen container on clean paper towel in client's bathroom, and follow procedure for collecting specimen of body fluids.

Container will be taken out of client's room, thus outer surface must not be contaminated.

b. Transfer specimen to container without soiling outside of container. After gloves are removed, place container in plastic bag, complete and apply biohazard label to outside of bag, and transport to laboratory. Perform hand hygiene and reglove if further procedures are to be performed.

10 Dispose of linen, trash, and disposable items.

Linen or refuse should be totally contained to prevent exposure of personnel to infective material.

a. Use sturdy moisture-impervious single bags to contain soiled articles. Use double bag if outer bag is torn or contaminated.

Heavy soiling can cause outer side of first bag to become contaminated.

b. Tie bags securely at top in knot.

11 Remove all reusable pieces of equipment. Clean any contaminated surfaces with disinfectant (see agency policy).

Items must be properly cleaned, disinfected, or sterilized for reuse.

12 Resupply room as needed. Have staff hand new supplies to you.

Limiting trips into and out of room reduces nurse and client's exposure to microorganisms.

13 Leave isolation room. Order for removing PPE depends on what is worn in room. This sequence describes steps to take if all barriers were required to be worn (CDC, 2005b).

a. Remove gloves (Procedural Guideline 4-1).

Prevents nurse from contacting contaminated glove's outer surface.

b. Remove eyewear or goggles.

c. Untie waist and neck strings of gown. Allow gown to fall from shoulders (see illustration). Remove hands from sleeves without touching outside of gown. Hold gown inside at shoulder seams and fold inside out. Discard disposable gown in trash bag.

Hands do not come in contact with soiled front of gown and therefore have not been soiled.

d. Remove mask. If mask secures over ears, remove elastic from ears, and pull mask away from face (see illustration). For a tie-on mask, while holding onto strings, untie *top* mask strings. Then hold strings while untying bottom strings. Pull mask away from face and drop into trash container. (Do not touch outer surface of mask.) If body fluids splash onto mask, dispose in biohazard waste container.

Ungloved hands will not be contaminated by touching only mask strings.

e. Perform hand hygiene.

STEPS	RATIONALE
f. Retrieve wristwatch and stethoscope (unless remains in room), and record vital signs on notepaper or clean paper towel.	Clean hands can contact clean items.
g. Explain to client when you plan to return to room. Ask if client requires any personal care items, books, etc., or has any requests or needs.	
h. Leave room, and close door, if necessary. (Close door if client is on airborne precautions.)	Keeping door open too long equalizes pressure in room and allows organisms to flow out.
14 See Completion Protocol (inside front cover).	

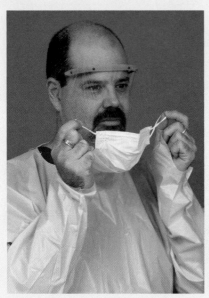

STEP 13c. Nurse removes mask.

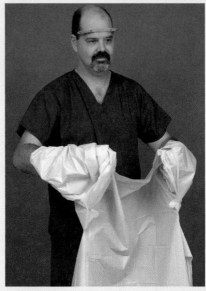

STEP 13d. Nurse removes gown.

EVALUATION

1 Ask client and family member to explain purpose of isolation in relation to diagnosed condition.

2 Monitor clinical status of neighboring clients.

Unexpected Outcomes and Related Interventions

1 Client avoids social and therapeutic discussions.

a. Confer with client, family, and/or significant other, and determine best approach to reduce client's sense of loneliness and depression.

b. Use therapeutic listening.

2 Infectious organism spreads to other clients.

a. Confer with physician, who may recommend an infectious disease consult.

b. Determine appropriate isolation precautions to take with other affected clients.

Recording and Reporting

• Procedures performed (including education) and client's response

• Type of isolation in use and the microorganism (if known)

• Client's response to social isolation

Sample Documentation

1320 Contact isolation in place for *Salmonella* in stool. Client incontinent of liquid stool. Wife at bedside, asking questions about barrier equipment. Discussed the method by which *Salmonella* is transmitted and explained the purpose of gown and gloves. Wife verbalized understanding when she requested gloves and gown to assist in cleanup.

Special Considerations
Pediatric Considerations

• Isolation creates sense of separation from family and loss of control. Strange environment confuses child. Preschoolers are unable to understand cause-effect relationship for isolation. Older children may be able to understand cause but still fantasize.

• Children require simple explanations, for example, "You need to be in this room to help you get better." All barriers to be used must be shown to child. Involve parents in any explanations. Nurses let children see their faces before applying masks so that children do not become frightened.

Geriatric Considerations

- Isolation can be a concern for older adults, especially those who have signs and symptoms of confusion or depression. Many times clients become more confused when confronted by a nurse using barrier precautions or when they are left in a room with the door closed. Assess need for closing door (negative airflow room) along with safety of client and additional safety measures required.
- Assess older adult for signs of depression: loss of appetite, decrease in verbal communications, or inability to sleep.

Home Care Considerations

- If client returns home with draining wound or productive cough, educate family on potential sources of contamination in the home and techniques for disposing of any biological wastes in accordance with state laws.
- Encourage clients to use vigilant hand washing and to avoid sharing personal care items with other family members.
- Have clients use a 5% (1:100 solution) bleach solution when performing household kitchen and bathroom cleaning of spills containing blood or other body fluids.

Long-Term Care Considerations

- Protective isolation is typically not used in long-term care settings.

SKILL 4.3 Special Tuberculosis Precautions

In 1989 the United States experienced a resurgence of TB. The increase in cases was due to the expansion of human immunodeficiency virus (HIV) infection, nosocomial transmission of *Mycobacterium tuberculosis* in health care settings, and increasing immigration from countries with a high incidence of TB (CDC, 2005). The current CDC guidelines for preventing and controlling TB focus on prompt detection, protecting close contacts of clients with contagious TB from contracting TB infection and disease, and applying effective infection-control measures in high-risk settings such as health care institutions. In 1994 the CDC released guidelines for stricter adherence to infection-control measures, including the use of TB precautions (CDC, 1994). Suspect TB in any client with respiratory symptoms lasting longer than 3 weeks. The risk of exposure is greatest before a diagnosis is made and isolation precautions are implemented. By the time persons with pulmonary TB seek medical attention, 30% to 40% of their close personal contacts have evidence of latent TB infection (CDC, 2005). Suspicious symptoms include fatigue, unexplained weight loss, dyspnea, fever and night sweats, and a cough that can sometimes be productive of blood. Isolation for clients with known or suspected TB includes a special, private acid-fast bacillus (AFB) isolation room (Box 4-1). Such rooms in existing facilities have negative pressure in relation to surrounding areas so that room air is exhausted directly to the outside or through special high-efficiency particulate air (HEPA) filters if recirculation is unavoidable. High-hazard procedures on clients with suspected or confirmed infectious TB must be performed in AFB treatment rooms.

OSHA and CDC guidelines require health care workers who care for active or suspected TB clients to wear N95 or P100 respirators (Figure 4-2). The respirators are high-efficiency particulate masks that have the ability to filter particles 1 μm in size with a filter efficiency of 95%

BOX 4-1 Tuberculosis Isolation

- TB isolation should be practiced for all clients with known or suspected TB. (Suspected TB is defined by agency policy and generally means any client with a positive AFB smear, a cavitating lesion seen on chest x-ray study, or identified as high risk by a screening tool.)
- Isolation must be in a single-client room designated as negative airflow and having at least six air exchanges per hour. Room air must be vented to the outside. The door must be closed to maintain negative pressure.
- Health care workers must wear an N95 particulate respirator mask or P100 respirator when entering an AFB isolation room. (Check agency policy for type of mask.)
- Workers must be fit-tested* before using a respirator for the first time. This ensures type and size of respirator appropriate for an individual.
- Workers must fit-check† the respirator's fit before each use.
- Respirator may be reused and stored according to agency policy.

AFB, Acid-fast bacillus.
*Procedure to determine adequate fit of respirator, usually by qualitative measure (wearers are exposed to a concentrated saccharin solution and asked if they can detect taste while wearing respirator).
†Procedure in which worker uses negative pressure to see if mask is properly sealed to face.

---

or higher. Health care employees who work in the rooms of TB clients must be fit-tested in a reliable way to obtain a face-seal leakage of 10% or less (CDC, 1994). Under National Institute for Occupational Safety and Health (NIOSH) criteria the minimally acceptable level of respiratory protection for TB is the N95 respirator. Hospital staff are trained in the wearing and storage of the respirator. OSHA also requires employers to provide training concerning transmission of TB, especially in areas where

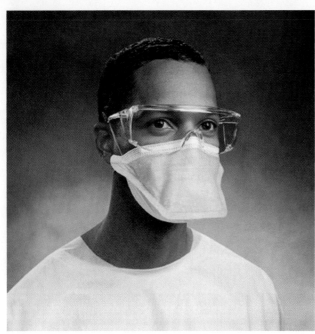

FIGURE 4-2 N95 respirator mask. (Courtesy Kimberly-Clark Health Care, Roswell, Ga.)

risk of exposure is high, such as in bronchoscopy procedural areas. Other requirements include annual TB skin testing for health care workers and appropriate follow-up when previously negative skin tests become positive (OSHA, 1993). In addition, the CDC now recommends health care workers receive a new blood test, the QuantiF-ERON-TB Gold test (QFT-G) (CDC, 2006b). This blood test aids in diagnosing M. *tuberculosis*, including latent TB. The advantages over traditional TB skin testing are that QFT-G does not boost responses measured by subsequent tests and the results are not subject to reader bias.

ASSESSMENT

1 Assess client's potential for infectious pulmonary or laryngeal TB (e.g., documentation of positive AFB smear or culture, signs or symptoms of TB, cavi-tation on chest x-ray study, history of a recent exposure, physician progress notes indicating plan to rule out TB).

2 Assess effectiveness of negative airflow in isolation room (e.g., use a flutter strip or smoke stick, consult with institution's plant engineering department). *Rationale: Determines that room has negative air pressure when flutter strip or smoke enters room.*

3 Consider type of care measures to be performed while in client's room. *Rationale: Allows nurse to organize all necessary equipment.*

PLANNING

Expected Outcomes focus on prevention of transmission of TB and client understanding of TB transmission.

1 Client describes how TB may be transmitted.
2 Staff or neighboring clients do not develop TB.

Delegation Considerations

Assessment of a client's status and type of care to perform may not be delegated. Basic care procedures performed under TB isolation can be delegated. The nurse directs personnel by:

• Clarifying for personnel precautions used under TB isolation, including fitting of mask.
• Instructing personnel on the type of clinical changes to report.

Equipment

• TB isolation room with negative airflow
• N95 or P100 respirator
• Clean gloves, gown, protective eyewear (based on client's clinical condition)
• Basic care items (e.g., medication equipment, hygiene items)

IMPLEMENTATION *for Special Tuberculosis Precautions*

STEPS	RATIONALE
1 See Standard Protocol (inside front cover).	
2 Before entering room, apply recommended mask. Be sure it fits snugly.	Reduces transmission of airborne droplet nuclei.
3 Explain purpose of AFB isolation to client, family, and others.	Improves ability of client to participate in care. TB cannot be transmitted through contact with clothing, bedding, food, or eating utensils.

STEPS	RATIONALE
4 Instruct client to cover mouth with tissue when coughing and to wear disposable surgical mask when leaving the room.	Reduces spread of droplet nuclei.
5 Provide care (see Skill 4.2).	
6 Leave the room, and close the door.	Maintains negative pressure in room.
7 Remove mask.	Most fitted respiratory devices are reusable.

> **COMMUNICATION TIP** TB is transmitted by inhalation of droplets that remain suspended in the air when client coughs, sneezes, speaks, or sings (CDC, 1994). Offer opportunity for questions.

8 Place reusable mask in labeled paper bag for storage, being careful not to crush mask. (Check agency policy for number of times it can be reused.)	Plastic bags seal in moisture.
9 See Completion Protocol (inside front cover).	

EVALUATION

1 Assess client's laboratory data for repeated AFB smears that may be negative.

2 Ask client and/or family to identify method of transmission for TB.

3 Be alert, and assess any suspected respiratory symptoms in neighboring clients.

Unexpected Outcomes and Related Interventions

1 Client fails to follow precautions for preventing transmission (e.g., fails to cover mouth when coughing, improperly disposes of soiled tissue).

a. Reexplain significant risk to family and friends.

b. Discuss client's concerns and feelings about the disease.

Recording and Reporting

- Procedures performed in isolation room and client's response
- Type of isolation precaution system

- Education given to client/family and their response to instruction
- Response of client/family to isolation

Sample Documentation

0800 Client on TB isolation, coughing productively blood-tinged sputum. Client having difficulty disposing of soiled tissues. Explained how TB can be transmitted to family members and other nurses. Client able to explain importance of disposing of soiled tissues in a container; verbalized concern about family exposure.

Special Considerations

Pediatric Considerations

- See Skill 4.2.

Geriatric Considerations

- See Skill 4.2

NCLEX® Style Questions

1 Covering the mouth when coughing reduces transmission of infection by:
1. Contact
2. Small droplet nuclei
3. Vector
4. Splashing

2 Put the following steps in order for removal of protective barriers, after leaving an isolation room:
1. Untie bottom mask strings.
2. Untie waist and neck strings of gown. Allow gown to fall from shoulders.
3. Remove gloves.
4. Remove eyewear or goggles.
5. Untie top mask strings.
6. Remove hands from gown sleeves without touching outside of gown; hold gown inside at shoulder seams, fold inside out, and then discard.
7. Pull mask away from face and drop into container.

3 Identify all of the following that classify as a case of a nosocomial or HAI:

1. An infected bedsore on a client admitted from a nursing home
2. A urinary tract infection (UTI) that develops after a Foley catheter placement
3. A client tested as HIV positive
4. The development of purulent drainage exiting from a central venous catheter insertion site
5. A *Staphylococcus* infection that develops in an incisional wound

4 When a nurse applies gloves when collecting a urine specimen, how does this technique break the chain of infection?

1. Blocks the portal of entry of a microorganism
2. Reduces susceptibility of the host
3. Controls a reservoir source of organism growth
4. Blocks the portal of exit

5 Which of the following breaks the chain of infection by controlling the reservoir source of microorganism growth?

1. Changing a soiled dressing
2. Cleaning a wound site
3. Avoiding sneezing
4. Disposing of used needles in a puncture-proof container

References for all chapters appear in Appendix D.

Basic Sterile Techniques

5

MEDIA RESOURCES

- **evolve** http://evolve.elsevier.com/Elkin

- **Video Clips**

- **Nursing Skills Online**

Surgical asepsis or sterile technique renders and maintains objects and areas free from pathogenic microorganisms (DeCastro, 2002). As in medical asepsis, hand hygiene with an appropriate cleanser or antiseptic is essential before beginning any surgical aseptic procedure. Surgical asepsis does require more precautions than medical asepsis (see Chapter 4). Strict adherence to the principles of sterile technique limits a client's risk for infection during invasive procedures, although infection can occur because of the presence of endogenous organisms on the skin and mucous membranes.

Although surgical asepsis is commonly practiced in operating rooms (ORs), labor and delivery (L&D) areas, and major diagnostic or special procedure areas, nurses also use surgical aseptic techniques at the client's bedside (Box 5-1) in three primary situations:

1. During procedures that require intentional perforation of a client's skin, such as insertion of an intravenous (IV) catheter
2. When the skin's integrity is broken, such as with a surgical incision or burn
3. During procedures that involve insertion of devices or surgical instruments into normally sterile body cavities (e.g., insertion of a urinary catheter)

A nurse in an OR follows a series of steps to maintain sterile technique, such as applying a mask, protective eyewear, and a cap; performing a surgical hand scrub; applying a sterile gown; and applying sterile gloves. In contrast, a nurse performing a sterile dressing change at a client's bedside or in the home may only perform hand hygiene and apply sterile gloves. Regardless of the procedures followed in different settings, the use of surgical asepsis depends on the nurse developing a surgical aseptic awareness. Always recognize the importance of strict adherence to aseptic principles. All health care providers involved in surgical asepsis have a responsibility to provide and maintain a safe environment by following aseptic principles (AORN, 2005).

BOX 5-1   Principles of Surgical Asepsis

- All items used within a sterile field must be sterile.
- A sterile barrier that has been permeated by punctures, tears, or moisture must be considered contaminated.
- After a sterile package is opened, a 2.5-cm (1-inch) border around the edges is considered unsterile.
- Tables draped as part of a sterile field are considered sterile only at table level.
- If there is any question or doubt of an item's sterility, the item must be considered unsterile.
- Persons wearing sterile barriers or sterile items contact only sterile areas and items. Unsterile persons or items contact only unsterile areas.
- Movement around and in the sterile field must not compromise or contaminate the sterile field.
- A sterile object or field out of the range of vision or an object held below a person's waist is contaminated.
- A sterile field is established immediately before the procedure, because there is a direct relationship between the time the sterile field is open and the presence of airborne contaminants.
- A sterile object or field becomes contaminated by prolonged exposure to air; stay organized, and complete any procedure as soon as possible.
- Open sterile items just before use. Do not cover a sterile field to be used at a later time.

Always have a client's full cooperation in treatment areas and at the bedside to minimize contamination of a work area. Prepare a client before a procedure, explaining how a procedure is to be performed and what a client can do to avoid contaminating sterile items (e.g., maintain position, avoid sudden body movements, refrain from touching sterile supplies, avoid coughing or talking over a sterile area). The nurse can be an excellent role model and client advocate in maintaining sterile technique. Reinforce aseptic principles if another caregiver breaks technique.

The Centers for Disease Control and Prevention (CDC) (1996) established standard precautions as the minimum standard for infection-control practice (see Chapter 4). The use of standard precautions calls for the wearing of masks in combination with eye protection devices such as goggles or glasses with solid side shields whenever splashes, spray, splatter, or droplets of blood or other potentially infectious fluids may be generated. These barriers keep the eyes, nose, and mouth free from exposure. Similarly, gowns are to be worn when there is risk of being splattered with blood or infectious materials.

EVIDENCE IN PRACTICE

Osborne S: Influences on compliance with standard precautions among operating room nurses, *Am J Infect Control* 31(7):415-423, 2003.

Researchers from Australia assessed OR nurses' attitudes and beliefs influencing their compliance with standard precautions. Using self-report measures, the study revealed that 72.1% of the nurses complied with standard precautions behaviors. The researchers cautioned that self-report data may overestimate actual compliance rates. The mean age for nurses who were noncompliant was greater than the mean age of OR nurses who reported being compliant. This suggests that older nurses may resist changing their behavior because of years of experience and tradition. Perceived barriers to compliance included lack of time, perceived "low-risk" clients, and personal protective equipment (PPE) interfering with care activities or not being available. This research suggests that nurses' perceptions of barriers significantly influence surgical asepsis compliance.

NURSING DIAGNOSES

The nursing diagnosis most directly related to clients requiring procedures involving sterile technique is **risk for infection.** Use of meticulous sterile technique reduces the incidence of wound infections in surgical clients. However, endogenous microorganisms can cause infections even when surgical asepsis has been carefully followed. **Ineffective protection** applies to clients who have latex allergies. Special precautions are needed during sterile aseptic procedures to avoid exposing clients to rubber products such as gloves.

SKILL 5.1   Applying Personal Protective Equipment

Certain surgical aseptic procedures performed at a client's bedside require the application of PPE such as a mask, cap, eyewear, gown, or gloves. For example, an agency may require a nurse to wear a mask during the changing of a central line dressing or to wear a mask and cap when changing the dressing on an extensive burn. Protective eyewear becomes important when there is the risk of being exposed to the splattering of blood or other body fluids. The skills for applying gloves and gowns can be found elsewhere in this text (see Chapter 4 and Skill 5.3).

Always assess a client's potential for acquiring an infection before applying a mask (e.g., does the client have a large open wound, or do you, as the nurse, have a respiratory infection?). If a mask is worn, it should be changed when it becomes moist or soiled (e.g., splattered with blood). Consider wearing a surgical cap to secure loose hair that might contaminate a sterile field. Follow standard precautions whenever using PPE.

ASSESSMENT

1 Review type of sterile procedure to be performed and consult agency policy regarding use of PPE. *Rationale: Not all sterile procedures require PPE. Ensures that nurse and client are properly protected.*

2 If you have symptoms of a respiratory infection, either avoid performing the procedure or apply a mask. *Rationale: A greater number of pathogenic microorganisms reside within the respiratory tract when infection is present.*

3 Assess the client's risk for infection (e.g., older adult, neonate, immunocompromised client). *Rationale: Some clients are at greater risk for acquiring an infection, so you must use additional protective barriers.*

PLANNING

Expected Outcomes focus on prevention of localized or systemic infection.

1 Client remains afebrile 24 to 48 hours after the procedure or during course of repeated procedures.

2 Client displays no signs of localized infection (e.g., redness, tenderness, edema, drainage) or systemic infection (e.g., fever, change in white blood cell [WBC] count) 24 hours after the procedure.

Delegation Considerations

The skill of applying PPE can be delegated. Instruct personnel to:

- Be available to hand off equipment or assist with client positioning during a sterile procedure.

Equipment

- Mask (different types are available for people with different skin sensitivities)
- Surgical cap (NOTE: Use only if hospital policy requires, or use to secure hair so as to prevent contamination of a sterile field)
- Hairpins, rubber bands, or both
- Protective eyewear (e.g., goggles or glasses with appropriate side shields)

IMPLEMENTATION *for Applying Personal Protective Equipment*

STEPS	RATIONALE
1 See Standard Protocol (inside front cover).	
2 Apply a cap:	
a. If hair is long, comb back behind ears and secure.	Cap must cover all hair entirely.
b. Secure hair in place with pins.	Long hair should not fall down or cause cap to slip and expose hair.
c. Apply cap over head as you would apply a hair net. Be sure all hair fits under cap's edges (see illustration).	
3 Apply a mask:	
a. Find top edge of mask, which usually has a thin metal strip along the edge.	Pliable metal fits snugly against bridge of nose.
b. Hold mask by top two strings or loops, keeping top edge above bridge of nose.	Prevents contact of hands with clean facial portion of mask. Mask will cover all of nose.

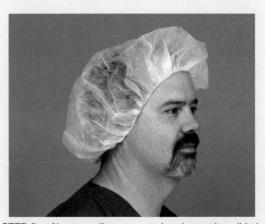

STEP 2c. Nurse applies cap over head, covering all hair.

STEPS	RATIONALE
c. Tie two top strings in a bow at top of back of head, over cap (if worn), with strings above ears (see illustration).	Position of ties at top of head provides a tight fit. Strings over ears may cause irritation.
d. Tie two lower ties in a bow snugly around neck with mask well under chin (see illustration).	Prevents escape of microorganisms through sides of mask as nurse talks and breathes.
e. Gently pinch upper metal band around bridge of nose.	Prevents microorganisms from escaping around nose.
4 Apply protective eyewear:	
a. Apply protective glasses, goggles, or face shield comfortably over eyes and check that vision is clear (see illustration).	Positioning can affect clarity of vision.
b. Be sure eyewear fits snugly around forehead and face.	Ensures eyes are fully protected.
5 Dispose of PPE.	
a. Remove gloves first, if worn (see Skill 5.3 for sterile gloves and Procedural Guideline 4-1 for clean gloves).	Prevents contamination of hair, neck, and facial area.
b. Remove eyewear, avoiding placing hands over soiled lens.	Reduces transmission of microorganisms.
c. Untie top strings of mask first, hold strings, untie bottom strings, and pull mask away from face while holding strings (see illustration).	Prevents top part of mask from falling down over nurse's uniform. Contaminated surface of mask could then contaminate uniform.
d. Do not touch outside surface of mask. Discard in plastic-lined receptacle.	Prevents contamination of hands.
e. Grasp outer surface of cap and lift from hair.	Minimizes contact of hands with hair.

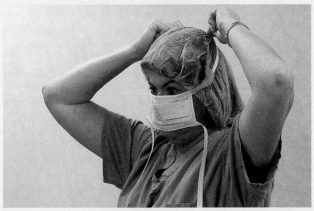
STEP 3c. Tie top strings of mask.

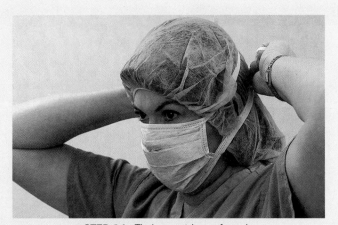
STEP 3d. Tie lower strings of mask.

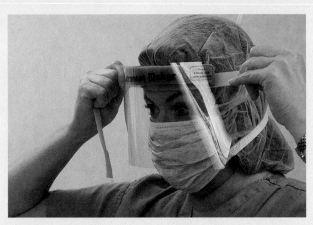
STEP 4a. Applying face shield over cap.

STEPS	RATIONALE
f. Discard cap in proper receptacle, and perform hand hygiene.	Reduces transmission of microorganisms.
6 See Completion Protocol (inside front cover).	

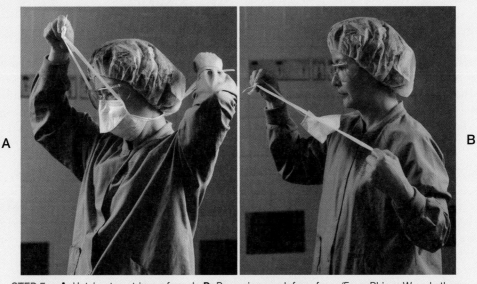

STEP 5c. **A,** Untying top strings of mask. **B,** Removing mask from face. (From Phipps W and others: *Medical-surgical nursing: concepts and clinical practice,* ed 6, St Louis, 1999, Mosby.)

EVALUATION

1 Following procedure, observe client for fever and signs of localized infection.

Unexpected Outcomes and Related Interventions

1 Client develops signs of infection.
a. Notify physician of findings.
b. Continue strict aseptic technique and hand hygiene.
c. Monitor temperature every 4 hours and as needed.

Recording and Reporting

- No recording or reporting is required for applying PPE.
- Record the procedure performed in the nurses' notes.

Special Considerations
Home Care Considerations

- Most procedures performed within the home are done using medical asepsis (see Chapter 4). However, more clients are receiving complicated procedures such as central line care. Consult agency policy for use of PPE in the home.

SKILL 5.2 Preparing a Sterile Field

- **Nursing Skills Online:** Infection Control, Lesson 3

Performing sterile aseptic procedures requires a work area in which objects can be handled with minimal risk of contamination. A sterile field provides a sterile surface for placement of sterile equipment. It is an area considered free of microorganisms and may consist of a sterile kit (Figure 5-1) or tray, a work surface draped with a sterile towel or wrapper, or a table covered with a large sterile drape (DeCastro, 2002). Sterile drapes establish a sterile field around a treatment site, such as a surgical incision, venipuncture site, or site for introduction of an indwelling urinary catheter. Drapes also provide a work surface for placing sterile supplies and for manipulating items with sterile gloves. Drapes are available in cloth, paper, and plastic. They may be wrapped in individual sterile packages or included within sterile kits or trays. An institution sometimes packages bundles containing sterile supplies. These bundles contain external and internal sterile (chemical) indicators that indicate the item has completed a sterilization process (Figure 5-2). After the bundle is opened, the inside surface of the linen cover can be used as a sterile field. Most drapes are fluid resistant. There are various styles, shapes, and sizes of drapes.

Many sterile items come prepackaged within containers that serve as both sterile fields and work areas. For example, a bladder catheterization kit and tracheal suction kit contain sterile items that can be moved with the tray and containers into which sterile solutions can be poured. After you create a sterile field, you are responsible to perform the procedure and to be sure the field is not contaminated.

ASSESSMENT

1 Verify that procedure requires surgical aseptic technique.
2 Assess client's comfort, oxygen requirements, and elimination needs before procedure. *Rationale: Certain sterile procedures may last a long time. Anticipate client's needs so that client can relax and avoid any unnecessary movement that might disrupt the procedure.*
3 Assess for latex allergies (see Skill 5.3). *Rationale: A focused review may reveal latex allergies even when no known allergies are indicated during the chart review.*
4 Check sterile package integrity for punctures, tears, discoloration, expiration date, and moisture. If using commercially packaged supplies or those prepared by agency, check sterilization indicator. *Rationale: Inspection of packaging ensures that only sterile items are presented to the sterile field (AORN, 2005).*

5 Anticipate number and variety of supplies needed for procedure. *Rationale: Ensures procedure is organized to prevent break in technique.*

PLANNING

Expected Outcomes focus on prevention of localized or systemic infection.

1 Client remains afebrile 24 to 48 hours after the procedure or during course of repeated procedures.
2 Client displays no signs of localized infection (e.g., redness, tenderness, edema, drainage) or systemic infection (e.g., fever, change in WBC count) 24 hours after the procedure.

Delegation Considerations

The skill of preparing a sterile field should not be delegated, except in the case of surgical technicians trained in surgical aseptic techniques. The nurse directs personnel to:

- Assist in positioning clients and obtaining necessary supplies.

Equipment

- Sterile gloves
- Sterile drape or kit that is to be used as a sterile field
- Sterile gown (see agency policy)
- Disposable cap and mask (see agency policy)
- Sterile equipment and solutions specific to the procedure
- Waist-high table or countertop surface
- Protective eyewear

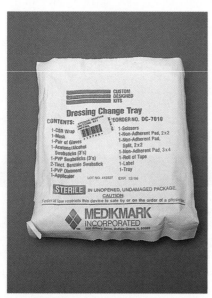

FIGURE 5-1 Sterile dressing kit.

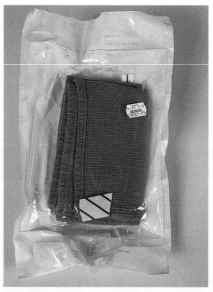

FIGURE 5-2 Tape with stripes changes color after sterilization.

IMPLEMENTATION *for Preparing a Sterile Field*

STEPS	RATIONALE
1 See Standard Protocol (inside front cover).	
2 Complete all priority care tasks before beginning procedure.	Sterile fields should be prepared as close as possible to time of use (AORN, 2005).
3 Ask visitors to step out of room briefly during procedure. Discourage movement by staff who will assist with procedure.	Traffic and movement increase potential for contamination through spread of microorganisms by air currents.
4 Apply cap, mask, protective eyewear, and/or gown as needed (consult agency policy) (see Skill 5.1).	
5 Select a clean, flat, dry work surface above waist level.	A sterile object below a person's waist is considered contaminated.
6 Check expiration dates on all kits, packs, and supplies to be sure they are sterile.	
7 Perform thorough hand hygiene.	Reduces transmission of microorganisms.
8 Prepare sterile work surface.	

> **COMMUNICATION TIP** Instruct the client not to touch the work surface or equipment during the procedure, and to remain still.

a. Sterile commercial kit or tray containing sterile items:	
(1) Place sterile kit or package containing sterile items on the work surface.	Once created, sterile field is sterile only at table level.
(2) Open outside cover and remove kit from dust cover. Place on work surface (see illustration).	Inner kit remains sterile.
(3) Grasp outer edge of tip of outermost flap.	Outer surface of package is considered unsterile. There is a 2.5-cm (1-inch) border around any sterile drape or wrap that is considered contaminated.
(4) Open outermost flap away from body, keeping arm outstretched and away from sterile field (see illustration).	Reaching over sterile field contaminates it.
(5) Grasp outer edge of first side flap.	Outer border is considered unsterile.

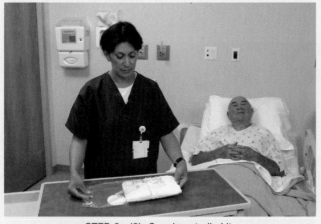

STEP 8a.(2) Opening sterile kit.

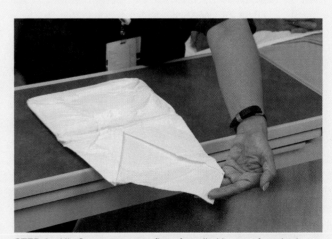

STEP 8a.(4) Open outermost flap of sterile kit away from body.

STEPS	RATIONALE
(6) Open side flap, pulling to side and allowing it to lie flat on table surface. Keep arm to the side and not extended over the sterile surface (see illustration).	Drape or flap should lie flat so it will not accidentally rise up and contaminate inner surface or the sterile items placed on its surface.
(7) Grasp outer edge of second side flap. Repeat Step (6) for opening second side flap (see illustration).	
(8) Grasp outer edge of last and innermost flap.	
(9) Stand away from sterile package and pull flap back, allowing it to fall flat on work surface (see illustration).	Reaching over sterile field contaminates it.
b. Sterile linen-wrapped package:	
(1) Place package on work surface above waist level.	Items placed below waist level are considered contaminated.
(2) Remove tape seal and unwrap both layers, following Steps 8a(2) through 8a(9) as with sterile kit (see illustration).	
(3) Use opened package wrapper as a sterile field.	Inner surface of wrapper is considered sterile.

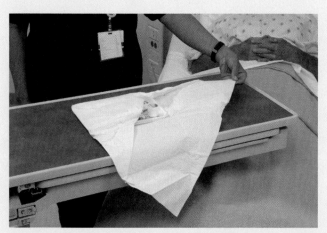

STEP 8a.(6) Open first side flap, pulling to side.

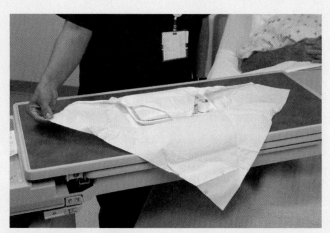

STEP 8a.(7) Open second side flap, pulling to side.

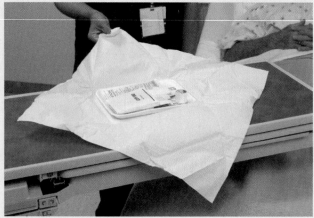

STEP 8a.(9) Open last and innermost flap, standing away from sterile field.

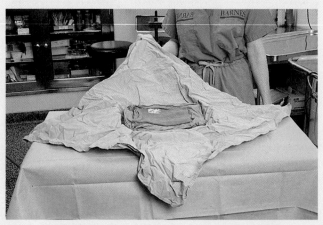

STEP 8b.(2) Open sterile linen-wrapped package.

STEPS	RATIONALE

c. Sterile drape:

(1) Place pack containing the sterile drape on work surface and open as described in Steps 8a(2) through 8a(9) for sterile package.

Ensures sterility of packaged drape.

(2) **Apply sterile gloves.**
(NOTE: This is an option depending on agency policy. You may touch outer 1-inch border of drape without wearing gloves.)

(3) Grasp folded top edge of drape with fingertips of one hand. Gently lift drape up from its wrapper without touching any object.

If a sterile object touches any nonsterile object, it becomes contaminated.

(4) Allow drape to unfold, keeping it above waist and the work surface and away from the body. (Carefully discard outer wrapper with other hand.)

Object held below person's waist or above chest is contaminated.

(5) With other hand, grasp the adjacent corner of drape. Hold drape straight over work surface (see illustration).

Drape can now be properly placed with two hands.

(6) Holding drape, first position the bottom half over top half of the intended work surface (see illustration).

Prevents nurse from reaching over sterile field.

(7) Allow top half of drape to be placed over bottom half of work surface (see illustration).

A flat sterile surface is now available for placement of sterile items.

9 Add sterile items to sterile field.

a. Open sterile item (following package directions) while holding outside wrapper in nondominant hand.

Frees dominant hand for unwrapping outer wrapper.

b. Carefully peel wrapper over nondominant hand (see illustration).

Item remains sterile. Inner surface of wrapper covers hand, making it sterile.

c. Being sure wrapper does not fall down on sterile field, place item onto field at an angle (see illustration). *Do not hold arm over sterile field.*

Secured wrapper edges prevent flipping wrapper and contaminating contents of sterile field (AORN, 2005).

NURSE ALERT Do not flip or throw objects onto sterile field.

---

d. Dispose of outer wrapper.

Prevents accidental contamination of sterile field.

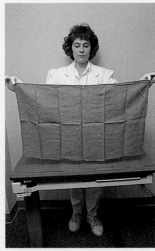

STEP 8c.(5) Hold corners of sterile drape up and away from body.

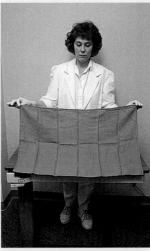

STEP 8c.(6) Position bottom half of sterile drape over top half of work surface.

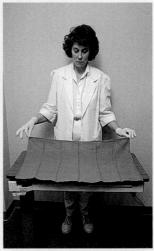

STEP 8c.(7) Allow top half of drape to be placed over bottom half of work surface.

STEPS

RATIONALE

10 Pour sterile solutions.

a. Verify contents and expiration date of solution.

b. Be sure receptacle for solution is located near or on sterile work surface edge. Sterile kits have cups or plastic molded sections into which fluids can be poured.

c. Remove sterile seal and cap from bottle in an upward motion.

d. With solution bottle held away from sterile field, and bottle lip 1 to 2 inches above inside of sterile receiving container, slowly pour entire contents of solution container (see illustration). Avoid splashing.

11 Proceed with intended sterile procedure.

12 See Completion Protocol (inside front cover).

Ensures proper solution and sterility of contents. Prevents reaching over sterile field.

Prevents contamination of bottle lip. Maintains sterility of inside of cap.

Edge and outside of bottle are considered contaminated. Slow pouring prevents splashing liquids, which causes fluid permeation of the sterile barrier, called *strike through*, resulting in contamination. Sterility of contents cannot be ensured if cap is replaced.

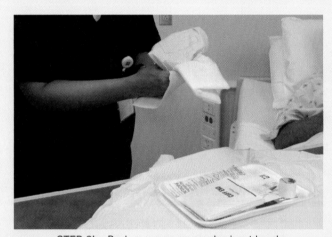

STEP 9b. Peel wrapper over nondominant hand.

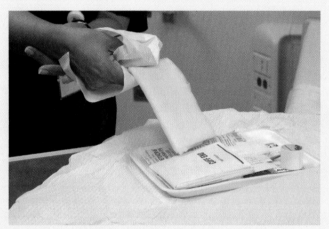

STEP 9c. Place sterile item on field.

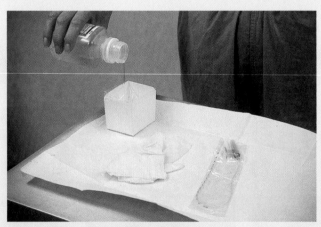

STEP 10d. Pouring solution into receiving container on sterile field.

EVALUATION

1 Observe for break in sterile technique.
2 Observe client for fever and signs of localized infection.

Unexpected Outcomes and Related Interventions

1 Client develops signs of infection.
a. Notify physician of findings.
b. Continue strict aseptic technique and hand hygiene.
c. Monitor temperature every 4 hours and as needed.
d. Encourage intake of fluids.

Recording and Reporting

- No recording or reporting is required for setting up sterile field.
- Record the procedure performed in the nurses' notes.

Special Considerations
Pediatric Considerations

- Children may be unable to cooperate during a sterile procedure depending on their level of developmental maturity.

- Instruct family members in how they may assist so that child does not contaminate sterile field.

Geriatric Considerations

- Memory and sensory deficits may impair client's ability to understand and cooperate with the procedure.

Home Care Considerations

- Adaptations may be made for some procedures, such as self-catheterization and home tracheostomy care. In some cases clients use medical asepsis rather than surgical technique.
- If possible, teach the client and family to perform sterile procedures well before discharge from acute care so that skills can be learned with professional assistance.
- Home visits should include assessing cleanliness of the environment, as well as assessing the understanding and ability of client and family to perform procedure safely.

SKILL 5.3 Sterile Gloving

- Nursing Skills Online: Infection Control, Lesson 4

Sterile gloves act as a barrier against the transmission of pathogenic microorganisms and are applied before performing any sterile procedure, such as a sterile dressing change or urinary catheter insertion. Always remember that sterile gloves do not replace hand hygiene.

You will use the open glove application method for most sterile procedures not requiring a sterile gown. Be careful not to contaminate the gloved hands by touching clean, contaminated, or possibly contaminated items or areas. If a glove becomes contaminated or torn, change it immediately. Keep your hands clasped about 12 inches in front of your body, above waist level, and below the shoulders until you are ready to perform a procedure.

It is important to choose not only the right size of glove but also the correct material. Many clients and health care workers have known allergies to latex, the natural rubber used in most gloves and other medical products (DeCastro, 2002). Box 5-2 lists individuals who are at risk for latex allergy. Latex proteins enter the body in various ways, through skin or mucous membranes, intravascularly, or via inhalation. The cornstarch powder used to make latex gloves slip on easily over the hands is a carrier of the latex proteins (Burt, 1998). This is one reason vigorous hand hygiene is necessary after glove removal. Studies have shown that individuals who are highly sensitive to latex develop local and systemic reactions when latex gloves are removed and the latex glove powder particles are suspended in the air, often for hours (Fleishman and Olmstead, 2000). The latex can then be inhaled or settle on clothing, skin, or mucous membranes. Reaction to latex can be mild to severe (Box 5-3). Choose latex-free or synthetic gloves when caring for individuals at high risk or with suspected latex sensitivity. Institutions have latex-free procedure kits available for use.

When choosing gloves, be sure they are tight enough that objects can be picked up easily but that they do not stretch so tightly over the fingers that they can easily tear. Sterile gloves are available in various sizes (e.g., 6, 6½, 7). There are also sterile gloves available in a "one-size-fits-all" style or in "small," "medium," and "large."

BOX 5-2 Individuals at Risk for Latex Allergy

- Spina bifida
- Congenital or urogenital defects
- History of indwelling catheters or repeated catheterizations
- History of using condom catheters
- High latex exposure (e.g., health care workers, housekeepers, food handlers, tire manufacturers, workers in industries that use gloves routinely)
- History of multiple childhood surgeries
- History of food allergies

Modified from Gritter M: The latex threat, *Am J Nurs* 98(9):26, 1998; and Kim KT and others: Implementation recommendations for making health care facilities latex safe, *AORN J* 67(3):615, 1998.

BOX 5-3 Levels of Latex Reactions

There are three types of common latex reactions, which (in order of increasing severity) include:

Irritant dermatitis: A nonallergic response characterized by skin redness and itching.

Type IV hypersensitivity: A cell-mediated allergic reaction to chemicals used in latex processing. Reaction can be delayed as long as 48 hours and includes redness, itching, and hives. Localized swelling, red and itchy or runny eyes and nose, and coughing may develop.

Type I allergic reaction: A true latex allergy that can be life threatening. Reactions vary based on type of latex protein and degree of individual sensitivity, including local and systemic. Symptoms include hives, generalized edema, itching, rash, wheezing, bronchospasm, difficulty breathing, laryngeal edema, diarrhea, nausea, hypotension, tachycardia, and respiratory or cardiac arrest.

Modified from Gritter M: The latex threat, *Am J Nurs* 98(9):26, 1998.

ASSESSMENT

1 Consider the type of procedure to be performed, and consult institutional policy on use of sterile gloves.
2 Consider client's risk for infection (e.g., preexisting condition, size or extent of area being treated). *Rationale: Directs nurse to follow added precautions (e.g., use of additional protective barriers) if necessary.*
3 Select correct size and type of gloves, then examine glove package to determine if it is dry and intact. *Rationale: Torn or wet package is considered contaminated.*
4 Inspect condition of hands for cuts, open lesions, or abrasions. Cover any lesions with an impervious dressing. *Rationale: Lesions harbor mircroorganisms. Presence of such lesions may contraindicate nurse's participation in procedure.*

5 Assess client for the following risk factors before applying latex gloves (see Box 5-3):
a. Previous reaction to the following items within hours of exposure: adhesive tape, dental or face mask, golf club grip, ostomy bag, rubber band, balloon, bandage, elastic underwear, IV tubing, rubber gloves, or condom.
b. Personal history of asthma, contact dermatitis, eczema, urticaria, or rhinitis.
c. History of food allergies, especially avocado, banana, peach, chestnut, raw potato, kiwi, tomato, or papaya.
d. Previous history of adverse reactions during surgery or dental procedures.
e. Previous reaction to latex product.
6 If client is expected to be at risk, check facility procedure for obtaining latex allergy cart. *Rationale: Contains nonlatex client care items.*

PLANNING

Expected Outcomes focus on prevention of localized or systemic infection, as well as latex reaction.

1 Client remains afebrile with no signs of localized infection 24 to 72 hours after the procedure or during the course of repeated procedures.
2 Client will not develop signs of latex sensitivity or allergic reaction.

Delegation Considerations

The skill of sterile gloving can be delegated. However, many procedures that require the use of sterile gloves cannot be delegated (see agency policy).

Equipment

- Package of correct-size sterile gloves: latex or synthetic nonlatex. (NOTE: Hypoallergenic, low-powder, or low-protein latex gloves may still contain enough latex protein to cause an allergic reaction [Burt, 1998].)

IMPLEMENTATION *for Sterile Gloving*

STEPS	RATIONALE
1 See Standard Protocol (inside front cover).	
2 Glove Application:	
a. Perform thorough hand hygiene.	Reduces transmission of microorganisms.
b. Place glove package near work area.	Ensures availability before procedure.
c. Open sterile gloves by carefully separating and peeling open adhered package sides (see illustration).	Prevents inner glove package from accidentally opening and touching contaminated objects.
d. Grasp inner glove package, and lay it on a clean, dry, flat surface at waist level. Open package, keeping gloves on wrapper's inside surface (see illustration).	Inner surface of glove package is sterile. Sterile object held below waist level is contaminated.
e. Identify right and left glove. Each glove has a cuff approximately 5 cm (2 inches) wide. Glove dominant hand first.	Proper identification of gloves prevents contamination by improper fit. Gloving of dominant hand first improves dexterity.

STEPS	RATIONALE

f. With thumb and first two fingers of nondominant hand, grasp edge of cuff of glove for dominant hand. Touch only glove's inside surface.

Inner edge of cuff will touch skin and is no longer considered sterile.

g. Carefully pull glove over dominant hand, leaving cuff and being sure cuff does not roll up wrist (see illustration). Be careful in working thumb and fingers into correct spaces.

h. With gloved dominant hand, slip fingers underneath second glove's cuff (see illustration).

Cuff protects gloved fingers; abducting thumb prevents contamination from contact with unsterile surface.

i. Carefully pull second glove over fingers of nondominant hand (see illustration).

> **NURSE ALERT** Do not allow fingers and thumb of gloved dominant hand to touch any part of exposed nondominant hand. Keep thumb of dominant hand abducted back.

j. Interlock fingers of gloved hands and hold away from body, above waist level, until beginning procedure (see illustration).

Prevents accidental contamination from hand movement.

3 Proceed with intended procedure.

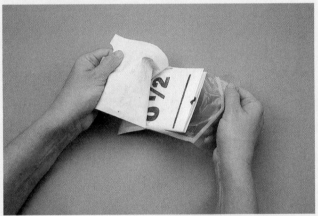

STEP 2c. Open outer glove package wrapper.

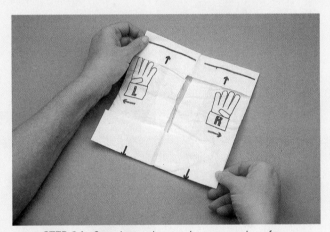

STEP 2d. Open inner glove package on work surface.

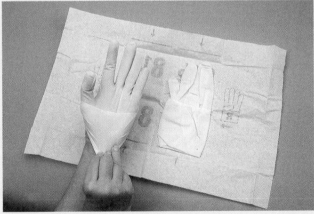

STEP 2g. Pick up glove for dominant hand and insert fingers; pull glove completely over dominant hand (example is for a left-handed person).

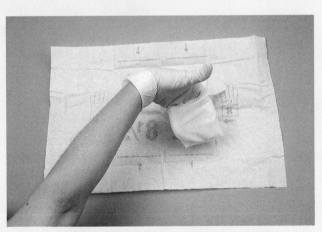

STEP 2h. Pick up glove for nondominant hand.

4 Glove Removal:

a. Grasp outside of one cuff with other gloved hand; avoid touching wrist. Pull glove off, turning it inside out (see illustration). Discard in proper receptacle.

b. Take fingers of bare hand and tuck inside remaining glove cuff. Peel glove off inside out. Discard in trash receptacle.

5 See Completion Protocol (inside front cover).

Outside of glove should not touch skin surface.

Fingers do not touch contaminated glove surface.

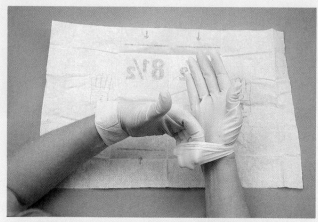

STEP 2i. Pull second glove over nondominant hand.

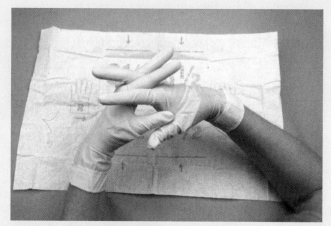

STEP 2j. Interlock gloved hands.

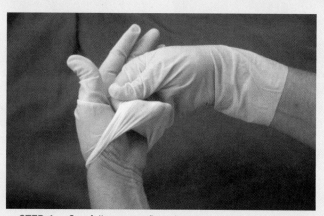

STEP 4a. Carefully remove first glove by turning it inside out.

EVALUATION

1 Evaluate client for signs and symptoms of infection (e.g., fever, development of wound drainage) for 48 hours after the procedure.

2 Evaluate client for signs of latex reaction.

2 Client develops signs of dermatitis or latex sensitivity.
a. Notify physician of findings.
b. Have dose of epinephrine and Solu-Medrol available, which may be needed for allergic reaction.

Unexpected Outcomes and Related Interventions

1 Client develops signs of infection.
a. Notify physician of findings. Wound cultures (see Chapter 13) and antibiotic therapy may be needed.
b. Apply standard precautions (see Chapter 4) and sterile technique (as appropriate).
c. Monitor temperature every 4 hours or per orders.

Recording and Reporting

- No recording or reporting is required for sterile gloving.
- Record the procedure performed in the nurses' notes.

NCLEX® Style Questions

1 Place an "S" next to the procedures requiring sterile (aseptic) technique and place an "M" next to those requiring only medical aseptic technique.
1. Urinary catheterization
2. Tracheal suctioning
3. Insertion of rectal suppository
4. Insertion of a feeding tube
5. Lumbar puncture
6. Sitz bath

2 The nurse has applied the first sterile glove on her right hand (dominant) without touching the sterile outer surface. She takes her gloved right hand and picks up the remaining glove at the top of the cuff and slips it over her left hand. Which of the following statements is correct?
1. The first glove is applied correctly but is contaminated while applying the second glove.
2. The first glove is applied incorrectly but the second glove is applied correctly.
3. The first glove is applied correctly and the second glove becomes contaminated.
4. Both gloves have been applied correctly.

3 When opening a sterile pack, which of the following will compromise the sterility of the contents?
1. Keeping the contents of the pack away from the table edge
2. Holding or moving the object below the waist
3. Opening the pack just before the procedure
4. Allowing movement around the sterile field that does not touch near the sterile field

4 Select all of the following clients that you might suspect to be at risk for a latex allergy:
1. A client who has had a surgical procedure
2. A health care worker who works in the OR
3. A client who reports frequent nausea and diarrhea after eating peaches
4. A client who develops hives after the taping of his surgical dressing
5. A health care worker who comes to work with coughing and respiratory congestion

References for all chapters appear in Appendix D.

6

Promoting Activity and Mobility

MEDIA RESOURCES

- **evolve** http://evolve.elsevier.com/Elkin
- **View Video!** Video Clips
- Nursing Skills Online

Regular physical activity and exercise contribute to both physical and emotional well-being (Huddleston, 2002; Konradi and Anglin, 2001). The benefits of physical activity include increased energy, improved sleep, better appetite, less pain, and improved self-esteem. It is useful to incorporate active exercises into activities of daily living (ADLs) (Box 6-1). Nurses make every effort to promote and maintain clients' functional mobility. Physical activities that clients are able to perform indicate their physical capacity, functional ability, and personal desires.

Three elements essential for mobility include: (1) the ability to move based on adequate muscle strength, control, coordination, and range of motion (ROM); (2) the motivation to move; and (3) the absence of barriers in the environment. To prevent injury to both client and caregiver, use of safe client handling techniques are essential. Evidence shows that many traditional techniques for client handling (e.g., manual client lifting, classes in body mechanics, back belts) are not effective in reducing caregiver injuries (Nelson and Baptiste, 2004). Instead, nurses should use evidence-based practices including client handling/equipment devices, ergonomic assessment protocols, and no-lift policies. Table 6-1 lists techniques designed to minimize caregiver injuries.

Immobilized clients, clients with chronic illnesses, and older adults are at a greater risk of developing complications of altered mobility that affect all body systems. Complications include muscle atrophy, loss of bone mass, joint contractures, pressure ulcers, cardiovascular and respiratory problems, constipation, urinary stasis, mental confusion, and depression (Jitramontree, 2001; Huether and McCance, 2004).

Bed rest is a medical intervention in which a client is restricted to bed for one of the following purposes: (1) decreasing oxygen requirements of the body, (2) reducing pain, or (3) allowing rest and recovery. Clients are at a higher risk for orthostatic or postural hypotension if they are older, immobilized, undergoing prolonged bed rest, or experiencing chronic illnesses (Dingle, 2003;

BOX 6-1 Examples of Incorporating Exercise into Activities of Daily Living

Upper Body
- Nodding head "yes": neck flexion
- Shaking head "no": neck rotation
- Reaching to bedside stand for book: shoulder extension
- Scratching back: shoulder hyperextension
- Brushing or combing hair: shoulder hyperextension
- Eating, bathing, and shaving: elbow flexion and extension
- Writing and eating: fingers and thumb flexion, extension, and opposition

Lower Body
- Walking: hip flexion, extension, and hyperextension; knee flexion and extension; ankle dorsiflexion; plantar flexion
- Moving to side-lying position: hip flexion, extension, and abduction; knee flexion and extension
- Moving from side-lying position: hip extension and adduction; knee flexion and extension
- While sitting, lifting knees up and straightening legs: strengthens muscles used for walking

TABLE 6-1 Preventing Lift Injuries in Health Care Workers

ACTION	RATIONALE
When planning to move a client, arrange for adequate help. If your institution has a lift team, use it as a resource.	A lift team is properly trained on techniques to prevent injury.
Use client handling equipment and devices (e.g., height adjustable beds, ceiling mounted lifts, friction-reducing slide sheets, air assisted devices) (Nelson and Baptiste, 2004).	These devices have shown promise in reducing a caregiver's muscular strain during client handling.
Encourage client to assist as much as possible.	Promotes client's abilities and strength while minimizing caregiver workload.
Keep back, neck, pelvis, and feet aligned. Avoid twisting.	Twisting increases risk of injury.
Flex knees, and keep feet about a shoulder width apart.	A broad base of support increases stability.
Position self close to client (or object being lifted).	Reduces horizontal reach and stress on back.
Use arms and legs (not back).	Leg muscles are stronger, larger muscles capable of greater work without injury.
Slide client toward yourself using a pullsheet or slide board. When transferring a client onto a stretcher or bed, a slide board is more appropriate.	Sliding requires less effort than lifting. Pullsheet minimizes shearing forces, which can damage client's skin.
Person with the heaviest load coordinates efforts of team involved by counting to three.	Simultaneous lifting minimizes the load for any one lifter.
Perfrom manual lifting as last resort and only if it does not involve lifting most or all of a client's weight (Nelson and Baptiste, 2004).	Lifting is a high-risk activity that causes significant biochemical and postural stressors.

Frederiks and others, 2003; Netea and others, 2002). Signs and symptoms of orthostatic hypotension include dizziness, light-headedness, nausea, tachycardia, pallor, and fainting. In these clients, moving to the dangling position (see Skill 6.3) may cause a gravity-induced drop in blood pressure. When a client stands, blood shifts from the thorax to the pelvis and lower extremities because of gravity. A drop in blood pressure results from the redistribution of blood (Phipps and others, 2007). The recommendation is to raise the head of the bed and allow a few minutes before dangling (Dingle, 2003; Kenny, 2000). Dangling a client before standing is an intermediate step that allows assessment of the individual before changing positions to maintain the safety of and prevent injury to the client.

EVIDENCE IN PRACTICE

Tinkoff A and others: Musculoskeletal problems of the neck, shoulder, and back and functional consequences in nurses, *Am J Ind Med* 41(3):170, 2002.

Musculoskeletal disorders are noted as the most prevalent and debilitating occupational health hazard among nurses.

The American Nurses Association (ANA, 2003) put forth a position statement calling for the use of assistive equipment and devices to reposition and transfer clients to promote a safe health care environment for nurses and their clients. The use of assistive equipment and continued use of proper body mechanics can significantly reduce the risk of musculoskeletal injuries (ANA, 2003). In addition, the Occupational Safety and Health Administration (OSHA, 2003) recommends that manual lifting of clients be minimized in all cases and eliminated when feasible. Many facilities are moving toward limited lift policies that minimize client handling by nurses and instead use lift devices to reduce on-the-job injuries. By becoming knowledgeable about safe, efficient lifting techniques and proper use of assistive equipment and devices, nurses can safely transfer clients without causing injury to the client or the nurse.

NURSING DIAGNOSES

Activity intolerance and **risk for activity intolerance** are situations in which clients experience altered vital signs (pulse, respiration, or blood pressure) in response to activity.

Impaired physical mobility is associated with pain or discomfort resulting from trauma or surgery, decreased strength and endurance, prolonged bed rest, or restrictive external devices such as casts, braces, drains, and intravenous (IV) tubing. **Risk for falls**, which includes use of assistive devices, multiple medications, orthostatic hypotension, and psychological factors such as fear of falling, results in a client's refusal to ambulate. **Risk for disuse syndrome** is a diagnosis that applies when inactivity is desired or unavoidable, increasing the risk for deterioration of cardiovascular, respiratory, musculoskeletal, and psychosocial body systems. A client with a nursing diagnosis of **acute pain** or **chronic pain** is susceptible to developing impaired mobility resulting from the nature and extent of discomfort.

SKILL 6.1   Assisting with Moving and Positioning Clients in Bed

- **Nursing Skills Online: Safety, Lesson 3**

A high-risk client-handling task for acute and long-term care settings is repositioning clients in bed (Nelson and Baptiste, 2004). Moving and positioning clients safely and effectively involves the use of ergonomics. Ergonomics involves fitting the task (e.g., moving a client up in bed) to the worker. When moving clients, be sure to elevate the bed, have additional care providers available, and use assistive devices such as slide boards when appropriate.

Correct body alignment involves positioning so that no excessive strain is put on clients' joints, tendons, ligaments, or muscles. Clients with impaired nervous or musculoskeletal system functioning, with increased weakness, or those restricted to bed rest benefit from repositioning (Hoeman, 2002). In general, clients should be repositioned as needed and at least every 2 hours if they are in bed and every 20 to 30 minutes if they are sitting in a chair. Additional variables influencing frequency of position changes include level of comfort, amount of spontaneous movement, presence of edema, loss of sensation, and overall physical and mental status (Hoeman, 2002). When positioning clients, be aware of potential pressure points (Figure 6-1). Dependent clients need a regularly scheduled program of assisted ROM exercises (see Skill 6.5).

Care must be taken to protect the skin from damage caused by shearing forces resulting from sliding rather than lifting the client (Figure 6-2). Shear injury occurs when the skin remains stationary and the underlying tissue shifts, resulting in tissue damage. This is especially important when the client is thin, has fragile skin, is nutritionally compromised, or is unable to move independently.

Use pillows and foam wedges for immobilized clients to position bony prominences, such as heels and ankles, off of excessive or extended pressure. The use of air or water mattresses is also recommended (see Chapter 26).

The immobilized client is at risk for many complications. One such complication is the development of deep vein thrombosis (DVT) of the lower extremities. In addition to repositioning, other measures to prevent DVTs may be initiated. Early ambulation is the most effective preventive measure. However, there are times when early ambulation is not an option. Early application of elastic stockings and sequential compression device (SCD) along with low–molecular-weight or low-dose heparin have been reported as successful in preventing the development of DVT (Phipps and others, 2007). Sequential compression stockings can be used alone or in conjunction with elastic stockings, depending upon the physician's preference (see Procedural Guideline 6-1 on p. 104).

FIGURE 6-1 A, Pressure points in lying position. **B,** Pressure points in sitting position.

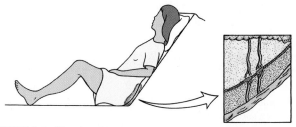

FIGURE 6-2 Shearing forces against sacrum cause tissue damage.

ASSESSMENT

1 Assess client's weight, age, level of consciousness, disease process, and ability to cooperate. *Rationale: Determines how many personnel will be needed to assist in moving client.*

2 Assess strength of muscles and mobility of joints to be used by observing client movement in bed and by applying gradual pressure to a muscle group (e.g., attempting to extend client's elbow). Compare strength in muscle groups, including arms and legs. *Rationale: Provides a baseline to determine client's ability to assist caregivers and to assess the client's progress toward improved activity tolerance and muscle endurance.*

3 Assess need for analgesic medication 30 to 60 minutes before position changes. *Rationale: Pain relief enhances client's ability to tolerate movement.*

4 Assess for tubes, incisions, and equipment. *Rationale: Will alter positioning procedure and types of positions used.*

5 Verify physician's orders before positioning client. *Rationale: Some positions may be contraindicated (i.e., spinal cord injuries, lung surgery).*

PLANNING

Expected Outcomes focus on mobility, self-care, and prevention of complications within the confines of the prescribed activity.

1 Client's skin remains intact without redness.

2 Client verbalizes a sense of comfort after each repositioning.

3 Client maintains changes in position in bed for at least 1 hour.

4 Client states two benefits of position changes and correct body alignment.

Delegation Considerations

Client assessment should not be delegated. The skill of moving and positioning clients with acute spinal cord or neurological trauma should not be delegated. The skill of moving and positioning clients without acute spinal cord or neurological trauma may be delegated. The nurse directs personnel by:

- Explaining how to adapt skill for specific client, such as allowing client to assist as much as possible and using additional personnel to change client's position safely.
- Reviewing what to observe and report back to nurse, such as reddened areas over pressure points, client's comfort, and ability of client to assist in changing position.

Equipment

- Pillows
- Footboard (optional)
- Trochanter roll
- Sandbag
- Hand rolls
- Side rails
- Friction-reducing device
- Sliding board
- Repositioning aid

IMPLEMENTATION *for Assisting with Moving and Positioning Clients in Bed*

STEPS	RATIONALE
1 **See Standard Protocol (inside front cover).** Review principles of body mechanics (see Table 6-1).	

> COMMUNICATION TIP Encourage client to assist as much as possible, discuss and review steps involved with client and family, and determine ways client can assist while being moved.

STEPS	RATIONALE
2 Raise bed to comfortable working height. Lower side rails as appropriate.	Raises level of work toward nurse's center of gravity.
3 Remove all pillows and devices used in previous position.	Reduces interference from bedding during positioning procedure.
4 Obtain extra help as needed.	Provides for client and nurse safety.
5 Adjust position of IV pole, tubes, and catheters.	Facilitates movement without tension and disruption.
6 Provide client with hearing aid and glasses if used.	Promoting client involvement motivates and speeds progress toward independence and provides a sense of control and security.
7 Position client.	
a. Moving a dependent client up in bed with two nurses and client's assistance:	
(1) Lower head of bed to lowest position. Place pillow near headboard.	Minimizes potential trauma from head contacting headboard.
(2) Assist client to supine position with knees flexed so that soles of one or both feet are flat on the bed.	Positions client to exert effort when moving up in bed.
(3) Face head of bed	Facing direction of movement prevents twisting nurse's body while moving client.

STEPS	RATIONALE
(4) Position one nurse at client's upper body. Nurse's arm nearest head of bed should be under client's head and opposite shoulder; other arm should be under client's closest arm and shoulder. Position other nurse at client's lower torso. The nurse's arms should be under client's lower back and torso.	Prevents trauma to client's musculoskeletal system by supporting shoulder and hip joints and evenly distributing weight.
(5) Place feet apart, with foot nearest head of bed behind other foot (forward-backward stance).	Wide base of support increases nurse's balance during shift in weight.
(6) Instruct client to flex neck, tilting chin toward chest.	Prevents hyperextension of neck when moving.
(7) If there is an overhead trapeze, have client grasp it.	Device will aid client pulling up in bed.
(8) Nurses flex knees and hips, bringing forearms closer to level of bed. Have client breathe out and lift with trapeze and/or push with feet on the count of three. Repeat if needed to move up farther in the bed.	Breathing out avoids Valsalva maneuver. Coordinates client's movement with nurse's lifting action.
(9) Ask client about level of comfort, and adjust as necessary.	
b. **Assisting dependent client to move up in bed with two nurses when client cannot assist:**	
(1) Remove pillow and lower head of bed to lowest position client can tolerate. Place pillow at head of bed.	Minimizes effort required to move client and minimizes potential trauma from head contact on headboard. NOTE: Clients with hypoxia may not tolerate lying flat.
(2) Roll client side to side, placing a repositioning aid under client that extends from shoulders to thighs.	Assists in moving client ergonomically and safely.
(3) With one nurse on each side of client, grasp repositioning aid firmly with hands near client's upper arms and hips. Pull device to move client up in bed (see illustration).	The closer nurses are to the client, the less stressful the task.

NURSE ALERT Review principles of body mechanics (see Table 6-1). This move requires at least two nurses and an assistive device when client is unable to assist. If client is very heavy, consider using more personnel.

---

(4) Nurses' knees are flexed with body facing the direction of the move. The foot away from the bed faces forward for a broader base of support (see illustration).

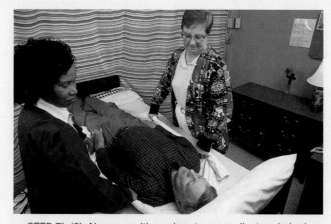

STEP 7b.(3) Nurses position selves to move client up in bed.

STEPS	RATIONALE

(5) Instruct client to rest arms on body, breathe out, and to lift head on the count of three.

(6) Lift client toward head of bed on the count of three. Repeat the move if necessary.

(7) Assist client as needed in shifting to attain position of comfort.

c. Positioning in semi-Fowler's and Fowler's position. For the semi-Fowler's position the head of the bed is raised 45 to 60 degrees. The high-Fowler's position, with the head of the bed raised 90 degrees, is recommended for eating.

Both positions improve breathing by decreasing pressure on the diaphragm as gravity pulls abdominal contents downward. These positions also facilitate visiting and diversional activities. In this position clients tend to slide toward the foot of the bed.

(1) Using two nurses, assist moving the client up in bed before raising the head of the bed (see Steps 7a and 7b).

Moving client up in bed before elevation of the head of the bed facilitates proper positioning.

(2) With client in supine position, raise the head of the bed to the appropriate level (45 to 90 degrees) (see illustration).

(3) Use pillows to support client's arms and hands if upper body is immobilized.

Minimizes development of dependent edema and prevents shoulder dislocation if client has upper extremity impairment.

(4) Position a pillow at lower back.

Supports lumbar vertebrae and decreases flexion of vertebrae.

(5) Place small pillow or roll under thigh.

Prevents hyperextension of knee and occlusion of popliteal artery from pressure from body weight.

(6) Place small pillow or roll under ankles.

Prevents prolonged pressure of mattress on heels.

> **NURSE ALERT** To keep feet in proper alignment, place footboard at bottom of client's feet, apply high-top sneakers on client's feet, or use other devices to maintain dorsiflexion.

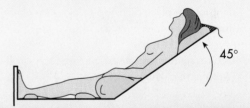

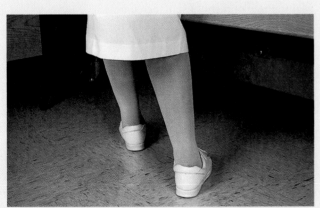

STEP 7b.(4) Nurse flexes knees with wide base of support.

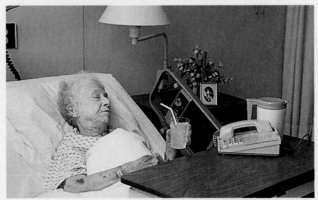

STEP 7c.(2) Raise head of bed to appropriate level.

STEPS	RATIONALE
d. Moving dependent client to 30-degree lateral (side-lying) position: This move removes pressure from bony prominences of entire back.	If client can move freely, a side-lying position with upper and lower shoulders aligned is acceptable.
(1) Lower head of bed flat if client can tolerate, keeping head of bed below 30-degree angle is desirable.	Reduces shear. Avoids working against gravity. Ensures that client will be in center of bed when turned.
(2) Place pillow near headboard.	
(3) Position client to side of bed opposite direction client is to be turned. Nurse stands on side of bed in direction client turns.	Provides room for client to turn.
(4) Prepare to turn client onto side. Flex client's knee that will not be next to mattress once turned. Place one hand on client's hip and one hand on client's shoulder.	Use of leverage makes turning to side easy.
(5) Roll client onto side rolling toward nurse.	Rolling decreases trauma to tissues. In addition, client is positioned so leverage on hip makes turning easy.
(6) Place pillow under client's head and neck.	Reduces lateral neck flexion. Decreases strain on sterno-cleidomastoid muscle.
(7) Bring dependent shoulder blade forward.	Prevents client's weight from resting directly on shoulder joint.
(8) Position both arms in slightly flexed position. Support upper arm with pillow level with shoulder; other arm, by mattress.	Improves ventilation by minimizing pressure on chest.
(9) Bring dependent hip slightly forward so that angle from hip to mattress is approximately 30 degrees.	The 30-degree lateral position reduces pressure on trochanter.
(10) Place small tuck-back pillow behind client's back. (Make by folding pillow lengthwise. Smooth area is slightly tucked under client's back.)	Provides support to maintain client on side.
(11) Place pillow under semiflexed upper leg keeping leg level at hip from groin to foot (see illustration).	Flexion prevents hyperextension of leg. Maintains leg in correct alignment. Prevents pressure on bony prominences.
(12) Place sandbag parallel to plantar surface of dependent foot or place high-top sneakers on client's feet.	Maintains dorsiflexion of foot. Prevents footdrop.
e. Logrolling to maintain neck and spinal alignment following injury or surgery:	
(1) Determine number of staff required to logroll client. (Minimum of three recommended.)	To prevent injury to client and/or caregivers, a minimum of three or four staff is recommended (Groeneveld, McKenzie, and Williams, 2001).
(2) Lower head of bed as much as client can tolerate.	Maintains alignment of spinal column.

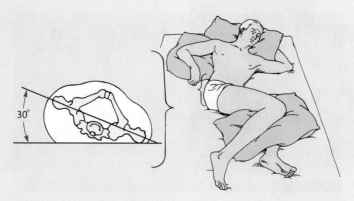

STEP 7d.(11) Thirty-degree lateral position with pillow placement.

STEPS	RATIONALE
(3) Place a pillow between the knees. (Use of a friction-reducing device [FRD] placed under client from shoulders to knees may facilitate turning.)	Prevents tension on the spinal column and adduction of the hip.
(4) Cross client's arms on chest.	Prevents injury to arms during turning.
(5) Position two nurses on side of bed to which the client will be turned. Position third nurse on other side of bed where pillows are to be placed (see illustrations).	Distributes weight equally between nurses.
(6) Fanfold or roll the FRD along side of client that will be turning.	Provides strong handles for nurse to grip FRD without slipping.
(7) With one nurse grasping FRD at client's shoulders and lower back and another at hips, roll client as one unit in a smooth, continuous motion on the count of three.	Maintains body in alignment, preventing twisting or tension of the spinal column (Groeneveld, McKenzie, and Williams, 2001).
(8) Nurse on opposite side of bed places pillows along length of client for support.	Maintains client in side-lying position.
(9) Gently lean client as a unit back toward pillows for support.	Ensures continued straight alignment of spinal column, preventing injury.
f. Moving dependent client to Sims' (semiprone) position: For this alternative to the lateral position, client lies somewhat forward onto abdomen.	This position is useful to discourage clients from rolling back to the supine position.
(1) Lower head of bed completely.	Provides for proper body alignment while client is lying down.
(2) Place client in supine position.	Prepares client for position.
(3) Position three nurses as in Step 7e. Roll client onto side, and position in lateral position. Turn partially onto abdomen, with dependent shoulder lifted out and arm placed at client's side.	Client is rolled only partially onto abdomen.
(4) Place small pillow under client's head.	Maintains proper alignment and prevents lateral neck flexion.
(5) Place pillow under flexed upper arm, supporting arm level with shoulder.	Prevents internal rotation of shoulder. Maintains alignment.
(6) Place pillow under flexed upper legs, supporting leg level with hip.	Prevents internal rotation of hip and adduction of leg. Flexion prevents hyperextension of leg. Reduces mattress pressure on knees and ankles.

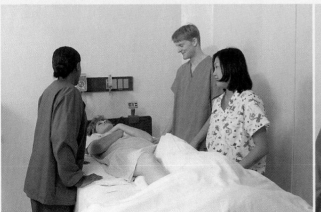
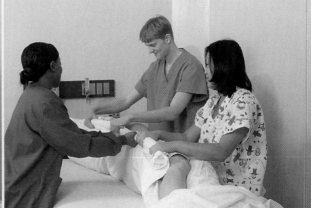

STEP 7e.(5) Logrolling a client.

STEPS	RATIONALE
(7) Place sandbags parallel to plantar surface of foot (see illustration), or apply high-top sneakers.	Maintains foot in dorsiflexion. Prevents footdrop.
g. Positioning dependent client in supine position:	
(1) Lower head of bed completely and using two nurses place client on back.	Supports normal curvature of lumbar spine.
(2) Place small rolled towel under lumbar area of back.	Provides support for lumbar spine.
(3) Place pillow under upper shoulders, neck, and head (see illustration).	Maintains correct alignment and prevents flexion contractures of cervical vertebrae.
(4) Place trochanter rolls or sandbags parallel to lateral surface of client's thighs (see illustration).	Prevents external rotation of hip.
(5) Place small pillow or roll under ankle to minimize pressure on heels.	Reduces pressure on heels, helping to prevent pressure sores.
(6) Place firm pillows against bottom of client's feet, or place high-top sneakers on client's feet.	Maintains feet in dorsiflexion. Prevents footdrop.
(7) Place pillows under pronated forearms, keeping upper arms parallel to client's body.	Reduces internal rotation of shoulder and prevents extension of elbows. Maintains correct body alignment.
(8) Place hand rolls in client's hands. Consider physical therapy referral for use of hand splints.	Reduces extension of fingers and abduction of thumb. Maintains thumb slightly adducted and in opposition to fingers.
h. Positioning client in prone position:	Prone positioning improves oxygenation in clients with severe pulmonary problems, such as adult respiratory distress syndrome (ARDS). This position is contraindicated in clients with spinal cord or facial trauma or surgery, obese clients, abdominal-pelvic surgery, hip and knee surgery, and those with increased intracranial pressure (IICP) (Marion, 2001).
(1) Lower head of bed completely and using two nurses roll client to one side.	
(2) Roll client over arm positioned close to body, with elbow straight and hand under hip. Position client on abdomen in center of bed.	Positions client correctly so alignment can be maintained.
(3) Turn client's head to one side, and support head with small pillow (see illustration).	Reduces flexion or hyperextension of cervical vertebrae.

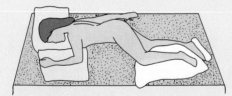

STEP 7f.(7) Sims' (semiprone) position. Note sandbag supporting right foot in dorsiflexion.

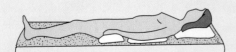

STEP 7g.(3) Pillow placement for supine position.

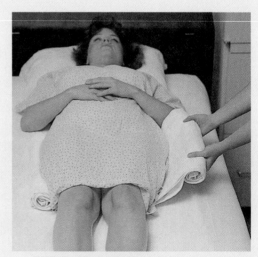

STEP 7g.(4) Positioning of trochanter roll.

STEPS	RATIONALE
(4) Place small pillow under client's abdomen below level of diaphragm (see illustration).	Reduces pressure on breasts of some female clients and decreases hyperextension of lumbar vertebrae and strain on lower back. Improves breathing by reducing mattress pressure on diaphragm.
(5) Support arms in flexed position level at shoulders.	Maintains proper body alignment. Support reduces risk of joint dislocation.
(6) Support lower legs with pillow to elevate toes (see illustration).	Prevents footdrop. Reduces external rotation of legs. Reduces mattress pressure on toes.
8 See Completion Protocol (inside front cover).	

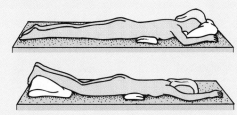

STEPS 7h.(3) and 7h.(4) Prone position with pillows in place.

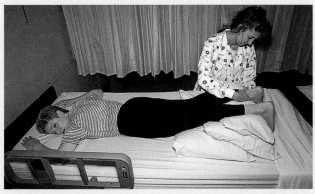

STEP 7h.(6) Prone position with pillows supporting lower legs.

EVALUATION

1 Inspect skin overlying pressure areas for erythema (redness) and blanching. Observe again in 60 minutes.
2 Ask client to describe level of comfort.
3 Observe client's body alignment and position.
4 Ask client to identify benefits of position changes and correct body alignment.

Unexpected Outcomes and Related Interventions

1 Client develops areas of abnormal reactive hyperemia, blistering, or skin irritation.
a. Change client's position more frequently.
b. Avoid prolonged pressure on any one pressure area.
c. Consider applying pressure relief support surface as indicated.
2 Client reports discomfort from stretching because of altered alignment.
a. Readjust position according to client's comfort level.
3 Client turns back to same position frequently and expresses discomfort with alternative positions.
a. Reinforce the rationale for position changes.
b. Provide diversional activities in various positions.
c. Identify client's perception of position preference and attempt to create incentive for compliance with alternative positions.

4 Client complains of respiratory distress.
a. Readjust client's position.

Recording and Reporting

- Describe client's previous position, new position, and use of supportive devices. Include skin assessment, tolerance to position, and instruction to client and family.

Sample Documentation

0800 Turned from back to left lateral position. Area of erythema approximately 3 cm in diameter noted over coccyx. Blanches easily. Urged not to lie on back.

1000 Found lying on back. Turned to right side and supported with pillows. Coccyx remains reddened, blanches to fingertip pressure.

Special Considerations
Pediatric Considerations

- Encourage children to be as active as their condition and restrictive devices allow. Materials or objects to stimulate activity and encouragement and participation of others must be available (Hockenberry and Wilson, 2007).

Geriatric Considerations

- Immobilized older adult clients are at higher risk of developing complications that affect all body systems including muscle atrophy, contractures, pressure ulcers, blood clots, pneumonia, constipation, urinary stasis, depression, and mental confusion (Jitramontree, 2001).
- Activity is especially important in older adults to maintain functional status (Meiner and Lueckenotte, 2006).
- In the presence of thin, fragile skin and/or nutritionally compromised state, lubricants or protective films or padding can reduce friction injury (see Chapter 23).

Home Care Considerations

- Teach family members body mechanics.
- In the absence of a hospital bed and equipment, creative adaptation will be required.
- Consider the need for a bed that places the bedridden client at caregiver's waist level.
- Teach caregivers to change client's position every 1 to 2 hours if possible, to maintain musculoskeletal alignment, and to reduce pressure on bony prominences. Develop a realistic turning schedule that is posted.

PROCEDURAL GUIDELINE 6-1

Applying Elastic Stockings and Sequential Compression Device

Delegation Considerations

The skill of applying elastic stockings and SCD may be delegated to assistive personnel (AP). The nurse initially determines the size of elastic stockings and assesses the client's lower extremities for any signs and symptoms of DVTs or impaired circulation.

- Inform AP to remove the SCD sleeves before allowing client to get out of bed.

Equipment

- Tape measure
- Powder or cornstarch (optional)
- Elastic support stockings, SCD (motor), disposable SCD sleeve(s), tubing assembly

Procedural Steps

1 **See Standard Protocol.**
2 Assess client for risk factors in Virchow's triad:
a. *Hypercoagulability* (i.e., clotting disorders, fever, dehydration)
b. *Venous wall abnormalities* (i.e., orthopedic surgery, varicose veins, atherosclerosis)
c. *Blood stasis* (i.e., immobility, obesity, pregnancy)
3 Observe for contraindications for use of elastic stockings or SCD:
a. Dermatitis or open skin lesions
b. Recent skin graft
c. Decreased circulation in lower extremities as evidenced by cyanotic, cool extremities and/or gangrenous conditions affecting the lower limb(s)

4 Assess condition of client's skin and circulation to the legs (i.e., presence of pedal pulses, edema, discoloration of skin, temperature, lesions, cuts).
5 Obtain physician's order.
6 Explain procedure and reasons for applying elastic stockings and SCD.
7 Use tape measure to measure client's legs to determine proper elastic stockings and SCD sleeve size. Follow manufacturer's directions.
8 Position client in supine position. Elevate head of bed to comfortable level.
9 It is optional to apply a small amount of powder or cornstarch to legs, provided client does not have sensitivity to either.
10 Apply elastic stockings:
a. Turn elastic stocking inside out by placing one hand into the sock, holding toe of sock with other hand, and pulling (see illustration).
b. Place client's toes into foot of elastic stocking, making sure that sock is smooth (see illustration).
c. Slide remaining portion of sock over client's foot, being sure that the toes are covered. Make sure the foot fits into the toe and heel position of the sock. Sock will now be right side out (see illustration).
d. Slide sock up over client's calf until sock is completely extended. Be sure sock is smooth and no ridges or wrinkles are present (see illustration).
e. Instruct client not to roll socks partially down.
11 Apply SCD sleeves:
a. Remove SCD sleeves from plastic, unfold, and flatten.
b. Arrange SCD sleeve under client's leg according to leg position indicated on inner lining of sleeve (see illustration).

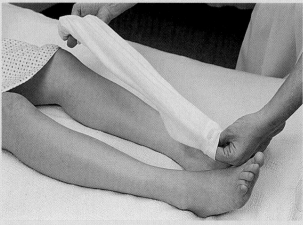

STEP 10a. Turn stocking inside out; hold toe and pull through.

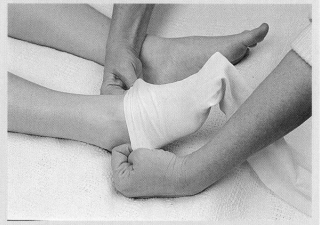

STEP 10c. Slide remaining portion of sock over foot.

PROCEDURAL GUIDELINE 6-1—cont'd

c. Place client's leg on SCD sleeve.

d. Back of ankle should line up with the ankle marking on inner lining of sleeve.

e. Position back of knee with the popliteal opening (see illustration).

f. Wrap SCD sleeves securely around client's leg.

g. Check fit of SCD sleeves by placing two fingers between client's leg and sleeve (see illustration).

12 Attach SCD sleeve's connector to plug on mechanical unit. Arrows on connector line up with arrows on plug from mechanical unit (see illustration).

13 Turn mechanical unit on. Green light indicates unit is functioning.

14 Monitor functioning SCD through one full cycle of inflation and deflation.

15 Follow completion protocol.

16 Remove SCD sleeves at least once per shift.

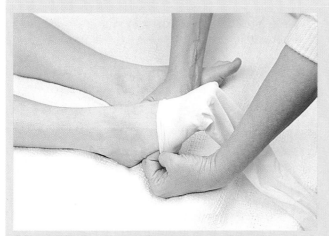

STEP 10b. Place toes into foot of stocking.

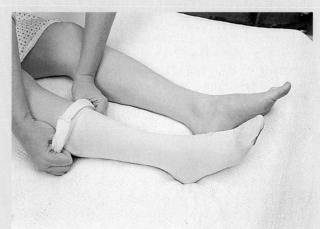

STEP 10d. Slide sock up leg until completely extended.

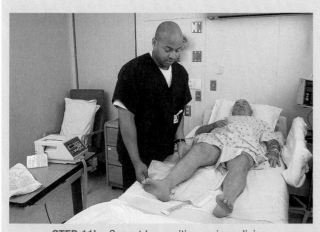

STEP 11b. Correct leg position on inner lining.

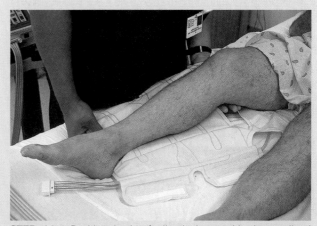

STEP 11e. Position back of client's knee with the popliteal opening.

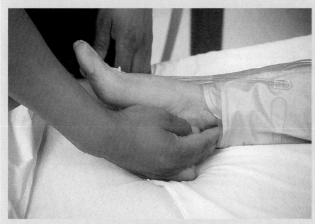

STEP 11g. Check fit of SCD sleeve.

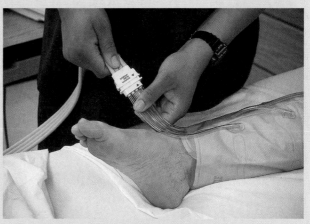

STEP 12 Align arrows when connecting to mechanical unit.

SKILL 6.2 Using Safe and Effective Transfer Techniques

Transferring is a nursing skill that assists the dependent client or the client with restricted mobility regain optimal independence as quickly as possible. It benefits the client psychologically by increasing social activity and mental stimulation and providing a change in environment (Konradi and Anglin, 2001). Thus mobilization plays a crucial role in the client's rehabilitation.

Transferring clients is another high-risk task for caregivers (Nelson and Baptiste, 2004). The nurse must be aware of the client's motor deficits, ability to aid in transfer, and body weight. As a rule of thumb, nurses should always consider mechanical lifts to help. If not available, consider a lift team to transfer clients safely. A lift team consists of two physically fit people competent in lifting techniques and who use client handling equipment to perform high-risk transfers (Nelson and Baptiste, 2004).

Many special problems must be considered in transfer. A client who has been immobile for several days or longer may be weak or dizzy or may develop orthostatic hypotension (a drop in blood pressure) when transferred. A client with neurological deficits may have paresis (muscle weakness) or paralysis unilaterally or bilaterally, which complicates safe transfer. A flaccid arm may sustain injury during transfer if unsupported. As a general rule, a nurse uses a transfer (gait) belt and obtains assistance for mobilization of such clients.

Client assessment is a key step prior to transfer. Client characteristics help nurses determine the safest equipment and best techniques to position and transfer clients (Nelson and others, 2003). Assessment guidelines developed by a Veterans Administration Hospital research team are included in this skill.

ASSESSMENT

1 Assess client's ability to bear weight, height and weight, and muscle strength of legs and upper arms. Compare right with left sides. *Rationale: Determines client's ability to assist nurse in handling and movement (Nelson and others, 2003).*
2 Assess joint mobility and limitations caused by contractures or discomfort. Assess for history of osteoporosis. *Rationale: Osteoporosis increases risk of pathological fractures with minimal stress.*
3 Assess vision, hearing, and altered sensation. Assess cognitive status, ability to follow verbal instructions, and appropriateness of response to simple commands. *Rationale: Determines the extent to which the client comprehends instructions and is able to assist during a transfer.*
4 Determine the position and functioning of IV tubing and poles, need for oxygen therapy, Foley catheter, surgical drains, and other drains or tubes. *Rationale: Prevents accidental removal of client's tubes and drains. Affects the way transfer is performed.*

5 Assess the need for prescribed analgesic medication before transfer. Plan activity for the period in which adequate pain relief is apparent without dizziness or excessive sedation. *Rationale: Analgesics enhance client's ability to tolerate movement. Peak levels vary according to the specific analgesic and route of administration.*
6 Assess vital signs. *Rationale: Vital sign changes such as increased pulse and respirations may indicate activity intolerance (see Chapter 11).*
7 Assess presence of weakness, dizziness, or orthostatic hypotension. *Rationale: Determines risk of fainting or falling during transfer.*
8 Consider type of equipment or assistive device needed. *Rationale: Ensures safer transfer.*

PLANNING

Expected Outcomes focus on improving the client's functional abilities and strength. It is also essential to promote body alignment and safety.

1 Client dangles legs or sits without dizziness, weakness, or orthostatic hypotension.
2 Client transfers without injury.
3 Client tolerates sitting in chair 30 to 40 minutes and is able to shift weight independently, at least every 15 minutes.
4 Client expresses benefit from change of environment while in the chair.

Delegation Considerations

The skills of effective transfer techniques may be delegated. The nurse supervises personnel during the transfer of clients who are transferred for the first time after prolonged bed rest, extensive surgery, critical illness, or spinal cord trauma. The nurse directs personnel by:
• Explaining how to adapt skill for specific client.
• Reviewing what to observe and report back to nurse such as client's ability to assist during transfer or client's report of discomfort or pain.

Equipment

• Nonskid shoes
• Bath blankets, pillows
• Transfer belt, sling or lap board (as needed)
• Slide board (friction-reducing board); air-assisted lateral transfer device
• Wheelchair: Position chair at 45-degree angle to bed, lock brakes, remove footrests, lock bed brakes
• Stretcher: Position at right angle (90 degrees) to bed, lock brakes on stretcher, lock brakes on bed
• Mechanical/hydraulic (Hoyer) lift: Use frame, canvas strips or chains, and hammock or canvas strips
• Ceiling lift and appropriate sling
• (Option: powered standing assist lift)

IMPLEMENTATION *for Using Safe and Effective Transfer Techniques*

STEPS	RATIONALE

1 See Standard Protocol (inside front cover).

2 Transferring client from bed to chair with bed in low position:

a. Position the chair or wheelchair so that the move will be toward client's stronger side. Chair should be at an appropriate distance to allow client participation and safety.

Facilitates balance and movement.

b. Lower bed to lowest position. Lower side rails, and turn client to one side with knees flexed.

c. Raise head of bed to highest position. Wait a few minutes and ask if client feels dizzy. Face client with feet comfortably apart and a broad base of support.

Minimizes onset of orthostatic hypotension (Dingle, 2003). Do not leave client unattended during dangling. Maximizes nurse's stability and balance and prevents twisting that could result in muscle strain.

d. Can client bear weight?

  (1) Fully—caregiver assistance not needed; standby for safety as needed.

  (2) Partially and patient is cooperative—Use stand and pivot technique:

    (a) Face client with feet comfortably apart and a broad base of support.

Maximizes nurse's stability and balance and prevents twisting that could result in muscle strain.

    (b) Assist client to sitting position. Have client use arm next to mattress and push while you help lift upper body as client's legs swing over edge of bed (see illustration).

Positions client on side of bed with minimal twisting effort by nurse.

    (c) Apply transfer or gait belt with handles. Option: Use powered standing assist lift.

Transfer belt allows nurse to maintain stability of client during transfer without injuring hands and reduces risk of falling once client stands (Hignett, 2003; Owens, Welden, and Kane, 1999; Nelson and Baptiste, 2004).

    (d) Assist client with putting on nonskid slippers or shoes and placing feet flat on the floor.

    (e) Spread feet apart. Flex hips and knees, aligning knees with client's knees (see illustration).

Flexion of knees and hips lowers nurse's center of gravity to object to be raised; aligning knees with client's allows for stabilization of knees when client stands.

COMMUNICATION TIP Psychological support and encouragement during transfer are important.

    (f) Grasp gait belt at handles.

Provides movement of client at center of gravity.

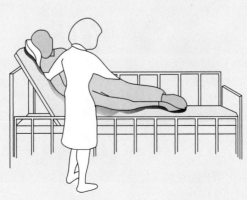

STEP 2d.(2)(b) Assisting client to sitting position.

STEPS	RATIONALE

> **NURSE ALERT** A gait belt or walking belt with handles should be used in place of the under-axilla technique. The under-axilla technique has been found to be physically stressful for nurses and uncomfortable for clients (Owens, Welden, and Kane, 1999).

(g) Rock client up to standing position on count of three while straightening hips and legs and keeping knees slightly flexed (see illustration). Unless contraindicated, instruct client to use hands to push up.

Rocking motion gives client's body momentum and requires less muscular effort to lift client.

(h) Maintain stability of client's weak leg with your knee.

Ability to stand can often be maintained in weak limb with support of knee to stabilize.

(i) Once standing, pivot client toward seat of chair. Have client then reach for arm of chair and assist with easing self into chair.

Clients should be asked to assist as much as possible with transfer (Nelson and Baptiste, 2004).

(j) Instruct client to use armrests on chair for support and ease into chair (see illustration).

Increases client's stability.

> **COMMUNICATION TIP** A useful tip is to tell the client, "When you feel the chair on the back of your knees, it is OK to sit down." This is especially helpful with clients who are fearful of falling.

(k) Flex hips and knees while lowering client into chair (see illustration).

(l) Observe client for proper alignment for sitting. Provide pillows to support affected (paralyzed) extremities.

(3) No. Client is cooperative but has no upper extremity strength. Use full-body sling lift and two nurses.

  (a) See step 3, p. 109.

(4) No. Client is cooperative and has upper extremity strength. Use seated transfer aid.

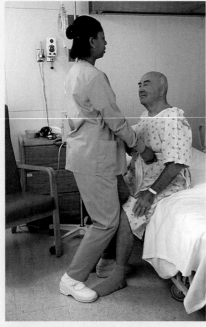

STEP 2d.(2)(e) Nurse flexes hips and knees, aligning with client's knees.

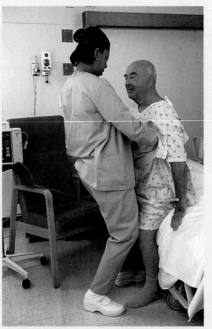

STEP 2d.(2)(g) Nurse rocks client to standing position.

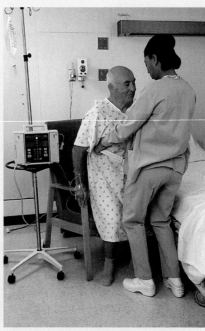

STEP 2d.(2)(j) Client uses armrest for support.

STEPS	RATIONALE
3 Using mechanical/hydraulic lift to transfer client from bed to chair (see illustration):	Research supports the use of mechanical lifts to prevent musculoskeletal injuries (Hignett, 2003).
a. Ask another caregiver to assist. Bring lift to bedside. Option: Use ceiling lift.	Before using lift, be thoroughly familiar with its operation.

> **COMMUNICATION TIP** A mechanical lift may frighten the client. Reassurance and ability to convey knowledge of procedure by caregivers will decrease anxiety.

STEPS	RATIONALE
b. Position chair near bed, and allow adequate space to maneuver lift.	Prepares environment for safe use of lift and subsequent transfer.
c. Raise bed to high position with mattress flat. Lower side rails on both sides, with nurse on each side.	Allows nurse to use proper body mechanics. Use two caregivers with a full body sling lift (Nelson and others, 2003).
d. Roll client on side away from nurse and lift.	Positions client for use of lift sling.
e. Place hammock or canvas strips under client to form sling. With two canvas pieces, lower edge fits under client's knees (wide piece), and upper edge fits under client's shoulders (narrow piece).	Two types of seats are supplied with mechanical/hydraulic lift: Hammock style is better for clients who are flaccid, weak, and need support; canvas strips can be used for clients with normal muscle tone. Hooks should face away from client's skin. Place sling under client's center of gravity and greatest portion of body weight.
f. Raise bed rail.	Maintains client safety.
g. Go to opposite side of bed, and lower side rail.	Keeps the device balanced and prevents injury from bumping against objects.
h. Roll client to opposite side, and pull hammock (strips) through.	Completes positioning of client on mechanical/hydraulic sling.
i. Roll client supine onto canvas seat.	Sling should extend from shoulders to knees (hammock) to support client's body weight equally.
j. Remove client's glasses, if appropriate.	Swivel bar is close to client's head and could break eyeglasses.
k. Place lift's horseshoe bar under side of bed (on side with chair).	Positions lift efficiently and promotes smooth transfer.

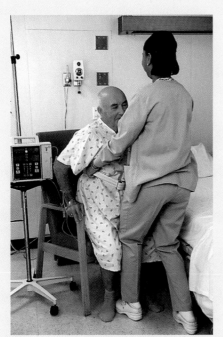

STEP 2d.(2)(k) Nurse eases client into chair.

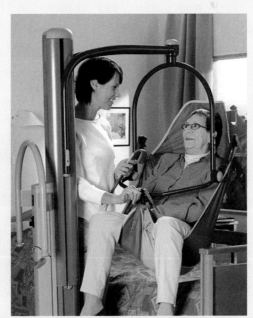

STEP 3 Mechanical (Hoyer) lift. (Courtesy Arjo, Morton Grove, Illinois.)

STEPS	RATIONALE
l. Lower horizontal bar to sling level by releasing hydraulic valve. Lock valve.	Positions hydraulic lift close to client. Locking valve prevents injury to client.
m. Attach hooks on strap (chain) to holes in sling. Short chains or straps hook to top holes of sling; longer chains hook to bottom of sling.	Secures hydraulic lift to sling.
n. Elevate head of bed.	Positions client in sitting position.
o. Fold client's arms over chest.	Prevents injury to client's arms.
p. Pump hydraulic handle using long, slow, even strokes until client is raised off bed.	Ensures safe support of client during elevation.
q. Use steering handle to pull lift from bed and maneuver to chair.	Moves client from bed to chair.
r. Roll base around chair.	Positions lift in front of the chair in which client is to be transferred.
s. Release check valve slowly (turn to left), and lower client into chair.	Safely guides client into back of chair as seat descends.

> **NURSE ALERT** Apply brakes on wheelchair. If transferring to a chair or commode, have another caregiver hold on to the chair or commode to prevent movement or slippage while client is lowered.

STEPS	RATIONALE
t. Close check valve as soon as client is down and straps can be released.	If valve is left open, boom may continue to lower and injure client.
u. Remove straps and mechanical/hydraulic lift.	Prevents damage to skin and underlying tissues from canvas or hooks.
v. Check client's sitting alignment, and correct if necessary.	Prevents injury from poor posture.
4 Transferring client from bed to stretcher:	
a. Lower head of bed as much as client can tolerate.	Maintains alignment of spinal column during transfer.
b. Can client assist?	
(1) Fully. Caregiver assistance not needed; stand by for safety as needed while client moves laterally to stretcher.	Nurse prevents fall between bed and stretcher.
(2) Partially or not at all. Client weighs more than 200 pounds. Use a mechanical lateral transfer aid or a friction-reducing device (see illustration) and three caregivers.	Transfer slide boards are made of smooth, low-friction material to ease sliding from bed to stretcher (Nelson and others, 2003).
(a) Cross client's arms on chest.	Prevents injury to arms during transfer.
(b) To place slide board under client, position two nurses on side of bed to which the client will be turned. Position third nurse on other side of bed.	Distributes weight equally between nurses.

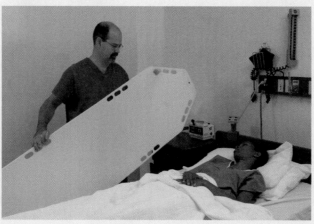

STEP 4b.(2) Slide board.

STEPS	RATIONALE
(c) Fanfold the drawsheet on both sides.	Provides strong handles in order to grip the drawsheet without slipping.
(d) Using the count of three, turn client onto side as one unit with a smooth, continuous motion.	Maintains body in alignment, preventing stress on any part of the body.
(e) Place slide board or friction-reducing device under client (see illustration).	Prevents friction from contact of skin with board.
(f) Gently roll client back onto slide board or device.	
(g) Line up the stretcher with the bed. Lock brakes on stretcher and bed.	Ensures the stretcher or bed does not move during transfer.
(h) Two nurses position themselves on side of stretcher, while third nurse positions self on side of bed without stretcher. The destination surface should be ½ inch lower.	Use of gravity to assist transfer makes lateral transfer easier.

> **NURSE ALERT** A nurse may also be positioned at head of client's bed to protect and support client's neck and head if client is weak or unable to assist.

(i) Fanfold drawsheet; using the count of three, the two nurses pull slide board or friction-reducing device with client onto stretcher while the third nurse holds the slide board in place (see illustration).	Slide board remains stationary and provides slippery surface to reduce friction and allows client to transfer easily to stretcher.

(3) Partially or not at all. Client weighs less than 200 pounds. Use friction-reducing device and two caregivers.

    (a) Follow Step 4b.(2) using only two caregivers.

5 See Completion Protocol (inside front cover).

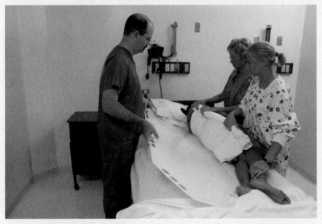

STEP 4b.(2)(e) Placing slide board under drawsheet.

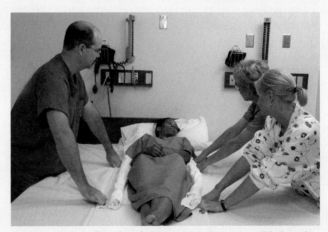

STEP 4b.(2)(i) Transfer of client to stretcher using slide board.

EVALUATION

1 Monitor vital signs. Ask if client feels dizzy.
2 Ask if client experienced pain or discomfort during transfer. Observe client's ability to bear weight (or avoid bearing weight if prescribed), ability to pivot, and number of personnel needed.
3 Monitor length of time client sits in chair and ability to shift weight every 15 minutes.
4 Ask client to describe response to environmental and position changes.

Unexpected Outcomes and Related Interventions

1 Client's weakness of lower extremities does not permit active transfer.
a. Consider physical therapy consultation.
b. Develop a plan for isotonic or isometric leg-strengthening exercises to be done while lying in bed or sitting in chair.
c. Use a transfer (gait) belt for balance and support.

2 Client tends to bear weight on non–weight-bearing leg.
a. Have another caregiver support affected leg as a reminder.
b. Use a transfer (gait) belt to facilitate balance and control.
3 Client sustains injury on transfer.
a. Evaluate incident that caused injury (e.g., assessment inadequate, change in client status, improper use of equipment).
b. Complete incident report according to institution policy.

Recording and Reporting

- Client's ability to bear weight and pivot, number of personnel needed to assist, and length of time in chair

Sample Documentation

0800 Transferred client from bed to chair with gait belt and assistance of one. Cooperative and able to stand erect with encouragement.

0815 Requested to return to bed. Stated, "I'm so tired, I just can't sit up any longer." Needed assistance of two with transfer back to bed. Knees buckled and legs were shaking during attempt to stand. Vital signs remained within normal limits.

Special Considerations
Pediatric Considerations

- Children's activities always require special safety precautions such as never leaving a child unattended, encouraging parent participation whenever possible, and ensuring activities are developmentally appropriate for age.

Geriatric Considerations

- Older persons who fear falling may be reluctant to move from bed to chair.
- Older adult clients who are depressed often prefer to stay in bed, especially if they are accustomed to being very independent and active and now need assistance.

Home Care Considerations

- Transfer ability at home is greatly enhanced by prior teaching of family, assessment of home for safety risks and functionality, and provision of applicable aids.
- Family should practice transfer in hospital to achieve success before taking client home.
- Alternatively, client (if living alone) practices activities as they will be performed at home. Clients are taught to transfer to armchairs for ease of rising and sitting.

SKILL 6.3 Assisting with Ambulation

In the normal walking posture, the head is erect; the cervical, thoracic, and lumbar vertebrae are aligned; the hips and knees have slight flexion; and the arms swing freely. Illness, surgery, injury, and prolonged bed rest can reduce activity tolerance so that assistance is required. Clients with hemiparesis (one-sided weakness) have difficulty with balance. Temporary or permanent damage to the musculoskeletal or nervous system may necessitate use of an assistive device such as a cane, crutches, or walker (see Skill 6.4). Clients with altered cardiovascular or respiratory function or prolonged bed rest may experience difficulty with ambulation, evidenced by chest pain, altered vital signs, dyspnea, orthostatic hypotension, or fatigue.

ASSESSMENT

1 Assess client's most recent activity experience, including distance ambulated and tolerance of activity. *Rationale: This facilitates realistic planning and identifies degree of assistance needed.*
2 Determine the best time to ambulate, considering other scheduled activities such as bathing. *Rationale: Rest is needed after activities requiring exertion and after meals.*
3 Check the availability of hand rails on the walls. Consider whether the assistance of one or two caregivers is required, and determine the need for assistive devices.

4 Assess client's motivation and ability to understand instructions and cooperate. *Rationale: Comparing this activity with client plans for the home environment often enhances motivation.*
5 Assess client's ability to bear weight. *Rationale: Determines degree of assistance client needs. For safety, another person may be needed initially to assist with client ambulation. Allow the client as much independence as possible.*
6 Assess for orthostatic hypotension and medications that may alter stability, including antihypertensive or narcotic medications. *Rationale: These drugs may cause hypotension, dizziness, or instability.*
7 Assess baseline vital signs before beginning ambulation. *Rationale: Post ambulation vital signs can be compared to baseline to determine client's activity tolerance and determine if client is experiencing orthostatic hypotension.*

PLANNING

Expected Outcomes focus on developing activity and rest patterns that support increased tolerance of activity. It is essential that these are tailored to each client's needs and abilities.
1 Client will ambulate without episode of injury.
2 Client is able to ambulate without excessive fatigue or dizziness.

3 Client maintains respirations, pulse, and blood pressure within 10% of resting values.

4 Client maintains erect posture while standing and walking.

Delegation Considerations

The skill of assisting the client with ambulation may be delegated. The nurse directs personnel by:

- Explaining how to adapt skill for specific client, such as obtaining an IV pole for a client with continuous IV fluids.

- Reviewing what to observe and report back to nurse, such as the distance the client was able to ambulate without fatigue.

Equipment

- Robe
- Nonskid footwear
- Portable IV pole (if needed)
- Transfer (gait) belt

IMPLEMENTATION *for Assisting with Ambulation*

STEPS	RATIONALE

1 See Standard Protocol (inside front cover).

> **COMMUNICATION TIP** Encourage client to move slowly at own pace, maintain erect posture, and look straight ahead.

2 Remove sequential compression stockings if present and assist client with putting on shoes or slippers with nonskid soles.	Prevents client from becoming tangled in cord. Shoes or slippers provide stable walking support.
3 Decide with client how far to ambulate.	Determines mutual goal.
4 Raise head of bed to highest position. Wait a few minutes and ask if client feels dizzy. Assist client in bed to a dangling position on side of bed. Have the client take a few deep breaths, until balance is gained. Have client move legs and feet while dangling (see illustration).	Allows a few minutes for circulation to equilibrate. Prevents orthostatic hypotension and potential injuries (Dingle, 2003; Kenny, 2000).
5 Ask if client feels dizzy or light-headed. If client appears light-headed, recheck blood pressure.	Allows nurse to detect orthostatic hypotension before ambulation begins.
6 Apply transfer (gait) belt around client's waist.	Transfer belt allows nurse to maintain stability of client during ambulation and reduces risk of falling (Hignett, 2003; Owens, 2000).
7 Assist client to stand at the bedside. Encourage to stand fully erect with shoulders back and looking ahead (not at the floor).	Standing at bedside allows client opportunity to stabilize before ambulating.

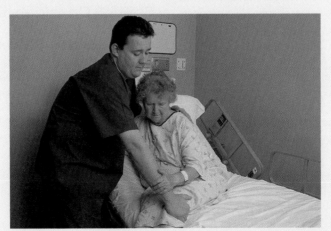

STEP 4 Client dangling. (From DeWit SC: *Fundamental concepts and skills for nursing,* ed 2, Philadelphia, 2005, Saunders.)

STEPS	RATIONALE
8 If client is unstable, seat client. Consider need for additional help. If client is very heavy, unstable, or fearful, use a sit-to-stand lift.	Provides added stability. Lift provides maximum safety for both client and caregiver if client is unstable.
9 If client has an IV line, place the IV pole on the same side as the site of infusion, and instruct client to hold and push the pole while ambulating.	
10 If a Foley catheter is present, client or caregiver carries the bag below the level of the bladder and prevents tension on the tubing.	Prevents reflux of urine from the bag back into bladder.
11 Take a few steps supporting client with one arm around the waist and the other under the elbow of the flexed arm. Grasp transfer (gait) belt handles. Option: use ambulation lift/ceiling lift with gait harness for more dependent clients who are now walking for first time after being in bed.	This provides balance and facilitates lowering client to the floor if client is unable to continue because of weakness or dizziness.
12 When ambulating in a hallway, position client between yourself and the wall. Encourage client to use hand rails if available.	The wall provides stable support for clients who start to fall away from nurse.
13 See Completion Protocol (inside front cover).	

EVALUATION

1 Observe ambulation and tolerance of ambulation, noting the frequency of rest periods.
2 Compare client's heart rate, respiratory rate, and blood pressure with baseline values immediately after ambulation and again after 5 minutes of rest.
3 Observe client's body alignment and balance while standing and walking.

Unexpected Outcomes and Related Interventions

1 Vital signs are altered: pulse more than 10% to 20% over resting rate or greater than 120 beats per minute; systolic blood pressure shows orthostatic changes; or dyspnea, labored breathing, and wheezing present. Client reports feelings of excessive fatigue or weakness.
a. Plan activity after adequate rest period.
b. Pace activity to proceed more slowly, and allow time to stop and rest at regular intervals. Sitting periodically may be helpful.
c. Assistive devices such as a cane or walker may decrease energy required (see Skill 6.4).
2 Client starts to fall.
a. Call for help.
b. Put both arms around client's waist from behind and spread feet apart for a broad base of support.
c. If necessary, ease client slowly to the floor, bending knees to prevent strain on back muscles.
d. Stay with client until assistance arrives to help lift client to wheelchair.

Recording and Reporting

• Record and report distance ambulated, client's tolerance, and any changes in vital signs.

Sample Documentation

1300 Ambulated 100 feet in hall with assistance of one. Gait steady. States, "I am so tired, I don't know if I can make it back to my room." BP 160/82, HR 120. Placed in wheelchair.

1305 Back in bed with assistance. BP 145/78, HR 92. Denies dizziness.

Special Considerations
Geriatric Considerations

• Older clients are often fearful of falling when ambulatory. Encouragement, reassurance, and assistance from family or caregiver decrease anxiety.
• Older adults may need more time in the morning to resume activity.

Assistive devices (i.e., canes, crutches, and walkers) are usually recommended for clients who cannot bear full weight on one or more joints of the lower extremities. Other indications for their use are instability, poor balance, or pain in weight bearing. It is important for the nurse to know the client's weight-bearing status and any specific movement precautions ordered by the physician. The wrong weight-bearing status or improper movement can cause further damage to the injured extremity (Phipps and others, 2007).

Non–weight-bearing status requires the client to support weight on the assistive device and the unaffected limb. The affected leg is kept off the floor at all times. Partial or touch-down weight bearing is similar to that for non–weight-bearing, but either limb can be advanced initially. Partial weight bearing more closely approximates normal walking except that less weight is placed on the affected limb. Total weight bearing allows the client to distribute equal weight between each limb with minimal weight on the assistive device. Muscle-strengthening exercises such as knee-and-foot extension (kicking leg straight out while sitting in a chair) or hip flexion (marching while sitting in a chair) and walking in parallel bars help the client increase strength and confidence before using an assistive device.

Rubber tips on the ends of assistive devices prevent slipping. Teach the client to lift rather than slide the device to reduce the possibility of catching the tips, which could cause the user to lose balance, trip, or fall. Personnel should attend to clients when using an assistive device until they are assured that the client's understanding and strength are sufficient for safe solo ambulation. Observing unaccompanied clients on their walks may reveal a need for attendance and/or additional or continued reminding about the amount of weight permitted or the distance covered.

CANES

Canes primarily increase the person's security and balance by broadening the base of support. Canes also absorb or take the body weight when necessary for mobility during partial weight-bearing periods. Instruction for use of cane-assisted ambulation is required to assess the client's balance, strength, and confidence. When canes are unilaterally used, they are most often used opposite the weak or injured side and are advanced forward with the injured or affected limb.

CRUTCHES

Persons using one or two crutches as aids for ambulation are frequently seen. The user's proficiency varies with age, condition, degree or extent of injury, musculoskeletal functions, and so on. Crutches may be a temporary aid for persons with sprains, in a cast, or following surgical treatments. Crutches may be routinely and continuously used for those with congenital or acquired musculoskeletal anomalies, neuromuscular weakness, or paralysis.

WALKERS

Constructed of aluminum or metallic alloys, walkers are lightweight aids strong enough to withstand prolonged use. Heights are adjustable for individual needs. The use of a walker facilitates partial, full, or non–weight bearing. Before using a walker, the client should understand the specific amount of weight bearing permitted or non–weight bearing to be maintained and how to use and care for the walker.

ASSESSMENT

1 Review client's chart, including medical history, previous activity level, and current activity order. *Rationale: Reveals client's current and previous health status.*

2 Assess client's physical readiness: vital signs; presence of confusion; and orientation to time, place, and person. *Rationale: Baseline vital signs offer a means of comparison after exercise. Level of orientation or confusion may reveal risk for fall.*

3 Assess ability to bear weight, ROM, and muscle strength or the presence of foot deformities. *Rationale: Determines if assistance is needed for client to ambulate safely.*

4 Assess client for any visual, perceptual, or sensory deficits. *Rationale: Determines if client can use assistive device safely.*

5 Assess environment for potential threats to client safety (e.g., bed brake, bed position, objects in pathway). Make sure floor is dry and area is well lighted. *Rationale: Provides for a safe, clutter-free environment.*

6 Assess client for discomfort. *Rationale: Determines if client needs prescribed analgesic before exercise.*

7 Assess client's understanding of technique of ambulation to be used. *Rationale: Allows client to verbalize concerns.*

8 Assess client's vital signs. *Rationale: Determines baseline to later evaluate activity tolerance.*

PLANNING

Expected Outcomes focus on improving mobility, minimizing activity intolerance, preventing risk for injury, minimizing fatigue, and improving client's knowledge.

1 Client demonstrates correct use of assistive device, gait pattern, and weight-bearing status.

2 Client rates discomfort or fatigue as 4 or less on a scale of 0 to 10 during ambulation.

3 Client performs activities with return of vital signs to baseline 3 to 5 minutes after rest.

4 Client independently performs all ADLs using assistive device safely.

Delegation Considerations

Teaching the client the use of assistive devices should not be delegated. The skill of ambulating with assistive devices may be delegated. The nurse directs personnel by:

- Explaining how to adapt skill for specific clients, such as weight-bearing status.
- Reviewing what to observe and report back to nurse, such as episodes of dizziness or fatigue.

Equipment

- Ambulation device (cane, crutches, walker)
- Well-fitting, nonskid flat shoes or slippers
- Robe; well-fitting pants or dress
- Transfer (gait) belt

IMPLEMENTATION *for Teaching Use of Cane, Crutches, and Walker*

STEPS	RATIONALE
1 See Standard Protocol (inside front cover).	

> **NURSE ALERT** Make sure that surface client will walk on is clean, dry, and well lighted. Remove objects that might obstruct the pathway.

STEPS	RATIONALE
2 Prepare client for procedure.	
a. Explain reasons for exercise and demonstrate specific gait technique to client or caregiver.	Teaching and demonstration enhance learning, reduce anxiety, and encourage cooperation.

> **NURSE ALERT** Care must be taken if the client has IV tubing or a Foley catheter. Obtain an IV pole with wheels that can be pushed as the client walks. Urinary catheter drainage bags must stay below the level of the bladder, so a second person may be needed to assist.

STEPS	RATIONALE
b. Decide with client how far to ambulate.	Determines mutual goal.
c. Schedule ambulation around client's other activities.	Helps minimize client fatigue.
d. Place bed in low position.	Reduces risk of injury.
e. Help client put on well-fitting, flat shoes or nonskid slippers.	
3 Apply transfer (gait) belt. Gait belt encircles client's waist and has handles for nurse to hold while client walks. Assist client to standing position and observe balance.	Providing constant contact by nurse reduces risk of fall or injury.
4 While standing next to client's side, have client take a few steps. When using an assistive device, stand next to the client's weak side with the device on the strong side. If client has weakness or paralysis, stand on affected side.	Position of the nurse offers stability.
5 Take a few steps forward with the client, assessing client's strength and balance.	Ensures client has satisfactory strength and balance to continue.
6 If client becomes weak or dizzy, return client to bed or chair, whichever is closer.	Prevents client from falling to floor.

> **COMMUNICATION TIP** Talk to the client about risks for falls. For example, "Some medications, tests, or procedures and long periods of staying in bed may make you feel dizzy or weak. Always ask someone to help you before trying to walk on your own." Let the client who has a fear of falling know that confidence can be regained with practice.

STEPS	RATIONALE
7 Make sure that the assistive device is the appropriate height and has rubber tips.	Rubber tips increase surface tension and reduce the risk of the device slipping.

> **COMMUNICATION TIP** Let the client know that use of the ambulation device may seem awkward at first. Independence will be gained after practice. Instruct the client to use good posture and always look ahead while using the ambulation device.

STEPS	RATIONALE

8 Cane (Same steps are taught whether standard or quad canes are used.)

a. Have client hold cane on uninvolved side 4 to 6 inches (10 to 15 cm) to side of foot. Cane should extend from greater trochanter to floor. Allow approximately 15 to 30 degrees elbow flexion (Hoeman, 2002).

Offers most support when on stronger side of body. Cane and weaker leg work together with each step. If cane is too short, client will have difficulty supporting weight and be bent over and uncomfortable. As weight is taken on by hands and affected leg is lifted off floor, complete extension of elbow is necessary.

b. Place cane forward 6 to 10 inches (15 to 25 cm), keeping body weight on both legs.

Distributes body weight equally.

c. Move involved leg forward, even with the cane (see illustration).

Body weight is supported by cane and uninvolved leg.

d. Advance uninvolved leg past cane.

Aligns client's center of gravity. Returns client body weight to equal distribution.

e. Move involved leg forward, even with uninvolved leg.

f. Repeat these steps.

9 Crutches

a. Crutch measurement includes three areas: client's height, distance between crutch pad and axilla, and angle of elbow flexion. Measurements may be taken with client standing or lying down. Make sure shoes are on before performing measurements.

Measurement promotes optimal support and stability. Radial nerves that pass under axilla are superficial. If crutch is too long, it can cause pressure on axilla. Injury to nerve causes paralysis of elbow and wrist extensors, commonly called crutch palsy. If crutch is too long, shoulders are forced upward and client cannot push body off the ground. If ambulation device is too short, client will be bent over and uncomfortable.

NURSE ALERT Instruct client to report any tingling or numbness in upper torso. This may mean crutches are being used incorrectly or that they are the wrong size.

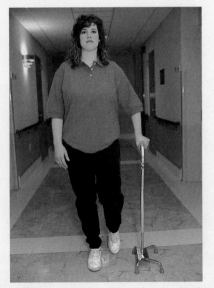

STEP 8c. Move involved leg forward even with the cane.

STEPS	RATIONALE

(1) *Standing:* Position crutches with crutch tips at point 4 to 6 inches (10 to 15 cm) to side and 4 to 6 inches in front of client's feet. Position crutch pads 1½ to 2 inches (4 to 5 cm) below axilla (Hoeman, 2002). Two or three fingers should fit between top of crutch and axilla (see illustration).

(2) *Supine:* Crutch pad should be 3 to 4 fingerwidths under axilla, with crutch tips positioned 6 inches (15 cm) lateral to client's heel (see illustration).

(3) Elbow flexion is verified with goniometer (see illustration). Handgrip should be adjusted so that client's elbow is flexed 15 to 20 degrees.

Low handgrips cause radial nerve damage. High handgrips cause client's elbow to be sharply flexed, and strength and stability of arms are decreased.

b. To use crutches, client supports self with hands and arms. Therefore strength in arm and shoulder muscles, ability to balance body in upright position, and stamina are necessary. Type of gait client uses in crutch walking depends on amount of weight client is able to support with one or both legs.

c. Have client stand up from a sitting position.

(1) Move to the edge of the chair, with the strong leg slightly under chair seat.

(2) Place both of the crutches in the hand on the affected side. If chair has armrests and is heavy and solid enough to avoid tipping, one armrest and both crutches may be used for bracing while rising. If the chair is lightweight, both armrests should be used for even bracing.

Balance can be lost or chairs tipped with uneven or one-sided pressure.

(3) Push down on the crutch hand rests while raising the body to a standing position.

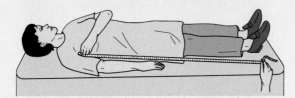

STEP 9a.(1) Top of crutch.

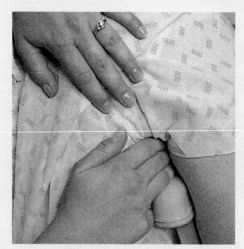

STEP 9a.(2) Measuring length of crutch.

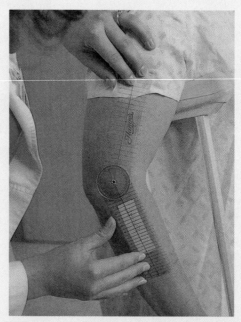

STEP 9a.(3) Goniometer determines elbow flexion.

STEPS	RATIONALE

d. Choose appropriate crutch gait (darkened areas in illustrations indicate moving foot).

  (1) *Four-point gait:*

    (a) Begin in tripod position (see illustration). Crutches are placed 6 inches (15 cm) in front and 6 inches to side of each foot. Posture should be erect head and neck, straight vertebrae, and extended hips and knees.

    (b) Move right crutch forward 4 to 6 inches (10 to 15 cm) (see illustration).

    (c) Move left foot forward to level of left crutch (see illustration).

    (d) Move left crutch forward 4 to 6 inches (see illustration).

    (e) Move right foot forward to level of right crutch (see illustration).

    (f) Repeat sequence.

Most stable of crutch gaits because it provides at least three points of support at all times. Requires weight bearing on both legs. Often used when client has paralysis, as in spastic children with cerebral palsy (Hockenberry and Wilson, 2007). May also be used for arthritic clients. Improves client's balance by providing wider base of support.

Crutch and foot position are similar to arm and foot position during normal walking.

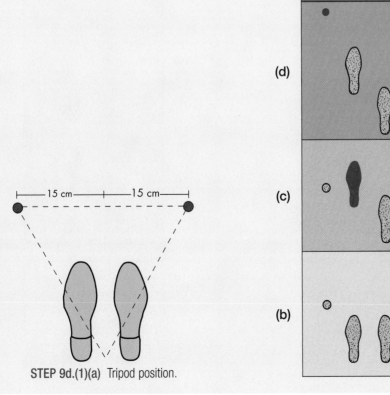

STEP 9d.(1)(a) Tripod position.

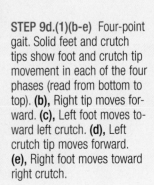

STEP 9d.(1)(b-e) Four-point gait. Solid feet and crutch tips show foot and crutch tip movement in each of the four phases (read from bottom to top). **(b),** Right tip moves forward. **(c),** Left foot moves toward left crutch. **(d),** Left crutch tip moves forward. **(e),** Right foot moves toward right crutch.

STEPS	RATIONALE

(2) *Three-point gait:* Requires client to bear all weight on one foot. Weight is borne on uninvolved leg, then on both crutches. Affected leg does not touch ground during early phase of three-point gait. May be useful for client with broken leg or sprained ankle.

(a) Begin in tripod position with weight borne on unaffected leg (see illustration).

    Improves client's balance by providing wide base of support.

(b) Advance both crutches and affected leg (see illustration).

(c) Move stronger leg forward (see illustration).

(d) Repeat sequence.

(3) *Two-point gait:* Requires at least partial weight bearing on each foot. Is faster than the four-point gait. Requires more balance because only two points support body at one time.

(a) Begin in tripod position (see illustration).

    Improves client's balance by providing wider base of support.

(b) Move left crutch and right foot forward (see illustration).

    Crutch movements are similar to arm movement during normal walking.

(c) Move right crutch and left foot forward (see illustration).

(d) Repeat sequence.

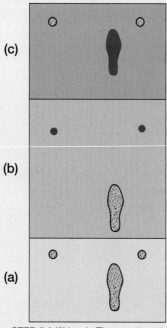

STEP 9d.(2)(a-c) Three-point gait with weight borne on unaffected right leg. Solid foot and crutch tips show weight bearing in each phase (read bottom to top).

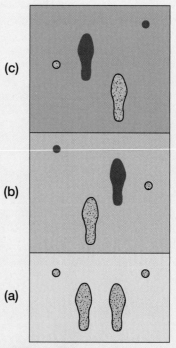

STEP 9d.(3)(a-c) Two-point gait. Solid areas indicate weight-bearing leg and crutch tips (read bottom to top).

STEPS	RATIONALE
(4) *Swing-to gait:*	Frequently used by clients whose lower extremities are paralyzed or who wear weight-supporting braces on their legs. This is the easier of the two swinging gaits. It requires the ability to bear body weight partially on both legs.
(a) Move both crutches forward.	
(b) Lift and swing legs to crutches, letting crutches support body weight.	
(c) Repeat two previous steps.	
(5) *Swing-through gait:* Requires that client have the ability to sustain partial weight bearing on both feet.	
(a) Move both crutches forward.	Increases client's base of support so that when the body swings forward, client is moving the center of gravity toward the additional support provided by crutches.
(b) Lift and swing legs through and beyond crutches.	
(6) *Climbing stairs with crutches:*	
(a) Begin in tripod position.	Improves client's balance by providing wider base of support.
(b) Client transfers body weight to crutches (see illustration).	Prepares client to transfer weight to unaffected leg when ascending first stair.
(c) Advance unaffected leg onto the step (see illustration).	Crutch adds support to affected leg. Client then shifts weight from crutches to unaffected leg.

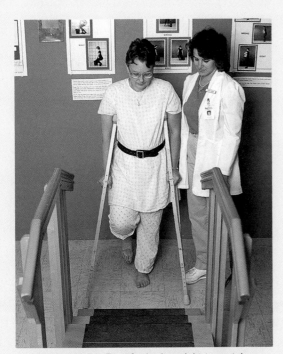

STEP 9d.(6)(b) Transfer body weight to crutches.

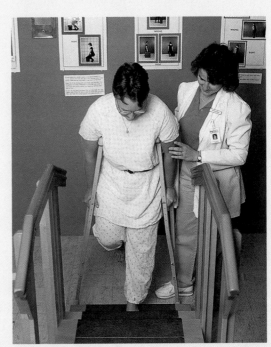

STEP 9d.(6)(c) Advance unaffected leg to stair.

STEPS	RATIONALE
(d) Align both crutches with the unaffected leg on the step (see illustration).	Maintains balance and provides wide base of support.
(e) Repeat sequence until client reaches top of stairs.	Improves client's balance by providing wider base of support.
(7) *Descending stairs with crutches:*	
(a) Begin in tripod position.	Prepares client to release support of body weight maintained by crutches.
(b) Transfer body weight to unaffected leg.	Maintains client's balance and base of support.
(c) Move crutches to stair below, and instruct client to transfer body weight to crutches and move affected leg forward.	Maintains balance and provides base of support.
(d) Move unaffected leg to stair below and align with crutches.	
(e) Repeat sequence until client reaches bottom step.	The non–weight-bearing client should be able to balance on one leg before transferring both crutches to the same hand.
(8) *Sitting in a chair:*	
(a) Transfer both crutches to the same hand and transfer weight to crutches and unaffected leg.	
(b) Grasp arm of chair with free hand and extend affected leg out while lowering into chair (see illustration).	
10 Walker	
a. Upper bar of walker should be slightly below client's waist. Elbows should be flexed at approximately 15 to 30 degrees when standing with walker, with hands on handgrips.	Walkers without wheels must be picked up and moved forward. Client must have sufficient strength to be able to move walker. A four-wheeled walker, which does not have to be picked up, is not as stable and may cause injury.

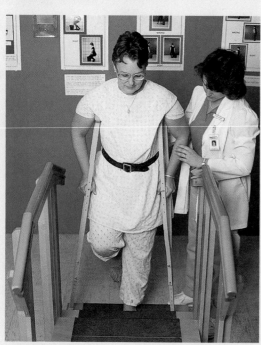

STEP 9d.(6)(d) Align crutches with unaffected leg.

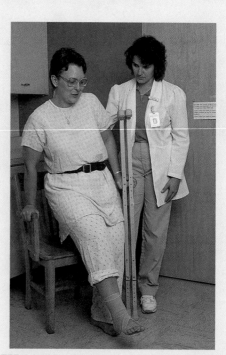

STEP 9d.(8)(b) Grasp arm of chair with free hand.

STEPS	RATIONALE

b. Assist client in ambulating.

(1) Have client stand in center of walker and grasp handgrips on upper bars.

Client balances self before attempting to walk. Position provides broad base of support between walker and client. Client then moves center of gravity toward the walker. Keeping all four feet of the walker on the floor is necessary to prevent tipping of the walker.

(2) Lift walker, moving it 6 to 8 inches (15 to 20 cm) forward, making sure all four feet of walker stay on the floor. Take a step forward with either foot. Then follow through with the other foot (see illustrations). If there is unilateral weakness after walker is advanced, instruct client to step forward with the weaker leg, support self with the arms, and follow through with the uninvolved leg. If client is unable to bear full weight on the weaker leg after advancing walker, have client swing the stronger leg through while supporting weight on hands. Instruct the client not to advance the lower extremity past the front bar of the walker.

Moving 6 to 8 inches simulates normal distance of steps. Providing constant contact of all four walker feet with the floor reduces the risk of injury or fall. Advancing with weaker extremity allows client to have maximal support of walker.

11 Have client take a few steps with the assistive device being used. If client is hemiplegic (one-sided paralysis) or has hemiparesis (one-sided weakness), stand next to client's unaffected side. Then support client by placing arm closest to client on gait belt.

Ensures client has satisfactory strength and balance to continue.

12 Take a few steps forward with client. Assess for strength and balance.

Allows client to rest.

13 If client becomes weak or dizzy, return to bed or chair, whichever is closer.

14 See Completion Protocol (inside front cover).

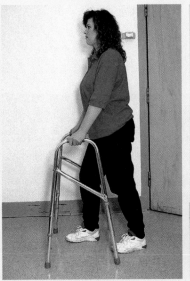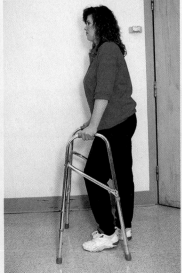

STEP 10b.(2) Lift walker, move it 6 to 8 inches, take step forward.

EVALUATION

1 Observe client using assistive device.

2 Inspect hands and axillae for redness, swelling, or skin irritation caused by using assistive device.

3 Ask client to rate level of discomfort or fatigue if present after ambulating.

4 Monitor client for postural hypotension, increased heart rate, decreased blood pressure, increased respirations, or shortness of breath during and after ambulation.

5 Ask client/family about the ease with which ADLs are performed using assistive device.

Unexpected Outcomes and Related Interventions

1 Client is unable to ambulate correctly.

a. Reassess client for correct fit of assistive device.

b. Have added assistance nearby to ensure safety.

c. Reassess comfort level.

d. Reassess muscle strength in uninvolved extremities. Alternative device may be needed.

e. Obtain physical therapy referral for gait training.

2 Client becomes dizzy and light-headed.

a. Call for assistance.

b. Have client sit or lie down on nearest chair or bed.

c. Assess client's vital signs.

d. Allow client to rest thoroughly before resuming activity.

e. Ask if client is ready to continue.

Recording and Reporting

• Record type of gait the client used, weight-bearing status, amount of assistance required, tolerance of activity, and distance walked in progress notes. Document instructions given to client and family.

• Immediately report any injury sustained during attempts to ambulate, alteration in vital signs, or inability to ambulate.

Sample Documentation

0900 Ambulated 20 feet correctly using quad cane, standby assist of one, and partial weight bearing on right lower extremity. Requested pain pills. Rates pain in right knee at 6 (scale 0 to 10). Returned to bed.

0930 Resting quietly in bed. Rates pain in right knee at 2 (scale of 0 to 10).

Special Considerations
Pediatric Considerations

• For rehabilitation of a small child who has not yet learned to walk or who is unsteady, special crutches with three or four legs provide needed stability to allow the child to maintain an upright posture and learn to walk (Hockenberry and Wilson, 2007).

Geriatric Considerations

• The older adult with arthritis may require additional time in the morning before resuming activities.

Home Care Considerations

• Client should be instructed in how to use the ambulation aid on various terrains (e.g., carpet, stairs, rough ground, inclines).

• Client should be instructed in how to maneuver around obstacles such as doors and how to use the aid when transferring, such as to and from a chair, toilet, tub, and car.

• Attach a "saddle bag" to client's walker to carry objects; caution client not to overfill to prevent forward tipping of walker.

PROCEDURAL GUIDELINE 6-2

Range-of-Motion Exercises

ROM exercises may be active, passive, or active assisted. They are active if the client is able to perform the exercise independently and passive if the exercises are performed for the client by the caregiver. In every aspect of ADLs, the nurse must encourage the client to be as independent as possible. Active and passive ROM exercises are encouraged and supervised every day by the nurse. Active ROM exercises can be incorporated into the client's ADLs (Table 6-2). Passive ROM can easily be incorporated into bathing and feeding activities. The nurse, in collaboration with the client, needs to develop a schedule for ROM activities.

Delegation Considerations

The skill of performing ROM exercises may be delegated. Clients with spinal cord or orthopedic trauma usually require exercise by nurses or physical therapists. The nurse directs personnel by:

• Explaining how to adapt skill for specific client, such as which joints need passive versus active ROM.

• Reviewing what to observe and report back to nurse, such as pain or fatigue during ROM.

Equipment

• No mechanical or physical equipment needed

Procedural Steps

1 See Standard Protocol (inside front cover).

2 Review client's chart for physical assessment findings, physician orders, medical diagnosis, medical history, and progress.

3 Obtain data on client's baseline joint function.

   a. Observe client's ability to perform ROM exercises during ADLs.

PROCEDURAL GUIDELINE 6-2—cont'd

b. Observe for limitations in joint mobility, redness or warmth over joints, joint tenderness, deformities, or crepitus produced by joint motion.

4 Determine client's or caregiver's readiness to learn. Explain all rationales for the ROM exercises, and describe and demonstrate exercises to be performed.

5 Assess client's level of comfort (on a scale of 0 to 10) before exercises.

> **NURSE ALERT** Consider premedicating client 30 minutes before ROM exercises begin, if necessary.

6 Use gloves if wound drainage or skin lesions are present.

7 Assist the client to a comfortable position, preferably sitting or lying down.

8 When performing active-assisted or passive ROM exercises (Table 6-3), support joint by holding distal and proximal areas adjacent to joint, cradling distal portion of extremity, or using cupped hand to support joint (see illustrations).

9 Complete exercises in head-to-toe sequence. Each movement should be repeated 5 times during exercise period. Inform client how these exercises are performed and how they can be incorporated into ADLs (see Table 6-2).

> **NURSE ALERT** If new resistance is noted within a joint, do not force joint motion. Consult with physician or physical therapist.

10 Observe client performing ROM activities.

11 Measure joint motion as needed.

12 Ask client to rate any discomfort on a scale of 0 to 10.

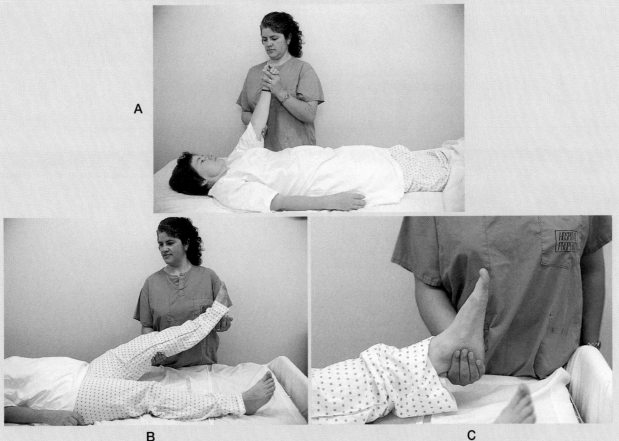

STEP 8 A, Support joint by holding distal and proximal areas adjacent to joint. **B,** Support joint by cradling distal portion of extremity. **C,** Use cupped hand to support joint.

TABLE 6-2 Incorporating Active Range-of-Motion Exercises into Activities of Daily Living

JOINT EXERCISED	ACTIVITY OF DAILY LIVING	MOVEMENT
Neck	Nodding head yes	Flexion
	Shaking head no	Rotation
	Moving right ear to right shoulder	Lateral flexion
	Moving left ear to left shoulder	Lateral flexion
Shoulder	Reaching to turn on overhead light	Flexion
	Reaching to bedside stand for book	Extension
	Applying deodorant	Abduction
	Combing hair	Flexion
Elbow	Eating, bathing, shaving, grooming	Flexion, extension
Wrist	Eating, bathing, shaving, grooming	Flexion, extension, abduction, adduction
Fingers and thumb	All activities requiring fine motor coordination (e.g., writing, eating, hobbies)	Flexion, extension, abduction, adduction, opposition
Hip	Walking	Flexion, extension
	Moving to side-lying position	Flexion, extension, abduction
	Moving from side-lying position	Extension, adduction
	Rolling feet inward	Internal rotation
	Rolling feet outward	External rotation
Knee	Walking	Flexion, extension
	Moving to and from side-lying position	Flexion, extension
Ankle	Walking	Dorisflexion, plantar flexion
	Moving toe toward head of bed	Dorsiflexion
	Moving toe toward foot of bed	Plantar flexion
Toes	Walking	Extension, flexion
	Wiggling toes	Abduction, adduction, extension, flexion

TABLE 6-3 Range-of-Motion Exercises

BODY PART	TYPE OF JOINT	TYPE OF MOVEMENT	RANGE (DEGREES)	PRIMARY MUSCLES
Neck, cervical spine	Pivotal	*Flexion:* Bring chin to rest on chest	45	Sternocleidomastoid
		Extension: Return head to erect position	45	Trapezius
		Hyperextension: Bend head back as far as possible	10	Trapezius
		Lateral flexion: Tilt head as far as possible toward each shoulder	40-45	Sternocleidomastoid
		Rotation: Turn head as far as possible in circular movement	180	Sternocleidomastoid, trapezius
Shoulder	Ball and socket	*Flexion:* Raise arm from side position forward to position above head	45-60	Coracobrachialis, deltoid
		Extension: Return head to erect position	180	Latissimus dorsi, teres major, triceps brachii
		Hyperextension: Move arm behind body, keeping elbow straight	45-60	Latissimus dorsi, teres major, deltoid
		Abduction: Raise arm to side to position above head with palm away from head	180	Deltoid, supraspinatus
		Adduction: Lower arm sideways and across body as far as possible	320	Pectoralis major
		Internal rotation: With elbow flexed, rotate shoulder by moving arm until thumb is turned inward and toward back	90	Pectoralis major, latissimus dorsi, teres major, subscapularis
		External rotation: With elbow in full circle, move arm until thumb is upward and lateral to head	90	Infraspinatus, teres major
		Circumduction: Move arm in full circle (circumduction is combination of all movements of ball-and-socket joint)	360	Deltoid, coracobrachialis, latissimus dorsi, teres major
Elbow	Hinge	*Flexion:* Bend elbow so that lower arm moves toward its shoulder joint and hand is level with shoulder	150	Biceps brachii, brachialis, brachioradialis
		Extension: Straighten elbow by lowering hand	150	Triceps brachii

TABLE 6-3 Range-of-Motion Exercises—cont'd

BODY PART	TYPE OF JOINT	TYPE OF MOVEMENT	RANGE (DEGREES)	PRIMARY MUSCLES
Forearm	Pivotal	*Supination:* Turn lower arm and hand so that palm is up	70-90	Supinator, biceps brachii
		Pronation: Turn lower arm so that palm is down	70-90	Pronator teres, pronator quadratus
Wrist	Condyloid	*Flexion:* Move palm toward inner aspect of forearm	80-90	Flexor carpi ulnaris, flexor carpi radialis
		Extension: Move fingers and hand posterior to midline	80-90	Extensor carpi radialis brevis, extensor carpi radialis longus, extensor carpi ulnaris
		Hyperextension: Bring dorsal surface of hand back as far as possible	80-90	Extensor carpi radialis brevis, extensor carpi radialis longus, extensor carpi ulnaris
		Abduction (radial deviation): Bend wrist laterally toward fifth finger with the hand prone.	up to 30	Flexor carpi radialis, extensor carpi radialis brevis, extensor carpi radialis longus
		Adduction (ulnar deviation): Bend wrist medially toward thumb with the hand prone.	30-50	Flexor carpi ulnaris, extensor carpi ulnaris
Fingers	Condyloid hinge	*Flexion:* Make fist	90	Lumbricales, interosseus volaris, interosseus dorsalis
		Extension: Straighten fingers	90	Extensor digiti quinti proprius, extensor digitorum communis, extensor indicis proprius
		Hyperextension: Bend fingers back as far as possible	30-60	Extensor digitorum
		Abduction: Bring fingers together	30	Interosseus dorsalis
		Adduction: Bring fingers together	30	Interosseus volaris
Thumb	Saddle	*Flexion:* Move thumb across palmar surface of hand	90	Flexor pollicis brevis
		Extension: Move thumb straight away from hand	90	Extensor pollicis longus, extensor pollicis brevis
		Abduction: Extend thumb laterally (usually done when placing fingers in abduction and adduction)	30	Abductor pollicis brevis and longus
		Adduction: Move thumb back toward hand	30	Adductor pollicis obliquus, adductor pollicis transversus
		Opposition: Touch thumb to each finger of same hand		Opponeus pollicis, opponeus digiti minimi
Hip	Ball and socket	*Flexion:* Move leg forward and up	90-120	Psoas major, iliacus, sartorius
		Extension: Move leg behind body	90-120	Gluteus maximus, semitendinosus, semimembranosus
		Hyperextension: Move leg behind body	30-50	Gluteus maximus, semitendinosus, semimembranosus
Knee	Hinge	*Abduction:* Move leg laterally away from body	30-50	Gluteus medius, gluteus minimus
		Adduction: Move leg back toward medial position and beyond if possible	30-50	Adductor longus, adductor brevis, adductor magnus
		Internal rotation: Turn foot and leg toward other leg	90	Gluteus medius, gluteus minimus, tensor fasciae latae
		External rotation: Turn foot and leg away from other leg	90	Obturatorius internus, obturatorius externus, quadratus femoris, piriformis, gemellus superior and inferior, gluteus maximus
		Circumduction: Move leg in circle	120-130	Psoas major, gluteus maximus, gluteus medius, adductor magnus
		Flexion: Bring heel back toward back of thigh	120-130	Biceps femoris, semitendinosus, semimembranosus, sartorius
		Extension: Return leg to floor	120-130	Rectus femoris, vastus lateralis, vastus medialis, vastus intermedius
Ankle	Hinge	*Dorsal flexion:* Move foot so that toes are pointed upward	20-30	Tibialis anterior
		Plantar flexion: Move foot so that toes are pointed downward	45-50	Gastrocnemius, soleus
Foot	Gliding	*Inversion:* Turn sole of foot medially	10 or less	Tibialis anterior, tibialis posterior
		Eversion: Turn sole of foot laterally	10 or less	Peroneus longus, peroneus brevis
Toes	Condyloid	*Flexion:* Curl toes downward	30-60	Flexor digitorum, lumbricalis pedis, flexor hallucis brevis
		Extension: Straighten toes	30-60	Extensor digitorum longus, extensor digitorum brevis, extensor hallucis longus
		Abduction: Spread toes apart	15 or less	Abductor hallucis, interosseus dorsalis
		Adduction: Bring toes together	15 or less	Adductor hallucis, interosseus plantaris

SKILL 6.5 Continuous Passive Motion Machine—for Client with Total Knee Replacement

Continuous passive motion (CPM) machines are designed to exercise many different joints, including the hip, ankle, shoulder, wrist, and fingers. Orthopedic surgeons routinely order a knee CPM machine postoperatively for a total knee arthroplasty (replacement). CPM may be initiated on the day of surgery or on the first postoperative day, according to the individual surgeon's preference. CPM machines are also often used in outpatient physical therapy or home health settings (Figure 6-3).

The purpose of the CPM machine is to mobilize the knee joint to prevent contracture, muscle atrophy, venous stasis, and thromboembolism. Passive movement of the joint can replace more strenuous exercises during the first few postoperative days. Properly used, CPM can decrease complications and shorten a client's hospital stay (Babis and others, 2001; Hammesfahr and Serafino, 2002).

The electronically controlled CPM machine flexes and extends the knee to a prescribed degree and at a set speed as ordered by the physician. A typical initial setting is 20 to 30 degrees of flexion and full extension (0 degrees) at 2 cycles per minute; however, this setting varies according to the client's condition and surgeon's preference (Ignatavicius and Workman, 2006).

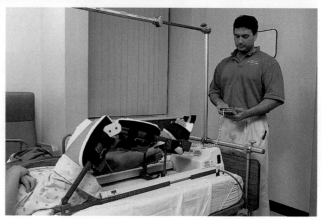

FIGURE 6-3 Use of CPM machine on knee.

ASSESSMENT

1 Check the machine's electrical cord and function of equipment. *Rationale: All electrical equipment in health care settings is routinely checked for safety. Routine observation of electrical cord and functioning of equipment each time it is used ensures electrical safety.*

2 Assess the setup of the machine before placing on bed: Check the stability of the frame, flexion/extension controls, speed controls, and on/off switch. *Rationale: Ensures that all pieces of the equipment are operational and will prevent damage to the client's knee.*

3 Assess the client's comfort on a scale of 0 to 10 before and during use. *Rationale: Determines if the client will be able to tolerate the CPM at the ordered flexion and extension.*

4 Assess client's baseline heart rate and blood pressure. *Rationale: Provides baseline to measure exercise tolerance.*

5 Assess the client's ability and willingness to learn about the CPM machine. *Rationale: Determines readiness to learn, reduces anxiety, and promotes client participation.*

6 Assess condition of skin at points where machine rubs/contacts leg and foot. *Rationale: Determines baseline for skin integrity.*

7 Assess client's ROM before therapy begins (see Procedural Guideline 6-2). *Rationale: Provides baseline to use as a measure for evaluation of effect of CPM.*

PLANNING

Expected Outcomes focus on improving joint ROM, maintaining physical mobility, and skin integrity.

1 Client increases length of time in CPM machine as ordered with no evidence of increased heart rate or increased blood pressure.

2 Client denies discomfort during or after CPM exercise.

3 Client increases flexion 6 to 7 degrees daily.

4 Client maintains intact skin throughout use of CPM.

Delegation Considerations

Assessment of the client's condition should not be delegated. Care of the client during CPM may be delegated.

- Instruct personnel to immediately report if the client reports pain.

Equipment

- CPM machine and sheepskin that is applied to the CPM machine
- Clean gloves

IMPLEMENTATION *for Continuous Passive Motion Machine—for Client with Total Knee Replacement*

STEPS	RATIONALE
1 See Standard Protocol (inside front cover).	
2 Provide analgesia as ordered 20 to 30 minutes before CPM is needed.	Assists client in tolerating exercise.
3 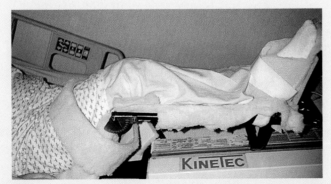 Apply gloves (if wound drainage is present).	
4 Demonstrate machine functioning before placing client's leg into the device.	Reduces anxiety and increases client cooperation.
5 Stop the machine in full extension. Place sheepskin on CPM machine.	This position allows correct fit of client's leg. Ensures all exposed hard surfaces are padded to prevent rubbing and chafing of client's skin.

COMMUNICATION TIP Discuss with client diversional activities that may be used during CPM.

STEPS	RATIONALE
6 Place client's leg in the machine, being sure to support above, below, and at knee.	Two nurses perform this step to prevent damage or injury to client or nurse.
7 Adjust CPM machine to client by lengthening and shortening appropriate section of the CPM frame.	Ensures a proper fit.
8 Center client's leg in the machine.	Avoids pressure on the lateral and medial aspects of the knee joint.
9 Align client's knee joint (bend of the knee) with the machine knee hinge, then position client's knee 2 cm below knee joint line of CPM machine.	This is extremely important because if the client's new knee is not properly aligned, the knee may be damaged (Babis and others, 2001).
10 Adjust the foot support to approximately 20 degrees of dorsiflexion to prevent footdrop.	Footdrop is an abnormal condition caused by damage of the perineal nerve and can cause abnormal gait.
11 When client's leg is in correct position, secure the Velcro straps across lower extremity (thigh) and top of foot (see illustration).	Correct placement of the thigh and foot straps prevents friction and skin breakdown.
12 Start CPM machine. Watch at least two full cycles of prescribed flexion and extension. Remove and discard gloves, if worn, and perform hand hygiene.	Ensures that CPM machine is fully operational at the preset flexion and extension modes.
13 Make sure client is comfortable. Provide client with the on/off switch. Instruct to use only if CPM machine seems to be malfunctioning.	Allows client to stop the machine if the degree of flexion/extension or speed changes, creating intolerable discomfort.
14 See Completion Protocol (inside front cover).	

STEP 11 Client's extremity correctly placed and secured to CPM machine.

EVALUATION

1 Ask client to keep a log of when the CPM machine is in use, with times and dates.
2 Observe client at the initial onset of an increase in the flexion of the machine.
3 Measaure HR or BP during CPM operation and when stopped.
4 Ask client to rate comfort level on a scale of 0 to 10.
5 Measure joint ROM achieved with CPM machine.
6 Observe skin every 2 hours for signs of breakdown.

Unexpected Outcomes and Related Interventions

1 Client cannot increase flexion.
a. Increase activities throughout the day to improve muscle strength (e.g., ambulation, physical therapy exercises).
b. Give "time-out" periods throughout the day to rest the leg.
c. Consider need for analgesia before CPM.
d. Sit client in chair, and have gravity assist with increasing knee flexion.
2 Client experiences increased pain when in CPM machine.
a. Reassess efficacy of current analgesia, and obtain new orders.
b. Release leg out of CPM machine until pain subsides.
c. Determine cause of increased pain.
3 Client develops reddened areas on heel from foot support.
a. Readjust foot in CPM machine at least every 2 hours.
b. Pad the foot support more.

Recording and Reporting

- Record joint exercised, degree of joint motion, time of CPM machine use, pain and need for analgesia, any joint abnormalities, and client's activity tolerance.
- Report immediately any resistance to range of joint motion; increased pain with CPM; and swelling, heat, or redness in joint.

Sample Documentation

1000 Medicated with two Tylenol with codeine #3 tabs 30 minutes before initiation of CPM. Functional CPM applied to left leg; able to tolerate 0 degrees extension and 40 degrees flexion at slow speed. Skin dry and intact, without evidence of breakdown.

Special Considerations

Geriatric Considerations

- Older adults who have chronic illnesses may need rehabilitation care to continue CPM because they are not able to manage the equipment in their home.
- Older adults have increased risk of skin breakdown because of decreased elasticity and increased fragility of the skin. Pressure from the CPM machine increases the risk of pressure ulcer development on the pressure points, especially the heel (Meiner and Lueckenotte, 2006).

Home Care Considerations

- Home care physical therapist may assist client/family in continuing CPM in the home.
- Be sure client/family have specific instructions regarding use of the CPM device; length of time for each session; expected outcomes; and what to do if the client experiences increased pain, the client is unable to tolerate the CPM sessions, or the equipment malfunctions (Branson and Goldstein, 2001).

Long-Term Care Considerations

- Because of insurance guidelines regarding length of stay in the hospital, most clients are discharged after a relatively short period. If the client needs additional physical therapy to maintain function of the new knee replacement and to increase flexion, client may be placed in a temporary rehabilitation or short- or long-term facility.
- Instruct client that CPM in extended care setting is needed to increase joint mobility and that client needs to actively participate in care.
- Additional physical therapy may be used in combination with CPM.

NCLEX® Style Questions

1 Mrs. Meander is an 80-year-old woman admitted for pneumonia. She is weak and frail and has an unsteady gait. A priority nursing diagnosis related to safety of this client would be:
1. Pain
2. Impaired skin integrity
3. Altered tissue perfusion
4. Risk for injury

2 You are transferring Mr. Simons, who can bear weight partially and is cooperative, from the bed to the chair for the first time. Which of the following techniques is the safest method of transfer for Mr. Simons and you?
1. Assistance is not needed.
2. Use the under-axilla technique to assist him out of the bed.
3. Transfer using a sling lift.
4. Transfer using a gait belt with stand and pivot technique.

3 Two AP ask for your assistance to transfer a 150 pound client from the bed to the stretcher. What are the appropriate responses? (Choose more than one response.)
1. "As long as we use proper body mechanics, no one will get hurt."
2. "The client only weighs 150 pounds; he can assist, so you should be able to transfer without my assistance."
3. "Use the slide board; it is more comfortable for the client, and it will protect you from injury."
4. "The three-person lift technique is recommended to ensure your safety and that of the client."

4 Mr. Williams has arrived on your unit after undergoing extensive abdominal surgery. He is awake and alert. He is refusing to be repositioned in bed. What would you assess first to determine Mr. Williams' refusal? Assess level of:
1. Consciousness
2. Pain
3. Motivation
4. Knowledge related to complications of immobility

5 Mrs. Black is admitted with an unstable spinal cord injury. The safest and most appropriate method of moving this client from side to side is to:
1. Use a slide board to move her from side to side.
2. Logroll with the assistance of at least three personnel.
3. Allow Mrs. Black to move herself so she gains independence.
4. Use a step-by-step method: Move the trunk, then hips, and finally the legs.

References for all chapters appear in Appendix D.

7

Promoting Hygiene

MEDIA RESOURCES

- **evolve** http://evolve.elsevier.com/Elkin
- **View Video!** Video Clips

Providing personal hygiene during illness or recovery promotes a client's comfort and well-being. Personal hygiene provides an opportunity for the nurse and client to interact about immediate and future emotional, social, and health-related concerns.

Because hygiene requires close contact with the client, the nurse needs to ensure as much privacy as possible and convey sensitivity and respect for personal beliefs and cultural customs (Box 7-1). Provide hygiene according to the client's usual routines and preferences. Some clients need encouragement to participate in self-care. Some clients lack the physical energy or functional status to perform self-care and need to be temporarily dependent on others to enhance the healing and recovery process. If the client cannot participate, the family or significant other may want to assist when appropriate. Family caregivers for a dependent client at home may desire to provide care or they may welcome a break from the responsibility. A full bath 3 times a week may be adequate for many older clients; optimal frequency depends on individual needs. Bathing older clients too frequently may contribute to dry skin and should be avoided.

Personal hygiene maintains skin integrity by promoting adequate circulation and hydration. The functions of intact skin include: (1) defense against infection; (2) awareness of touch, pain, heat, cold, and pressure; and (3) control of body temperature. The nurse bathes clients and changes linens when any body part becomes soiled. Problems such as incontinence, wound drainage, or diaphoresis may require frequent bathing. In addition to cleansing the skin, bathing a client has several benefits (Box 7-2).

Normally the skin is elastic, well hydrated, firm, and smooth. With age the skin becomes thinner, dry, less vascular, more fragile, and prone to bruising and tears. Bathing is an excellent opportunity to assess the skin for common skin problems (Table 7-1).

BOX 7-1 Cultural Considerations for Personal Hygiene

- For Middle-Eastern and East-Asian women, avoid uncovering the lower torso and exposing the arms.
- Orthodox Jews, Amish, Hindus, and Muslims consider touching unrelated males and females taboo. Therefore males should care for males, and females should care for females. Family members should perform personal care involving the lower torso if gender-appropriate caregivers are not available. Among Hindus and Muslims the right hand is reserved for eating and praying and the left hand is used only for cleaning gender-private areas.
- Chinese, Japanese, Koreans, and Hindus consider the upper body cleaner than the lower parts.
- Hindus consider it irreverent to show any negative nonverbal communication when washing older adults' feet (Galanti, 2004).

BOX 7-2 Benefits of Bathing

- *Cleansing the skin:* Removal of perspiration, some bacteria, sebum, and dead skin cells minimizes skin irritation and reduces the chance of infection.
- *Stimulating circulation:* Muscle activity, warm water, and stroking extremities enhance circulation.
- *Promoting range of motion (ROM):* Movement of extremities assists in maintaining joint function.
- *Reducing body odors:* Secretions and excretions from axillae and perineal areas result in body odors that are eliminated by bathing.
- *Improving self-image:* Promotes relaxation and feeling clean and comfortable. Care of hair and teeth enhances appearance and sense of well-being.

EVIDENCE IN PRACTICE

Sheppard CM, Brenner PS: The effects of bathing and skin care practices on skin quality and satisfaction with an innovative product, *J Gerontol Nurs* 26(10):36, 2000.

Researchers compared the Bag Bath/Travel Bath with traditional bathing techniques for effects on skin dryness in older adults. The researchers were interested in finding a bathing product to benefit older adults who are at risk for dry skin. The Bag Bath/Travel Bath, which contains a no-rinse surfactant, a humectant to trap moisture, and an emollient, significantly reduced overall skin dryness, especially skin flaking and scaling. There are now several commercial body cleansing systems available that contain the same ingredients as the Bag Bath/Travel Bath.

NURSING DIAGNOSES

Bathing/hygiene self-care deficit is appropriate when the focus of care is helping the client move toward independence in bathing. **Dressing/grooming self-care deficit** is appropriate when the focus is to improve a client's ability to provide self-care with oral hygiene or hair care. **Risk for impaired skin integrity** is considered when the client has reduced sensation, immobility, impaired circulation, incontinence, inadequate nutrition, or fragile skin. **Impaired skin integrity** is an appropriate diagnosis in the presence of pressure ulcers, vascular ulcerations, and blisters. **Impaired oral mucous membrane** is appropriate for oral ulcerations, erythema, and irritation. **Imbalanced nutrition: less than body requirements** is appropriate when a client's appetite and intake are diminished because of altered mucous membranes. **Disturbed body image** is often appropriate when the client loses interest in grooming or experiences hair loss.

TABLE 7-1 Common Skin Problems and Related Interventions

PROBLEM	INTERVENTIONS
Dry skin: flaky, rough texture to skin, which may crack and become infected.	Bathe less frequently; rinse away all soap or use a waterless cleanser rather than soap; increase fluid intake; use moisturizing lotion.
Acne: inflammatory papulopustular skin eruption, usually involving bacterial breakdown of sebum, typically on face, neck, shoulders, and back.	Wash hair daily. Wash skin twice daily with warm water and soap to remove oils and cosmetics (if used); cosmetics that can accumulate in pores should be used sparingly. Topical antibiotics, if prescribed, may minimize problems.
Hirsutism: excessive growth of body and facial hair, especially in women; may cause negative body image by giving women a male appearance.	Shaving is safest method; electrolysis and laser permanently remove hair by destroying hair follicles; tweezing and bleaching are temporary measures; depilatories may remove unwanted hair but may cause infection, rashes, or dermatitis.
Rashes: skin eruption from overexposure to sun or moisture or from allergic reaction; may be flat, raised, localized, or systemic; may be associated with pruritus (itching).	Wash and rinse thoroughly; apply antiseptic spray or lotion to prevent further itching and aid in healing process; warm or cold soaks relieve inflammation.
Contact dermatitis: inflammation of skin characterized by abrupt onset with erythema, pruritus, pain, and scaly, oozing lesions; usually results from contact with substance difficult to identify and eliminate.	Wash and rinse thoroughly. Identify and avoid contributing agents; provide linens rinsed and sterilized to minimize irritation.
Abrasion: scraping or rubbing away of epidermis that results in localized bleeding and later weeping of serous fluid; easily infected.	Wash with mild soap and water; observe dressings for retained moisture, which can increase risk of infection.

SKILL 7.1   Complete Bathing

The extent of the bath and the methods used depend on the client's ability to participate, the condition of the client's skin, and in some settings, time of day (Box 7-3). A partial bath consists of bathing only body parts that would cause discomfort or odor if left unbathed, such as hands, face, breasts, perineal area, and axillae. Clients who cannot tolerate a complete bath and self-sufficient clients unable to reach all body parts may be given a partial bed bath. A tub bath or shower is used to give a more thorough bath. In the tub or shower, washing and rinsing all body parts is easier; however, safety is of primary concern, and nursing personnel must provide safety measures for clients with limited strength, mobility, or altered mental capacity.

ASSESSMENT

1 Assess degree of assistance needed for bathing. Factors may include vision, ability to sit without support, hand grasp, range of motion (ROM) of extremities, and cognitive ability.

2 Assess client's tolerance of activity, level of discomfort with movement, and presence of shortness of breath or chest pain with exertion. *Rationale: Determines the type of cleansing bath appropriate for the client.*

3 Assess client's preferences for time of day, products used, usual frequency of bathing, and type of bath.

4 Identify any problems affecting skin condition:
a. Excessive moisture from diaphoresis or incontinence
b. Drainage or excretions from lesions or body cavities
c. Presence of external devices (e.g., catheters, drains, dressings, restraints)
d. Rashes or skin damage related to pruritus and scratching
e. Skin dehydration *Rationale: Determines extent of hygiene and toiletry items or other equipment to have available for the client.*

BOX 7-3 Client Hygiene: AM and PM Care

In the morning when the client wakes and before breakfast:
- Assist the client with toileting.
- Assist the client with washing hands and face and oral care.
- Make sure the client's environment is neat and set up for breakfast.

In the evening before the client goes to sleep:
- Assist the client with toileting.
- Assist the client with washing hands and face and oral care.
- Make sure that the client's bed is clean, dry, and wrinkle free with adequate blankets for warmth.
- Offer the client a back massage to promote comfort and relaxation.
- Make sure the client's environment is neat and free of hazards and that the call button is within reach.

---

5 Identify any prescribed limitations of activity or positioning required by client's illness or treatment plan. *Rationale: Determines client's safety needs to prevent injury.*

6 Assess room environment for temperature level. *Rationale: Protects the client from discomfort.*

PLANNING

Expected Outcomes focus on promoting comfort, mobility, and self-care abilities.

1 Client's skin is clean and free of excretions, drainage, and odor.

2 Client maintains functional ROM of hands and shoulders.

3 Client demonstrates ability to wash face, hands, and chest independently.

4 Client expresses comfort and relaxation.

NOTE: This procedure assumes client is totally dependent. When client is able to assist, encourage and allow as much involvement as possible.

Delegation Considerations

Assessment of the client's skin, pain level, and ROM should not be delegated. The skill of bathing may be delegated. The nurse directs personnel by:

- Consulting with the nurse if there may be a change in type of bath (complete, partial assist, tub, shower) that is planned.
- Notifying the nurse of any skin integrity problems so the nurse can inspect areas of breakdown or potential breakdown.
- Encouraging the client to maintain independence or increase participation as much as possible during bath and, if appropriate, involve the family or significant other.
- Informing the nurse of concerns regarding changes in comfort level or activity tolerance noticed during bathing.

Equipment

- Washcloths and towels
- Bath blanket
- Soap and soap dish
- Toilet tissue or peri-wipes
- Warm water
- Toiletry items (e.g., deodorant, powder, lotion)
- Clean hospital gown or client's own pajamas
- Laundry bag
- Clean gloves (when body secretions are present)
- Washbasin

IMPLEMENTATION *for Complete Bathing*

STEPS	RATIONALE

1 See Standard Protocol (inside front cover).

> **COMMUNICATION TIP** Talk to the client throughout the bath, using a reassuring tone of voice so the client feels safe and comfortable during bathing. Inform the client of the next step as you proceed, even if the client is unable to respond.

2 Offer client bedpan or urinal. — *Provides comfort and prevents interruption of bath.*

a. If client is incontinent, check perineum for fecal material. If present, enclose it in a fold of underpad and remove as much as possible with disposable wipes first.

b. Cleanse anal area from front to back (see illustration), with special attention to folds of buttocks, using as many washcloths as necessary to cleanse and rinse thoroughly. — *Washing from front to back prevents transmission of microorganisms from anus to urethra or genitalia.*

c. Dry area completely.

d. Remove and discard underpad, and replace with a clean one.

e. Remove gloves.

3 Place bath blanket over client, and remove top sheet without exposing client. Have client hold top of bath blanket while removing linen. — *Blanket provides warmth and privacy.*

4 Place soiled linen in laundry bag, taking care not to allow soiled linen to contact uniform.

5 Remove client's gown or pajamas. If an extremity is injured or has limited mobility, begin removal from unaffected side first. For clients with an intravenous (IV) line, use a gown with sleeves that have shoulder straps if possible. — *Reduces risk of increased pain or injury.*

a. When the gown does not have shoulder snaps, remove the gown from arm *without* IV, and slide it off the shoulder and arm toward the wrist, keeping the IV carefully secured (see illustration). — *Reduces risk of accidental dislodgement of IV.*

b. Remove the bag from the IV pole (see illustration).

c. Slide IV bag and tubing through sleeve (see illustration).

d. Rehang the bag, check flow rate, and regulate if necessary (see illustration). — *Manipulation of tubing and container may disrupt flow rate.*

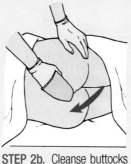

STEP 2b. Cleanse buttocks from front to back.

STEPS	RATIONALE

e. If IV pump is in use, with the assistance of a registered nurse (RN), turn pump off, clamp tubing, remove tubing from pump, and proceed as before. Insert tubing into pump, unclamp tubing, and turn pump on at correct rate. Observe flow rate, and regulate if necessary. Discard gloves.

Sterility, patency, and correct rate of infusion must be maintained.

> **NURSE ALERT** For debilitated clients at risk of falls, provide safety by using side rails as appropriate if at any time it is necessary to leave the client unattended. Check temperature of bath water throughout the bath, and change as needed to maintain warmth.

6 Fill washbasin two-thirds full with warm water. Adjust water temperature to be comfortably warm to your wrist, then allow the client to test temperature tolerance. Place washbasin and supplies within easy reach.

Warm water promotes comfort, relaxes muscles, and prevents chilling.

7 Remove pillow. Place one bath towel under client's head and another over chest.

Removing pillow facilitates bathing ears and neck. Towels absorb moisture.

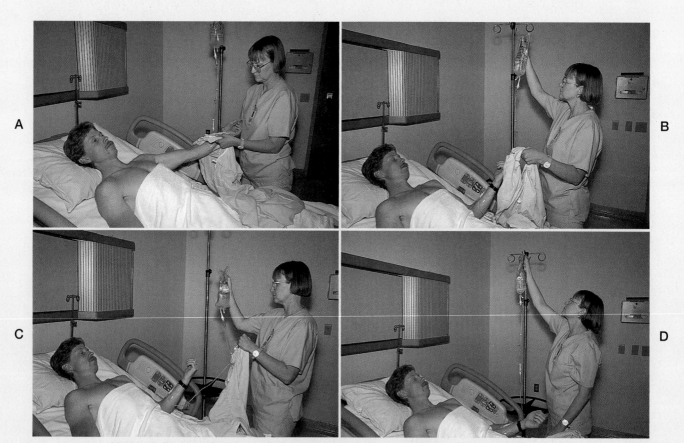

STEP 5 **A,** Remove client's gown. **B,** Remove IV bag from pole. **C,** Slide IV tubing and bag through arm of client's gown. **D,** Rehang IV bag.

STEPS	RATIONALE

8 Immerse washcloth in water, wring thoroughly, and form mitt (see illustration).

Mitt retains heat better and prevents loose ends from dripping or annoying client.

9 Wash face.

a. Wash client's eyes with plain warm water using a clean area of cloth for each eye, bathing from inner to outer canthus (see illustration). Dry around eyes gently and thoroughly.

Soap irritates eyes. Bathing inner to outer canthus prevents secretions from entering nasolacrimal duct. Using a clean area of the cloth reduces the possibility of infection transmission.

b. Wash, rinse, and dry forehead, cheeks, nose, neck, and ears without using soap. Ask men if they want to be shaved (see Skill 7.3).

Soap can be used if client prefers; however, soap tends to dry face, which is exposed to air more than other body parts. If client has a preferred face wash, it may be used.

> **NURSE ALERT** Clients who are unconscious have lost the normal blink reflex of the eye, which increases their risk for corneal drying, corneal abrasions, and eye infections. There will be a physician's order or agency policy to instill eye drops or ointment to help keep the client's eyes moist. Reassess eyes every 2 to 4 hours for dryness. In the absence of a blink reflex, keep the eyelids closed and covered with an eye patch or shield. Avoid taping the eyelid, which can injure tissues (American Society of Health-Systems Pharmacists, 2002).

10 Wash trunk and upper extremities.

a. Expose client's arm. Place bath towel lengthwise under arm. Bathe with minimal soap and water using long, firm strokes from distal to proximal (fingers to axilla).

Promotes venous blood return to heart.

b. Raise and support arm above head (if possible) to wash, rinse, and dry axilla thoroughly (see illustration).

Raising arm promotes ROM and facilitates thorough cleansing.

c. Move to the opposite side of the bed and repeat Steps 10a and 10b. Apply deodorant or powder sparingly to underarms, following client preference.

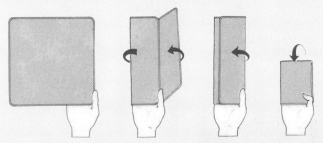

STEP 8 Steps for folding washcloth to form a mitt.

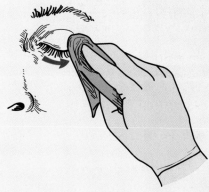

STEP 9a. Wash eye from inner to outer canthus.

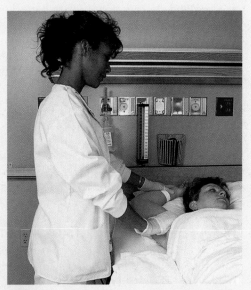

STEP 10b. Positioning the arm to wash the axilla.

STEPS	RATIONALE
d. Cover client's chest with bath towel, and fold bath blanket down to umbilicus. Bathe chest using long, firm strokes, lifting breast upward if necessary. Rinse and dry well.	Skin under breasts is vulnerable to excoriation if not kept clean and dry.
11 Wash the abdomen.	
a. Place bath towel over chest and abdomen, and fold bath blanket down to just above pubic region. Bathe, rinse, and dry abdomen with special care to umbilicus and skinfolds of abdomen and groin.	Keeping skinfolds clean and dry helps prevent odor and skin irritation.
12 Wash legs.	
a. Expose client's leg nearest to you, leaving perineum covered.	
b. Place bath towel under leg, supporting leg at knee and with foot flat on bed.	
c. Place client's foot in a basin to soak while washing and rinsing. If client is unable to support leg, assistance will be needed or soaking omitted.	
d. Wash and dry leg using long, firm strokes from ankle to knee, then knee to thigh (see illustration). Wash between toes of the foot. Rinse and dry thoroughly.	

> **NURSE ALERT** Do not soak the feet of clients with diabetes mellitus or peripheral vascular disease. This may lead to maceration (excessive softening of the skin) and infection (ADA, 2001). Use short, light strokes when washing the legs of a client at risk of deep vein thrombosis (DVT, i.e., blood clots). Long, firm strokes can dislodge a clot, resulting in an embolism.

STEPS	RATIONALE
e. Raise side rail (if used), move to opposite side, lower side rail, and repeat with other leg and foot. If skin is dry, apply lotion.	Promotes good body mechanics for the nurse.
f. Cover with bath blanket, and raise side rail (if used). Change bath water.	Provides client warmth and safety.
13 Wash back.	
a. Place client in side-lying position. Place towel lengthwise along client's side and keep client covered as much as possible.	
b. Wash, rinse, and dry back from neck to buttocks using long, firm strokes. Remove and discard gloves.	

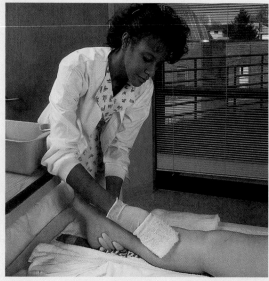

STEP 12d. Washing the leg.

STEPS	RATIONALE

14 Wash perineum.

a. Allow client to provide self-care with or without supervision.

b. Dependent female:

   (1) Position waterproof pad under client's buttocks with client supine. Drape client with bath blanket to expose perineum only.

   (2) Wash labia majora using washcloth, soap, and warm water. Gently retract labia and wash groin from front to back (perineum toward rectum). Using a separate part of the washcloth, repeat on the opposite side.

            Washing from front to back prevents contamination of urethral meatus with fecal matter.

   (3) Gently separate labia, and expose urethra and vagina. Wash from pubic area toward rectum, cleansing thoroughly (see illustration).

            Facilitates cleansing of labial folds and perineum.

> **NURSE ALERT** Avoid tension on indwelling catheter if present, and clean area around it thoroughly. Make sure catheter is secure and positioned over (not under) the thigh. Also provide urinary catheter care (see Skill 9.4).

   (4) Rinse and dry perineum thoroughly. Assess for redness, swelling, discharge, irritation, or skin breakdown.

c. Dependent male:

   (1) Gently grasp shaft of penis, and if client is not circumcised, retract foreskin.

            Gentleness reduces risk of having an erection. Secretions and microorganisms tend to collect under foreskin.

   (2) Wash tip of penis at urethral meatus first. Using circular motion, cleanse away from meatus (see illustration). Replace foreskin to its natural position.

            Discharge may indicate presence of infection or inflammation. Replacing foreskin prevents constriction of the penis, which may result in edema.

   (3) Rinse washcloth thoroughly. Gently cleanse shaft of penis and scrotum, washing underlying skinfolds. Rinse and dry.

            Minimizes risk of discomfort from secretions or moisture.

15 Cover client with bath blanket and remove gloves.

16 Apply body lotion to skin as needed and apply topical moisturizing agents to dry, flaky, or scaling areas. Replace gown.

            Dry skin results in reduced pliability and cracking. Moisturizers help prevent skin breakdown (AHCPR, 1992).

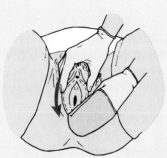

STEP 14b.(3) Cleanse from the perineum to rectum (front to back).

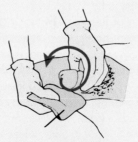

STEP 14c.(2) Wash the penis in a circular motion.

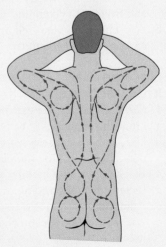

STEP 18b. Massage in a circular motion upward from buttocks.

STEPS	RATIONALE
17 Perform hand hygiene, dispose of water, and store basin appropriately.	
18 Massage back.	
a. Position client prone if possible. Side-lying position is also frequently used.	
b. Using lotion, begin at sacral area and massage in circular motion, stroking upward from buttocks to shoulders and upper arms and over scapulae with smooth, firm strokes (see illustration). Keep hands on skin, and continue massage pattern for 3 to 4 minutes.	Massage stimulates circulation.
c. Knead skin by grasping tissue between thumb and fingers. Knead upward along each side of spine and around muscles of neck, avoiding bony prominences.	

> **NURSE ALERT** Evidence suggests that firm massage over bony prominences may result in decreased blood flow and tissue damage in some clients (AHCPR, 1992).

STEPS	RATIONALE
d. End massage with long stroking movements, and tell client you are ending massage.	Long strokes promote comfort and relaxation.
e. Observe and report any redness or skin breakdown, paying particular attention to bony prominences.	
f. Remove excess lotion from back with bath towel.	Excess lotion could promote maceration of skin.
19 Assist client with grooming, oral hygiene, shaving, hair care, and application of makeup (if desired).	
20 Make client's bed (see Skill 7.5).	
21 See Completion Protocol (inside front cover).	

EVALUATION

1 Observe areas on skin for erythema, exudate, drainage, or breakdown.
2 Measure ROM in hands, arms, and shoulders, and compare with baseline.
3 Assess vital signs if client is experiencing distress or restlessness.
4 Observe for improved ability to assist with self-bathing and hygiene to determine progress.
5 Ask client to view self in mirror and comment on appearance and comfort.

Unexpected Outcomes and Related Interventions

1 Client's skin on lower extremities is dry, flaky, and itchy.
a. Limit the frequency of baths to every other day or less.
b. Use antibacterial soap sparingly. Use a mild soap that is nondrying, and rinse thoroughly.
c. Blot skin dry after bathing, and apply lotion to skin.
d. Increase hydration status.
e. Administer antipruritics as ordered to control itching.
f. Use distraction techniques to remove focus from itching.
2 The client's skin has evidence of rashes, redness, scaling, or cracking.

a. Evaluate the need for a change in frequency of bathing and soap product used.
b. Collaborate with the physician regarding application of ointments or creams to provide a protective barrier and help maintain moisture within the skin.
c. For obese clients with fungal growth between skinfolds, consider antifungal powders to minimize moisture and treat irritations.
3 The rectum, perineum, or genital region is inflamed, is swollen, or has foul-smelling discharge.
a. Bathe area frequently enough to keep clean and dry.
b. Apply protective barrier or antiinflammatory cream.
c. Report to physician.

Recording and Reporting

- Routine documentation may include completion of flow sheet. Record observations made during the bath, which may include type of bath given, client's ability to assist or cooperate, condition of client's skin, and any nursing interventions for improving skin integrity.
- Record client's response to bathing and any concerns voiced by client regarding self-care needs.

Sample Documentation

0900 Client cooperative with turning during bed bath. Stated he felt "very weak." Both legs dry and flaking. Client complained of severe itching. Bath oil added to bath water. Emollient lotion applied after bath. States itching is less now.

Special Considerations

Pediatric Considerations

- Infants chill easily, so keep body covered and work quickly.
- Use only mild soap for bathing infants and children (Hockenberry and Wilson, 2007).
- Always try to maintain a child's usual bathing routine (Hockenberry and Wilson, 2007).

Geriatric Considerations

- Older adults may chill easily.
- Older adults with limited mobility need assistance in perineal care. Using a side-lying position increases client's comfort and provides nurse with opportunity to provide perineal care and inspect surrounding skin.
- Older adults with urinary incontinence need meticulous skin care to reduce skin irritation from urine and feces.

Home Care Considerations

- Type of bath chosen depends on assessment of the home, availability of running water, and condition of bathing facilities.
- In home setting, set up equipment according to established routines. Client is best resource for what works in terms of convenience and saving time.
- The two types of bath for the homebound client are the complete bed bath and the partial bed bath (during which only critical parts of the body are washed, and which may take place at the sink or in the tub or shower).
- Adhesive strips on bottom of tub or shower, hand rails, chairs, or stools in tub or shower help protect client from falls and injury. Client also may use portable shower seat.

Long-Term Care Considerations

- Skin-related problems in long-term care may include methicillin-resistant *Staphylococcus aureus* (MRSA) infections, pressure ulcers, and dermatitis (Meiner and Lueckenotte, 2005).
- Residents in long-term care facilities should be encouraged to do as much of their own personal care as they are able and to wear their own clothes.

PROCEDURAL GUIDELINE 7-1

Commercial Bag Bath or Cleansing Pack

Delegation Considerations

The use of a bag bath can be delegated.

- Direct personnel to notify the nurse of any skin integrity problems.

Equipment

- Prepackaged, disposable bathing systems are available over the counter (OTC) for use in the home and in health care agencies. Each bath kit contains 8 to 10 disposable cloths premoistened with a cleansing solution that does not require rinsing or towel drying.

Procedural Steps

1 See Standard Protocol (inside front cover).

2 Assess condition of the skin (see Skill 7.1).

3 Warm bath bag or pack in a microwave, following package directions.

4 Use a single towel for each body part cleansed. Follow the same order as the total or partial bed bath. No rinsing is needed.

5 Allow the skin to air dry for 30 seconds. It is permissible to lightly cover client with a bath towel to prevent chilling. No towel drying is needed.

6 **See Completion Protocol (inside front cover).**

NOTE: If there is excessive soiling (e.g., in the perineal region), an extra bag bath may be necessary, or conventional washcloths, water, and towels may also be used.

SKILL 7.2 Oral Care for the Debilitated or Unconscious Client

Oral hygiene maintains the comfort and integrity of oral cavity mucosa and helps control plaque-associated oral diseases. Adequate daily oral hygiene includes brushing, flossing, and rinsing. Many factors influence oral hygiene (Box 7-4). For dependent or chronically ill clients, encouragement to attend to oral hygiene helps create a general sense of comfort and improves appetite (Figure 7-1). Frequency of oral care should be based on the condition of the oral cavity and client's comfort. Oral hygiene may be required as often

as every 1 to 2 hours. For unconscious clients, first assess the client's gag reflex and determine the type of suction apparatus needed to prevent aspiration.

Treatment for oral infections (mucositis) or tissue damage may include the use of oral rinses. These mouth rinse mixtures generally include some combination of alcohol-free antifungals, a commercial oral rinse or normal saline for cleaning, a topical anesthetic such as lidocaine for pain, and ice chips (Lecours, 2001). Research has shown that twice daily rinsing

BOX 7-4 Factors Influencing Oral Hygiene

- Client lacks upper-extremity strength or dexterity to perform oral hygiene (e.g., is paralyzed, has limited ROM).
- Client is unable or unwilling to attend to personal hygiene needs (e.g., is unconscious, depressed, confused).
- Client is diabetic and prone to dryness of mouth, gingivitis, periodontal disease, and loss of teeth.
- Client is prone to dehydration or has a fever, or is NPO (unable to take food or fluids). Thick secretions develop on tongue and gums. Lips become cracked and reddened.
- Radiation therapy causes soreness, mild erythema, swollen mucosa, dysphagia, dryness, taste changes, and possible oral infection.
- Chronic inflammatory disease may be caused by bacteria, viral or fungal infections, or ineffective oral hygiene.
- Chemotherapy causes ulcerations and inflammation of mucosa and possible oral infection. Chemical injury may result from irritating substances such as alcohol, tobacco, acidic foods, or side effects of medications, including chemotherapy, antibiotics, steroids, and antidepressants. Mucositis (inflammation of the mucous membranes in the mouth) is a common complication in clients receiving radiation or chemotherapy (Lecours, 2001).
- Trauma to oral cavity from oral tubes, suctioning, hot foods, broken teeth, or ill-fitting dentures causes swelling, ulcerations, inflammation, and possible bleeding. Mouth breathing and use of oxygen may result in dry mucous membranes.

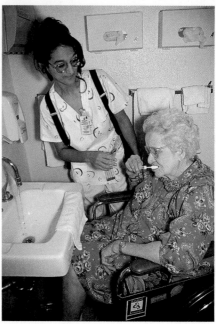

FIGURE 7-1 Nurse observes client's toothbrushing technique.

with an essential oil–containing mouth rinse is an effective adjunct to flossing (Bauroth and others, 2003). Check physician's orders or agency policy for products to use.

Clean dentures as regularly as natural teeth to prevent gingival infection and irritation (Procedural Guideline 7-2, p. 145). Loose dentures can cause discomfort and make it difficult for clients to chew food and speak clearly. Loose dentures may result from weight loss. Dentures can be easily lost or broken. Store dentures in an enclosed, labeled cup and soak when not worn (e.g., during surgery or a diagnostic procedure). Reinsert dentures as soon as possible. The change in appearance when they are not worn may be of major concern to the client.

Unconscious clients are at risk because of the absence of saliva movement and production, which leads to large numbers of gram-negative bacteria in the oral cavity. Critically ill clients with endotracheal tubes and who are on mechanical ventilation are at risk for ventilator-associated pneumonia if the saliva is aspirated. Many clients have no gag reflex. Proper hygiene requires keeping the mucosa moist and removing secretions. Foam stick toothettes have been found to stimulate mucosal tissues but are ineffective in removing tooth debris (Grap and others, 2003).

ASSESSMENT

1 Apply gloves and assess for presence or absence of gag reflex by placing tongue blade or suction tip on back of tongue. *Rationale: Clients with no gag reflex are at risk for aspiration. Suction equipment must be available.*

2 Inspect lips, teeth, gums, buccal mucosa, palate, and tongue, using tongue depressor and penlight if necessary (see Chapter 12). Observe for color, texture, moisture, lesions or ulcers, and condition of teeth (or dentures). Ask if areas of tenderness exist. *Rationale: Every effort should be made to prevent or minimize oral problems.*

3 Identify presence of oral problems, then remove gloves. *Rationale: Any oral problems put clients at risk for infection or nutritional deficiencies.*

a. Dental caries: discoloration of tooth enamel

b. Gingivitis: inflammation of gums

c. Periodontitis: receding gum lines, inflammation, gaps between teeth, rough or jagged teeth

d. Halitosis: bad breath

e. Cracked lips

f. Dry, cracked, coated tongue

PLANNING

Expected Outcomes focus on promoting comfort, preventing aspiration, and promoting integrity of oral mucous membranes.

1 Client's oral mucous membranes and gums are smooth, moist, pink, and intact.

2 Client maintains clean dental surfaces.

3 Client verbalizes comfort and displays no restlessness or facial grimacing during oral care.

4 The family or significant other demonstrates proper oral hygiene regimen.

Delegation Considerations

The nurse should assess oral structures and the gag reflex to rule out risk of aspiration and identify special considerations or equipment that will be needed. The skills of oral care and toothbrushing may be delegated. The nurse directs personnel by:

- Informing them of client's level of consciousness, presence or absence of gag reflex, proper positioning, and type of suction apparatus needed
- Instructing care provider to report any changes in oral mucosa

Equipment

- Soft-bristled toothbrush
- Sponge toothette for edentulous client
- Fluoridated toothpaste
- Essential oil antiseptic mouth rinse
- Water or normal saline (check agency policy)
- Padded tongue blade
- Emesis basin
- Face towel
- Paper towels
- Suction equipment (optional): suction machine or small bulb syringe
- Clean gloves
- Water-soluble lubricant
- Oral airway (uncooperative client or client with bite reflex)

IMPLEMENTATION *for Oral Care for the Debilitated or Unconscious Client*

STEPS	RATIONALE
1 **See Standard Protocol (inside front cover).**	
2 Position unconscious client in side-lying position with bed flat and head turned toward mattress. Place towel under chin. Have emesis basin available.	Side-lying position minimizes risk of aspiration. Dependent or debilitated client may be positioned with head of bed elevated if not in danger of aspirating.
3 Remove dentures or partial plates if present.	Provides clear access to oral cavity. Some clients tend to bite on any object placed in mouth.
4 Separate upper and lower teeth gently with padded tongue blade between back molars (see illustration). Wait until client is relaxed with mouth open, then insert blade with smooth, quick motion *and without using force.* Option: insert oral airway.	

> **NURSE ALERT** Suction should be on and ready for use if gag reflex is absent (see Chapter 31). Suctioning of excess oral secretions reduces the risk of aspiration.

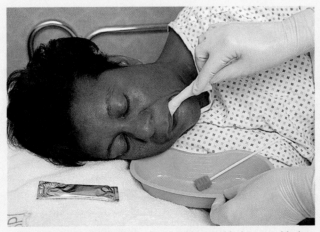

STEP 4 Gently separate the teeth with a padded tongue blade.

STEPS	RATIONALE
5 Brush teeth with toothpaste using a gentle up-and-down motion. Clean chewing and inner tooth surfaces first. Clean outer tooth surfaces. Brush roof of mouth, gums, and inside cheeks. Gently brush tongue but avoid stimulating gag reflex (if present). Moisten brush with water or essential oil antiseptic mouth rinse to rinse thoroughly. Bulb syringe may also be used to rinse. Repeat rinse several times.	Brushing action removes food particles between teeth and along chewing surfaces. Swabbing helps remove secretions and crusts from mucosa and moistens mucosa. Rinsing removes debris. Using essential oil antiseptic mouth rinse a minimum of twice daily is at least as effective as flossing daily in reducing plaque and gingivitis (Bauroth and others, 2003).
6 For clients without teeth, use a Toothette moistened in water or normal saline to clean oral cavity. Rinse with essential oil antiseptic mouth rinse.	Less traumatic to gum mucosa.
7 Suction secretions as they build up.	Removes fluid in posterior pharynx that can potentially be aspirated.
8 Apply a thin layer of water-soluble jelly to lips (see illustration).	Lubricates lips and prevents drying and cracking.
9 **See Completion Protocol (inside front cover).**	

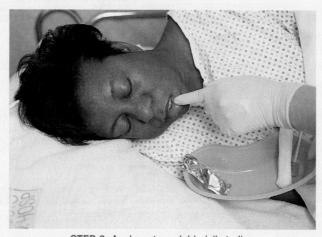

STEP 8 Apply water-soluble jelly to lips.

EVALUATION

1 Inspect oral mucous membranes for moistness, color, smoothness, and intact appearance.
2 Inspect dental surfaces for cleanliness.
3 Observe for restlessness or grimace during care. Ask client if mouth feels more comfortable.
4 Observe client, spouse, or significant other providing oral hygiene regimen.

Unexpected Outcomes and Related Interventions

1 Mucosa, tongue, or gums remain coated with thick secretions.
a. Provide mouth care more frequently if secretions are thick or if oral ulcers are present (Lecours, 2001).
b. To loosen and remove thick mucus, use Toothette or soft toothbrush for cleaning and rinse with normal saline or a solution of tepid water.
c. Increase hydration.

2 Lips are cracked or inflamed.
a. Lubricate lips more frequently with water-soluble lubricant.
3 Client has gurgles in back of throat from accumulation of liquid and is unable to clear throat or cough.
a. Suction back of throat to clear airway and prevent aspiration.

Recording and Reporting

• Routine documentation may include completion of a flow sheet.
• Record observations made during oral care, including:
  • Condition of mucous membranes and lips, including presence of bleeding, ulcerations, dry mucosa, or crusting
  • Client's level of consciousness and ability to cooperate and/or swallow
  • Whether suction is necessary for oral care and if the client's gag reflex is present

Sample Documentation

0700 Mouth care given. Mucous membranes moist, pink, no inflammation. Lips dry, cracked. Moisturizing gel applied to lips. Client unresponsive. No gag reflex elicited. Oral pharynx suctioned frequently during oral care.

Special Considerations

Pediatric Considerations

- Remind children about performing oral care; supervision and/or assistance are often needed (Hockenberry and Wilson, 2007).
- Teach proper oral hygiene and the importance of regular dental care to parents and care providers (Hockenberry and Wilson, 2007).

Geriatric Considerations

- Older adults are more prone to oral injury and periodontal disease. Good oral hygiene practices can help older adults preserve their ability to eat.
- Clients unable to grasp a toothbrush need an enlarged handle placed on toothbrush (e.g., push handle through center of a plastic ball).

- Clients with diabetes require visits to the dentist a minimum of every 6 months.
- Older adults, especially those at risk for oral problems, may need soft, bland, nonacidic foods.

Home Care Considerations

- During the initial admission visit, the professional nurse documents the condition of the client's mouth, teeth, and gums, thus providing a baseline for assessment of the client's ability to comply with special diets and fluid intake and to carry out oral hygiene practices.
- On regular visits, assess for signs and symptoms of infection or irritation, including reddened, bleeding oral lesions.
- Provide special care to clients undergoing head and neck radiation, because gums may be dry and swollen and may interfere with proper denture fit.

Long-Term Care Considerations

- Residents of long-term care facilities continue to require regular dental care and examinations and need to have their dentures evaluated for proper fit.

PROCEDURAL GUIDELINE 7-2

Care of Dentures

Delegation Considerations

The skill of denture care may be delegated.

Equipment

- Soft-bristled toothbrush or denture toothbrush
- Denture cleaning agent or toothpaste
- Denture adhesive (optional)
- Glass of water
- Emesis basin or sink
- Washcloth
- Clean gloves
- Denture cup (if dentures are to be stored after cleaning)

Procedural Steps

1. **See Standard Protocol (inside front cover).**
2. Ask client if dentures fit and if there is any gum or mucous membrane tenderness or irritation.
3. Ask client about preferences for denture care and products used.
4. Encourage client to independently provide denture care if able. If client is unable, it is important for the nurse to provide care.
5. Provide denture care during routine mouth care.
6. Fill emesis basin with tepid water or, if using sink, place washcloth in bottom of sink and fill sink with an inch of water.
7. Ask client to remove dentures. Alternatively, apply gloves, grasp upper plate at front with thumb and index finger wrapped in gauze, and pull downward. Gently lift lower denture from jaw, and rotate one side downward to remove from client's mouth. Hold dentures over emesis basin or sink lined with washcloth and containing 1 inch of water.

8. Apply cleaning agent to brush, and brush surfaces of dentures using back-and-forth motion to cleanse biting surfaces and short strokes from top of denture to biting surfaces. Use short strokes to clean inner tooth surfaces. Use back-and-forth motion to clean undersurface of dentures (see illustration).
9. Rinse thoroughly in tepid water.
10. Some clients use an adhesive to seal dentures in place. Apply a thin layer to undersurface before inserting.
11. If client needs assistance with insertion of dentures, moisten upper denture and press firmly to seal it in place. Then insert moistened lower denture. Ask if dentures feel comfortable.
12. Some clients prefer to have their dentures stored to give the gums a rest and to reduce risk of infection. Keeping dentures moist will prevent warping and facilitate easier insertion. Store in a secure place to prevent loss.
13. **See Completion Protocol (inside front cover).**

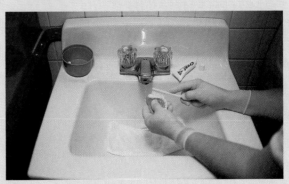

STEP 8 Cleansing denture in sink.

SKILL 7.3 Hair Care—Shampooing and Shaving

Brushing, combing, and shampooing are basic measures for all clients unable to provide self-care. Many agencies have a beauty shop where clients can go for professional hair care. Fever, malnutrition, some medications, emotional stress, and depression affect the condition of hair. Diaphoresis leaves hair oily and unmanageable. Excessively dry or oily hair may be associated with hormone changes. Dry, brittle hair occurs with aging and excessive use of shampoo. African-Americans' hair may be quite dry. Lanolin conditioners may be used to maintain conditioning.

Certain chemotherapy agents and radiation therapy may cause alopecia (hair loss). Many clients choose to wear a wig and others prefer head scarves or turbans. The average growth of healthy hair is ½ inch per month. Table 7-2 describes common hair and scalp conditions and nursing interventions.

Frequency of shampooing depends on the hair's condition and the person's personal preferences. Dry hair requires less frequent shampooing than oily hair or hair of people who exercise actively. Hospitalized clients who have excess perspiration or treatments that leave blood or solutions in the hair may need a shampoo. Positioning with the neck hyperextended over the sink's edge is contraindicated for clients who have had neck injuries or back pain. Clients may be placed on a stretcher with their head extended over a sink. Bedridden clients use a plastic shampoo trough that drains into a bedside container.

Dependent clients with beards or mustaches need assistance keeping the facial hair clean, especially after eating. Shaving of facial hair is a task most men prefer to do for themselves daily. Food particles easily collect in the hair. Because some religions and cultures forbid cutting or shaving any body hair, be sure to obtain those clients' consent (Galanti, 2004).

ASSESSMENT

1 Determine any restrictions that may be necessary. Often a physician's order is required to wash a client's hair. If exposure to moisture is contraindicated, use dry shampoo. *Rationale: Contraindications include increased intracranial pressure (IICP); cerebrospinal fluid (CSF) leaks; open incisions of face, head, or neck; cervical neck injuries; tracheostomy; facial edema; and respiratory distress.*

2 Inspect condition of hair and scalp. Note distribution of hair, oiliness, and texture. Inspect scalp for abrasions, lacerations, lesions, inflammation, and infestation. *Rationale: Determines the need for conditioners or medicated shampoo.*

3 Before shaving client, assess for risk for bleeding. Review medical history and laboratory values: platelet count, prothrombin time (PT), and activated partial thromboplastin time (aPTT). *Rationale: Use an electric razor for clients with leukemia, hemophilia, or disseminated intravascular coagulation (DIC) and clients receiving anticoagulant therapy (heparin, Coumadin or Lovenox) or taking high doses of aspirin. Use an electric razor for clients with risk for bleeding.*

4 If client prefers to shave himself, assess ability to manipulate razor to determine how much assistance will be needed.

5 Ask if there are any product preferences or personal items to be used.

PLANNING

Expected Outcomes focus on comfort and promoting self-concept.

1 Client expresses increased sense of comfort.
2 Client verbalizes improved self-image.

TABLE 7-2 Common Hair and Scalp Conditions and Related Interventions

PROBLEM	INTERVENTIONS
Alopecia (hair loss): chemotherapeutic agents kill cells that rapidly multiply, including both tumor and normal cells.	Some clients wear scarves. Some clients prefer hairpieces. Referral may be needed for professional consultation for long-term interventions.
Dandruff: scaling of scalp accompanied by itching; if severe, may involve eyebrows.	Shampoo regularly with medicated shampoo.
Pediculosis	
Head lice: parasites attached to hair strands. Eggs look like oval particles. Bites or pustules may be found behind ears and at hairline. May spread to furniture and other people.	Shampoo with a medicated shampoo to kill lice or permethrin (Nix) available as a creme rinse. Repeat 12 to 24 hours later. Caution against use of products containing Lidone, because the ingredient is toxic. Change bed linens, and follow isolation precautions for pediculosis according to agency policy.
Body lice: parasites tend to cling to clothing. Client itches. Hemorrhagic spots may appear on skin where lice are sucking blood. Lice may lay eggs on clothing and furniture.	For body lice, apply a medicated lotion for lice, and repeat according to instructions on product. Follow appropriate agency isolation precautions.
Crab lice: found in pubic hair, are grayish white with red legs, and may spread via sexual contact.	For pubic lice, shave hair off affected area, use medicated product for lice, and notify sexual partner of proper treatment.

Delegation Considerations

Assessment of the client's condition may not be delegated. The skills of shampooing and shaving can be delegated. In the presence of neck or back pain or trauma or injury to the cervical spine, the nurse directs personnel by:

- Indicating how to properly position clients with mobility restriction
- Instructing caregiver to report how the client tolerated the procedure and any concerns identified needing assessment by the professional nurse

Equipment

- Brush
- Comb
- Shampoo board
- Shampoo
- Conditioner (optional)
- Towels (two or more)
- Razor
- Shaving cream
- Basin of very warm water

IMPLEMENTATION *for Hair Care—Shampooing and Shaving*

STEPS	RATIONALE

1   See Standard Protocol (inside front cover).

2   Shampoo for client confined to bed:

> **NURSE ALERT** In the presence of head lice, caregiver should wear disposable gown and gloves.

> **NURSE ALERT** Use caution in providing hair care when clients have neck pain or neck or back injury. A physician's order is usually required.

a. Place a towel and waterproof pad under client's shoulders, neck, and head.

b. Brush and comb client's hair by separating hair into small sections, releasing tangles with fingers. Moistening with water or mineral oil may help free tangles.

   Anchoring tangled hair at scalp prevents painful pulling of scalp.

c. Position client supine with head and shoulders at top edge of bed. Place plastic trough under head and washbasin at end of trough spout (see illustration). Be sure spout extends beyond edge of mattress.

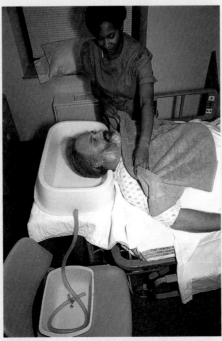

STEP 2c. Client with waterproof pad under shoulders, neck, and head.

STEPS	RATIONALE
d. Place bath towel over client's shoulders. Obtain warm water, testing temperature with your wrist. Allow client to feel water temperature for comfort.	Prevents accidental burn to scalp.
e. Slowly pour warm water from water pitcher over hair until it is completely wet (see illustration). Protect client's face with towel or washcloth over eyes, as needed. If hair contains matted blood, put on gloves and apply hydrogen peroxide to dissolve clots. Then rinse hair with saline.	
f. Apply small amount of shampoo, and work up a lather with both hands. Start at hairline, and work toward back of neck. Lift head slightly to wash back of head. Massage scalp gently.	
g. Rinse thoroughly, and repeat if necessary until hair is free of soap. Dry using a second towel if needed or use hair dryer (if available).	
h. Assist client to a comfortable position, and complete styling of hair. Braids may be helpful for clients with very long hair.	
3 Caring for coarse, curly hair:	
a. Shampooing coarse, curly hair is identical to shampooing wavy or straight hair, but the hair should be conditioned after washing.	Coarse, curly hair, seen, for example, in African-American clients, does not retain moisture as other types of hair do. Shampooing may be necessary only once a week (Crute, 1997).
b. To untangle wet, coarse, curly hair, use the wide teeth of a comb. Beginning at the nape of the neck, comb small subsections of the hair starting at the hair ends. Continue to work through small sections until hair is free of tangles.	Working on small sections of the hair keeps fragile hair from becoming entangled.

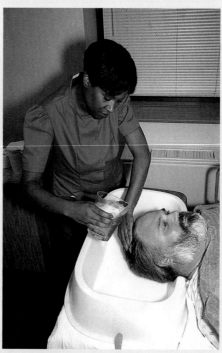

STEP 2e. Pour water over hair.

STEPS	RATIONALE

c. To comb through dry hair it is best to lubricate the hair by applying a conditioner and loosening any tangles with your fingers. Then, using a wide-tooth comb, start on either side of the head and insert the comb with the teeth upward to the hair near the scalp. Comb through the hair in a circular motion by turning the wrist while lifting up and out. Continue until the hair is combed through, and then comb into place using hands to shape.

Coarse, curly hair can be very dry and fragile and will be damaged if not combed carefully. Dry areas of the hair may require further lubrication with a leave-in conditioner and/or styling lotion (Crute, 1997).

4 Shaving beard:

a. 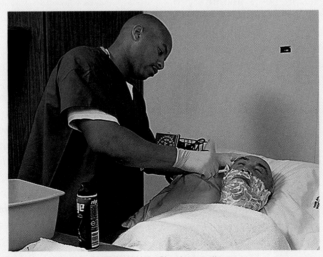 Assist client to sitting position if possible, and place towel over chest and shoulders.

b. Place a warm, moist washcloth over client's face for several seconds.

Softens beard.

c. Shave using appropriate tools available.

(1) Apply shaving cream, using product client prefers. With a disposable razor at a 45-degree angle, shave in direction of hair growth using short strokes. Hold skin taut with nondominant hand (see illustration). Ask client to tell you if it becomes uncomfortable. Dip razor blade in water as shaving cream accumulates on blade's edge.

Skin sensitivity can occur with some products. Holding skin taut helps prevent razor cuts and discomfort during shaving.

(2) Apply conditioner for electric razor. Turn electric razor on and shave across side of face using a gentle downward stroke in direction of hair growth.

d. If necessary, gently comb mustache or beard. Allow client to use mirror and direct areas to trim with scissors.

Allows client to make decisions about care and maintain independence.

e. Rinse and dry face. Remove gloves. Apply aftershave if desired.

Provides a positive effect for comfort and self-esteem.

5   See Completion Protocol (inside front cover).

STEP 4c.(1) Shaving a client.

EVALUATION

1 Offer a mirror, and ask how client feels and looks.
2 Inspect condition of shaved area of skin for nicks, cuts, or areas of dryness.

Unexpected Outcomes and Related Interventions

1 Client has small nicks or cuts on skin.
a. Apply pressure and if necessary a small dressing or Band-Aid.
2 Client has areas of skin surface that appear dry.
a. Use moisturizing shaving foam next time, and apply moisturizing lotion to skin.

Recording and Reporting

- Routine documentation may include completion of a flow sheet. It is usually not necessary to document hair care unless it is included on the agency's checklist.

Special Considerations

Pediatric Considerations

- African-American children require special hair care, possibly including some type of hair dressing specified by their parents. Do not use petroleum jelly (Hockenberry and Wilson, 2007).

Geriatric Considerations

- Hair growth declines sharply between 50 and 60 years.
- Usually the facial hair of older clients does not grow quickly. Thus a shave might not be necessary each day.

Home Care Considerations

- Assess room temperature, availability of water, and most satisfactory position for the client.
- Provide extra protection from wetness for clients with casts.
- Construct a trough by arranging a plastic shower curtain or tablecloth under the client's head and then tapering the cloth to form a narrow end that can drain into a bucket or basin next to the client's bed.
- In the home setting, one of the nurses greatest challenges is to find ways the client can shampoo the hair without causing injury. For example, a client with a long leg cast may need to wash the hair at a sink until it is safe to shower or until the cast is removed and tub baths can be resumed.
- Caution clients about using chemicals and hot combs for straightening hair. Such practices can cause considerable damage to the hair. Misuse can result in scalp burns, hair loss, and allergic reactions that can cause severe skin rashes, urticaria, and conjunctivitis (Crute, 1997).

SKILL 7.4   Foot and Nail Care

Foot and nail care prevents infection, odors, and injury to soft tissues. Alterations may result from biting nails or trimming them improperly, exposure to harsh chemicals, or wearing ill-fitting shoes (ADA, 2001). Changes also occur in the shape, color, and texture of nails that may result from various nutritional, infectious, and circulatory disorders (Table 7-3).

Many older clients may have poor vision, hand tremors, obesity, or limited joint mobility that contributes to difficulties with foot and nail care (Meiner and Lueckenotte, 2005). Older clients may also have excessive dryness of the skin and poor circulation.

Clients with peripheral vascular disease, such as diabetes, may have inadequate arterial or venous circulation or both. These clients are at high risk for neuropathy, a degeneration of peripheral nerves with loss of sensation. Thus, the clients cannot sense pressure or pain from foot lesions. Inspect the feet of clients with altered sensation daily. These injuries are easily infected and heal slowly because of inadequate circulation (ADA, 2001).

ASSESSMENT

1 Identify client's risk for foot or nail problems.
a. Reduced visual acuity, lack of coordination, and inability to bend. *Rationale: Normal physiological changes of aging interfere with client's ability to care for nails and feet.*
b. History of diabetes. *Rationale: Neurovascular changes reduce sensation and circulation to peripheral tissues. Break in skin integrity places these clients at high risk for skin infection (ADA, 2001).*
c. History of cardiac or renal conditions with increased tissue edema, particularly in dependent areas (e.g., feet). *Rationale: Edema reduces blood flow to neighboring tissues.*
d. History of a stroke. *Rationale: Muscle weakness or paralysis of one lower extremity and altered walking patterns increase friction and pressure on the affected foot. Loss of sensation prevents client from being aware of foot problem.*
2 Inspect all surfaces of toes, feet, and nails. Pay particular attention to areas of dryness, inflammation, or cracking. Also inspect areas between toes, heels, and soles of feet. *Rationale: Changes in skin increase risk for infection.*

TABLE 7-3 Common Foot and Nail Problems and Related Interventions

PROBLEM	PREVENTION	INTERVENTIONS
Callus: thickened epidermis, usually flat, painless, and on underside of foot; caused by friction or pressure.	Wear proper footwear, and always wear clean socks or stockings.	Soak callus in warm water to soften. Creams or lotions can help prevent reformation. Refer diabetic client to a podiatrist.
Corns: caused by friction and pressure from shoes, mainly on toes, over bony prominence; usually cone shaped, round, raised, and tender; may affect gait (Figure 7-2).	Wear proper footwear; pain is aggravated by tight shoes. Always wear clean socks or stockings.	Surgical removal may be necessary. Use oval corn pads carefully, because they increase pressure on toes and reduce circulation.
Plantar warts: fungating lesions on sole of foot caused by papillomavirus (Figure 7-3).	Warts are contagious. Avoid going barefoot, especially in public places.	Treatment ordered by physician may include applications of acid, burning, or freezing for removal.
Athlete's foot: fungal infection of foot; scaling and cracking of skin occur between toes and on soles of feet; may have small blisters containing fluid. Apparently induced by tight footwear (Figure 7-4).	Feet should be well ventilated. Avoid tight footwear. Dry feet well after bathing; apply powder. Wear clean socks.	Treat with medicated powder or cream. Refer to physician if condition does not improve with medicated products.
Ingrown nails: toenail or fingernail grows inward into soft tissue around nail; may be painful (Figure 7-5).	Cut with a nail clipper and file toenails straight across after bathing when they are soft. If nails are thick or vision is poor, have toenails trimmed by a podiatrist.	Treat with frequent warm soaks in antiseptic solution. Surgical removal of portion of nail that has grown into skin may be necessary. Refer diabetic clients to a podiatrist.
Fungus infection: thick, discolored nails with yellow streaks.	Keep feet and nails clean and dry. Check feet and nails daily.	Refer to podiatrist.

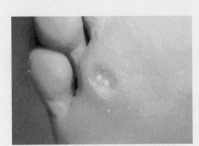

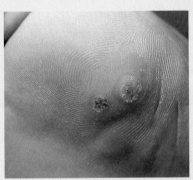

FIGURE 7-2 Corn. (From Weston WL, Lane AT: *Color textbook of pediatric dermatology,* ed 3, St Louis, 2002, Mosby.)

FIGURE 7-3 Plantar warts. (From Zitelli BJ, Davis HW: *Atlas of pediatric physical diagnosis,* ed 3, St Louis, 1997, Mosby.)

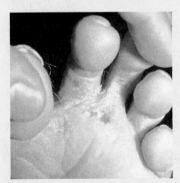

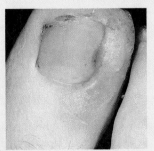

FIGURE 7-4 Ahtlete's foot, tinea pedis. (From Greenberger NJ, Hinthorn DR: *History taking and physical examination: essentials and clinical correlates,* St Louis, 1993, Mosby. Courtesy Dr Loren Amundson, University of South Dakota, Sioux Falls, SD.)

FIGURE 7-5 Ingrown toenail. (From Habif TP: *Clinical dermatology: a color guide to diagnosis and therapy,* ed 2, St Louis, 1990, Mosby.)

3 Palpate the dorsalis pedis pulse of both feet simultaneously, comparing the strength of pulses. Note color and warmth of toes and feet. Observe for capillary refill of nails of less than 3 seconds. *Rationale: Circulatory alterations may change integrity of nails and increase client's chance of localized infection when a break in skin integrity occurs.*

> **NURSE ALERT** A physician's order is required for trimming nails, especially when impaired circulation is suspected (e.g., diabetes mellitus, peripheral vascular disease, leg ulcers).

4 Assess sensation in the feet by checking for light touch or discrimination between warm and cold. *Rationale: Changes in sensation impair ability to respond to pressure or pain.*

5 Determine client's ability to perform self-care. *Rationale: Limited vision, lack of coordination, and inability to reach feet influence degree of assistance required.*

6 Assess client's foot and nail care practices for existing foot problems (e.g., home remedies such as cutting corns with razor blade or scissors, applying adhesive tape on foot, or using oval corn pads on toes). *Rationale: OTC liquid preparations to remove corns may cause burns and ulcerations.*

7 Assess type of footwear worn by clients, including type and cleanliness of socks worn, type and fit of shoes, and restrictive garters or knee-high hose. *Rationale: Improper footwear and constrictive clothing contribute to foot problems (ADA, 2001).*

PLANNING

Expected Outcomes focus on self-care practices that maintain healthy nails and feet and promote circulation and comfort.
1 Client maintains nail integrity and cleanliness.
2 Client correctly demonstrates nail care.
3 Client walks steadily in appropriate footwear.
4 Client identifies ways to minimize sources of pressure or irritation when walking.

Delegation Considerations

The skill of foot and nail care may be delegated *except* for diabetic clients or clients with peripheral vascular disease or circulatory compromise. The nurse directs personnel by:
- Instructing to report any breaks in skin, redness, numbness, swelling, or pain.

Equipment

- Basin (appropriate size for soaking)
- Washcloth
- Bath or face towel
- Nail clippers (check agency policy)
- Orange stick (optional)
- Emery board or nail file
- Clean gloves

IMPLEMENTATION *for Foot and Nail Care*

STEPS	RATIONALE
1 See Standard Protocol (inside front cover).	
2 Soak feet and fingers.	

> **NURSE ALERT** Soaking the feet of clients with diabetes mellitus or peripheral vascular disease is not recommended. Soaking may lead to maceration (excessive softening of the skin), ulceration, or infection (ADA, 2001).

STEPS	RATIONALE
a. Explain that soaking requires 10 to 20 minutes.	Softens tissues to assist with removal of dead cells.
b. Assist ambulatory client to sit in chair with disposable bath mat under feet. If confined to bed, assist to a semi-Fowler's position with a waterproof pad and bath towel under feet.	

> **COMMUNICATION TIP** Encourage inspection of feet as part of foot care routine. "Let's look at your feet to see if there are any problem areas."

STEPS	RATIONALE
c. Fill washbasin and emesis basin with warm water. Test temperature of water with back of hand.	Clients with decreased sensation to feet are unable to detect temperature of water.
d. Place washbasin on bath mat or towel, and help client place one foot in basin. Place emesis basin on over-bed table in front of client. Place call light within client's reach. Offer diversional activity.	Clients with muscular weakness or tremors may have difficulty positioning feet.
3 Foot and nail care:	
a. Allow client's feet and fingers to soak for 10 to 20 minutes. If necessary, rewarm water after 10 minutes.	Softening of corns, calluses, and cuticles ensures easy removal of dead cells and easy manipulation of cuticle.

STEPS	RATIONALE

b. Begin care on fingernails. Clean gently under nails with orange stick while immersing fingers (see illustration).

c. Remove from basin and dry thoroughly.

Thorough drying slows fungal growth and prevents maceration of tissues. Friction removes dead skin layers.

d. Unless contraindicated, trim nails with nail clippers; clip nails straight across and even with tops of fingers (see illustration). Shape nails with emery board or file.

Cutting straight across prevents splitting of nail margins and formation of sharp nail spikes that can irritate lateral nail margins.

> **NURSE ALERT** If client has circulatory problems, do not cut nails; file the nails only. Clients with severe hypertrophy of nails or diabetes may be referred to podiatrist.

e. Push cuticle back gently with orange stick.

Reduces incidence of inflamed cuticles.

f. Move over-bed table away from client.

Provides easier access to feet.

g. Remove feet from basin and scrub callused areas with washcloth.

Warm water softens nails and thickened epidermal cells, reduces inflammation of skin, and promotes local circulation.

h. Clean gently under nails with orange stick. Remove feet from basin and dry thoroughly.

Removal of debris reduces chance of infection.

i. Clean and trim toenails as in Steps 3d and 3e. Do not file corners of toenails.

Shaping corners of toenails damages tissues.

4 Apply a thin coat of plain petroleum jelly or unscented lotion to feet and hands. Do not apply lotion between toes.

Excess lotion can promote growth of microorganisms (ADA, 2006).

5 Wash and thoroughly dry minor cuts. Only mild antiseptics (e.g., Neosporin ointment) are applied as prescribed. Remove gloves. Notify physician of any cuts.

With impaired circulation, cuts are more likely to heal more slowly, and there is a risk for infection.

6 Encourage client to avoid wearing elastic stockings, knee-high hose, or constricting garters and to avoid crossing legs at knees and ankles.

Impairs circulation to the lower extremities.

7 Instruct client to wear well fitting shoes and to inspect shoes daily for foreign objects, roughness, or structural tears.

Reduced circulation is accomplished by reduced sensation, allowing injuries to go untreared unless detected by inspections. Foreign objects can cause foot sores.

8 **See Completion Protocol (inside front cover).**

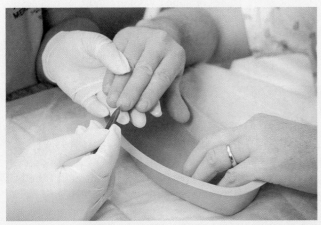

STEP 3b. Cleanse under fingernails.

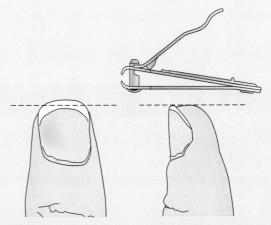

STEP 3d. Use a nail clipper to clip fingernails straight across.

EVALUATION

1 Inspect nails and surrounding skin surfaces after soaking and nail trimming. Note any remaining rough areas.

2 Ask client to explain and demonstrate nail care.

3 After toenail care, observe client's walk in appropriate footwear.

Unexpected Outcomes and Related Interventions

1 Nails are discolored, rough, and concave or irregular in shape. Cuticles and surrounding tissues are inflamed and tender to touch. Localized areas of tenderness are present on feet, with calluses or corns at points of friction.

a. Repeat nail and foot care to relieve inflammation and remove layers of cells from calluses or corns. Referral to a podiatrist may be needed.

b. Change in footwear or corrective foot surgery may be needed for permanent improvement in corns or calluses.

2 Client unable to explain or perform foot care.

a. Provide repeated opportunities for client to practice nail care.

b. Refer to podiatrist for regular follow-up care.

3 Client complains of pain while walking and has unsteady gait.

a. Special footwear may be required, or client may need referral to a podiatrist.

Recording and Reporting

- Record foot care and condition of the feet and nails, including areas of inflammation, infection, ulceration, or injury.
- Record teaching given to clients about foot care and evidence of understanding of information.
- Record client's ability to care for own feet.

Sample Documentation

0900 Right great toe red, inflamed, and tender. States this was first noted before admission 1 week ago. Feet soaked for 10 minutes in warm water and dried thoroughly. Lotion applied. Toe inflammation reported to RN.

Special Considerations
Pediatric Considerations

- Keep the nails of infants and children short and clean (Hockenberry and Wilson, 2007).
- It is best to cut an infant's nails with manicure scissors with rounded tips while the infant is sleeping (Hockenberry and Wilson, 2007).

Geriatric Considerations

- Changes in aging skin of the feet include thinning of epidermis and subcutaneous fat and dryness because of decreased activity of oil and sweat glands. Nails become opaque, tough, scaly, brittle, and hypertrophied.
- Limited exercise can result in laxity of foot ligaments and musculature and lead to instability and impaired mobility.
- Common foot problems of older adults include heel pain caused by tearing of plantar fascia and foot musculature, metatarsalgia (pain beneath metatarsal head), hammer toes and claw toes, bunions, corns and calluses, ingrown toenails, fungal infections, arthritis, and neuropathies that cause diminished sensation in foot (Meiner and Lueckenotte, 2005).

Home Care Considerations

- Moleskin applied to areas of feet that are under friction is less likely to cause local pressure than corn pads; wrapping small pieces of lamb's wool around toes reduces irritation of soft corns between toes.
- Assess use of bathroom sink for soaking client's hands and tub for soaking feet.

SKILL 7.5 Bedmaking—Occupied Bed

Safety and comfort are primary considerations for bedmaking. Change a client's bed when linens become soiled. Straighten out and tighten the sheets periodically throughout the day to keep them wrinkle free.

The typical hospital bed has a firm mattress on a metal frame with three sections that allow the head and foot of the bed to raise and lower separately. Beds usually operate by electricity. In some settings they may be operated with a crank at the foot of the bed. Beds also can be raised to a height that facilitates good body mechanics for client care and lowered for client safety when getting into and out of bed. A variety of special beds and mattresses exist for special purposes (see Chapter 25).

Bedmaking may be done with the client out of the bed (unoccupied) (Procedural Guideline 7-3, p. 158) or in the bed (occupied). An unoccupied bed is left open with the top sheets fanfolded down. A postoperative surgical bed is prepared for clients returning from the operating room (OR) or procedural area. The bed is left with the top sheets fanfolded lengthwise and not tucked in to facilitate the client's transfer from a stretcher. A closed bed, which is made with the top sheets left up, is used after a client is discharged and housekeeping cleans the unit.

MAKING AN OCCUPIED BED

Bedrest presents many risks; occupied bedmaking is limited to those clients who cannot tolerate being out of bed. In addition some clients have activity or positioning restrictions ordered by their health care provider. If a client is confined to bed, perform bedmaking in a way that conserves time and the client's energy. If a client experiences severe pain with movement, an analgesic administered 30 to 60 minutes before the procedure is helpful in controlling pain and maintaining comfort. Even though the client is unable to get out of bed, encourage self-help if possible, which helps maintain the client's strength and mobility.

ASSESSMENT

1 Determine if the client has been incontinent or if drainage is present from dressings, IV, or drainage tubes. *Rationale: This determines the need for clean gloves and placement of waterproof pads.*

PLANNING

Expected Outcomes focus on the client's safety and comfort.
1 Client has a clean, safe bed throughout hospitalization.

2 Client verbalizes a sense of comfort while in bed.
3 Client's skin remains free of irritation.

Delegation Considerations

The skill of bedmaking is delegated to AP. The nurse directs personnel by:
- Explaining client's activity restrictions
- Explaining what to do if the client becomes fatigued or short of breath
- Instructing care provider to immediately report any unexpected concerns (e.g., excess wound drainage, dislodged IV tubing)

Equipment

- Linen bag or hamper
- Bath blanket (if available)
- Bottom sheet (flat or fitted)
- Drawsheet (optional)
- Waterproof pads (optional)
- Top sheet
- Blanket
- Mattress pad (needs to be changed only when soiled)
- Spread
- Pillowcase
- Clean gloves

IMPLEMENTATION *for Bedmaking—Occupied Bed*

STEPS	RATIONALE
1 See Standard Protocol (inside front cover).	
2 Lower head of bed to flat position, if tolerated by client. Lower side rail on nurse's side; leave far side rail up.	Promotes good body mechanics when applying linens and facilitates access to clients.
3 Loosen all top linens. Remove spread and blanket separately, leaving client covered with top sheet or bath blanket. Fold spread and blanket in quarters, and place on a chair if they are clean and are to be reused. Place soiled linens directly into a soiled linen bag.	
4 Assist client to turn toward you in a side-lying position. Slide pillow over so it remains under client's head. Check that any tubing is not being pulled. Raise the side rail.	Uses good body mechanics and provides safety, security, privacy, and warmth.
5 Go to the opposite side of the bed. Loosen all bottom linens. Fanfold or roll bottom sheet, drawsheet, and any pads toward and under the client (see illustration). Clean and dry mattress if necessary.	Reduces transmission of organisms and keeps new linen dry.

COMMUNICATION TIP Talk with clients during bedmaking, and show interest by listening to them. Periodically use eye contact and respond to them directly. Encourage bed-bound clients to assist as much as possible and to report any discomfort or the need to rest. Interact throughout the entire procedure even if there is no evidence of a response. Clients often can hear even when they cannot speak or respond.

6 Apply clean linens to exposed half of bed.
a. Place clean fitted bottom sheet on bed with seam side down.

STEPS	RATIONALE
b. Place flat sheets with the center of the sheet on bed, seam side down with bottom hem even with the foot end of mattress.	
c. Open sheet toward client, unfolding lengthwise to cover mattress (see illustration).	
d. Tuck top of sheet under head end of mattress.	
7 Miter top corner of flat bottom sheet at head of bed (see Procedural Guideline 7-3).	Mitered corners are more secure and do not loosen easily.
8 Tuck remaining portion of sheet under mattress, working from top to bottom. Keep linens smooth.	
9 If needed, place folded drawsheet and/or waterproof pads (absorbent side up) on center of bed with seam side down. Fanfold toward client. Keep clean and soiled linen separate.	Provides additional protection to bed linen.
10 Keeping client covered, assist client to logroll toward you over layers of linen (see illustration).	
11 Raise side rail on the side client is facing.	
12 Go to other side of bed, and lower side rail.	
13 Assist client in positioning over folds of linen. Remove soiled linen by rolling into a ball toward foot of bed. Hold linen away from uniform and place in a disposable bag or hamper.	Reduces transmission of microorganisms.

> **NURSE ALERT** Use thoughtful judgment and avoid leaving client alone with side rail down if safety is a potential concern.

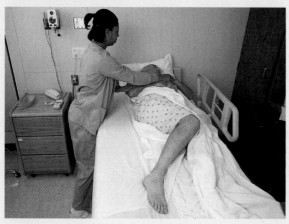

STEP 5 Old linen tucked alongside client.

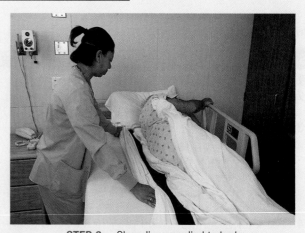

STEP 6c. Clean linen applied to bed.

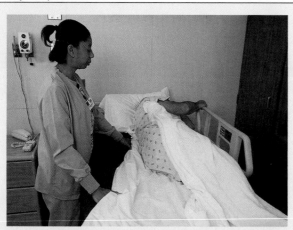

STEP 10 Client rolling over layers of linen toward nurse.

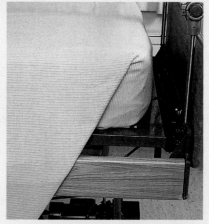

STEP 22 Modified mitered corner.

STEPS	RATIONALE
14 Remove gloves if worn, and dispose of them properly. Perform hand hygiene.	
15 Gently slide clean linen from beneath the client toward you, and smooth the clean linen out over mattress. Assist client to rolling back to supine position.	Minimizes friction of linen being pulled across skin.
16 Miter the top corner of bottom sheet as in Step 7.	
17 Grasp side of flat bottom sheet tightly. Keeping it taut, tuck it under mattress.	
18 Repeat with drawsheet, proceeding from middle to top to bottom.	
19 Smooth waterproof pads that are on top of drawsheet.	
20 Place a clean top sheet and blanket or spread over client; leave several inches of sheet at top to be folded down.	
21 With client grasping clean top linens, slide out used top sheet or bath blanket. Cuff top sheet over blanket and spread.	Prevents exposure of client. Gives a neat appearance to bed and keeps client's face off blanket.
22 Make a modified mitered corner with top linens at foot of bed (see Procedural Guideline 7-3, Step 15). Miter the corner as before, but do not tuck in lower edge of triangle (see illustration).	
23 Loosen linen at client's feet to form toe pleats. Adjust to client's comfort.	Allows for movement of client's feet, prevents top linen from forcing feet into plantar flexion, and prevents pressure ulcers from developing.
24 Remove pillow and replace pillowcase.	
25 **See Completion Protocol (inside front cover).**	

EVALUATION

1 Observe client's linens for cleanliness and tightness.
2 Ask if client is comfortable after bed is made.
3 Observe client's skin for signs of irritation.

Unexpected Outcomes and Related Interventions
1 Client is not comfortable in bed.
a. Check that linens are clean and dry. Tighten them.
b. Assist client with changing position in bed.
2 Client's skin appears red and irritated.
a. Reposition client frequently. Consider use of pressure-relieving mattress (see Chapter 25).
b. Keep client's bedding clean and dry.

Recording and Reporting
- Bedmaking is usually not documented. Some agencies require the nurse to record this activity on a flow sheet.

Special Considerations
Pediatric Considerations
- Infants and children must be kept in cribs and use bedding that meets the U.S. Consumer Product Safety Commission (CPSC) guidelines (Hockenberry and Wilson, 2007).

Geriatric Considerations
- Older adults have fragile skin and require more protection. Be sure bed linens are clean, dry, and free of wrinkles.
- Encourage older adults to spend as much time out of bed as possible.
- Use drawsheets and waterproof pads with caution. Accumulation of moisture creates a risk for skin maceration and breakdown.

Home Care Considerations
- Assess the primary caregiver's ability and willingness to maintain a clean environment for the client.
- Assess home laundry facilities to plan with the primary caregiver the frequency with which linens could reasonably be laundered.
- Assess the amount of linen in the home to establish with the primary caregiver the number of changes of sheets that could be reserved for the client's use.

PROCEDURAL GUIDELINE 7-3
Unoccupied Bedmaking and Surgical Bed

Delegation Considerations

Bedmaking is delegated to AP.

Equipment

- Linen bag
- Mattress pad (change only when soiled)
- Bottom sheet (flat or fitted), drawsheet (optional), waterproof pads (optional), top sheet, blanket, bedspread, pillowcases
- Bedside chair or table
- Clean gloves (if linen is soiled)
- Washcloth
- Antiseptic cleanser

Procedural Steps

1 **See Standard Protocol (inside front cover).**
2 Assist to bedside chair or recliner, or encourage ambulation if appropriate.
3 Raise bed to comfortable working position with side rails lowered.
4 Gloves will be necessary if linen is soiled with body fluids. Remove soiled linen and place in laundry bag, taking care not to contact uniform. Avoid shaking or fanning linen.
5 Reposition mattress, and wipe off any moisture using a washcloth moistened in antiseptic solution. Dry thoroughly. Remove gloves and perform hand hygiene.
6 Apply all bottom linen on one side of bed before moving to opposite side.

7 Place fitted sheet smoothly over mattress. If using a flat unfitted sheet, place it seam side down, with vertical center fold lengthwise down middle of bed. Place the lower edge even with bottom edge of mattress. Pull remaining top portion of sheet over top edge of mattress.
8 Miter top corner of bottom sheet:
a. Face head of bed diagonally. Lift the corner of the mattress with the hand that is away from the head of the bed.
b. With the other hand, tuck top edge of bottom sheet smoothly under mattress so that side edges of sheet above and below mattress meet if brought together.
c. Pick up the top edge of sheet approximately 45 cm (18 inches) from the top of mattress (see illustration).
d. Lift sheet and lay it on top of mattress to form a neat triangular fold, with lower base of triangle even with mattress side edge (see illustration).
e. Tuck lower edge of sheet, which is hanging free below the mattress, under mattress. Tuck with palms down without pulling triangular fold (see illustration).
f. Hold portion of sheet covering side of mattress in place with one hand. With the other hand, pick up top of triangular linen fold and bring it down over side of mattress. Tuck this portion under mattress. Tuck remaining portion of unfitted sheet under mattress moving toward foot of bed (see illustration).

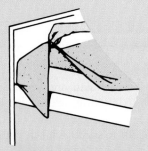

STEP 8c. Top edge of sheet picked up.

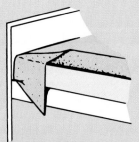

STEP 8d. Sheet on top of mattress in triangular fold.

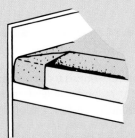

STEP 8e. Lower edge of sheet tucked under mattress.

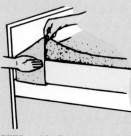

STEP 8f. Triangular fold placed over side of mattress.

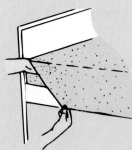

STEP 15 Modified mitered corner.

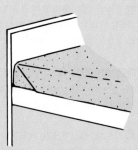

STEP 20c. Fanfold linen over to far side of bed.

PROCEDURAL GUIDELINE 7-3—cont'd

9 Optional: Apply waterproof pad or drawsheet, laying center fold along middle of bed lengthwise. Smooth pad or drawsheet over bottom sheet, and tuck under mattress.

10 Move to the opposite side of the bed. Apply fitted sheet smoothly over each mattress corner. For an unfitted sheet, miter top corner of bottom sheet (steps 8a.-f.), making sure corner is taut.

11 Grasp remaining edge of unfitted bottom sheet, and tuck tightly under mattress while moving from head to foot of bed.

12 Smooth pad or drawsheet over mattress, and tuck excess edge under mattress, keeping palms down.

13 Place top sheet over bed with vertical center fold lengthwise down middle of bed. Open sheet out from head to foot, being sure top edge of sheet is even with top edge of mattress. Optional: Spread a blanket or spread evenly over bed in same fashion.

14 Standing on one side at foot of bed, lift mattress corner slightly with one hand, and with other hand tuck top sheet and blanket or spread under mattress.

15 Make modified mitered corner with top sheet, blanket, and spread. After triangular fold is made, leave tip of triangle untucked (see illustration on p. 156).

16 Go to other side of bed. Complete Step 15 to make a modified corner at foot of bed.

17 Make a horizontal toe pleat with all top layers of linen:
a. Stand at foot of bed and fanfold in sheet 5 to 10 cm (2 to 4 inches) across bed.
b. Pull sheet up from bottom to make fold approximately 15 cm (6 inches) from bottom edge of mattress.

18 At the top of the bed make a cuff by turning edge of top sheet down over top edge of blanket and spread.

19 Apply clean pillowcase. Open the bed by fanfolding top covers to the foot of the bed. Leave the bed in low position.

20 Surgical bed (variation):
a. Fold all linen from foot of bed toward center of mattress, even with the foot of the mattress.
b. Fold corners toward opposite side of bed, forming a triangle.
c. Fanfold linen toward you on the side of the bed away from where client will be transferred (see illustration).

21 Leave all side rails down and bed in high position to match the height of the stretcher.

22 **See Completion Protocol (inside front cover).**

NCLEX® Style Questions

1 When planning care for Julia, a 45-year-old woman who has hirsutism, which of the following interventions is most important in relation to this condition?
1. Wash hair daily and skin twice daily with warm water and soap to remove oils. Use topical antibiotics if prescribed.
2. Wash thoroughly; apply antiseptic spray or lotion to prevent itching and aid in healing.
3. Wash with mild soap and water. Observe for signs of infection.
4. Shave facial hair as desired by client to enhance body image.

2 Place the following steps of bathing a client in the correct sequence.
1. Inspect skin condition to assess for lesions or body fluids.
2. Provide back care and apply lotion to moisturize dry, flaky, or scaling areas on the back.
3. Bathe client in systematic fashion: face, upper extremities, chest, abdomen.
4. Wash perineum, cleansing from front to back.
5. Assist client with toileting (bedpan or urinal) as needed.
6. Apply clean gloves.

3 Which of the following clients is most likely to require special attention for being able to perform oral care?
1. A 34-year-old woman with mucositis who is being treated with chemotherapy for cancer
2. A 45-year-old female with shoulder pain caused by rheumatoid arthritis
3. A 32-year-old diabetic with healthy teeth and well-controlled blood sugars
4. An 82-year-old alert and cooperative client recovering from dehydration and electrolyte imbalance whose lips are cracked and peeling

4 A 62-year-old diabetic who gives herself insulin is admitted with uncontrolled diabetes. Which of the following physiological changes is characteristic of diabetic clients and must be considered when performing skin hygiene measures?
1. Severe physical pain
2. Reduced blood flow to peripheral tissues
3. Edema associated with cardiac or renal conditions
4. Muscle weakness causing unsteady gait

5 An 88-year-old client is confined to bed with heart failure and is receiving oxygen. When providing AM care, which of the following interventions should the nurse complete first?
1. Making the bed
2. Bathing head to toe
3. Caring for dentures
4. Assisting with toileting

References for all chapters appear in Appendix D.

8

Promoting Nutrition

MEDIA RESOURCES

- **evolve** http://evolve.elsevier.com/Elkin
- **View Video!** Video Clips
- Nursing Skills Online

Adequate nutrients in the form of water, carbohydrates, proteins, lipids, vitamins, and minerals are ingested, digested, and absorbed to maintain body tissue and provide energy. Digestion is the mechanical and chemical process by which food is broken down into its simplest form for absorption. The body absorbs nutrients to provide the energy to perform basic bodily functions and the energy needed for activity and injury.

The 2005 U.S. Department of Health and Human Services (USDHHS) and U.S. Department of Agriculture (USDA) *Dietary Guidelines for Americans* contains 23 general recommendations based on 18 specific population recommendations (Box 8-1). The USDA also published the new Food Guide Pyramid, MyPyramid (Figure 8-1). MyPyramid incorporates the principles of the new *Dietary Guidelines for Americans*. In contrast to the previous food guide pyramid, MyPyramid does not make specific recommendations by food group in the actual graphic. It was designed to be simple and to be used as a guide for Americans to formulate their own healthy food choices. The pyramid, used in conjunction with the website http://www.mypyramid.gov, provides nutritional recommendations based on a person's age, sex, and physical activity level.

In addition, *Healthy People 2010* developed recommendations in the form of an official strategy for improving our nation's health (USDHHS, 2005). Examples of some of the nutritional focus areas include food safety, achieving a healthy weight to reduce disease risk; and utilizing the *Dietary Guidelines for Americans* (USDHHS, 2005). Early recognition of malnourished or at-risk clients has strong positive influences on health outcomes (Box 8-2). Clients who receive nothing by mouth (NPO) and receive only intravenous (IV) fluids for as few as 3 to 5 days are at nutritional risk. In addition, nutritional problems often occur in chronic disease, eating disorders, critical illness, metabolic diseases, and obesity (Hammond, 2003). Prevention and early detection of malnutrition are the most effective treatments. Studies have identified that a large proportion of adult hospitalized clients are either malnourished or at risk (Bickford and others, 1999).

An effective method to detect malnutrition early is routine nutritional screening. Nutritional screening is the process of identifying characteristics known to be associated with nutrition problems. The purpose of the screening is to quickly identify individuals at nutritional risk. A nutritional screening tool incorporates objective and subjective data. Objective data commonly included in nutritional screening tools includes height, weight, weight change, primary diagnosis, disease stage, and the presence of comorbidities (ASPEN, 2002). The Joint Commission on Accreditation of Healthcare Organizations' (JCAHO, 2006) standards require the identification of clients who are nutritionally at risk by means of an initial screening mechanism. This screening must be completed within 24 hours of admission to a hospital, within 14 days of admission to a long-term care facility, or within a facility-defined period of time in ambulatory care and home care settings (JCAHO, 2006).

At-risk clients undergo a more thorough assessment of their nutritional status (Box 8-3). Nutritional assessment differs from nutritional screening in that nutritional assessment, commonly performed by a registered dietitian or nutrition professional, is an in-depth evaluation that incorporates medical history, a detailed dietary history, physical examination, anthropometric measurements, and laboratory data (ADA, 1994). It includes an assessment of body compartments as well as an analysis of structure and function of organ systems and their effect on metabolism (ASPEN, 2002). Nurses and dietitians working together can develop a plan of care to meet nutritional needs based on nutritional assessment, the client's food preferences, and any cultural or religious requirements.

BOX 8-1 Dietary Guidelines for Americans 2005

Good Nutrition
- Eat a variety of foods and fluids within the common basic food groups in order to receive adequate amounts of vitamins, minerals, and other important nutrients.
- Limit intake of saturated fat, trans fat, cholesterol, added sugar, salt, and alcohol.

Physical Activity
- Perform physical activity at least 30 minutes daily.
- Lower the amount of sedentary activities such as watching TV and sitting in front of computer.
- Good examples of physical activity are aerobic exercises, resistance exercises, and stretching.

Weight Management
- Maintain body weight within a healthy or acceptable range.
- To prevent weight gain, increase physical activity level and decrease intake of high-calorie foods or beverages.

Adapted from US Department of Health and Human Services and US Department of Agriculture: *Dietary guidelines for Americans 2005,* ed 6, Washington, DC, 2005, US Government Printing Office.

BOX 8-2 Clients at High Nutritional Risk

Diagnoses/Conditions
- Alcoholism
- Anorexia
- Burns
- Cancer
- Cognitive dysfunction
- Dysphagia
- Human immunodeficiency virus (HIV)
- Inflammatory bowel disease
- Malabsorption syndromes
- Metabolic disorders
- Psychosocial disorders
- Renal/hepatic/pancreatic dysfunction
- Sepsis
- Trauma

Surgeries/Therapies
- Bowel resection
- Chemotherapy
- Gastric surgery
- Head and neck resection
- Liver or bile duct surgery
- Multiple medications
- Radiation therapy

BOX 8-3 Components of a Nutritional Assessment

Medical History
- Illnesses, conditions, or medications that require a change in the kind and/or amount of food eaten

Dietary History
- 24-hour food recall
- Protein and calorie intake greater or less than body requirements
- Pattern of three or more drinks of beer, liquor, or wine almost every day
- Psychological status, food allergies, religious beliefs, economic limitations, and social support
- Physical ability to purchase food, cook, and feed self

Physical Assessment
- Height and usual weight
- Dentition status
- Weight gain or loss of 10 pounds in the past 6 months
- Ideal body weight
- Frame size

Anthropometrics*
- Triceps skinfold (TSF)
- Midarm circumference (MAC)
- Midarm muscle circumference (MAMC)† or estimated skeletal muscle mass

Laboratory Tests
- Fasting blood glucose
- Renal labs (blood urea nitrogen [BUN], creatinine)
- Visceral proteins (albumin, transferrin, prealbumin)
- Complete blood count (CBC—hemoglobin, hematocrit)
- Electrolytes (Na, K, Cl)
- Lipid profile (cholesterol, low-density lipoprotein [LDL], high-density lipoprotein [HDL], triglycerides)
- Liver function tests (alanine aminotransferase [ALT], aspartate aminotransferase [AST])

*These anthropometric measurements are not usually done in the clinical setting and should be done only by trained professionals.
†MAMC = MAC (cm) − [TSF (cm) × 3.14]

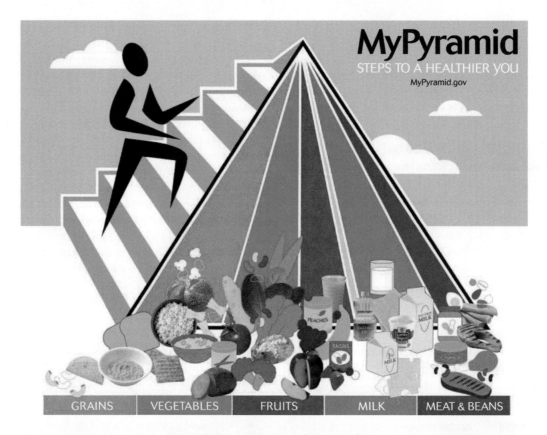

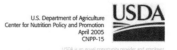

FIGURE 8-1 Food Guide Pyramid. (From US Department of Agriculture: *USDA's food guide pyramid*, Washington, DC, 2005, US Government Printing Office; available at http://www.mypyramid.gov.)

Height and weight are routinely obtained for each client on hospital admission (Procedural Guideline 8-1). This information is compared to standards for height-weight relationships. Body mass index (BMI) measures weight corrected for height and serves as an alternative to traditional weight charts. Calculation of BMI is achieved by dividing the client's weight in kilograms by his or her height in meters squared. For example, a person who weighs 68 kg and is 61 inches tall (1.54 m) would have a BMI of 28.7. The BMI has limited utility in individuals with increased lean muscle mass or with large frames. It is also more relevant for determining obesity than for assessing malnutrition. A BMI of less than 18.5 or greater than 30 places a client at high risk of illness (USDHHS, 2006).

Another method of weight assessment is through a comparison to ideal body weight (IBW). One method of calculating IBW is as follows: For women IBW equals 100 pounds plus 5 additional pounds for each inch of height over 60 inches (5 feet); for men IBW can be estimated with a baseline of 106 pounds plus 6 additional pounds for each inch of height over 60 inches.

Weight should not be considered as a sole determinant of nutritional status because weight alone does not reveal body composition. Weight gain among individuals with disease may reflect tumor or fluid retention while masking loss of lean body mass. Body composition measurement techniques provide an opportunity to distinguish loss of lean body mass in disease states.

Laboratory and biochemical tests assist in nutritional assessment; however, there is no one test that is diagnostic for malnutrition. Some of the basic laboratory tests to study nutritional status include plasma protein values such as serum albumin, prealbumin, and transferrin. Serum albumin value is a widely used indicator of protein stores. However, it is not specific for malnutrition and is affected by many factors, such as dehydration, hemorrhage, steroids, and surgery. Although serum albumin is a poor marker for nutritional screening, it is an excellent indicator of prognosis in many disease states, as well as for surgical patients (Vanek, 1998).

Cholesterol level is also helpful. A total cholesterol level less than 160 mg/dL may indicate malnutrition. A complete blood count (CBC) is useful for nutritionally related anemia. Low values for hemoglobin and hematocrit may indicate nutritional deficiency. Further testing is indicated to determine if anemia is related to nutritional intake (Cunningham, 2003).

Dietary intake information identifies existing and potential nutritional excesses and deficits. In a full diet history, information that reflects both diet and general health is included. Information should include the client's usual intake of foods and liquids and information about preferences, allergies, and food availability. In some situations, a 24-hour or 3- to 7-day food diary may be kept to calculate nutritional intake and compare it with daily requirements.

There are multiple factors affecting a client's nutritional needs. Initial assessment includes age; socioeconomic status; personal food preference; use of alcohol or illegal drugs; vitamin, mineral, or herbal supplements; prescription or over-the-counter (OTC) drugs, and nutritional knowledge level. Eating patterns and food choices are also significantly affected by ethnicity, culture, and religious influences. Cultural awareness helps in incorporating preferences into dietary recommendations (Box 8-4).

Clinical observation involves physical assessment of body systems for signs of nutritional decline (Table 8-1). Most nutritional problems develop slowly over weeks and months. Because improper nutrition affects all body systems, clues to malnutrition require careful analysis of data from the physical assessment.

Nurses have the most client contact time and are in a key position to educate clients about nutrition. Early identification of potential problems helps to avoid more serious problems. The nurse's role as educator often involves providing information about community resources, referral to a dietitian, supporting healthy changes, and monitoring progress.

Nutritional screening has been identified as a vital step preceding the nutrition care process. The nutritional assessment builds on the information collected as part of the nutritional screening. The ultimate goal of the assessment is to develop an effective nutrition plan of care that can address issues identified as part of the assessment and screening (Shopbell and others, 2001).

BOX 8-4 Selected Examples of Cultural or Religious Beliefs Related to Food

- The theory of hot and cold foods predominates in many cultures. Filipinos, Caribbean Islanders, Mexicans, and Latinos may plan their meals based on these beliefs. Food classification as hot or cold varies slightly from culture to culture. Mexicans believe hot is warmth, strength, and reassurance, whereas cold is menacing and weak. Classification has nothing to do with spiciness. Hot foods include rice, grains, alcohol, beef, lamb, chili peppers, chocolate, and cheese. By contrast, cold foods include beans, citrus fruits, dairy products, most vegetables, honey, raisins, chicken, fish, and goat. Foods can be made hot or cold through methods of preparation.
- Orthodox Judaism requires adherence to kosher food preparation methods and prohibits eating pork, predatory fowl, shellfish (i.e., crab, shrimp), blood, and mixing of milk or dairy products with meat dishes. No cooking is done on the Sabbath (sundown Friday through sundown Saturday). For all Jewish sects no leavened bread is eaten during Passover.
- Muslims also prohibit the intake of pork and sometimes practice dietary guidelines similar to kosher, called halal.
- The Church of Jesus Christ of Latter-Day Saints (Mormons) prohibits the use of alcohol, tobacco, and caffeine.
- Seventh-Day Adventists encourage a vegetarian diet and prohibit intake of pork, shellfish, and alcohol.

TABLE 8-1 Clinical Signs of Nutritional Status

BODY AREA	SIGNS OF GOOD NUTRITION	SIGNS OF POOR NUTRITION
General appearance	Alert, responsive	Listless, apathetic, cachectic.
Weight	Normal for height, age, body build	Overweight or underweight (special concern for underweight).
Posture	Erect, arms and legs straight	Sagging shoulders, sunken chest, humped back.
Muscles	Well-developed, firm, good tone, some fat under skin	Flaccid, poor tone, undeveloped, tender, "wasted" appearance, cannot walk properly.
Nervous control	Good attention span, not irritable or restless, normal reflexes, psychological stability	Inattentive, irritable, confused, burning and tingling of hands and feet (paresthesia), loss of position and vibratory sense, weakness and tenderness of muscles (may result in inability to walk), decrease or loss of ankle and knee reflexes.
Gastrointestinal (GI) function	Good appetite and digestion, normal regular elimination, no palpable (perceptible to touch) organs or masses	Anorexia, indigestion, constipation or diarrhea, liver or spleen enlargement.
Cardiovascular function	Normal heart rate and rhythm, no murmurs, normal blood pressure for age	Rapid heart rate (above 100 beats per minute, tachycardia), enlarged heart, abnormal rhythm, elevated blood pressure.
General vitality	Endurance, energetic, sleeps well, vigorous	Easily fatigued, no energy, falls asleep easily, looks tired, apathetic.
Hair	Shiny, lustrous, firm, not easily plucked, healthy scalp	Stringy, dull, brittle, dry, thin and sparse, depigmented, can be easily plucked. May indicate protein, zinc, vitamin B_{12}, or essential fatty acid deficiency.
Skin (general)	Smooth, slightly moist, good color	Rough, dry, scaly, pale, pigmented, irritated, bruises, petechiae, delayed wound healing, xanthoma (yellowish papules), presence of decubitus ulcers. May indicate vitamin A, zinc, protein, vitamin C, or essential fatty acid deficiency.
Face and neck	Skin color uniform, smooth, healthy appearance, not swollen	Greasy, discolored, scaly, swollen, skin dark over cheeks and under eyes, lumpiness or flakiness of skin around nose and mouth. May indicate protein and calorie malnutrition.
Lips	Smooth, good color, moist, not chapped or swollen	Dry, scaly, swollen, redness and swelling (cheilosis), or angular lesions (stomatitis) at corners of the mouth or fissures or scars. May indicate iron, vitamin B_6, niacin, or riboflavin deficiency.
Gums	Good pink color, healthy, red, no swelling or bleeding	Spongy, bleed easily, marginal redness, inflamed, gums receding. May indicate vitamin C, folic acid, or vitamin B_{12} deficiency.
Tongue	Good pink color or deep reddish in appearance, not swollen or smooth, surface papillae present, no lesions	Swelling, scarlet and raw, magenta color, beefy (glossitis), hyperemic and hypertrophic papillae, atrophic papillae.
Teeth	No cavities, no pain, bright, straight, no crowding, well-shaped jaw, clean, no discoloration	Unfilled caries, absent teeth, worn surfaces mottled (fluoresis), malpositioned. May indicate protein and calorie malnutrition or excessive fluoride usage.
Eyes	Bright, clear, shiny, no sores at corner of eyelids, membranes moist and healthy pink color, no prominent blood vessels or mound of tissue or sclera, no fatigue circles beneath	Pale conjunctival membranes, redness of membranes (injection), dryness, Bitot's spots, redness and fissuring of eyelid corners (angular palpebritis), dryness of eye membrane (conjunctival xerosis), dull appearance of cornea (corneal xerosis), soft cornea (keratomalacia). May indicate vitamin A, iron, folic acid, riboflavin, or vitamin B–complex deficiency.
Neck (glands)	No enlargement	Thyroid enlarged. May indicate iodine deficiency.
Nails	Firm, pink	Spoon-shaped (koilonychia), brittle, ridged, blue lunula. May indicate iron, chromium, or vitamin A deficiency and excess copper.
Legs and feet	No tenderness, weakness, or swelling; good color	Edema, tender calf, tingling, weakness, muscle wasting. May indicate protein and energy malnutrition and deficiencies of thiamin, selenium, calcium, vitamin D, and potassium.
Skeleton	No malformation	Bowlegs, knock-knees, chest deformity at diaphragm, beaded ribs, prominent scapulae.

Adapted from Hammond K: Dietary and clinical assessment. In Mahan L, Escott-Stump S: *Krause's food nutrition and diet therapy,* Philadelphia, 2003, Saunders.

EVIDENCE IN PRACTICE

Perry L, Love C: Screening for dysphagia and aspiration in acute stroke: a systematic review, *Dysphagia* 16:7-18, 2001.

Clients at risk for dysphagia (difficulty swallowing) should be formally screened so that steps can be taken to decrease the risk of aspiration. Clients who have suffered stroke, have Alzheimer's disease, undergone head and neck surgery, and have Parkinson's disease are examples. Dysphagia screening is recommended as part of a multidisciplinary approach to nutrition management. The malnutrition occurring in these individuals is secondary to insufficient protein, calorie, and micronutrient intake. Registered nurses (RNs), registered dietitians, physicians, or speech language pathologists can perform these screenings in clients. Early screening and treatment of dysphagia leads to more cost-effective treatment, improved quality of care, and optimal nutritional outcome.

THERAPEUTIC DIETS

Therapeutic diets require a physician's order and are used for many disease states, complementing and at times even replacing drug therapy. For example, clients with diabetes mellitus have inadequate production or effectiveness of insulin, resulting in high levels of plasma glucose. Type 2 diabetes mellitus, also called non–insulin dependent diabetes mellitus (NIDDM), accounts for 90% to 95% of individuals with diabetes. This type of diabetes is often managed with diet, exercise, or an oral hypoglycemic agent to balance plasma glucose. The diet is individualized according to the client's age, build, weight, and activity level. Protein provision of approximately 15% to 20% of daily intake is recommended to meet client needs and prevent renal risk (Franz and others, 2004). Fats are moderately controlled (30% or less), complex carbohydrates make up the majority of the diet (50% to 55%) rather than simple carbohydrates, and a daily intake of 25 to 30 g of fiber is recommended (AHA, 2006).

Therapeutic diets may also be modified in consistency or texture. After surgery clients may initially require a liquid diet for 1 to 2 days. A mechanical soft diet is used for clients without teeth; a high-fiber, high-residue diet is used in clients with constipation. When there are no restrictions, the order may be diet as tolerated (DAT) or regular diet. Other examples of therapeutic diets include diets low in fat or cholesterol, low in protein, and low in sodium (Table 8-2). For specific information about special diets see the agency dietary manual or contact a dietitian.

NURSING DIAGNOSES

Imbalanced nutrition: less than body requirements is the nursing diagnosis for clients when the focus is increasing the quantity or quality of nutritional intake. **Feeding self-care**

TABLE 8-2 Diets of Modified Consistency

DIET	DESCRIPTION
Clear-liquid	Foods that are clear and liquid at room or body temperature. For example, chicken broth, tea, soda, gelatin, and apple or cranberry juice, which leave little residue and are easily absorbed. Is commonly ordered for short-term use (24 to 48 hours) postoperatively, prior to diagnostic tests, and after episodes of vomiting or diarrhea.
Full-liquid	Consists of foods that are liquid at room or body temperature and are easily digested and absorbed. Includes foods allowed on clear-liquid diet plus milk and some milk-containing foods, such as creamed, strained soups and ice cream. Is commonly ordered before or after surgery for clients who are acutely ill from infection or for clients who cannot chew or tolerate solid foods. Determine if clients are lactose tolerant.
Pureed	Includes easily swallowed foods that do not require chewing. May be ordered for clients with head and neck abnormalities or who have had oral surgery. Diets can be modified for low sodium, fat, or calorie control.
Mechanical or dental-soft	Consists of lightly seasoned foods that do not need chewing, such as chopped or ground foods. Avoids tough meats, nuts, bacon, and fruits with tough skins or membranes. May be ordered for clients who have chewing problems or mild GI problems. Used as transition diet from liquids to regular.
Soft	Includes foods that are low in fiber, easily digested, easy to chew, and simply cooked. Does not permit fatty, rich, and fried foods. Is sometimes referred to as low-fiber diet.
High-fiber	Includes sufficient amounts of indigestible carbohydrate to relieve constipation, increase gastrointestinal (GI) motility, and increase stool weight.
Diet as tolerated	Commonly ordered postoperatively. Permits clients' preferences and situations to be considered, and allows for postoperative diet progression.
Sample Therapeutic Diets	
Restricted fluid intake	Required in severe heart failure and kidney failure.
Sodium-restricted	Allows low levels of sodium by food selection and may include a 4-g (no added salt), 2-g (moderate), 1-g (strict), or 500-mg (very strict) diet. May be ordered for clients with congestive heart failure (CHF), renal failure, cirrhosis, or hypertension.
Fat-modified	Low total and saturated fat and low cholesterol. Cholesterol intake limited to less than 300 mg daily and fat intake to 30% to 35% by eliminating or reducing fatty foods for hypercholesterolemia, malabsorptive disorders, diarrhea, and steatorrhea.
Diabetic	Ordered as essential treatment for clients with diabetes mellitus. Provides clients with a diet recommended by American Diabetes Association (ADA), which allows for clients to select set amount of food from basic food groups.

Grodner M, Lon S, DeYoung S: *Foundations and clinical applications of nutrition*, ed 3, St Louis, 2004, Mosby.

deficit relates to the inability of clients to prepare food or feed themselves because of mobility or because of coordination, visual, or mental problems. **Impaired swallowing** is related to an altered gag reflex or inability to cough, weakened muscles of chewing, or mechanical alterations such as cancer of the upper airway, an obstructing tumor, or an esophageal fistula (abnormal opening between the esopha-gus and adjacent body cavity). **Risk for aspiration** is appropriate for clients who have difficulty swallowing or who are relearning to swallow after neurological damage or surgery. **Imbalanced nutrition: more than body requirements** is appropriate when clients are more than 10% to 20% over the desired weight range for their height.

SKILL 8.1 Feeding Dependent Clients

- **Nursing Skills Online: Safety, Lesson 4**

Some hospitalized clients are unable to feed themselves adequately because of the severity of their illness or the fatigue and debilitation associated with their condition. Others are limited by loss of arm or hand movement, impaired vision, brain injury, or the need to remain in a flat or prone position. When assisting the client with feeding, the nurse encourages the client to ingest an adequate volume of food at a comfortable pace. It is important to encourage independence when possible with the use of adaptive devices or finger foods and with comfortable and safe positioning for swallowing. Sitting and talking during mealtime is important because mealtime is often viewed as a social time for clients.

ASSESSMENT

1 On admission and weekly, measure client's weight and assess pertinent laboratory values indicative of nutritional balance.

2 Assess food tolerance, cultural and religious preferences, and food likes and dislikes. *Rationale: Determines if certain foods will improve oral intake and desire to feed independently.*

3 Confirm client's diet with physician orders to ensure the client receives proper diet. *Rationale: Clients with chronic diseases, such as cardiac or renal disease, may need alterations in nutrient content or flavoring. After surgical procedures the client may progress from a clear liquid diet to a regular diet as the client's ability to digest or tolerance of more complex nutrients returns.*

4 Place a tongue blade on the back of the client's tongue to determine the presence of a gag reflex. *Rationale: Clients who do not gag are at risk for aspiration (see Skill 8.2).*

5 Assess client's ability to swallow by placing fingers at level of larynx and asking client to swallow saliva. *Rationale: Movement of larynx can normally be palpated.*

6 Assess level of consciousness, ability to cooperate, mobility/activity orders, and physical limitations. *Rationale: Determines appropriate positioning for meals and level of assistance required.*

7 Assess need for toileting, hand washing, and oral care before feeding. *Rationale: Reduces interruptions and improves appetite during the meal.*

PLANNING

Expected Outcomes focus on increased independence with eating, improved nutritional intake, and safe intake of food.

1 Client's body weight remains stable or trends toward the desired level.

2 Client's nutrition-related laboratory values trend toward normal. (Note serum prealbumin and hemoglobin values.)

3 Client demonstrates increased ability to self-feed or open items on tray as appropriate.

4 Client coughs appropriately when eating with no new signs of respiratory compromise.

5 Client uses adaptive utensils appropriately as indicated.

6 Client improves quality of nutritional intake.

Delegation Considerations

The skill of assisting the client with oral nutrition may be delegated. The nurse directs personnel by:

- Explaining how to position client to avoid any swallowing problems
- Reviewing to observe for coughing, gagging, or difficulty in swallowing and to report information back to the nurse

Equipment

- Meal tray
- Over-bed table
- Adaptive utensils if appropriate (Figure 8-2)
- Damp washcloth (optional)
- Oral hygiene supplies (optional)

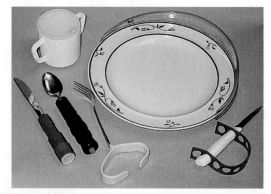

FIGURE 8-2 Adaptive equipment. *Clockwise from upper left:* Two-handled cup with lid, plate with plate guard, utensils with splints, and utensils with enlarged handles.

IMPLEMENTATION *for Feeding Dependent Clients*

STEPS	RATIONALE
1 See Standard Protocol (inside front cover).	
2 Offer toileting and hand washing before meal.	Increases level of comfort.
3 Offer toothbrush or mouthwash before meal.	May improve appetite in client with stomatitis or other oral hygiene problems.
4 Check the environment for distractions. Reduce the noise level if possible.	
5 Position client appropriately for safe eating within limitations of ability.	Positioning helps improve swallowing and digestion and avoids aspiration.
a. Up in chair	
b. High-Fowler's position in bed (see illustration)	
c. Side-lying position if flat in bed	
6 Assess tray for completeness and correct diet.	Prevents intake of incomplete or incorrect diet.
7 Assist client with setting up meal tray if client is unable to do so: Open packages, cut up food, apply seasonings/condiments, butter bread, and place napkin.	Reduces effort needed to self-feed.
8 Place adaptive utensils on tray if indicated, and instruct in their use.	
9 If client is visually impaired, identify food location on plate as if it were a clock (e.g., the chicken is at 12 o'clock) (see illustration).	Visually impaired client may feed self when given adequate information about tray.
10 Pace feeding to avoid client fatigue. Ask client the order in which he or she wishes to eat food. Interact with client during mealtime. Verbally encourage self-feeding attempts.	Gives client some control of situation and avoids embarrassment about limitations. Social interaction may improve appetite.

> **COMMUNICATION TIP** Use simple verbal prompts and touch, for example, "Here is your bread" (place bread in the client's hand). Pantomime desired behaviors, such as drinking a beverage.

STEPS	RATIONALE
11 Assist client with washing hands and repositioning as desired.	
12 Monitor intake and output (I&O) (see Skill 9.1) and calorie count.	Physician's orders may require identifying the specific number of calories consumed. The dietitian usually completes this; however, the nurse is vital in the recording of percentages of menu items consumed.
13 See Completion Protocol (inside front cover).	

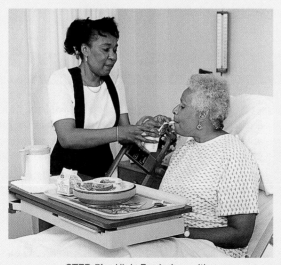

STEP 5b. High-Fowler's position.

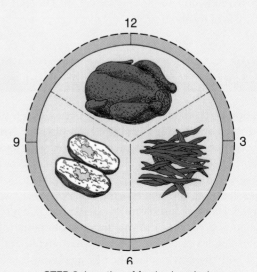

STEP 9 Location of food using clock.

EVALUATION

1 Monitor body weight daily or weekly.
2 Monitor laboratory values as ordered.
3 Observe client's technique for self-feeding: certain items, part or all of meal.
4 Observe client for choking, coughing, gagging, or food left in the mouth during eating.
5 Observe use of adaptive utensils.
6 Observe amount of food on tray after meal.

Unexpected Outcomes and Related Interventions

1 Client refuses to eat food offered.
a. Determine if client has other food preferences, cultural influences, or religious restrictions.
b. Determine if client's ability and desire to eat is better at other times of the day.
2 Client chokes on food.
a. Use suction equipment if necessary to clear food from airway.
b. If choking occurs repeatedly, stop feeding and notify physician.
3 Food sits on side or back of mouth (see Skill 8.2).
a. Initiate interventions to assist dysphagic clients with eating (see Skill 8.2).

Recording and Reporting

- Record the food and fluids actually consumed (for calorie count and I&O) and the degree of participation/independence. Describe client's ability to swallow and any choking that occurs.
- Report any choking or food tolerance/intolerance and significant changes to the dietitian.

Sample Documentation

0800 Able to feed self 5 bites with encouragement. Reported, "That is all I can do." Remaining breakfast fed to client. No difficulty swallowing or coughing noted. Consumed 70% of meal.

Special Considerations
Pediatric Considerations

- Food allergies are common in infancy because the immature intestinal tract is more permeable to proteins. Food allergies may be prevented by avoiding cow's milk for the first 6 months.
- Age affects the requirements for essential nutrients. Periods of rapid growth increase the need for calories, protein, vitamins, and minerals. A child requires more calories per kilogram of body weight than an adult.

Geriatric Considerations

- Changes in taste perception, oral mucus and saliva production, and dentition with aging may affect the client's food choices and ability to chew or swallow. Assess the client's food patterns for nutrient, calorie, and fluid adequacy.
- Older adults may have difficulty eating because of physical symptoms or lack of teeth or dentures.
- Thirst sensation may diminish in older adults, leading to inadequate fluid intake or dehydration.

Home Care Considerations

- Homebound older adults may benefit from Meals on Wheels, which can provide as many as three meals per day depending on the client's community (Meals on Wheels, 2006).
- Clients who are unable to feed themselves independently may eat better if other family members participate at mealtimes to avoid social isolation.

Long-Term Care Considerations

- Institutionalized older adults often have nutrition issues related to poor appetite, infections, weight loss, pressure ulcers, and polypharmacy. In 2005 the American Dietetic Association (ADA) published a position statement endorsing liberalized diets for older adults in long-term care (Niedert, 2005).

SKILL 8.2 Aspiration Precautions

Aspiration in the adult client usually occurs as a result of difficulties in swallowing (dysphagia). Swallowing dysfunction, better known as dysphagia, is associated with multiple myogenic, neurogenic, and obstructive causes (Box 8-5). Dysphagia is a decreased ability to voluntarily pass fluids and/or solids from the mouth to the stomach. Swallowing is a complex event, requiring both voluntary and involuntary movements. It requires the coordination of cranial nerves and the muscles of the tongue, pharynx, larynx, and jaw. Clients with neuromuscular diseases involving the brain, brain stem, cranial nerves, or muscles of swallowing should

be assessed for swallowing difficulties before feeding. Notify the care provider immediately if a client complains of difficulty swallowing or displays the following characteristics:

- Cough and/or voice change (hoarseness) after swallowing
- Weak involuntary cough or delayed cough (as long as 2 minutes after swallowing)
- Abnormal lip closure and slowed tongue movement; tongue weakness
- Slow, weak, or uncoordinated speech
- Regurgitation and pocketing of food

BOX 8-5 Causes of Dysphagia

Myogenic
- Aging
- Dermatomyositis
- Muscular dystrophy
- Myasthenia gravis
- Polymyositis

Neurogenic
- Amyotrophic lateral sclerosis (Lou Gehrig disease)
- Cerebral palsy
- Diabetic neuropathy
- Guillain-Barré syndrome
- Multiple sclerosis
- Parkinson's disease
- Stroke

Obstructive
- Anterior mediastinal masses
- Benign peptic stricture
- Candidiasis
- Cervical spondylosis
- Esophageal webs
- Extrinsic structural lesions
- Head and neck cancer
- Inflammatory masses
- Lower esophageal ring
- Trauma/surgical resection
- Zenker's diverticulum

Other
- Connective tissue disorders
- Gastrointestinal (GI) or esophageal resection
- Rheumatological disorders
- Vagotomy

"Silent aspiration" occurs without a cough and poses a serious problem if left untreated. Silent aspiration accounts for 40% to 70% of aspiration in clients with dysphagia. If a client continues to aspirate, NPO status should be maintained. Dysphagia may lead to other medical complications including aspiration of food, aspiration pneumonia, and malnutrition.

There are many dysphagia screening tools, such as a registered dietitian dysphagia screening tool, a standardized swallowing assessment, or Smithard's bedside swallowing assessment. Subsequent to the identification of a swallowing problem, an order for a swallow evaluation should be obtained. Speech pathologists are trained to perform evaluation of swallowing and to recommend appropriate interventions. A speech therapist or radiologist may conduct a videofluoroscopic swallow study (VFSS) to assess level of dysphagia. The client is given pureed, liquid, and solid-consistency barium in varied amounts while the swallowing mechanism is visualized (Bastian, 1998).

After dysphagia is identified, several steps are taken to decrease risk of aspiration. Maintaining an upright position to enhance the effects of gravity is important. When feeding the client with weakness on one side, as in clients with hemiparesis, place food on the unaffected side of the mouth and observe the swallowing event closely for delays. Providing verbal coaching throughout the swallowing process can greatly help the client swallow more effectively.

A priority for dysphagic clients is the initiation of safe oral nutrition and hydration (Westergren, 2006). Changes in food consistencies and/or liquid consistencies, or even elimination of oral intake and initiation of tube feedings, are common diet modifications (Table 8-3). Liquid or pureed foods are sometimes the only consistency tolerated by clients with mechanical disorders that cause dysphagia, such as cancer and surgical resection. Clients with oropharyngeal dysphagia, caused by myasthenia gravis or muscular dystrophy, have more success with semi-solid consistencies that are easy to chew (Groher, 1997). Liquids often have to be thickened with a commercial thickener to decrease transit time and allow for protection of the airway (Dorner, 2002).

Liquids pose an increased risk for aspiration. Thickeners added to food or fluids increase the consistency and thus allow the client more control of the volume of fluid in the mouth. There are four levels of liquid consistencies: thin liquids (low viscosity), nectar-like liquids (medium viscosity), honey-like liquids (honeylike viscosity) and spoon-thick liquids (pudding-like viscosity) (NDDTF, 2002). After a client is placed on a thickened liquids diet, careful monitoring and assistance are needed at each meal or snack to prevent the client from choking or aspirating.

ASSESSMENT

1 Perform nutritional screening. *Rationale: Clients with aspiration from dysphagia may alter their eating pattern or choose foods that do not provide adequate nutrition (Perry and McLaren, 2003).*

2 Identify client's risk for aspiration (see Box 8-5). *Rationale: Clients with neurological problems, clients who exhibit poor lip and tongue control, and clients who had tongue or neck surgeries are at increased risk for aspiration.*

3 Observe client during mealtime for signs of dysphagia, and allow client to attempt to feed self. Note presence of fatigue at the end of the meal. *Rationale: Detects abnormal eating patterns, such as frequent clearing of throat or prolonged eating time. Fatigue increases risk of aspiration.*

4 Ask client about any difficulties with chewing or swallowing various textures of food.

5 Assess client's swallowing reflex before feeding by placing fingers on client's throat at level of the larynx, then asking client to swallow saliva. *Rationale: Movement of the larynx normally can be palpated.*

6 Place identification on client's chart or Kardex indicating dysphagia. *Rationale: Identification reduces risk of client receiving oral nutrition without supervision.*

TABLE 8-3 National Dysphagia Diet Stages

STAGE	DESCRIPTION	EXAMPLES
NDD-1: Dysphagia Pureed	Uniform Cohesive "Pudding-like" texture	Smooth hot cereal cooked to a "pudding" consistency Mashed potatoes Pureed meat Liquids and water thickened with thickening agent Pureed vegetables Yogurt
NDD-2: Dysphagia Mechanically Altered	Moist Soft textured Easily forms a bolus	Cooked cereals Dry cereals moistened with milk Canned fruit (except pineapple) Moist ground meat Well-cooked chopped vegetables Cooked noodles in sauce/gravy
NDD-3: Dysphagia Advanced	Regular foods (except very hard, sticky, or crunchy foods)	Moist breads (with butter, jelly, etc.) Well-moistened cereals Peeled soft fruits (banana, peach, plum) Tender, thin-sliced meat Baked potato (with no skin) Tender cooked vegetables
Regular	All foods	No restrictions

Modified from National Dysphagia Diet Task Force (NDDTF): *National dysphagia diet: standardization for optimal care*, Chicago, 2002, American Dietetic Association.
NDD, National Dysphagia Diet.

PLANNING

Expected Outcomes focus on adequate food and fluid intake to prevent malnutrition and dehydration while avoiding aspiration.

1 Client exhibits no symptoms of aspiration or new respiratory distress.
2 Client maintains adequate nutritional intake.

Delegation Considerations

The skill of instituting aspiration precautions may not be delegated. The nurse directs personnel by:

- Reviewing what to observe, such as choking, coughing, change in voice, or vomiting, and instructing personnel to immediately report these to the nurse.

Equipment

- Upright chair
- Thickener agent
- Tongue blade
- Penlight
- Suction equipment

IMPLEMENTATION *for Aspiration Precautions*

STEPS	RATIONALE
1 See Standard Protocol (inside front cover).	
2 Using a penlight and tongue blade, gently inspect mouth for pockets of food.	Pockets of food in the mouth can indicate difficulty swallowing.
3 Elevate head of client's bed so that hips are flexed at a 90-degree angle and head is flexed slightly forward, or help client to the same position in the chair.	Reduces risk of aspiration.
4 Observe client consume various consistencies of foods and liquids. Add thickener to thin liquids to create the consistency of honey (if necessary).	Thin liquids such as water and fruit juice are difficult to control in the mouth and are more easily aspirated (Goulding and Bakheit, 2000).
5 Place ½ to 1 teaspoon of food or 10 to 15 ml of liquid on unaffected side of the mouth, allowing utensil to touch the mouth or tongue.	

NURSE ALERT Avoid asking client to talk while eating.

STEPS	RATIONALE
6 Place hand on throat to gently palpate swallowing event as it occurs (see illustration). Swallowing twice is often necessary to clear the pharynx.	
7 Provide verbal coaching and positive reinforcement while feeding client.	Verbal cueing keeps client focused on swallowing. Positive reinforcement enhances client's confidence in ability to swallow.
8 Observe for coughing, choking, gagging, and drooling of food; suction airway as necessary.	These are indications that suggest dysphagia and risk for aspiration (Westergren, 2006).
9 Maintain upright position for 15 to 30 minutes after eating.	Helps avoid aspiration or regurgitation.
10 Provide mouth care after meals.	This dislodges any food or fluids that may have accumulated inside client's cheeks.
11 Advance diet to thicker foods that require more chewing and finally to thin liquids as tolerated.	Dietitian and/or speech pathologist can direct safest advancement of diet.
12 **See Completion Protocol (inside front cover).**	

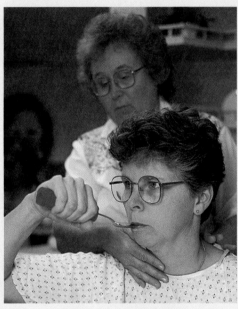

STEP 6 Palpate swallowing.

EVALUATION

1 Observe contents of client's mouth during meal for food pocketing.

2 Observe client for a continuous (not prolonged or delayed) swallowing event.

3 Observe client for coughing or choking during meal.

4 Monitor I&O, calorie count, and food eaten from tray.

5 Monitor daily or weekly weight (see Procedural Guideline 8-1).

Unexpected Outcomes and Related Interventions

1 Client begins coughing, choking, or turning blue.

a. Stop feeding client.

b. Position client in high-Fowler's position or, if unable, position on side.

c. Suction airway until clear.

d. Notify physician for possible study to evaluate for aspiration.

2 On inspection, food is found pocketed in client's cheeks.

a. Teach client to use the tongue or to massage the cheek externally to move food to a more functional area of the mouth.

Recording and Reporting

• Record client's tolerance of various food textures, amount of assistance required, position during meal, absence or presence of any symptoms of dysphagia, and amount eaten.

• Report any coughing, gagging, choking, or swallowing difficulties to nurse in charge or physician.

Sample Documentation

1200 Fed half of pureed diet and 4 oz juice with 1 teaspoon of thickener added with much encouragement. Refused additional food. No coughing or aspiration noted.

Special Considerations

Pediatric Considerations

- Swallowing is an automatic reflex for the first 3 months of life, and the infant has no voluntary control until approximately 6 weeks of age.
- Coordinated muscle action typical of the adult type of swallowing gradually develops with neural and muscular development.
- By 6 months of age the infant is capable of swallowing, holding food in the mouth, or spitting it out at will (Hockenberry and Wilson, 2007).

Geriatric Considerations

- Degenerative changes in the esophagus result in a decline in its motility, leading to dysphagia, heartburn, or vomiting and decreased food intake from fear of a recurrence of symptoms (Meiner and Lueckenotte, 2006).

Long-Term Care Considerations

- It is estimated that 40% to 60% of nursing home residents have some degree of dysphagia, which can lead to aspiration pneumonia, chronic malnutrition, decreased quality of life, and frustration for residents, family, and staff (Shanley and O'Loughlin, 2000).

PROCEDURAL GUIDELINE 8-1

Obtaining Height and Weight on Platform or Chair Scale

Obtaining Body Weights

A person's general level of health is reflected in the ratio of height to weight. Standardized tables can help reveal the normal expected weight for a client at a given height. Rapid weight gain of 2 pounds in a day can indicate fluid retention problems. A loss of 5% of body weight in a month or 10% of body weight in 6 months is significant. The JCAHO requires all hospitalized and home care clients to have height-weight measurement (JCAHO, 2006).

Obtaining an accurate body weight is important because it is one parameter used to evaluate and treat many diseases, including congestive heart failure (CHF), fluid overload, and renal failure. When monitoring weight for therapeutic purposes, care must be taken in using the same scale at or near the same time of the day, weighing the same amount of clothing or linen, and weighing client after emptying drainage bags (e.g., colostomy bag, catheter bag). Weight of drainage alters body weight (500 ml equals 1 pound). A chair scale should be used if client cannot stand independently. A bed scale should be used if client is unable to bear weight. Some of the new models of beds have scales built into their structures. Obtaining a client's weight on this type of scale requires following the manufacturer's instructions.

Infants may be weighed on a calibrated beam balance scale (Figure 8-3) or electronic scale. The infant is best weighed unclothed.

Delegation Considerations

The skill of obtaining height and weight may be delegated. The nurse directs personnel by:
- Explaining which weight device (i.e., platform or chair scale) to use for specific client
- Reviewing to observe client's intolerance (e.g., dizziness, lightheadedness) and to report information back to the nurse

Equipment
- Appropriate scale: standing, chair, or stretcher/bed scale

Procedural Steps
1 See Standard Protocol (inside front cover).
2 Determine client's ability to bear weight and safely stand on a scale. If client is alert but unable to stand, a chair scale may be used. If client is not alert or is critically ill, a bed scale is the safest means to obtain a weight.
3 Empty any pouches or drainage devices attached to client that contain drainage.

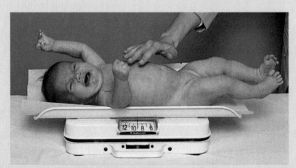

FIGURE 8-3 Weighing an infant. (From Wong DL: *Whaley & Wong's nursing care of infants and children,* ed 7, St Louis, 2003, Mosby.)

PROCEDURAL GUIDELINE 8-1—cont'd

4 Weigh client.

a. Platform or chair scale:

(1) Place platform or chair scale at client's bedside.

(2) Balance and calibrate scale to 0 pounds/kilograms. Balance beam should be in the middle of mark; digital scale should read 0.

(3) Ask client to step up onto platform scale and stand still (see illustration), or assist client with sitting on chair scale (see illustration).

(4) Adjust balance on scale until it is in middle of mark or until digital scale displays a reading (see illustration).

(5) With the client standing erect with good posture and without shoes, swing the metal rod attached to the back of the scale over the crown of the head (see illustration).

(6) With the rod horizontal to the measuring stick, measure height in inches or centimeters.

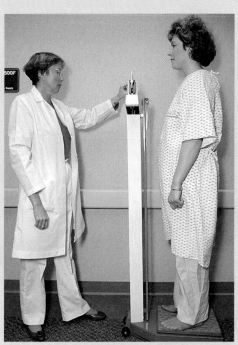

STEP 4a.(3) Standing weight.

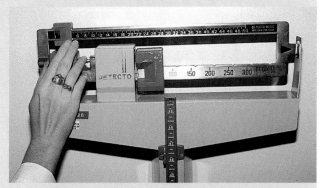

STEP 4a.(4) Balance the scale by moving the weight.

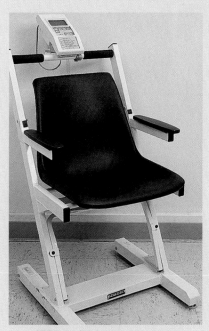

STEP 4a.(3) Using chair scale.

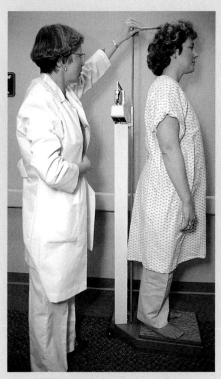

STEP 4a.(5) Measuring height.

PROCEDURAL GUIDELINE 8-1—cont'd

b. Bed scale:

(1) Place sling with same type and amount of linen and a client gown on arms of scale.

(2) Calibrate scale to 0 with linens and gown.

(3) Roll client onto side. Place sling under client (see illustration), using good body mechanics (see Chapter 6).

> **NURSE ALERT** To ensure client safety, obtain additional personnel and raise side rails as needed.

(4) Attach scale, and elevate until clear of bed (see illustration).

(5) Instruct client to remain still, if possible.

(6) Read digital weight on scale (see illustration).

(7) Lower client onto bed, roll over sling, then remove sling and scale from client's bed.

5 Compare weight obtained with previous weight.

6 Record weight on appropriate form (see agency policy).

7 **See Completion Protocol (inside front cover).**

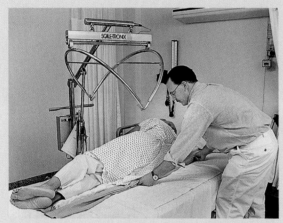

STEP 4b.(3) Place sling under client.

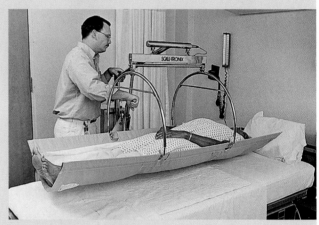

STEP 4b.(4) Elevate sling.

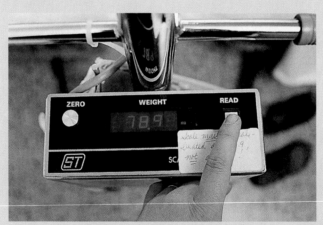

STEP 4b.(6) Read digital weight.

NCLEX® Style Questions

1 What is the most accurate assessment data reflecting the nutritional status of a postoperative client?
1. Skin integrity
2. The BMI
3. Prealbumin levels
4. Hydration

2 What is the BMI of a 5-foot woman who weighs 180 pounds?
1. 25
2. 30
3. 35
4. 40

3 Which cholesterol level indicates malnutrition?
1. 160 mg/dL
2. 170 mg/dL
3. 180 mg/dL
4. 190 mg/dL

4 Which of the following is a responsibility that should not be delegated?
1. Nutrition screening
2. Obtaining weight
3. Feeding
4. Aspiration precautions

5 Dysphagia can result from all of the following except:
1. Stroke
2. Hypertension
3. Guillain-Barré syndrome
4. Parkinson's disease

6 A client who is 2 days postoperative has normal GI function but is unable to chew due to facial surgery would benefit most from:
1. Clear-liquid diet
2. High-fiber diet
3. Soft diet
4. Pureed diet

References for all chapters appear in Appendix D.

9

Assisting with Elimination

MEDIA RESOURCES

- **evolve** http://evolve.elsevier.com/Elkin
- **View Video!** Video Clips
- Nursing Skills Online

Elimination is a basic function most people take for granted. Nurses routinely assist clients with elimination needs. It is important to understand the many factors that influence elimination. Most people believe elimination is a very private activity. The sights, sounds, and odors associated with elimination may be embarrassing and may prompt clients to decrease fluid intake to minimize the need to void or to ignore the urge to defecate for as long as possible. Clients with limited mobility have difficulty meeting elimination needs. Those with difficulty lowering to and rising from a sitting position may need assistance with an elevated toilet seat. Clients who have difficulty ambulating may need assistance using a bedside commode, bedpan, and/or urinal to prevent fecal and/or urinary incontinence. Some clients become incontinent of stool or urine as a result of neurological or cognitive dysfunction. Equipment such as an external collection device helps to maintain continence in men. However, there are no effective devices for women (Lekan-Rutledge and others, 2003).

Emotional factors affect elimination. Anxiety may result in urinary frequency and urgency or urinary retention. Anxiety, fear, and anger may accelerate peristalsis, resulting in diarrhea and gaseous distention. Persons suffering from depression may have decreased peristalsis, resulting in reabsorption of water from the stool and subsequent constipation.

Nurses are responsible for assisting clients with elimination. Because urine and feces are irritating to the skin, clients with elimination disorders require good skin care. Monitoring elimination status through the careful measurement of intake and output (I&O) keeps the nurse and other health care personnel informed about the client's fluid status.

EVIDENCE IN PRACTICE

Marklew A: Urinary catheter care in the intensive care unit, *Nurs Crit Care* 9(1):21, 2004.

Webster J and others: Water or antiseptic for periurethral cleaning before urinary catheterization: a randomized controlled trial, *Am J Infect Control* 29(6):389, 2001.

Urethral catheterization is a common procedure for clients with urinary retention or incontinence. Several complications are associated with urinary catheters, including urinary tract infection (UTI).

External meatal cleansing prevents the onset of UTIs and is routine in the care of clients with indwelling catheters. It is now generally accepted that using disinfectants and antibacterial agents as a part of meatal care is ineffective in decreasing the risk of catheter-related infection. Instead, cleansing of the external urethral meatus with soap and water is an essential part of catheter care. It is also recommended that external catheters be considered as an alternative to indwelling catheterization because there is a lower incidence of associated UTIs.

NURSING DIAGNOSES

Many different nursing diagnoses may pertain to clients with altered elimination. **Toileting self-care deficit** is appropriate for clients when the focus is to promote independence with toileting activities. **Constipation** applies with decreased frequency of stool passage and/or passage of hard, dry stool re-lated to inadequate dietary fiber, limited physical activity, or altered routines. **Risk for constipation** is appropriate when assessment reveals factors in the client's history that pose a risk for constipation. **Perceived constipation** results when a client expects a daily bowel movement and at the same time uses laxatives, enemas, or suppositories to achieve this.

Diagnoses such as **diarrhea** and **bowel incontinence** apply for clients who develop problems with normal defecation. Numerous nursing diagnoses relate to urinary incontinence, the involuntary loss of urine (e.g., **urge, stress,** and **total urinary incontinence**). The nursing diagnoses of **risk for impaired skin integrity, impaired skin integrity,** and **impaired tissue integrity** may be appropriate for incontinent clients.

The client may also develop or be at risk for **deficient fluid volume** or **excess fluid volume.** Additional diagnoses associated with the care of indwelling catheters may be **deficient knowledge** and **risk for infection.**

SKILL 9.1 Monitoring Intake and Output

Measuring and recording I&O is an important nursing responsibility. Intake to be measured and recorded includes liquids taken orally, by feeding tube, and parenterally. Output includes urine, vomitus, liquid stool, nasogastric drainage, and drainage from surgical tubes. Physicians often order I&O measurement as a routine practice after surgery or for select medical conditions. Nurses can initiate I&O measurement when they assess a client who has problems in maintaining an adequate fluid balance (e.g., change in drinking habits or increased urinary output). At specified times, usually every 8 hours, nurses total and evaluate a client's I&O. Significant alterations are identified by comparing 24-hour totals over several days. Because fluid imbalance can occur at any time, remain aware of I&O for all clients, even when documentation is not required.

Record I&O as soon as you complete measurements. If more than one client is in the same room, each must have measuring receptacles labeled with name and bed location. When possible, assistance from the alert client or family facilitates accurate I&O measurements.

ASSESSMENT

1 Identify medications that alter urine output. *Rationale: Diuretics cause water, sodium, and potassium excretion, resulting in an increased output; steroids (e.g., prednisone, cortisone) cause sodium and water retention and potassium excretion, resulting in a decreased output (Lewis, Heitkemper, and Dirkson, 2003).*

2 Monitor laboratory reports such as hematocrit (Hct) and urine specific gravity. *Rationale: Increased Hct value suggests fluid volume deficit (FVD); decreased Hct value suggests fluid volume excess (FVE). Increased specific gravity suggests dehydration; decreased specific gravity suggests fluid overload.*

3 Identify clients with conditions that alter fluid balance:

a. Fever. *Rationale: Prolonged fever increases insensible water loss from the lungs.*

b. Diarrhea and/or vomiting. *Rationale: Excessive fluid loss resulting from diarrhea results in losses of sodium, potassium, chloride, and bicarbonate, causing a fluid and electrolyte imbalance (see Chapter 28).*

c. Surgical wound drainage or chest tube drainage. *Rationale: May lead to excessive plasma or whole blood loss.*

d. Gastric suction. *Rationale: Loss of fluids may result in FVD.*

e. Major burns. *Rationale: Fluid volume loss is directly proportional to amount and depth of burn injury. Major fluid shifts can occur at specific intervals following severe burns.*

f. Congestive heart failure (CHF), renal disease, or endocrine disorders. *Rationale: Diseases of the heart, kidneys, and metabolism pose a risk for fluid and electrolyte imbalance.*

4 Identify clients with impaired swallowing, altered level of consciousness (LOC), and impaired mobility. *Rationale: Clients have risk for insufficient fluid intake.*

5 Weigh the client daily at the same time, on the same scale, in the same clothes. *Rationale: Fluid changes are reflected in sudden weight changes. Weight loss greater than 2% suggests FVD. Weight gain greater than 2% may indicate inadequate FVE. Differences in weight gain frequently occur before edema is present.*

6 Assess signs and symptoms of dehydration and fluid overload (see Chapter 28).

7 Assess the client's and family's knowledge of the purpose of I&O measurement and ability to participate actively in

measurement. *Rationale: Identifying the gap between the known and unknown helps to focus the teaching process (Lewis, Heitkemper, and Dirkson, 2003).*

PLANNING

Expected Outcomes focus on maintaining fluid balance, encouraging adequate fluid intake, and achieving normal laboratory values and body weight.

1 Client maintains fluid balance, as evidenced by intake approximately 600 ml greater than output, with total 24-hour output of at least 1500 ml.
2 Client's hematocrit and urine specific gravity are within normal limits (WNL).
3 Client's weight remains within 2% of baseline.

Delegation Considerations

The skills of evaluating I&O totals at the end of the shift, assessing trends in 24-hour total over several days, monitoring and recording of intravenous (IV) therapy, **recording** chest tube and wound drainage, and **administering** tube feedings may not be delegated. The nurse directs personnel by:
- Informing when to measure and record oral intake and output.
- Instructing personnel to observe and report any significant alteration in intake or changes in color, amount, or odor of output, including episodes of incontinence.

Equipment
- Sign alerting all personnel of I&O measurement
- Daily I&O record
- Graduated measuring containers (Figure 9-1)

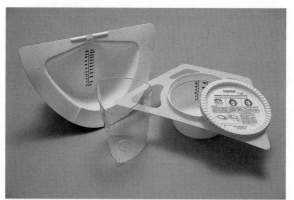

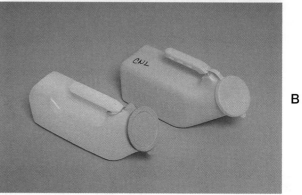

FIGURE 9-1 Graduated measuring containers and urinals. **A,** *Left to right:* "hat" receptacle, specipan, and graduated measuring container. **B,** Urinals.

- Bedpan, urinal, bedside commode, or specipan or "hat" (receptacle that fits inside commode)
- Clean gloves

IMPLEMENTATION *for Monitoring Intake and Output*

STEPS	RATIONALE
1 See Standard Protocol (inside front cover).	
2 Explain to client and family the reasons for needing accurate I&O measurements.	Accurate measurements help to identify fluid imbalance.

> **COMMUNICATION TIP** Tell client or family exactly what is to be measured and where to record it. Have client or family demonstrate ability to measure and record accurately.

STEPS	RATIONALE
3 Measure and record all fluid intake.	Provides comprehensive and accurate fluid balance assessment.
a. Liquids with meals may include gelatin, custards, ice cream, popsicles, and sherbets (any substance that becomes liquid at room temperature). Ice chips are recorded as 50% of measured volume (e.g., 100 ml ice equals 50 ml water).	
b. Liquid medicines such as antacids are counted as fluid intake, as are liquids taken with medicines.	

STEPS	RATIONALE

c. Enteral nutrition (tube feedings) (see Chapter 31).

d. IV fluid, blood components (see Chapter 27), and total parenteral nutrition (TPN) solutions.

4 Instruct client and family to call nurse to empty contents of urinal, urine "hat," or commode each time it is used. Also monitor and record incontinence, vomiting, and excessive perspiration.

Family can be valuable partners in preventing lost I&O measurements. Urine leakage on a pad can be weighed (1 ml of urine weighs 1 g) and counted as intake.

> **NURSE ALERT** Report urine output less than 30 ml/hr. Urine output less than 30 ml/hr may indicate decreased renal perfusion (Lewis, Heitkemper, and Dirkson, 2003).

5 Inform client and family that Foley catheter drainage bag, wound drainage device, or gastric drainage are closely monitored, measured, and recorded and that the nurse or assistive personnel (AP) are responsible for this. Each client must have a graduated container clearly marked with name and bed location and used only for the client indicated.

Prevents client or family from disrupting drainage systems.

6 Measure drainage at the end of the shift using appropriate containers and noting characteristics of drainage: color, consistency, amount, and odor. If splashing is anticipated, wear mask, eye protection, and/or gown.

Provides comprehensive and accurate assessment over standard time frames. Dark, concentrated urine suggests dehydration; colorless urine may indicate overhydration (Lewis, Heitkemper, and Dirkson, 2003).

> **NURSE ALERT** Empty full urinary drainage bag prior to ambulation.

a. Measure urine using a urinal, or specipan or "hat" into which the client voids, or a graduated container.

b. Measure urine output from Foley catheter into clean graduated container (see illustration). Do not touch edge of graduated container or floor with tip of port while draining and before recapping. If tip of port becomes contaminated, cleanse with antiseptic swab.

Contaminated port creates source for infection that could spread through drainage system to client.

c. Observe color and consistency of urine in Foley drainage tubing. Some clients may have a special device that is emptied into the larger container hourly.

Drainage in tubing is representative of current output. Characteristics of drainage in the bag are often noticeably different based on changes over time.

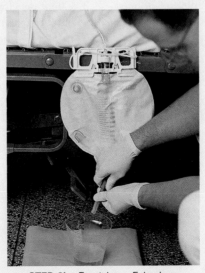

STEP 6b. Emptying a Foley bag.

STEPS	RATIONALE

d. Measure chest tube drainage by marking and recording the time on the collection chamber at specific intervals (see Chapter 29).

e. Measure and record output from all other sources, such as nasogastric suction (see Chapter 30).

f. Measure Jackson-Pratt Hemovac drainage using a medicine cup (see illustration) (see Chapter 21).

Drainage is usually less than 30 ml in volume.

g. Measure larger drainage pouches with a 240-ml graduated container (see illustration).

7 See Completion Protocol (inside front cover).

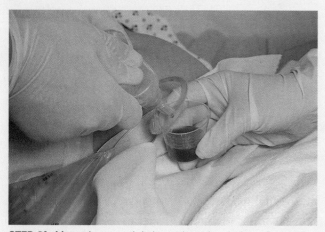

STEP 6f. Measuring wound drainage through a Jackson-Pratt drain.

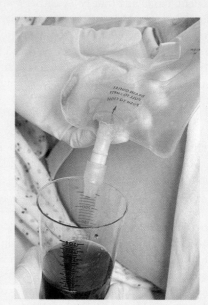

STEP 6g. Measuring wound drainage.

EVALUATION

1 Monitor total I&O at the end of each shift and 24 hours for any imbalance.

2 Monitor laboratory test reports for serum Hct values and specific gravity.

3 Compare daily weights, noting increase or decrease greater than 2% within 48 hours.

Unexpected Outcomes and Related Interventions

1 Client develops FVE (see Chapter 28), as evidenced by intake greater than output and weight gain greater than 2% over 24 to 48 hours, a low Hct value, and decreased specific gravity.

a. Assess other signs of FVE (see Chapter 28).

b. Anticipate fluid restriction.

c. Administer diuretics as ordered.

d. Weigh client daily.

e. Notify physician of changes in client's physical assessment.

2 Client develops FVD (see Chapter 28), as evidenced by output greater than intake, weight loss greater than 2% in 24 to 48 hours, a high Hct value, and increased specific gravity.

a. Assess other signs and symptoms of FVD (see Chapter 28).

b. Administer fluid replacement as ordered.

c. Weigh client daily.

d. Notify physician of changes in client's physical assessment.

Recording and Reporting

• Document I&O total on the specified I&O summary form in the client's chart every 8 hours or as ordered (Figure 9-2).

• Document any changes or clinical signs in nurse's notes.

• Report immediately to physician any urine output less than 30 ml/hr or significant changes in daily weight.

Sample Documentation

1500 Client states she feels as though she cannot eat or drink anything; refused lunch. 300 ml PO fluid intake in 8 hours; temperature 38.5° C. Urine dark amber, output 200 ml this shift. Physician notified.

1530 1000 ml NS started IV in back of right hand with #18 angiocath. Infusing per pump at 125 ml/hr without signs of swelling or redness. Client denies discomfort at site.

Special Considerations

Pediatric Considerations

- Infants and young children have a greater need for water and are more vulnerable to alterations in fluid and electrolyte balance than other age groups (Hockenberry and Wilson, 2007).
- Infants ingest and excrete a greater amount of fluid per kilogram of body weight than do older children (Hockenberry and Wilson, 2007).
- Obtain accurate I&O for infants and young children by weighing diapers (1 g weight equals 1 ml urine) or by using urine collection bags.

Geriatric Considerations

- Older adults are more susceptible to fluid imbalances with fever, chronic illness, gastroenteritis, or trauma.
- Incontinence may be discovered when I&O is monitored; however, incontinence is not a function of age (Meiner and Lueckenotte, 2006).

Home Care Considerations

- Assess client's or primary caregiver's ability to maintain accurate I&O measurement at home.
- Demonstrate measuring, recording, and weighing, and request return demonstration from client or home caregiver.

Long-Term Care Considerations

- Promote continuity between acute care and long-term care facilities.
- Clients in long-term care facilities can take an active part in their care if they are taught to measure and record I&O.

SKILL 9.2 Providing a Bedpan and Urinal

A client restricted to bed uses a bedpan or urinal for elimination. Women use bedpans to pass urine and feces. Men use bedpans for defecation and typically use urinals for urination.

Two types of bedpans are available (Figure 9-3). The regular and most commonly used bedpan has a curved, smooth upper end and a tapered lower end. A fracture pan, designated for clients with body or leg casts or clients restricted from raising their hips (e.g., after a total joint replacement), slips easily under a client. The upper end (wide end) of either pan fits under the client's buttocks toward the sacrum, with the lower end (tapered end) fitting just under the upper thighs.

ASSESSMENT

1 Assess client's normal elimination habits: routine pattern, effect of certain foods/fluids and eating habits on bowel elimination, effect of stress and level of activity on normal bowel elimination patterns, current medications, and normal fluid intake. *Rationale: Managing a client's elimination problems depends on a thorough understanding of normal elimination and factors that may create alterations.*

2 Assess client to determine level of mobility, including ability to sit upright and ability to lift hips or turn. *Rationale: Determines if client can assist in positioning on bedpan or if totally dependent on nurse. Determines type of bedpan needed.*

3 Auscultate bowel sounds, and palpate abdomen and bladder for distention. Ask client if flatus is being passed. *Rationale: Abnormal bowel sounds, passage of flatus, or a distended bladder indicates bowel or urinary elimination alterations.*

4 Assess client's level of comfort. Especially note presence of rectal or abdominal pain or presence of hemorrhoids or skin irritation surrounding anus. *Rationale: Pain limits client's ability to assist with positioning. Rectal or abdominal pain reduces client's ability to bear down during defecation.*

5 Determine if a urine or stool specimen is to be collected. *Rationale: Ensures that nurse gathers necessary supplies before placing client on bedpan.*

6 Assess characteristics of urine and feces, including color, amount, consistency, and odor. *Rationale: Provides baseline to determine elimination status.*

PLANNING

Expected Outcomes focus on the management of bowel and urinary elimination.

1 Client successfully defecates while on bedpan.
2 Client's perineal and perianal skin remain intact without redness or irritation.
3 Client eliminates without pain.

Delegation Considerations

The skill of providing a bedpan and urinal may be delegated. The nurse directs personnel by:

- Informing personnel about correct positioning guidelines for clients with mobility restrictions or clients who have therapeutic equipment such as wound drains, IV catheters, or traction.
- Instructing personnel to provide personal hygiene as necessary after defecation and urination.

Intake and Output Summary

Patient Label	P.O. Intake	Tube Feedings	Hyperalimentation	I.V. Primary	I.V.P.B.	Blood/Blood Products	Other:	Urine	Emesis	G.I. Suction	Drainage	Other: Chest tube
Date: 6-10-XX												
2200–0600	120				50			325			50	75
0600–1400	800							700			75	50
1400–2200	650				50			500			30	50
24Hr. Subtotal	1570				100			1525			155	175
Total Intake/Output	1670							1855				
Date:												
2200–0600												
0600–1400												
1400–2200												
24Hr. Subtotal												
Total Intake/Output												
Date:												
2200–0600												
0600–1400												
1400–2200												
24Hr. Subtotal												
Total Intake/Output												
Date:												
2200–0600												
0600–1400												
1400–2200												
24Hr. Subtotal												
Total Intake/Output												
Date:												
2200–0600												
0600–1400												
1400–2200												
24Hr. Subtotal												
Total Intake/ Output												
Date:												
2200–0600												
0600–1400												
1400–2200												
24Hr. Subtotals												
Total Intake/Output												
Date:												
2200–0600												
0600–1400												
1400–2200												
24Hr. Subtotals												
Total Intake/Output												

FIGURE 9-2 I&O summary.

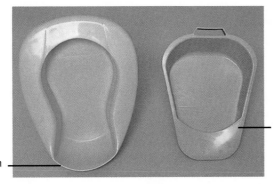

Open rim

FIGURE 9-3 Type of bedpans. *Left,* Regular bedpan; *right,* fracture bedpan.

Open rim

Equipment
- Clean gloves
- Bedpan (regular or fracture) (see Figure 9-3)
- Urinal
- Graduated container (used for measuring volume if on I&O)
- Bedpan cover
- Toilet tissue
- Specimen container (if necessary) or plastic bag, clearly labeled with date, client's name, and identification number
- Washbasin, washcloths, towels, and soap
- Clean drawsheet (if necessary)

IMPLEMENTATION *for Providing a Bedpan and Urinal*

STEPS	RATIONALE
1 See Standard Protocol (inside front cover).	
2 Bedpan.	
a. Provide privacy by closing curtains around bed or door of room.	
b. Place bedpan under warm, running water for a few seconds, then dry. Be careful that pan is not too hot.	Metal pans are very cold. Warming helps client to relax anal spincter.
c. Raise side rail on opposite side of bed.	Protects client from falling out of bed. Client can use side rail to grasp onto and assist self to move in bed.
d. Raise bed horizontally according to nurse's height.	Promotes use of good body mechanics and reduces muscle strain for nurse and client.
e. Have client assume supine position.	Position eases eventual pan placement.

> **NURSE ALERT** Observe for presence of drains, IV fluids, and traction. These devices may impede a client from assisting with the procedure and may also require more staff to assist placing the client on a bedpan.

> **COMMUNICATION TIP** Be matter-of-fact in your approach and tone of voice. Maintain a pleasant facial expression. Use terms the client will understand.

STEPS	RATIONALE
3 Place client who can assist on bedpan.	
a. Raise client's head 30 to 60 degrees.	Prevents hyperextension of back and provides support to upper torso when client raises hips.
b. Remove upper bed linens just enough so they are out of the way, but do not unduly expose client. Place bedpan in accessible location.	Maintains client's privacy and comfort.
c. Instruct client in how to flex knees and lift hips upward.	Little effort should be required of the client, whose body weight is supported by lower legs, feet, upper torso, and arms.

STEPS	RATIONALE
d. Place hand, palm up and closest to client's head, under client's sacrum to assist lifting. As client raises hips, use other hand to slip bedpan under client (see illustration). Be sure open rim of bedpan is facing toward foot of bed (see Figure 9-3). *Do not shove bedpan under client's hips.*	Ensures that bedpan is placed high enough under buttocks so feces enter pan. Incorrect placement of bedpan can cause spillage and discomfort for client. Shoving bedpan under client increases risk of friction injury to underlying skin and tissues.
e. *Optional:* if using a fracture pan, slip it under the client as the hips are raised. Be sure open rim of bedpan is facing toward foot of bed.	Requires less maneuvering by client.
f. Raise head of bed to 30 degrees or to level of comfort (unless contraindicated). Have client bend knees or raise knee gatch (if not contraindicated).	This approximates the normal position for elimination.
4 Place client who is immobile or has mobility restrictions on bedpan.	
a. Lower head of bed flat or head slightly raised (if tolerated by medical condition).	Assists client for whom it is unsafe to exert effort when lifting hips, who must remain flat, or who is unable to lift hips to roll onto bedpan.
b. Remove top linens as needed to turn client while minimizing exposure.	Maintains privacy and comfort.
c. Assist client with rolling onto one side, backside toward you.	Facilitates bedpan placement.
d. Place bedpan firmly against client's buttocks and down into mattress. Be sure open rim of bedpan is facing toward foot of bed (see illustrations).	Incorrect placement can cause client discomfort and spillage of contents.

NURSE ALERT Use a fracture pan if the client has had total hip replacement. An abduction pillow must be placed between the legs when turning to prevent dislocation of the new joint.

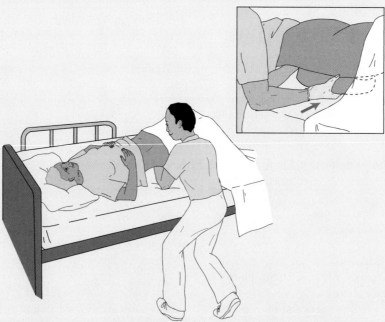

STEP 3d. The client raises the hips and buttocks off the bed as the bedpan is slid underneath. (From Sorrentino SA: *Mosby's textbook for nursing assistants,* ed 5, St Louis, 2000, Mosby.)

STEPS	RATIONALE
e. Keeping one hand against bedpan, place other hand around client's far hip. Ask client to roll back onto bedpan. *Do not shove bedpan under client.*	Positions client squarely on pan with minimal exertion. Shoving bedpan under client increases risk of friction injury to underlying skin and tissues.
f. Raise client's head 30 degrees or to level of comfort (unless contraindicated). Have client bend knees or raise knee gatch (if not contraindicated).	This approximates the normal position for elimination.
5 Maintain client's comfort and safety. Cover client for warmth.	Discomfort may prevent defecation.
6 Keep call bell and toilet tissue within easy reach for client, and place bed in lowest position.	
7 Ensure that bed is in lowest position and upper side rails are up.	Promotes client safety and enables the client to reposition as needed.
8 Remove and discard gloves.	Reduces transmission of microorganisms.
9 Allow client to be alone, but monitor status and respond promptly.	Provides privacy. Sitting on bedpan is uncomfortable. Monitor status because client may not be able to call for assistance.
10 Remove bedpan.	
a. Position client's bedside chair close to working side of bed.	Provides area to place bedpan after removal from client. Prevents spillage that could occur if full bedpan were placed on bed surface.
b. Maintain privacy; determine if client is able to wipe own perineal area. If nurse must wipe perineal area, use several layers of toilet tissue or perineal wipes. For female clients, cleanse from mons pubis toward rectal area.	Cleansing from an area of lesser contamination to greater contamination reduces spread of microorganisms.

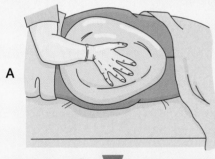

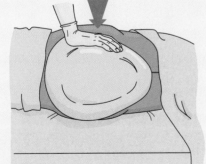

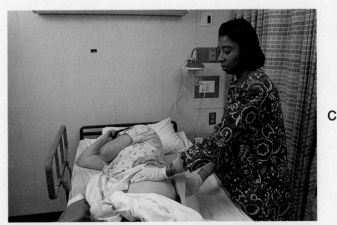

STEP 4d. A, Position the client on one side, and place the bedpan firmly against the buttocks. **B,** Push down on the bedpan and toward the client. **C,** Nurse places the bedpan in position. (**A** and **B** from Sorrentino SA: *Mosby's textbook for nursing assistants,* ed 5, St Louis, 2000, Mosby.)

STEPS	RATIONALE
c. Deposit contaminated tissue in bedpan. However, if you need to measure I&O or need a specimen, discard contaminated tissue in the commode. Allow client to perform hand hygiene after wiping perineal area.	Ensures accurate I&O recording.
d. For mobile client: Ask client to flex knees, placing body weight on lower legs, feet, and upper torso; lift buttocks up from bedpan. At same time, place hand farthest from client on side of bedpan and place other hand (closest to client) under sacrum completely lifted off bedpan. Place bedpan on bedside chair and cover.	Covering bedpan prevents spillage of contents.
e. For immobile client: Lower head of bed. Assist client with rolling onto side and off of bedpan. Hold bedpan flat and steady while client is rolling off it, otherwise spillage will occur. After client is completely lifted off bedpan, place it on bedside chair and cover.	
11 Change any soiled linens and return client to comfortable position.	
12 Position bed in lowest position. Ensure that call bell, phone, drinking water, and desired personal items are within reach.	Reduces risk of client fall.
13 Obtain stool or urine specimen as ordered. Empty bedpan into toilet or in special receptacle in appropriate utility room. Spray faucet attached to most institution toilets allows bedpan to be rinsed thoroughly.	Empty bedpan as soon as possible to prevent spread of offensive odor. Client uses same bedpan each time. If it becomes too soiled, replace with a clean one.

> **NURSE ALERT** Before emptying the bedpan, note the color and appearance of urine and stool. Measure the amount if I&O is being recorded (see Skill 9.1) and check for whether a specimen is needed (see Skills 13.1 and 13.2).

14 Remove and discard gloves.

15 Providing a urinal for a male client:

a. Provide privacy by closing curtain or door.

b. Assist client into appropriate position: on side, back, or sitting with head of bed elevated, or assist to standing position.	Men find it easier to void and empty bladder while standing.

> **NURSE ALERT** Always determine mobility status and risk for orthostatic hypotension before having a client stand to void.

c. If possible, client should hold urinal. If client needs assistance, position penis completely in urinal and hold urinal in place or assist client in holding urinal.	Penis is placed completely within urinal to avoid urine spills.

d. After the client has finished voiding, observe urine. Empty and cleanse urinal (use spray faucet attached to institution toilet). Return urinal to client for future use.

e. Urinals may be attached to the side rail for easy access.

f. Allow client to perform hand hygiene after voiding.

16 See Completion Protocol (inside front cover).

EVALUATION

1 Observe client's ability to use bedpan or urinal.

2 Observe and record the appearance and characteristics of stool, including color, odor, consistency, frequency, amount, shape, and constituents.

3 Observe and record the appearance, odor, and amount of urine.

4 Observe skin integrity in the perineal and perianal area.

5 Evaluate client's activity tolerance and level of comfort.

Unexpected Outcomes and Related Interventions

1 Client is unable to void using a bedpan or urinal.

a. Provide sensory stimulation that promotes voiding, such as running water in the sink or warm water over perineum, stroking the inner thigh, placing hand in warm water, or providing a drink (if not contraindicated).

b. Male clients may need to stand in order to void. Obtain adequate assistance if client is at risk of falling.

2 Client is unable to defecate using a bedpan.

a. Assist to as normal a position as possible. Have client massage upper abdomen from right to left to promote peristalsis.

b. Provide reading materials, and allow ample time and privacy for the process.

c. Consider use of a bedside commode rather than the bedpan if client is able to be up in a chair. Transfer client to commode as you would a chair. Client can sit on frame of commode in normal squatting position.

d. Collaborate with physician to consider client's need to have a stool softener or laxative ordered.

3 Client is incontinent.

a. Identify detailed information about episodes of incontinence, including how often, amount, and circumstances involved.

b. Offer bedpan or urinal more frequently (e.g., every 2 hours).

c. If client experiences the urge but cannot wait, place urinal within client's reach.

d. Male clients may benefit from an external catheter (see Skill 9.3).

Recording and Reporting

• Describe feces and urine, including odor, consistency, amount, and any other pertinent characteristics.

• If I&O measurement is being monitored in client, include output data on flow sheet (see Figure 9-2).

• Record client's elimination patterns; report alterations to physician.

Sample Documentation

0800 C/O abdominal cramping. Large, loose, light-brown stool evacuated on bedpan.

Special Considerations
Pediatric Considerations

• Infants and young children who are not toilet trained will not be able to use a bedpan or urinal (Hockenberry and Wilson, 2007).

• Older children may be embarrassed or self-conscious when asked to use a bedpan or urinal (Hockenberry and Wilson, 2007).

Geriatric Considerations

• The aging process alters defecation and micturition (Meiner and Lueckenotte, 2006). The older client may require the bedpan or urinal more frequently and more quickly or may not perceive the need to void or defecate.

• The older client may have a greater need for the "normal" position to empty the bowel or bladder because of long-ingrained cultural practices.

• Teach the older client the importance of diet and exercise in elimination.

Home Care Considerations

• Assess client and family for ability to carry out bowel and bladder care.

• Assess environment for accessibility of facilities and safety features such as elevated toilet seat.

Long-Term Care Considerations

• Provide personnel with a history of the client's elimination patterns to facilitate bowel and bladder care.

• Stress to personnel the importance of maintaining professional, respectful attitudes toward both cognitively impaired and alert clients requiring assistance with urine and bowel elimination.

SKILL 9.3 Applying an External Catheter

The application of an external urinary drainage device is a convenient, safe method of draining urine in male clients. The external catheter is suitable for incontinent or comatose clients who have complete and spontaneous bladder emptying. The external catheter is a soft, pliable rubber sheath that slips over the penis (Figure 9-4). External catheters have elastic adhesive provided to secure them in place. The catheter may be attached to a leg drainage bag or a standard urinary drainage bag.

Monitor an external catheter at least every 4 hours to detect potential problems such as skin irritation or inflammation of the urinary meatus. Change a catheter once every

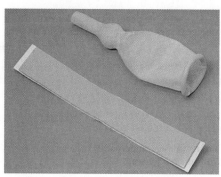

FIGURE 9-4 External catheter without adhesive.

24 hours for aseptic purposes. Cleanse the urethral meatus and penis thoroughly and inspect for signs of skin irritation with each catheter change.

ASSESSMENT

1 Assess urinary elimination patterns, ability to urinate voluntarily, and continence. *Rationale: Incontinent clients are at risk for skin breakdown and thus are candidates for external catheters.*

2 Assess mental status of client and client's knowledge of the purpose of an external catheter. *Rationale: Reveals need for client instruction. Teaching can include self-application.*

3 Assess condition of penis. *Rationale: Provides a baseline to compare changes in condition of skin after application of the external catheter.*

PLANNING

Expected Outcomes focus on promoting dryness and preventing continual exposure of skin to urine.

1 Client is continent with external catheter intact.
2 Penile shaft is free of skin irritation, breakdown, or swelling.
3 Client can explain the purpose of the procedure and what to expect.

Delegation Considerations
Assessment of the skin of the client's penile shaft and whether client has latex allergy should not be delegated. The skill of applying a condom catheter can be delegated. The nurse directs personnel by:

• Clarifying how to apply the adhesive strip that secures the condom catheter because methods for applying the catheter differ among manufacturers (see manufacturer's instructions).

• Instructing personnel to report to the nurse if swelling, redness, skin irritation, or breakdown is present.

Equipment
• Condom catheter kit (rubber condom catheter sheath of appropriate size, strip of elastic adhesive, skin preparation)
• Urinary collection bag with drainage tubing or leg bag and straps
• Skin preparation (tincture of benzoin)
• Basin with warm water and soap
• Towels and washcloth(s)
• Bath blanket
• Clean gloves
• Scissors

IMPLEMENTATION *for Applying an External Catheter*

STEPS	RATIONALE
1 See Standard Protocol (inside front cover).	
2 Provide privacy by closing room door or bedside curtain. Be sensitive to privacy needs.	
3 Raise bed to appropriate working height. If side rails are raised, lower side rail on working side.	
4 Assist client into supine position with a bath blanket over upper torso and lower extremities; expose only genitalia for procedure.	Promotes comfort and draping prevents unnecessary exposure of body parts.
5 Prepare urinary drainage collection bag and tubing. Clamp off drainage bag port. Secure collection bag to bed frame; bring drainage tubing up between side rails and bed frame. Be sure tubing is not pulled when side rails are raised. *Optional:* Prepare leg bag for connection to external catheter.	Provides easy access to drainage equipment. Positioning keeps drainage bag below level of client's bladder.
6 Provide perineal care (see Skill 7.1), and dry thoroughly.	Prevents skin breakdown from exposure to secretions. Rubber sheath rolls onto clean, dry skin more easily.

STEPS	RATIONALE

> **NURSE ALERT** Clip hair at base of penis. In some cases shaving the hair at the base of the penis may be necessary. Hair adheres to condom and is pulled during condom removal or may get caught in rubber as external catheter is applied.

7 Apply skin preparation to length of penile shaft and allow to dry. In an uncircumcised male, return foreskin to normal position. Do not apply preparation to glans of penis.

Skin preparation has an alcohol base. Evaporation prevents irritation. Ensuring foreskin in normal position prevents foreskin from tightening around penile shaft, which impedes circulation to penis and causes trauma to tissue.

8 With nondominant hand, grasp penis along shaft. With dominant hand, hold condom sheath at tip of penis and smoothly roll sheath onto penis (see illustration).

Ensures proper condom application.

> **NURSE ALERT** Allow 2.5 to 5 cm (1 to 2 inches) of space between tip of glans penis and end of condom catheter.

9 Apply adhesive.
a. Spiral wrap penile shaft with strip of elastic adhesive. Strip should be spiral wrapped and not overlap itself (see illustration).

Condom must be secured firmly so it is snug and stays on but not tight enough to cause constriction of blood flow. With some brands of catheters, the adhesive strip is applied before the condom is applied.

b. For newer catheters that are self-adhesive, apply catheter as in Steps 7 and 8, then apply gentle pressure on penile shaft for 10 to 15 seconds to secure catheter.

10 Connect drainage tubing to end of condom catheter. Be sure condom is not twisted. Catheter can be connected to a large-volume bag or leg bag (see illustration).

Allows urine to be collected and measured. Keeps client dry. Twisted condom obstructs urine flow.

11 Place excess coiling of tubing on bed and secure to bottom sheet.

Prevents looping of tubing and promotes free drainage of urine.

12 Lower bed, and place side rails accordingly.

Promotes safety.

> **NURSE ALERT** Do not apply standard adhesive tape, Velcro, or elastic strips around the penis; this could interfere with circulation and cause necrosis of penis.

13 See Completion Protocol (inside front cover).

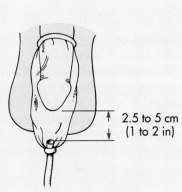

STEP 8 Condom catheter.

2.5 to 5 cm (1 to 2 in)

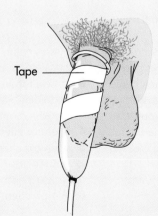

Tape

STEP 9a. Tape applied in spiral fashion.

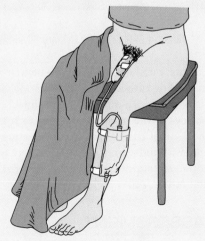

STEP 10 Leg bag.

EVALUATION

1 Observe urinary drainage.

2 Inspect penis with condom catheter in place within 30 minutes after application. Look for swelling and discoloration. Ask client if there is any discomfort.

3 Inspect skin on penile shaft for signs of breakdown or irritation at least daily when condom is removed during bath and when reapplied.

4 Determine client's understanding of the procedure.

Unexpected Outcomes and Related Interventions

1 Urination is reduced in amount or frequency.
a. Check for bladder distention.
b. Observe whether urine is pooling at tip of condom, bathing the penis in urine; reapply as necessary.
c. Check for kinks in tubing or in condom catheter.
2 Skin around penis is reddened and excoriated.
a. Reassess for possible latex allergy.
b. Remove external catheter, and notify physician.
c. Do not reapply until penis and surrounding skin are free from irritation.
3 Condom does not stay on.
a. Reapply as necessary.
b. Reassess condom size.
4 Penile swelling or discoloration occurs.
a Remove catheter, and allow swelling to decrease.
b. Notify physician.

Recording and Reporting

• Record condom application; condition of penis, skin, and scrotum; urinary output and voiding pattern; and client response to external catheter application.

Sample Documentation

0900 Urinary dribbling constant for 1 week. Perineal area reddened, even with frequent washing, drying, and application of barrier lubricant. Skin of penis intact without edema. Self-adhesive external catheter applied; connected to leg drainage bag.

1000 Voided 200 ml in leg bag without discomfort. Penis without swelling or discoloration.

Special Considerations

Geriatric Considerations

• Evaluate clients with neuropathy carefully before application of an external catheter and at more frequent intervals, at least twice daily.

• The skin on the penis will be very delicate on an older adult and prone to tearing; use extreme caution with adhesives.

• External catheters are not recommended in clients with prostatic obstruction.

Home Care Considerations

• External catheters may contribute to UTIs; therefore teach the family signs and symptoms of infection, and emphasize medical asepsis.

• Encourage use of a leg bag during the day and a bedside drainage bag at night.

• Loose-fitting clothing may be needed to promote adequate drainage.

• Explain to the family that long-term use of external catheters may result in skin breakdown.

Long-Term Care Considerations

• Teach personnel signs and symptoms of UTI and complications associated with external catheter use.

SKILL 9.4 Catheter Care

• **Nursing Skills Online:** Urinary Elimination, Lesson 5

Clients with altered urinary elimination may require an indwelling catheter (see Chapter 33). The catheter potentially provides a direct route for infection from the client's bladder to the outside. The urinary tract is the most common site of nosocomial (hospital-acquired) infections. Clients with indwelling catheters require regular catheter care with soap and water to reduce the risk of UTIs (Webster and others, 2001).

ASSESSMENT

1 Assess the urethral meatus and surrounding tissues for inflammation, swelling, secretions, or encrustations at the catheter insertion site. *Rationale: Determines presence of infection and status of hygiene.*

2 Assess color, clarity, and odor of urine. *Rationale: Urine that is cloudy and has a strong odor may indicate UTI.*

3 Assess for any complaints of pain or discomfort in lower abdomen. *Rationale: May indicate inflammation of urinary tract mucosa caused by bacterial invasion (Lewis, Heitkemper, and Dirkson, 2003).*

4 Monitor client's temperature. *Rationale: Fever may indicate a UTI.*

5 Monitor client's fluid intake. *Rationale: Decreased fluid intake inhibits the natural flushing of urinary system and increases the possibility of bacterial growth.*

6 Assess client's understanding of catheter care. *Rationale: Identifies the need for client instruction.*

PLANNING

Expected Outcomes focus on promoting perineal cleanliness and absence of UTI.

1 Urine is clear, and volume is adequate.
2 Urethral meatus is free of secretions and encrustations.
3 Client is afebrile.
4 Client verbalizes feeling of comfort after procedure.

Delegation Considerations

The skill of catheter care for clients with trauma or surgical procedures that involve the perineal area may not be delegated. Routine catheter care may be delegated and incorporated into perineal care. The nurse directs personnel by:

- Instructing personnel to report to the nurse catheter drainage (color, odor, amount).
- Instructing personnel to report to the nurse condition of catheter (leaks, secretions or encrustation at catheter insertion site), and condition of perineum (presence of inflammation, discharge, contamination from fecal discharge).
- Informing personnel how to follow positioning guidelines for clients with mobility restrictions.

Equipment

- Soap, washcloth, towel, basin, and warm water
- Clean gloves
- Bath blanket
- Waterproof pad

IMPLEMENTATION for Catheter Care

STEPS	RATIONALE
1 See Standard Protocol (inside front cover).	
2 Close bedside curtain or door. Be sensitive to client's needs.	Maintains client's privacy and comfort.
3 Raise bed to working height. If side rails are raised, lower side rail on working side.	Promotes proper use of body mechanics.
4 Position client, and cover with bath blanket, exposing only perineal area.	Reduces client embarrassment. Ensures easy access to perineal area.
a. Female in dorsal recumbent position.	
b. Male in supine position.	
5 Place waterproof pad under client.	
6 Provide routine perineal care (see Skill 7.1), being sure all perineal folds are cleansed thoroughly.	Removes secretions that harbor microorganisms.
7 Hold the catheter securely near the meatus with the gloved nondominant hand. Using a clean washcloth, soap, and water, take the dominant hand and wipe in a circular motion along the length of the catheter for about 10 cm (4 inches). Avoid placing tension on or pulling on the exposed catheter tubing.	Reduces presence of secretions, drainage, or fecal matter on exterior of catheter surface, decreasing risk of bacterial growth. External meatal cleansing reduces the risk for UTI (Cravens, 2000; Webster and others, 2004). Tension causes urethral trauma. Pulling on the catheter tubing may lead to accidental removal.
8 Replace as necessary the anchor device used to secure the catheter tubing to the client's leg or abdomen (see Skill 33.1).	Anchoring of catheter reduces pressure on the urethra, reducing the possibility of tissue injury. Local irritation to the urethra predisposes tissues to bacterial invasion.
9 Check drainage tubing and bag to ensure that:	
a. Tubing is coiled and secured onto bed linen.	
b. Tubing is not looped or positioned above level of bladder.	Ensures free flow of urine and prevents backflow into bladder.
c. Tubing is not kinked or clamped.	Ensures bladder drainage.
d. Collection bag is positioned on lower bed frame with urine flowing freely from tubing (see Skill 33.1).	Any interruption with the free flow of urine may cause UTI.
10 Empty collection bag as necessary or at least every 8 hours (see Skill 9.1).	Urine in collection bag provides a medium for bacteria growth.
11 Remove and discard gloves.	
12 See Completion Protocol (inside front cover).	

EVALUATION

1 Observe color, clarity, and amount of urine.
2 Inspect the catheter insertion site for secretions and encrustations.
3 Monitor the client's temperature.
4 Ask client about feelings of discomfort or burning.

Unexpected Outcomes and Related Interventions

1 Urethral or perineal irritation is present.
a. Assess for leaking of catheter, and replace as needed.
b. Ensure that the catheter is anchored correctly (see Skill 33.1).
c. Notify physician if securing catheter does not improve urethral irritation.
2 Client develops a UTI as evidenced by fever and by cloudy and concentrated urine.
a. Assess other signs of UTI.
b. Increase fluid intake to at least 1500 ml/day.
c. Monitor body temperature.
d. Notify physician of findings.

Recording and Reporting

• Record in nurses' notes condition of the perineum, including any secretions or encrustations at catheter insertion site and characteristics of the urine.

Sample Documentation

1000 Incontinent of large amount liquid brown stool after breakfast. Perineal area cleansed and catheter care given. No inflammation of perineum. No secretions or encrustations at catheter insertion site. Urine in catheter tubing and bag light amber and clear, draining well.

Special Considerations
Pediatric Considerations
• Describe the procedure to children at their level of understanding. You may also need to explain the procedure to the parents of young children.

Geriatric Considerations
• The older adult client may exhibit atypical symptoms of a UTI such as change in mental status (Meiner and Lueckenotte, 2006).
• Older adults are at high risk for nosocomial (hospital-associated) infections because of age-related changes in the immune system (Lewis, Heitkemper, and Dirkson, 2003).

Home Care Considerations
• Teach client and family importance of routine catheter care using soap and water (Promfret, 2000).
• Teach client and family signs and symptoms to report to nurse or physician.

SKILL 9.5 Administering an Enema

• Nursing Skills Online: Bowel Elimination/Ostomy, Lesson 2

An enema is the instillation of a solution into the rectum and sigmoid colon. The primary reasons for an enema include promotion of defecation in constipated clients or emptying the bowel before diagnostic procedures or abdominal surgeries. Clients should not rely on enemas to maintain bowel regularity because they do not treat the cause of irregularity or constipation. Frequent enemas disrupt normal defecation reflexes, resulting in dependence on enemas for elimination.

The volume and type of fluid instilled lubricates or breaks up the fecal mass, stretches the rectal wall, and initiates defecation. An oil-retention enema lubricates the rectum and colon, softens the feces, and facilitates defecation. An oil-retention enema can be used alone or as adjunct therapy to manual removal of a fecal impaction. An impaction involves presence of a fecal mass too large or hard to be passed voluntarily. Either constipation or diarrhea can suggest the presence of an impaction.

Cleansing enemas promote complete evacuation of feces from the colon by stimulating peristalsis through infusion of large volumes of solution. When "enemas until clear" is ordered in preparation for surgery or diagnostic testing, the water expelled may be colored but should not contain solid fecal material. Check agency policy, but usually clients should receive only three consecutive enemas to prevent fluid and electrolyte imbalance.

Medicated enemas contain pharmacological agents to reduce dangerously high serum potassium levels, as with a sodium polystyrene sulfonate (Kayexalate) enema, or to reduce bacteria in the colon before bowel surgery, as with a neomycin enema.

A carminative enema, such as the Harris or return-flow enema, relieves accumulated flatus. Always administer a small amount (100 to 200 ml) of enema solution into the client's rectum and colon. As the container is lowered, the solution flows back through the enema tubing to the container. Flatus will also return. You can slowly repeat raising and lowering the container numerous times to reduce flatus and increase peristalsis.

ASSESSMENT

1 Assess last bowel movement, bowel sounds, presence of hemorrhoids, mobility, and presence of abdominal pain

or cramping. *Rationale: Determines factors indicating need for enema and influences type of enema used. Also, establishes baseline for bowel function. Hemorrhoids may obscure the rectal opening and cause discomfort or bleeding with evacuation.*

2 Assess medical record for presence of increased intracranial pressure (IICP), glaucoma, or recent rectal or prostate surgery. *Rationale: Conditions contraindicate use of enemas.*

3 Determine client's level of understanding of purpose of enema.

4 Review physician's order for enema and clarify reason for enema administration. *Rationale: Order by physician is usually required for hospitalized client. Used to determine how many enemas client will receive and type of enema to be given.*

PLANNING

Expected Outcomes focus on establishing a normal pattern of bowel elimination and normal consistency of stools.

1 Client verbalizes relief of abdominal discomfort.
2 Stool is evacuated.
3 Abdomen is soft and nondistended.

Delegation Considerations

The skill of enema administration may be delegated. The nurse directs personnel by:

- Instructing how to position clients with therapeutic equipment such as drains, IV catheters, or traction.
- Instructing how to position clients with mobility restrictions.
- Instructing to immediately report to the nurse any symptoms of client intolerance of procedure, such as increasing abdominal pain, abdominal cramping, distention, or presence of rectal bleeding.

Equipment

- Clean gloves
- Water-soluble lubricant
- Waterproof absorbent underpads
- Toilet tissue

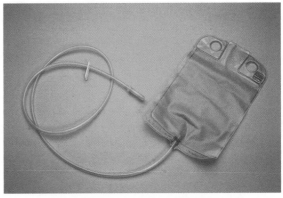

FIGURE 9-5 Enema bag with tubing.

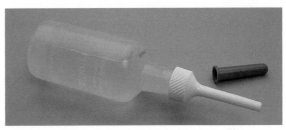

FIGURE 9-6 Prepackaged enema container with rectal tip.

- Bedpan, bedside commode, or access to toilet
- Washbasin, washcloths, towel, and soap
- Bath blanket
- IV pole

Enema Bag Administration

- Enema container (Figure 9-5)
- Tubing and clamp (if not already attached to container)
- Correct volume of warmed (tepid) solution (adult: 750 to 1000 ml; adolescent: 500 to 700 ml; school-age child: 300 to 500 ml; toddler: 250 to 350 ml; infant: 150 to 250 ml)

Prepackaged Enema

- Prepackaged enema container with rectal tip (Figure 9-6)

IMPLEMENTATION *for Administering an Enema*

STEPS	RATIONALE
1 See Standard Protocol (inside front cover).	
2 Provide privacy by closing door of room or curtain around bed. Be sensitive to client's needs.	Promotes client comfort and privacy.
3 Raise bed to appropriate working height for nurse; raise side rail on client's left side.	Promotes proper body mechanics and client safety.
4 Assist client into left side-lying (Sims') position with right knee flexed. Encourage client to remain in position until procedure is completed. Children may also be placed in dorsal recumbent position.	Allows enema solution to flow downward by gravity along natural curve of sigmoid colon and rectum, thus improving retention of solution.

STEPS	RATIONALE

> **NURSE ALERT** Clients with minimal sphincter control may not be able to retain all of enema solution and will require placement of a bedpan under the buttocks. Administering enema with client sitting on toilet is unsafe because curved rectal tubing can abrade rectal wall.

> **COMMUNICATION TIP** Adapt explanation of procedure to developmental level of client. If client is confused, use simple explanation and have personnel assist with positioning.

5 Place waterproof pad absorbent side up under hips and buttocks.

Prevents soiling of linen.

6 Cover client with bath blanket, exposing only rectal area, and clearly visualize anus.

Provides warmth, reduces exposure of body parts, and allows client to feel more relaxed and comfortable. Presence of hemorrhoids obscures anal opening and increases discomfort with bowel elimination.

7 Place bedpan or commode in easily accessible position. If client will be expelling contents into toilet, ensure toilet is available and place client's slippers and bathrobe in easily accessible location.

Bedpan is used if client unable to get out of bed.

8 Administer enema.

a. Administer enema in prepackaged disposable container:

(1) Remove plastic cap from rectal tip. Tip may be already lubricated. Apply more lubricant if needed.

Lubrication provides for smooth insertion of tip without rectal irritation or trauma.

(2) Gently separate buttocks and locate anus. Instruct client to relax by breathing out slowly through mouth.

Breathing out promotes relaxation of external rectal sphincter. Presence of hemorrhoids obscures location of anus.

(3) Insert lubricated tip of container gently into rectum, angling towards umbilicus.
Adult: 7.5 to 10 cm (3 to 4 inches) (see illustration)
Adolescent: 7.5 to 10 cm (3 to 4 inches)
Child: 5 to 7.5 cm (2 to 3 inches)
Infant: 2.3 to 3.75 cm (1 to 1.5 inches)

Gentle insertion prevents trauma to rectal mucosa.

(4) Squeeze bottle continuously until all of solution has entered rectum and colon. Instruct client to retain solution until urge to defecate.

Hypertonic solutions require only small volumes to stimulate defecation. Intermittent squeezing results in return of solution to bottle.

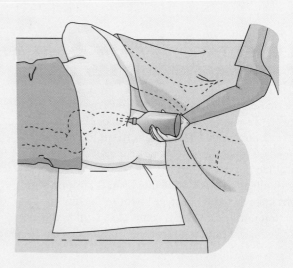

STEP 8a.(3) The tip of the commercial enema is inserted into the rectum. (From Sorrentino SA: *Mosby's textbook for nursing assistants,* ed 5, St Louis, 2000, Mosby.)

STEPS	RATIONALE

b. Administer enema in standard enema bag:

(1) Add warmed solution to enema bag: Warm tap water as it flows from faucet. Check temperature of solution by pouring small amount of solution over inner wrist.

Hot water can burn intestinal mucosa. Cold water can cause abdominal cramping and is difficult to retain.

(2) Raise container, release clamp, and allow solution to flow long enough to fill tubing.

Removes air from tubing.

(3) Reclamp tubing.

(4) Lubricate 6 to 8 cm (2.5 to 3 inches) of tip of tubing with lubricant.

Eases tube insertion through anus.

(5) Gently separate buttocks and locate anus. Instruct client to relax by breathing out slowly through mouth

Breathing out promotes relaxation of external anal sphincter.

(6) Insert tip of rectal tube slowly by pointing tip in direction of client's umbilicus (see illustration). Length of insertion varies:
   Adult: 7.5 to 10 cm (3 to 4 inches)
   Adolescent: 7.5 to 10 cm (3 to 4 inches)
   Child: 5 to 7.5 cm (2 to 3 inches)
   Infant: 2.3 to 3.75 cm (1 to 1.5 inches)

Careful insertion prevents trauma to rectal mucosa from accidental lodging of tube against rectal wall. Forceful insertion beyond recommended length could cause bowel perforation.

NURSE ALERT   If tube does not pass easily, do not force. Consider allowing a small amount of fluid to infuse and then try to slowly reinsert tube. The instillation of fluid may relax the sphincter and provide added lubrication.

---

(7) Hold tubing in rectum constantly until end of fluid instillation.

Bowel contraction can cause expulsion of rectal tube.

(8) With container at client's hip level, open regulating clamp and allow solution to enter slowly.

Rapid infusion can stimulate evacuation of tubing and cause cramping.

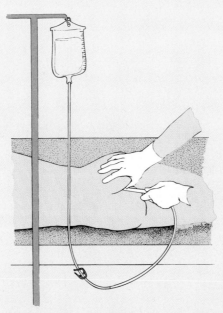

STEP 8b.(6) Insertion of rectal tube into rectum.

STEPS	RATIONALE
(9) Raise height of enema container slowly to appropriate level above anus: 30 to 45 cm (12 to 18 inches) for high enema; 30 cm (12 inches) for regular enema (see illustration); 7.5 cm (3 inches) for low enema. Instillation time varies with volume of solution administered (e.g., 1 L may take 10 minutes). Hang container on IV pole.	Allows for continuous, slow instillation of solution. Raising container too high causes rapid infusion and possible painful distention of colon. High pressure can cause rupture of bowel in infant.
(10) Lower container or clamp tubing if client complains of cramping or if fluid escapes around rectal tube.	Temporary cessation of infusion minimizes cramping and promotes ability to retain all the solution.
(11) Clamp tubing after all the solution is instilled. Tell client that the procedure is completed and that you will be removing rectal tube.	Clients may misinterpret the sensation of removing the tube as loss of control.
9 Place layers of toilet tissue around tube at anus and gently remove tubing.	Provides for client's comfort and cleanliness.
10 Explain to client that feeling of distention is normal. Ask client to retain solution as long as possible until urge to defecate occurs. Have client lie quietly in bed. (For infant or young child gently hold buttocks together for a few minutes.)	Solution distends bowel. Length of retention varies with type of enema and client's ability to contract rectal sphincter. Longer retention promotes more effective stimulation of peristalsis and defecation.
11 Discard prepackaged enema container or tubing in proper receptacle. Rinse out reusable container thoroughly with warm soap and water.	
12 Assist client to bathroom or commode if possible. If necessary to use the bedpan, assist to as near the normal position for evacuation as possible	Normal squatting position promotes defecation.
13 Observe character of feces and solution (caution client against flushing toilet before inspection).	
14 Assist client as needed to wash anal area with warm soap and water.	Fecal contents can irritate skin. Hygiene promotes client's comfort.
15 See Completion Protocol (inside front cover).	

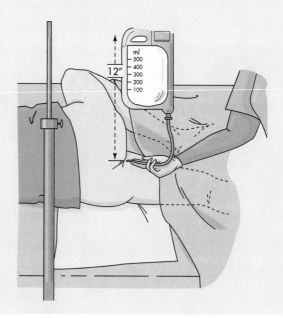

STEP 8b.(9) An enema is given in Sims' position. The IV pole is positioned so that the enema bag is 12 inches above the anus. (From Sorrentino SA: *Mosby's textbook for nursing assistants,* ed 5, St Louis, 2000, Mosby.)

EVALUATION

1 Ask client if abdominal discomfort was relieved.
2 Inspect color, consistency, and amount of stool and characteristics of fluid passed.
3 Assess for abdominal distention.

Unexpected Outcomes and Related Interventions

1 Client is unable to hold enema solution.
a. If this occurs during instillation, slow rate of infusion.
b. Position on bedpan while administering the solution.
2 Severe cramping, bleeding, or sudden severe abdominal pain occurs and is unrelieved by temporarily stopping or slowing flow of solution.
a. Stop enema.
b. Notify physician.
3 With an order for "enemas until clear," after three enemas the water is highly colored or contains solid fecal material.
a. Notify physician.

Recording and Reporting

• Record type of enema given; client's signs and symptoms; response to enema; and results, including color, amount, and appearance of stool.

Sample Documentation

2000 Last BM 5 days ago. C/O abdominal fullness and rectal pressure. Abdomen distended, firm; 1000-ml soap suds enema given with "mild" abdominal cramping during administration. Solution returned with large amount of dark-brown, soft-formed stool.

2100 States, "I feel better now." Abdomen soft, nondistended. Resting in bed with side rails up ×2.

Special Considerations
Pediatric Considerations

• Infants and children do not usually receive prepackaged hypertonic enemas because the solutions can cause rapid fluid shifts (Hockenberry and Wilson, 2007).
• The use of oral stool softeners is the initial recommended treatment of constipation in children.

Geriatric Considerations

• Older adults may become fatigued more quickly and are at greater risk for fluid and electrolyte imbalances; therefore caution is needed when administering enemas "until clear."
• Teach older adults and their caregivers dietary and activity measures to avoid constipation.
• Older adults may have difficulty in retaining enema solution.

Home Care Considerations

• Assess client's and family's ability and motivation to administer enema in the home, and provide instruction as needed.
• Assess client's ability to manipulate equipment to self-administer enema.
• Instruct client and family not to exceed number and volume of enemas.

Long-Term Care Considerations

• Teach long-term care personnel signs and symptoms (diaphoresis, pallor, shortness of breath, palpitations) that require stopping enema administration and to report immediately to the nurse.

NCLEX® Style Questions

1 While receiving a soaps suds enema, the client states, "I am beginning to feel like I have to go to the bathroom." Which of the following techniques would best help the client overcome the urge to defecate?
1. Ask the client to hold his or her breath.
2. Clamp the tubing.
3. Hold the client's buttocks together firmly.
4. Raise the fluid container.
2 When a client is suspected of having hardened feces because of prolonged constipation, which of the following type of enemas would the nurse anticipate being prescribed?
1. Soap suds
2. Kayexalate
3. Oil retention
4. Tap water

3 The nurse is helping the client on bedrest eat lunch when he needs to use the urinal. After the client uses the urinal, the most appropriate action for the nurse would be to:
1. Assist the client to wash his hands.
2. Take the client's vital signs.
3. Continue to help the client eat lunch.
4. Record I&O.
4 What intervention should be included on the care plan for a client with an external catheter?
1. Limit the client's intake to 800 ml daily.
2. Assess the skin on the penis for irritation.
3. Use adhesive tape to secure the condom.
4. Retract the foreskin before the catheter is applied.

5 The nurse is calculating the client's I&O for an 8-hour shift. The client had 2 pieces of toast, 4 ounces of apple juice, and 8 ounces of coffee for breakfast. At 0900 the client urinated 500 ml. The client has an IV of D5W at 125 ml per hour. During the afternoon, the client had 6 ounces of ice chips and 12 ounces of cola and voided 200 ml. At 1400 the client's Jackson-Pratt was emptied of 20 ml serosanguineous drainage. In addition, the client vomited two times, 250 ml each time.

What was the client's total I&O for the 8-hour shift? Intake_____ Output_____

References for all chapters appear in Appendix D.

Promoting Comfort and Pain Control

10

MEDIA RESOURCES

- *evolve*   http://evolve.elsevier.com/Elkin

Pain is an unpleasant sensory and emotional experience. It is also complex because it is highly subjective and individualized. Pain results from disease, trauma, and certain therapies, or it has no identifiable cause (American Pain Society [APS], 2003). A person's behavioral, emotional, and cognitive responses define their pain experience. Pain is tiring and drains a person's physical, emotional, and mental energy. The client is the only one who knows whether pain is present and what the experience is like; therefore it is important to partner with clients to find the best individualized pain therapies.

Pain is the most common reason a person seeks health care. Clients experience various forms of stress, undergo painful procedures, and experience painful illnesses. In addition, the experience of staying in a health care environment and the symptoms of diseases disrupt a client's comfort level. Assisting clients with acquiring comfort is a challenge. One of the nurse's responsibilities is to create comfortable environments for clients and to apply principles of pain management to assist clients in gaining comfort.

Adequate pain management is a priority for health care agencies. Clients expect good pain control. Accrediting organizations such as the Joint Commission on Accreditation of Healthcare Organizations have established standards for timely and effective pain management (JCAHO, 2006). The Agency for Healthcare Research and Quality (AHRQ), the American Pain Society (APS), and the World Health Organization (WHO) also have written guidelines for pain management. The American Nurses Association's (ANA's) *Code of Ethics* (2001) states, "The nurse promotes, advocates for and strives to protect the health, safety and rights of the client." This statement ethically obligates nurses to provide clients with adequate pain control.

PHYSIOLOGY OF PAIN

Promoting comfort and controlling pain are two of the most important goals of nursing practice. Nurses are most effective in managing clients' pain if they understand the physiology of pain. Pain physiology involves four stages: transduction, transmission, perception, and modulation. Transduction is the conversion of mechanical, chemical, or thermal noxious energy (e.g., burns, trauma to skin, pressure) to electrical energy in sensory nerves that then initiates an action potential (nerve stimulus). Transmission is the movement of impulses along sensory nerves via the spinal cord to the brain. Perception is the process whereby the brain interprets the stimuli to be noxious and thus begins to respond to the stimuli. Modulation involves brain activation of descending spinal cord pathways that block pain transmission. Because pain is complex, a combination of therapies can effectively minimize or relieve pain. Pharmacological therapies block pain transmission at receptor sites and alter perception within the brain. Nonpharmacological therapies offer different sources of stimuli that distract and relax a client so as to alter pain perception. This chapter describes both pharmacological and nonpharmacological therapies.

EVIDENCE IN PRACTICE

Good M and others: Relaxation and music reduce pain after gynecologic surgery, *Pain Manag Nurs* 3(2):61-70, 2002.

Pain management is an active area of research. There is great emphasis on trying to understand the types of therapies clients find most beneficial. Nonpharmacologial pain therapies offer promising results. For example, Good and others tested relaxation, chosen music, and the combination of relaxation and music on pain experienced by 311 clients undergoing gynecological surgery. The clients were tested for pain sensation and distress during ambulation and rest on postoperative days 1 and 2. Clients who received any one of the interventions had significantly less pain than those clients who received no nonpharmacological intervention on both days. The three interventions were similar in their effect on pain. Clients who received the interventions plus patient-controlled analgesia (PCA) had less pain than clients who used PCA alone. Nurses should always try nonpharmacological interventions as an appropriate pain management therapy.

NURSING DIAGNOSES

Acute pain and **chronic pain** are nursing diagnoses that focus on pain control. In contrast, there are numerous nursing diagnoses that apply to a client's response to pain. **Impaired physical mobility** related to pain applies to clients who have limited independent physical movement resulting from painful conditions. **Fatigue** related to pain applies to clients who experience a decreased capacity for physical and mental work. **Risk for disuse syndrome** is a state in which a client is at risk for deterioration of body systems and deconditioning resulting from inactivity. Severe pain can be one causative factor. **Disturbed sleep patterns** related to pain applies to clients who suffer a disruption in the amount and quality of sleep as a result of unrelieved discomfort. Other nursing diagnoses may include **anxiety, ineffective coping,** or **powerlessness** when pain compromises a client's emotional resources. **Impaired social interaction** and **spiritual distress** apply to clients whose social awareness and spiritual health have been exhausted by chronic pain. **Deficient knowledge** may apply to clients requiring instruction regarding use of nonpharmacological therapies, PCA, and local anesthetic pump devices. **Risk for infection** and **risk for injury** are potential nursing diagnoses for clients receiving epidural analgesia.

SKILL 10.1 Nonpharmacological Pain Management

Nonpharmacological or complementary therapies are quite effective in offering pain relief. Examples of nonpharmacological therapies include distraction, removing painful stimuli, massage, guided imagery (see Skill 10.2), cutaneous stimulation, music, biofeedback, meditation, hypnosis, and relaxation techniques (see Skill 10.2) (Rakel and Barr, 2003). Nurses use these therapies to lessen the reception and perception of pain (Table 10-1). For example, massage involves gentle application of touch and movement to muscles, tendons, and ligaments without manipulation of the joints. A proper massage blocks pain impulse perception and helps relax muscles.

Treatment approach that uses both pharmacological and nonpharmacological therapies is most effective in pain management (Berry and others, 2001). Nonpharmacological therapies should be used along with and not instead of pharmacological interventions, and vice versa. Those who benefit most from nonpharmacological therapies include clients who find such therapies appealing, express anxiety or fear, benefit from avoiding or reducing drug therapy, are likely to have a prolonged interval of postoperative pain, and have incomplete pain relief from drug therapies (AHCPR, 1992a).

ASSESSMENT

1 Ask clients if they are in pain. Clients from various cultures may not admit to having pain; additional pain assessment techniques may be necessary. *Rationale: A clinician must accept a client's report of pain (APS, 2003). In clients of differing cultures, watch for nonverbal indicators of pain such as grimacing, clenching teeth, etc., and ask significant others if they believe the client is in pain.*

TABLE 10-1   Nonpharmacological Interventions for Pain*

INTERVENTIONS	COMMENTS
Physical	
Progressive muscle relaxation	Reduces mild to moderate pain. Requires 3 to 5 minutes of staff time for instruction.
Massage	Effective for reduction of mild to moderate discomfort. May be firm, gentle, or light stroking of the body part involved or the opposite extremity. Requires 3 to 10 minutes of staff time.
Transcutaneous electrical nerve stimulation (TENS)	Effective in reducing mild to moderate pain by stimulating the skin with mild electrical current. Electrodes are placed over or near the site of pain. Requires special equipment. Requires physician order.
Heat/cold application	Selection of heat versus cold varies with the situation. Moist heat relieves stiffness of arthritis and relaxes muscles. Cold applications reduce acute pain associated with inflammation from arthritis or from acute injury. Requires physician order.
Psychological/Cognitive	
Music	Simple relaxation. Best taught preoperatively. Both client-preferred and "easy listening" music effective for mild to moderate pain.
Biofeedback	Reduces mild to moderate pain and operative site muscle tension. Requires client to have high cognitive level of function. Requires skilled personnel and special equipment.
Imagery	Reduces mild to moderate pain. Requires skilled personnel.
Education	Effective for reduction of all types of pain. Should include sensory and procedural information and instruction aimed at reducing activity-related pain. Requires 5 to 15 minutes of staff time.

*Should be used with analgesic medication.

2 Assess characteristics of a client's pain. Use the **PQRSTU** of pain assessment:

P: Precipitating/aggravating factors (for example, "What starts your pain or makes it worse?"). Consider client's experience with over-the-counter (OTC) drugs (including herbals and topicals) that have helped to reduce pain in the past.

Q: Quality (for example, "Tell me what your pain feels like").

R: Region/Radiation (for example, "Show me where your pain is").

S: Severity; use a valid pain rating scale (Figure 10-1).

T: Timing; ask client if pain is constant, intermittent, continuous, or a combination. Does pain increase during specific times of day or during certain activities?

U: How is pain affecting U (client) in regards to daily activities, work, and relationships?

Rationale: Provides important baseline to determine efficacy of nursing measures. An appropriate pain rating scale should be reliable, easily understood, and easy to use (McCaffery and Pasero, 1999).

3 Examine site of client's pain or discomfort. Inspect (discoloration or swelling) and palpate (change in temperature, area of altered sensation, areas that trigger pain, painful area, and range of motion [ROM] of involved joints) the area. Percussion and auscultation may further help to assess cause of pain. *Rationale: This may reveal the nature of the pain and appropriate interventions.*

4 Identify possible factors for the discomfort/pain. Pain may be acute (postoperative, associated with labor of childbirth, traumatic wounds, burns) or chronic (associated with cancer, migraine headaches, low back pain,

joint pain). *Rationale: Causative factors influence the choice of interventions most likely to be successful.*

5 Assess factors that influence perception of pain (e.g., past pain history and ability to cope, depression, fatigue, loneliness, anxiety, helplessness, fear). *Rationale: These factors significantly reduce clients' ability to cope with pain.*

6 Assess clients' culturally determined beliefs about pain. *Rationale: Culture influences the meaning pain holds for a client and how a client reacts to discomfort.*

7 Assess client's response to pharmacological treatment. *Rationale: Determines extent to which therapies have been successful.*

8 Assess physical, behavioral (Box 10-1), and emotional signs and symptoms of pain, including vocalizations of moaning, grimacing, irritability or change in usual behavior, decreased activity, abnormal gait, guarding of body part, diaphoresis, decreased gastrointestinal (GI) motility, nausea, vomiting, insomnia, anorexia, fatigue, depression, hopelessness or anger, and concomitant symptoms (symptoms that occur with pain, e.g., headache or constipation). *Rationale: Signs and symptoms may reveal source and nature of pain. Nonverbal responses to pain are especially useful in assessing pain in clients who are cognitively impaired or nonverbal. Before assuming that a change in behavior is caused by pain, complete a physical assessment. This will rule out other possible causes for change in behavior such as pneumonia, urinary tract infection (UTI), constipation, or medication side effect. After these are ruled out, a trial of short-acting pain medications should be initiated and the client's behavior observed (Wentz, 2001).*

9 In cognitively impaired clients, obtain a proxy pain intensity rating from the primary caregiver (e.g., family member, friend). *Rationale: Proxy ratings (ratings by someone who knows client) may closely approximate the client's pain intensity.*

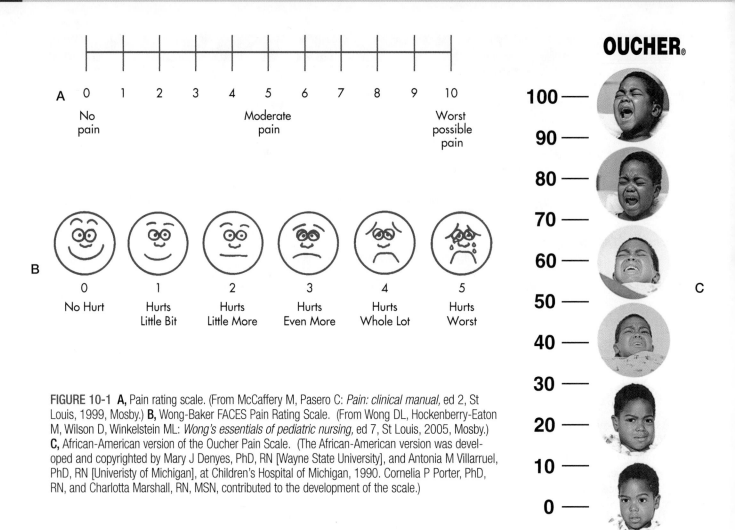

OUCHER®

A 0 1 2 3 4 5 6 7 8 9 10

No pain   Moderate pain   Worst possible pain

B

0	1	2	3	4	5
No Hurt	Hurts Little Bit	Hurts Little More	Hurts Even More	Hurts Whole Lot	Hurts Worst

100 —
90 —
80 —
70 —
60 —
50 —
40 —
30 —
20 —
10 —
0 —

C

FIGURE 10-1 **A,** Pain rating scale. (From McCaffery M, Pasero C: *Pain: clinical manual,* ed 2, St Louis, 1999, Mosby.) **B,** Wong-Baker FACES Pain Rating Scale. (From Wong DL, Hockenberry-Eaton M, Wilson D, Winkelstein ML: *Wong's essentials of pediatric nursing,* ed 7, St Louis, 2005, Mosby.) **C,** African-American version of the Oucher Pain Scale. (The African-American version was developed and copyrighted by Mary J Denyes, PhD, RN [Wayne State University], and Antonia M Villarruel, PhD, RN [Univeristy of Michigan], at Children's Hospital of Michigan, 1990. Cornelia P Porter, PhD, RN, and Charlotta Marshall, RN, MSN, contributed to the development of the scale.)

BOX 10-1 Behavioral Indicators of Pain

- *Facial expression:* grimace, frowning, clenched teeth, tightly closed eyes
- *Vocalizations:* moaning, crying, gasping
- *Posture:* bent, leaning, guarding
- *Gait:* favors one side, uneven
- *Activity level:* pacing, restlessness, increased hand and finger movements, inactivity
- *Muscles:* tense, guarded
- *Behavior:* change in usual activities
- *Emotions:* irritable, withdrawn
- *Change in ADLs:* eating, sleeping, dressing, conversing, interacting with others

10 Assess for factors such as noise, temperature, or bright lights that may aggravate the client's perception or tolerance of pain. *Rationale: Environmental factors may intensify perception of discomfort.*

11 Consider physician's orders regarding activity or positioning restrictions. *Rationale: Affects choices used in positioning and massage.*

12 Assess client's music preferences (vocal, instrumental, both), style of music (classical, jazz, other), and favorite artist. *Rationale: Assists in selection of individualized music for relaxation. In older adults at risk for agitation, music can be effective in reducing agitation (Gerdner, 2001).*

PLANNING

Expected Outcomes focus on attaining comfort and pain relief and improving client's ability to participate in routine activities.

1 Client understands and uses identified pain rating scale appropriately with client and health care providers mutually agreeing on pain intensity goal.

2 Client is relaxed and comfortable as evidenced by self-reported reduction in pain severity; slow, regular respirations; calm facial expression; calm tone of voice; relaxed muscles; and relaxed posture.

3 Client's behavioral symptoms such as inactivity, anorexia, depression, or fatigue will improve (e.g., initiates walking, food intake increases, begins to socially interact).

Delegation Considerations

Assessment of the client's pain should not be delegated. The skill of nonpharmacological pain management may be delegated. The nurse instructs personnel to:

- Eliminate environmental conditions that enhance pain.
- Provide client with appropriate rest periods.
- Adapt interventions based on any positioning or ambulation restrictions (e.g., administer massage in side-lying versus prone position).

Equipment

- Pain rating scale
- Night-light
- Client's preferred reading material
- Music: compact disk (CD), audiotape, or radio
- Massage: lotion or oil, folded sheet, bath towel

IMPLEMENTATION *for Nonpharmacological Pain Management*

STEPS	RATIONALE
1 See Standard Protocol (inside front cover).	
2 Prepare client's environment: • Temperature suited to client • Lighting • Sound • Eliminate unnecessary interruptions and coordinate care activities; allow for rest.	Temperature and sound extremes can enhance client's perception of pain. Bright or very dim lighting can aggravate pain sensation. Fatigue increases pain perception.
3 Teach client how to use pain rating scale (Box 10-2). Explain range of intensity scores and how they relate to measure of pain.	Accurate reporting by client improves pain assessment and treatment.
4 Set pain intensity goal with client.	Pain is unique to each individual. When able, client sets individual goal for tolerable pain severity.
5 Give pain-relieving medications as ordered (see Skill 10.3) at least 30 minutes before trying a nonpharmacological intervention.	When analgesics reach their peak effect, other pain-relief measures may be more effective.
6 Remove or reduce painful stimuli.	
a. Assist client with attaining comfortable position within normal body alignment.	Turning and repositioning reduces stimulation of pain and pressure receptors. Also maximizes response to pain-relieving interventions.
b. Use pillows as needed for alignment and support and to position off of pressure areas (see illustration).	Repositioning reduces strain on muscles and pressure areas, resulting in less stimulation of pain receptors.
c. Smooth wrinkles in bed linens.	Reduces irritation to skin.
d. Loosen any constrictive bandage or device (e.g., blood pressure cuff, elastic wrap bandages, band of elastic hose, identification band).	Bandage or device encircling extremity may apply pressure and restrict circulation.

BOX 10-2 Teaching the Client and Family How to Use a Pain Rating Scale

- Show and briefly explain available pain rating scales, and ask which one the client prefers. Offer vertical and horizontal scales as options.
- Explain the purpose of the scale: "This scale allows us to know the level of your pain and how it changes over time as we provide you comfort measures."
- Explain the parts of the scale, for example, 0 means no pain, whereas 10 means the worst pain you can imagine.
- Discuss pain as a broad concept that is not restricted to a severe or intolerable sensation. Discomfort, hurt, and ache are also considered pain sensations.

- Verify the client understands the concept of pain; ask client to give an example of pain experienced in the past.
- Ask the client to practice using the pain rating scale with present pain, or select one of client's examples. Also, ask to rate worst pain and average pain in past 24 hours.
- Set mutual goal for comfort and function/recovery.

Modified from McCaffery M, Pasero C: *Pain: clinical manual*, ed 2, St Louis, 1999, Mosby.

STEPS	RATIONALE
7 Reduce or eliminate emotional factors that increase the pain experience.	Fear or anxiety may cause muscle tension and vasoconstriction, which intensify the pain experience.
a. Accept the client, and acknowledge the client's report of pain.	Relieves client's anxiety.

> **COMMUNICATION TIP** This is a good time to use open-ended statements, such as, "Tell me what having pain has been like for you," or "What makes your pain feel better (or worse)?"

STEPS	RATIONALE
b. Explain the cause of pain (if known).	Giving information reduces anxiety from the unknown.
c. Spend time to allow client to talk about pain; answer questions and listen attentively.	Conveys a sense of caring and interest in client's welfare.
d. Answer call lights promptly.	Clients in pain expect caregivers to respond quickly when pain worsens.
8 Splint over the site of pain (e.g., using a pillow or folded blanket).	Splinting reduces pain by minimizing muscle movement.
a. Explain purpose of splinting.	Improves client's ability to deep breathe, cough, and move.
b. Place pillow or blanket over site of discomfort, then assist client to place hands firmly over area.	Splinting immobilizes painful area.
c. Have client hold area firmly while coughing, deep breathing, and turning.	Splinting decreases movement and subsequent pain during activity.
9 Administer a massage:	
a. Adjust bed to high, comfortable position, and lower side rails (if raised).	Ensures proper body mechanics and prevents strain on nurse's back muscles.
b. Place client in comfortable position such as prone or side-lying.	Enhances relaxation and exposes area to be massaged.

> **NURSE ALERT** Clients with respiratory difficulties may lie on side with head of bed elevated.

STEPS	RATIONALE
c. Turn on soft pleasing music of client's preference.	Promotes relaxation.
d. Drape client to expose only area to be massaged.	Maintains client's privacy and warmth.
e. Verify that client is not allergic to lotion, then warm lotion in hands or in basin of warm water. (NOTE: If you choose to massage head and scalp, defer use of lotion until completed.)	Warm lotion is soothing, and warmth helps to produce local muscle relaxation.

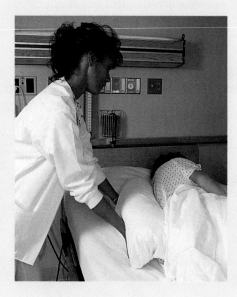

STEP 6b. Positioning client in side-lying lateral position for comfort.

STEPS	RATIONALE

f. Choose stroke technique based on desired effect:

Ensures fuller relaxation of body part.

> **NURSE ALERT:** Clients who are heavily medicated or unable to communicate verbally need very gentle massage because they cannot inform the nurse if massage becomes uncomfortable.

(1) Effleurage (see illustration): Massaging upward and outward from vertebral column, and back again

Gliding stroke, used without manipulating deep muscles, smoothes and extends muscles, increases nutrient absorption, and improves lymphatic and venous circulation.

(2) Pétrissage (see illustration)

Use on tense muscle groups to "knead" muscles, promote relaxation, and stimulate local circulation.

(3) Friction

Strong circular strokes bring blood to surface of skin, thereby increasing local circulation and loosening tight muscle groups.

g. Encourage client to slowly breathe deeply and relax during massage.

Potentiates effects of massage.

h. Standing behind client, touch scalp and temples.

Avoids startling the client.

i. Supporting client's head, use friction to rub muscles at base of head.

Strong circular strokes stimulate local circulation and relaxation.

j. Massage hands and arms, as appropriate:

Releases tension in hands and arms. Anxious behaviors may be significantly reduced with hand massage (Mok and Woo, 2004).

(1) Support hand, and apply friction to palm using both thumbs.

(2) Support base of finger, and work each finger in corkscrewlike motion.

(3) Complete hand massage using effleurage strokes from fingertips to wrist.

(4) Knead muscles of forearm and upper arm between thumb and forefinger.

Encourages relaxation; enhances circulation and venous return.

k. After determining client has no neck injury or condition that contraindicates neck manipulation, massage neck as appropriate.

Massage may be contraindicated after spinal cord injuries or surgery to head and neck because of risk of causing further injury.

(1) Place client prone unless contraindicated.

Provides access to neck muscles.

(2) Knead each neck muscle between thumb and forefinger.

Reduces tension that often localizes in neck muscles.

(3) Gently stretch neck by placing one hand on top of shoulders and other at base of head and gently moving hands away from each other.

Helps relax neck muscles.

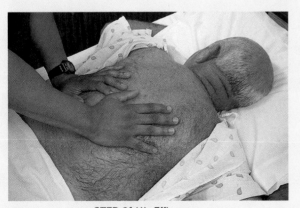

STEP 9f.(1) Effleurage.

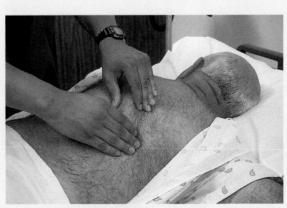

STEP 9f.(2) Pétrissage.

STEPS	RATIONALE
l. Massage back as appropriate:	
(1) Keep client in prone position unless contraindicated: Side-lying is an option.	
(2) Do not allow hands to leave client's skin.	Continuous contact with skin's surface is soothing and stimulates circulation to tissues. Breaking contact with skin can startle client.
(3) Apply hands first to sacral area; massage in circular motion. Stroke upward from buttocks to shoulders. Massage over scapulas with smooth, firm stroke. Continue in one smooth stroke to upper arms and laterally along sides of back down to iliac crest (see illustration). Continue massage pattern for 3 minutes.	General firm pressure applied to all muscle groups promotes relaxation.
(4) Use effleurage along muscles of spine in upward and outward motion.	Massage follows distribution of major muscle groups.
(5) Use pétrissage on muscles of each shoulder toward front of client.	Area often tightens because of tension.
(6) Use palms in upward and outward circular motion from lower buttocks to neck.	Brings blood to surface of skin.
(7) Knead muscles of upper back and shoulder between thumb and forefinger.	These muscles are thick and can be vigorously massaged.
(8) Use both hands to knead muscles up one side of back, then other.	
(9) End massage with long stroking effleurage movements.	Most soothing of massage movements.
m. Massage feet, as appropriate:	
(1) Place client supine; determine if client is easily ticklish.	If client is ticklish, massage may become a source of discomfort.
(2) Hold foot firmly. Support ankle with one hand or support sides of foot with each hand while performing massage.	Maintains joint stability during massage.
(3) Make circular motions with thumb and fingers around bones of ankle and top of foot.	Relaxes muscles.
(4) Trace space between tendons with firm finger pressure, moving from toe to ankle.	
(5) Massage sides and top of each toe. Use top of fist to make circular motions on bottom of foot.	

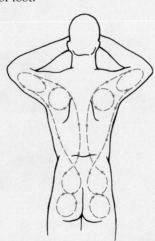

STEP 9l.(3) Circular massage of the back.

STEPS	RATIONALE
(6) Knead sides of foot between index finger and thumb.	
(7) End massage with firm, sweeping motions over top and bottom of foot.	Light strokes may tickle and be uncomfortable.
(8) If using lotion, wipe feet dry to prevent slipping when standing.	Reduces risk of fall.
n. Tell client you are ending massage. Ask client to inhale deeply and exhale. Then caution client to move slowly after resting a few minutes.	Returns client to a more awake and alert state. When deeply relaxed, client may experience dizziness on arising too rapidly.
o. Wipe excess oil or lotion from client's back with towel.	Excess lotion or oil can irritate skin and cause breakdown.
p. Return bed to low position, and raise side rails (if appropriate) when massage is finished.	Prevents client falls.
q. Perform hand hygiene.	Reduces transmission of microorganisms.
10 Use distraction to reduce client's attention to pain.	The reticular activating system (RAS) in the brain is essential for concentration. The RAS inhibits painful stimuli if a person receives sufficient or excessive sensory input. Distraction with sensory stimuli meaningful to a client helps that person ignore pain.
Possible distractions include:	
a. Music: Provide a music intervention session for approximately 30 minutes, in a location where the client spends majority of time. Set volume or loudness at a comfortable level (Gerdner, 2001). Offer earphones if desired. Increase volume if pain increases.	Music produces an altered state of consciousness through sound, silence, space, and time.
b. Prayer	Prayer is an effective coping resource that helps minimize physical and psychological symptoms of distress.
c. Describing pictures or discussing pleasant memories	Reminiscing is an effective distraction, allowing client to focus on pleasant experiences that were pain free.
11 After nonpharmacological interventions, be sure client is left in a comfortable and clean environment.	Promotes client's comfort, rest, sleep, and ability to participate in usual routines.
12 See Completion Protocol (inside front cover).	

EVALUATION

1 Within 1 hour of an intervention, ask client to verbalize how well the pain has been relieved and what his or her pain intensity is now (0 to 10).
2 Observe client's facial expression, body language, position, mobility, and relaxation.
3 Ask client to describe ability to rest, sleep, eat, and participate in usual activities.

Unexpected Outcomes and Related Interventions

1 Client's pain intensity is greater than desired, client describes worsening of pain, or client displays nonverbal behavior reflecting pain.
a. Perform a complete pain re-assessment.
b. Implement alternative nonpharmacological pain-relief measures.
c. Ask family members what might be helpful.
d. Consult with physician about analgesic necessity.

2 Client experiences adverse reaction to medication.
a. Assess adverse reaction effects on client.
b. Notify physician.
c. Be prepared to administer antidote (e.g., antiemetic, antihistamine, opioid-reversing agent).
d. Monitor for effectiveness of antidote.

Recording and Reporting

• Pain documentation should be on a regular (every 4 to 12 hours) basis (agency dependent).
• Report inadequate pain relief (not reaching goal), a reduction in client function, and/or adverse effects from pain interventions (pharmacological and nonpharmacological). Box 10-3 lists suggestions for how to communicate with physicians about pain.
• Record findings of ongoing assessment, interventions completed (including notification of physician, if done), and client's response to interventions.

BOX 10-3 Nurse-Physician Pain Communication

1 Identify physician by name.
2 Give your name.
3 State the general nature of the call.
4 Identify the client by name and diagnosis.
5 State the pain management goal: rating and activities.
6 Summarize the current pain rating and effect of pain on activities.
7 List the current analgesic doses and relevant side effects.
8 Identify nonpharmacological measures used and their effect.
9 Suggest a solution (on the basis of a clinical practice guideline or your own expertise).

Modified from McCaffery M, Pasero C: *Pain: clinical manual*, ed 2, St Louis, 1999, Mosby.

Sample Documentation

0700 Rates pain in left shoulder at 6 (scale 0 to 10). Pain is intermittent and nonradiating. Grimaces during turning, holds shoulder when shifting position. Tylenol #3, 2 tablets administered. Positioned on right side, provided back massage, and turned on requested jazz music for 30 minutes.

0730 Muscles less tensed; turning more easily on own. Pain intensity rated a 4.

Special Considerations

Pediatric Considerations

- The FACES Pain Rating Scale and Oucher Pain Scale are specifically designed to measure pain intensity in children (see Figure 10-1) (Wong and Baker, 1988; Beyer and others, 1992).
- Children may not report pain because they may have misconceptions about the cause of their pain or fear the consequences (e.g., receiving an injection).
- Infants and children experience pain but may respond differently than adults. For example, they may cry and thrash about, have a shortened attention span, suck or rock, or be quiet and withdrawn. Others may become active when they are in pain. Variations in activity levels

are related to the child's personality and development (Hockenberry and Wilson, 2007).
- Parents are a helpful source of information when assessing a child's pain and planning pain-relief therapies.

Geriatric Considerations

- Older adults tend to have inadequately managed pain because of concerns regarding adverse effects of pain medications (Herr, 2002).
- Older adults may require more instruction to adequately understand the pain management tool selected.
- Pain is not a natural part of aging, although older adult clients are at risk for experiencing more pain-causing conditions (American Geriatrics Society, 2002).
- Older adults with pain may underreport pain (Herr, 2002). Explain the importance of honesty in reporting pain.
- Use terms other than *pain*, such as *hurt* or *pressure*, when assessing older adult clients because they may reserve the word *pain* for severe discomfort.
- Most forms of touch such as massage are pleasurable to older adults. Use with caution in clients with bone metastases or osteoporotic bones (Meiner and Lueckenotte, 2006).
- Reminiscence (e.g., sharing stories from the past) is an effective form of distraction in older adults.

Home Care Considerations

- Consider the client's home living conditions, such as the type of bed and environmental stimuli. A supportive bed and quiet environment will enhance sleep and promote pain management.
- Assess the pain management attitudes of family care providers (significant others). Without family care providers' participation, a client may not achieve successful pain management.

Long-Term Care Considerations

- Teach assistive personnel (AP) how to deliver specific nonpharmacological therapies and how to recognize potential nonverbal pain behaviors.

SKILL 10.2 Relaxation and Guided Imagery

The ability to relax physically promotes mental relaxation. Relaxation techniques such as guided imagery and progressive relaxation exercises provide clients with self-control when pain occurs. Clients who use relaxation techniques successfully achieve physiological and behavioral changes (e.g., decreased pulse, blood pressure, and muscle tension). For effective relaxation, the client needs to participate and cooperate. Teach relaxation only when the client is not in acute discomfort or severe pain and thus is able to concentrate. Explain the techniques in detail. It often takes several

teaching sessions before clients effectively reduce pain. A client can practice relaxation training at any time and usually with no side effects. Relaxation techniques are especially useful for chronic pain, labor pain, and relief of procedure-related pain.

Guided imagery is a form of relaxation. It involves using focused concentration to effectively reduce pain perception and minimize reaction to pain. In guided imagery a client draws upon personal memories, dreams, and visions to create an image in the mind, concentrates on that image, and gradually becomes less aware of pain. The goal of imagery is to have the client use one or several of the senses to create a desired image. This image creates a positive psychophysiological response. There is evidence that addition of relaxation and guided imagery are safe interventions that decrease pain, anxiety, and medication use (Antall and Kresevic, 2004).

Involve clients in choosing images that they find pleasant. This requires a careful nursing assessment (Kwekkeboom and others, 2003). Otherwise, you may mistakenly describe images of objects or things that the client fears or dislikes. For example, a scene of rolling waves at the seashore may be restful to one client but frightening to another. You may use imagery with progressive relaxation or massage or as a distraction. For competence in guided imagery, certification is available nationally through the Academy for Guided Imagery (AGI).

ASSESSMENT

1 Assess character of client's pain, including severity (see Skill 10.1). *Rationale: Establishes baseline to evaluate efficacy of relaxation measures.*

2 Assess facial expressions and verbal indications of discomfort or distress (e.g., grimacing, frowning, tone of voice, moaning). *Rationale: Provide criteria to determine efficacy of relaxation measures.*

3 Observe body position and movement, including restlessness, muscle tension, hand and finger movements, pacing, rhythmical or rubbing motions, and immobilization. *Rationale: Indicates physical or psychological distress and establishes baseline to measure efficacy of intervention.*

4 Assess underlying probable cause of pain. *Rationale: Determines if relaxational approaches are appropriate to use.*

5 Examine site of client's pain or discomfort. Inspect for discoloration, swelling, and drainage; palpate for change in temperature, area of altered sensation, painful area, areas that trigger or reduce pain, and range of joint motion. *Rationale: Clinical observations clarify nature of pain. Site of pain may indicate specific types of pain-relief measures.*

6 Review physician's orders. *Rationale: In some acute settings a medical order is needed to perform nonpharmacological therapies.*

7 Review any restrictions on client's mobility or positioning. *Rationale: Influences approach used in positioning client.*

8 Assess client's willingness to receive nonpharmacological relief measure. *Rationale: Clients have the right to decide about their own care. Active participation increases effectiveness.*

> **NURSE ALERT** It is helpful the first time to administer an analgesic before implementing relaxation techniques so that client can gain a level of comfort needed to practice noninvasive approaches.

9 Assess client's language level and identify descriptive terms that you will use when guiding client through relaxation.

PLANNING

Expected Outcomes focus on alleviating or reducing discomfort, increasing client's sense of control, and empowering client in pain relief.

1 Client achieves comfort as demonstrated by regular, deep respirations; relaxed body position; and calm facial expression and tone of voice.

2 Client achieves comfort with a pain intensity score at or below pain intensity goal.

3 Client demonstrates and describes guided imagery and relaxation techniques.

Delegation Considerations

The assessment of the appropriateness of relaxation and guided imagery for clients may not be delegated. The exercises of relaxation and guided imagery may be delegated. The nurse directs personnel by:

- Identifying and explaining which techniques work best for the client.
- Making clear the expected client response.
- Instructing personnel to report a worsening of client's condition.

Equipment

- Relaxation audiotape, tape player, or disk and DVD player

IMPLEMENTATION *for Relaxation and Guided Imagery*

STEPS	RATIONALE
1 See Standard Protocol (inside front cover).	
2 Explain purpose of each technique and what will be expected of client during activity.	Proper explanation of activity results in enhanced client participation.
3 Plan time to perform technique when client is able to concentrate.	Increases success with techniques.
4 Prepare environment by: • Controlling lighting in room • Controlling distractions by visitors/staff • Keeping comfortable room temperature • Closing curtains around client's bed or closing door	A darkened comfortable room, with minimal distractions, helps client attend to technique and may help reduce anxiety.

STEPS	RATIONALE
5 Progressive Relaxation	
a. Have client assume comfortable sitting position (if tolerated) or position of client preference.	Enhances client's ability to relax.
b. Instruct client to take several slow, deep diaphragmatic breaths.	Increased oxygen can lessen anxiety and prevent shortness of breath with relaxation. Breaths should be diaphragmatic and deep to avoid hyperventilation.
c. Have client close eyes, if desired.	Client may be less easily distracted.
d. After client establishes a regular breathing pattern, coach the client to locate any area of muscular tension:	Will focus on removing areas of distress.
(1) Alternating tightening and relaxing all muscle groups for 6 to 7 seconds, beginning at feet and working upwards toward head.	Alternating tension and relaxation in muscle groups heightens awareness of the difference.
(2) Tightening muscles during inhalation and relaxing muscles during exhalation.	Relaxation is integrated response associated with diminished sympathetic nervous system arousal; decreased muscle tension is desired outcome. Relaxation decreases pulse, respiration rates, and blood pressure and reduces anxiety.
(3) As each muscle group relaxes, ask client to enjoy relaxed feeling and allow mind to drift and think how nice it is to be relaxed. Have client breathe deeply.	Distracts client from perceiving pain. Enhances relaxation response.
(4) Calmly explain during exercise that client may feel sensations of tingling, heaviness, floating, or warmth as relaxation occurs.	Prevents anxiety should sensation occur without warning.
(5) Ask client to continue slow, deep breaths.	Allows opportunity to enjoy feelings of relaxation.
e. When finished, have client inhale deeply, exhale, and then initially move about slowly after resting a few minutes.	Returns client to a more awake and alert state. When deeply relaxed, client may feel dizzy on arising too quickly.
6 Deep Breathing	
a. Instruct client to sit comfortably with feet uncrossed. If client is unable to sit, move to a supine position with small pillow under head.	Encourages relaxation.
b. Place one of client's hands on the chest and the other hand on the abdomen.	Allows client to focus on chest and then abdomen.
c. Instruct client to inhale deeply through the nose, allowing the abdomen to rise and the hand to move outward.	Provides steady timing of inhalation and focuses the client on stretching abdominal muscles.
d. Tell client that when the abdomen is partially expanded, continue to breathe and allow chest to expand, moving the upper hand outward.	Affords maximal inhalation.
e. Pause for a few seconds. Then have client exhale slowly through pursed lips. Repeat for 4 to 6 minutes.	Permits optimal exchange of oxygen and carbon dioxide. Provides slow, controlled release of air.
7 Guided Imagery	
a. Direct client through exercise:	
(1) Instruct client to imagine that inhaled air is ball of healing energy.	Development of specific images assists in removal of pain perception.
(2) Imagine inhaled air travels to area of pain.	Client's ability to concentrate decreases pain perception.
b. Alternatively nurse may direct imagery:	
(1) Have client begin with slow deep breathing.	Encourages relaxation.
(2) Suggest client think about going to a pleasant place (e.g., beach, field of flowers).	Directs imagery after selection of restful place by nurse and client.
(3) Direct client to experience all sensory aspects of restful place (e.g., for beach: warm breeze, warm sand between toes, blue sky, rhythmic sound of waves, smell of salt air, gulls gliding in the air).	Helps client concentrate and relax through stimulation of numerous senses.

STEPS	RATIONALE
(4) Direct client to continue deep, slow, rhythmic breathing.	Promotes relaxation through muscle relaxation.
(5) Direct client to count to three, inhale, and open eyes.	Prevents dizziness after exercise.
(6) End the experience: "Experience the comfort and relaxation. When you open your eyes, you will feel alert and renewed. Breathe deeply. Be aware of where you are now, stretch gently, and when you are ready, open your eyes." Suggest client move about slowly initially.	
8 See Completion Protocol (inside front cover).	

EVALUATION

1 Observe character of respirations, body position, facial expression, tone of voice, mood, mannerisms, and verbalization of discomfort.
2 Use pain rating scale to evaluate comfort level.
3 Observe client perform relaxation technique.
4 Ask client to demonstrate relaxation technique at a time of low stress.

Unexpected Outcomes and Related Interventions

1 Client is not able to concentrate on technique because of intense pain.
a. Fully assess pain.
b. Consider a different technique or combination.
c. Administer an analgesic before attempting relaxation techniques again.
d. Ensure environment is conducive to technique.
2 Client is unable to perform relaxation technique.
a. Reinstruct client and demonstrate procedure.
b. Coach client through relaxation procedure.
c. Try different relaxation intervention.

Recording and Reporting

- Record in nurses' notes client's assessment findings, including pain rating before procedure, type of relaxation technique, preparation given to client, pain rating after relaxation, and client's behavioral responses to technique.
- Incorporate pain-relief technique into nursing care plan.
- Report client's response to relaxation to the staff at change of shift.
- Report any unusual responses to techniques (e.g., uncontrolled or aggravated pain) to nurse in charge or physician.

Sample Documentation

2000 Moaning, moving about in bed frequently; reports a severe frontal headache (7 on scale of 0 to 10) worsened by bright lights. Headache is constant. States cannot sleep. Tylenol #3, 2 tablets administered orally. Participated in deep breathing exercise and a 10-minute progressive relaxation exercise.

2045 States frontal headache is relieved (3 on scale of 0 to 10), now only intermittent. Lying supine in bed, quiet, eyes closed.

2200 Guided imagery practiced for 5 minutes in preparation for sleep. States feeling "much more relaxed and comfortable now." Verbalizes plans to practice this regularly using "favorite fishing spot" as setting.

Special Considerations
Pediatric Considerations

- Relaxation works for all ages and should be suited to the child's developmental level (e.g., a pacifier can be used for an infant, listening to music on a CD player with headphones for a teen).
- Because children have active imaginations, relaxation can be a useful adjuvant to pain control.
- Parents can provide comfort by their conversation and by holding and cuddling their child (AHCPR, 1992b; Hockenberry and Wilson, 2007).

Geriatric Considerations

- Visual, hearing, cognitive, and motor impairments may make it difficult for older adults to be able to effectively use relaxation or guided imagery (AHCPR, 1992b). However, do not assume techniques will not work. Assess clients carefully.
- In a survey of 1597 older adults, Astin and others (2000) found 41% used complimentary therapies; 6.5% used guided imagery. Of those using guided imagery, 82% reported improvement in symptoms.

Home Care Considerations

- Family members may need to collaborate planning time to reduce noise and other stimuli in the home to promote client's relaxation.
- Discuss nonpharmacological interventions with client's family and friends.

SKILL 10.3 Pharmacological Pain Management

Analgesics are the most common treatment for pain. Although analgesics effectively relieve pain, nurses still tend to undertreat clients. Undertreatment occurs because of incorrect drug information, concerns about addiction, anxiety over errors in using opioids, and administration of less medication than was ordered (Gunnarsdottir and others, 2003). Nurses must understand the drugs available for pain relief and their pharmacological effects.

There are three types of analgesics: (1) nonopioids, (2) opioids (traditionally called narcotics), and (3) adjuvants or coanalgesics (e.g., anticonvulsants, antidepressants, muscle relaxants, antiarrhythmics). Nonopioid analgesics, including acetaminophen, tramadol (Ultram), and nonsteroidal antiinflammatory drugs (NSAIDs), relieve mild to moderate pain (Table 10-2). Ketorolac (Toradol) is an injectable analgesic NSAID that is comparable to morphine in potency and used for severe pain. NSAIDs act by inhibiting the synthesis of prostaglandins, reducing inflammation, and decreasing transmission and perception of peripheral nerve stimuli. NSAIDs do not depress the central nervous system (CNS), nor do they interfere with bowel or bladder function.

Opioid analgesics are generally used for severe pain. The term *opioid* is preferred to *narcotic* because the word narcotic generally infers illegal use of substances. Opioids relieve pain by binding to receptor sites in the nervous system. Opioid analgesics include codeine, morphine, hydromorphone (Dilaudid), fentanyl, oxycodone, propoxyphene (Darvon), and other natural and synthetic medications. Meperidine (Demerol) is no longer a drug of choice because of its potential for causing seizures.

Opioids affect the higher centers of the CNS. Morphine and other opioids depress vital nervous system functions such as respirations (rate and depth), although this is rare (Wheeler and others, 2002). Respiratory depression is only clinically significant if there is a decrease in the rate *and* depth of respirations from the client's baseline assessment (McCaffery and Pasero, 1999). Clients who are breathing deeply rarely have clinical respiratory depression. It is important to note that sedation *always* occurs before respiratory depression. Clients can also experience side effects such as nausea, vomiting, constipation, and altered mental processes. Except for constipation, these side effects usually stop once the client has been receiving opioids around the clock (ATC) for 4 to 7 days. One way to maximize pain relief while minimizing drug toxicity is to give the medication on a regular ATC basis rather than on an as-needed (prn) basis. ATC administration ensures a more constant blood level of analgesic. The APS (2003) recommends ATC administration if pain is anticipated for the majority of the day.

Adjuvants or coanalgesics such as sedatives, anticonvulsants, steroids, antidepressants, antianxiety agents, and muscle relaxants have analgesic properties to enhance pain control. For example, corticosteroids relieve pain associated with inflammation and bone metastasis. Adjuvants also relieve symptoms associated with pain, including nausea, anxiety, and depression. Although adjuvants enhance pain control, they have *no* direct analgesic effect. Adjuvants are given alone or with analgesics, especially for treatment of chronic pain (Gordon, 2003). Many adjuvants are more effective than opioids in relieving neuropathic pain. The drugs can cause drowsiness and impaired coordination or mental alertness. Do not automatically attribute these side effects to opioids. Always assess a client carefully to determine the source of side effects.

The proper use of analgesics requires careful assessment and critical thinking in the application of pharmacological principles. Remember that each client's response to an analgesic is highly individualized.

ASSESSMENT

1 Perform complete pain assessment as for Skill 10.1. *Rationale: Assesses character of pain and type of analgesic to administer.*

2 Check last time medication was administered, as well as dose, route, and degree of relief experienced. *Rationale: Determines if next dose can be administered and whether dose adjustment is necessary.*

3 Determine if client has allergies to medications.

4 Determine an analgesic's prescribed route, frequency, and indication for pain relief. Nonopioids can be alternated or given with opioids. Injectable medications generally act within 15 to 30 minutes. Immediate-release oral medications may take 1 hour to be effective, whereas some extended-release preparations may take as long as 2 hours to be effective. Oral analgesics usually have a longer duration of action than injectables. *Rationale: Allows for planning pain-relief measures with client activities, anticipating peak and duration of analgesic, and evaluating effectiveness of analgesic.*

TABLE 10-2 Commonly Used* Nonopioids and Their Maximum Doses per 24 Hours	
MEDICATIONS	**MAXIMUM DOSE PER 24 HOURS**
Acetaminophen (Tylenol, Anacin-3, Panadol, Tempra)	4000 mg
Aspirin (acetylsalicylic acid) (ASA, Aspergum, Bayer Aspirin, Ecotrin, Empirin, Nuprin, Excedrin)	4000 mg
Ibuprofen (Motrin, Advil, and others)	3200 mg

*All may be purchased without a prescription.

5 Know the comparative potencies of analgesics in oral and injectable form. Refer to an equianalgesic chart. *Rationale: If nurses on succeeding shifts choose different routes for the same doses, the client will not receive the same level of pain control.*

PLANNING

Expected Outcomes focus on elimination or reduction of pain and return to optimal functioning with minimal side effects.

1 Client understands and uses pain rating scale appropriately with client and health care providers mutually agreeing on pain intensity goal.

2 Client achieves comfort with a pain intensity at or below pain intensity goal.

3 Clients who are unable to state a pain intensity goal have a goal set at 4 or below (0 to 10 scale) because this level has been shown to minimally affect function (Feldt, 2000).

4 Client is able to adequately function and perform activities of daily living (ADLs, e.g., walking, working, eating, sleeping, interacting).

5 Client does not experience intolerable or unmanageable adverse effects from the analgesic.

Delegation Considerations

The skill of analgesic administration may not be delegated. The nurse directs personnel by:

- Explaining the behaviors and physical changes associated with pain and to report their occurrence immediately
- Reviewing comfort measures to use to support pain relief

Equipment

- Prescribed medication
- Pain scale (0 to 10 range)
- Necessary administration device (see Chapters 16, 17, and 18)
- Controlled substance record (for opioids only)

IMPLEMENTATION *for Pharmacological Pain Management*

STEPS	RATIONALE
1 See Standard Protocol (inside front cover).	
2 Prepare selected analgesic, following "six rights" for administration of medications (see Chapter 15).	Ensures safe and appropriate medication administration.
3 Identify client by comparing name on medication administration record (MAR) with name on arm band and asking client's name, hospital number, and/or birthdate.	Ensures right client receives analgesia. At least two client identifiers (neither to be the client's room number) are to be used whenever administering medications (JCAHO, 2007).
4 Administer analgesic or adjuvant (see Chapters 16, 17, and 18) at appropriate time.	An NSAID is as effective as an opioid for some clients but not others. An oral analgesic usually brings the same relief as an injectable. Know the nature of your client's pain.

> **NURSE ALERT** If a client is unable to swallow or has a gastrostomy or jejunostomy tube in place, remember that with the exception of methadone the extended-release opioid formulations may not be crushed for administration. Some capsules may be opened and contents mixed in applesauce or other soft food, but they may not be crushed.

a. As soon as pain occurs	Pain is easier to prevent than to treat.
b. Before pain increases in severity	Higher levels of pain may not respond to ordered analgesic.
c. Before pain-producing procedures or activities	Reduces or blocks pain transmission in the CNS, allowing procedure to be completed with less discomfort.
d. Routinely, ATC	Maintains analgesic within therapeutic range ATC, reducing pain intensity and minimizing side effects. The ATC schedule avoids the low plasma concentrations that permit breakthrough pain.
5 Include nonpharmacological comfort measures in addition to analgesics (see Skills 10.1 and 10.2).	Increases effectiveness of pharmacological agents; treats nonphysiological aspects of pain.
6 Administer nursing care measures during times of peak effects of analgesics. Consider duration of action of analgesics when planning activities as well.	Effects vary depending on the type of medication used; allows for anticipation of next dose; permits evaluation of effectiveness of analgesic; maximizes effectiveness of nursing measures to prevent complications.
7 Monitor for adverse effects.	Anticipation of adverse effects leads to more timely intervention.

STEPS	RATIONALE

> **NURSE ALERT** Clients receiving ATC opioids should also receive stimulant laxatives. Opioids decrease intestinal propulsion (peristalsis) but not intestinal motility (churning); thus stool softeners alone are ineffective. Recommend stimulant laxatives.

8 See Completion Protocol (inside front cover).

EVALUATION

1 Ask client to rate pain intensity using appropriate pain scale both at rest and with activity.
2 Evaluate PQRSTU aspects of pain (see Skill 10.1).
3 Observe client's position, mobility, relaxation, and ability to rest, sleep, eat, and participate in usual activities.
4 Observe for adverse side effects of medications.

Unexpected Outcomes and Related Interventions

1 Client's pain intensity is greater than desired.
a. Evaluate the dose of medication administered.
b. Try an alternative nonpharmacological intervention.
c. Consult with physician if alternative analgesic or adjuvant can be given.
2 Client continues to show nonverbal behaviors reflecting pain.
a. Try a different nonpharmacological intervention.
b. Consult with physician if different analgesic or adjuvant can be given.
c. Discomfort that is unrelieved or is worse may indicate need for additional diagnostic, medical, or surgical intervention or a change in the pain management plan.

Recording and Reporting

- Record client's pain rating (before and 30 minutes after medication), behavioral response to analgesic, and additional comfort measures given. Incorporate pain-relief techniques in nursing care plan.
- Record medication, dose, route, and time given in MAR.
- Report unsuccessful or untoward client response to analgesics to physician.

Sample Documentation

0800 Reports severe continuous aching pain of 9 (scale 0 to 10) in lower back. Pain worsens upon turning and sitting. Finds some relief on left side. Morphine 5 mg given IV push. Positioned on left side with legs supported and back in alignment. Gentle massage provided to lower back.

0830 States, "I feel better now; the pain is still there but less than before." Rates pain 5 (scale 0 to 10).

Special Considerations
Pediatric Considerations

- Children (except infants under 3 to 6 months of age) metabolize drugs more rapidly than adults; younger children may require higher doses of opioids to achieve the same analgesic effect (Hockenberry and Wilson, 2007).
- Children should not have to endure pain, such as from intramuscular (IM) injections, to achieve pain relief. Use the least traumatic route of administration.
- The effectiveness of an analgesic is enhanced by offering a supportive attitude toward a child. Reinforce the cause and effect of the analgesic; then you can condition the child to expect pain relief (provided the regimen is effective) (Hockenberry and Wilson, 2007).

Geriatric Considerations

- Cognitive impairment or dementia affects an older adult's ability to report pain severity on a pain scale. Instead, be alert for subtle behaviors that indicate pain (see Box 10-1).
- Older adults may have liver or kidney impairment, resulting in faster onset and prolonged effect of analgesics because of reduced metabolism and excretion of these drugs. Physician's order should titrate dosage and frequency of analgesic administration to the client's response to the specific analgesic agent (Buffum and Buffum, 2000; American Medical Directors' Association, 1999). Rule of thumb: Start low, and go slow.
- Avoid IM analgesic administration in older adults because IM injections hurt and because analgesic uptake from the muscle into the cardiovascular system is unpredictable, thus affecting therapeutic and side effect profile (Waitman, 2001; Perin, 2000).
- Avoid a combination of opioids.
- Specific analgesics to avoid in older adults because of cardiovascular, CNS, renal, and/or liver toxicity include propoxyphene hydrochloride (Darvon, Darvocet) and meperidine (Demerol).
- Because of renal and liver decline associated with the aging process, maximum daily doses of NSAIDs and acetaminophen may need to be lower.
- If an older adult client is cognitively impaired and had a procedure that usually causes pain, the nurse should consult with the physician about ordering an appropriate analgesic ATC instead of prn.

Home Care Considerations

- Family members may need to understand the importance of ATC analgesic administration to maximize effect.
- Encourage family members to accept and acknowledge the client's report of pain.
- Family members who manage a client's pain while at home need to have access to health care providers on a 24-hour basis.

Long-Term Care Considerations

- In a study surveying 113 nursing directors of long-term care facilities, respondents were asked to rate how well they believed pain was managed among their residents. The percentage of directors who believed pain was suboptimally managed was 52% for chronic pain; 24% for pain in the terminally ill; 18% for residents with acute, short-term pain; and 13.5% for residents with postoperative pain. The three most common sources of pain were arthritis, back pain, and cancer pain. Obstacles to pain management included lack of specific knowledge about pain management among nurses and physicians, lack of a standardized treatment approach, and physicians' attitudes toward treating pain (Tarzian and Hoffmann, 2004).
- Careful assessment of concurrent medical conditions that may affect pharmacological management of pain is essential.
- Because many older adults are also receiving several drugs for a variety of conditions, drug-drug interactions are a possibility.
- A variety of medical conditions require a variety of physicians. Facilitate communicating information about prescribed medications among physicians.

SKILL 10.4 Patient-Controlled Analgesia

PCA is an interactive method of pain management that permits client control over pain through self-administration of analgesics (Pasero, 2003b). It is a safe method of analgesic administration for conditions such as postoperative, traumatic, labor and delivery (L&D), sickle cell crisis, cancer, and end-of-life pain. A client depresses the button on a PCA device to deliver a regulated dose of analgesic. Thus clients using PCA must be able to understand how, why, and when to self-administer medication and be able to physically depress the device (APS, 2003). Clients with acute postoperative pain and chronic (e.g., cancer) pain benefit from PCA. Common routes of PCA administration include subcutaneous and intravenous (IV).

Occasionally nurse-controlled analgesia (NCA) is ordered, whereby the nurse caring for the client depresses the button after first assessing the client. In addition, family-controlled analgesia (FCA) is used in children with cognitive or physical disabilities (Lehr and BeVier, 2003). In FCA one person is chosen as the client's primary pain manager (Pasero and McCaffery, 2005). In 2004 the JCAHO issued a "sentinel event alert" on *unauthorized* PCA administration. Nurses must advise clients, family, and other visitors that PCA is for client use only (JCAHO, 2004). PCA is not recommended in situations in which oral analgesics could easily manage pain (APS, 2003).

A PCA device may be electronic or nonelectronic, consisting of an infusion device, a prefilled drug reservoir, and tubing that delivers the medication from the infuser through the client-control module to tubing connected to the client's IV line. PCA devices are individually programmed to automatically deliver a specific physician-prescribed continuous infusion (basal rate) of medication, a bolus dose (client initiated), or both. The system is designed to deliver no more than a specified number of doses either every hour or every 4 hours (depending on the pump) to avoid overdoses. A typical PCA prescription relies on a series of "loading" doses (e.g., 3 to 5 mg of morphine, repeated every 5 to 10 minutes until initial pain diminishes). A low-dose basal infusion (0.5 to 1 mg/hr) at night allows uninterrupted sleep. A preprogrammed delay time or "lockout" (usually 6 to 16 minutes) between client-initiated doses prevents overdosing. In addition, the total amount of opioid that the client may receive in 1 or 4 hours can be limited. Use continuous basal infusions with caution in opioid-naive clients (clients who have used opioids ATC less than approximately 1 week) during the first 24 to 48 hours postoperatively. These clients are more likely to develop respiratory depression from a combination of opioids and anesthetics.

PCA has several advantages. It allows more constant serum levels of the opioid and thus avoids the peaks and troughs of a large bolus. Clients receive better pain relief and fewer side effects from opioids, because blood levels are maintained at a level of minimum effective analgesia concentration for the individual. When used postoperatively, fewer complications arise because earlier and easier ambulation occurs as a result of effective pain relief. Increased client control and independence are other advantages. Because the device provides medication on demand as soon as the client feels the need, the total amount of opioid use can be reduced. PCA allows the client to manage pain with minimal nursing intervention. Clients are not dependent on the nursing staff for pain management.

Concerns involving PCA use are client-related, pump failure, and operator errors. Clients may not understand how PCA therapy works, mistake the PCA button for a nurse call button, or have family members operate the demand button. The pump may fail to deliver drug on demand, have a faulty alarm or low battery, or lack free-flow protection. Operators may incorrectly program the dose, concentration, or rate. They also may fail to clamp or unclamp tubing, improperly load syringe or cartridge, fail to monitor for side effects/overdose, or not respond to alarms (Leavitt, 2003). PCA requires careful, ongoing monitoring.

Recently, researchers tested a new pain therapy based on the concept of PCA. Patient-controlled oral analgesia (PCOA) was tested on clients recovering from total knee replacement (Riordan and others, 2004). Although used on only a small group of clients, the therapy is promising. PCOA involves clients wearing a pouch containing a single dose of oral analgesic and then self-administering the medication when needed. Clients who used PCOA self-reported better pain control than clients who received medications from nursing staff.

ASSESSMENT

1 Check physician's orders for name of medication, dosage, frequency of medication (continuous, demand, or both), and lockout settings. Verify that client is not allergic to prescribed medication. *Rationale: Ensures right drug is administered to client.*

2 Assess client's cognitive ability. *Rationale: Determines appropriateness of client to be able to use PCA for pain management.*

3 For cognitively impaired or non–English-speaking clients, assess nonverbal pain responses. *Rationale: Because client cannot verbalize pain intensity, nonverbal responses help the nurse to determine the presence of pain.*

4 Assess character of client's pain, including behavioral and emotional signs and symptoms (see Skill 10.1). *Rationale: Establishes baseline to determine client's response to analgesia.*

5 Assess environment for factors that add to or heighten pain. *Rationale: Elimination of irritating stimuli may be effective in further reducing pain perception.*

6 Assess existing IV infusion line (peripheral or central) for patency and condition of venipuncture site for infiltration or inflammation. *Rationale: IV line must be patent with fluid infusing for medication to reach venous circulation safely and effectively. The PCA should never be attached to an IV line with blood running or to IV lines with cardiovascular drugs infusing. If necessary, start another IV site.*

7 Determine client's physical ability to manipulate PCA device. *Rationale: Determines if client can safely self-manage PCA.*

8 Assess if client has history of sleep apnea. *Rationale: PCA may be contraindicated in postoperative clients with sleep apnea because of risk for respiratory depression.*

PLANNING

Expected Outcomes focus on proper use of the PCA device and adequate pain control without oversedation and with no or manageable adverse effects.

1 Client reports pain relief with a pain intensity score at or below pain intensity goal.

2 Client exhibits relaxed facial expression and body position.

3 Client correctly operates PCA device.

4 Client remains alert and oriented.

5 Client increasingly participates in self-care activities.

Delegation Considerations

The skill of PCA administration may not be delegated. The nurse directs personnel by:

- Explaining the signs of sedation and unrelieved pain to report to the nurse when they occur
- Instructing personnel to report any new symptom or change in client status to the nurse
- Cautioning personnel to never administer a PCA dose for the client

Equipment

- PCA system and tubing (Figure 10-2)
- Identification label and time tape (may already be attached and completed by pharmacy)
- 18- or 20-gauge needle (if not using needleless system)
- Alcohol swab
- Adhesive tape
- Clean gloves
- Have opioid reversal agent (e.g., Narcan) closely available

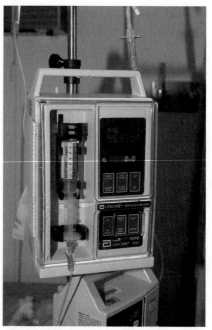

FIGURE 10-2 PCA device.

IMPLEMENTATION *for Patient-Controlled Analgesia*

STEPS	RATIONALE
1 See Standard Protocol (inside front cover).	
2 Before initiating analgesia, explain purpose and demonstrate function of PCA to client and family, including:	Ensures client understands how to manipulate device and implications of therapy. Clients want to know the type of drug, information about side effects, reassurance the device is safe, reassurance they cannot overdose or become addicted, and instructions on device technique (Chumbley and others, 2002).
a. Type of medication in PCA device.	
b. Device administers self-initiated small but frequent amounts of medication as needed to provide comfort and minimize side effects from analgesia.	Helps client to understand the value of controlling pain. Small dosing with client-controlled administration produces constant serum drug levels rather than peaks and troughs associated with prn nurse-administered therapy (Pasero, 2003b).

> **COMMUNICATION TIP** Advise client, "Giving yourself a dose of pain medication before you reposition, walk, or cough and deep breathe will help you perform activities more easily."

STEPS	RATIONALE
c. Device is programmed to deliver ordered type and dose of pain medication, lockout interval, and 1- or 4-hour maximum dose limit.	Confirms with client the safety of a PCA device.
d. Allowing client to push medication demand button on PCA unit. Explain that this is to be done when client feels discomfort, instead of calling nurse.	Gives client control of pain.

> **COMMUNICATION TIP** Explain to client, "Press the PCA button to deliver a small dose of pain medication into your IV. Because you are administering your pain medication, you will not need to wait for a nurse to draw up and administer a pain shot; therefore your pain will decrease sooner. There is a lockout time between doses so you cannot give yourself an overdose."

STEPS	RATIONALE
e. That the lockout time between demand doses prevents overdose.	Relieves client's fear of possible overdose.
f. Infuser will be on IV pole or attached to bed, clothing, or wrist.	
g. To notify the nurse for possible side effects (be specific as to possible effects), problems in attaining pain relief, changes in severity or location of pain, alarm sounding, or questions that arise.	Ensures nurse's more timely response to developing problems.
3 Check infuser and client-control module for proper function.	Avoids medication error and injury to client.
4 Program computerized PCA pump as ordered to deliver prescribed medication dose and lockout interval.	Ensures safe, therapeutic drug administration.
5 Position client to ensure venipuncture or central line site is accessible.	Ensures unimpeded flow of infusion.
6 Follow the "six rights" of drug administration (see Chapter 16). Identify client by comparing name on MAR with name on client's identification bracelet. Ask client to state name.	Ensures client's safety. At least two client identifiers (neither to be the client's room number) are to be used whenever administering medications (JCAHO, 2007).
7 Attach drug reservoir to infusion device and prime tubing.	Locks system and prevents air from infusing into IV tubing. Wearing gloves reduces potential contact with blood when working with IV line.
8 Attach 18- or 20-gauge needle to exit tubing adapter of client-control module or attach needleless system adapter.	Connects device with IV line.

STEPS	RATIONALE
9 Wipe injection port of main IV line with alcohol if closed port is being used.	Alcohol is a topical antiseptic that minimizes entry of microorganisms during needle insertion.
10 Insert needleless adapter or needle into injection port nearest client.	Establishes route for medication to enter main IV line.
11 Secure connection with tape and immobilize PCA tubing.	Prevents dislodging of needle or needleless adapter from port. Facilitates client's ability to ambulate.
12 Administer loading dose of analgesia as prescribed.	A one-time dose may be given manually by nurse or programmed into PCA pump to establish a level of analgesia.
13 Discard gloves and supplies in appropriate containers. Perform hand hygiene.	Reduces transmission of infection.
14 If client is having pain, demonstrate use of PCA system; if not, have client repeat instructions given earlier.	Repeating instructions reinforces learning. Return demonstration helps nurse determine client's level of understanding and ability to manipulate device.
15 To discontinue PCA:	
a. Obtain necessary PCA information from pump for documentation, including amount infused and amount to discard.	Ensures correct documentation of Schedule II drugs.
b. [hand icon] Turn pump off.	
c. Disconnect PCA tubing from IV maintenance line, but maintain IV access.	Ensures continued IV therapy.
d. Dispose of empty cassette or syringe according to institutional policy.	Control and dispensation of opioids are regulated by the Controlled Substances Act.
e. If PCA is discontinued before device is completely empty, record drug wastage on PCA medication record per institutional policy. Note date, time, amount of drug wasted, and reason for wastage. Wastage must be witnessed and record signed by two registered nurses (RNs).	Complies with documentation of Schedule II drugs.
16 See Completion Protocol (inside front cover).	

EVALUATION

1 Use pain rating scale to determine if pain intensity has decreased.

2 Monitor clients frequently (at least every 2 hours during the first 24 hours of therapy) if sedation at a level of 3 is detected (Box 10-4) (Pasero and McCaffery, 2005).

3 Observe client for signs of adverse reactions, especially excessive sedation.

4 Have client demonstrate dose delivery.

5 Evaluate number of attempts (number of times client pushed the button) and delivery of demand doses (number of times drug actually given), as well as basal dose, if ordered, according to agency policy (usually every 4 to 8 hours).

6 Observe client initiate self-care activities.

Unexpected Outcomes and Related Interventions

1 Client verbalizes continued or worsening discomfort or displays nonverbal behaviors indicating pain.

a. Perform complete pain reassessment.

BOX 10-4 Sedation Scale

S = Sleeping; easy to arouse
1 = Awake and alert
2 = Slightly drowsy; easily aroused
3 = Frequently drowsy; arousable; drifts off to sleep during conversation
4 = Somnolent; minimal or no response to physical stimulation

Modified from McCaffery M, Pasero C: *Pain: clinical manual*, ed 2, St Louis, 1999, Mosby.

---

b. Evaluate number of attempts and deliveries initiated by client.

c. Evaluate for possible complications other than pain condition for which client is being treated.

d. Inspect IV site for possible catheter occlusion or infiltration, and check tubing for possible kinking.

e. Check that maintenance IV fluid is continuously running.

f. Evaluate pump for operational problems.

g. Check to see if client manipulates PCA button correctly.

h. Consult with physician, who may need to adjust the dosage parameters because blood levels of analgesics need to remain stable to be effective. A continuous rate of administration may be needed to provide coverage during hours of sleep, the PCA dose may need to be increased, or an adjuvant may need to be added.

NURSE ALERT Do not increase demand or basal dose *and* decrease the interval time (e.g., from 10 to 5 minutes) simultaneously because this will increase the risk for oversedation, respiratory depression, and other adverse effects.

---

   i. Use nonpharmacological comfort measures.
2 Client is sedated and not readily arousable.
   a. Stop PCA.
   b. Elevate head of bed 30 degrees, unless contraindicated.
   c. Instruct client to take deep breaths.
   d. Notify physician.
   e. Apply ordered oxygen at 2 L/min via nasal cannula.
   f. Measure vital signs, including pulse oximetry.
   g. Ask family members if they depressed PCA button without client knowledge.
   h. Review MAR for other possible sedating drugs.
   i. Prepare to administer opioid-reversing agent.

Recording and Reporting

- Record drug, concentration, dose (basal and/or demand), time started, and lockout time on appropriate medication form. Many institutions have a separate flow sheet for PCA documentation.
- Dose calculation includes adding demand and continuous dose together. The following example is documented on a PCA flow sheet (Figure 10-3). A PCA pump of hydrocodone 0.5 mg/ml is initiated at 1400 with the following parameters: PCA demand dose, 0.5 mg; continuous dose, 0.25 mg/hr; with a lockout interval of 10 minutes. At 1800 the total amount of drug (1 mg from continuous/basal dose of 0.25 mg/hr and 7 mg from PCA demand doses administered by the client) was 8 mg. In addition, the volume (ml) of drug needs monitoring. The cumulative volume column alerts the nurse to the need for a new reservoir and to the possible diversion of opioids (volume administered and volume remaining in reservoir should equal total beginning volume).

Sample Documentation

1700 Reports no pain when lying still, but has burning abdominal incisional pain; intensity of 4 (goal is 4) when turning. Sleeping at intervals but arouses easily. Respiratory rate is 16, regular and deep. IV PCA infusing in left forearm without signs of infiltration.

Special Considerations
Pediatric Considerations

- Client-controlled analgesia is effective in pain control in children who can understand the concept. When selecting a child for PCA use, consider the developmental and cognitive level and motor skills. PCA use is usually safe and effective for clients as young as 8 to 9 years old (Lehr and BeVier, 2003).
- Remind family members not to push the button for the child. Some facilities have allowed parents with specific guidelines and training to push the button for children too young or unable to control PCA device on their own. This practice remains controversial (Hockenberry and Wilson, 2007).
- Delivery of the PCA dose on the upstroke of the button (review device insert) prevents accidental depression of the button when the child falls asleep (Lehr and BeVier, 2003).

Geriatric Considerations

- Older adults appear more sensitive to analgesic properties and side effects of opioids (American Geriatrics Society, 2002). Older adults' reduced renal and liver function slows opioid metabolism and excretion. This causes a faster peak effect and a longer duration of action of the opioid (APS, 2003). Physician's order should start with a low dose and titrate upward slowly.
- If an older adult becomes confused while using a PCA device, the dose should be lowered, the lockout lengthened, or a nonopioid analgesic added to reduce the opioid dose (Pasero, 1999).

Home Care Considerations

- PCA should not be used in clients physically or cognitively unable to activate device.
- Home care nurses should be available to client and family members through regular telephone contact and scheduled nursing visits.
- Provide instruction regarding appropriate dosage adjustment and potential errors.
- Notify physician if after dosage adjustments pain intensity remains unacceptable.

Long-Term Care Considerations

- PCA pumps are generally not found in a long-term care facility, but when used should have the same precautions as for hospital use. PCA is often used with clients under hospice care.

Barnes-Jewish Hospital
BJC HealthCare™

CONTROLLED DRUG RECORD

ADDRESSOGRAPH

PATIENT NAME *SAM JACKSON*	DIVISION *2 MAIN*	CONTROL NUMBER **183003**

IV/PCA	EPIDURAL
☐ Morphine 1 mg/ml in NS, 100 ml in Casette ☐ Meperidine 10 mg/ml in NS, 100 ml in Cassette ☒ Hydromorphone 0.5 mg/ml in NS, 100 ml in Cassette ☐ Fentanyl 50 mcg/ml, 50 ml in Cassette ☐ Lorazepam 1 mg/ml in D5W, 40 ml in Cassette ☐ Other: Drug/Diluent _____ 　　Concentration _____ mg/ml 　　Total Volume _____ ml	☐ Hydromorphone _____ mg/ml in NS 250 ml ☐ Morphine 0.04 mg/ml in NS 250 ml ☐ Fentanyl _____ mcg/ml/Bupivacaine _____ % in NS 250 ml ☐ Bupivacaine 0.8 mg/ml and Sufentanil 0.4 mcg/ml in 100 ml NS ☐ Other: Drug/Diluent _____ 　　Concentration _____ mg/ml 　　Total Volume _____ ml

ROUTE: ☐ Central Line ☐ Peripheral ☐ Epidural

METHOD: ☐ PCA ☐ Large Volume Infusion

DRUG DISPENSED BY: ☐ Pharmacy ☐ PYXIS

DISPENSING PHARMACIST SIGNATURE *M. Smith, PhD.*	DATE *1-18-07*	TIME *1330*
DRUG STARTED BY: NURSE SIGNATURE *Jill St. John*	DATE *1-18-07*	TIME *1400*

STOP HERE, DETACH THIS SECTION AND ROUTE TO PHARMACY

DOCUMENT EVERY 8 HOURS

DATE/TIME	BASAL RATE	BOLUS RATE	VOLUME CC/ML INFUSED	CUMULATIVE VOLUME CC/ML INFUSED	AMOUNT MG/MCG INFUSED	CUMULATIVE MG/MCG INFUSED	ATTEMPTS/ DELIVERED	NURSE SIGNATURE
1-18 1800	0.25	0.50	16cc	16cc	8 mg	8 mg	20 / 14	J. Wills, RN
1-18 2200	0.25	0.50	8cc	24cc	4 mg	12 mg	10 / 6	J. Wills, RN
— PUMP DISCONTINUED								J. Wills, RN

☒ WASTAGE ☐ RETURNED	DATE *1-18-07*	TIME *1800*	VOLUME *76 cc*
NURSE SIGNATURE: #1 *J. Wills, RN*		NURSE SIGNATURE: #2 *Susan Crow, RN*	
PRINTED NURSE NAME #1 *J. Wills, RN*		PRINTED NURSE NAME #2 *S. Crow, RN*	

MUST BE COMPLETED BEFORE RETURNED TO PHARMACY

FIGURE 10-3 PCA flow sheet. (Courtesy Barnes-Jewish Hospital, St Louis, Mo.)

SKILL 10.5 Epidural Analgesia

The administration of analgesics into the epidural space has become an increasingly popular technique for managing acute pain during labor, following surgery, and for chronic pain, especially for clients with cancer. Block and others (2003) reviewed more than 100 scientific studies to find that epidural analgesia provides better postoperative pain relief than use of parenteral (IV, subcutaneous, or IM) opioids. This was true for all time points (e.g., for each day after surgery). Epidural opioids reduce the total amount of opioids required to control pain, thus producing fewer side effects.

The epidural space is a potential space that contains a network of vessels, nerves, and fat located between the vertebral column and the dura mater, the outermost protective layer of the spinal cord (Figure 10-4). Drugs administered in the epidural space distribute (1) by diffusion through the dura mater into the cerebrospinal fluid (CSF), where they act directly on receptors in the dorsal horn of the spinal cord; (2) via blood vessels in the epidural space and deliver systemically; and/or (3) by absorption by fat in the epidural space, creating a depot where the drug is slowly released systemically (Pasero, 2003a). When an opioid injected epidurally diffuses slowly into the CSF of the subarachnoid space and binds to opiate receptors in the dorsal horn of the spinal cord, the binding blocks pain impulse transmission to the cerebral cortex.

Opioids and local anesthetics, separately or in combination, are used in epidural analgesia. Opioids are delivered close to their site of action (CNS) and thus require much smaller doses to achieve pain relief. Common opioids given epidurally include morphine, hydromorphone (Dilaudid), fentanyl, and sufentanil. These opioids differ by their "fat loving" and "water loving" properties that affect absorption rate and duration of action. Fentanyl and sufentanil are fat loving, causing them to have a quicker onset and shorter duration of action (2 hours). Morphine and hydromorphone

are water loving, resulting in longer onset and duration of action (as long as 24 hours with a single bolus dose).

For epidural catheter placement, place the client in the lateral side-lying or sitting position with shoulders and hips in alignment and hips and head flexed. An anesthesiologist or nurse anesthetist places a catheter in the epidural space below the second lumbar vertebra, where the spinal cord ends (Figure 10-5). However, epidurals may also be placed at the thoracic level of the spinal cord. Catheters intended for temporary or short-term use are not sutured in place and exit from the insertion site on the back. A catheter intended for permanent or long-term use is "tunneled" subcutaneously and exits on the side of the body (Figure 10-6) or on the abdomen. Tunneling reduces infection and catheter dislodgement.

Although the use of epidural opioids for control of pain has many advantages for the client, it also requires astute nursing observation and care. For example, no other supplemental opioids or sedatives should be administered when clients are on PCA. The combined effect can cause respiratory depression. Because of its anatomical location, the epidural catheter can migrate through the dura and disrupt spinal nerves and vessels. Catheter migration into the subarachnoid space can produce dangerously high medication levels. You must frequently monitor the client's level of analgesia. In many hospitals, anesthesiologists and nurse anesthetists are the only health care professionals who may initiate an epidural opioid infusion or administer a bolus. Some hospitals have nurses who have successfully com-

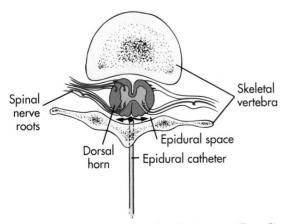

FIGURE 10-4 Anatomical drawing of epidural space. (From Sinatra S: Spinal opioid analgesia: an overview. In Sinatra RS and others, editors: *Acute pain management,* St Louis, 1992, Mosby.)

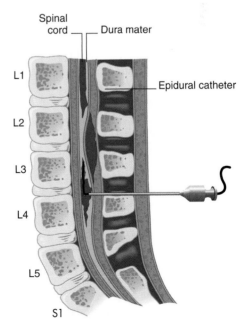

FIGURE 10-5 Placement of epidural catheter. (From Lewis SM, Heitkemper MM, Dirksen SR: *Medical-surgical nursing,* ed 6, St Louis, 2004, Mosby.)

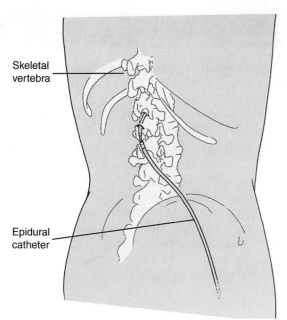

Skeletal
vertebra

Epidural
catheter

FIGURE 10-6 Tunneled epidural catheter.

pleted a certification program that enables them to begin the epidural opioid infusion or administer a bolus after the catheter has been placed (check agency policy).

ASSESSMENT

1 Assess level of client's comfort and character of client's pain (see Skill 10.1). *Rationale: Establishes baseline pain level.*

2 Assess presenting medical/surgical condition, and appropriateness for epidural analgesia. *Rationale: Certain conditions may make epidural analgesia the treatment of choice: postoperative states, clients with trauma or advanced cancer, women in labor, and clients predisposed to cardiopulmonary complications because of preexisting medical condition or surgery.*

3 For cognitively impaired or non–English-speaking clients, assess nonverbal pain responses. *Rationale: Because client cannot verbalize pain intensity, nonverbal responses help the nurse to determine the presence of pain.*

4 Check to see if client receives anticoagulants. *Rationale: Anticoagulation may contraindicate placement of epidural catheter because of the inability to apply pressure at the epidural insertion site and risk of bleeding (Horlocker and others, 2003).*

> NURSE ALERT Contraindications to epidural analgesia include coagulopathies, abnormal clotting studies, history of multiple abscesses, and sepsis. Additional contraindications may include skeletal or spinal abnormalities.

5 Assess if client takes herbals and if so which ones. *Rationale: Herbals may interfere with clotting and could predispose to bleeding at the epidural insertion site.*

6 Assess client's history of drug allergies.

7 Assess environment for factors that may contribute to pain.

8 Assess sedation level of client by assessing level of wakefulness or alertness, ability to follow commands, and drowsiness (see Box 10-4). *Rationale: Establishes a baseline before first dose. Sedation always precedes respiratory depression from opioids (Young-McCaughan and Miaskowski, 2001).*

9 Assess rate, pattern, and depth of respirations and blood pressure. *Rationale: Establishes baseline. Vasodilation can occur, and hypotension, including orthostatic hypotension, is common. Respiratory depression may also occur.*

10 Assess initial motor and sensory function (see Chapter 12). Test sensation in lower extremities. Have clients flex both feet and knees and raise each leg off the bed (Bird and Wallis, 2002). Give special attention to clients with preexisting sensory or motor abnormalities. *Rationale: Establishes a baseline. Excess analgesia causes adverse neurological effects. Preexisting conditions may mask sensory/motor changes from analgesia.*

11 Check to see if epidural catheter is secured to client's skin from the back, side, or front. *Rationale: Prevents accidental catheter dislodgement.*

12 Assess catheter insertion site for redness, warmth, tenderness, swelling, and drainage. *Rationale: Establishes baseline. Local inflammation and superficial skin infection at insertion site can develop. Purulent drainage is a sign of infection. Clear drainage may indicate CSF leaking from punctured dura. Bloody drainage may indicate catheter entered blood vessel.*

13 Check physician's order for medication, dosage, and infusion method. *Rationale: Ensures right client receives right infusion.*

14 If continuous infusion, check infusion pump for proper calibration and operation. *Rationale: Ensures client will obtain prescribed analgesic dose.*

15 If continuous infusion, check patency of tubing. Keep IV line patent until 24 hours after epidural analgesia has ended. *Rationale: Kinked tubing will interrupt analgesic infusion. Patent IV line allows for IV access in case medications need to be given to counteract adverse reactions.*

PLANNING

Expected Outcomes focus on elimination or reduction of pain and prevention of complications of epidural analgesia.

1 Client verbalizes pain relief within 30 to 60 minutes of initiation of epidural infusion with a pain intensity score at or below pain intensity goal.

2 Client's epidural dressing remains dry and intact.

3 Client does not have headache while epidural catheter is in place or as long as 72 hours after removal.

4 Client experiences no redness, warmth, exudate, tenderness, or swelling at catheter insertion site during time epidural catheter is in place. The client is afebrile.

5 Client's respirations are regular, of adequate depth, and equal to or greater than 8 breaths per minute.

6 Client remains normotensive and heart rate remains at or above client's baseline.

7 Client is awake, alert, and oriented to person, place, and time.

8 Client voids without difficulty; averages 30 to 60 ml per hour.

9 Client has no or minimal pruritus and no paresthesias of lower extremities.

10 Catheter and injection cap or infusion pump tubing are securely taped and labeled.

Delegation Considerations

The skill of epidural analgesia administration should not be delegated. The nurse directs personnel by:

- Instructing personnel to pay attention to the insertion site when repositioning or ambulating clients to prevent catheter disruption.
- Instructing personnel to report any catheter disconnection immediately.
- Instructing personnel to immediately report to the nurse any change in client status or comfort level.

Equipment

- Clean gloves
- Prediluted preservative-free opioid or local anesthetic as prescribed by physician and prepared for use in IV infusion pump (usually prepared by pharmacy)
- Infusion pump and compatible tubing without Y ports (Some infusion pumps have tubing color-coded for intraspinal use)
- Filter needle
- Antiinfective swab
- Syringe
- Tape
- Label (for injection port)

IMPLEMENTATION *for Epidural Analgesia*

STEPS	RATIONALE
1 See Standard Protocol (inside front cover).	
2 Identify client by comparing name on MAR with name on arm band and asking client's name, hospital number, and/or birthdate.	Ensures right client receives epidural analgesia. At least two client identifiers (neither to be the client's room number) are to be used whenever administering medications (JCAHO, 2007).
3 Explain purpose and function of epidural analgesia and expectations of client during procedure (e.g., having client call for assistance to get out of bed).	Proper explanation of therapy enhances client cooperation.
4 Attach "epidural line" label to the epidural infusion tubing.	Labeling helps to ensure medication analgesic is administered into correct line and the epidural space.
5 Use tubing *without* Y ports for continuous infusions.	Use of tubing without Y ports prevents accidental injection or infusion of other medication meant for vascular space into epidural space.
6 Administer continuous infusion:	
a. Attach container of diluted preservative-free medication to infusion pump tubing and prime the tubing (see Chapter 27).	Tubing filled with solution and free of air bubbles avoids an air embolus.
b. Attach proximal end of tubing to pump and distal end to epidural catheter. Tape all connections. Give ordered bolus or start infusion. (See Chapter 27 for use of infusion pump.)	Pump propels fluid through tubing. Taping maintains a secure closed system to prevent infection. A filter may be needed on tubing (check agency policy).
c. Check infusion pump for proper calibration and operation. Press "on" button. Some institutions require two nurses to check settings.	Maintains patency and ensures client receives proper medication dose.
7 Administer bolus dose of analgesic:	
a. Following procedure in Chapter 17, draw up prediluted, preservative-free opioid solution through filter needle.	Preservative may be toxic to nerve tissue (Cosentino, 2000).
b. Change from filter needle to regular 20-gauge needleless adapter or needle.	Prevents infusion of microscopic glass particles and allows medication to be injected.
c. Clean injection cap with antiinfective. (Do not use alcohol.)	Cleaning agent prevents introduction of microorganisms into CNS. Alcohol causes pain and is toxic to neural tissue.
d. Dry the injection cap with sterile gauze.	Reduces possible injection of povidone-iodine.
e. Insert needleless adapter or needle attached to syringe into injection cap. Aspirate.	Aspiration of more than 1 ml of clear fluid or bloody return means catheter may have migrated into subarachnoid space or into a blood vessel (Pasero, 1999). Do not inject drug. Notify anesthesiologist or nurse anesthetist immediately.

STEPS	RATIONALE
f. Inject opioid at a rate of 1 ml over 30 seconds.	Slow injection prevents client discomfort by lowering the pressure exerted by fluid as it enters the epidural space (Cox, 2001).
g. Remove needle or syringe from injection cap. There is no need to flush with saline.	The catheter is in a space, not a blood vessel.
8 Dispose of uncapped adapter/needle and syringe in sharps container.	
9 Explain that nurses will be monitoring client's response to epidural analgesic routinely. Also instruct client on signs or problems to report to nurse.	Builds trust to encourage client to be a partner in care.

> **COMMUNICATION TIP** Explain to client, "Some potential side effects of epidural analgesia that we will be watching you for include excessive sleepiness or sedation, slowing of your respirations, inability to pass urine, and itching. Please let a nurse know if you experience any of these problems. Also let a nurse know if your pain level increases or if your epidural catheter feels wet or starts to peel off."

STEPS	RATIONALE
10 Before removal of epidural catheter, check for presence of therapeutic anticoagulation.	Removal of epidural catheter while a client is anticoagulated increases the risk of a spinal hematoma because of anticoagulation and inability to compress vessels (Horlocker and others, 2003).
11 See Completion Protocol (inside front cover).	

EVALUATION

1 Evaluate client's comfort level; use pain rating scale to determine if pain intensity has decreased.
2 Inspect dressing for drainage or disruption.
3 Assess for reports of headache and note nonverbal signs of headache.
4 Monitor temperature and assess catheter insertion site for redness, warmth, exudate, tenderness, or swelling.
5 Observe respiratory rate, rhythm, depth, and pattern; sedation level; and skin color. Monitor respiratory rate and depth at least every 1 to 2 hours depending on institutional policy.
6 Observe respiratory rate, rhythm, and pattern every 2 hours for 12 to 24 hours after epidural bolus of opioid to an opioid-naive client (Pasero, 1999).

7 Monitor blood pressure and pulse. Assist client when changing positions.
8 Assess sedation level, level of consciousness (LOC), and orientation.
9 Assess intake and output (I&O) and client's voiding pattern. If voiding in amounts less than 150 ml at a time and experiencing frequency, palpate for bladder distention and consider intermittent catheterization.
10 Assess client's sensation, beginning in lower extremities and moving up to trunk. Have client flex both feet and knees and then raise each leg off the bed. Ask client if numbness or tingling is felt in lower extremities.
11 Assess client for pharmacological side effects: nausea, vomiting, pruritus, presence of tinnitus, or mouth numbness (Bird and Wallis, 2002).

Unexpected Outcomes and Related Interventions

1 Client states pain is still present.
a. Check all tubing, connections, and pump settings.
b. Confer with physician regarding adequacy of medication dose.
2 Client is sedated or not easily arousable.
a. Stop epidural infusion.
b. Administer opioid-reversing agent per physician order.
c. Monitor continuously until client is easily arousable.

> **NURSE ALERT** Keep an ampule of naloxone (Narcan), 0.4 mg/ml, an opioid antagonist, at the bedside to use in case of emergency to counteract respiratory depression (respiratory rate less than or equal to 8 breaths per minute and reduced depth). Dilute naloxone with 9 ml of preservative-free saline, and administer 0.5 ml intravenously over 2 minutes and assess respirations (see agency policy). Titrate to effect. When respiratory rate is 10 breaths per minute or above and depth is adequate, naloxone may be discontinued; however, continue to observe client because respiratory depression may reappear and thus require more naloxone (Pasero and McCaffery, 2000). If 0.8 mg of naloxone produces no effect, consider other causes. Naloxone may reverse the opioid's effect but will also reverse pain control. Client may require alternative medication for pain relief.

3 Client experiences periods of apnea, or respirations are fewer than 8 breaths per minute, shallow, or irregular.

a. Instruct client to take deep breaths.

b. Stop or reduce rate of epidural infusion and notify physician.

c. Prepare to administer opioid-reversing agent per physician order.

d. Monitor every 15 minutes until respirations are 8 or more and of adequate depth; continue for 2 hours observing for return of respiratory depression. Naloxone has a shorter half-life than immediate-release opioids.

4 Client reports sudden headache. Clear drainage is present on epidural dressing or more than 1 ml of fluid can be aspirated from catheter.

a. Stop infusion or bolus doses.

b. Notify physician.

5 Blood is present on epidural dressing or can be aspirated from catheter.

a. Stop infusion.

b. Notify physician.

6 Redness, warmth, tenderness, swelling, or exudate is noted at catheter insertion site.

a. Notify physician.

7 Client experiences minimal urinary output, urinary frequency or urgency, bladder distention, pruritus, or nausea and vomiting.

a. Consult with physician about reducing opioid dose and discuss treatment for side effects.

Recording and Reporting

- Record drug, dose, and time given (if injection) or time begun and ended (if continuous infusion) on appropriate medication record. Specify concentration and diluent.
- With continuous infusion, obtain and record pump readout hourly for first 24 hours after infusion is begun and then every 4 hours. Review pump settings and usage with staff on next shift.
- Record regular periodic assessments of client's status in nurses' notes or on appropriate flow sheet (Figure 10-7), including vital signs, I&O, sedation level, pain severity score, neurological status, appearance of epidural site, presence or absence of adverse reactions to medication, and presence or absence of complications resulting from placement and maintenance of epidural catheter.
- Report any adverse reactions or complications to physician.

Sample Documentation

0800 Fentanyl 2000 mcg in 500 ml 0.9 NS infusing at 15 ml/hr into epidural catheter via infusion pump. Respiratory rate 10 with moderate depth and regular pattern. States abdominal surgical pain is 5 (scale 0 to 10), compared with previous 7.

1000 Respiratory rate 6 with shallow depth and periods of apnea, O_2 saturation 90%, HR 70, BP 110/70. Arouses with verbal stimulation. Epidural infusion stopped. Narcan 0.2 mg IV push given in titrated doses. Anesthesiologist notified.

1005 Respiratory rate 8, shallow depth, regular pattern, O_2 saturation 94%, HR 78, BP 118/72. Alert, awake, oriented ×3.

1020 Respiratory rate 12, moderate depth, regular pattern. HR 82, BP 124/78. Rates abdominal surgical incision pain 4 on 0 to 10 scale.

Special Considerations
Pediatric Considerations

- Epidural analgesia may be used in all pediatric age groups.
- Dose of analgesic is by milligram or microgram per kilogram.
- Epidural analgesia in infants and children is used for acute pain conditions such as sickle cell crisis and heel cord tendon release in muscular dystrophy (Hockenberry and Wilson, 2007).
- During epidural analgesia, infants and children require continuous cardiac, respiratory, and oxygen saturation monitoring.

Geriatric Considerations

- Because older adult clients often receive medications for hypertension, evaluating for hypotension during epidural analgesia is essential.

Home Care Considerations

- Clients needing home therapy will be discharged with a tunneled catheter.
- Assess the client's fine motor skills, cognitive function, stage of disease and prognosis, and ability of family/significant other to care for catheter before considering catheter placement and home care.
- Teach client and caregiver the proper dosage and technique for administration of medication. Evaluate client's or family member's technique for catheter care and administering medication. Reinforce instructions.
- Explain pain assessment using the pain scale. Observe family member assess client's pain.
- Explain available drug and dosage for breakthrough pain. Inform client how to contact clinician for increase in dosage if highest level prescribed is ineffective.
- Teach client and caregiver aseptic technique for medication administration and for all catheter care procedures, including dressing changes. Instruct client to change dressing every week (policy varies among home health agencies). Teach signs and symptoms of infection and signs and symptoms to report to nurse or physician (see Box 10-3).
- Provide client and family list of all supplies needed for procedures and where to purchase.
- Teach client and caregiver about signs and symptoms of adverse reactions to medications and interventions used to treat side effects.

MEMORIAL MEDICAL CENTER
Springfield, Illinois

EPIDURAL ANALGESIA FLOW SHEET

Analgesic Drug Used:

_____ Duramorph (_____mcg/ml)
__✓__ Fentanyl (_10_ mcg/ml)
_____ Hydromorphone (_____mcg/ml)
_____ Sufentanil (_____mcg/ml)

Device In Use:
_____ Abbott PCA (mcg units)
_____ Bard PCA (ml units)

Date	5/3	5/3													
Time	09	13													
Mode: B = Bolus / P = PCA / C = Continuous / P+C = PCA + Continuous	P+C	P+C													
Manual Bolus by MD (Drug/Dose)	3mcg	—													
Volume in Bag	100	60													
Volume Infused	—	40													
Concentration	0.0	0.0	0.0	0.0	0.0	0.0	0.0	0.0	0.0	0.0	0.0	0.0	0.0	0.0	0.0
PCA Dose (ml)	1.0	1.0													
Delay (min)	20	20													
Basal Rate	10	10													
One Hour Limit	13	13													
Sedation Level	2	3													
Analgesic Level	7	3													
Complications	—	—													
Initials	JD	JD													
RN Signature	J Davenport, RN														

Sedation Level
1=wide awake   4=mostly sleeping
2=drowsy   5=awakens only when aroused
3=dozing intermittently

Analgesic Level
1 2 3 4 5 6 7 8 9 10
no   worst
pain   pain
                            imaginable

Complications
1=nausea   5=headache
2=vomiting   6=respiratory depression
3=pruritis   7=ileus
4=unable to void

Record of Waste & Spoilage				
Date	Quantity	Describe in Detail	Signature #1	Signature #2

White copy to chart   Yellow copy to Pharmacy   Pink copy to Anesthesia Pain Service   Page 1 of 1

FIGURE 10-7 Epidural and analgesia documentation form. (Courtesy Memorial Medical Center, Springfield, Ill.)

- Urinary retention: Teach how to perform straight intermittent catheterization.
- Pruritus: Advise client to wear clean, lightweight cotton clothing; keep room cool; use cool moist compresses; lubricate skin; and apply cornstarch.

Long-Term Care Considerations
- Epidural pain management is rarely used in long-term care settings.

SKILL 10.6 Local Anesthetic Infusion Pump for Analgesia

During surgery for joint replacement, surgeons may apply an infusion pump (Figure 10-8) to deliver a local anesthetic (Marcaine) to the surgical site through a one-way catheter. Local anesthesia provides pain relief directly to the surgical site. Clients may still require oral analgesics, but the total dose is often reduced (Pasero, 2000). The pump has both a demand (4 to 6 ml per bolus) and a continuous rate (2 to 4 ml/hr) feature. Continuous flow reservoirs hold 100 ml, whereas the client-controlled units have a 60-ml reservoir. The device is left in for about 48 hours. The nurse teaches the client how to remove the catheter at home. This pump is meant for one-time use only. Nursing care involves assessment of catheter connections, evaluation of local anesthetic side effects, and client teaching.

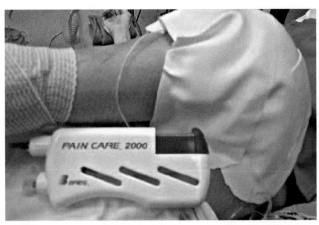

FIGURE 10-8 Local anesthetic infusion pump. (Courtesy Breg, Inc., Vista, Calif.)

ASSESSMENT

1 Perform complete pain assessment as for Skill 10.1, including nonverbal behaviors and type of activities influenced by pain (e.g., sleeping, eating, moving affected extremity).

2 Review surgeon's operative report for position of catheter. *Rationale: Confirms catheter location.*

3 Read label on device. *Rationale: Informs you about type of anesthetic, concentration, volume, flow rate, date and time prepared, and name of person who prepared it.*

4 Assess surgical dressing and site of catheter insertion. *Rationale: Dressing should be dry and intact. If not, stop infusion and notify physician. Catheter may not be properly placed.*

5 Assess catheter connections. *Rationale: Connections should be firmly attached. If tubing becomes detached, do not reattach because infection could occur. Notify physician.*

6 Assess for blood backing up in tubing. If present, stop infusion and notify physician. *Rationale: Indicates possible displacement of catheter into blood vessel.*

7 Determine extremity activity level from physician orders. *Rationale: Excessive activity may displace catheter.*

8 Assess for signs of Marcaine toxicity: hypotension, dizziness, tremor, severe itching, swelling of the skin or throat, irregular heartbeat, palpitations, confusion, ringing in the ears, muscle twitching, numbness around the mouth, metallic taste, seizures. *Rationale: Ensures prompt treatment of complication.*

PLANNING

Expected Outcomes focus on pain relief and improvement in client's ability to resume activity.

1 Client verbalizes full or partial pain relief with a pain intensity score at or below pain intensity goal.

2 Client achieves reduction of nonverbal pain behaviors such as grimacing, clenching teeth, or rocking.

3 Client is free of adverse drug reactions.

4 Client sleeps and eats better, is more active, and communicates easily with family and friends.

5 Surgical dressing remains dry and intact.

Delegation Considerations

The skill of managing local infusion pump analgesia should not be delegated. The nurse directs personnel by:

- Informing them to pay attention to the insertion site when providing care, to avoid dislocation.
- Instructing them to report any catheter disconnection immediately.
- Instructing them to notify nurse immediately of a change in client's status or level of comfort.

Equipment

- Pump in place from surgery
- Clean gloves
- Sterile 4 × 4 gauze pads

IMPLEMENTATION *for Local Anesthetic Infusion Pump for Analgesia*

STEPS	RATIONALE
1 See Standard Protocol (inside front cover).	
2 Remove catheter:	Prevents exposure to body fluids.
a. Remove surgical dressing.	
b. Have client in relaxed position.	Relaxes joint muscles, reducing traction from muscle tension, and provides distraction.
c. Explain to client what he or she will feel when you remove the catheter.	Helping client to anticipate nature of discomfort can relive anxiety.
d. Place 4 × 4 gauze over site. Grasp catheter firmly and pull outward from skin with steady motion	If resistance is felt, stop pulling. Reposition extremity and try again. If tubing continues to stretch and demonstrates resistance, stop pulling, cover area with sterile dressing, and notify physician.
e. Look for mark on end of catheter tip.	Indicates complete removal of catheter.

STEPS	RATIONALE
f. After catheter is removed, place a new sterile gauze dressing over the area and apply pressure for at least 2 minutes.	Prevents hematoma formation.
g. Place catheter in plastic bag using standard precautions.	Client is to bring catheter to physician's office on first visit.
3 Remind client of physician's follow-up appointment.	Improves likelihood of client adherence.
4 See Completion Protocol (inside front cover).	

EVALUATION

1 Ask client to rate pain intensity using appropriate pain scale both at rest and with activity.
2 Observe client's position, mobility, relaxation, and ability to rest, sleep, eat, and participate in usual activities.
3 Observe for signs of adverse drug reaction.
4 Inspect condition of surgical dressing.

Unexpected Outcomes and Related Interventions

1 Client verbalizes pain intensity greater than previously determined goal or demonstrates nonverbal behaviors indicative of pain. Catheter may be displaced or clogged, or surgical site may be developing complications.
a. Check reservoir for presence of medication.
b. Notify physician.
2 Client reports symptoms of Marcaine toxicity. Possible hypersensitivity to local anesthetic, displacement of catheter into vein, or pump failure (releasing too much drug into site).
a. Stop pump, and call surgeon immediately.

Recording and Reporting

- Record drug, concentration, date inserted, and if continuous or demand feature in medication record.
- Record client's pain rating, response to anesthetic, and additional comfort measures given.
- Record additional analgesics necessary to control pain.
- Record any adverse reactions to local anesthetic.

Sample Documentation

1000 Returns from OR after right total knee replacement. Dressing dry and intact. Local anesthetic pump in place, catheter connections intact, receiving continuous 0.125% Marcaine infusion at 3 ml/hr. Client currently rates knee pain at 3 (scale 0 to 10).

Special Considerations
Pediatric Considerations

- Local infusion pumps are not yet used in the pediatric population.

Geriatric Considerations

- No special considerations are necessary unless client is mentally compromised. Continuous dosing may be administered, but demand doses require a mentally competent adult.

Home Care Considerations

- If device is on demand (not continuous), instruct client to depress button every 6 hours.
- Instruct client to notify health care provider if pain meets or exceeds pain intensity goal.
- Have client notify physician if excessive fluid or bleeding on the dressing occurs.
- Provide written instructions regarding the possible adverse reactions to Marcaine that should be reported to physician immediately.
- Provide written and verbal instruction as to how and when to discontinue device when at home. Catheter should be placed in a plastic bag and brought with client to first follow-up physician visit.
- Provide instructions regarding extremity movement.

NCLEX® Style Questions

1 Jay Mabry is completing a massage for a client, Mr. Riddle. He tells Mr. Riddle to inhale deeply and exhale and to then move slowly as he sits up in bed. The nurse ends the massage in this way to prevent:
1. Muscle cramping
2. Intravascular clotting
3. Valsalva maneuver
4. Postural hypotension

2 In a 7 PM nurses' note summary, the nurse writes, "Epidural catheter in place; dressing has 5-cm-wide circle of clear drainage." The nurse's findings indicate which of the following?
1. Infection
2. CSF leak
3. Epidural catheter migrated into blood vessel
4. Proper function of catheter

3 It is important to understand that nonpharmacological therapies to promote comfort should be used in which of the following situations?
1. With analgesics
2. In place of analgesics
3. On an ATC basis
4. With severe pain only

4 Review each of the clinical cases below and identify the client most at risk for respiratory depression from opioid use.
1. Respirations 20, deep; pulse 82 at baseline. Respirations 14, deep; pulse 76 after analgesia.
2. Respirations 18, deep; sedation level 2 at baseline. Respirations 14, shallow; sedation level 4 after analgesia.
3. Respirations 18, deep; sedation level 1 at baseline. Respirations 10, deep; sedation level 3 after analgesia.
4. Respirations 16, deep; sedation level 3 at baseline. Respirations 14, shallow; sedation level 2 after analgesia.

5 As the nurse, you would suspect Marcaine toxicity in a client connected to a local infusion pump when observing which of the following symptoms:
1. Hypotension, dizziness, and severe itching
2. Reduced sensation in lower extremities, urinary urgency, and distended bladder
3. Reduced respiratory rate and depth with increase in sedation level
4. Orthostatic hypotension and tingling in extremities

6 Ms. Lemar has been receiving morphine via a continuous epidural infusion for longer than 12 hours. When you enter the room you find the client difficult to arouse, with respirations fewer than 8 breaths per minute. Your first nursing action should be to:
1. Stop the epidural infusion.
2. Monitor the client continuously until client arouses.
3. Instruct the client to take deep breaths.
4. Notify physician.

References for all chapters appear in Appendix D.

11

Vital Signs

MEDIA RESOURCES

- **evolve** http://evolve.elsevier.com/Elkin
- **View Video!** Video Clips
- **Nursing Skills Online**

Temperature, pulse, respirations, and blood pressure are the vital signs, which indicate the body's ability to regulate body temperature, maintain blood flow, and oxygenate body tissues. Oxygen saturation is an additional vital sign obtained through pulse oximetry that reflects the ability of the cardiac and respiratory system to maintain adequate oxygenation. Pain assessment is considered a fifth vital sign (see Chapter 10). Frequently pain is the symptom that leads clients to seek health care.

Vital signs indicate clients' responses to physical, environmental, and psychological stressors. Vital signs may reveal sudden changes in a client's condition. A change in one vital sign (e.g., pulse) can reflect changes in the other vital signs (temperature, respirations, blood pressure, and oxygen saturation). The nurse's findings aid in determining whether it is necessary to assess specific body systems more thoroughly. The nurse must measure vital signs correctly, understand and interpret the values, begin interventions as needed, and report findings appropriately. Keeping clients informed of their vital signs promotes understanding of their health status.

Analysis and interpretation of vital signs are needed to make decisions about nursing interventions. In addition, the nurse uses clinical judgment to determine which vital signs to measure, when measurements should be made (Box 11-1), and when measurements can be safely delegated. For example, after assessing an abnormal respiratory rate, the nurse also auscultates lung sounds. In certain situations, vital sign assessment may be limited to measurement of a single vital sign for the purpose of monitoring a specific aspect of a client's condition. For example, after administering an antihypertensive medication, the nurse measures the client's blood pressure to evaluate the drug's effect.

TEMPERATURE

Body tissues and cell processes function best within a relatively narrow temperature range between 36° C and 38° C (96.8° F and 100.4° F). The temperature range of a normal adult depends on age, physical activity, status of hydration, and state of health, including the presence of infection (Table 11-1). Temperature fluctuates in a 24-hour cycle, being lowest between 1 AM and 4 AM, rising steadily throughout the day, and peaking at about 6 PM. Body temperature is physiologically regulated by vasodilation, vasoconstriction, shivering, and sweating. A client's behavior can adjust body temperature by avoiding temperature extremes, adding or removing external clothing or coverings, and ingesting fluids and drugs. Average body temperature varies depending on the measurement site used. Each site and type of thermometer has unique techniques, contraindications, or limitations and norms (Table 11-2). The measurement of body temperature is aimed at obtaining a representative average of the core body tissues. Sites reflecting core temperatures include rectal, tympanic, esophageal, pulmonary artery, and urinary bladder. These sites tend to be more reliable indicators of body temperature than sites reflecting surface temperatures, which are the skin, oral, and axillary sites. Several types of thermometers are commonly available to measure body temperature (Box 11-2). Temperature can be measured on a Celsius or Fahrenheit scale. Although some electronic thermometers can display both Celsius and Fahrenheit readings, conversion charts are also available to convert from one system to the other. To ensure accuracy and client safety, each type of thermometer must be used correctly and appropriately.

PULSE

The pulse is a palpable bounding of blood flow caused by pressure wave transmission from the left ventricle to the aorta, large arteries, and peripheral arteries. Assessing the pulse provides indications of heart function and tissue perfusion (circulation). In adults the radial pulse is the site for routine pulse assessment (Figure 11-1). The brachial or apical pulse is the site for routine pulse assessment in infants.

Normally the pulse is easily palpable, regular in rhythm, and ranges between 60 and 100 beats per minute in adults. When palpated, a normal pulse does not fade in and out and is not easily obliterated by pressure. Pulse abnormalities include bradycardia (pulse less than 60 beats per minute), tachycardia (pulse greater than 100 beats per minute), and arrhythmia (irregular pulse rate). *Weak, feeble,* and *thready* are descriptive words for a pulse of low volume that is difficult to palpate. *Bounding* is the term used to describe a pulse that is very strong. Strength (amplitude) of pulses may be rated by the following scale: 4+, bounding; 3+, full; 2+, normal; 1+, weak; 0, absent. Changes in the pulse reflect the client's metabolic rate and physiological responses to stress, exercise, blood loss, and pain. If abnormalities are identified, such as an irregular rhythm or an inability to palpate the radial pulse, an apical pulse must be obtained (Figure 11-2). The apical pulse, the most accurate noninvasive measure of heart rate and rhythm, is obtained using a

---

BOX 11-1 When to Take Vital Signs

1. On admission to a health care facility.
2. When assessing client during home health visits.
3. In a hospital or care facility on a routine schedule according to a physician's or health care provider's order or institution's standards of practice.
4. Before and after a surgical procedure or invasive diagnostic procedure.
5. Before, during, and after a transfusion of blood products.
6. Before, during, and after the administration of medications or application of therapies that affect cardiovascular, respiratory, and temperature-control functions.
7. When the client's general physical condition changes (e.g., loss of consciousness, increased severity of pain).
8. Before and after nursing interventions influencing a vital sign (e.g., before and after a client previously on bed rest ambulates, before and after client performs range-of-motion [ROM] exercises).
9. When the client reports specific symptoms of physical distress (e.g., feeling "funny" or "different").

TABLE 11-1 Vital Signs: Normal Ranges

VITAL SIGNS	NORMAL RANGES
Temperature	36-38° C; 98.6-100.4° F
Oral/tympanic	37.0° C; 98.6° F
Rectal	37.5° C; 99.5° F
Axillary	36.5° C; 97.7° F
Pulse	Adult: 60-100 beats per minute, strong and regular
Respirations	Adult: 12-16 breaths per minute, deep and regular
Blood Pressure*	Systolic: less than 120 mm Hg; diastolic: less than 80 mm Hg; average blood pressure 120/80 mm Hg
Pulse Pressure	30-50 mm Hg

*In some clients, blood pressure is consecutively measured lying, sitting, and standing or in both arms. In normal individuals the change from lying to standing causes a decrease in systolic blood pressure of less than 15 mm Hg (Barkauskas and others, 2002). Record the position and extremity, and compare the measurements for significant differences.

TABLE 11-2 Advantages and Limitations of Selected Temperature Measurement Sites

ADVANTAGES	LIMITATIONS
Oral	
Easily accessible—requires no position change.	Causes delay in measurement if client has recently ingested hot/cold fluids or foods, smoked, or received oxygen by mask or nasal cannula.
Comfortable for client.	
Provides accurate surface temperature reading.	Not used with clients who have had oral surgery, trauma, history of epilepsy, or shaking chills.
Reflects rapid change in core temperature.	
Reliable route to measure temperature in intubated clients.	Not used with infants or small children or with confused, unconscious, or uncooperative clients.
	Risk of body fluid exposure.
Tympanic	
Easily accessible site.	More variability of measurement than with other core temperature devices.
Minimal client repositioning required.	Requires removal of hearing aid before measurement.
Obtained without disturbing, repositioning, or waking client.	Requires disposable sensor cover available only in one size.
Used for clients with tachypnea without affecting breathing.	Otitis media and cerumen impaction distort readings.
Provides accurate core reading because eardrum is close to hypothalamus; sensitive to core temperature changes.	Not used with clients who have had surgery of the ear or tympanic membrane.
	Does not accurately measure core temperature changes during and after exercise.
Very rapid measurement (2 to 5 seconds).	Does not obtain continuous measurement.
Unaffected by oral intake of food, fluids, or smoking.	Affected by ambient temperature devices (e.g., incubators, radiant warmers, facial fans).
	Anatomy of ear canal makes it difficult to position correctly in neonates, infants, and children younger than 3 years (Holtzclaw, 2002).
Axillary	
Safe and noninvasive.	Long measurement time (3 minutes).
Used with newborns and unconscious clients.	Requires continuous positioning by nurse.
	Measurement lags behind core temperature during rapid temperature changes.
	Not recommended to detect fever in infants and young children.
	Requires exposure of thorax, which can result in temperature loss, especially in newborns.
	Affected by exposure to the environment, including time to place thermometer (Maxton, Justin, and Gilles, 2004).
Rectal	
Argued to be more reliable when oral temperature cannot be obtained.	Lags behind core temperature during rapid temperature changes (Maxton, Justin, and Gilles, 2004).
	Not used for clients with diarrhea or clients who have had rectal surgery or bleeding tendencies.
	Requires positioning and may be a source of client embarrassment and anxiety.
	Risk of body fluid exposure.
	Requires lubrication.
	Readings may be influenced by impacted stool (Maxton, Justin, and Gilles, 2004).
	Not used for routine vital signs in newborns.
Skin	
Inexpensive.	Measurement lags behind other sites during temperature changes, especially during hyperthermia.
Provides continuous reading.	
Safe and noninvasive.	Sometimes affected by environmental temperature.
Used for neonates.	Diaphoresis or sweat can impair adhesion.
Temporal Artery	
Easy to access without position change.	Inaccurate with head covering or hair on forehead.
Very rapid measurement.	Affected by skin moisture such as diaphoresis or sweating.
No risk of injury to client or nurse.	Not used if continuous measurement is required.
Eliminates need to disrobe or unbundle client.	
Comfortable for client.	
Used in premature infants, newborns, and children.	
Reflects rapid change in core temperature.	
Sensor cover not required.	

BOX 11-2 Types of Thermometers

Electronic Thermometers

- A rechargeable battery-powered display unit with a thin wire cord and a temperature-processing probe covered by a disposable cover.
- Within 1 minute after placement, the thermometer displays a digital temperature reading.
- Separate probes are used for oral temperature measurement (blue tip) and rectal temperature measurement (red tip) (see illustration A).

Tympanic Electronic Thermometers

- The tympanic membrane reflects core body temperature because it shares its blood supply with the hypothalamus, the body's temperature-control center in the brain.
- The probe consists of an otoscope-like speculum with an infrared sensor tip that detects heat radiated from the tympanic membrane of the ear (see illustration B).
- Within 2 to 5 seconds after placement in the ear canal and depressing the scan button, a digital reading appears on the display unit. A sound signals when the peak temperature has been measured.

Chemical Dot Single-Use or Reusable Thermometers

- Thin strips of plastic with a temperature sensor at one end and chemically impregnated dots formulated to change color at different temperatures (see illustration C).
- Chemical dots on the thermometer change color to reflect temperature reading, usually within 60 seconds.
- Useful for screening temperatures, especially in infants, during invasive procedures, and in orally intubated critical care clients (Potter and others, 2003).
- Not appropriate for monitoring fever in acutely ill clients or monitoring temperature therapies.
- Chemical dot thermometers may underestimate oral temperature by 0.4° C or more in 50% of adults (Potter and others, 2003).
- Easy to store, disposable, and can be used for clients requiring isolation.
- Can be used at axillary or rectal site if covered by a plastic sheath with a placement time of 3 minutes.

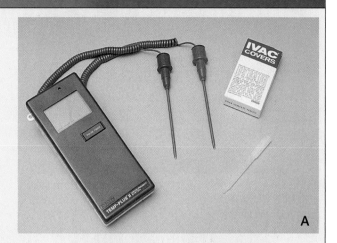

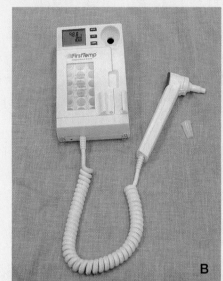

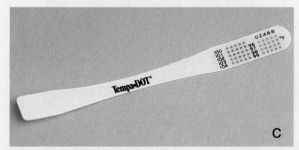

A, Electronic thermometer with disposable plastic sheath. **B,** Electronic tympanic membrane thermometer. **C,** Chemical dot disposable single-use thermometer.

stethoscope (see Chapter 12). Familiarity and practice using a stethoscope improve assessment skills (Box 11-3). The stethoscope magnifies the sounds as they are transmitted from the chest wall, through the tubing, to the listener. In adults, the apical pulse is auscultated (heard with a stethoscope) by placing the diaphragm over the point of maximum impulse at the fifth intercostal space on the left midclavicular line (Figure 11-3).

RESPIRATIONS

Movement of air between the environment and the lungs involves three interrelated processes. Ventilation is the mechanical movement of air in and out of the lungs. Diffusion involves the movement of respiratory gases (oxygen and carbon dioxide) between the alveoli and red blood cells (RBCs). Perfusion involves distribution of blood through the pulmonary capillaries.

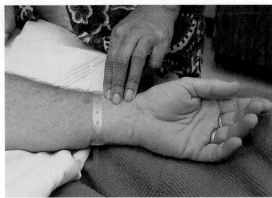

FIGURE 11-1 Palpating the right radial pulse. (From Sorrentino S, Gorek B: *Basic skills for nursing assistants in long-term care,* St Louis, 2005, Mosby.)

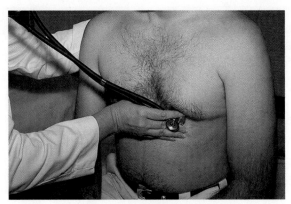

FIGURE 11-2 Assessing apical pulse.

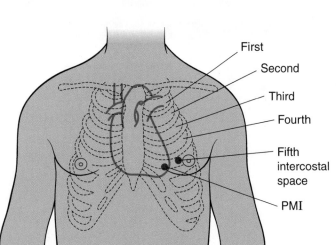

FIGURE 11-3 Point of maximum impulse is at fifth intercostal space.

These three processes are evaluated by observing the rate, depth, and rhythm of respiratory movements. Rate refers to the number of times the person breathes in and out in 1 minute. Depth of respirations is estimated by observing the movement of the chest during inspiration and can be described as deep or shallow. Rhythm of respirations is normally regular; however, irregular respiration patterns may occur (Table 11-3).

Breathing patterns are determined by observing the client's chest or the abdomen. Diaphragmatic breathing results from the contraction and relaxation of the diaphragm and is most visible in the abdomen. Healthy men and children usually demonstrate diaphragmatic breathing (Figure 11-4), whereas women breathe more with the thorax, most apparent in the upper chest. Labored respirations usually involve the accessory muscles of respiration in the neck. The breathing cycle consists of a period of inspiration followed by a period of expiration. When something such as a foreign

body interferes with the movement of air into the lungs, the intercostal spaces retract during inspiration. A longer expiration phase is evident when the outward flow of air is obstructed (e.g., asthma). If a client is experiencing dyspnea, a subjective experience of inadequate or difficult breathing, lung sounds should be auscultated. Dyspnea is associated with increased effort to inhale and exhale and active use of intercostal and accessory muscles. Orthopnea is difficulty breathing while lying flat and is relieved by sitting or standing. Lung sounds are assessed if the client has excessive secretions, complains of chest pain, or has sustained trauma to the chest (see Chapter 12).

BLOOD PRESSURE

Blood pressure is the force exerted by the blood against the arterial walls. The systolic blood pressure is the peak pressure occurring during the heart's contraction as blood is forced under high pressure into the aorta. The diastolic blood pressure is the pressure present when the ventricles are relaxed and there is minimal pressure exerted against the arterial wall. The pulse pressure is the difference between the systolic and diastolic pressure; for a blood pressure of 120/80, the pulse pressure is 40.

Blood pressure reflects many factors within the circulatory system, including cardiac output, peripheral resistance, blood volume, blood viscosity, and vessel wall elasticity. For example, a decreased cardiac output related to congestive heart failure (CHF) or a low blood volume related to dehydration results in a low blood pressure. An increase in peripheral resistance related to stress or arteriosclerosis (loss of elasticity of the vessel walls) results in a high blood pressure. Drug therapy can decrease or increase blood pressure by acting on any one or all of the factors regulating the circulatory system.

A diagnosis of prehypertension in nonpregnant adults is made when an average of two or more diastolic readings on at least two subsequent visits is 80 to 89 mm Hg (Joint National Committee, 2003) (Table 11-4). One blood pressure

Labels in Figure 11-3
First
Second
Third
Fourth
Fifth intercostal space
PMI

Box 11-3 Learning to Use a Stethoscope

1 Place earpieces in both ears with tips of earpieces turned toward the face. Lightly blow against the diaphragm (flat side of chestpiece). Now place the earpieces in both ears with the tips turned toward the back of the head, and again blow against the diaphragm. Compare comfort in the ears and amplification of sounds with earpieces in both directions. Most people find pointing earpieces toward the face more comfortable and effective.

2 If the stethoscope has both a diaphragm (flat side) and a bell (bowl shaped with a rubber ring) (see illustration A), put earpieces in ears and lightly blow against the diaphragm. The chestpiece can be turned to allow sound to be carried through either side (bell or diaphragm) of the chestpiece. If sound is faint, lightly blow into the bell. Then turn the chestpiece, and blow again against both the diaphragm and the bell. The diaphragm is used for higher-pitched heart sounds, bowel sounds, and lung sounds (see illustration B). The bell is used for lower-pitched heart sounds and vascular sounds (see illustration C).

3 With earpieces in place and using the diaphragm, move the diaphragm lightly over the hair on your arm. The bristling sound mimics a sound heard in the lungs. When listening for significant sounds hold the diaphragm firmly and still, eliminating extraneous sounds.

4 Place the diaphragm over the front of your chest directly on your skin, and listen to your own breathing, comparing the bell and the diaphragm. Repeat the process while listening to your heartbeat. Ask someone to speak in a conversational tone, and note how the speech detracts from hearing clearly. When using a stethoscope, both the client and the examiner should remain quiet.

5 With the earpieces in your ears, gently tap the tubing. Note that this also generates extraneous sounds. When listening to a client, maintain a position that allows tubing to extend straight and hang free. Movement may allow tubing to rub or bump objects, creating extraneous sounds. Kinked tubing muffles sounds.

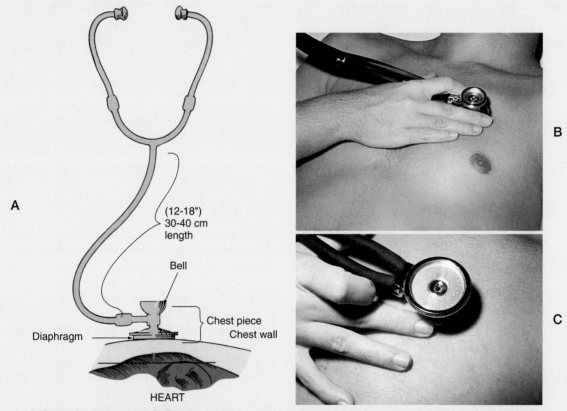

A, Parts of a stethoscope. **B,** The diaphragm is placed firmly and securely when auscultating high-pitched lung and bowel sounds. **C,** The bell must be placed lightly on the skin to hear low-pitched vascular and heart sounds.

recording does not qualify as a diagnosis of hypertension. Prehypertension places clients at high risk for the development of hypertension. In these clients early intervention by adoption of healthy lifestyles reduces the risk for or prevents hypertension. Factors that increase the risk for hypertension include obesity, increased sodium intake, smoking, and lack of exercise.

Two methods are available to determine blood pressure: auscultatory and oscillometric. The auscultatory method detects the sounds of the rush of blood (Korotkoff phases) as blood resumes its flow through the artery. The auscultatory method is performed manually with the use of a sphygmomanometer and a stethoscope or electronically with an auscultatory blood pressure machine. The electronic auscul-

TABLE 11-3 Alterations in Breathing Pattern

ALTERATION	DESCRIPTION
Apnea	Respirations cease for several seconds. Persistent cessation results in respiratory arrest.
Biot's respiration	Respirations are abnormally shallow for two to three breaths followed by irregular period of apnea.
Bradypnea	Rate of breathing is regular but abnormally slow (less than 12 breaths per minute).
Cheyne-Stokes respiration	Respiratory rate and depth are irregular, characterized by alternating periods of apnea and hyperventilation. Respiratory cycle begins with slow, shallow breaths that gradually increase to abnormal rate and depth. The pattern reverses, and breathing slows and becomes shallow, climaxing in apnea before respiration resumes.
Hyperpnea	Respirations are increased in depth. Hyperpnea occurs normally during exercise.
Hyperventilation	Rate and depth of respirations increase. Hypocarbia may occur.
Hypoventilation	Respiratory rate is abnormally low, and depth of ventilation may be depressed. Hypercarbia may occur.
Kussmaul's respiration	Respirations are abnormally deep but regular.
Tachypnea	Rate of breathing is regular but abnormally rapid (greater than 20 breaths per minute).

TABLE 11-4 Classification of Blood Pressure for Adults Age 18 Years and Older

CATEGORY	SYSTOLIC* (mm Hg)		DIASTOLIC* (mm Hg)
Normal	less than 120	or	less than 80
Prehypertension*	120-139	or	80-89
Stage 1 hypertension	140-159	or	90-99
Stage 2 hypertension	160 or greater	or	100 or greater

Modified from Joint National Committee: The seventh report of the Joint National Committee on prevention, detection, evaluation, and treatment of high blood pressure, *JAMA* 289:2560-2571, 2003.

*Based on the average of two or more readings taken at each of two or more visits after an initial screening. Client not taking antihypertensive drugs and not acutely ill. When systolic and diastolic blood pressures fall into different categories, the higher category should be selected to classify the individual's blood pressure status. For example, 160/92 mm Hg should be classified as Stage 2 hypertension.

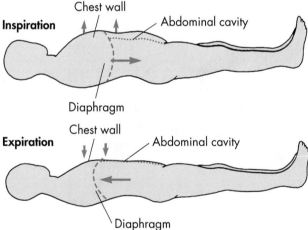

FIGURE 11-4 Illustration of a diaphragmatic and chest wall movement during inspiration and expiration.

tatory blood pressure machine uses a microphone to detect the Korotkoff phases.

A sphygmomanometer includes a pressure manometer, an occlusive cloth or vinyl cuff that encloses an inflatable rubber bladder, and a pressure bulb with a release valve that inflates the bladder. It can be portable or wall mounted. The manometer has a glass-enclosed circular gauge containing a needle that registers millimeter calibrations. The needle of the gauge should point to zero when not in use and move freely when the cuff pressure is released. The metal parts of the gauge are subject to temperature expansion and contraction; routine maintenance for calibration is required.

The cloth or disposable vinyl compression cuff of the sphygmomanometer contains an inflatable bladder. The cuff is placed around the arm or thigh. Cuffs come in several different sizes, and the blood pressure measurement is not accurate unless the correct size blood pressure cuff is used (Figure 11-5). Many adults require a large cuff. The bladder, enclosed by the cuff, should encircle at least 80% of the arm of an adult; the cuff width should be at least 40% greater than the arm circumference (Pickering and others, 2005). The cuff is quickly inflated until blood flow ceases. The cuff is slowly deflated while the needle begins to fall. Korotkoff phases are auscultated by placing the stethoscope over the artery distal to the blood pressure cuff. In some clients, the sounds are clear and distinct, whereas in others, only the beginning and ending sounds are heard (Figure 11-6). The blood pressure is recorded with the systolic and diastolic numbers written as a fraction. The systolic pressure is the first heart sound. Before the sounds cease, they may become distinctly muffled (second sound). The diastolic pressure is the last sound heard. In adults the systolic and diastolic blood pressure readings

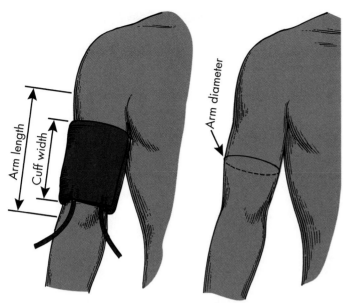

FIGURE 11-5 Proper cuff size: Length of bladder is 80% of arm circumference; cuff width is at least 40% larger than arm diameter.

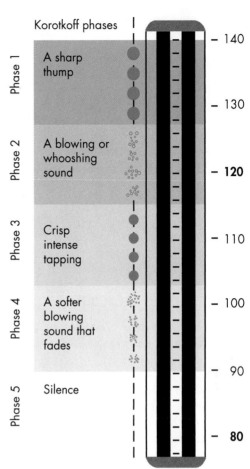

Korotkoff phases		
Phase 1	A sharp thump	— 140 — 130
Phase 2	A blowing or whooshing sound	**120**
Phase 3	Crisp intense tapping	— 110
Phase 4	A softer blowing sound that fades	— 100 — 90
Phase 5	Silence	— **80**

FIGURE 11-6 Sounds auscultated during blood pressure measurement can be differentiated into five Korotkoff phases. In this example the blood pressure is 140/90.

are identified and recorded by the pressures corresponding to the first of two consecutive sounds heard and the disappearance of sounds (not muffling), respectively. Confirm the last sounds by continuing to listen for 10 to 20 mm Hg below the last sound heard. The nurse promotes accuracy in measurement by being aware of the various factors that influence accurate blood pressure values when a stethoscope and sphygmomanometer are used (Table 11-5).

Many different styles of auscultatory and oscillometric electronic blood pressure machines are available to determine blood pressure automatically (Figure 11-7). The oscillometric method of obtaining blood pressure relies on an electronic sensor to detect the vibrations caused by the rush of blood through the artery. When the cuff is deflated, some oscillometric blood pressure machines determine the initial burst of oscillations and translate the information into a systolic pressure reading. The diastolic measurement is made when the oscillations are lowest, just before they stop. Other oscillometric blood pressure machines record the mean blood pressure and compute systolic and diastolic blood pressure from a programmed formula.

Electronic blood pressure machines are used when frequent blood pressure assessment is required, such as in critically ill or potentially unstable clients, during or after invasive procedures, or when therapies require frequent monitoring (e.g., trials of new drugs). Electronic blood pressure machines can be found in public areas such as shopping malls or in clients' homes. Although electronic blood pressure machines are fast and they free the nurse for other activities, they do have disadvantages (Box 11-4). Auscultatory electronic blood pressure machines are sensitive to external noise and are less precise on clients with obese upper extremities (Jones and others, 2003).

TABLE 11-5 Common Mistakes in Blood Pressure Assessment

ERROR	EFFECT
Bladder or cuff too wide	False-low reading
Bladder or cuff too narrow or too short	False-high reading
Cuff wrapped too loosely or unevenly	False-high reading
Deflating cuff too slowly	False-high diastolic reading
Deflating cuff too quickly	False-low systolic and false-high diastolic reading
Arm below heart level	False-high reading
Arm above heart level	False-low reading
Arm not supported	False-high reading
Stethoscope that fits poorly or impairment of the examiner's hearing, causing sounds to be muffled	False-low systolic and false-high diastolic reading
Stethoscope applied too firmly against antecubital fossa	False-low diastolic reading
Inflating too slowly	False-high diastolic reading
Repeating assessments too quickly	False-high systolic reading
Inaccurate inflation level	False-low systolic reading
Multiple examiners using different Korotkoff sounds for diastolic readings	False-high systolic and false-low diastolic reading

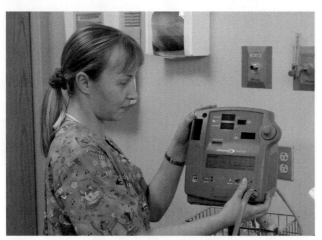

FIGURE 11-7 Electronic blood pressure machines vary in appearance.

EVIDENCE IN PRACTICE

Armstrong RS: Nurses' knowledge of error in blood pressure measurement technique, *Int J Nurs Pract* 8:118-126, 2002.

Confidence in their blood pressure measurement technique was reported by over 88% of the acute care nurses surveyed in this study. Despite confidence, 71% correct was the highest score for any other survey question. Only 14% of the nurses knew that incorrect arm positions can significantly affect blood pressure measurement. The results of this study suggest that ongoing education is necessary to maintain skills and knowledge. Critical areas of potential error should be reviewed routinely: cuff selection, extremity positioning, inflation/deflation rate, rounding off, and detection of Korotkoff sounds.

NURSING DIAGNOSES

Hyperthermia is the nursing diagnosis when a client's body temperature is above the upper range of normal (over 38° C or 100.4° F). Conversely, **hypothermia** is the nursing diagnosis for a body temperature below the lower value of 36° C (96.8° F). **Risk for imbalanced body temperature** is an appropriate nursing diagnosis for a client who demonstrates risk factors for hypothermia or hyperthermia because the client is unable to maintain a body temperature within a normal range. Clients at risk include those at the extremes

BOX 11-4 Advantages and Limitations of Electronic Blood Pressure Measurement

Advantages
- Ease of use
- Ability to use a stethoscope not required
- Efficient when frequent repeated measurements are indicated
- Allows blood pressure to be measured frequently, as often as every 15 seconds, with accuracy
- Not sensitive to outside noise (oscillometric device)

Limitations
- Expensive
- Requires source of electricity and space to position machine
- Sensitive to outside motion interference and cannot be used in clients with seizures, tremors, or shivers
- Not accurate for clients with irregular heart rate or hypotension (blood pressure less than 90 mm Hg systolic), or in situations of reduced blood flow
- Accuracy standards for electronic blood pressure manufacturers are voluntary (Jones and others, 2003)
- Vulnerable to error among older adult and obese clients (Jones and others, 2003)

of age (older adults and the young) and the extremes in weight (obese and malnourished) and those with exposure to environmental extremes.

Decreased cardiac output is manifested by decreased blood pressure, decreased or irregular peripheral pulses, and/or difficulty breathing. Decreased cardiac output to meet body demands increases the **risk for activity intolerance,** which should be considered when an individual has insufficient energy to endure or complete required or desired daily activities.

Ineffective airway clearance is appropriate for clients who are unable to clear secretions or obstructions and maintain airway patency. **Ineffective breathing pattern** is appropriate when the client's rate, depth, and rhythm of respirations or chest and abdominal movements are not adequate for gas exchange to occur. **Impaired gas exchange** refers to altered oxygen or carbon dioxide exchange in the lungs or at the cellular level. The lowered oxygen level is assessed by observing any circumoral, nail bed, or mucous membrane cyanosis; tachycardia; dizziness; and mental confusion.

SKILL 11.1 Assessing Temperature, Pulse, Respirations, and Blood Pressure

- **Nursing Skills Online: Vital Signs, Lessons 3 and 4**

The nurse routinely obtains a baseline measurement of vital signs at initial contact with a client to provide a means for comparison with subsequent vital sign values. This skill routinely includes temperature measurement with an electronic thermometer using the oral, tympanic, rectal, or axillary sites; palpating the radial pulse; and auscultating an upper extremity blood pressure.

ASSESSMENT

1 Consider normal daily fluctuations in vital signs. *Rationale: Body temperature tends to be lowest in early morning, peak in late afternoon, and gradually decline during the night. When temperatures are taken between 5 PM and 7 PM, fever is more accurately assessed. Blood pressure varies throughout the day, with lower blood pressure during sleep, highest blood pressure in the afternoon, a decrease in evening, and an increase beginning at 4 AM to 6 AM. Blood pressure can drop 10% to 20% during nighttime sleep (Joint National Committee, 2003).*

2 Identify client's medications or treatments that may influence vital signs. *Rationale: Antiarrhythmics, cardiotonics, antihypertensives, vasodilators, and vasoconstrictors affect blood pressure and pulse rate. Antiinflammatory drugs, steroids, warming or cooling blankets, and fans affect temperature. Oxygen and bronchodilators affect respiratory assessment.*

3 Identify factors affecting the client that influence vital signs. *Rationale: Exercise increases metabolism and heat production, resulting in increased temperature, pulse, respirations, and blood pressure. Vital signs also tend to increase through hormonal and neural stimulation related to anxiety and pain. Anxiety raises blood pressure as much as 30 mm Hg.*

4 Identify factors likely to interfere with accuracy of vital signs. *Rationale: Smoking and intake of hot or cold food and fluid affect oral temperature. Caffeine and nicotine increase pulse rate. Coffee increases blood pressure within 15 minutes and can last as long as 3 hours (Joint National Committee, 2003). Blood pressure and pulse rate are immediately increased by smoking, which lasts as long as 15 minutes (Joint National Committee, 2003). Talking to a client when blood pressure is being assessed increases readings 10% to 40% (Thomas and others, 2002).*

5 Identify clinical conditions that influence blood pressure. *Rationale: High blood pressure is associated with rapid intravenous (IV) infusion of fluids or blood products, increased intracranial pressure (IICP), cardiovascular disease, and renal disease. Low blood pressure is associated with rapid vasodilation, shock, hemorrhage, and dehydration.*

6 Assess pertinent laboratory values, including complete blood count (CBC) and arterial blood gases (ABGs). *Rationale: Low values for hemoglobin, hematocrit (Hct), and RBC count are associated with decreased oxygen transport to tissues and hypoxia. ABG levels reflect adequacy of oxygenation and ventilation. Low hemoglobin levels, decreased oxygenation, and decreased ventilation can increase pulse rate, blood pressure readings, and respiratory rate. A white blood cell (WBC) count greater than 12,000/mm3 in a nonpregnant adult suggests the presence of infection, which can lead to hyperthermia; a WBC count less than 5000/mm3 suggests that the body's ability to fight infection is compromised, which can lead to ineffective thermoregulation.*

7 Determine previous baseline vital signs from client's record. *Rationale: Allows the nurse to assess for change in condition by comparing future vital sign measurements.*

8 Determine appropriate temperature site for client, considering advantages and disadvantages of each site (see Table 11-2).

9 Determine blood pressure device most appropriate for client. *Rationale: Electronic blood pressure device can be used when frequent measurements are required.*

PLANNING

Expected Outcomes focus on identifying abnormalities and restoring homeostasis.

1 Client's vital signs are within normal range for client's age group.

2 Client identifies factors that influence vital signs.

3 A baseline is established for clients with chronic diseases that alter vital signs, such as arteriosclerosis.

4 Client states strategies to reduce personal risk factors for hypertension.

Delegation Considerations

The skill of vital sign measurements for stable clients may be delegated. The nurse directs personnel by:

- Explaining any precautions needed in positioning client during vital sign measurements, the appropriate route or limb and type of device for assigned client to measure vital signs, and frequency of specific vital sign measurements
- Reviewing usual vital sign values of client and significant changes or abnormalities to report to the nurse

Equipment

- Thermometer (select based on site used; see Table 11-2)
- Disposable probe covers
- Water-soluble lubricant (for rectal measurements only)
- Stethoscope
- Sphygmomanometer
- Blood pressure cuff of appropriate size
- Alcohol swab
- Watch that displays seconds
- Vital signs flow sheet

IMPLEMENTATION *for Assessing Temperature, Pulse, Respirations, and Blood Pressure*

STEPS	RATIONALE
1 See Standard Protocol (inside front cover).	
2 Assist client to comfortable position either lying or sitting. When obtaining blood pressure, avoid injured arm or arm with IV infusion, previous breast or axilla surgery, cast, or arteriovenous (AV) shunt for renal dialysis.	Good circulation facilitates accuracy in blood pressure measurement. Blood pressure measurement temporarily disrupts circulation.

STEPS	RATIONALE

3 Assess oral temperature (electronic):

a. Remove thermometer pack from charging unit; attach oral (blue tip) probe stem to thermometer unit. Grasp top of probe stem, being careful not to apply pressure on the ejection button. Slide disposable plastic probe cover over thermometer probe stem until cover locks in place (see illustration).

Charging provides battery power. Ejection button releases plastic cover from probe stem. Probe cover prevents transmission of microorganisms between clients.

b. Ask client to open mouth; then gently place thermometer probe under tongue in posterior sublingual pocket lateral to center of lower jaw (see illustration). Ask client to hold thermometer probe with lips closed.

Heat from superficial blood vessels in sublingual pocket produces temperature reading. With electronic thermometer, temperatures in right and left posterior sublingual pockets are significantly higher than in area under front of tongue.

c. Leave thermometer probe in place until audible signal indicates completion and client's temperature appears on digital display; remove thermometer probe from under client's tongue. Inform client of temperature reading, and record measurement.

Probe must stay in place until signal occurs to ensure accurate reading.

d. Push ejection button on thermometer probe stem to discard probe cover into an appropriate receptacle. Return thermometer stem to storage position of thermometer unit. Return thermometer to charger.

Returning thermometer probe stem automatically causes digital reading to disappear. Storage position protects stem. Charger maintains battery charge of unit.

4 Assess tympanic temperature:

a. Assist client in assuming a comfortable position with head turned toward side, away from nurse. If client lies on one side, use upper ear. Note if there is an obvious presence of earwax in client's ear canal.

Ensures comfort and facilitates visualization of the ear canal. Heat trapped in lower ear will cause false-high temperature reading. Lens cover of speculum must not be impeded by earwax, which can obstruct optical pathway.

b. Remove thermometer handheld unit from charging base, being careful not to apply pressure to ejection button. Slide disposable speculum cover over otoscope-like tip until it locks in place. Be careful not to touch lens cover.

Ejection button releases disposable probe cover from thermometer tip. Soft disposable speculum cover prevents transmission of microorganisms between clients. Dust or fingerprints on lens can obstruct optical pathway.

c. If holding handheld unit with right hand, obtain temperature from client's right ear; left-handed persons should obtain temperature from client's left ear.

The less acute angle of approach the better the probe will seal inside the auditory canal.

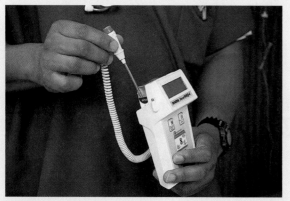

STEP 3a. Inserting thermometer stem into plastic probe cover.

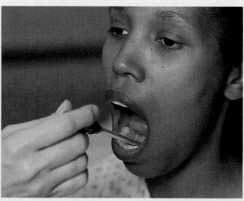

STEP 3b. Probe under tongue in posterior sublingual pocket.

STEPS	RATIONALE

d. Insert speculum into ear canal following manufacturer's instructions for tympanic probe positioning.

  (1) Pull ear pinna backward, up, and out for an adult.

  (2) Move thermometer in figure-eight pattern.

  (3) Fit speculum tip snug in ear canal and do not move.

  (4) Point speculum tip toward nose.

Note an obvious presence of earwax in the client's ear canal; if present, switch to other ear or choose alternative site.

Correct positioning of probe with respect to ear canal allows maximum exposure of the tympanic membrane. The ear tug straightens the external auditory canal, allowing maximum exposure of tympanic membrane. Some manufacturers recommend moving the speculum tip in a figure-eight pattern that allows the sensor to detect maximum tympanic membrane heat radiation. Gentle pressure seals the ear canal from ambient air temperature, which can alter readings as much as 2.8° C or 5° F.

e. As soon as the probe is in place, depress scan button on handheld unit. Leave thermometer probe in place until audible signal occurs and client's temperature appears on digital display (see illustration).

Signal indicates infrared energy has been detected.

f. Carefully remove speculum from auditory meatus. Push ejection button on thermometer stem to discard speculum cover into appropriate receptacle.

g. If temperature is abnormal, repeat measurement in other ear, or wait 2 to 3 minutes to repeat in same ear. Consider an alternative site or instrument.

Time allows ear canal to regain usual temperature.

h. Inform client of temperature reading. Return handheld unit to charging base.

Returning handheld unit to charging base will cause digital reading to disappear and protect sensor tip from damage.

5 Assess rectal temperature (electronic):

a. Draw curtain around bed and/or close room door. Assist client to side-lying Sims' position with upper leg flexed. Move aside bed linen to expose only anal area. Keep client's upper body and lower extremities covered with sheet or blanket.

Maintains client's privacy, minimizes embarrassment, and promotes comfort.

b. Remove thermometer pack from charging unit, and attach rectal thermometer probe stem (red tip) to thermometer unit. Grasp top of probe stem, being careful not to apply pressure on ejection button. Slide disposable plastic probe cover over thermometer probe stem until cover locks in place.

Ejection button releases plastic cover from probe. Probe cover prevents transmission of microorganisms between clients.

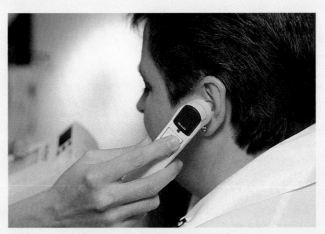

STEP 4e. Tympanic membrane thermometer with probe cover positioned in client's ear.

STEPS	RATIONALE

c. Squeeze liberal portion of lubricant on tissue. Dip thermometer probe end into lubricant, covering 2.5 to 3.5 cm (1 to 1½ inches) for adult.

Lubrication minimizes trauma to rectal mucosa during insertion. Tissue avoids contamination of remaining lubricant in container.

d. With nondominant hand, separate client's buttocks to expose anus. Ask client to breathe slowly and relax.

Fully exposes anus for thermometer insertion. Relaxes anal sphincter for easier thermometer insertion.

e. Gently insert thermometer into anus in direction of umbilicus 3.5 cm (1½ inches) for adult. Do not force thermometer.

Ensure adequate exposure against blood vessels in rectal area.

> **NURSE ALERT** If thermometer cannot be adequately inserted into rectum, or resistance is felt during insertion, remove thermometer and consider an alternative method for obtaining temperature.

f. When positioned, hold thermometer probe in place until audible signal indicates completion and client's temperature appears on digital display; remove thermometer probe from anus.

Probe must stay in place until signal occurs to ensure accurate reading.

g. Push ejection button on thermometer probe stem to discard probe cover into appropriate receptacle. Inform client of temperature measurement. Return thermometer stem to storage position of thermometer unit. Return thermometer base to charge.

Returning thermometer probe stem automatically causes digital reading to disappear. Storage position protects stem. Charger maintains battery charge of unit.

h. Wipe client's anal area with soft tissue to remove lubricant or feces, and discard tissue. Remove and dispose of gloves in appropriate receptacle.

6 **Assess axillary temperature (electronic):**

a. Draw curtain around bed and/or close room door. Assist client to supine or sitting position. Move clothing or gown away from shoulder and arm.

Maintains client's privacy, minimizes embarrassment, and promotes comfort. Exposes axilla for correct thermometer probe placement.

b. Remove thermometer pack from charging unit. Attach oral thermometer probe stem (blue tip) to thermometer unit. Grasp top of thermometer probe stem, being careful not to apply pressure on ejection button. Slide disposable plastic probe stem cover over thermometer stem until cover locks in place.

Ejection button releases plastic cover from probe.

c. Raise client's arm away from torso and inspect for skin lesions and excessive perspiration; dry area if needed. Insert thermometer probe into center of axilla, lower arm over thermometer, and place arm across client's chest (see illustrations).

Maintains proper placement of thermometer against blood vessels in axilla.

> **NURSE ALERT** In an infant or young child it may be necessary to hold the arm against the child's side when using the axillary method. If infant is in a side-lying position, the lower axilla will record the higher temperature.

> **NURSE ALERT** Do not use axilla if skin lesions are present because local temperature may be altered and area may be painful to touch.

d. When positioned, hold thermometer probe in place until audible signal indicates completion and client's temperature appears on digital display; remove thermometer probe from axilla. Inform client of temperature reading, and record measurement.

Thermometer probe must stay in place until signal occurs to ensure accurate reading.

STEPS	RATIONALE
e. Push ejection button on thermometer probe stem to discard probe cover into appropriate receptacle. Return thermometer probe stem to storage position of thermometer unit. Return thermometer to charger.	Returning thermometer stem automatically causes digital reading to disappear. Maintains battery charge.
7 Assess pulse:	
a. If client is supine, place client's forearm straight alongside or across lower chest or upper abdomen with wrist extended straight (see illustration). If sitting, bend client's elbow 90 degrees and support lower arm on chair or on nurse's arm.	Relaxed position of lower arm permits full exposure of artery to palpation.
b. Place tips of first two or middle three fingers of hand over groove along radial or thumb side of client's wrist (see illustration). Slightly extend or flex client's wrist with palm down until strongest pulse is noted.	Fingertips are most sensitive parts of hand to palpate arterial pulsation. Nurse's thumb has pulsation that may interfere with accuracy.

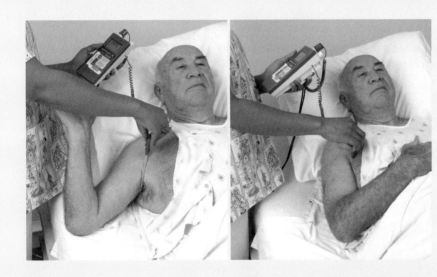

STEP 6c. Thermometer placed in axilla.

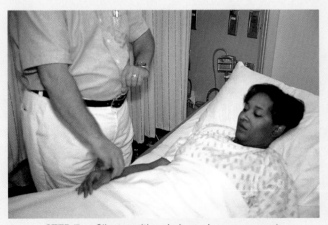

STEP 7a. Client position during pulse assessment.

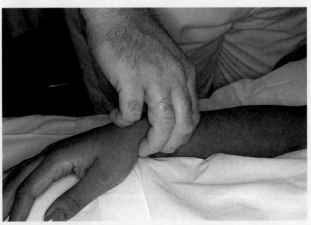

STEP 7b. Hand placement for pulse assessment.

STEPS	RATIONALE
c. Lightly compress against radius, obliterate pulse initially, then relax pressure so pulse becomes easily palpable.	Pulse is more accurately assessed with moderate pressure. Too much pressure can impede blood flow and impair pulse.
d. Determine strength of pulse. Note whether thrust of vessel against fingertips is bounding, strong, weak, or thready.	Strength reflects volume of blood ejected against arterial wall with each heart contraction.
e. After pulse can be felt regularly, look at watch's second hand and begin to count rate; when sweep hand hits number on dial, start counting with zero, then one, two, and so on.	Rate is determined accurately only after nurse is assured pulse can be palpated. Timing begins with zero. Count of one is first beat palpated after timing.
If pulse is regular, count rate for 30 seconds and multiply total by 2.	It requires 30 seconds to determine if the pulse is regular in rhythm.
If pulse is irregular, count rate for 60 seconds. Assess frequency and pattern of irregularity and compare radial pulses bilaterally.	Inefficient contraction of heart fails to transmit pulse wave, interfering with cardiac output, resulting in irregular pulse. Longer time period ensures more accurate count. A marked difference between radial pulses may indicate arterial flow is compromised in one extremity and action should be taken immediately.

> **NURSE ALERT** If pulse is irregular, assess for a pulse deficit. Count apical pulse (see Chapter 12) while colleague counts radial pulse. Begin apical pulse, initiating counting by a signal to simultaneously assess pulses for a full minute. If pulse count differs by more than 2 beats per minute, a pulse deficit exists, which may indicate alteration in cardiac output.

8 Assess respirations:	
a. Without changing the position of your hand on the pulse, observe one complete respiratory cycle (one inspiration and one expiration) (see illustration).	Maintaining the same position keeps client from being aware that you are counting respirations. Inconspicuous assessment prevents client from consciously or unintentionally altering rate and depth of breathing. Viewing an entire respiratory cycle promotes accurate measurement.
b. After cycle is observed, look at watch's second hand and begin to count rate; when sweep hand hits number on dial, begin time frame, counting one with first full respiratory cycle.	Timing begins with count of one. Respirations occur more slowly than pulse; thus timing does not begin with zero.

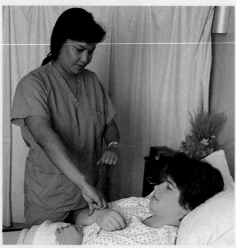

STEP 8a. Assessing respirations after pulse count.

STEPS	RATIONALE

c. If rhythm is regular, count number of respirations in 30 seconds and multiply by 2. If rhythm is irregular, less than 12 respirations per minute, or greater than 16 respirations per minute, count for 1 full minute.

Respiratory rate is equivalent to number of respirations per minute. Suspected irregularities require assessment for at least 1 minute (see Table 11-3).

d. Note depth of respirations by observing degree of chest wall movement while counting rate. Obtain a more objective assessment of depth by palpating chest wall or auscultating the posterior chest during respiratory excursion (see Chapter 12) after rate is counted. Depth is shallow, normal, or deep.

Character of ventilatory movement may reveal specific disease state, restricting volume of air from moving into and out of the lungs.

> **NURSE ALERT** Position of discomfort may cause client to breathe more rapidly. Respiratory rate less than 12 breaths per minute or greater than 16 breaths per minute and shallow and slow respirations (hypoventilation) may require immediate intervention.

e. Note rhythm of ventilatory cycle. Normal breathing is regular and uninterrupted. Sighing should not be confused with abnormal rhythm. Periodically people unconsciously take single deep breaths or sighs to expand small airways prone to collapse.

Character of ventilations can reveal specific types of alterations.

f. Observe for evidence of dyspnea (increased effort to inhale and exhale). Ask client to describe subjective experience of shortness of breath compared with usual breathing pattern.

Clients with chronic lung disease may experience difficulty breathing all the time and can best describe their own discomfort from shortness of breath.

> **NURSE ALERT** Occasional periods of apnea are a symptom of underlying disease in the adult and must be reported to the physician or nurse in charge. Irregular respirations and short episodes of apnea are normal in a newborn.

9 Manually auscultate upper extremity blood pressure:

a. Determine the best site for blood pressure assessment. Avoid applying cuff to extremity when IV fluids are being infused; when an AV shunt or fistula is present; when breast or axillary surgery has been performed on that side; or when extremity has been traumatized, diseased, or requires a cast or bulky bandage. The lower extremities may be used when the brachial arteries are inaccessible (see Procedural Guideline 11-1).

Inappropriate site selection may result in poor amplification of sounds, causing inaccurate readings. Application of pressure from inflated bladder temporarily impairs blood flow and can further compromise circulation in extremity that already has impaired blood flow.

b. Select appropriate cuff size (see Figure 11-5).

Use of improper size cuff can cause false-high or false-low readings (see Table 11-5). If cuff is too small, it tends to come loose as it is inflated.

c. Expose upper arm by removing restrictive clothing.

Ensures proper cuff application. Tight clothing causes congestion of blood and can falsely elevate blood pressure readings.

d. With client sitting or lying, position client's forearm at heart level, supported if needed with palm turned up (see illustration). If sitting, client should be instructed to keep feet flat on floor without legs crossed.

If arm is extended and not supported, client may perform isometric exercise that can increase diastolic pressure 10%. Placement of arm above the level of the heart causes false-low readings. Placement of arm lower than the level of the heart causes false-high readings. Even in the supine position a diastolic increase of as much as 3 to 4 mm Hg can occur for each 5 cm the arm is below the level of the heart (Netea and others, 2003).

STEPS	RATIONALE

> **NURSE ALERT** Client should be seated or lying in a quiet environment, free from temperature extremes, for at least 5 minutes before blood pressure is obtained. Eliminate extraneous noise, such as television and conversation. Noise interferes with accuracy. Falsely elevated readings will be obtained if client moves, talks, or coughs during blood pressure measurement (Joint National Committee, 2003).

e. Palpate brachial artery (see illustration).

f. Position cuff 2.5 cm (1 inch) above site of brachial pulsation (antecubital space). Apply bladder of cuff above artery by centering arrows marked on cuff over artery. If there are not any center arrows on cuff, estimate the center of the bladder and place this point over artery. With cuff fully deflated, wrap cuff evenly and snugly around upper arm (see illustration).

Inflating bladder directly over brachial artery ensures proper pressure is applied during inflation. Loose fitting cuff causes false-high readings.

g. Position manometer gauge vertically at eye level. Observer should be no farther than 1 m (approximately 1 yard) away.

Looking up or down at gauge can result in distorted readings.

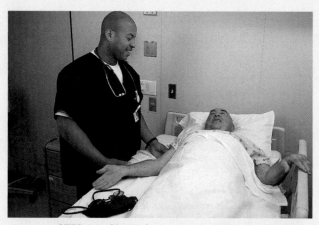

STEP 9d. Client's forearm supported in bed.

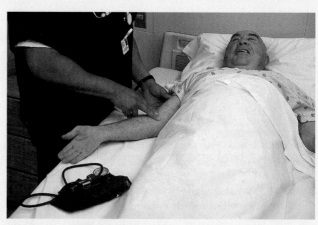

STEP 9e. Palpating the brachial artery.

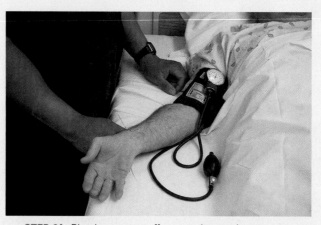

STEP 9f. Blood pressure cuff wrapped around upper arm.

STEPS	RATIONALE

h. Measure blood pressure.

(1) Two-Step Method:

(a) Relocate brachial pulse. Palpate artery distal to the cuff with fingertips of nondominant hand while inflating cuff. Note point at which pulse disappears and continue to inflate cuff to a pressure 30 mm Hg above that point. Note the pressure reading. Slowly deflate cuff, and note point when pulse reappears. Deflate cuff fully and wait 30 seconds.

Estimating systolic pressure prevents false-low readings, which may result from the presence of an auscultatory gap (inaudible sounds below the actual systolic pressure). Palpation determines maximal inflation point for accurate reading. If unable to palpate artery because of weakened pulse, use ultrasonic stethoscope (see Chapter 12). Completely deflating cuff prevents venous congestion and false-high readings.

(b) Place stethoscope earpieces in ears, and be sure sounds are clear, not muffled.

Ensures earpiece follows angle of ear canal to facilitate hearing.

(c) Relocate brachial artery, and place bell or diaphragm of stethoscope over it. Do not allow chestpiece to touch cuff or clothing (see illustration).

Proper stethoscope placement ensures the best sound reception. The bell provides better sound reproduction. The diaphragm is easier to secure with fingers and covers a larger area. Stethoscope improperly positioned causes muffled sounds that often result in false-low and false-high diastolic readings.

(d) Close valve of pressure bulb clockwise until tight.

Tight closure prevents air leak during inflation.

(e) Quickly inflate cuff to 30 mm Hg above palpated systolic pressure (see illustration).

Rapid inflation ensures accurate measure of systolic pressure.

(f) Slowly release pressure bulb valve, and allow needle to fall at rate of 2 to 3 mm Hg/sec. Make sure there are no extraneous sounds.

Too rapid or slow a decline in pressure can cause inaccurate readings. Noise interferes with precise hearing of Korotkoff phases.

NURSE ALERT If you hear sounds immediately, release the pressure, wait 60 seconds, and estimate systolic pressure at higher reading. Reinflate the cuff to 30 mm Hg above the sound first heard. Reinflation of a partially deflated cuff is uncomfortable for client and may render an inaccurate reading.

(g) Note point on manometer when first clear sound is heard. The sounds will slowly increase in intensity.

First Korotkoff phase reflects systolic blood pressure.

(h) Continue to deflate cuff gradually, noting point at which sound disappears in adults. Note pressure to nearest 2 mm Hg. Listen for 10 to 20 mm Hg after the last sound, and then allow remaining air to escape quickly.

Beginning of the fifth Korotkoff phase is an indication of diastolic pressure in adults (Joint National Committee, 2003). The fourth Korotkoff phase involves distinct muffling of sounds, and in children it is recorded as the diastolic pressure (Joint National Committee, 2003).

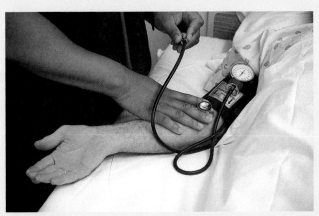

STEP 9h.(1)(c) Stethoscope over brachial artery to measure blood pressure.

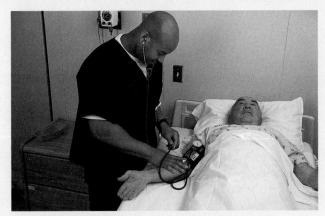

STEP 9h.(1)(e) Inflating the blood pressure cuff.

STEPS	RATIONALE

(2) One-Step Method:
  (a) Place stethoscope earpieces in ears, and be sure sounds are clear, not muffled.
  (b) Relocate brachial artery, and place diaphragm of stethoscope over it. Do not allow chest-piece to touch cuff or clothing.
  (c) Close valve of pressure bulb clockwise until tight.
  (d) Quickly inflate cuff to 30 mm Hg above client's usual systolic pressure.
  (e) Slowly release pressure bulb valve, and allow manometer needle to fall at rate of 2 to 3 mm Hg/sec. Note point on manometer when you hear the first sound. The sound will slowly increase in intensity.
  (f) Continue to deflate cuff gradually, noting point at which sound disappears in adults. Note pressure to nearest 2 mm Hg. Listen for 20 to 30 mm Hg after the last sound, and then allow remaining air to escape quickly.
i. The Joint National Committee (2003) recommends the average of two sets of blood pressure measurements, 2 minutes apart. Use the second set of blood pressure measurements as the client's baseline.

j. Remove cuff from client's arm unless measurement must be repeated
k. Inform client of the blood pressure. If possible, discuss risk factors for high blood pressure. If blood pressure is elevated, inquire as to any factors that may have affected blood pressure, including general health, life stress, or diet changes. If client takes blood pressure medication, determine if anything has interfered with prescribed regimen.

Rationale column:

Ensures each earpiece follows angle of ear canal to facilitate hearing.
Proper stethoscope placement ensures optimal reception.

Tightening of valve prevents air leak during inflation.

Inflation above systolic level ensures accurate measures of systolic pressure.
Too rapid or slow a decline in pressure release causes inaccurate readings. The first Korotkoff sounds reflect systolic pressure.

Beginning of the fifth Korotkoff sound is an indicator of diastolic pressure in adults (Joint National Committee, 2003). Fourth Korotkoff sound involves distinct muffling of sounds and is an indication of diastolic pressure in children (Joint National Committee, 2003).
Two sets of blood pressure measurements help prevent false positives based on a client's sympathetic response. Averaging minimizes the effect of anxiety, which often causes a first reading to be higher than subsequent measures (Joint National Committee, 2003).
Continuous cuff inflation causes arterial occlusion, resulting in numbness and tingling of client's arm.

> **COMMUNICATION TIP** This is a good time to discuss with client the benefits of exercise and weight control in reducing the risks for hypertension and coronary artery disease (CAD) or lowering an existing blood pressure elevation.

10 See Completion Protocol (inside front cover).

EVALUATION

1 Compare vital signs with client's baseline and normal expected ranges.
2 Ask client to identify factors that influence vital signs.
3 Identify a baseline for clients with chronic diseases that alter vital signs.
4 Ask client to describe strategies to reduce personal risk factors for hypertension.

Unexpected Outcomes and Related Interventions

1 Client has a temperature 1° C or more above normal range.
a. Assess for additional related data suggesting local or systemic infection, including pain or tenderness; purulent drainage; local area of redness or unusual warmth; loss of appetite; headache; hot, dry skin; flushed face; thirst; general malaise; or chills.

b. Reduce external covering on client's body to promote heat loss. Do not induce shivering.

c. If fever persists or reaches unacceptable level as defined by physician, administer antipyretics and antibiotics as ordered and apply hypothermia blanket.

2 Client has a temperature 1° C or more below normal range.

a. Remove any wet clothes and replace with dry garments; cover client with warm blankets.

b. Close room doors or windows to eliminate drafts.

c. Monitor apical pulse rate and rhythm (see Chapter 12), because hypothermia may cause bradycardia, cardiac arrhythmias, and electrolyte imbalances.

3 Client has a weak, thready, or difficult-to-palpate radial pulse.

a. Assess both radial pulses, and compare findings. Assess for swelling in surrounding tissues or any encumbrance (e.g., dressing, cast) that may impede blood flow.

b. Observe for symptoms associated with altered peripheral tissue perfusion, including pallor or cyanosis of tissue distal to pulse and cold extremities.

4 Client has pulse greater than 100 beats per minute (tachycardia).

a. Auscultate the apical pulse (see Chapter 12).

b. Identify related data (e.g., pain, fear or anxiety, recent exercise, low blood pressure, blood loss).

c. Observe for symptoms associated with abnormal cardiac function, including dyspnea, fatigue, chest pain, orthopnea, syncope, palpitations (unpleasant awareness of pulse), jugular vein distention, edema of dependent body parts, cyanosis, or pallor of skin (see Chapter 12).

5 Client has pulse less than 60 beats per minute (bradycardia).

a. Auscultate the apical pulse (see Chapter 12).

b. Observe for factors that may alter heart rate and regularity, including medications such as cardiotonics and antiarrhythmics; it may be necessary to withhold prescribed medications until the physician can evaluate the need to alter the dosage.

6 Client has irregular rhythm.

a. Auscultate the apical pulse (see Chapter 12), and identify the pattern of irregularity. Assess for a pulse deficit.

b. Clients with an irregular rhythm may require an electrocardiogram (ECG) or 24-hour heart monitor per physician's order to detect heart abnormalities.

7 Client has abnormal respiratory rate, depth, or pattern of dyspnea with complaints of feeling short of breath.

a. Observe for related factors, including obstructed airway; noisy respirations; cyanosis of nail beds, lips, mucous membranes, and skin; restlessness; irritability; confusion; dyspnea (labored breathing); shortness of breath; productive cough; and abnormal breath sounds (see Chapter 12). Consider possible effects of anesthesia or medications such as opioid analgesics.

b. Assist client to a supported sitting position (semi-Fowler's or high-Fowler's unless contraindicated), which improves ability to take a deep breath.

8 Client has blood pressure above acceptable range. NOTE: A diagnosis of hypertension involves two or more elevated readings on separate occasions.

a. Assess blood pressure in other arm and compare findings. Recheck or have another nurse recheck readings in 1 to 2 minutes. Verify correct selection and placement of blood pressure cuff.

b. Observe for related symptoms. Although symptoms may not be apparent unless blood pressure is extremely high, client may have a headache (usually occipital), flushing of face, or nosebleed; older adult client may notice fatigue.

9 Client is hypotensive when blood pressure is not sufficient for adequate perfusion and oxygenation of tissues.

a. Compare to baseline. A systolic reading of 90 mm Hg may be an acceptable value for some persons and cause no ill effects.

b. Observe for symptoms associated with hypotension related to decreased cardiac output, which include tachycardia; weak, thready pulse; weakness, dizziness, or confusion; pale, dusky, or cyanotic skin; or cool, mottled skin over extremities.

10 Client blood pressure is inaudible or difficult to obtain.

a. Determine that no immediate crisis is present by obtaining respiratory rate and pulse rate.

b. Use alternative sites or procedures to obtain blood pressure: Auscultate blood pressure in lower extremity (see Procedural Guideline 11-1), use a Doppler ultrasonic instrument, or implement palpation method to obtain systolic blood pressure.

Recording and Reporting

• Record vital signs promptly on vital sign flow sheet, computer database, or nurses' notes. Record associated findings and related factors in narrative form in nurses' notes. Record position of client, pulse, and method and site of blood pressure and temperature measurements.

• Record measurements of vital signs after administration of specific therapies in narrative form in nurses' notes.

Sample Documentation

2300 Blood pressure 104/56 right arm, supine, dropping from baseline of 124/72. Radial pulse 112, weak, thready. Respirations 24, regular. Temperature 36.8° C tympanic. Reports dizziness. Skin pale. Denies dyspnea, nausea, or pain. Physician notified. Orders received.

Special Considerations
Pediatric Considerations

• Axillary temperature cannot be relied on to detect fevers in infants and young children.

• Temperature is best taken as the last vital sign with children who cry or become restless.

- Children often have a sinus arrhythmia, which is an irregular heartbeat that speeds up with inspiration and slows down with expiration. Breath holding in a child affects pulse rate.
- Apical or brachial pulse is best site for assessing infant's or young child's heart rate and rhythm.
- Acceptable average respiratory rate for newborns is 35 to 40 breaths per minute; infant (6 months) is 30 to 50 breaths per minute; toddler (2 years) is 25 to 32 breaths per minute; and child is 20 to 30 breaths per minute.
- Blood pressure is not a routine part of assessment in children younger than 3 years. Average width of blood pressure cuff bladder for infant is 2.4 to 3.2 inches; for child, cuff bladder is 4.8 to 5.4 inches.

Geriatric Considerations

- The temperature of older adults is at the lower end of the acceptable temperature range. Temperatures considered within normal range may reflect a fever in an older adult (Sund-Levander and others, 2002).
- A decrease in sweat gland reactivity in the older adult results in higher threshold for sweating at high temperatures, which can lead to hyperthermia.
- Older adults are at high risk for hypothermia because of diminished sensation to cold, abnormal vasoconstrictor responses, and impaired shivering.
- Once elevated, the pulse rate of an older adult takes longer to return to normal resting rate.

- Older adults have a reduced heart rate with exercise because of a decreased responsiveness to catecholamines (Stanley, Blair, and Beare, 2005).
- A change in lung function with aging results in respiratory rates that are generally higher in older adults, with a normal range of 16 to 25 breaths per minute.
- Older adults who have lost upper arm mass, especially the frail elderly, require special attention to selection of smaller blood pressure cuff.
- Skin of older adults is more fragile and susceptible to cuff pressure when blood pressure measurements are frequent. More frequent assessment of skin under cuff or rotation of blood pressure sites is recommended.
- Older adults are instructed to change position slowly and wait after each change to avoid postural hypotension and to prevent injuries.

Home Care Considerations

- Assess family's financial ability to afford a sphygmomanometer for performing blood pressure evaluations on a regular basis.
- Consider an electronic blood pressure cuff with large digital display for home if client or caregiver has hearing or vision difficulties.
- Clients taking certain prescribed cardiotonic or antiarrhythmic medications should learn to assess their own pulse rates to detect side effects of medications.

PROCEDURAL GUIDELINE 11-1

Obtaining Blood Pressure from Lower Extremity by Auscultation

- Nursing Skills Online: Vital Signs, Lesson 5

Delegation Considerations

The skill of obtaining blood pressure from a lower extremity may be delegated. The nurse directs personnel by:
- Explaining how to best position client
- Reviewing client's baseline measure and instructing to report blood pressure findings to the nurse

Equipment

- Stethoscope
- Sphygmomanometer
- Large-leg blood pressure cuff, wide and long enough to allow for larger girth of thigh

Procedural Steps

1 See Standard Protocol (inside front cover).
2 Assist client to prone position to access the popliteal artery. If client is unable to assume prone position, assist client to supine position with knee slightly flexed.
3 Move aside bed linen and any constrictive clothing to ensure proper cuff application.
4 Locate and palpate the popliteal artery just below the thigh in the back of the knee in the popliteal space.

5 Apply blood pressure cuff with the bladder over the posterior aspect of the midthigh, 2.5 cm (1 inch) above popliteal artery (see illustration). Make sure the cuff is wide and long enough to allow for the larger girth of the thigh.
6 Obtain blood pressure using auscultatory method. Systolic pressure in the legs is usually 10 to 40 mm Hg higher than the brachial artery, but the diastolic pressure is the same.
7 See Completion Protocol (inside front cover).

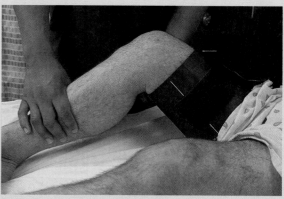

STEP 5 Lower extremity blood pressure cuff positioned above popliteal artery at midthigh.

PROCEDURAL GUIDELINE 11-2
Electronic Blood Pressure Measurement

Delegation Considerations

The use of an electronic blood pressure machine may be delegated unless the client is considered unstable or needs to be closely monitored for evaluating response to medications. The nurse directs personnel by:

- Explaining about frequency of blood pressure measurement, appropriate limb, and cuff size for blood pressure measurement
- Reviewing usual values for client and what to report to the nurse

Equipment

- Electronic blood pressure machine
- Source of electricity
- Blood pressure cuff of appropriate size as recommended by manufacturer

Procedural Steps

1 **See Standard Protocol (inside front cover).**
2 Determine appropriateness of using electronic blood pressure measurement. Clients with irregular heart rates, peripheral vascular disease, seizures, tremors, and shivering are not candidates for this device.
3 Determine best site for cuff placement (see Skill 11.1).
4 Assist client to comfortable position, either lying or sitting. Plug machine into source of electricity. Place electronic blood pressure machine near client, ensuring that the connector hose (between cuff and machine) is adequate.
5 Locate on/off switch and turn machine on to enable device to self-test computer systems.
6 Select appropriate cuff size for client extremity (Table 11-6) and appropriate cuff for machine. Electronic blood pressure cuff and machine must be matched by the manufacturer and cannot be interchanged.
7 Expose extremity by removing restrictive clothing that can cause congestion of blood and distention of vessel walls. Do not place blood pressure cuff over clothing.
8 Prepare blood pressure cuff by manually squeezing all the air out of the cuff and connecting cuff to connector hose.
9 Wrap cuff snugly around extremity, verifying that only one finger can fit between cuff and client's skin. Make sure the "artery" arrow marked on the outside of the cuff is correctly placed (see illustration).
10 Verify that connector hose between cuff and machine is not kinked. Kinking prevents proper inflation and deflation of cuff.
11 Following manufacturer's directions, set the frequency control for automatic or manual, then press the start button. The first blood pressure measurement will pump the cuff to a peak pressure of about 180 mm Hg. After this pressure is reached, the machine

begins a deflation sequence that determines the blood pressure. The first reading determines the peak pressure inflation for additional measurements.

> **NURSE ALERT** If unable to obtain blood pressure with electronic device, verify machine connections (e.g., plugged into working electrical outlet, hose-cuff connections tight, machine on, correct cuff). Repeat electronic measurement. If still unable to obtain blood pressure, use auscultatory technique (see Skill 11.1).

12 When deflation is complete, digital display will provide most recent values and flash time in minutes that has elapsed since measurement occurred (see illustration).
13 Set frequency of blood pressure measurements, as well as upper and lower alarm limits for systolic, diastolic, and mean blood pressure readings. Intervals between blood pressure measurements may be set from 1 to 90 minutes. The nurse determines frequency and alarm limits based on client's acceptable range of blood pressure, nursing judgment, and physician order. Additional readings can be determined at any time by pressing the start button. Pressing the cancel button immediately deflates the cuff.

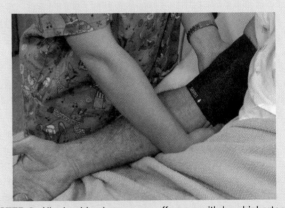

STEP 9 Aligning blood pressure cuff arrow with brachial artery.

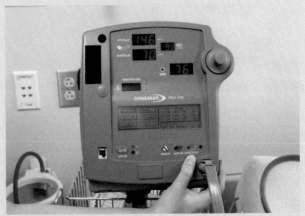

STEP 12 Monitor displays reading. Verify electronic alarm settings.

TABLE 11-6 Proper Cuff Size for Electronic Monitor*

CUFF TYPE	LIMB CIRCUMFERENCE (cm)
Small adult	17-25
Adult	23-33
Large adult	31-40
Thigh	38-50

*It is mandatory for the 12- to 24-foot cord to be used for adult monitoring.

Continued

PROCEDURAL GUIDELINE 11-2—cont'd

14 If frequent blood pressure determinations are required, the cuff may be left in place. Remove cuff at least every 2 hours to assess underlying skin integrity, and if possible, alternate blood pressure sites. Clients with abnormal bleeding tendencies are at risk for microvascular rupture form repeated inflations. When electronic blood pressure machine is no longer required, clean blood pressure cuff and machine according to facility policy to reduce transmission of microorganisms.

15 Compare electronic blood pressure readings with auscultatory blood pressure as ordered, usually every 1 to 2 hours, to verify accuracy of the electronic blood pressure device.

16 **See Completion Protocol (inside front cover).**

SKILL 11.2 Measuring Oxygen Saturation with Pulse Oximetry

- Nursing Skills Online: Airway Management, Lesson 2

Pulse oximetry is a noninvasive measurement of arterial oxygen saturation (Sao_2) that assesses the level of oxygen in the blood available to the body tissues. Sao_2 reflects the percentage of hemoglobin that is bound with oxygen in the arteries and is expressed as a percentage; for example, an Sao_2 of 96% indicates that 96% of the hemoglobin molecules are carrying oxygen molecules. The more the hemoglobin is saturated with oxygen, the higher the Sao_2. Normally the Sao_2 is greater than 90% in adults. The pulse oximeter is a device that measures pulse saturation (Spo_2), a reliable estimate of Sao_2 (Grap, 2002). For an Sao_2 over 70% the Spo_2 is accurate to 2%. The measurement of Spo_2 is simple, is painless, and has fewer risks than obtaining an ABG level, which is an invasive procedure. Pulse oximetry is indicated in clients who have an unstable oxygen status or in those who are at risk for alterations in oxygenation.

A pulse oximeter includes a probe with a light-emitting diode (LED) connected by cable to an oximeter (Figure 11-8). Light waves emitted by the LED are absorbed and then reflected back by oxygenated and deoxygenated hemoglobin molecules. The reflected light is processed by the oximeter, which calculates Spo_2. In adults the oximeter sensor is applied to the finger, toe, earlobe, or bridge of the nose. In addition, sensors for infants and children can be applied to the palm or the sole of the foot. The nurse selects the appropriate sensor site for the client's condition (Box 11-5). Spo_2 can be assessed continuously, intermittently, or with spot checks, depending on the client's condition.

ASSESSMENT

1 Identify client conditions that alter oxygen saturation (e.g., clients recovering from conscious sedation, clients requiring oxygen therapy, clients with chronic respiratory conditions, clients with chest wall injury or chest pain).

BOX 11-5 Characteristics of Pulse Oximeter Sensors and Sites

Reusable Sensors
Digit Sensors
- Easy to apply; conform to various sizes
- Yield strong correlation with Sao_2
- Clip-on sensor probe may not fit properly on obese clients

Earlobe Sensors
- Clip-on is smaller and lighter, although more positional than digit sensor
- Research suggests greater accuracy at lower saturations (Grap, 2002)
- Yield strong correlation with Sao_2
- Good when uncontrollable or rhythmic movements are present (e.g., hand tremors seen with Parkinson's disease)
- Vascular bed least affected by decreased blood flow (Grap, 2002)

Disposable Sensors
- Can be applied to variety of sites: earlobe of adult or nose bridge, palm, or sole of infant
- Less restrictive for continuous Spo_2 monitoring
- Expensive
- Contain latex
- Skin under adhesive may become moist and harbor pathogens
- Available in variety of sizes; pad can be matched with infant weight

---

FIGURE 11-8 Finger probe sensor connected to pulse oximeter.

BOX 11-6 Factors Affecting Determination of Pulse Oxygen Saturation

Interference with Light Transmission

- Outside light sources can interfere with the oximeter's ability to process reflected light.
- Carbon monoxide (caused by smoke inhalation or poisoning) artificially elevates Spo$_2$ by absorbing light similar to oxygen.
- Client motion can interfere with the oximeter's ability to process reflected light.
- Jaundice may interfere with the oximeter's ability to process reflected light.
- Intravascular dyes (methylene blue) absorb light similar to deoxyhemoglobin and artificially lower saturation.

Reduction of Arterial Pulsations

- Peripheral vascular disease (Raynaud's disease, atherosclerosis) can reduce pulse volume.
- Hypothermia at assessment site decreases peripheral blood flow.
- Pharmacological vasoconstrictors (epinephrine, phenylephrine, dopamine) will decrease peripheral pulse volume.
- Low cardiac output and hypotension decrease blood flow to peripheral arteries.
- Peripheral edema can obscure arterial pulsation.

2 Identify client medications or treatments that may influence oxygen saturation. *Rationale: Oxygen therapy, respiratory therapy such as postural drainage and percussion, and bronchodilators will affect the client's ability to ventilate and perfuse lung tissue.*

3 Review factors that influence oxygen saturation. *Rationale: Any abnormalities in the type or amount of hemoglobin affect the ability of oxygen to be carried to the tissues (Box 11-6).*

4 Identify client factors likely to interfere with accuracy of pulse oximeter. *Rationale: Skin pigmentation affects the ability of Spo$_2$ to predict Sao$_2$. Darker pigments can result in false-high readings.*

5 Assess pertinent laboratory values, including hemoglobin and ABGs if available. *Rationale: Anemia affects the ability of oxygen to attach to the hemoglobin molecule. ABG levels measure Sao$_2$, which serves as a standard and provides a basis for comparison to assist in the assessment of respiratory status.*

6 Determine client-specific site appropriate to place pulse

oximeter sensor by measuring capillary refill (see Chapter 12). If less than 3 seconds, select alternative site; note presence of moisture or nail polish. *Rationale: Site must have adequate local circulation for sensor to detect hemoglobin molecules that absorb emitted light. Changes in Spo$_2$ are reflected in the circulation of finger capillary bed within 30 seconds and earlobe capillary bed within 5 to 10 seconds. Moisture, dark nail polish, and acrylic nails impede sensor detection of emitted light and produce falsely elevated Spo$_2$ levels (Grap, 2002).*

7 Determine previous baseline Spo$_2$ from client's record. *Rationale: Baseline information provides basis for comparison and assists in assessment of current status and evaluation of interventions.*

PLANNING

Expected Outcomes focus on monitoring and maintaining adequate oxygenation when client is at risk for hypoxemia.

1 Sao$_2$ level greater than 90% is maintained, with or without oxygen therapy, during sleep, after removal of secretions with suctioning, and with exertion of ambulating in the hall for 5 minutes. (NOTE: Acceptable level must be individualized for each client.)

2 Skin integrity beneath pulse oximeter sensor is maintained.

Delegation Considerations

The skill of measuring oxygen saturation with a pulse oximeter can be delegated. The nurse directs personnel by:

- Explaining appropriate site and probe sensor for measurement of oxygen saturation
- Identifying client-specific factors that can falsely lower Spo$_2$
- Reviewing to observe for changes in client's vital signs and to report Spo$_2$ measurements of less than 90%

Equipment

- Oximeter
- Oximeter sensor appropriate for client and recommended by the oximeter manufacturer (see Box 11-5)
- Acetone or nail polish remover
- Vital signs flow sheet

IMPLEMENTATION *for Measuring Oxygen Saturation with Pulse Oximetry*

STEPS	RATIONALE
1 See Standard Protocol (inside front cover).	
2 Select site, which may include ear, nail bed, or bridge of nose. If finger is selected, remove finger nail polish and acrylic nail (if worn) with acetone or polish remover.	Opaque coatings decrease light transmission, and nail polish containing blue pigments can absorb light emissions and falsely alter saturation (Grap, 2002).

NURSE ALERT Mixing probes from different manufacturers can result in burn injury to the client. If client has a latex allergy or latex sensitivity, avoid adhesive sensor, which contains latex.

STEPS	RATIONALE

3 Determine capillary refill at site. If less than 3 seconds, select alternative site.

Cold temperature with vasoconstriction or vascular disease may decrease circulation, impede refill, and prevent sensor from measuring Spo_2.

4 Position client comfortably. If finger is chosen as monitoring site, support lower arm. Instruct client to keep sensor probe site still.

Movement interferes with Spo_2 determination. Pressure of sensor probe's spring tension on finger or earlobe may be uncomfortable.

5 Attach sensor to selected site (see illustration), making sure photodetectors of light sensors are aligned opposite each other. Instruct client that clip-on probe will feel like a clothespin on a finger but will not hurt.

Pulse waveform/intensity display enables detection of valid pulse or presence of interfering signal. Pitch of audible beep is proportional to Spo_2 value. Double-check pulse rate to ensure oximeter accuracy. Pressure of sensor's spring tension on a finger may be uncomfortable.

6 After sensor is in place, turn on oximeter by activating power. Observe pulse waveform/intensity display and audible beep. Compare oximeter pulse rate with client's radial pulse.

Ensures oximeter accuracy.

COMMUNICATION TIP Inform client that oximeter alarm will sound if the sensor falls off or if client moves the sensor.

NURSE ALERT Do not attach probe to finger, ear, or bridge of nose if area is edematous or skin integrity is compromised. Do not attach sensor to fingers that are hypothermic. Do not place sensor on same extremity as electronic blood pressure cuff. Blood flow to finger will be temporarily interrupted when cuff inflates and cause inaccurate blood pressure reading that triggers alarm.

NURSE ALERT If oximeter pulse rate, client's radial pulse rate, and apical pulse rate are different, reevaluate oximeter sensor placement and reassess pulse rates.

---

7 Leave sensor in place until oximeter reaches constant value and pulse display reaches full strength during each cardiac cycle. Read Spo_2 on digital display.

Reading may take 10 to 30 seconds, depending on site selected.

8 If continuous Spo_2 monitoring is planned, verify Spo_2 alarm limits, which are preset by the manufacturer at a low of 85% and a high of 100%. Limits for Spo_2 and pulse rate should be determined as indicated by client's condition. Verify that alarms are on. Assess skin integrity under sensor every 2 hours. Relocate sensor at least every 4 hours, and more frequently if skin integrity is altered.

Spring tension of sensor or sensitivity to disposable sensor adhesive can cause skin irritation and lead to disruption of skin integrity.

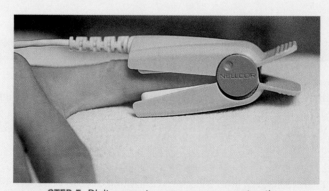

STEP 5 Digit sensor to measure oxygen saturation.

STEPS	RATIONALE

9 If intermittent or spot-checking SpO_2 measurements are planned, remove sensor probe and turn oximeter power off. Store sensor probe in appropriate location.

Sensor probes are expensive and vulnerable to damage.

10 See Completion Protocol (inside front cover).

EVALUATION

1 Compare SpO_2 levels whenever oxygen therapy is initiated or discontinued, before and during sleep, before and after removal of secretions with suctioning, and during activity.

2 Assess skin integrity under sensor every 2 hours.

Unexpected Outcomes and Related Interventions

1 Client's SpO_2 is less than 90%.

a. Observe for signs and symptoms of decreased oxygenation: cyanosis, restlessness, altered respiratory patterns, and tachycardia.

b. Reposition probe and reevaluate waveform. If SpO_2 is unacceptable, notify physician or nurse in charge. An ABG may be ordered to validate SpO_2 reading.

c. Observe for and minimize factors that decrease SpO_2, such as lung secretions, increased activity, altered neurological status, and hyperthermia.

d. Assist client to a position that maximizes ventilation effort (e.g., placing an obese client in a high-Fowler's position) and verify appropriate oxygen delivery system and liter flow.

2 Pulse rate indicated on oximeter is less than radial or apical pulse rate.

a. Change sensor site. Clients who have cold hands or peripheral vascular disease may have decreased blood flow to extremity.

b. Assess apical and radial pulse along with other signs and symptoms that would indicate compromised cardiac status or decreased peripheral blood flow.

Recording and Reporting

- Record SpO_2 on vital sign flow sheet or nurses' notes; include type and amount of oxygen therapy used by client during assessment. Assessment of SpO_2 after administration of specific therapies is documented in narrative form in nurses' notes.

- Report abnormal SpO_2, as well as signs and symptoms of oxygen desaturation, to nurse in charge or physician.

Sample Documentation

1715 Continuous pulse ox on right index finger. Sensor relocated to left index finger. Capillary refill R = L, 2 seconds. Skin intact, no redness noted. SpO_2 93% with 3 L O_2 via nasal cannula. RR 24, client denies dyspnea, remains in semi-Fowler's position.

Special Considerations
Pediatric Considerations

- Infant and toddler sensors attached to adhesive sensor pads are available and conform to fingers, palm of hand, and sole of foot.

- Earlobe and bridge of nose sensors are not used for infants and toddlers.

Geriatric Considerations

- Identifying an acceptable sensor site may be difficult on older adults because of the likelihood of peripheral vascular disease, cold-induced vasoconstriction, and anemia.

- Older adults require more frequent assessment of skin under sensor site because of tissue fragility and decreased elasticity caused by aging.

Home Care Considerations

- Pulse oximetry is used in home care to noninvasively monitor oxygen therapy or changes in oxygen therapy.

NCLEX® Style Questions

1 Four hours postoperatively, Ms. Coburn's vital signs are BP 130/64 mm Hg, HR 102, RR 16, SpO_2 90%, tympanic temperature 100.2° F. What vital sign requires immediate attention?
   1. Heart rate
   2. Oxygen saturation
   3. Respiratory rate
   4. Temperature

2 Ms. Augsten is a 72-year-old woman who arrives at the outpatient clinic complaining of a headache. Her blood pressure is 170/88 mm Hg in the right arm and 188/92 mm Hg in the left arm. She reports that she ran out of her blood pressure medication last week and has not been able to afford to refill her prescription. What is your priority nursing action?
   1. Allow the client to relax for 15 minutes and reevaluate the blood pressure measurements.

2. Contact the social worker for financial assistance.
3. Notify the physician.
4. Retake the blood pressure in the left arm with a different size cuff.

3 Mrs. Williams arrives with her 4-year-old son, Carl, at her scheduled visit with her primary care provider. You obtain vital signs and conduct an initial screening assessment of Carl. You note that his skin is warm and dry, and his left ear is red and draining fluid. Mrs. Williams states Carl has not wanted to eat or drink for the past 2 days. What vital sign is a priority and how should it be obtained?

1. Blood pressure, left arm
2. Heart rate, radial pulse
3. Oxygen saturation, ear sensor
4. Temperature, left ear

4 Mr. Best is recovering from pneumonia and receiving oxygen via 4-L nasal cannula. The nursing assistant obtains his routine vital signs and reports a respiratory rate of 26 and an oxygen saturation of 92%. What information about Mr. Best would be most helpful in determining your priority nursing action?

1. Activity just before vital signs
2. Baseline vital signs
3. Complaints of dyspnea
4. Medication list

5 Mr. Bailey is a conditioned athlete and arrives at the clinic with a complaint of light-headedness. His vital signs are BP 82/56 mm Hg, HR 68, RR 16, temperature 96.6° F tympanic, and pulse ox 100%. What is your priority nursing action?

1. Ask him if he has had anything to eat recently.
2. Notify the physician.
3. Obtain blood pressure in other arm.
4. Repeat temperature measurement using oral thermometer.

References for all chapters appear in Appendix D.

Health Assessment

MEDIA RESOURCES

- **evolve** http://evolve.elsevier.com/Elkin

Nurses perform systematic assessments on a regular basis in nearly every health care setting. In acute care settings, a brief assessment at the beginning of each shift identifies any changes in a client's status for comparison with the previous assessment. This routine assessment takes 10 to 15 minutes and reveals information that adds to the client's database (Box 12-1). In nursing homes and home care settings, nurses complete similar assessments weekly, monthly, or more frequently when a client's health status changes.

Nurses perform a more comprehensive assessment when a client is admitted to a health care agency. This assessment involves a detailed review of a client's condition and includes a nursing history and a behavioral and physical examination. The health history involves an interview with a client to gather subjective data about any presenting conditions. A physical assessment includes a head-to-toe review of each body system that offers objective information about the client. The client's condition and response affect the extent of the examination. After gathering data, the nurse groups significant findings into patterns of data that reveal actual or potential nursing diagnoses (see Chapter 1). Each abnormal finding directs the nurse to gather additional data. Initial assessment and examination provide a baseline for the client's functional status and serve as a comparison for future assessment findings. In addition, the information is useful in selecting the best nursing measures to manage the client's health problems.

Nurses are often the first to detect changes in clients' conditions. For this reason, the ability to think critically and interpret client behaviors and physiological changes is essential. The skills of physical assessment are powerful tools for detecting subtle, as well as obvious, changes in a client's health. During the physical assessment is an ideal time to offer client teaching and encourage promotion of health practices, such as breast (Box 12-2) and genital (Box 12-3) self-examination. The American Cancer Society (ACS, 2004) recommends guidelines for early detection.

BOX 12-1   Checklist for Routine Shift Assessment

1 **Mental and Neurological Status**
   a. Level of consciousness (LOC)/responsiveness
   b. Alertness/orientation
   c. Pupils equal, round, and reactive to light and accommodation (PERRLA)
   d. Mood
   e. Behavior
2 **Vital Signs**
   a. Blood pressure
   b. Pulse
   c. Respiration
   d. Temperature
   e. Pain and comfort level
3 **Motor Sensory Function**
   a. Range of motion (ROM)
   b. Movement
   c. Strength
   d. Presence of numbness or tingling
4 **Integument (Skin/Mucous Membranes)**
   a. Color
   b. Temperature
   c. Turgor
   d. Moisture
   e. Edema
   f. Integrity

5 **Cardiopulmonary System**
   a. Heart sounds
   b. Apical rate and rhythm
   c. Lung sounds
   d. Breathing pattern
   e. Peripheral pulses
   f. Capillary refill
6 **Gastrointestinal (GI) System**
   a. Bowel sounds
   b. Abdominal palpation
   c. Degree of abdominal distention
   d. Bowel elimination problems (e.g., diarrhea, constipation, flatulence)
7 **Wounds**
   a. Cleanliness
   b. Presence of swelling, redness, infection, or drainage
   c. Bandage/dressing
8 **Invasive Tubes (e.g., Intravenous [IV] Lines, Nasogastric [NG] Tubes, Wound Drains, Catheters)**
   a. Device and location
   b. IV line: Correct fluid/medicine infusing
   c. Patency and position
   d. Presence of redness, swelling, or tenderness at site
   e. Drainage rate or infusion rate
   f. Date of last tubing change

ASSESSMENT TECHNIQUES

Inspection, palpation, percussion, auscultation, and olfaction are the five basic assessment techniques. Each skill enables the nurse to collect a broad range of physical data about clients. Nurses need experience to recognize normal variations among clients, as well as ranges of normal for an individual. Remember, cultural diversity is one factor that influences both normal variations and potential alterations that may be found during the assessment. It is very important to take the time needed to carefully assess each body part. Hurrying can cause the nurse to overlook significant signs and make incorrect conclusions about a client's condition.

Inspection is the visual examination of body parts or areas. An experienced nurse learns to make multiple observations, almost simultaneously, while becoming very perceptive of any abnormalities. The secret is to always pay attention to the client. Watch all movements, and look carefully at the body part being inspected. It is important to recognize normal physical characteristics of clients of all ages before trying to distinguish abnormal findings.

Inspection requires good lighting and full exposure of body parts. Inspect each area for size, shape, color, symmetry, position, and the presence of abnormalities. If possible, inspect each area compared with the same area on the opposite side of the body. When necessary, use additional light, such as a penlight, to inspect body cavities such as the mouth and throat. *Do not hurry. Pay attention to detail.* Verify and clarify all abnormalities with subjective client data. In other words, ask the client for further information about each abnormality or change.

Palpation uses the sense of touch. Through palpation the hands make delicate and sensitive measurements of specific physical signs. Palpation detects resistance, resilience, roughness, texture, temperature, and mobility. Palpation is often used with or after visual inspection. The nurse uses different parts of the hand to detect specific characteristics. For example, the dorsum (back) of the hand is sensitive to temperature variations. The pads of the fingertips detect subtle changes in texture, shape, size, consistency, and pulsation of body parts. The palm of the hand is especially sensitive to vibration. The nurse measures position, consistency, and turgor by lightly grasping the body part with the fingertips.

Assist the client to relax and position comfortably because muscle tension during palpation impairs the ability to palpate correctly. Asking the client to take slow, deep breaths enhances muscle relaxation. Palpate tender areas last. Ask the client to point out areas that are more sensitive and note any nonverbal signs of discomfort. Clients appreciate clean, warm hands; short fingernails; and a gentle approach. Palpation is either light or deep and is controlled by the amount of pressure applied with the fingers or hand. Light palpation precedes deep palpation. Consider the client's condition, the area being palpated, and the reason for using palpation. For example, when a client is admitted to the emergency department after an automobile accident,

BOX 12-2 Breast Self-Examination

BSE should be done once a month so that you become familiar with the usual appearance and feel of your breast. Familiarity makes it easier to notice any changes in the breast from one month to another. Early discovery of a change from what is "normal" is the main idea behind BSE.

For women who menstruate, the best time to do BSE is 2 or 3 days after a period ends, when the breasts are least likely to be tender or swollen. For women who no longer menstruate, pick a day, such as the first day of the month, to remind yourself to do BSE.

Procedure

1 Stand before a mirror. Inspect both breasts for anything unusual, such as any discharge from the nipples, puckering, dimpling, or scaling of the skin.

The next two steps are designed to emphasize any change in the shape or contour of the breasts. As you do them, you should be able to feel your chest muscles tighten.

2 Watching closely in the mirror, clasp hands behind your head and press head forward.

3 Next, press hands firmly on hips and bow slightly toward the mirror as you pull your shoulders and elbows forward.

The next part of the examination may be done in the shower. Gliding fingers over soapy skin makes it easier to appreciate the texture underneath.

4 Raise your left arm. Use three or four fingers of your right hand to explore your left breast firmly, carefully, and thoroughly. Beginning at the outer edge, press the flat part of your fingers in small circles, moving the circles slowly around the breast. Gradually work toward the nipple. Be sure to cover the entire breast. Pay special attention to the area between the breast and the armpit, including the armpit itself. Feel for any unusual lump or mass under the skin.

5 Gently squeeze the nipple and look for a discharge. Repeat the exam on your right breast.

6 Steps 4 and 5 should be repeated lying down. Lie flat on your back, left arm over your head, and a pillow or folded towel under your left shoulder. This position flattens the breast and makes it easier to examine. Use the same circular motion described earlier. Repeat on your right breast.

Call your physician if you find a lump or other abnormality.

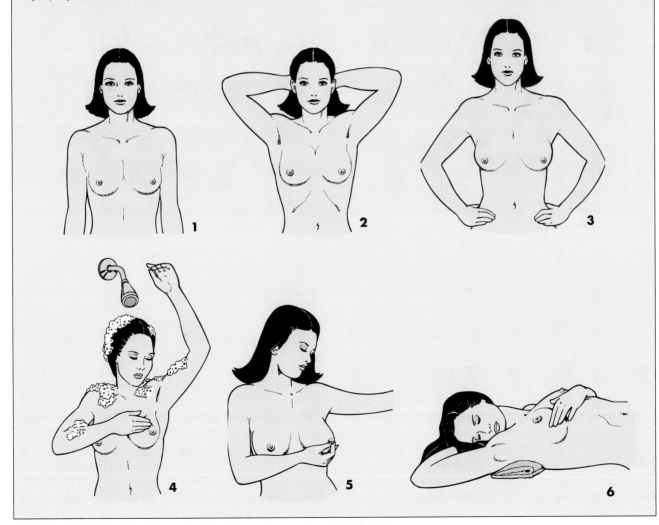

From Seidel HM and others: *Mosby's guide to physical examination,* ed 6, St Louis, 2006, Mosby.

Box 12-3 Genital Self-Examination

All men 15 years and older should perform this examination monthly. Perform the examination after a warm bath or shower when the scrotal sac is relaxed. Call your physician if you find a lump or any other abnormality.

Penile Examination

1. Stand naked in front of a mirror and hold the penis in your hand and examine the head. Pull back the foreskin if uncircumcised.
2. Inspect and palpate the entire head of the penis in a clockwise motion, looking carefully for any bumps, sores, or blisters.
3. Look for any bumpy warts.
4. Look at the opening at the end of the penis for discharge.
5. Look along the entire shaft of the penis for the same signs.
6. Separate pubic hair at the base of the penis and carefully examine the skin underneath.

Testicular Examination

1. Look for swelling or lumps in the skin of the scrotum while looking in the mirror.
2. Use both hands, placing the index and middle fingers under the testicles and the thumb on top.
3. Gently roll the testicle, feeling for lumps, thickening, or a change in consistency (hardening).
4. Find the epididymis (a cordlike structure on the top and back of the testicle; it is not a lump).
5. Feel for small, pea-sized lumps on the front and side of the testicle. The lumps are usually painless and are abnormal.

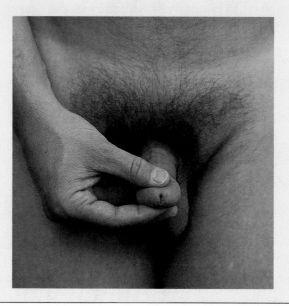
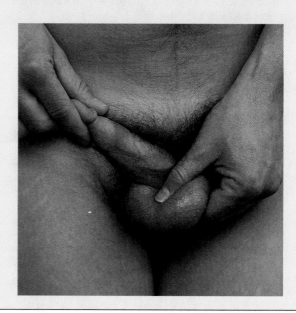

From Seidel HM and others: *Mosby's guide to physical examination,* ed 6, St Louis, 2006, Mosby.

consider the factors surrounding the client's injury and inspect the chest wall carefully before performing any palpation around the area of the ribs.

For light palpation, apply pressure slowly, gently, and deliberately, depressing about 1 cm (½ inch). Check tender areas further, using light intermittent pressure. After light palpation, deeper palpation may be used to examine the condition of organs (Figure 12-1). Depress the area being examined approximately 1 inch (2 cm). Caution is the rule. Bimanual palpation involves one hand placed over the other while applying pressure. The upper hand exerts downward pressure as the other hand feels the subtle characteristics of underlying organs and masses. Seek the assistance of a qualified instructor before attempting deep palpation.

Percussion involves tapping the body with the fingertips to evaluate the size, borders, and consistency of body organs and to discover fluid in body cavities. Percussion identifies the location, size, and density of underlying structures. To percuss, you strike the body's surface with a finger to create a vibration (Figure 12-2). Sounds are heard as percussion tones arise from vibrations in body tissues (Seidel and others, 2006). The character of sound depends on the density of underlying tissues. The technique requires practice and skill and is typically used by advanced practice nurses (APNs).

Auscultation is listening with a stethoscope to sounds produced by the body. To auscultate correctly, listen in a quiet environment for both the presence of sound and its characteristics. To be successful in auscultation, the nurse must first recognize normal sounds from each body structure, including the passage of blood through an artery, heart sounds, and movement of air through the lungs. These sounds vary according to the location in which they can most easily be heard. Likewise, nurses become familiar with areas that normally do not emit sounds. It is important for

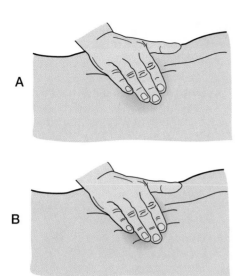

FIGURE 12-1 **A,** During light palpation, gentle pressure against underlying skin and tissues can be used to detect areas of irregularity and tenderness. **B,** During deep palpation, depress tissue to assess condition of underlying organs.

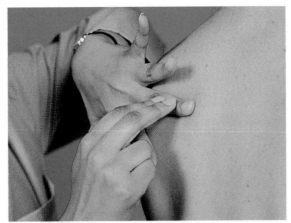

FIGURE 12-2 Indirect percussion. (From Barkauskas VH and others: *Health and physical assessment,* ed 3, St Louis, 2002, Mosby.)

you to listen to many normal sounds in order to recognize abnormal sounds when they arise.

To auscultate, the nurse needs good hearing acuity, a good stethoscope, and knowledge of how to use the stethoscope properly (see Chapter 11). Nurses with hearing disorders may purchase stethoscopes with greater sound amplification and may need to ask colleagues to verify some findings through auscultation. It is essential to place the stethoscope directly on the client's skin because clothing obscures and changes sound.

Through auscultation there are four characteristics of sound:

Frequency: Number of sound wave cycles generated per second by a vibrating object. The higher the frequency, the higher the pitch of a sound and vice versa.

Loudness: Amplitude of a sound wave. Auscultated sounds are described as either loud or soft.

Quality: Sounds of similar frequency and loudness from different sources. Terms such as *blowing* or *gurgling* describe quality of sound.

Duration: Length of time that sound vibrations last. Duration of sound is short, medium, or long. Layers of soft tissue dampen the duration of sounds from deep internal organs.

Olfaction uses the sense of smell to detect abnormalities that go unrecognized by any other means. Some alterations in body function and certain bacteria create characteristic odors (Table 12-1).

PREPARATION FOR ASSESSMENT

The process of assessment begins the moment you see the client and continues with each encounter. Always know the client's health history and the reason for seeking care.

Also be alert for any changes or problems that may have developed since the last assessment.

Preparation of the environment, equipment, and client facilitates a smooth assessment. To promote client comfort and efficiency it is essential to provide privacy for the client. In a health care facility, close the door or pull privacy curtains. In the home, examine the client in the bedroom. A comfortable environment includes a warm, comfortable temperature; a loose-fitting gown or pajamas for the client; adequate direct lighting; control of outside noises; and precautions to prevent interruptions by visitors or health care personnel. If possible, place the bed or exam table at waist level so that you can access the client easily.

Preparing the Client

Prepare the client both physically and psychologically for an accurate assessment. A tense, anxious client may have difficulty understanding, following directions, or cooperating with your instructions. To prepare the client:

1 Make the client comfortable by allowing the opportunity to empty the bowel or bladder (a good time to collect needed specimens).

2 Provide privacy. This may involve asking friends or family to step out of the room.

3 Minimize client's anxiety and fear by conveying an open, receptive, and professional approach. Using simple terms, thoroughly explain what will be done, what the client should expect to feel, and how the client can cooperate. Even if the client appears unresponsive, it is still important to explain your actions.

4 Provide access to body parts while draping areas that are not being examined.

5 Reduce distractions. Turn down volume or turn off television/radio.

TABLE 12-1 Assessment of Characteristic Odors

ODOR	SITE OR SOURCE	POTENTIAL CAUSES
Alcohol	Oral cavity	Ingestion of alcohol
Ammonia	Urine	Urinary tract infection (UTI)
Body odor	Skin, particularly in areas where body parts rub together (e.g., underarms, beneath breasts)	Poor hygiene, excess perspiration (hyperhidrosis), foul-smelling perspiration (bromhidrosis)
Feces	Wound site	Wound abscess
	Vomitus	Bowel obstruction
	Rectal area	Fecal incontinence
Fetid, sweet odor	Tracheostomy or mucous secretions	Infection of bronchial tree (*Pseudomonas* bacteria)
Foul-smelling stools in infant	Stool	Malabsorption syndrome
Halitosis	Oral cavity	Poor dental and oral hygiene, gum disease
Musty odor	Casted body part	Infection inside cast
Stale urine	Skin	Uremic acidosis
Sweet, fruity ketones	Oral cavity	Diabetic acidosis
Sweet, heavy, thick odor	Draining wound	*Pseudomonas* (bacterial) infection

6   Eliminate drafts, control room temperature, and provide warm blankets.

7   Help the client assume positions during the assessment so that body parts are accessible and the client stays comfortable. A client's ability to assume positions will depend on physical strength and limitations. Some positions are uncomfortable or embarrassing; keep a client in position no longer than is necessary.

8   Pace assessment according to the client's physical and emotional tolerance.

9   Use a relaxed voice tone and facial expressions to put the client at ease.

10   Encourage the client to ask questions and report discomfort felt during the examination.

11   Have a third person of the client's gender in the room during assessment of genitalia. This prevents the client from accusing you of behaving in an unethical manner.

12   At the conclusion of the assessment, ask the client if there are any concerns or questions.

PHYSICAL ASSESSMENT OF VARIOUS AGE-GROUPS

Children and Adolescents

1   Routine assessment of children focuses on health promotion and illness prevention, particularly for care of well children with competent parenting and no serious health problems (Hockenberry and Wilson, 2007). Focus on growth and development, sensory screening, dental examination, and behavioral assessment.

2   Children who are chronically ill, disabled, in foster care, or foreign-born adopted may require additional assessments because of their unique health risks.

3   When obtaining histories of infants and children, gather all or part of information from parents or guardians.

4   Parents may think they are being tested or judged by the examiner. Offer support during examination, and do not pass judgment.

5   Call children by their preferred name, and address parents as "Mr. and Mrs. Brown" rather than by first names.

6   Open-ended questions often allow parents to share more information and to describe more of the child's problems.

7   Older children and adolescents respond best when treated as adults and individuals and often can provide details about their health history and severity of symptoms.

8   The adolescent has a right to confidentiality. After talking with parents about historical information, arrange to be alone with the adolescent to speak privately and to perform the examination.

Older Adults

1   Do not assume that aging is always accompanied by illness or disability. Most older adults are able to adapt to change and maintain functional independence (Burke and Laramie, 2004).

2   Allow extra time, and be calm, relaxed, and unhurried with older adults.

3   Provide adequate space for an examination, particularly if the client uses a mobility aid.

4   Plan the history and examination, taking into account the older adult's energy level, physical limitations, pace, and adaptability. You may need more than one session to complete the assessment (Burke and Laramie, 2004).

5   Measure performance under the most favorable of conditions. Take advantage of natural opportunities for assessment (e.g., during bathing, grooming, and mealtime) (Burke and Laramie, 2004).

6   Sequence an examination to keep position changes to a minimum. Be efficient throughout the examination to limit client movement.

7   Be sure an examination of an older adult includes review of mental status.

EVIDENCE IN PRACTICE

Vahabi M: Breast cancer screening methods: a review of the evidence, *Health Care Women Int* 24(9):790, 2003.

A recent survey of research studies about the effectiveness of breast self-examination (BSE) and scheduled mammography was conducted. Results found that mammography screening for women age 40 years and older at least every 2 years was still favored as a method of breast cancer detection. Many women found their own breast cancers, so the need for BSE continues to be important for all women.

SKILL GUIDELINES

1 Prioritize the assessment based on a client's presenting signs and symptoms or health care needs. For example, when a client develops sudden shortness of breath, first assess the lungs and thorax. If a client is acutely ill, you may choose to assess only the involved body systems. Use judgment to ensure that an examination is relevant and inclusive.

2 Organize the examination. Compare both sides of the body for symmetry. If a client becomes fatigued, offer rest periods. Perform painful or intrusive procedures near the end of the exam.

3 Use a head-to-toe approach following the sequence of inspection, palpation, and auscultation (except for abdominal assessment). This sequence facilitates an effective assessment.

4 Encourage the client to actively participate. Clients usually know about their physical condition. Often the client can let you know when certain findings are normal or when there have been actual changes.

5 Always identify the client using at least two client identifiers, other than the room number. Using an arm band and having the client state name (if able) are standards (JCAHO, 2007). In long-term care settings arm bands are not used; however, pictures are available for identification. *Caution:* clients with difficulty hearing or altered level of consciousness (LOC) may answer to name other than their own.

6 Respect the client's race, gender, age, and cultural beliefs. These important variables often influence assessment findings and exam approaches. Consider also a client's health beliefs, use of alternative therapies, nutritional habits, relationships with family, and comfort with close physical contact (Box 12-4).

7 Follow standard precautions for infection control. During an assessment you may have contact with body fluids and discharge. Always wear gloves when there are lesions, wounds, or breaks in the skin. In some circumstances you will need to wear a gown.

8 Record quick notes to facilitate accurate documentation.

9 Use assessment skills during each client contact, including activities such as bathing, administration of medications, other therapies, or while conversing with a client.

10 Integrate health promotion and education into physical assessment activities. There are "teachable moments" when you can share findings and educate clients about health promotion.

11 Record a summary of the assessment using appropriate medical terminology and in the sequence that findings are gathered. Use commonly accepted medical abbreviations to keep notes concise.

BOX 12-4 Cultural Awareness of Touch During Physical Examination

Physical contact with a client can convey a variety of meanings, depending on the client's cultural background. Consider these guidelines, but remember that each client is an individual and may respond differently.
Hispanics: Highly tactile, very modest (men and women); may ask for health care provider of same gender; women may refuse to be examined by male health care provider
Asians/Pacific Islanders: Avoid touching (patting head is strictly taboo); touching during an argument equals loss of control (shame); public display of affection toward members of same gender is permissible (but not toward members of opposite gender)
African-Americans: May not like to be touched without permission; may exercise level of distrust or caution initially in care provider
Native Americans: Shake hands lightly; may not like to be touched without permission; nonverbal communication is important

Data from Meiner SE and Lueckenotte AG: *Gerontologic nursing*, ed 3, St Louis, 2006, Mosby; Seidel HM and others: *Mosby's guide to physical examination*, ed 6, St Louis, 2006, Mosby.

NURSING DIAGNOSES

It is important to be aware of previously established nursing diagnoses. The client may present with many nursing diagnoses. However, the following are easily screened for during an assessment.

Impaired skin integrity or **risk for impaired skin integrity** is appropriate when the client is at risk for or has experienced skin breakdown. Influencing factors may include immobility, moisture from incontinence, inadequate nutrition, or circulatory alterations. **Ineffective airway clearance** is appropriate when the client is unable to clear secretions or has obstructions of the respiratory tract. **Ineffective breathing pattern** involves altered inhalation or exhalation and may include either hypoventilation or hyperventilation. Influencing factors may include pain, anxiety, and decreased muscle strength or energy. **Activity intolerance** applies when physical energy is inadequate for the completion of desired activities because of altered cardiac function. Activity intolerance may also be related to prolonged immobility, weakness, and muscle atrophy. **Decreased cardiac output** is appropriate when there is a need to reduce cardiac workload or improve cardiac performance.

Assessment of a client's discomfort may identify the diagnoses of **acute** or **chronic pain.** Abdominal pain is one of the most common symptoms found in hospitalized clients. **Constipation** or **diarrhea** may be associated with abdominal pain or cramping and altered peristalsis resulting in either infrequent hard stools or frequent unformed stools and fluid loss. **Ineffective tissue perfusion** involves a chronic deficit in blood supply to the extremities and is appropriate when findings reveal alteration in arterial or venous circulation.

Disturbed thought processes is appropriate when the client lacks orientation to time, place, person, and/or event or demonstrates an abnormality in any of the six components of the mental health examination. **Acute confusion** is appropriate when the client has an abrupt onset of global, transient changes and disturbances in attention, cognition, sleep-wake cycle, and psychomotor activity (Ladwig and Ackley, 2006). **Impaired memory** is appropriate when the client experiences the inability to remember or recall information or behavioral skills (Ladwig and Ackley, 2006).

Risk for injury is appropriate when the client has muscle weakness or altered LOC. **Impaired physical mobility** may apply when the client is in the postoperative period and when the procedure, surgery, or disease causes pain. Clients found to have breaks in the skin or open wounds are at **risk for infection.**

SKILL 12.1   General Survey

The general survey begins a review of the client's primary health problems, and it includes assessment of the client's vital signs, height and weight, general behavior, and appearance. The survey provides information about characteristics of an illness, a client's hygiene, skin and body image, emotional state, recent changes in weight, and developmental status. The survey reveals important information about the client's behavior that can influence how the nurse communicates instructions to the client and continues the assessment.

ASSESSMENT

1 Note if client has had any acute distress: difficulty breathing, pain, or anxiety. If such signs are present, defer general survey until later and focus immediately on body system affected. *Rationale: Signs establish priorities regarding what part of the examination to conduct first.*

2 Review graphic sheet for previous vital signs and consider factors or conditions that may alter values (see Chapter 11). *Rationale: Provides baseline data about client's vital signs.*

3 Determine client's primary language. If you identify a need for an interpreter, determine availability of professional interpreter. It is best to have an interpreter of the same gender, who is older and more mature. Have the interpreter translate verbatim if possible. *Rationale: Facilitates client understanding and promotes accuracy of information provided by client.*

4 Reconfirm (after reviewing history) primary reason client seeks health care. *Rationale: Keeps assessment focused on client to ensure that client's expectations are addressed.*

5 Identify client's normal height and weight. If a sudden gain or loss in weight has occurred, determine amount of weight change and period of time in which it occurred. Assess if client has recently been dieting or following exercise program. *Rationale: Generally, weight of 10% to 20% above standard indicates excess body fat (Moore, 2001); however, fluid retention is one factor that must be ruled out. A person's weight can fluctuate daily because of fluid loss or retention (1 L of water weighs 1 kg or 2.2 pounds).*

6 Review client's past fluid intake and output (I&O) records. *Rationale: Fluid and electrolyte balance affects health and function in all body systems (see Chapter 9).*

7 Identify client's general perceptions about personal health. *Rationale: Assessment of client's general appearance and client's own perceptions may reveal specific problem areas.*

8 Assess for evidence of latex allergy, which may include contact dermatitis or systemic reactions (see Chapter 4). *Rationale: Gloves will be worn during certain aspects of the assessment. Repeated exposure may result in more serious reactions, including asthma, itching, and anaphylaxis (Ball and Bindler, 2006; Seidel and others, 2006).*

PLANNING

Expected Outcomes focus on accurate assessment data.

1 Client demonstrates alert, cooperative behaviors without evidence of physical or emotional distress during assessment.

2 Client provides appropriate subjective data related to physical condition.

Delegation Considerations

The general survey should not be delegated to assistive personnel (AP). Measuring height and weight, oral intake, urinary output, and vital signs (not the initial set or when client is unstable) and reporting a client's subjective signs and symptoms may be delegated. The nurse directs personnel by:

• Instructing personnel to report all monitoring data to the nurse.

Equipment

• Stethoscope
• Sphygmomanometer and cuff
• Thermometer
• Digital watch or wristwatch with second hand
• Tape measure
• Clean gloves (use nonlatex if necessary)
• Tongue blade

IMPLEMENTATION *for General Survey*

STEPS	RATIONALE
1 See Standard Protocol (inside front cover).	
2 Prepare the client. Tell client you will be doing a routine check for areas of concern. Ask if any area you examine hurts when touched.	Gains client's cooperation. Pain is an important finding during assessment.
3 Throughout the assessment note the client's verbal and nonverbal behaviors. Determine client's LOC and orientation by observing and talking to client (Box 12-5).	Behaviors may reflect specific physical abnormalities. Dementia and LOC influence ability to cooperate.

> **NURSE ALERT** Timing of recent medications, especially pain medication and sedatives, may cause client to be groggy or less responsive.

STEPS	RATIONALE
4 Obtain temperature, pulse, respirations, and blood pressure unless routinely taken within past 3 hours, or repeat if a serious potential change is noted (e.g., change in LOC or difficulty breathing [see Chapter 11]). Inform client of vital signs.	Vital signs provide important information regarding physiological changes in relation to oxygenation and circulation.
5 Observe the following aspects of appearance: gender, race, and age. Note the client's physical features.	Gender influences type of examination performed and manner in which assessments are made. Different physical characteristics and predisposition to illnesses are related to gender and race.
6 If uncertain whether client understands a question, rephrase or ask a similar question.	Inappropriate response from a client may be caused by language barriers, deterioration of mental status, preoccupation with illness, or decreased hearing acuity.
7 If a client's responses are inappropriate, ask short, to-the-point questions regarding information the client should know, for example, "Tell me your name," "What is the name of this place?" "Tell me where you live," "What day is this?" or "What season of the year is this?"	Measures client's orientation to person, place, and time. This may be noted in documentation as "Oriented ×3." If disoriented in any way, include subjective and/or objective data rather than just documenting "disoriented."
8 If client is unable to respond to questions of orientation, offer simple commands, for example, "Squeeze my fingers" or "Move your toes."	LOC exists along a continuum that includes full responsiveness, inability to consciously initiate meaningful behaviors, and unresponsiveness to stimuli.

BOX 12-5 Possible Symptoms of Dementia

Learning and Retaining New Information
- Trouble remembering recent conversations, events, and appointments
- Frequently misplaces objects

Handling Complex Tasks
- Difficulty following a complex train of thought
- Difficulty performing tasks that require many steps

Reasoning Ability
- Unable to develop plan to address problems at work or home
- Displays uncharacteristic disregard for rules of social conduct

Spatial Ability and Orientation
- Difficulty driving
- Difficulty in organizing objects around the house
- Difficulty finding way around familiar places

Language
- Increasing difficulty with expressing self
- Difficulty following conversations

Behavior
- Appears more passive and less responsive
- More irritable and suspicious than usual
- Misinterprets visual and auditory stimuli

STEPS	RATIONALE

NURSE ALERT When client responds inappropriately to questions or requests, or family members comment on client's change in memory or confusion, perform a more specialized assessment for cognitive function such as the Mini-Mental State Examination (MMSE) (Box 12-6). When a client exhibits a marked change in mental status, notify the physician immediately.

9 Assess affect and mood. Note if verbal expressions match nonverbal behavior and if appropriate to situation.

Reflects client's mental and emotional status, consciousness, and feelings.

10 Observe client interaction with spouse or partner, older adult child, or caregiver. Be alert for indications of fear, hesitancy to report health status, or willingness to let caregiver control assessment interview. Does partner or caregiver have a history of violence, alcoholism, or drug abuse? Is the person unemployed, ill, or frustrated with caring for client? Note if client has any obvious physical injuries.

Abuse is often first suspected in clients who have suffered obvious physical injury or neglect, show signs of malnutrition, or have bruises on the extremities or trunk. Evidence of abuse is often identified first by health care providers, because clients are often unable to tell family or friends. Partners or caregivers may have history of abusive or addictive behaviors.

11 Observe for signs of abuse:

a. For a child: Blood on underclothing, pain in genital area, or difficulty sitting or walking. Physical injury inconsistent with parent's or caregiver's account of how injury occurred.

Indicative of child sexual abuse (Ball and Bindler, 2006). Suggestive of child physical abuse.

b For a female client: Injury or trauma inconsistent with reported cause or obvious injuries to face or neck (black eyes, broken nose, lip lacerations, broken teeth, strangulation marks, burns).

May indicate domestic abuse.

c. For an older adult: Injury or trauma inconsistent with reported cause, injuries in unusual locations (such as neck or genitalia), pattern injuries (left when an object with which a person is struck leaves an imprint), parallel injuries (such as bilateral bruises on the upper arms suggesting the person was held and shaken) and burns (shaped like a cigarette, iron, rope, or immersion with a clear line of demarcation).

Prolonged interval between injury and time medical care was sought are signs indicative of older adult abuse or neglect (Gray-Vickery, 2001).

NURSE ALERT A pattern of findings indicating abuse usually mandates a report to a social service center (refer to state guidelines). Obtain an immediate consultation with physician, social worker, and other support staff to facilitate placement in a safer environment.

BOX 12-6 MMSE Sample Items

Orientation to Time
"What is the date?"

Naming
"What is this?" [Point to a pencil or pen.]

Registration
"Listen carefully, I am going to say three words. You say them back after I stop. Ready? Here they are . . . (HOUSE [pause], CAR [pause], LAKE [pause]. Now repeat those words back to me."
    Repeat up to 5 times, but score only the first trial.

Reading
"Please read this and do what it says." [Show examinee the words on the stimulus form: CLOSE YOUR EYES.]

STEPS	RATIONALE
12 Assess posture, noting alignment of the shoulders and hips. Observe whether the client has a slumped, erect, or bent posture.	May reflect musculoskeletal problem, mood, or presence of pain.
a. Assess body movements. Are they purposeful? Are there tremors of the extremities? Are any body parts immobile? Are movements coordinated or uncoordinated?	May indicate neurological or muscular problem or emotional stress (see Skill 12.6).
13 Assess speech. Is it understandable and moderately paced? Is there an association with the person's thoughts?	May reflect neurological impairment, injury or impairment of mouth, improperly fitting dentures, or differences in dialect and language.
14 Observe hygiene and grooming for presence or absence of makeup, type of clothes (hospital or personal), and cleanliness.	Grooming may reflect activity level before examination, resources available to purchase grooming supplies, client's mood, and self-care practices. May also reflect culture, lifestyle, and personal preferences.
a. Observe the color, distribution, quantity, thickness, texture, and lubrication of hair.	Changes in hair distribution may reflect hormonal changes, changes from aging, poor nutrition, or use of certain hair care products.
b. Inspect the condition of nails (hands and feet).	Changes may indicate inadequate nutrition or grooming practices, nervous habits, or systemic diseases.
c. Assess the presence or absence of body odor.	Body odor may result from physical exercise, deficient hygiene, or physical or mental abnormalities. Inadequate oral hygiene or unhealthy teeth may cause bad breath.
15 Inspect exposed skin and ask if client has noted any changes in the skin, including:	Incidence of melanoma, an aggressive form of skin cancer, has increased significantly. It is more than 10 times higher among whites than blacks (ACS, 2004). The cancer can spread to other parts of the body quickly. Early detection and prompt treatment are critical (Box 12-7).
a Pruritus, oozing, bleeding	
b. Change in the appearance of a mole, bump, or nodule; change in sensation, itchiness, tenderness, or pain	
c. Petechiae (pinpoint-size, red or purple spots on the skin caused by small hemorrhages in the skin layers)	Petechiae may indicate serious blood clotting disorder, drug reaction, or liver disease.
16 Inspect skin surfaces. Compare color of symmetrical body parts, including areas unexposed to sun. Look for any patches or areas of skin color variation.	Changes in color can be indicative of pathological alterations (Table 12-2).

> **NURSE ALERT** Be alert for basal cell carcinomas, such as an open sore that does not heal, shiny nodule, a pink or reddish growth, or a scar-like area. These are often seen in sun-exposed areas, which frequently occur in sun-damaged skin.

BOX 12-7 Malignant Melanoma

The ABCD Rule of Melanoma: This simple mnemonic helps you remember the characteristics that should alert you to the possibility of malignant melanoma.

- **A** **A**symmetry of lesion
- **B** **B**orders: irregular
- **C** **C**olor blue/black or variegated
- **D** **D**iameter greater than 6 mm

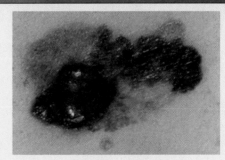

Typical melanoma.

Illustration from Zitelli B, Davis H: *Atlas of pediatric physical diagnosis*, ed 4, St Louis, 2002, Mosby.

STEPS	RATIONALE
17 Carefully inspect color of face, oral mucosa, lips, conjunctivae, sclera, palms of hands, and nail beds.	You can more readily identify abnormalities in areas of body where melanin production is lowest.

> **NURSE ALERT** When assessing the skin of a client with bandages, cast, restraints, or other restrictive devices, note areas of pallor and decreased temperature, which may indicate impaired circulation. Immediate release of pressure from the restrictive device may be necessary.

STEPS	RATIONALE
18 Use ungloved fingertips to palpate skin surfaces to feel texture and moisture of intact skin.	Changes in texture may be the first indication of skin rashes in dark-skinned clients. Hydration, body temperature, and environment may affect the skin. Older adults are prone to xerosis, presenting as dry, scaly skin (Burke and Laramie, 2004).
a. Using dorsum (back) of hand, palpate for temperature of skin surfaces. Compare symmetrical body parts. Compare upper and lower body parts. Note distinct temperature differences and localized areas of warmth.	Skin on dorsum of hand is thin, which allows detection of subtle temperature changes. Cool skin temperature often indicates decreased blood flow. A stage I pressure ulcer may cause warmth and erythema (redness) of an area. Environmental temperature and anxiety may also affect skin temperature.
b. Assess skin turgor by grasping fold of skin on the sternum, forearm, or abdomen with the fingertips. Release skinfold, and note ease and speed with which skin returns to place (see illustration).	With reduced turgor, skin remains suspended or "tented" for a few seconds before slowly returning to place, indicating decreased elasticity and possible dehydration. With altered turgor it is essential to provide measures for prevention of pressure ulcers.

TABLE 12-2 Pathological Color Changes

COLOR CHANGES	LIGHT SKIN	DARK SKIN
Cyanosis: related to hypoxia (late sign of decreased oxygen), heart or lung disease, cold environment	Blue tinge, especially in conjunctivae, nail beds, earlobes, oral membranes, soles, and palms; may be seen in base of tongue	Ashen-gray lips and tongue
Peripheral cyanosis: results from low cardiac output or local vasoconstriction (bluish discoloration of lips and nail beds)		
Ecchymoses: bruising related to bleeding into skin, often from trauma	Purple to yellowish green areas resulting from bleeding into skin, usually related to trauma	Difficult to see except in mouth or conjunctivae
Erythema: related to increased blood flow (fever, irritation)	Redness easily seen anywhere on body	Difficult to assess; palpate for warmth or edema
Jaundice: related to deposits of bilirubin in tissue, liver disease	Yellow staining in sclerae of eyes, skin, fingernails, soles, palms, and oral mucosa	Most reliably assessed in sclerae, hard palate, palms, and soles
Pallor: related to decreased perfusion (blood flow, anemia, shock)	Loss of rosy glow in skin, especially face	Ashen-gray appearance in black skin
Petechiae: minute hemorrhages into skin	Purple pinpoints most easily seen on buttocks, abdomen, and inner surfaces of arms or legs	Usually invisible except in oral mucosa, conjunctivae, or eyelids and covering eyeballs

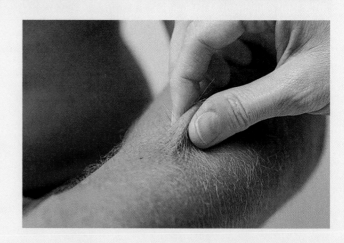

STEP 18b. Assessment of skin turgor. (From Seidel HM and others: *Mosby's guide to physical examination,* ed 5, St Louis, 2003, Mosby.)

STEPS	RATIONALE

19 Inspect character of any secretions; note color, odor, amount, and consistency (e.g., thin and watery or thick and oily). Remove gloves.

Description of secretions helps to indicate whether infection is present or the wound is healing.

20 Assess condition of skin for pressure areas, paying particular attention to regions at risk for pressure (e.g., sacrum, greater trochanter, heels, occipital area, clavicles). If you see areas of redness, place fingertip over area and apply gentle pressure, then release. Look at skin color.

Normal reactive hyperemia (redness) is a visible effect of localized vasodilation, the body's normal response to lack of blood flow to underlying tissue. Affected area of skin will normally blanch with fingertip pressure. An exception is a stage I pressure ulcer, which will not blanch with pressure. If pressure is not relieved, tissue damage can occur in as little as 90 minutes because of tissue hypoxia (Chapter 22).

> **NURSE ALERT** With evidence of normal reactive hyperemia, reposition the client and develop a turning schedule if client is dependent (see Chapter 6).

21 When you detect a lesion, use adequate lighting to inspect color, location, texture, size, shape, and type (Box 12-8). Note also grouping (e.g., clustered or linear) and distribution (localized or generalized).

Observation of the lesion allows for accurate description and identification.

  a. Use gloves if lesion is moist or draining. Gently palpate any lesion to determine mobility, contour (flat, raised, or depressed), and consistency (soft or hard).

Gentle palpation prevents rupture of underlying cysts. Gloves reduce transmission of microorganisms.

  b. Note if client reports tenderness during palpation.

Tenderness may indicate inflammation or pressure on body part.

  c. Measure size of lesion (height, width, depth) with centimeter ruler.

Provides for baseline to assess changes in lesion over time.

22 With gloves still on, inspect and palpate intravenous (IV) site for evidence of inflammation (redness, heat, swelling, drainage, tenderness) or infiltration (puffiness, pallor, coolness). Note when site is due to be changed.

Agency policy will indicate how often tubing and site changes are performed to prevent infections. Presence of infiltration or phlebitis requires IV therapy to be discontinued (see Chapter 27).

23 Check the IV fluid and any added medications (apply six rights of medication administration). Note the type of fluids, rate of infusion, and expiration date of fluids and tubing.

Infusion rate that is too rapid may result in fluid volume excess (FVE); a rate too slow can result in inadequate fluid replacement. Changing the fluids and tubing according to agency policy helps prevent IV-related infections (Eggimann and others, 2002).

24 See Completion Protocol (inside front cover).

EVALUATION

1 Observe throughout the assessment for evidence of physical or emotional distress, which may alter assessment data.

2 Compare assessment findings with previous observations to identify changes.

3 Ask the client if there is information about physical condition that has not been discussed.

Unexpected Outcomes and Related Interventions

1 Client demonstrates acute distress such as shortness of breath, acute pain, or severe anxiety.

  a. Respond immediately by obtaining vital signs, reposition client with head of bed elevated, apply oxygen, or give medication as appropriate.

  b. Notify charge nurse or physician if orders are needed for relief of acute symptoms.

BOX 12-8 Types of Skin Lesions

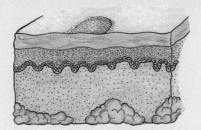

Macule: flat, nonpalpable, change in skin color, smaller than 1 cm (e.g., freckle, petechia)

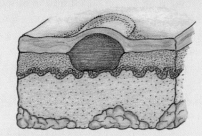

Papule: palpable, circumscribed, solid elevation in skin, smaller than 0.5 cm (e.g., elevated nevus)

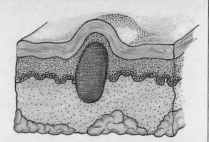

Nodule: elevated solid mass, deeper and firmer than papule, 0.5 to 2.0 cm (e.g., wart)

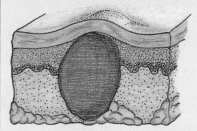

Tumor: solid mass that may extend deep through subcutaneous tissue, larger than 1 to 2 cm (e.g., epithelioma)

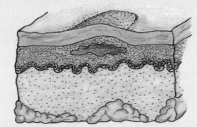

Wheal: irregularly shaped, elevated area or superficial localized edema, varies in size (e.g., hive, mosquito bite)

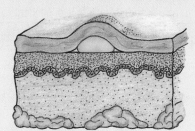

Vesicle: circumscribed elevation of skin filled with serous fluid, smaller than 0.5 cm (e.g., herpes simplex, chickenpox)

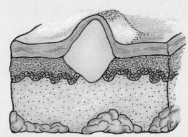

Pustule: circumscribed elevation of skin similar to vesicle but filled with pus, varies in size (e.g., acne, staphylococcal infection)

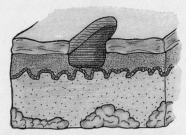

Ulcer: deep loss of skin surface that may extend to dermis and frequently bleeds and scars, varies in size (e.g., venous stasis ulcer)

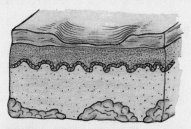

Atrophy: thinning of skin with loss of normal skin furrow with skin appearing shiny and translucent, varies in size (e.g., arterial insufficiency)

2 Client has abnormal skin condition (dry texture, reduced turgor, lesions, or erythema).

a. Identify contributing factors, and prevent continued irritation or damage as appropriate (see Chapter 22).

3 Client is unwilling or unable to provide adequate information relating to identified concerns.

a. Seek information from family members if present, and review client's record for baseline data.

Recording and Reporting

- Record client's vital signs on vital sign flow sheet.
- Document changes in LOC, mood, speech, and body movements on neurological flow sheet.

- Describe abnormal skin conditions, noting size, location, color, whether raised or indented, and presence or absence of drainage.
- Describe abnormal sensations such as pruritus, pain, or burning. Include specific location and record bilateral comparison. Include client's subjective descriptions of sensations (use client quotes). Determine if sensation changes are related to inappropriately applied therapy (e.g., cast or dressings).
- Report any skin breakdown and draining lesions to physician and/or clinical specialist.
- Record condition of IV site on IV flow sheet, including presence or absence of redness, tenderness, swelling, or leakage.

Sample Documentation

0830 Reports a "painful bottom." A 2-cm flat, round, erythematous area is noted on the sacrum. Area does not blanch following palpation. Skin integrity is intact with normal turgor. Repositioned to left side and will be repositioned every 2 hours.

Special Considerations
Pediatric Considerations

- Measurement of physical growth including height, weight, length, and head circumference are key elements in evaluation of a child's health status (Zuguo and others, 2004).
- Weigh infants nude. Children may be weighed in light underclothes or gown.
- A child's interactions with parents provide valuable information regarding the child's behavior.

Geriatric Considerations

- An older adult's presenting signs and symptoms can be deceiving. An older adult has a diminished physiological reserve that may mask the usual, or "classic," signs and symptoms of a disease. In older adults signs and symptoms are often blunted or atypical (Burke and Laramie, 2004).
- Postural hypotension is common in older clients. Vital signs should be checked in lying, sitting, and standing positions, especially when positional dizziness and light-headedness are reported.
- Common skin changes with aging include dryness, wrinkling, reduced elasticity, and "liver spots" in areas exposed to sun. Common lesions include seborrheic keratosis (pigmented macular-papular lesion that can be warty, scaly, or greasy); cherry angioma (bright ruby-red or purplish papular lesion); skin tags (soft pinkish-tan to light-brown pedunculated lesions); and senile lentigines (gray-brown irregular macular lesions on sun-exposed areas) (Burke and Laramie, 2004).
- Inspection of the feet is critically important in the presence of impaired circulation, impaired vision, and diabetes. Common podiatric conditions include ulceration, fungal infection, calluses, bunions, and plantar warts (Gareth, 2002).

Home Care Considerations

- In the home the focus may be on the client's ability to perform basic self-care tasks. Be sure that the home assessment builds on all health concerns identified in other settings.
- The home health nurse takes a small portable scale to monitor weight changes.
- Older adults may report problems with sense of smell during examination. Stress the importance of installing house smoke detectors and checking/dating food labels for possible spoilage.

Long-Term Care Considerations

- The Minimum Data Set (MDS) is a tool used for a comprehensive assessment of residents in long-term care settings. It provides a total picture of a resident and an ongoing comprehensive assessment of each resident, emphasizing functional ability and both a physical and psychosocial profile. Only a registered nurse (RN) can be the assessment coordinator. Contributions are made by licensed practical or vocational nurses (LPNs or LVNs), the dietary supervisor, social worker, recreational therapist, physical therapist, and occupational therapist (Tabloski, 2006).

SKILL 12.2   Assessing the Head and Neck

An examination of the head and neck includes assessment of the head, ears, eyes, nose, mouth, and sinuses. Assessment of the head and neck uses inspection, palpation, and auscultation, with inspection and palpation often used simultaneously.

ASSESSMENT

1 Assess for history of headache, dizziness, pain, or stiffness. *Rationale: Headaches and dizziness may be a sign of stress, a symptom of another underlying problem such as high blood pressure, or a result of injury.*

2 Determine if the client has a history of eye disease, diabetes, or hypertension. *Rationale: Common conditions predispose clients to visual alterations requiring physician referral.*

3 Ask if the client has experienced blurred vision, flashing lights, or reduced visual field. *Rationale: These common symptoms indicate visual problems..*

4 Ask if the client has experienced ear pain, itching, discharge, vertigo, tinnitus (ringing in the ears), or change in hearing. *Rationale: These signs and symptoms indicate infection or hearing loss.*

5 Review client's occupational history. *Rationale: Client's occupation can create a risk of injury, potential for eye fatigue, or prolonged noise exposure.*

6 Ask if the client has a history of allergies, nasal discharge, epistaxis (nosebleeds), or postnasal drip. *Rationale: History is useful in determining source of nasal and sinus drainage.*

7 Determine if the client smokes or chews tobacco. *Rationale: Tobacco users have greater risk for mouth and throat cancer (ACS, 2004).*

PLANNING

Expected Outcomes focus on identifying altera-tions in the head and neck.

1 Client will recognize warning signs and symptoms of eye, ear, sinus, and mouth disease.
2 Client will take appropriate safety precautions for occu-pational injury related to the head and neck.

Delegation Considerations

Assessment skills of the head and neck should not be delegated to AP. For clients with abnormal findings of the head and neck, instruct personnel to observe for nasal discharge and nasal bleeding and report all monitoring data to the nurse.

Equipment

- Stethoscope
- Clean gloves (use nonlatex if necessary)
- Tongue blade
- Pen light

IMPLEMENTATION *for Assessing the Head and Neck*

STEPS	RATIONALE
1 **See Standard Protocol (inside front cover).**	
2 Inspect the head.	
a. Note head position and facial features.	Head tilting to one side may indicate hearing or visual loss.
b. Note the client's facial features for symmetry.	Neurological disorders such as paralysis may affect the symmetry of the face.
3 Assess the eyes.	
a. Inspect position of eyes, color, condition of conjunctivae, and movement.	Asymmetrical positioning may reflect trauma or tumor growth. Differences in color may be congenital; changes in color of conjunctivae may be because of local infection or symptomatic of another abnormality (e.g., pale conjunctiva is associated with anemia).
b. Assess client's near vision (ability to read newspaper or magazines) and far vision (ability to follow movement or read clock, television, or signs at a distance).	If client has visual acuity or visual field loss, make adjustments to support self-care measures (e.g., feeding, bathing and hygiene, dressing) and teaching.

> **NURSE ALERT** Clients with visual field problems may be at risk for injury because they can-not see objects in front of them.

c. Inspect pupils for size, shape, and equality (see illustration).	Normal pupils are round, clear, and equal in size and shape.
d. Test pupillary reflexes. To test reaction to light, dim room light. As client looks straight ahead, move penlight from side of client's face and direct light on pupil. Observe pupillary response of both eyes (consensual response), noting briskness and equality of reflex (see illustrations).	

2 3 4 5 6 7 8 9

STEP 3c. Pupil size in millimeters.

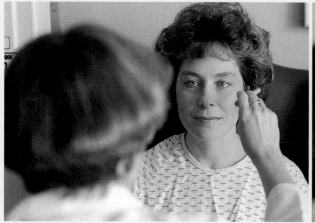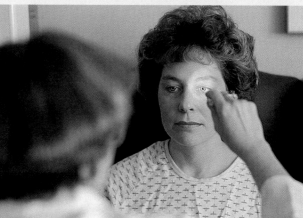

STEP 3d. A, To check pupil reflexes, first hold penlight to side of client's face. **B,** Illuminate pupil to cause pupil to constrict.

STEPS	RATIONALE

4 Assess hearing. Note client's response to questions and presence or use of a hearing aid. If hearing loss is suspected, ask client to repeat random numbers with two equally accented syllables (e.g., nine, four). Repeat, gradually increasing voice intensity until client correctly repeats the numbers.

Seidel and others (2006) report that clients normally hear numbers clearly when whispered, responding correctly at least 50% of the time. For client with obvious hearing impairment, speak clearly and concisely, stand so that client can see face, and speak toward client's good ear, using a low pitch, and without yelling.

> **NURSE ALERT** If hearing deficit is present, have a qualified nurse inspect client's ears because impaired hearing may be caused by impacted cerumen, external otitis, or swelling in ear canal because of allergic reaction to material in hearing aid.

5 Assess the sinuses. If there is nasal discharge, assess color, amount, odor, and associated symptoms (e.g., sneezing, nasal congestion, mouth breathing).

Helps to rule out the presence of infection, allergy, or drug use.

6 In clients with a nasogastric (NG), nasointestinal (NI), or nasotracheal (NT) tube, inspect the nares for excoriation or inflammation. Stabilize tube as needed.

Swallowing or coughing reflex causes movement of tubes against nares, and pressure against tissues and mucosa can result in tissue erosion.

7 Assess the mouth. Use a tongue blade to depress the tongue and inspect the oral mucosa, tongue, teeth, and gums for hydration, discoloration, and obvious lesions (see illustration). Determine if client wears dentures or retainers and if they are comfortable. You may remove dentures to visualize and palpate gums.

Tongue blade retracts tongue and inside of mouth for better visualization. Ill-fitting dentures and retainers chronically irritate mucosa and gums and may pose a risk for mouth cancer.

8 Inspect and palpate the neck. Ask the client if there is a history of neck pain or difficulty with movement of the neck.

This determines that all neck structures are present, including neck muscles, lymph nodes of the head and neck, thyroid gland, and trachea. May indicate muscle strain, head injury, local nerve injury, or swollen lymph nodes.

a. Neck muscles: Inspect neck for bilateral symmetry of muscles. Ask client to flex and hyperextend neck and turn head side to side.

Detects muscle weakness, strain, and range of motion (ROM).

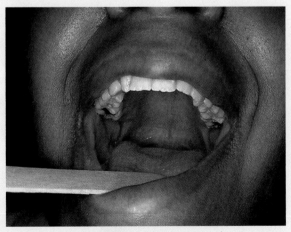

STEP 7 Inspect mouth.

STEPS	RATIONALE

b. Lymph nodes:
   (1) With client's chin raised and head tilted slightly, inspect area where lymph nodes are distributed and compare both sides (see illustration).

Lymph nodes may be enlarged from infection or from various diseases such as cancer.

   (2) To examine lymph nodes, have client relax with neck flexed slightly forward. To palpate, face or stand to the side of client and use pads of middle three fingers of hand. Palpate gently in a rotary motion for superficial lymph nodes (see illustration).

This position relaxes tissues and muscles.

   (3) Note if lymph nodes are large, fixed, inflamed, or tender.

Large, fixed, inflamed, or tender lymph nodes indicate local infection, systemic disease, or neoplasm.

9 **See Completion Protocol (inside front cover).**

STEP 8b.(1) Lymphatic drainage system of the head and neck. If the group of nodes is often referred to by another name, the second name appears in parentheses. (From Seidel HM and others: *Mosby's guide to physical examination*, ed 5, St Louis, 2003, Mosby.)

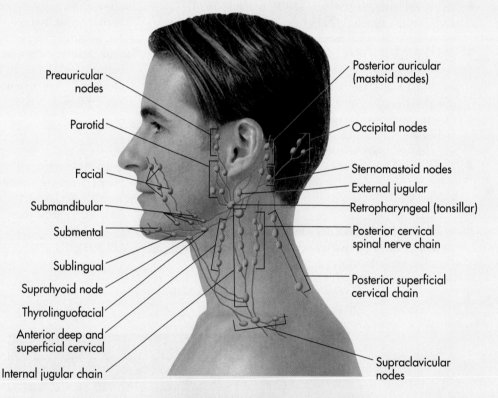

Preauricular nodes
Parotid
Facial
Submandibular
Submental
Sublingual
Suprahyoid node
Thyrolinguofacial
Anterior deep and superficial cervical
Internal jugular chain

Posterior auricular (mastoid nodes)
Occipital nodes
Sternomastoid nodes
External jugular
Retropharyngeal (tonsillar)
Posterior cervical spinal nerve chain
Posterior superficial cervical chain
Supraclavicular nodes

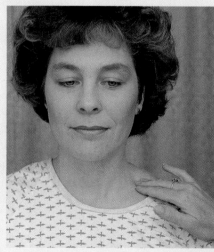

STEP 8b.(2) Palpation of cervical lymph nodes.

EVALUATION

1 Compare assessment with previous observations to identify changes.

2 Ask the client to describe common symptoms of eye, ear, sinus, or mouth disease.

3 Ask the client to list occupational safety precautions.

Unexpected Outcomes and Related Interventions

1 Client demonstrates yellow nasal discharge, sneezing, and complaint of sinus pain.

a. Reposition into semi-Fowler's or other comfortable position to relieve sinus pain.

b. Monitor temperature for fever.

c. Notify physician if these are new findings.

2 Client complains of severe headache and dizziness when standing.

a. Respond immediately by obtaining vital signs, especially blood pressure.

b. Return client to bed in position of comfort to minimize dizziness and relieve headache.

c. Identify contributing factors (stress, pain, or elevated blood pressure).

d. Notify physician.

Recording and Reporting

• Record any abnormal findings such as hearing or visual loss, pain and its location, and current infection in nurses' notes or flow sheet.

• If client has a sinus infection and mucus is purulent, consult with physician about obtaining a specimen if appropriate (see Chapter 13). Record amount, color, consistency, and odor of mucus.

• Report increased headache, dizziness, or visual changes immediately to charge nurse or physician.

Sample Documentation

1200 Copious, green, thick nasal discharge noted. Complains of frontal "headache." Blood pressure 110/70. Head of bed raised to 60 degrees. Physician notified.

Special Considerations
Pediatric Considerations

• Infants may resist eye examination by closing eyes. Holding them in an upright position over their caregivers' shoulders may cause eyes to open (Ball and Bindler, 2006).

• Any problems with ocular alignment or visual impairment requires immediate referral to a pediatrician or pediatric ophthalmologist (American Academy of Pediatrics, 2003).

• Headaches in children are usually caused by loss of sleep, poor nutrition, eye fatigue, and allergies. Children as young as 3 years of age can develop severe migraine headaches, but the symptoms are vague and difficult to diagnose (Rosenblum and others, 2001).

Geriatric Considerations

• Older adults commonly have loss of peripheral vision caused by changes in the lens.

• Instruct clients older than age 65 to have regular hearing checks.

• Measurement of visual acuity helps determine level of assistance client requires with daily living activities and ability of client to safely ambulate and function independently within home.

SKILL 12.3 Assessing the Thorax and Lungs

Assessment of respiratory function is one of the most critical assessment skills because alterations can be life threatening. Routine assessment is essential; changes in respirations or breath sounds can occur quickly as a result of a variety of factors, including immobility, infection, and fluid overload. Assessment includes auscultation, which assesses the movement of air through the tracheobronchial tree. Recognizing the sounds created by normal airflow allows you to detect sounds caused by obstruction of the airways. Auscultation of the lungs requires familiarity with landmarks of the chest (Figure 12-3). During the assessment, keep a mental image of the location of the lung lobes. To locate the position of each rib, locate the angle of Louis by palpating the "speed bump" on the sternum where the second rib connects with the sternum. Count the ribs and intercostal spaces from this point. Auscultation involves listening to breath sounds using a stethoscope; the sounds are best heard when the person breathes deeply through the mouth.

Adventitious sounds (abnormal sounds) result from air passing through fluid, mucus, or narrowed airways; alveoli suddenly reinflating; or an inflammation between the pleural linings. The four types of adventitious sounds include crackles (rales), gurgles (rhonchi), wheezes, and pleural friction rubs (Table 12-3). Note the location and characteristics of the sounds, as well as diminished breath sounds or the absence of breath sounds (found with collapsed or surgically removed lobes).

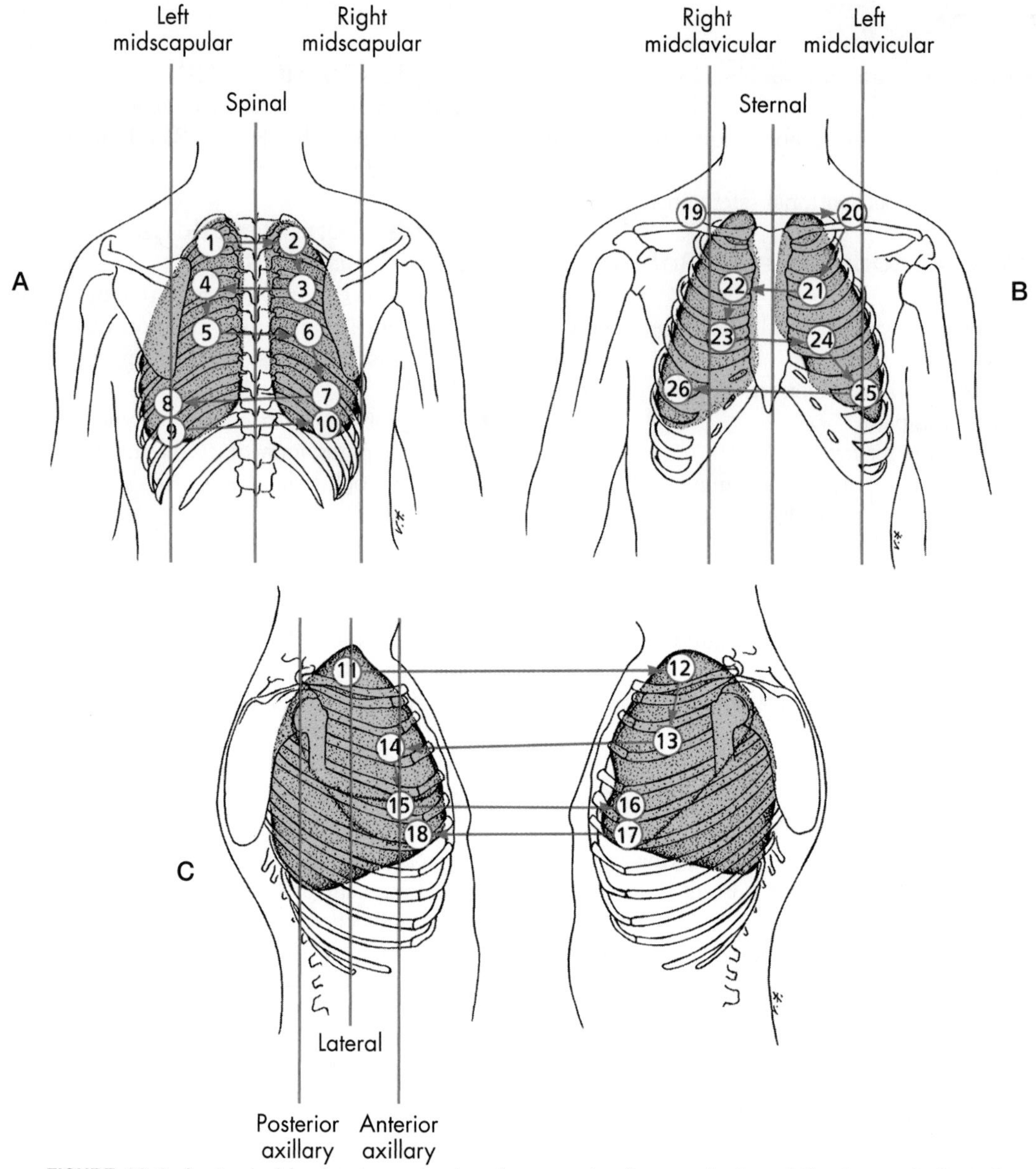

Left midscapular
Right midscapular
Spinal

A

Right midclavicular
Left midclavicular
Sternal

B

C

Lateral

Posterior axillary
Anterior axillary

FIGURE 12-3 Anatomical landmarks and order of progression for examination of the thorax. **A,** Posterior thorax. **B,** Anterior thorax. **C,** Lateral thorax.

ASSESSMENT

1 Assess history of tobacco or marijuana use, including type of tobacco, duration of use, and amount in pack years. Pack years equal number of years smoking times the number of packs per day (e.g., 4 years times ½ pack per day equals 2 pack years). If client has quit, determine the length of time since smoking stopped. *Rationale: Smoking is a risk factor linked with the incidence of lung cancer, heart disease, and chronic lung disease (emphysema and chronic bronchitis) and responsible for 87% of all lung cancers in the United States (ACS, 2004).*

2 Ask if client experiences any of the following: persistent cough (productive or nonproductive), sputum production, chest pain, shortness of breath, orthopnea, dyspnea during exertion, activity intolerance, or recurrent attacks of pneumonia or bronchitis. *Rationale: Warning signs of lung cancer include persistent cough, bloody sputum, and recurrent lung infections.*

3 Check for history of allergies to pollens, dust, or other airborne irritants, as well as to any foods, drugs, or chemical substances. Determine if client works in environment containing pollutants such as asbestos, coal dust, or chemical irritants. Does client have exposure to secondhand cigarette smoke? *Rationale: Clients with chronic respiratory disease, particularly asthma, have symptoms aggravated by change in temperature and humidity, irritating fumes or smoke, emotional stress, and physical exertion. Allergic response may be associated with wheezes on auscultation, dyspnea, cyanosis, and diaphoresis.*

4 Review history for known or suspected human immunodeficiency virus (HIV) infection, substance abuse, low

TABLE 12-3   Adventitious Sounds

SOUND	SITE AUSCULTATED	CAUSE	CHARACTER
Crackles (also called rales)	Are most commonly heard in dependent lobes: right and left lung bases	Random, sudden reinflation of groups of alveoli	Are fine, short, interrupted crackling sounds heard during inspiration, expiration, or both; vary in pitch: high or low; may or may not change with coughing*; sound like crushing cellophane
Rhonchi	Are primarily heard over trachea and bronchi; if loud enough, can be heard over most lung fields	Fluid or mucus in larger airways, causing turbulence	Are low-pitched, continuous sounds heard more during expiration; may be cleared by coughing; sounds like blowing air through milk with a straw
Wheezes	Can be heard over all lung fields	Severely narrowed bronchus	Are high-pitched, musical sounds heard during inspiration or expiration; do not clear with coughing
Pleural friction rub	Is heard best over anterior lateral lung field (if client is sitting upright)	Inflamed pleura, parietal pleura rubbing against visceral pleura	Has grating quality heard best during inspiration; does not clear with coughing

Data from Seidel HM and others: *Mosby's guide to physical examination,* ed 6, St Louis, 2006, Mosby.

income, and residence in nursing home. *Rationale: Known risk factors for exposure to and/or development of tuberculosis (TB).*

5 Ask if client has history of cough, hemoptysis (bloody sputum), weight loss, fatigue, night sweats, and/or fever. *Rationale: Signs and symptoms for both TB and HIV infection.*

6 Review family history for cancer, TB, allergies, or chronic obstructive pulmonary disease (COPD). *Rationale: Reveals family or genetic predisposition for the development of respiratory problems.*

PLANNING

Expected Outcomes focus on identifying alterations in respiratory function.

1 Respirations are passive, diaphragmatic or costal, and regular (12 to 20 breaths per minute in adult) with symmetrical expansion.

2 Breath sounds are clear to auscultation in all lung fields.

Delegation Considerations

The skill of assessing the lungs and thorax should not be delegated to AP. Reporting respiratory distress, difficulty breathing, and changes in rate and depth, as well as measuring the client's respirations after respirations are stabilized, may be delegated.

- In clients with respiratory difficulty, instruct personnel to keep head of bed elevated for client to breathe and report any changes to the nurse.

Equipment

- Stethoscope

IMPLEMENTATION *for Assessing the Thorax and Lungs*

STEPS	RATIONALE

1   **See Standard Protocol (inside front cover).**

2   Position client sitting upright. For bedridden client, elevate head of bed 45 to 90 degrees.

Promotes full lung expansion during examination.

a.   If client is unable to tolerate sitting, use the supine position or side-lying position.

Clients with chronic respiratory disease may need to sit up throughout the examination because of shortness of breath. Assistance of another caregiver may be required to position unresponsive clients.

b.   Remove gown or drape first from posterior chest, keeping front of chest and legs covered. As examination progresses, remove gown from area being examined.

Avoids unnecessary exposure and provides full visibility of thorax. Allows direct placement of diaphragm or bell of stethoscope on client's skin, which enhances clarity of sounds.

c.   Explain all steps of procedure, encouraging client to relax and breathe normally through the mouth.

Anxiety may alter respiratory function. Breathing through the mouth decreases extraneous sounds from air passing through the nose.

3   *Posterior thorax:*

a.   If possible, stand behind client to inspect thorax for shape, deformities, position of the spine, slope of the ribs, retraction of intercostal spaces during inspiration, and bulging of intercostal spaces during expiration.

Allows for identification of any factors that may impair chest expansion and any symptoms of respiratory distress. In a child, shape of chest is almost circular, with anteroposterior (AP) diameter in 1:1 ratio. In adult, chest is twice as wide as deep, with 2:1 lateral to anterior/posterior diameter. Chronic lung disease results in 1:1 ratio. This is referred to as a "barrel chest." Clients with breathing problems assume postures that improve ventilation.

> **NURSE ALERT** Localized chest pain may be evidenced by the client holding the chest wall during breathing. Assess the nature of pain, including onset, severity, precipitating factors, quality, region, and radiation.

---

b.   Determine the rate and rhythm of breathing. Have client relaxed.

This is a good time to count respirations, with client relaxed and unaware of inspection. Awareness could alter respirations.

c.   Systematically palpate posterior chest wall, costal spaces, and intercostal spaces, noting any masses, pulsations, unusual movement, or areas of localized tenderness (see Figure 12-3, A, for numbered areas to systematically palpate). If suspicious mass or swollen area is detected, palpate for size, shape, and typical qualities of lesion. Do not palpate painful areas deeply.

Palpation assesses further characteristics and confirms or supplements findings from assessment. Localized swelling or tenderness may indicate trauma to ribs or underlying cartilage. A fractured rib fragment could be displaced.

d.   Standing behind client, place thumbs along the spinal processes at the tenth rib, with the palms lightly contacting the posterolateral surfaces (see illustration A). The nurse's thumbs should be about 2 inches (5 cm) apart, with the thumbs pointing toward the spine and the fingers pointing laterally. Press hands toward client's spine to form small skinfold between thumbs. After exhalation, client takes deep breath. Note movement of thumbs (see illustration B), and note symmetry of chest wall movement. Normally thumbs separate 1½ to 2 inches (3 to 5 cm) during chest excursion.

Palpation of chest excursion assesses depth of client's breathing. This technique is a good measure to evaluate client's ability to perform deep breathing exercises (see Chapter 29). Limited movement on one side may indicate that client is voluntarily splinting during ventilation because of pain. Avoid allowing the hands to slide over the skin, which gives a false measure of excursion.

STEPS	RATIONALE
e. Auscultate breath sounds. Have client take slow deep breaths with the mouth slightly open. For adult, place diaphragm of stethoscope firmly on chest wall over intercostal spaces (see illustration). Listen to entire inspiration and expiration at each stethoscope position (see Figure 12-3, A). Systematically compare breath sounds over right and left sides. If sounds are faint, ask client to breathe a little deeper temporarily.	Assesses movement of air through tracheobronchial tree (Table 12-4). Recognition of normal airflow sounds allows detection of sounds caused by mucus or airway obstruction. Sounds are characterized by length of inspiratory and expiratory phases. Gurgles (rhonchi) caused by fluid or mucus in larger airways can be diminished or eliminated by effective coughing. Crackles (rales) and wheezes do not change with coughing.
f. If you auscultate adventitious sounds, have client cough. Listen again with stethoscope to determine if sound has cleared with coughing (see Table 12-3).	Coughing may clear adventitious sound.
4 *Lateral thorax:*	
a. Instruct client to raise arms, and inspect chest wall for same characteristics as reviewed for posterior chest.	Improves access to lateral thoracic structures. Allows for location of abnormalities in lateral lung fields.
b. Extend palpation and auscultation of posterior thorax to lateral sides of chest, except for excursion measurement (see Figure 12-3, C).	Locates abnormalities in lateral lung fields.
5 *Anterior thorax:*	
a. Inspect accessory muscles of breathing: sternocleidomastoid, trapezius, and abdominal muscles, noting effort to breathe.	Extent to which accessory muscles are used reveals degree of effort to breathe. Generally these muscles are not used for breathing.

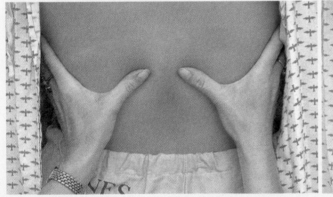 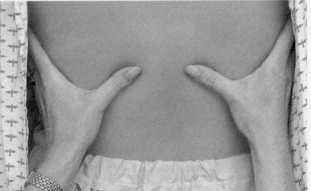

STEP 3d. A, Position of hands for palpation of posterior thorax excursion. **B,** As client inhales, movement of chest excursion separates nurse's thumbs.

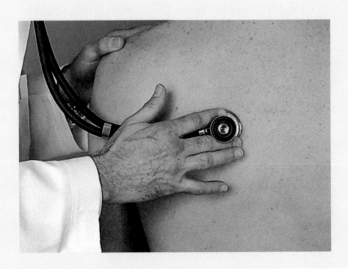

STEP 3e. Use of diaphragm of stethoscope to auscultate breath sounds. (From Seidel HM and others: *Mosby's guide to physical examination,* ed 5, St Louis, 2003, Mosby.)

STEPS	RATIONALE
b. Inspect width or spread of angle made by costal margins and tip of sternum. Angle is usually larger than 90 degrees between margins.	Indicates congenital, acquired, or traumatic alterations that may influence client's chest expansion.
c. Observe the client's breathing pattern, observing symmetry and degree of chest wall and abdominal movement. Respiratory rate and rhythm are more often assessed on the anterior chest wall.	Assesses client's effort to breathe: symmetrical, passive movement indicates no respiratory distress.
d. Palpate anterior thoracic muscles and ribs for lumps, masses, tenderness, or unusual movement.	Localized swelling or tenderness may indicate trauma to underlying ribs or cartilage.
e. Palpate anterior chest excursion. Place hands over each lateral rib cage, with thumbs approximately 2 inches (5 cm) apart and angled along each costal margin. As client inhales deeply, thumbs should normally separate approximately 1½ to 2 inches (3 to 5 cm), with each side expanding equally.	Assesses depth of client's breathing and ability to perform deep breathing exercises. Certain abnormalities are evident if expansion is not symmetrical.
f. With client sitting, auscultate anterior thorax. Begin above the clavicles, and move across and then down (see Figure 12-3, B).	A systematic pattern of assessment comparing sides helps identify abnormal sounds.
6 See Completion Protocol (inside front cover).	

TABLE 12-4 Normal Breath Sounds

TYPE	DESCRIPTION	LOCATION	ORIGIN
Bronchial	Loud and high-pitched sounds with hollow quality. Expiration lasts longer than inspiration (3:2 ratio).	Best heard over trachea	Created by air moving through trachea close to chest wall
Bronchovesicular	Medium-pitched and blowing sounds of medium intensity. Inspiratory phase is equal to expiratory phase.	Best heard posteriorly between scapulae and anteriorly over bronchioles lateral to sternum at first and second intercostal spaces	Created by air moving through large airways
Vesicular	Soft, breezy, low-pitched sounds. Inspiratory phase is 3 times longer than expiratory phase.	Best heard over lung's periphery (except over scapula)	Created by air moving through smaller airways

EVALUATION

1 Compare respiratory findings (depth, regularity, and breath sounds) with findings of previous shift to identify changes.

2 Have client identify factors leading to lung disease.

Unexpected Outcomes and Related Interventions

1 Client demonstrates hypoventilation, cyanosis, and/or altered LOC.

a. Stay with the client and call for help.

b. Position client in semi-Fowler's or other comfortable position.

c. Consult physician about need to initiate oxygen therapy.

d. Monitor vital signs.

e. Notify physician; arterial blood gases (ABGs) may need to be drawn for blood gas analysis.

2 Client has copious mucus production, audible inspiratory wheezing, or congested cough with thick, tenacious mucus.

a. Assist client to cough by splinting chest; teach to inhale slowly through nose, exhale, and cough; encourage expectoration of sputum.

b. Auscultate breath sounds before and after cough to evaluate cough effectiveness.

c. Encourage increased fluid intake (if permitted).

d. If unable to clear airway by coughing, suctioning is indicated (see Chapter 29).

e. Monitor vital signs.

f. Notify physician.

3 Client demonstrates weakness, fatigue, dyspnea, altered vital signs, or dizziness with exertion.

a. Provide bed rest and limited activity to conserve oxygen.

b. Assess response to activity.

c. Plan interventions alternately with periods of rest.

d. Monitor for restlessness, anxiety, confusion, and respiratory status.

Recording and Reporting

- Record in nurses' notes or on flow sheet the client's respiratory rate and character; adventitious breath sounds, including type, location, and presence on inspiration, expiration, or both; and changes noted after coughing.
- If client has a productive cough and mucus is purulent, obtain order for a specimen (see Chapter 13). Record amount, color, consistency, and odor of mucus.
- Report increased dyspnea and acute respiratory distress immediately to nurse in charge or physician.

Sample Documentation

0730 Inspiratory wheezing noted over anterior upper lobes bilaterally. Respirations 26 and regular. C/O shortness of breath even at rest. Head of bed raised to 90 degrees. M.D. notified.

Special Considerations
Pediatric Considerations

- Infants and young children have thin chest walls, allowing breath sounds from one lung to be heard over entire chest (Ball and Bindler, 2006).
- Children younger than 7 years of age normally exhibit noticeable abdominal or diaphragmatic movement. Older children and adults exhibit more costal or thoracic movement. Use stethoscope bell to auscultate breath sounds in children. Breath sounds are louder in children because of their thin chest walls.
- In children, observe for use of accessory muscles, which is a sign of respiratory distress and may involve intercostal, suprasternal, supraclavicular, or sternal muscles (Hockenberry and Wilson, 2007).
- Head bobbing and nasal flaring are signs of significant respiratory distress in infants (Hockenberry and Wilson, 2007).

Geriatric Considerations

- Older adults have a costal angle (anteriorly) of slightly less than 90 degrees. The AP diameter may be increased from kyphosis.
- In older adults, chest expansion is reduced because of calcification of rib cartilage and partial contraction of inspiratory muscles.
- Older adults should be vaccinated against the flu in the early fall (Burke and Laramie, 2004).

SKILL 12.4 Cardiovascular Assessment

A client who presents with signs or symptoms of heart (cardiac) problems, such as chest pain, may be suffering a life-threatening condition requiring immediate attention. In this situation the nurse must act quickly and decide on the portions of the examination that are absolutely necessary. When a client's condition is stable, a more thorough assessment can reveal baseline heart function and any risks for heart disease. Clients tend to seek information about heart disease because it remains a leading cause of death in the United States. The heart, neck vessels, and peripheral circulation are assessed together because the systems work together.

Inadequate tissue perfusion results in an inadequate delivery of oxygen and nutrients to cells, a condition called ischemia. This is caused by constriction of the vessels or by occlusion (blockage) from clot formation. The effects of the ischemia depend on the duration of the problem and the metabolic needs of the tissues. Ischemia results in pain. If lack of oxygen to tissues is unrelieved, tissue necrosis (death) occurs. An embolus is a blood clot that breaks loose and travels through the circulation. If the clot obstructs circulation to the lungs or the brain, it can be life threatening. The nurse's assessment can determine the integrity of the circulatory system.

The nurse assesses the heart after examining the lungs because the client is already in a suitable position with the chest exposed. Assessment then proceeds to the neck vessels and ends with the peripheral circulation. The nurse uses inspection, palpation, auscultation, and percussion during the examination.

ASSESSMENT

1 Assess client for history of smoking, alcohol intake, caffeine intake (coffee, tea, soft drinks, chocolate), use of "recreational" drugs, exercise habits, and dietary patterns and intake. *Rationale: These can contribute to risk factors for cardiovascular disease. Additionally, caffeine and alcohol may cause tachycardia.*

2 Determine if client is taking medications for cardiovascular function (e.g., antiarrhythmics, antihypertensives, antianginals) and if client knows their purpose, dosage, and side effects. *Rationale: Allows you to assess client's compliance with and understanding of drug therapies. Medications for cardiovascular function cannot be taken intermittently.*

3 Ask if client has experienced dyspnea, chest pain or discomfort, palpitations, excess fatigue, cough, leg pain or cramps, edema of the feet, cyanosis, fainting, or orthopnea. Ask if symptoms occur at rest or during exercise. *Rationale: These are the cardinal symptoms of heart disease. Cardiovascular function may be adequate during rest but not during exercise.*

4 If client reports chest pain, determine onset (sudden or gradual), precipitating factors, quality, region, severity, and if pain radiates. Anginal pain is usually a deep pressure or ache that is substernal and diffuse, radiating to one or both arms, neck, or jaw. *Rationale: Symptoms may reveal acute coronary syndrome or coronary artery disease (CAD).*

5 Assess family history for heart disease, diabetes, high cholesterol levels, hypertension, stroke, or rheumatic heart disease. *Rationale: Family history of these conditions increases risk for heart and vascular disease.*

6 Ask client about a history of heart trouble (e.g., heart failure, congenital heart disease, CAD, hypertension, diabetes), heart surgery, or vascular disease (hypertension, phlebitis, varicose veins). *Rationale: Knowledge reveals client's level of understanding of condition. A preexisting condition influences the examination techniques to use and the expected findings.*

7 Ask if client experiences leg cramps, numbness or tingling in extremities, sensation of cold hands or feet, or pain in legs. Also determine if client has noted any swelling or cyanosis of feet, ankles, or hands. *Rationale: These are common signs and symptoms of peripheral vascular disease.*

8 If client experiences leg pain or cramping in lower extremities, ask if it is relieved or aggravated by walking or standing for long periods or occurs during sleep. *Rationale: Relationship of symptoms to exercise can help determine if problem is vascular or musculoskeletal. Musculoskeletal pain is not usually relieved when exercise ends.*

PLANNING

Expected Outcomes focus on identifying alterations in cardiovascular function.

1 Heart is in normal sinus rhythm (NSR) with rate from 60 to 100 beats per minute (adolescent through adult), without extra sounds or murmurs.

2 Point of maximal impulse (PMI) is palpable at fifth intercostal space at left midclavicular line in children older than age 7 and in adults (Figure 12-4). PMI is at fourth intercostal space at left midclavicular line in children younger than age 7 (Hockenberry and Wilson, 2007) (Figure 12-5).

3 Client describes changes in own behavior that may improve cardiovascular function.

4 Client describes schedule, dosage, purpose, and benefits of medications being taken for cardiovascular function.

5 Blood pressure is within normal limits for client (see Chapter 11).

6 Carotid pulse is localized, strong, elastic, and equal bilaterally. No change occurs during inspiration or expiration and without carotid bruit. This indicates a patent vessel.

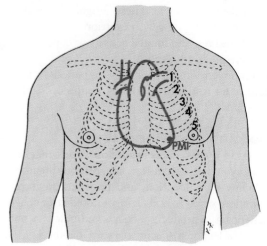

FIGURE 12-4 Location of PMI in adult.

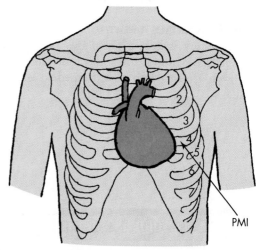

FIGURE 12-5 Location of PMI in child younger than 7 years old. (From Hockenberry MJ and Wilson D: *Wong's nursing care of infants and children,* ed 8, St Louis, 2007, Mosby.)

7 Venous pressure is normal, with jugular veins distended when client lies supine and flattened when client is in sitting position.

8 Peripheral pulses are equal and strong (2+), extremities are warm and pink, with capillary refill less than 2 seconds. There is no dependent edema. Peripheral hair growth is normal, and the skin is free of lesions.

Delegation Considerations

Comprehensive cardiovascular assessment should not be delegated to AP. You may delegate counting the apical and peripheral pulses if the client is stable. Assessment of peripheral pulse is important in specialty areas such as vascular surgery and orthopedics. The nurse instructs personnel to:

• Recognize skin temperature and color changes of affected extremities along with changes in peripheral pulses and report any changes to the nurse.

Equipment
- Stethoscope
- Doppler stethoscope (optional)
- Conducting gel (if a Doppler stethoscope is used)

IMPLEMENTATION *for Cardiovascular Assessment*

STEPS	RATIONALE
1 **See Standard Protocol (inside front cover).**	
2 Assist client to be as relaxed and comfortable as possible.	An anxious or uncomfortable client can have mild tachycardia, which will confound findings.
3 Have client assume semi-Fowler's or supine position.	Provides adequate visibility and access to left thorax and mediastinum. Client with heart disease often experiences shortness of breath while lying flat.
4 Explain procedure. Avoid facial gestures reflecting concern.	Client with previously normal cardiac history may become anxious if you show concern.
5 Be sure that room is quiet.	Subtle, low-pitched heart sounds are difficult to hear.
6 Assess the heart.	
a. Form a mental image of the exact location of the heart (see illustration). The base of the heart is the upper portion, and the apex is the bottom tip. The surface of the right ventricle composes most of the heart's anterior surface.	Visualization improves ability to assess findings accurately and determine possible source of abnormalities.
b. Find the angle of Louis, felt as a ridge in the sternum approximately 2 inches (5 cm) below the suprasternal notch (between the sternal body and manubrium). Slip fingers down each side of angle to feel adjacent ribs. The intercostal spaces are just below each rib.	Provides examiner with landmarks for locating and assessing heart sounds.
c. Find the following anatomical landmarks (see illustration for Step 6a):	Familiarity with landmarks allows you to describe findings more clearly and ultimately may improve assessment.
(1) The aortic area is at the second intercostal space, right of the sternum *(1)*.	
(2) The pulmonic area is at the second intercostal space, left of the sternum *(2)*.	
(3) The second pulmonic area is found by moving down left side of sternum to third intercostal space *(3)*, also referred to as Erb's point.	

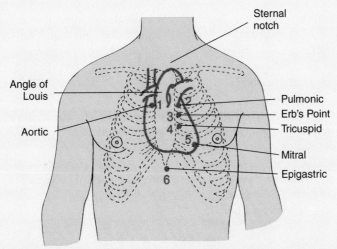

STEP 6a. Anatomical sites for assessment of cardiac function.

STEPS	RATIONALE

(4) The tricuspid area *(4)* is located at the fourth left intercostal space along the sternum.

(5) The mitral area is found by moving fingers laterally to client's left to locate fifth intercostal space at left midclavicular line *(5)*.

(6) The epigastric area *(6)* is at the inferior tip of the sternum.

d. Stand to the client's right, and look first at the precordium with the client supine. Note any visible pulsations and more exaggerated lifts. Inspect closely at the area of the apex.

May reveal size and symmetry of the heart. The apical impulse may be visible at the midclavicular line in the fifth intercostal space. The apical impulse (PMI) may become visible only when the client sits up, bringing the heart closer to the anterior wall. It is easily obscured by obesity.

e. Locate the PMI by palpating with fingertips along fifth intercostal space in midclavicular line. Note a light, brief pulsation in an area ½ to 1 inch (1 to 2 cm) in diameter at the apex.

In the presence of serious heart disease, the PMI will be located to the left of the midclavicular line related to enlarged left ventricle. In chronic lung disease the PMI may be to the right of the midclavicular line as a result of enlarged right ventricle.

NURSE ALERT A stronger than expected impulse may be a heave or lift, which may indicate increased cardiac output or left ventricular hypertrophy.

---

f. If palpating PMI is difficult, turn client onto left side.

Maneuver moves the heart closer to the chest wall.

g. Inspect the epigastric area, and palpate the abdominal aorta. Note a localized strong beat.

Rules out reduced blood flow or diffuse pulse, which may indicate a number of abnormalities.

h. Auscultate heart sounds. Begin by having client sit up and lean slightly forward; then have client lie supine; and end the examination with client in a left lateral recumbent position (see illustrations). In a female client it may be necessary to lift the left breast to hear heart sounds more effectively.

Different positions help to clarify type of sounds heard. Sitting position is best to hear high-pitched murmurs (if present). Supine is common position to hear all sounds. Left lateral recumbent is best position to hear low-pitched sounds.

(1) While auscultating sounds, ask client not to speak but to breathe comfortably. Begin with the diaphragm of the stethoscope; then alternate with the bell. Use very light pressure for the bell. Inch the stethoscope along; avoid jumping from one area to another. Do not try to hear all heart sounds at once.

Auscultation requires the examiner to isolate each heart sound at all auscultation sites.

(2) Begin at the apex or PMI; move systematically to the aortic area, pulmonic area, Erb's point, tricuspid area, and mitral area (see illustration for Step 6a). (NOTE: Some examiners use reverse sequence.) S$_1$ is best heard at the apex and is simultaneous with the carotid pulse.

At normal slow rates S$_1$ is high pitched and dull in quality and sounds like "lub." This sound precedes the systolic phase of heart contraction.

(3) Listen for S$_2$ at each site. This sound is best heard at the aortic area. Heart sounds will vary by pitch, loudness, and duration, depending on the auscultatory site.

Normal sounds S$_1$ and S$_2$ are high pitched and best heard with diaphragm. S$_2$ precedes the diastolic phase and sounds like "dub."

(4) After both sounds are heard clearly as "lub-dub," count each combination of S$_1$ and S$_2$ as one heartbeat. Count the number of beats for 1 minute.

Determines apical pulse rate.

STEPS	RATIONALE

(5) Assess heart rhythm by noting the time between S_1 and S_2 (systole) and then the time between S_2 and the next S_1 (diastole). Listen to the full cycle at each auscultation area. Note regular intervals between each sequence of beats. There should be a distinct pause between S_1 and S_2.

Failure of heart to beat at regular intervals is an arrhythmia, which interferes with heart's ability to pump effectively.

(6) When heart rate is irregular, compare apical and radial pulses (Table 12-5). Auscultate the apical pulse, and then immediately palpate the radial pulse. A colleague can assess the radial pulse while the nurse assesses the apical pulse.

Determines if a pulse deficit (radial pulse is slower than apical) exists. Deficit indicates that ineffective contractions of the heart fail to send pulse waves to the periphery.

7 Assess neck vessels.

a. To assess carotid arteries, have client remain in sitting position.

Allows easier mobility of neck to expose artery for inspection and palpation.

b. Inspect neck on both sides for obvious arterial pulsations. Ask client to turn head slightly away from artery being examined. Sometimes pulse wave can be seen.

Carotids are the only sites to assess quality of pulse wave. Experience is required to evaluate wave in relation to events of cardiac cycle.

c. Palpate each carotid artery separately with index and middle fingers around medial edge of sternocleidomastoid muscle. Ask client to raise chin slightly, keeping the head straight (see illustration). Note rate and rhythm, strength, and elasticity of artery. Also note if the pulse changes as client inspires and expires.

If both arteries were occluded simultaneously, client could lose consciousness from reduced circulation to brain. Turning head improves access to artery. Change during respiratory cycle may indicate a sinus arrhythmia.

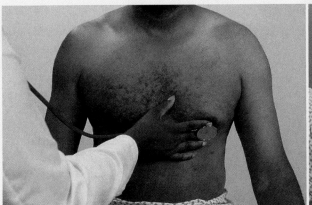
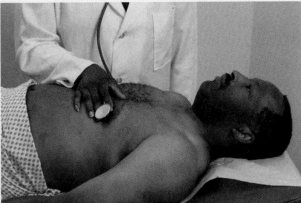
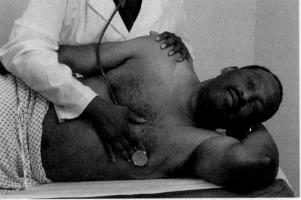

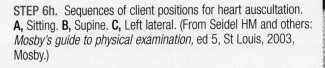

STEP 6h. Sequences of client positions for heart auscultation. **A,** Sitting. **B,** Supine. **C,** Left lateral. (From Seidel HM and others: *Mosby's guide to physical examination,* ed 5, St Louis, 2003, Mosby.)

STEPS	RATIONALE

> **NURSE ALERT** Do not vigorously palpate or massage the artery. Stimulation of carotid sinus may cause a reflex drop in heart rate and blood pressure.

d. Place bell of stethoscope over each carotid artery, auscultating for blowing sound (bruit) (see illustration). Ask client to hold breath for a few heartbeats so the respiratory sounds will not interfere with auscultation (Seidel and others, 2006).

Narrowing of carotid artery's lumen by arteriosclerotic plaques causes disturbance in blood flow. Blood passing through narrowed section creates turbulence and emits blowing or swishing sound.

e. To assess jugular venous pressure, position client supine and raise head of bed or place pillows so client's head is raised 45 degrees. Observe for level of venous filling and visible jugular pulsation (see illustration) and measure between highest point of jugular pulsation and angle of Louis.

Normal veins are flat when the client is sitting and pulsations become evident as the client's head is lowered. Jugular venous pressure exceeding 1 inch (2.5 cm) indicates fluid overload.

> **NURSE ALERT** Visible jugular pulsation suggests need for immediate treatment.

TABLE 12-5 Common Types of Arrhythmias

TYPE	DEFINITION	CAUSE
Atrial fibrillation	Rapid, random contractions of atria cause irregular ventricular beats at 120 to 150 beats per minute.	Atria discharge very rapidly, with some impulses not reaching ventricles. This condition occurs in rheumatic heart disease and mitral stenosis. It causes reduced cardiac output.
Premature ventricular contraction	Premature beat occurs before regularly expected heart contraction.	Ventricle contracts prematurely because of electrical impulse bypassing normal conduction pathway. It may occur so early that it is difficult to detect as second beat. It may be followed by a pause.
Sinus arrhythmia	Pulse rate changes during respiration, increasing at peak of inspiration and declining during expiration.	Blood is momentarily trapped in lungs during inspiration, causing fall in heart's stroke volume.
Sinus bradycardia	Pulse rhythm is regular, but rate is slower than normal at 40 to 60 beats per minute.	Sinoatrial node fires less frequently. This is common in well-conditioned athletes and with use of antiarrhythmic medications.
Sinus tachycardia	Pulse rhythm is regular, but rate is accelerated to more than 100 beats per minute.	Exercise, emotional stress, and caffeine or alcohol ingestion are common factors that cause increased firing of sinoatrial nodes.

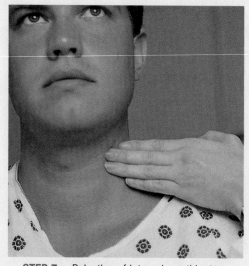

STEP 7c. Palpation of internal carotid artery.

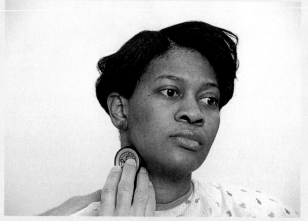

STEP 7d. Auscultation for carotid artery bruit. (From Seidel HM and others: *Mosby's guide to physical examination,* ed 5, St Louis, 2003, Mosby.)

STEPS	RATIONALE

8 Assess peripheral vascular area.

a. Inspect lower extremities for changes in color and condition of the skin (Table 12-6). Note skin and nail texture, hair distribution, venous patterns, edema, and scars or ulcers. Compare skin color lying and standing.

Changes may reflect impaired peripheral circulation.

b. Palpate edematous areas, noting mobility, consistency, and tenderness.

Assists in determining extent of edema. Edema results from fluid in tissues. Inadequate venous return causes edema in the sacrum if client is confined to bed or in the feet and ankles if sitting.

c. Assess for pitting edema by pressing area firmly for 5 seconds, then releasing. Depth of indentation determines severity (see illustration).

In some settings a tape measure may be used to observe the extent of edema by measuring the circumference of the extremity daily.

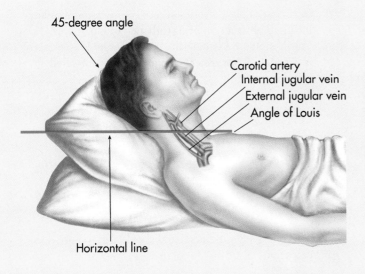

STEP 7e. Position of client to assess jugular vein distention. (From Thompson J and others: *Mosby's manual of clinical nursing,* ed 5, St Louis, 2001, Mosby.)

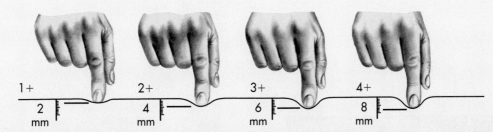

STEP 8c. Assessing for pitting edema. (From Cannobio MM: *Cardiovascular disorders,* St Louis, 1990, Mosby.)

TABLE 12-6 Signs of Venous and Arterial Insufficiency

ASSESSMENT CRITERION	VENOUS	ARTERIAL
Color	Normal or cyanotic	Pale; worsened by elevation of extremity; dusky red when extremity lowered
Edema	Often marked	Absent or mild
Pulse	Normal	Decreased or absent
Skin changes	Brown pigmentation around ankles	Thin, shiny skin; decreased hair growth; thickened nails
Temperature	Normal	Cool (blood flow blocked to extremity)

STEPS	RATIONALE

d. Check capillary refill by grasping client's fingernail or toenail and noting color of nail bed. Next, apply gentle, firm pressure to the nail bed. Release quickly, watching for color change. Circulation is restored and normally returns to pink color in less than 2 seconds.

Cold environmental temperature with vasoconstriction and vascular disease can delay refill. Local pressure from a cast or bandage may also deter refill.

e. Ask if the client experiences pain or tenderness, and then palpate for heat, firmness, or localized swelling of the calf muscle, which are signs of deep vein thrombosis (DVT).

Clients who have been immobilized for several days and those who have bone or joint disease, surgical correction of joint or bone, or pain are at risk for altered tissue perfusion (Glover, 2005). Some clients have DVTs and only complain of calf pain (Bartley, 2005; Urbano, 2001).

> **NURSE ALERT** Homans' sign is no longer a reliable indicator for the presence or absence of DVT (Bartley, 2005; Day, 2003; Glover, 2005; Urbano, 2001) and should not be considered a reliable parameter. Trauma to the vein or muscle, reduced mobility, and increased blood clotting are reliable risk factors. If the calf is swollen, red, or tender, notify client's physician for further assessment and evaluation.

f. Starting at the most distal part of each extremity, palpate each peripheral artery for equality, comparing side to side; elasticity of vessel wall (depress and release artery, noting ease with which it springs back to shape); and strength of pulse (force of blood against arterial wall) using the following rating scale (Seidel and others, 2006):

   0 No pulse palpable
   1+ Diminished, pulse barely palpable, weak and thready, and easy to obliterate
   2+ Normal pulse, easy to palpate
   3+ Full, easy to palpate and not easily obliterated
   4+ Strong, bounding against fingertips, and cannot be obliterated

Comparison of both arteries allows you to determine any localized obstruction or disturbance in blood flow. Pulses should be symmetrical side to side. If asymmetry is noted, look for other factors related to impaired circulation.

g. Palpate radial pulse by lightly placing tips of first and second fingers in groove formed along radial side of forearm, lateral to flexor tendon of wrist (see illustration).

Pulse is relatively superficial and should not require deep palpation.

h. Palpate ulnar pulse by placing fingertips along ulnar side of forearm (see illustration).

Palpated when arterial insufficiency to hand is expected or when nurse assesses that radial occlusion (e.g., during ABG sampling) might affect circulation to hand (see Chapter 29).

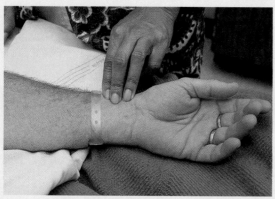

STEP 8g. Palpation of radial pulse.

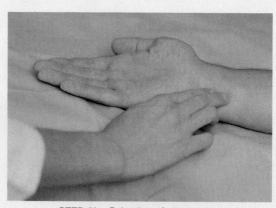

STEP 8h. Palpation of ulnar pulse.

STEPS	RATIONALE
i. Palpate brachial pulse by locating groove between biceps and triceps muscles above elbow at antecubital fossa (see illustration). Place tips of first two fingers in muscle groove.	Artery runs along medial side of extended arm, requiring moderate palpation.
j. Have client lie supine with feet relaxed, and palpate dorsalis pedis pulse. Gently place fingertips between great and first toe; slowly move fingers along groove between extensor tendons of great and first toe until pulse is palpable (see illustration).	Artery lies superficially and does not require deep palpation. Pulse may be congenitally absent.
k. If the dorsalis pedis pulse is difficult to palpate or it is not palpable, use a Doppler instrument over the pulse site. (1) Apply conducting gel to the client's skin over the pulse site or onto transducer tip of probe. (2) Turn Doppler on. Gently apply ultrasound probe to the skin, changing Doppler angle until pulsation is audible. Adjust volume as needed. Wipe off gel from client and Doppler.	Doppler amplifies sounds, allowing you to hear low-velocity blood flow through peripheral arteries.
l. Palpate posterior tibial pulse by having client relax and slightly extend feet. Place fingertips behind and below medial malleolus (ankle bone) (see illustration).	Artery is easily palpable with foot relaxed.
m. Palpate popliteal pulse by having client slightly flex knee with foot resting on table or bed. Instruct client to keep leg muscles relaxed. Palpate deeply into popliteal fossa with fingers of both hands placed just lateral to midline. Client may also lie prone to achieve exposure of artery (see illustration).	Flexion of knee and muscle relaxation improve accessibility of artery. Popliteal pulse is one of the more difficult pulses to palpate.

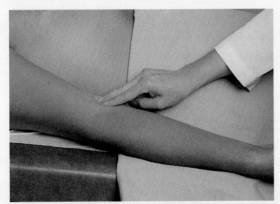

STEP 8i. Palpation of brachial pulse.

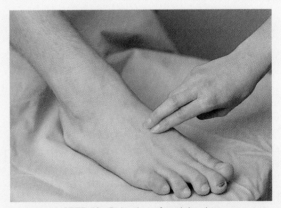

STEP 8j. Palpation of pedal pulse.

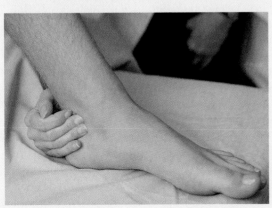

STEP 8l. Palpation of posterior tibial pulse.

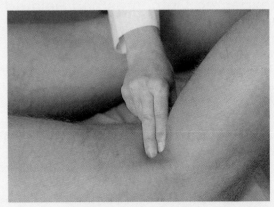

STEP 8m. Palpation of popliteal pulse with client prone.

STEPS	RATIONALE
n. With client supine, palpate femoral pulse by placing first two fingers over inguinal area below inguinal ligament, midway between pubic symphysis and anterosuperior iliac spine (see illustration). **9 See Completion Protocol (inside front cover).**	Supine position prevents flexion in groin area, which interferes with artery access.

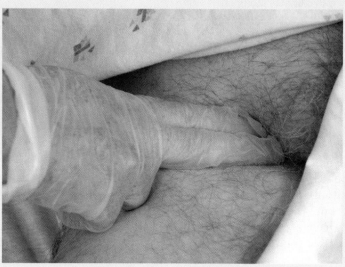

STEP 8n. Palpation of femoral pulse.

EVALUATION

1 Compare findings with normal assessment characteristics of heart and vascular system.
2 If heart sounds are not audible or pulses are not palpable, ask another nurse to confirm assessment.
3 Compare pulses and capillary refill bilaterally with previous shift assessment.
4 Compare presence and extent of edema with previous shift assessment.
5 Ask client to describe behaviors that increase risk for heart and vascular disease.

Unexpected Outcomes and Related Interventions

1. Pulsations, vibrations, or both are palpable. These result from a valvular problem, murmur, or both.
a. Be prepared to assist with an electrocardiogram (ECG) and obtain vital signs.
2 PMI is found left of the midclavicular line, suggesting cardiomegaly.
a. Be prepared to assist with an ECG and obtain vital signs.
3 Heart rate is irregular and/or the rate is less than 60 beats per minute or more than 100 beats per minute.
a. Check blood pressure. If low, arrhythmia is contributing to inadequate cardiac output.

b. Observe for sensations or reports of dizziness or feeling "faint."
c. Notify physician.
4 Pulse deficit is present.
a. Be prepared to assist with an ECG and obtain vital signs.
5 Client is unable to explain risks for heart or vascular disease.
a. Provide additional education.
6 Previously palpable pedal pulses are diminished or absent.
a. Notify physician.
b. Elevate extremity.
7 Client's lower extremities have pale, cool, thin, and shiny skin, with reduced hair growth and thickened nails, indicating chronic arterial insufficiency.
a. Instruct client in proper foot care.
b. Refer to podiatrist for nail trimming.
c. Inspect feet for signs of impaired skin integrity.

Recording and Reporting

- Document quality (clear or muffled), intensity (weak or pounding), rate, and rhythm (regular, regularly irregular, or irregularly irregular) of heart sounds and peripheral pulses on nurses' notes or flow sheet.
- Document activity level and subjective data related to fatigue, shortness of breath, and chest pain.

- Document preferred position for rest, medications and/or treatments used, and client's response.
- Report immediately to physician any irregularities in heart function and indications of impaired arterial blood flow.
- Report to charge nurse or physician any changes in peripheral circulation, which may indicate circulatory compromise that can result in permanent nerve damage or tissue death if untreated.

Sample Documentation

0730 Apical pulse rate 104 and irregular. Pulse deficit 6/min. BP 110/70. Denies chest pain or other discomfort. Resting quietly in bed without complaints of distress. Notified M.D. of pulse deficit.

Special Considerations
Pediatric Considerations

- Perform cardiac assessment on infant or toddler while quiet, before more uncomfortable procedures.

- Capillary refill in infants is usually less than 1 second.
- It is not uncommon for children to have third heart sounds (S_3). Sinus arrhythmia occurs normally in many children (Hockenberry and Wilson, 2007).
- Children have louder, higher-pitched heart sounds because of their thin chest walls.
- Children cannot increase their stroke volume, only their heart rate, causing a lack of oxygen to tissues (Ball and Bindler, 2006).

Geriatric Considerations

- PMI may be difficult to find in an older adult because AP diameter of the chest deepens.
- Accidental massage of the carotid sinus during palpation of the carotid artery can be a particular problem for older adults, causing a sudden drop in heart rate from vagal nerve stimulation (Ebersole, Hess, and Luggen, 2004).

SKILL 12.5 Assessing the Abdomen

Abdominal assessment is complex because of the multiple organs located within and near the abdominal cavity. This area of the body is associated with many health complaints, and many people are embarrassed by bowel or bladder dysfunction, reproductive problems, or urinary elimination problems. Abdominal pain is one of the most common symptoms clients report when seeking medical care. Abdominal pain can be caused by alterations in organs such as the stomach, gallbladder, or intestines; or the pain may be the result of spinal or muscular injury. An accurate assessment requires matching the client's history with a careful assessment of the location of physical symptoms (Table 12-7).

To perform an effective abdominal assessment you need detailed knowledge of the underlying structures involved, including the lower pelvis, kidneys, rectum, genitalia, liver, gallbladder, stomach, spleen, intestines, and reproductive organs (Figure 12-6). An abdominal assessment is routine after abdominal surgery and for any client who has undergone invasive diagnostic tests of the gastrointestinal (GI) tract (see Chapter 14).

The order of an abdominal assessment differs from that of other assessments. You begin with inspection and follow with auscultation. It is important to auscultate before palpation because these maneuvers may alter the frequency and character of bowel sounds.

ASSESSMENT

1 If client has abdominal or low back pain, assess the character of pain in detail (location, onset, frequency, precipitating factors, aggravating factors, type of pain, severity, course). *Rationale: Knowing pattern of characteristics of pain helps determine its source.*

2 Carefully observe client's movement and position, such as lying still with knees drawn up, moving restlessly to find a comfortable position, or lying on one side or sitting with knees drawn up to chest. *Rationale: Positions assumed by the client may reveal nature and source of pain (e.g., peritonitis, renal stone, pancreatitis). Clients with appendicitis often lie on side or back with knees flexed to reduce pain (Phipps and others, 2003).*

3 Assess client's normal bowel habits: frequency of stools; character of stools; recent changes in character of stools; measures used to promote elimination, such as laxatives, enemas, dietary intake; and eating and drinking habits. *Rationale: These data, compared with information from physical assessment, may help to identify cause and nature of elimination problems.*

4 Determine if client has had abdominal surgery, trauma, or diagnostic tests of the GI tract. *Rationale: Surgery or trauma to abdomen may result in altered position of underlying organs. Diagnostic tests may change character of stool.*

5 Determine whether client has had any nausea, vomiting, or cramping, especially in past 24 hours. *Rationale: Changes may indicate alterations in upper GI tract (e.g., stomach, gallbladder) or lower colon.*

6 Assess for difficulty in swallowing, belching, flatulence, bloody emesis (hematemesis), black or tarry stools (melena), heartburn, diarrhea, or constipation. *Rationale: Indicative of GI alterations.*

7 Determine if client takes antiinflammatory medications (e.g., aspirin, steroids, nonsteroidal antiinflammatory drugs [NSAIDs]), or antibiotics. *Rationale: These medications may cause GI upset or bleeding.*

TABLE 12-7   Common Causes of Abdominal Pain

CONDUCTION	PHYSICAL ALTERATION	PHYSICAL SIGNS AND SYMPTOMS
Appendicitis	Obstruction of the appendix associated with inflammation, perforation, and peritonitis.	Sharp pain directly over the irritated peritoneum 2-11 hours after onset. Often pain localizes at McBurney's point in the right lower quadrant between the anterior iliac crest and the umbilicus. Associated with rebound tenderness.
Constipation	Disruption in normal bowel pattern, which may occur with opiod use or inadequate fiber and fluid intake.	Generalized discomfort accompanied by distention and palpation of a hard mass in the left lower quadrant. Nausea and vomiting may begin after several days.
Crohn's disease	A chronic inflammatory lesion of the ileum. Cause is unknown.	Steady colicky pain in the right lower quadrant, with cramping, tenderness, flatulence, nausea, fever, and diarrhea. Often associated with bloody stools, weight loss, weakness, and fatigue.
Gastroenteritis	Inflammation of the stomach and intestinal tract.	Generalized abdominal discomfort accompanied by nausea, vomiting, and diarrhea.
Pancreatitis	Inflammation of the pancreas associated with alcoholism and gallbladder disease.	Steady epigastric pain close to the umbilicus radiates to the back. Associated with abdominal rigidity and vomiting. Pain is unrelieved by vomiting.
Paralytic ileus	Obstruction of the small bowel that occurs after abdominal surgery or use of anticholinergic medications.	Generalized severe abdominal distention, nausea, and vomiting.
Peptic ulcers	Damage of gastrointestinal (GI) mucosa at any area of the GI tract. May be caused by bacterial infection or nonsteroidal antiinflammatory drugs (NSAIDs). Believed to be unrelated to stress. Aggravated by smoking and excessive alcohol use.	Localized midepigastric pain with heartburn that develops 2 hours or more after meals, when the stomach is empty. Eating may relieve the pain. Acidic liquid, such as orange juice or coffee, may aggravate the pain.

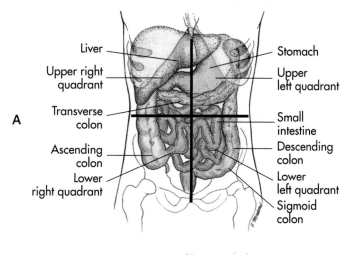

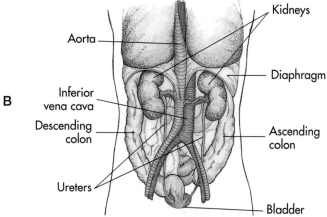

FIGURE 12-6 A, Anterior view of abdomen divided by quadrants. **B,** Posterior view of abdominal sections.

8 Inquire about family history of cancer, kidney disease, alcoholism, hypertension, or heart disease. *Rationale: Data may reveal risk for significant abdominal alterations (e.g., chronic alcohol ingestion can cause GI and liver problems).*

9 Determine if female client is pregnant. *Rationale: Pregnancy may cause nausea and vomiting, as well as changes in abdominal shape and contour.*

10 Review client's history for health care occupation, hemodialysis, IV drug use, household or sexual contact with hepatitis B virus (HBV) carrier, sexually active heterosexual person (more than one sex partner in previous 6 months), sexually active homosexual or bisexual man, or international traveler in area of high HBV prevalence. *Rationale: These are risk factors for HBV exposure. Abdominal findings for hepatitis include jaundice, hepatomegaly, anorexia, abdominal discomfort, tea-colored urine, and clay-colored stool (Seidel and others, 2006).*

PLANNING

Expected Outcomes focus on identifying alterations in the abdomen.

1 Abdomen is soft and symmetrical with smooth and even contour. No mass, distention, or tenderness is palpable. No forceful visible pulsations are noted.

2 Bowel sounds are active and audible in all four quadrants.

3 Client denies discomfort or worsening of existing discomfort after examination.

4 Client is able to list warning signs of colon cancer.

Delegation Considerations

The skill of abdominal assessment should not be delegated to AP. The RN instructs personnel to:

- Report the development of abdominal pain and changes in the client's bowel habits or dietary intake to the nurse.

Equipment

- Stethoscope
- Tape measure
- Examination light
- Marking pen

IMPLEMENTATION *for Assessing the Abdomen*

STEPS	RATIONALE
1 See Standard Protocol (inside front cover).	
2 Prepare client.	
a. Ask if client needs to empty bladder or defecate.	Palpation of full bladder can cause discomfort and feeling of urgency and make it difficult for client to relax.
b. Keep upper chest and legs draped.	Expose only areas to be examined.
c. Be sure that room is warm.	Provides for client comfort.
d. Expose area from just above the xiphoid process down to the symphysis pubis.	Exposes areas to be examined during abdominal assessment.
e. Have client lie supine or in a dorsal recumbent position with arms down at sides and knees slightly bent. A small pillow may be placed under client's knees.	Placing the arms under the head or keeping knees fully extended can cause the abdominal muscles to tighten. Tightening of muscles prevents adequate palpation.

> **NURSE ALERT** Observe respirations as position is changed. If abdomen is distended, lying flat increases respiratory difficulty because of pressure on the diaphragm (Tryniszewski, 2005).

STEPS	RATIONALE
f. Maintain conversation during assessment except during auscultation. Explain steps calmly and slowly.	If client relaxes there is improved accuracy of findings.
g. Ask client to point to tender areas.	Painful areas are assessed last. Manipulation of body part can increase client's pain and anxiety and make remainder of assessment difficult to complete.
3 Identify landmarks that divide abdominal region into quadrants. Boundary begins at the tip of xiphoid process to symphysis pubis with line crossing and intersecting the umbilicus, dividing abdomen into four equal sections (see Figure 12-6).	Location of findings by common reference point helps successive examiners to confirm findings and locate abnormalities.
4 Inspect skin of abdomen's surface for color, scars, venous patterns, rashes, lesions, silvery white striae (stretch marks), and artificial openings. Observe lesions for characteristics described in Skill 12-1.	Scars reveal evidence that client has past trauma or surgery. Striae indicate stretching of tissue from growth, obesity, pregnancy, ascites, or edema. Venous patterns may reflect liver disease (portal hypertension). Artificial openings indicate bowel or urinary diversion.
5 If bruising is noted, ask if client self-administers injections (e.g., heparin, insulin).	Frequent injections can cause bruising and hardening of underlying tissues.

> **NURSE ALERT** Bruising may also indicate physical abuse, accidental injury, or bleeding disorders.

STEPS	RATIONALE
6 Inspect the contour, symmetry, and surface motion of the abdomen. Note any masses, bulging, or distention. (Flat abdomen forms a horizontal plane from xiphoid process to symphysis pubis. Round abdomen protrudes in convex sphere from horizontal plane. Concave abdomen sinks into muscular wall. All are normal.)	Changes in symmetry or contour may reveal underlying masses, fluid collection, or gaseous distention. An everted (pouch extends outward) umbilicus may indicate distention. A hernia can also cause the umbilicus to protrude upward.

STEPS	RATIONALE

7 If abdomen appears distended, note if distention is generalized. Look at the flanks on each side.

Distention may be caused by one or more of the nine *F's* (fat, flatus, feces, fluids, fibroid, full bladder, false pregnancy, fatal tumor, and fetus) (Seidel and others, 2006). If gas causes distention, flanks do not bulge. If fluid causes distention, flanks bulge. A tumor may cause a unilateral bulging or distention. Pregnancy causes symmetrical bulge in lower abdomen.

8 If distention is suspected, measure size of abdominal girth by placing tape measure around abdomen at level of umbilicus (see illustration). Use marking pen to indicate where tape measure was applied.

Consecutive measurements will show any increase or decrease in abdominal distention. Make all subsequent measurements at same level of umbilicus to provide objective means to evaluate changes. Use a water-based pen to make a mark on abdomen for subsequent measurements.

9 If NG or intestinal tube is connected to suction, turn off momentarily.

Sound of machine obscures bowel sounds.

10 To auscultate bowel sounds, place the diaphragm of the stethoscope lightly over each of the four abdominal quadrants. Ask client not to talk. Listen until you hear repeated gurgling or bubbling sounds in each quadrant (minimum of once in 5 to 20 seconds). Describe sounds as normal, hyperactive, hypoactive, or absent. Listen 5 minutes over each quadrant before deciding that bowel sounds are absent (see illustration).

Normal bowel sounds occur irregularly every 5 to 15 seconds. Absence of sounds indicates cessation of gastric motility. Hyperactive bowel sounds not related to hunger or a recent meal may indicate diarrhea or early intestinal obstruction. Hypoactive or absent bowel sounds may indicate paralytic ileus or peritonitis (Tryniszewski, 2005). It is common for bowel sounds to be hypoactive postoperatively for 24 hours or more, especially after abdominal surgery.

> **NURSE ALERT** Severe paralytic ileus may be accompanied by nausea and vomiting, increasing distention, and inability to pass flatus.

11 Place the bell of the stethoscope over the epigastric region of the abdomen and each quadrant. Auscultate for vascular (whooshing) sounds.

Determines presence of turbulent blood flow (bruit) through thoracic or abdominal aorta.

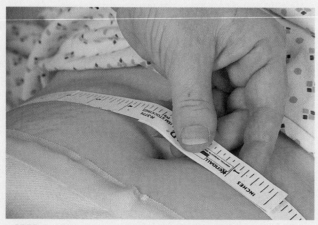

STEP 8 Measuring abdominal girth at the level of the umbilicus

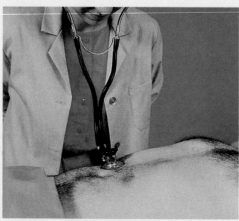

STEP 10 Auscultation of bowel sounds. (From Barkauskas VH and others: *Health and physical assessment,* ed 3, St Louis, 2002, Mosby.)

> **NURSE ALERT** If aortic bruit is auscultated, suggesting presence of an aneurysm, stop assessment and notify physician immediately. Percussion or palpation over abdominal bruit can cause rupture of an already weakened vessel wall in the presence of an abdominal aneurysm.

12 Ask client if abdomen feels unusually tight, and determine if this is a recent development.

Continued sensation of fullness helps to detect distention. A feeling of fullness after a heavy meal causes only temporary distention. Tightness is not felt with obesity.

13 Lightly palpate over each abdominal quadrant, laying the palm of the hand with fingers extended and approximated lightly on the abdomen. Keep the palm and forearm horizontal. The pads of the fingertips depress the skin approximately ½ inch (1 cm) in a gentle dipping motion (see illustration).

Detects areas of localized tenderness, degree of tenderness, and presence and character of underlying masses. Palpation of sensitive area causes guarding (voluntary tightening of underlying abdominal muscles).

> **NURSE ALERT** Palpate painful areas last. Avoid quick jabs. To avoid tickling, place the client's hand on the abdomen with the nurse's hand on the client's.

  a. Note muscular resistance, distention, tenderness, and superficial masses or organs while observing client's face for signs of discomfort.

  b. Note if abdomen is firm or soft to touch.

Client's verbal and nonverbal cues may indicate discomfort from tenderness. Firm abdomen may indicate active obstruction with fluid or gas building up.

Soft abdomen is normal or reveals that obstruction is resolving.

14 Just below umbilicus and above symphysis pubis, palpate for a smooth, rounded mass. While applying light pressure, ask if client has sensation of need to void.

Detects presence of dome of distended bladder.

> **NURSE ALERT** Routinely check for distended bladder if client has been unable to void, client has been incontinent, or an indwelling Foley catheter is not draining well.

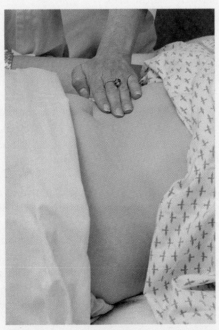

STEP 13 Light palpation of the abdomen.

STEPS	RATIONALE
15 If masses are palpated, note size, location, shape, consistency, tenderness, mobility, and texture.	Descriptive characteristics help to reveal type of mass.
16 When tenderness is present, test for rebound tenderness by pressing slowly and deeply into the involved area and then letting go quickly. Note if pain is aggravated.	Results are positive if pain increases. May indicate peritoneal irritation such as appendicitis (Seidel and others, 2006).
17 See Completion Protocol (inside front cover).	

EVALUATION

1 Observe throughout the assessment for evidence of discomfort.
2 Compare assessment findings with previous assessment to identify changes.
3 Ask client to describe signs and symptoms of colon cancer.

Unexpected Outcomes and Related Interventions

1 Abdomen is asymmetrical, with palpable mass and hypoactive bowel sounds.
a. Report to the physician because findings may indicate enlarged liver, spleen, or tumor.
2 Abdomen protrudes symmetrically, with skin taut; client complains of tightness and/or bowel sounds are absent. GI motility has ceased. Client is vomiting.
a. Keep client on "nothing by mouth" (NPO) status, and encourage ambulation.
b. Notify physician; findings may indicate an obstruction.
c. Gastric decompression with insertion of NG tube may become necessary.
3 Hyperactive bowel sounds are evident with GI motility. Commonly they result from anxiety, diarrhea, overuse of laxatives, inflammation of the bowel, or reaction of the intestines to certain foods.
a. Client may need to be NPO.
b. Contact physician if client may need antidiarrheal medications.
4 Rebound abdominal tenderness is found.
a. Avoid palpating area.
b. Notify physician if this is a new finding.
c. Keep client on NPO status until physician can evaluate.
5 Bladder is palpable over symphysis pubis. Bladder is distended.
a. Facilitate voiding by placing client in sitting position or encouraging client to bear down.
b. If unable to void, urinary catheterization may be necessary.
6 Internal organs (liver, spleen) are enlarged or tender.
a. Do not continue to palpate area.
b. Enlargement may be because of cancerous involvement, hepatitis, or cirrhosis.
c. Notify physician.
d. Keep client NPO until physician evaluates.

7 Abdominal girth is increased and fluid has built up within peritoneal cavity.
a. Notify physician.
b. Place client on NPO status.

Recording and Reporting

- Document quality of bowel sounds, presence of distention, abdominal circumference, and presence of tenderness on nurse's notes or flow sheet.
- Record client's ability to void and defecate, including description of output.
- Record content of any client instruction.
- Report serious abnormalities, such as absent bowel sounds, presence of mass, or acute pain, to nurse in charge and physician.

Sample Documentation

0800 Abdomen is distended. No passage of flatus since surgery, and bowel sounds are hypoactive over all 4 quadrants. Encouraged to sip on warm fluids and ambulate frequently. Denies nausea, vomiting, or pain at this time.

Special Considerations
Pediatric Considerations

- Most common palpable mass in child is feces, usually felt in right lower quadrant (Ball and Bindler, 2006; Hockenberry and Wilson, 2007).
- Have a child stand erect and then lie supine during inspection of abdomen. Normal abdomen of infants and young children is cylindrical in erect position and flat in supine position. School-age children may have a rounded abdomen until 13 years of age when standing.
- Infants and children, until age 7, are abdominal breathers.
- In infants and children skin is usually taut and without wrinkles or creases.

Geriatric Considerations

- Older adults often lack abdominal tone; underlying organs are more easily palpable (Reuben and others, 2005).
- A weakened intestinal musculature and decreased peristalsis affect the large intestine.
- Constipation, nausea, flatulence, and heartburn are common.
- Older adults may have increased fat deposits over the abdomen.

SKILL 12.6 Musculoskeletal and Neurological Assessment

The nurse uses the skills of inspection and palpation during the musculoskeletal and neurological assessment. Initial assessment (see Skill 12.1) involves a general inspection of gait, posture, and body position. A more thorough assessment of major bone, joint, and muscle groups, and sensory, motor, and cranial nerve function is indicated in the presence of abnormalities. The assessment can be performed while the nurse examines other body systems. For example, while assessing head and neck structures, the nurse also assesses neck ROM and examines selected cranial nerves. The nurse integrates assessment into routine activities of care, for example, while bathing or positioning the client. Always assess a client who reports pain, loss of sensation, or impairment of muscle function.

Prolonged illness or immobility may result in muscle weakness and atrophy. Neurological assessment is often conducted simultaneously because muscles may be weakened as a result of nerve involvement.

ASSESSMENT

1 Review client history (particularly with female clients) for risk of osteoporosis, including heavy alcohol use, cigarette smoking, constant dieting, calcium intake less than 500 mg daily, thin and light body frame, females who have never been pregnant (nulliparous), menopause before age 45, postmenopausal status, bilateral oophorectomy (ovary removal), family history of osteoporosis, or European American, Asian, or Native American descent. *Rationale: These factors increase the risk for osteoporosis.*

2 Ask client to describe history of alteration in bone, muscle, or joint function (e.g., recent fall, trauma, lifting heavy objects, bone or joint disease with sudden or gradual onset) and location of alteration. *Rationale: Assists in assessing nature of musculoskeletal problem. Osteoporosis-related fractures occur in half of all postmenopausal women; of those, 15% will suffer from hip fractures (U.S. Preventive Services Task Force, 2003).*

3 Assess nature and extent of client's musculoskeletal pain: location, duration, severity, predisposing and aggravating factors, relieving factors, and type of pain. If pain or cramping is reported in the lower extremities, ask if it is relieved or aggravated by walking. Assess the distance walked and characteristics of pain before, during, and after activity. *Rationale: Alterations in bone, joints, or muscle are frequently accompanied by pain. Pain has implications not only for comfort but also for ability to perform activities of daily living (ADLs). Pain caused by certain vascular conditions tends to increase with activity.*

4 Determine how client's alteration influences ability to perform ADLs (e.g., bathing, feeding, dressing, toileting, ambulating) and social functions (e.g., household chores, work, recreation, sexual activities). *Rationale: Level of nursing care is determined by extent to which client can perform self-care. Type and degree of restriction in continuing social activities influence topics for client education.*

5 Assess height decrease of woman older than 50 by subtracting current height from recall of maximum adult height. *Rationale: Measurement may be useful in screening for osteoporosis. A loss of height is frequently the first clinical sign of osteoporosis (Pachucki-Hyde, 2001).*

6 Ask if client has noted signs of reduced sensation or weakness in extremities. *Rationale: These signs indicate neurological changes.*

7 Determine if the client is taking analgesics, antipsychotics, antidepressants, or nervous system stimulants. *Rationale: These medications alter LOC or cause behavioral changes.*

8 Determine if the client has a history of seizures/convulsions; characteristics of any symptoms; and relationship to time of day, fatigue, or emotional stress. *Rationale: Seizure activity often originates from central nervous system (CNS) alteration. Characteristics of seizure help determine its origin.*

9 Screen client for headache; tremors; dizziness; numbness; or tingling of body part, visual changes, weakness, pain, or changes in speech. *Rationale: These symptoms commonly result from CNS dysfunction. Identifying patterns may assist in diagnosis.*

10 Discuss with spouse, family member, or friends any recent changes in client's behavior (e.g., increased irritability, mood swings, memory loss, change in energy level). *Rationale: Behavioral changes may result from intracranial pathology.*

11 Assess client for history of change in vision, hearing, smell, taste, or touch. *Rationale: Major sensory nerves originate from brain stem. These symptoms may help localize nature of problem.*

12 Review past history for head or spinal cord injury, hypertension, or psychiatric disorder. *Rationale: These factors may cause neurological symptoms or behavioral changes to develop, focusing assessment on possible cause.*

PLANNING

Expected Outcomes focus on identifying deficits in musculoskeletal and neurological function.

1 Client demonstrates erect posture, strong grasp, and steady gait, with arms swinging freely at side.

2 There is bilateral symmetry of extremities in length, circumference, alignment, position, and skinfolds (Seidel and others, 2006).

3 Full active ROM is present in all joints with good muscle tone and absence of contractures, spasticity, or muscular weakness.

4 Client is alert and oriented to person, place, and time. Behavior and appearance are appropriate for condition/situation.

5 Client demonstrates normal pupil reaction to light and accommodation (Skill 12.2); external ocular muscles intact; facial sensation intact; symmetrical facial expressions; soft palate and uvula midline and rise upon phonation; gag reflex intact; speech clear without hoarseness; no difficulty swallowing.

6 Client distinguishes between sharp and dull sensations and light touch on symmetrical areas of extremities.

7 Gait coordinated and steady. Romberg's test negative.

Delegation Considerations

Assessment of musculoskeletal and neurological function should not be delegated to AP. The nurse instructs personnel to:

- Report any problems noted in ROM, muscle strength, or client's report of reduced sensation.
- Take precautions during ROM exercises to avoid forcing a joint beyond the client's current ROM.
- Be aware of clients at risk for falls and provide with instructions for clients with muscular weakness who require special assistance with transfer and ambulation.

Equipment

- Tape measure
- Cotton balls or cotton-tipped applicators
- Penlight
- Opposite tip of cotton swab or tongue blade broken in half
- Tongue blade
- Tuning fork

IMPLEMENTATION *for Musculoskeletal and Neurological Assessment*

STEPS	RATIONALE
1 **See Standard Protocol (inside front cover).**	
2 Prepare client.	
a. Integrate musculoskeletal and neurological assessment during other portions of physical assessment or during care.	As in assessment of integument, you can conduct an assessment as the client moves in bed, rises from chair, walks, or goes through movements required during complete physical examination. Integration with care conserves client's energy and allows observation of client performing activities more naturally.
b. Plan time for short rest periods during assessment.	Movement of body parts and various maneuvers may fatigue client. It is particularly important to consider rest periods with older adults and very ill clients.
3 Musculoskeletal Assessment	
a. Observe ability to use arms and hands for grasping objects.	Assesses coordination and muscle strength.
b. Assess muscle strength of upper extremities by applying gradual increase in pressure to muscle group.	Upper and lower extremity on client's dominant side is normally stronger than that on nondominant side. Pain, rather than weakness, may cause reduced muscle strength; however, long-term pain can lead to muscle weakening.
c. To assess hand grasp strength, have client grasp fingers of both your hands and squeeze them as hard as possible. To avoid discomfort, cross your hands.	It is common for client's dominant hand to be slightly stronger than nondominant hand. By crossing hands, client's right hand grasps your right hand.
d. Place hand on lower arm or leg and have client move major joint (e.g., elbow, knee) against resistance (e.g., flex elbow). Have client maintain resistance until told to stop. Compare symmetrical muscle groups. Note weakness, and compare right with left.	Compares strength of symmetrical muscle groups. Rate muscle strength on scale of 0 to 5. Grade as follows: 0 No voluntary contraction 1 Slight contractility, no movement 2 Full ROM, passive 3 Full ROM, active 4 Full ROM against gravity, some resistance 5 Full ROM against gravity, full resistance
e. If muscle weakness is identified, measure muscle size with tape measure placed around body of muscle. Compare with same muscle on opposite side of body.	Indicates degree of atrophy.
f. Observe position for sitting, supine, prone, or standing. Muscles and joints should be exposed and free to move to allow for accurate measurement.	Each joint or muscle group may require different position for measurement.

STEPS	RATIONALE
g. Inspect gait as client walks and stands. Observe for foot dragging, shuffling or limping, balance, presence of obvious deformity in lower extremities, and position of trunk in relation to legs.	Gait is more natural if client is unaware of nurse's observation. Observations may indicate a neuromusculoskeletal disorder.
h. Stand behind client, and observe postural alignment (position of hips relative to shoulders) (see illustration A). Look sideways at cervical, thoracic, and lumbar curves (see illustration B).	Abnormal curves of posture include lordosis (swayback, increased lumbar curvature), kyphosis (hunchback, exaggerated posterior curvature of thoracic spine), and scoliosis (lateral spinal curvature). Postural changes may indicate muscular, bone, or joint deformity; pain; or muscular fatigue. Head should be held erect.

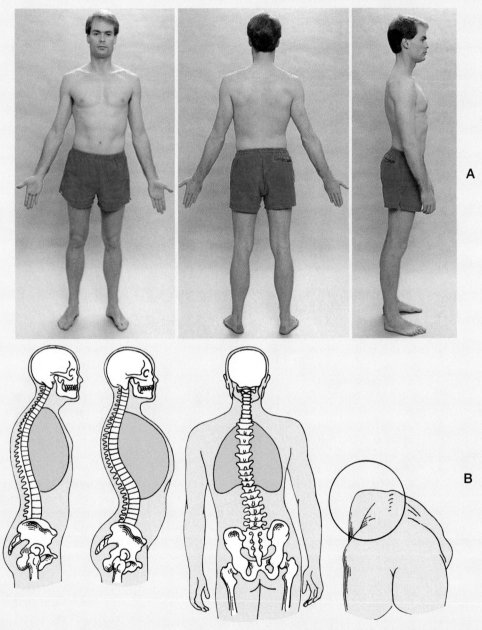

A

B

STEP 3h. A, Inspection of overall body posture: *1,* anterior view; *2,* posterior view; *3,* lateral view. (From Seidel HM and others: *Mosby's guide to physical examination,* ed 5, St Louis, 2003, Mosby.) **B,** Spinal deformities: *1,* kyphosis; *2,* lordosis; *3,* scoliosis; *4,* scoliosis with client bending forward.

STEPS	RATIONALE
i. Make a general observation of the extremities. Look at overall size, gross deformity, bony enlargement, alignment, and symmetry.	General review helps to pinpoint areas requiring in-depth assessment.
j. Gently palpate bones, joints, and surrounding tissue in involved areas. Note any heat, tenderness, edema, or resistance to pressure.	May reveal changes resulting from trauma or chronic disease. Do not attempt to move joint when fracture is suspected or when joint is apparently "frozen" by lack of movement over a long period of time.
k. Ask client to put major joint through its full ROM (Table 12-8). Observe equality of motion in same body parts.	Assessment of client's normal ROM provides baseline for assessing later changes after surgery or inactivity.
(1) *Active motion.* (Client needs no support or assistance and is able to move joint independently.) Instruct client in moving each joint through its normal range. It may be necessary to demonstrate movements and ask client to mimic your movements.	Identifies muscle strength and detects limited ROM.
(2) *Passive motion.* (Joint has full ROM, but client does not have the strength to move it independently.) Have client relax and move the same joints passively until the end of the range is felt. Support extremity at joint.	Clients with deformities, reduced mobility, joint fixation, or weakness may require passive motion assessment. Determines ability to perform joint motion in the presence of muscle weakness.

TABLE 12-8 Assessing Range of Motion*

BODY PART	ASSESSMENT PROCEDURE	ROM
Upper Extremities		
Shoulders	Raise both arms to a vertical position at the sides of the head.	Flexion
	Place both hands behind the neck, with elbows out to the sides.	External rotation and abduction
	Place both hands behind the small of the back.	Internal rotation
	Have client make small circles with hands with arms extended at shoulder level.	Circumduction
Elbows	Bend and straighten the elbows.	Flexion and extension
	Place hands at waist with elbows flexed.	Flexion
Wrists	Flex and extend wrist.	Flexion and extension
	Bend wrist to radial then ulnar side.	Radial and ulnar deviation
	Turn palm upward, then downward.	Supination and pronation
Hands	Make a fist with both hands; open hand.	Flexion and extension
	Extend and spread fingers and thumb outward; bring back together.	Adduction and abduction
Lower Extremities		
Hips (with client supine)	With knees extended, raise one leg upward.	Flexion: Expect 90 degrees
	Repeat with knee flexed.	Abduction: Expect 45 degrees
	Swing legs laterally.	Adduction: Expect 30 degrees
	With knee flexed, hold the ankle and rotate the leg inward and outward.	Internal and external rotation: Expect 40-45 degrees
Knees (with client sitting)	Raise the foot, keeping the knee in place.	Extension: Expect full extension and up to 15 degrees hyperextension
Ankles	With foot held off the floor, point toes, then bring toes back toward the knee.	Plantar flexion: Expect 45 degrees
		Dorsiflexion: Expect 20 degrees
Toes	Turn foot inward and then outward.	Inversion and eversion: Expect to reach 5 degrees
	Bend toes down and back.	Expect to reach 40 degrees

*This may be done actively by the client (active range of motion [AROM]) or passively by the nurse (passive range of motion [PROM]).

STEPS	RATIONALE
l. Palpate joint for swelling, stiffness, tenderness, and heat; note any redness.	Indicates acute or chronic inflammation. ROM may cause pain or injury.
m. Assess muscle tone in major muscle groups. Normal tone causes mild, even resistance to movement through entire ROM.	If muscle has increased tone (hypertonicity), any sudden movement of joint is met with considerable resistance. Hypotonic muscle moves without resistance. Muscle feels flabby.

4 Neurological Assessment

STEPS	RATIONALE
a. Assess LOC and orientation by asking client to identify name, location, day of week, and year; note behavior and appearance.	A fully conscious client responds to question spontaneously. As consciousness declines, client may show irritability, short attention span, or unwillingness to cooperate. As consciousness continues to deteriorate, client becomes disoriented to name, time, and place. Behavior and appearance reveal information about client's mental status.
b. Assess cranial nerves. (1) CN III (oculomotor), IV (trochlear), VI (abducens) by assessing extraocular movement functioning. Ask client to follow movement of your finger through the six cardinal positions of gaze; measure pupillary reaction to light reflex and accommodation (see Skill 12.2) using penlight.	These cranial nerves are those most likely affected by increased intracranial pressure (ICP), which causes changes in response of pupil or size of pupil; pupils may change shape (more oval) or react sluggishly. ICP impairs movement of external ocular muscles. Accommodation is ability of the eye to adjust vision from near to far.
(2) CN V (trigeminal) by applying light sensation with a cotton ball to symmetrical areas of face.	Sensations should be symmetrical; unilateral decrease or loss of sensation may be caused by CN V lesion.
(3) CN VII (facial) by noting facial symmetry. Have client frown, smile, puff out cheeks, and raise eyebrows.	Expressions should be symmetrical; drooping of upper and lower face may be caused by Bell's palsy; asymmetry may be caused by cerebrovascular accident (CVA).
(4) CN IX (glossopharyngeal) and CN X (vagus) by having client speak and swallow. Ask client to say "ah" while using tongue blade and penlight. Check for midline uvula and symmetrical rise of uvula and soft palate. Use tongue blade, and place on posterior tongue to elicit gag reflex.	Damage to CN IX causes loss of gag reflex, hoarseness, and nasal voice. A unilateral paralysis is observed when palate fails to rise and uvula pulls toward normal side.
c. Assess extremities for sensation. Begin by having client close eyes.	Perform all sensory testing with client's eyes closed so that client is unable to see when or where a stimulus strikes the skin.
(1) *Pain:* Ask client to indicate when sharp or dull sensation is felt as you alternately apply sharp and blunt ends of tongue blade to skin surface. Apply in symmetrical areas of extremities.	Client should be able to distinguish sharp or dull sensations. Impaired sensations may indicate disorders of the spinal cord or peripheral nerves.
(2) *Light touch:* Apply light wisp of cotton to different points along skin's surface in symmetrical areas of extremities.	Client should be able to distinguish when touched.
(3) *Vibration:* Apply stem of vibrating tuning fork to distal joints of toes and fingers. Have client voice when and where vibration is felt and when sensation stops.	Loss of vibratory sensation occurs with peripheral neuropathy.
(4) *Position:* Grasp finger or toe, holding it by its sides with your thumb and index finger. Alter moving finger or toe up and down. Ask client to state when finger is up or down. Repeat with toes.	Client should be able to distinguish movements of a few millimeters. Decreased/absent position sense may occur in spinal anesthesia, paralysis, or other neurological disorders.
d. Assess motor and cerebellar function. (1) *Gait:* Have client walk across the room, turn, and come back. Note use of assistive devices.	Neurological and musculoskeletal disorders may impair gait and balance.

(2) *Romberg's test*: Have client stand with feet together, arm at sides, both eyes open and closed (for 20 to 30 seconds). Protect client's safety by standing at side; observe for swaying.

Romberg's test should be negative; slight swaying is considered normal.

e. Assess deep tendon reflexes (DTRs).

(1) In clients with back pain or surgery, CVA, or spinal cord compression, it is appropriate to monitor DTRs (Seidel and others, 2006). In most settings this is not part of the routine shift assessment.

Muscle spasticity and hyperactive reflexes may result from disorders such as stroke and paralysis. Diminished DTRs and muscle weakness may suggest lower motor neuron disorders such as amyotrophic lateral sclerosis (ALS) or Guillain-Barré syndrome.

(2) For each reflex tested, compare sides and assign a grade on the following scale:

0 No response
1+ Sluggish or diminished response
2+ Normal, active, or expected response
3+ More brisk than expected; slightly hyperactive
4+ Very brisk; hyperactive, with clonus.

Clonus is described as repeated spasms of muscular contraction and relaxation

(3) *Knee reflex*: Palpate the patellar tendon just below the patella. Tap the pointed end of the reflex hammer briskly on the tendon.

Knee reflex is the most common DTR assessment performed. The normal response is knee extension (see illustration).

(4) *Plantar response (Babinski's reflex)*: Using the handle end of the reflex hammer, stroke the lateral aspect of the sole, from the heel to the ball of the foot.

The toes should flex inward and downward (see illustration).

(5) After stroking the soles of feet, if Babinski's reflex is present, the great toe will dorsiflex, accompanied by fanning of the other toes.

Indicates CNS dysfunction. Dorsiflexion of the great toes and fanning of the others is normal in a child younger than age 2 (Hockenberry and Wilson, 2007).

5 See **Completion Protocol (inside front cover).**

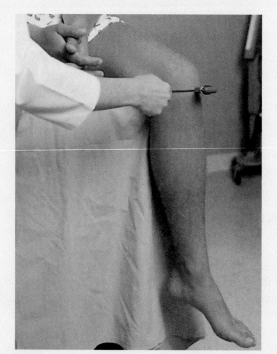

STEP 4e.(3) Position for testing patellar tendon reflexes. Lower leg will normally extend.

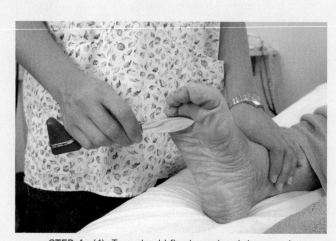

STEP 4e.(4) Toes should flex inward and downward.

EVALUATION

1 Compare muscle strength and ROM with previous assessment.

2 Compare neurological status with previous assessment.

3 Evaluate level of client's discomfort after procedure.

Unexpected Outcomes and Related Interventions

1 Joints are prominent, swollen, and tender with nodules or overgrowth of bone in distal joints, indicating signs of arthritis.

a. Instruct client in proper ROM.

b. Determine client's knowledge regarding antiinflammatory medications.

2 Reduced ROM in one or more major joints.

a. Assess for pain during movement, with joint unstable, stiff, painful, or swollen or with obvious deformity.

b. Notify physician.

c. Reduce mobility in extremity until cause of abnormal joint motion is determined.

3 Client demonstrates weakness in one or more major muscle groups, or gait demonstrates unsteady balance with shuffling or stumbling of feet.

a. Notify physician.

b. Provide for client safety when ambulating.

4 Client has changes in mental status and pupillary response or other neurological deficits.

a. Notify physician immediately.

b. Place on fall precautions.

c. Monitor vital signs and client's LOC closely.

Recording and Reporting

- Record posture, gait, muscle strength, and ROM in nurses' notes or appropriate assessment flow sheet.
- Record LOC, orientation, pupillary response, sensation and reflex responses in nurses' notes or appropriate assessment flow sheet.
- Report acute pain or sudden muscle weakness to nurse in charge or physician.
- Report any change in LOC or change in size or reaction of pupil to the nurse in charge or physician.

Sample Documentation

1530 Out of bed to chair, ambulated without difficulty. Strong, stable gait noted. No complaints of weakness, dizziness, or pain.

Special Considerations
Pediatric Considerations

- Examine infants carefully for musculoskeletal anomalies resulting from genetic or fetal insults. An examination includes review of posture, generalized movement, symmetry and skin creases of the extremities, muscle strength, and hip alignment.
- Normally the back of a newborn is rounded or C-shaped from the thoracic and pelvic curves.
- Scoliosis, lateral curvature of the spine, is an important childhood problem, especially in females apparent at puberty. (For closer examination, have child stand erect, wearing only underclothes. Observe from behind, looking for asymmetry of shoulders and hips. Then observe from the back as the child bends forward.) Uneven dress hems or pant leg hems or uneven fit of clothing at the waist may be noted.
- Watching a child during play can reveal information about musculoskeletal function.

Geriatric Considerations

- Older adult's gait normally has smaller steps and a wider base of support.
- Older adults tend to assume a stooped, forward-bent posture, with hips and knees somewhat flexed and arms bent at the elbows and the level of the arms raised (Ebersole, Hess, and Luggen, 2004).
- In older adults, joints often become swollen and stiff, with reduced ROM resulting from cartilage erosion and fibrosis of synovial membranes.
- Older adults may develop kyphosis because of osteoporosis.
- Functional assessment is a measure of older person's ability to perform basic self-care tasks (Burke and Laramie, 2004). When client is unable to perform self-care easily, determine the need for assistive devices.

NCLEX® Style Questions

1 In conducting a general survey of a client the nurse knows that the survey should include which of the following? Select all that apply.
1. Appearance
2. Obtaining peripheral pulses
3. Observing specific body systems
4. Conducting a detailed history
5. Behavior
6. Pupillary response
7. Posture

2 In teaching a client about skin lesions, the nurse knows that teaching has been successful when the client identifies which lesion as abnormal?
1. A symmetrical lesion
2. A lesion with regular edges and borders
3. One that is blue/black or varied in color
4. One that is less than 7 mm in diameter

3 On respiratory assessment the nurse notes high-pitched, musical sounds on auscultation. The nurse interprets these sounds as:
1. Normal
2. Rhonchi
3. Crackles
4. Wheezes

4 The nurse determines the client has a palpable vibration during cardiovascular assessment. After documenting this finding the nurse should:
1. Reposition the client for comfort.
2. Report the finding to the physician.
3. Initiate fluid restriction.
4. Do nothing as this is a normal finding.

5 Place the following components of the abdominal assessment in the correct order:
1. Palpation
2. Inspection
3. Auscultation

6 An infant has a history of vomiting and diarrhea. Assessment findings reveal dry mucous membranes, decreased urine output, weight loss of 1 pound over the past 2 days, and urine specific gravity of 1.040. Based on this data, an appropriate nursing diagnosis is:
1. Excess fluid volume
2. Total urinary incontinence
3. Deficient fluid volume
4. Ineffective feeding pattern

7 Which of the following does the nurse document as an abnormal finding during a neurological assessment?
1. Pupils equal, round, and reactive to light and accommodation
2. DTR reflex very brisk
3. Negative Romberg's test
4. Uvula rises symmetrically

References for all chapters appear in Appendix D.

Laboratory Tests

13

MEDIA RESOURCES

- **evolve** http://evolve.elsevier.com/Elkin
- **Video Clips**
- **Nursing Skills Online**

Laboratory test results aid in the diagnosis of health care problems, provide information about the stage and activity of a disease process, and measure client's response to therapy. Proficiency and judgment in obtaining specimens minimize client discomfort, ensure client safety, and ensure accuracy and quality of diagnostic procedures. Nurses are accountable for correctly collecting specimens, monitoring client outcomes, and ensuring that these tests are collected in a timely manner. When there are questions about laboratory tests, consult the institution's procedure manual or call the laboratory.

Normal values for laboratory tests are found in reference books. However, each laboratory also establishes its own values for each test, which are printed on the agency's laboratory slips. It is important to know the significance of abnormal findings. Discuss only major deviations with the health care provider immediately.

Confidentiality is an important issue associated with testing. Agencies must have clearly written and enforced policies regarding disclosure of test results while maintaining confidentiality within the health care system (USDHHS, 2003).

When collecting any specimen, know the purpose of the test, how much of the specimen is needed, what collection container is appropriate, and how it is to be transported to the laboratory (Parini, 2000). Clients may experience embarrassment or discomfort when giving a sample of body excretions or secretions. It is important to handle excretions discreetly and to provide the client with as much privacy as possible.

With clear instructions many clients are able to obtain their own specimens of urine, stool, and sputum, thus avoiding unnecessary exposure. Consider the words you use because many clients, especially children, would not understand the terms *void*, *urine*, or *stool*. Be sure the words and instructions are clearly understood.

Cultural considerations are important when collecting specimens. Customs may affect the client's response and willingness to participate in various diagnostic procedures. Southeast Asians consider the blood as a vital life force that should not be wasted. Introduction of a swab or tongue blade into the mouth to collect specimens may be threatening to Southeast Asians who believe that diseases can be introduced through the mouth and that the head is the seat of one's life force. Muslims and Hindus designate that only the left hand is to be used for tasks related to urine and stool (Lawrence and Rozmus, 2001).

Whenever possible, use same gender caregivers when collecting vaginal, rectal, or urinary specimens from clients whose cultural values demand modesty and distinct separation of gender roles. Provide privacy both when giving instructions and collecting the specimen.

A laboratory requisition is needed for each specimen to instruct laboratory personnel on the test to be performed on each specimen and to facilitate accurate reporting of the results. Each requisition includes client identification (name and numbers), the date and time the specimen is obtained, the name of the test, and the source of specimen/culture for each container (JCAHO, 2006).

Before specimen collection, at least two client identifiers are needed, neither of which may be the client's room number or physical location (JCAHO, 2007). After the specimen is collected, and in the presence of the client, the container itself (not the lid) must be labeled with the same two identifiers (e.g., client name and hospital identification number), specimen source, collection date and time, series number (if more than one specimen), and anatomical site if appropriate (e.g., wound culture from knee versus abdominal incision). In some agencies bar codes are used to label specimens.

All who handle body fluids are at risk for exposure to body fluids. The use of hand hygiene and clean gloves are necessary when collecting a specimen. A plastic bag marked "biohazard" is used to enclose the specimen for delivery to the laboratory (Figure 13-1). Specimens are delivered promptly to the laboratory. Specimens left at room temperature are at risk for additional bacterial growth, thereby altering the results of the test.

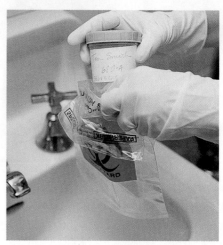

FIGURE 13-1 Enclose all specimens in a biohazard plastic bag.

EVIDENCE IN PRACTICE

Roark DC, Miguel K: RFID: bar coding's replacement, *Nurs Manage* 37(2):28, 2006.

Identification errors are the most common serious laboratory errors. One of the most important factors in safe and effective collection of laboratory specimens is ensuring that caregivers perform the right test and obtain the right specimen from the right client. Misidentification of specimens may lead to incorrect diagnoses and unnecessary or inappropriate treatments.

New technologies provide simple and accurate identification systems to ensure client safety and meet the basic requirement of two client identifiers. One option is the bar code on the client's identification bracelet, which is scanned when a specimen is collected. A second option is a radio frequency identification device (RFID), which is a wireless networking technology using a microchip with a radio antenna in an electronic tag on the client's arm band. A third option uses a bar code implanted under the client's skin, which transmits a unique code to a special scanner using radio waves. Additional detailed medical information is accessed from an accompanying database.

NURSING DIAGNOSES

Anxiety may be related to anticipating embarrassment, discomfort, or pain as a specimen is obtained. **Fear** may be related to anticipation of unfavorable or unknown test results. **Risk for infection** applies when skin or tissue integrity is altered.

- Nursing Skills Online: Specimen Collection, Lessons 1 and 2; Urinary Catheterization, Lesson 4

A urinalysis provides information about kidney or metabolic function, nutrition, and systemic diseases. Urine is collected using a variety of methods depending upon the purpose of the urinalysis and the presence or absence of a urinary catheter. Regardless of the method of collection, guidelines for assessment, planning, and evaluation are similar. Routine urinalysis includes measurement of nine or more elements (Table 13-1).

Types of Urine Tests and Specimens

A *random urine specimen for routine urinalysis* is collected using a specimen "hat" (Figure 13-2), which is placed under a toilet seat to collect voided urine. Approximately 120 ml of urine is then placed in a specimen container, properly labeled, and sent to the laboratory.

A *culture and sensitivity (C&S) of urine* is performed to identify urinary tract infection (UTI) (culture) and to determine the most effective antibiotic for treatment (sensitivity). Use sterile technique to ensure that any microorganisms present originate in the urine and not from the client's skin, hands, or the environment. Specimens for C&S are collected either as a clean-voided midstream specimen or under sterile conditions from a urinary catheter. Urine collected by these methods may also be analyzed for the same components as the routine urinalysis.

A *timed urine specimen for quantitative analysis* requires urine to be collected over 2 to 72 hours. The 24-hour timed collection (see Procedural Guideline 13-1) is most common and allows for measurement and quantitative analysis of elements such as amino acids, creatinine, hormones, glucose, and adrenocorticosteroid excreted.

Chemical properties of urine are tested by immersing a specially prepared strip of paper (Chemstrip) into a clean urine specimen. The test detects the presence of glucose, ketones, protein, or blood *not* normally present in the urine (see Procedural Guideline 13-2). When the screening test for the presence of substances in the urine is positive, additional laboratory tests are used to determine the client's diagnosis or to measure the effectiveness of treatment. This type of screening is used when more detailed laboratory testing is not readily available, for example, in a physician's office or clinic and in the outpatient, long-term care, or home setting. It may also be done for pregnant women on admission to the hospital in labor.

ASSESSMENT

1 Assess client's understanding of need for the specimen. *Rationale: This determines the need for health teaching. Client's understanding of purpose promotes cooperation.*

2 Assess client's ability to assist with urine specimen collection: able to position self and hold container. *Rationale: This determines client's level of assistance required.*

3 Determine if fluid, dietary requirements, or medications need to be administered in conjunction with test. *Rationale: Certain substances affect excretion and levels of urinary constituents.*

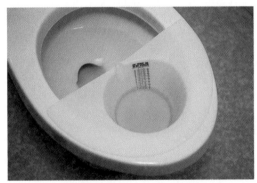

FIGURE 13-2 Specimen "hat."

TABLE 13-1 Elements Measured in Routine Urinalysis		
ELEMENT	**NORMAL VALUE**	**SIGNIFICANCE**
pH value	4.6-8.0 (average 6.0)	Indicates acid-base balance.
Protein level	Not normally present	Presence suggests renal disease or damage.
Glucose level	Not normally present	Elevated in diabetes.
Ketones	Not normally present	Present with dehydration, starvation, and poorly controlled diabetes mellitus.
Blood	< 2 red blood cells (RBCs)	Elevated with kidney disease or damage, trauma, and surgery.
Specific gravity	1.005-1.030 (usually 1.010-1.025)	Reflects urine concentration. Increased with dehydration; decreased with overhydration; altered with kidney damage and abnormal antidiuretic hormone (ADH) secretion.
White blood cell (WBC) count	0 to 4 per low-power field	Elevated with UTI.
Bacteria	Not normally present	Presence indicates urinary tract infection (UTI).
Casts	Not normally present	Presence indicates kidney abnormality.

Pagana KD, Pagana TJ: *Mosby's diagnostic and laboratory tests reference,* ed 7, St Louis, 2005, Mosby.

Specific amounts of fluid may be required for concentration/dilution tests. Drugs such as cortisone preparations, diuretics, and anesthetics increase glucose levels. Anticoagulants increase risk of blood in the urine.

4 Assess for signs and symptoms of UTI (frequency, urgency, dysuria, hematuria, flank pain, cloudy urine with sediment, foul odor, fever). *Rationale: Indicators of UTI.*

5 Assess client's current urinary elimination pattern. *Rationale: Possible indicator of UTI. Knowledge of frequency of urination facilitates effective planning of specimen collection.*

PLANNING

Expected Outcomes focus on the collection of an appropriate uncontaminated specimen by nurse or client with client knowledgeable of the purpose of the specimen examination.

1 Client explains procedure for specimen collection.

2 Client explains purpose of specimen analysis.

3 Client's specimen is appropriate and free of contaminants, such as toilet tissue or stool.

Delegation Considerations

The skill of collecting urine specimens may be delegated. The nurse directs personnel by:

- Explaining when to collect specimen
- Reviewing to observe the amount and appearance of urine specimen and if the urine is not clear (e.g., contains blood, cloudiness, or excess sediment) to report this information back to the nurse

Equipment

- Completed identification labels (with appropriate client identifiers)
- Completed laboratory requisition including appropriate client identification, date, time, name of test, and source of culture
- Small plastic bag for delivery of specimen to laboratory (or container as specified by agency)

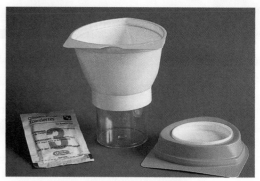

FIGURE 13-3 Clean-voided urine kit.

Clean-Voided Urine Specimen

- Clean gloves
- Commercial kit for clean-voided urine (Figure 13-3) containing:
  - Cotton balls or antiseptic towelettes
  - Antiseptic solution (usually chlorhexidine or povidone-iodine solution)
  - Sterile water or normal saline
  - Sterile specimen container
  - Sterile gloves
- Soap, water, washcloth, and towel
- Bedpan (for nonambulatory client) or specimen "hat" (for ambulatory client)

Sterile Urine Specimen from Urinary Catheter

- Clean gloves
- 3-ml safety syringe with 1-inch needle (21 to 25 gauge) for culture; 20-ml safety syringe with 1-inch needle (21 to 25 gauge) for routine urinalysis
- Clamp or rubber band
- Alcohol, chlorhexidine, or other disinfectant swab
- Specimen container (nonsterile for routine urinalysis; sterile for culture)

IMPLEMENTATION *for Urine Specimen Collection—Midstream, Sterile Urinary Catheter*

STEPS	RATIONALE
1 See Standard Protocol (inside front cover).	
2 Explain to client and/or family member reason specimen is needed, how client can assist (when applicable), and how to obtain a specimen that is free of tissue and stool.	Promotes cooperation and client participation. In some cases client can collect clean-voided specimen independently.
3 Collect clean-voided urine specimen.	
a. Give client or family member towel, washcloth, and soap to cleanse perineum, or assist client (after application of clean gloves) with cleansing perineum. If client is bedridden, this may be done with the client positioned on the bedpan to facilitate access to the perineum.	Clients usually prefer to wash their own perineal area when possible.

STEPS	**RATIONALE**

b. Using surgical asepsis, open outer package of commercial specimen kit.

Maintains sterility of specimen container.

c. Apply sterile gloves.

Prevents introduction of microorganisms into urine specimen from nurse's hands.
Cotton ball or gauze pad is used to cleanse perineum.

d. Pour antiseptic solution over cotton balls (unless kit contains prepared gauze pads in antiseptic solution).

e. Open specimen container, maintaining sterility of inside of specimen container, and place cap with sterile inside surface up. Do not touch inside of cap or container.

Contaminated specimen is the most frequent reason for inaccurate reporting of urine cultures and sensitivities.

f. Perform urine collection by assisting or allowing client to independently cleanse perineum and collect specimen. The amount of assistance needed varies with each client; provide assistance if necessary.

Maintains client's dignity and comfort.

> **COMMUNICATION TIP** Inform client that antiseptic solution will feel cold. Tell female to wipe from front to back. Tell uncircumcised male client to retract foreskin for effective cleansing of urinary meatus and during voiding.

(1) Male:

(a) Hold penis with one hand; using circular motion and antiseptic towelette, cleanse meatus, moving from center to outside (see illustration).

Reduces number of microorganisms at urethral meatus and moves from areas of least to most contamination.

(b) If agency procedure indicates, rinse area with sterile water and dry with cotton balls or gauze pad.

Prevents contamination of specimen with antiseptic solution.

(c) After client has initiated urine stream into toilet or bedpan, pass urine specimen container into stream and collect 30 to 60 ml of urine (see illustration).

Initial urine flushes microorganisms that normally accumulate at urinary meatus and prevents collection in specimen.

(2) Female:

(a) Spread labia minora with fingers of nondominant hand. Using a new antiseptic swab, cotton ball, or gauze *each time*, cleanse the area from front to back over the urinary meatus and along each side.

Provides access to urinary meatus.

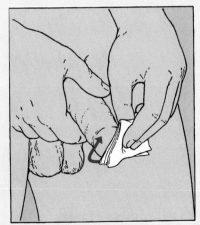

STEP 3f.(1)(a) Cleanse penis with circular motion. (Modified from Grimes D: *Infectious diseases,* Mosby's clinical nursing series, St Louis, 1991, Mosby.)

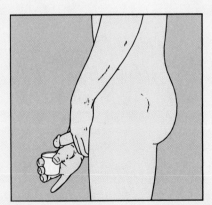

STEP 3f.(1)(c) Position of male for collecting midstream urine specimen.

STEPS	RATIONALE

(b) Use the dominant hand to cleanse from front (above urethral orifice) to back (toward anus) *three times* (begin with center, then do left and right sides (see illustration).

Prevents contamination of urinary meatus with fecal material.

(c) If agency procedure indicates, rinse area with sterile water and dry with cotton.

Prevents contamination of specimen with antiseptic solution.

(d) While continuing to hold labia apart, client initiates urine stream into the toilet or bedpan; after stream is achieved, pass specimen container into stream and collect 30 to 60 ml of urine.

Initial urine flushes out microorganisms that normally accumulate at the urinary meatus and provides uncontaminated urine from the bladder itself.

g. Remove specimen container before flow of urine stops and before releasing penis or labia. Client finishes voiding into bedpan or toilet.

Prevents contamination of specimen with skin flora.

h. Replace cap securely on specimen container, touching only outside.

Retains sterility of inside of container and prevents spillage of urine.

i. Cleanse urine from exterior surface of container. Remove and dispose of sterile gloves.

Prevents transfer of microorganisms to others.

NURSE ALERT	Indicate on the laboratory slip if client is menstruating.

---

4 Collect urine from an indwelling urinary catheter.

a. Explain that although a syringe with a needle is to be used to remove the urine from the catheter, client will not experience discomfort.

Minimizes anxiety when nurse manipulates catheter and aspirates urine with syringe and needle.

b. Explain that catheter will need to be clamped for 10-30 minutes before obtaining a urine specimen and why it is not obtained from drainage bag.

c. Clamp drainage tubing with clamp or rubber band for as long as 30 minutes below the site chosen for withdrawal (see illustration).

Permits collection of fresh, sterile urine in catheter tubing.
Amount of time depends upon amount of urine client produces.

d. At the appropriate time, position client so catheter port is easily accessible. Cleanse self-sealing diaphragm with disinfectant swab, allowing it to dry.

Prevents entry of microorganisms into catheter.

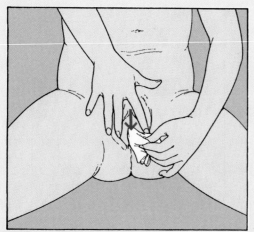

STEP 3f.(2)(b) Cleanse from front to back, holding labia apart. (Modified from Grimes D: *Infectious diseases,* Mosby's clinical nursing series, St Louis, 1991, Mosby.)

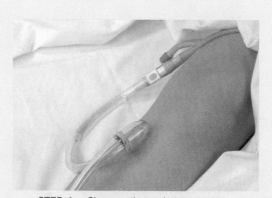

STEP 4c. Clamp catheter drainage tubing.

STEPS	RATIONALE
e. Insert needle of syringe at 45-degree angle just above where catheter is attached to drainage tube at built-in sampling port in silastic, silicone, or plastic catheter (see illustration).	Ensures entrance of needle into catheter lumen and prevents accidental puncture of lumen leading to balloon that holds catheter in place in bladder. Accidental aspiration of water from lumen can result in catheter slipping out of bladder.
f. Withdraw 3 ml for culture or 20 ml for routine urinalysis.	Allows collection of urine without contamination. Obtains proper volume for testing.
g. Transfer urine from syringe into clean urine container for routine urinalysis, or into a sterile urine container for culture.	Prevents contamination of urine during transfer procedure.
h. Place lid tightly on container.	Prevents contamination of specimen by air and loss by spillage.
i. Unclamp catheter, and allow urine to flow into drainage bag. Ensure urine flows freely.	Allows urine to drain by gravity and prevents stasis of urine in bladder, which can cause discomfort and potential damage to the kidneys.
5 Securely attach properly completed identification label to the side of specimen container (not the lid).	
6 Send specimen and requisition to laboratory within 20 minutes. Refrigerate if delay cannot be avoided.	Delay of analysis may alter test results significantly (National Committee for Clinical Laboratory Standards [NCCLS], 2001).
7 **See Completion Protocol (inside front cover).**	

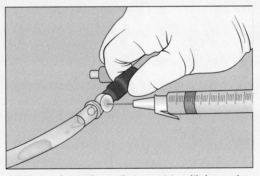

STEP 4e. Accessing catheter port to withdraw urine.

EVALUATION

1 Ask client to identify steps in specimen collection procedure.

2 Ask client to state purposes of specimen collection.

3 Inspect clean-voided specimen for contamination with toilet tissue or stool.

4 Observe urinary drainage system to be sure it is intact and patent.

Unexpected Outcomes and Related Interventions

1 Client is unable to void, or urine does not collect in drainage tube.

a. Offer fluids (if permitted) to enhance urine production.

2 Client's urine specimen is contaminated with stool and tissue.

a. Reinforce importance of obtaining specimen free of contaminants.

b. Collect a new specimen, and assist client with specimen collection; place specimen "hat" as close to front of commode as possible.

3 Lumen that leads to balloon holding catheter in bladder is punctured.

a. Notify provider and prepare for insertion of new catheter.

b. Obtain new specimen.

Recording and Reporting

- Record method used to obtain specimen, date and time collected, type of test ordered, laboratory receiving specimen, characteristics of specimen, and client's tolerance to procedure of specimen collection.
- Report any abnormal findings.

Sample Documentation

1135 Clean-voided specimen of 130 ml dark amber urine obtained. Specimen sent to lab. Reports frequent urge to void, burning sensation with voiding, and voiding small amounts.

Special Considerations

Pediatric Considerations

- It is not possible to obtain a midstream urine collection on a non–toilet-trained child; consequently, urine for culture should be obtained by use of a sterile plastic urine-collecting bag that adheres to the perineum.

Geriatric Considerations

- Older adults may need assistance in positioning to obtain specimen. In confused clients, assistive personnel (AP) may be necessary to hold client's hands while sample is being obtained.
- The older client may need a written reminder placed on the bathroom mirror to collect all urine.

Home Care Considerations

- When a specimen for culture is collected at home, the specimen is kept on ice until it reaches the laboratory to minimize bacterial growth before applying it to a culture medium in a laboratory setting.

PROCEDURAL GUIDELINE 13-1

Collecting 24-Hour Timed Urine Specimens

Delegation Considerations

The skill of collecting a timed urine specimen may be delegated. The nurse directs personnel by:

- Explaining the time to begin specimen collection, how to store collected urine, where to place signs that a timed urine collection is in progress, and to save all urine
- Reviewing what to observe for and to report the presence of blood, mucus, or foul odors present in the specimen or if there is a break in the collection procedure

Equipment

- Large collection bottle with cap that usually contains a chemical preservative for urine
- Bedpan, urinal, or specimen "hat"
- Graduated measuring cup, if intake and output (I&O) are to be recorded
- Basin large enough to hold collection bottle surrounded by ice if immediate refrigeration is required
- Instructional signs that remind client and staff of timed urine collection
- Clean disposable gloves
- Completed identification labels (with appropriate client identifiers)
- Completed laboratory requisition, including appropriate client identification, date, time, name of test, and source of culture
- Small plastic bag for delivery of specimen to laboratory (or container as specified by agency)

Procedural Steps

1. **See Standard Protocol (inside front cover).**
2. Explain the reason for specimen collection, how client can assist, and that urine must be free of feces and toilet tissue.

3. Place signs indicating timed urine specimen collection on client's door and toileting area. If client leaves unit for another test or procedure, be sure that personnel in that area collect and save all urine.
4. If possible, have client drink two to four glasses of water about 30 minutes before timed collection to facilitate ability to void at the appropriate time for the test to begin.
5. Discard the first specimen as test begins. Print time that test began on laboratory requisition. For accurate results the client must begin the test with an empty bladder.
6. Measure volume of each voiding if I&O is being recorded. Then place all voided urine in labeled specimen bottle with appropriate additive.

> **NURSE ALERT** It is essential for all urine to be collected for accurate test results. Restart timed period if urine is accidentally lost, discarded, or contaminated.

7. Unless instructed otherwise, keep specimen bottle in specimen refrigerator or in container of ice in bathroom to prevent decomposition of urine.
8. Encourage client to drink two glasses of water 1 hour before timed urine collection ends.
9. Encourage client to empty bladder during last 15 minutes of urine collection period.
10. At end of collection period, send labeled specimen to laboratory with appropriate requisition.
11. Remove signs, and inform client that specimen collection period is completed.
12. **See Completion Protocol (inside front cover).**

PROCEDURAL GUIDELINE 13-2

Urine Screening for Glucose, Ketones, Protein, Blood, and pH

Delegation Considerations

The skill of urine screening for glucose, ketones, protein, blood, and pH may be delegated. The nurse directs personnel by:

- Explaining when to obtain the specimen (e.g., before meals, following a "double-voided" specimen)
- Reviewing the need to report to the nurse the results of the test or any blood, mucus, or odor in the specimen

Equipment

- Specimen "hat," bedpan, urinal, or commode
- Watch with second hand or digital counter
- Clean disposable gloves
- Reagent test strip (check expiration date on container)
- Test strip color chart

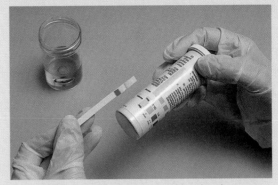

STEP 6 Compare multistix with color chart.

Procedural Steps

1 **See Standard Protocol (inside front cover).**
2 Determine if a "double-voided" specimen is needed for glucose testing. If required, ask client to void and then drink a glass of water.
3 Ask client to collect a fresh random urine sample (see Skill 13.1), or if required the "double-voided" specimen. If client is catheterized, a 5-ml specimen from catheter is adequate.
4 Immerse end of reagent test strip into urine container. Remove the strip immediately, and tap it gently against container's side to remove excess urine.

5 Hold strip in horizontal position to prevent mixing of chemical reagents.
6 Precisely time the number of seconds specified on container, then compare color of strip with color chart on container (see illustration).
7 Remove and discard gloves.
8 When appropriate, discuss test results with client.
9 **See Completion Protocol (inside front cover).**

SKILL 13.2 Testing for Gastrointestinal Alterations—Gastroccult Test, Stool Specimen, and Hemoccult Test

- Nursing Skills Online: Specimen Collection, Lessons 3 and 4

The collection of gastric secretions may involve obtaining a specimen via a nasogastric (NG) or nasointestinal (NI) tube. When a client has emesis, the nurse tests the material for the presence of blood. Analysis of stool or gastric secretions from the gastrointestinal (GI) tract provides useful information about pathological conditions such as the presence of tumors, infection, and malabsorption problems. Clients can often assist in providing stool specimens. A meat-free, high-residue diet for 24 hours before testing is desirable to prevent false positive results.

The term *occult blood* refers to blood that is not visible but is present in microscopic amounts. Tests done to detect the presence of occult blood in stool (guaiac test) or emesis and gastric secretions (Gastroccult test) reveal bleeding in the esophagus, stomach, small intestine, or large intestine. The tests verify the presence of blood when the nurse notices red or black coloration of stool or gastric contents, or a coffee-grounds appearance of gastric contents in emesis or with NG suction (see Chapter 30).

Hemoccult testing is useful for screening for the presence of occult (invisible) blood in the stool for conditions such as colon cancer, bleeding GI ulcers, and localized gastric or intestinal irritation. The stool may appear bloody following a diet including red meat. Hemoccult testing differentiates between blood and other questionable substances in stool. When blood is present, further testing is indicated to determine the source of the bleeding.

ASSESSMENT

1 Assess client's medical history for GI disorders (e.g., history of bleeding, hemorrhoids, colitis, malabsorption disorders).
2 Determine client's ability to cooperate with procedure and collect specimen.
3 Assess female client's menstrual cycle. *Rationale: A woman who is menstruating may have a stool specimen contaminated with blood.*
4 Review medications for drugs that can contribute to GI bleeding. *Rationale: Anticoagulants, steroids, nonsteroidal antiinflammatory drugs (NSAIDs), ascorbic acid (vitamin C), antiinflammatory agents, and alcohol commonly cause bleeding tendency or irritation of GI mucosa.*

5 Check physician's orders for dietary restrictions before testing. *Rationale: Diets rich in red meats, green leafy vegetables, poultry, and fish may produce false-positive guaiac results.*

PLANNING

Expected Outcomes focus on the collection of an appropriate specimen, with client knowledgeable of the purpose of the specimen test.
1 Client will discuss the purpose of test.
2 Client will maintain a high-residue diet that is free of red meat for specified period.
3 Client's specimen is appropriate for testing analysis.

Delegation Considerations
Assessment of the client's condition should not be delegated. The skills of obtaining and testing gastric secretions from an NG or nasoenteral tube may not be delegated. The skill of obtaining stool specimens may be delegated. The nurse directs personnel by:
- Explaining when to obtain stool specimen
- Reviewing with personnel to report immediately if blood is detected, not to discard stool from a positive test, and to report immediately if blood is observed in client emesis or NG tube drainage

Equipment
- Clean gloves
- Soap, water, washcloth, and towel

Gastroccult Test
- Facial tissues
- Emesis basin
- Wooden applicator or 3-ml syringe
- 60-ml bulb or catheter tip syringe
- Cardboard Gastroccult slide and developing solution (Figure 13-4)

Stool Specimens
- Plastic container with lid
- Two tongue blades
- Paper towel
- Bedpan, specimen "hat," or bedside commode
- "Save stool" signs (24-hour timed specimen)
- Sterile test tube and swab (for culture)
- Completed identification labels (with appropriate client identifiers)
- Completed laboratory requisition, including appropriate client identification, date, time, name of test, and source of culture
- Small plastic bag for delivery of specimen to laboratory (or container as specified by agency

Hemoccult (Guaiac Test)
- Paper towel
- Wooden applicator
- Cardboard Hemoccult slide and Hemoccult developing solution (Figure 13-5)

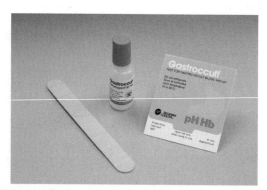

FIGURE 13-4 Cardboard Gastroccult slide and developing solution.

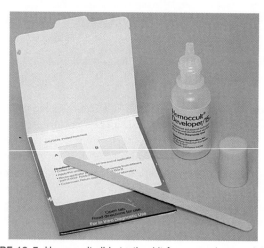

FIGURE 13-5 Hemoccult slide testing kit for measuring occult blood.

IMPLEMENTATION *for Testing for Gastrointestinal Alterations—Gastroccult Test, Stool Specimen, and Hemoccult Test*

STEPS	RATIONALE

1 **See Standard Protocol (inside front cover).**

2 Arrange for dietary and/or medication restrictions as indicated.

3 Discuss reason specimen is needed, how client can assist in collecting an uncontaminated specimen (for stool specimen), and how gastric specimen will be obtained.

Promotes client cooperation.

4 Perform Gastroccult test.

> **NURSE ALERT** Gastroccult and Hemoccult slides and developers are *not* interchangeable.

a. To obtain specimen of gastric contents from NG or nasoenteral tube, position client in high-Fowler's position in bed or chair.

Minimizes chance of aspiration of gastric contents. Position relieves pressure on abdominal organs. If client is nauseated, flat position in bed or one in which client cannot sit straight may cause abdominal discomfort.

b. Verify NG tube placement (see Chapter 30).

Ensures aspiration of gastric contents.

c. Collect gastric contents via NG or nasoenteral tube by disconnecting tube from suction or gravity drainage. Attach bulb- or catheter-tipped syringe. Aspirate 5 to 10 ml.

Only small amount of specimen is needed for pH and occult blood testing.

d. To obtain sample of emesis, use a 3-ml syringe or wooden applicator to gather sample.

e. Using applicator or syringe, apply 1 drop of gastric sample to Gastroccult blood test slide.

Sample must cover test paper for test reaction to occur.

f. Apply 2 drops of commercial Gastroccult developer solution over sample and 1 drop between positive and negative performance monitors (see illustration).

g. Verify that performance monitor turns blue after 30 seconds.

Indicates proper function of the testing paper.

h. After 60 seconds compare color of gastric sample with that of performance monitors.

If sample turns blue, test is positive for occult blood. If sample turns green, test is negative for occult blood.

i. Explain test results to client.

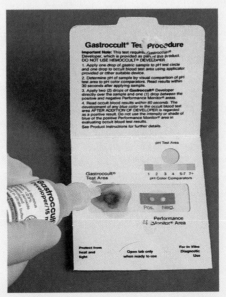

STEP 4f. Apply developing solution to Gastroccult test area.

STEPS	RATIONALE

j. Dispose of test slides, wooden applicator, and 1-ml syringe in proper receptacle.

Reduces spread of infection.

k. If needed, reconnect NG tube to drainage system, suction, or clamp as ordered.

NG tube serves to decompress abdomen by promoting drainage.

5 Collect stool specimen.

a. Assist client as needed into bathroom or to commode or bedpan. Instruct client to void into toilet or urinal before collecting specimen in container. Provide a clean, dry bedpan or specimen "hat" in which to defecate.

Feces must not be mixed with urine, water, or toilet tissue. Urine inhibits fecal bacterial growth. Toilet tissue contains bismuth, which interferes with test results.

b. If needed, assist client in washing after toileting, and leave in a comfortable position.

c. Transport specimen container with stool to bathroom or utility room and gather specimen.

(1) **Culture.** Remove swab from sterile test tube, gather bean-sized piece of stool, and return swab to tube. If stool is liquid, soak cotton swab in it and return to tube.

Stool is touched only by sterile swab to prevent introduction of bacteria.

(2) **Timed stool specimen.** All of each stool is placed in waxed cardboard containers for specific time ordered and kept in specimen refrigerator.

Tests for dietary products and digestive enzymes such as fat content or bile require analysis of all feces over select time period.

   (a) For timed test, place signs that read "Save all stool (with appropriate date or time)" over client's bed, on bathroom door, and above toilet.

Helps prevent any accidental disposal of stool.

   (b) After specimen going to the laboratory is obtained, immediately place lid on container tightly.

Prevents spread of microorganisms by air or contact with other articles.

(3) **All other tests, including Hemoccult (guaiac) test.** Obtain specimen by using tongue blades and transfer portion of stool to container (2.5 cm [1 inch] of formed stool or 15 ml of liquid stool).

6 Perform Hemoccult test.

a. Use tip of wooden applicator to obtain small portion of feces.

b. Open flap of Hemoccult slide. Use tip of wooden applicator to obtain a small portion of feces and apply thin smear of stool on paper in first box.

Guaiac paper inside box is sensitive to fecal blood content.

c. Obtain a second fecal specimen from different portion of stool and apply thinly to slide's second box (see illustration).

Occult blood from upper GI tract is not always equally dispersed through stool. Findings of occult blood are more conclusive when entire specimen is found to contain blood.

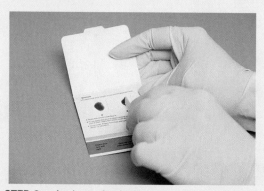

STEP 6c. Apply stool to both spots on Hemoccult slide.

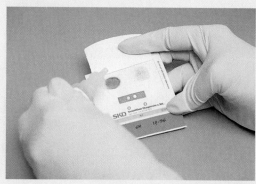

STEP 6d. Apply developing solution to Hemoccult slide.

STEPS	RATIONALE
d. Close slide cover, and turn slide over to reverse side. Open cardboard flap, and apply 2 drops of Hemoccult developing solution on each box of guaiac paper (see illustration).	Developing solution penetrates underlying fecal specimen. Blood is indicated by change in color of guaiac paper.
e. Read results of test after 30 to 60 seconds. Note color changes.	Bluish discoloration indicates occult blood (guaiac positive). No change in color of guaiac paper indicates negative results.

6 See Completion Protocol (inside front cover).

EVALUATION

1 Observe quantity, character, and color of stool, emesis, or gastric secretions.
2 Compare test findings with normal expected results.
3 Ask client to explain the purpose of the test.

Unexpected Outcomes and Related Interventions

1 Occult blood test results are positive.
a. Continue to monitor client.
b. Notify physician.

Recording and Reporting

- Record results of test in appropriate records (check agency policy); include characteristics of stool/gastric contents in nurses' notes.
- Report positive results to physician.

Sample Documentation

1600 Large, liquid, dark brown stool tested positive for occult blood. Physician notified. Client informed that test is to be repeated ×2.

Special Considerations
Home Care Considerations

- Clients are instructed to collect Hemoccult specimens at home and return them to the clinic or physician's office. To collect stool specimen, a piece of plastic wrap can be draped over the toilet. If possible the specimen should not be contaminated with urine. The client prepares slide with feces, closes cardboard slide, and returns it to the office or clinic.

SKILL 13.3 Blood Glucose Monitoring

A blood glucose meter is an effective and efficient method for assessing glucose control in the client with diabetes mellitus. In the health care setting, the monitor used may be different from the type the client uses at home. The client needs to know about the general principles for accurate glucose monitoring and reporting of results. It is often helpful to request that a family member bring the meter from home to assess the client's skill. Blood glucose monitoring (BGM) checks glucose levels in a sample of capillary blood, usually obtained from the fingertip. The results are used to direct lifestyle changes, such as diet, medication, and physical activity. Regular BGM is an essential component of any diabetes self-management program (AADE, 2006).

Most glucose meters require a skin puncture to obtain a sample of capillary blood. The sample is placed on a test strip and the meter calibrates the level of glucose in the sample. Immediate feedback on glucose levels helps clients prevent or recognize and quickly treat abnormal glucose levels according to the care provider's instructions.

There are two types of meters: *reflectance meters* and *sensor-type meters*. With the older reflectance type, a drop of blood reacts with an enzyme on the test strip and changes the color of the strip. Many of these meters are being replaced with the sensor-type meters. Sensor-type meters measure the electronic charge generated by the reaction of the glucose and an enzyme and display an actual glucose reading in mg/dl format. Most meters on the market today are the sensor-type meter. Today's meters are portable, lightweight, and run on batteries. They all provide fast results, usually in a minute or less and some even in 5 seconds (ADA, 2006b). Although all meters use a drop of whole blood on a test strip, some read the plasma glucose level or have been programmed to calculate the plasma glucose level. A meter that provides plasma glucose levels will have results that are closer to the laboratory's results (AADE, 2003). Many of the meters for home use have memory capability and can store 100 to 450 glucose readings.

Most meters now allow for the use of alternate site or forearm capillary blood testing. Many feel that this is less painful than finger-stick testing. Alternate site testing is most accurate and correlates best to finger-stick testing at times when blood glucose levels are not changing rapidly, such as checking fasting blood glucose levels. When blood glucose levels are changing at a rapid level, such as after meals or if the client is experiencing hypoglycemic symptoms, it is best to use the fingertip testing site.

Lancets and automatic lancing devices are part of glucose monitoring kits. Most lancet devices come with short and long lancet covers to provide different degrees of penetration, and many have adjustable covers or caps (ADA, 2006b). A disposable needle needs to be placed in the lancet device for finger and alternate site testing. It is recommended that the disposable needle be changed after each use and disposed of in an appropriate container, such as a home sharps container or #2 plastic container.

Glucose meters vary in size, shape, weight, ease of use, size of display readout, size of blood sample required, and other features. Larger voice-activated meters are available for clients with visual impairment. Glucose monitors and supplies are readily available and competitively priced. Medicare and many third-party payers now cover some or all of the cost of supplies for home monitoring if the client is eligible. Setting goals for blood glucose levels needs to take into consideration the capacity and motivation of the client to achieve the goals, the age of the client, other illnesses, and the potential danger that hypoglycemia causes for the client (Cunningham, 2001). In otherwise healthy individuals with diabetes, blood glucose levels often are to remain as close to possible to the normal range. The frequency and timing of BGM should be dictated by the particular needs and goals of the client (ADA, 2006a).

This skill describes the technique used to measure blood glucose with a plasma-calibrated, sensor-type glucose meter. Specific steps in using meters will vary, depending on the make and model of the equipment used. Manufacturers' instructions should always be followed.

ASSESSMENT

1 Assess understanding of the procedure and the purpose and importance of BGM. *Rationale: Gives the caregiver a baseline on which to provide necessary teaching. Adults learn best when the teaching and learning relate to what the client already knows.*

2 Review all medications that the client is receiving. *Rationale: Drugs such as corticosteroids, diuretics, and anesthetics increase blood glucose levels. Anticoagulants increase risk for local ecchymosis and/or excessive bleeding from puncture site.*

3 Determine if specific conditions need to be met before or after glucose level is checked (e.g., fasting or postprandial status, medication administration including insulin). *Rationale: Dietary intake, especially of carbohydrates, alters blood glucose levels. Pre-meal doses of short- or rapid-acting insulin are based on current blood glucose levels.*

4 Assess area of skin to be used as puncture site. Inspect fingers or forearms for edema, inflammation, or open cuts or sores. Avoid areas of bruising and/or open lesions and the hand on the side of a mastectomy. *Rationale: The puncture site should not be edematous, inflamed, or recently punctured because these factors cause increased interstitial fluid and blood to mix, which increases the risk for infection (Malarkey and McMorrow, 2005). The sides of the fingertips have fewer nerve endings and good vascularity.*

5 Review the physician's order for timing and frequency of blood glucose measurement. *Rationale: Test schedule is based on the client's physiological status, risk for glucose imbalance, and any established facility protocols.*

PLANNING

Expected Outcomes focus on minimizing tissue damage at the puncture site, achieving accurate results, and maintaining blood glucose levels within the client's goal range.

1 Puncture site shows no evidence of excessive or prolonged bleeding or tissue damage.

2 Blood glucose measurements are accurate and within the established goal range for the client.

3 Client can verbalize procedure for self-monitoring of blood glucose and provide feedback on possible causes of results that are out of the target range.

Delegation Considerations

Assessment of the client's condition may not be delegated. When the client's condition is stable, the skill of obtaining and testing a sample of blood for blood glucose level may be delegated. The nurse directs personnel by:

- Explaining what sites to use for the puncture and when to obtain glucose levels
- Reviewing expected values and reminding to report all unexpected glucose levels to the nurse

Equipment

- Antiseptic swab
- Lancet device (a specific device may be used for a specific meter)
- Sterile lancet
- Blood glucose meter (e.g., OneTouch®, FreeStyle Freedom™)
- Blood glucose test strips appropriate for meter brand being used
- Clean gloves

IMPLEMENTATION *for Blood Glucose Monitoring*

STEPS	RATIONALE

1 **See Standard Protocol (inside front cover).**

2 Instruct client to wash hands and forearm (if applicable) thoroughly with soap and warm water. Rinse and dry.

Reduces presence of microorganisms. Warmth promotes vasodilation at puncture site. Establishes practice for client when test is performed at home.

3 Position client comfortably in chair or in semi-Fowler's position in bed.

Ensures easy accessibility to puncture site.

> **NURSE ALERT** Blood glucose meters that are available vary. Follow the manufacturer's directions and agency policy.

4 Remove reagent strip from vial, and tightly seal cap.

Protects strips from accidental discoloration caused by exposure to air or light.

5 Check the code on the test strip vial.

Code on test strip must match code entered into the glucose meter.

6 Insert the test strip into the meter. Do not bend the strip. The meter will automatically turn on.

A bent strip will not measure blood sample accurately.

7 The meter will display a code on the screen. Match the code displayed with the code from the test strip vial. Press the proper button on the meter to confirm matching codes. The meter is ready for use.

Codes must match for meter to operate.

> **NURSE ALERT** Meters will have different messages that confirm meter is ready for testing and blood can now be applied.

8 Prepare the lancet device. NOTE: Some meters recommend this step be completed before preparing the test strip.

a. Remove cap from lancet device. Insert new lancet.

Never reuse a lancet device due to risk of infection.

b. Twist off the protective disk on the tip of the lancet. Replace the cap of the lancet device.

c. Cock the lancet device, adjusting for proper puncture depth.

Each client will vary as to depth of insertion needed for lancet to produce blood drop.

9 Obtain blood sample.

a. Wipe finger or forearm lightly with alcohol swab. Choose a vascular area for puncture site. In stable adults, select lateral side of finger; be sure to avoid central tip of finger, which has more dense nerve supply (Malarkey and McMorrow, 2005).

Removes any remaining resident microorganisms. Too much alcohol can cause blood to hemolyze. Side of finger is less sensitive to pain and has a dense nerve supply. Alternate sites should not be used when clients are hypoglycemic, prone to hypoglycemia (during peak activity of an injected basal insulin or as long as 2 hours after injecting rapid-acting insulin), after exercise, during illness, or when blood glucose levels are rapidly increasing or decreasing (AADE, 2003).

b. Hold area to be punctured in a dependent position while gently massaging finger toward puncture site (Malarkey and McMorrow, 2005).

Increases blood flow to area before puncture.

c. Hold the tip of lancet device against the area of skin chosen for a test site (see illustration). Press the release button on the device. Some devices allow you to see the blood sample forming. Remove the device.

Placement ensures lancet will enter skin properly.

d. With some devices, a blood sample will begin to appear (see illustration). Otherwise, gently squeeze or massage fingertip until a round drop of blood forms.

Adequate size blood sample is needed to test glucose.

STEPS	RATIONALE

10 Obtain test results.

a. Be sure meter is still on. Bring the test strip in the meter to the drop of blood (see illustration). The blood will be wicked onto the test strip. (Follow specific meter directions to be sure a full sample is obtained.)

Blood enters strip and glucose device will show message on screen to signal enough blood is obtained.

> **NURSE ALERT** Do not scrape blood onto the test strips or apply blood to wrong side of test strip. This will prevent proper glucose measurement.

b. The blood glucose test result will appear on the screen (see illustration). Some devices will beep when completed.

11 Turn meter off. Dispose of test strip and lancet in proper receptacle.

Meter is battery powered. Proper disposal reduces risk of needlestick injury and spread of infection.

12 Discuss test results with client, and encourage questions.

13 See Completion Protocol (inside front cover).

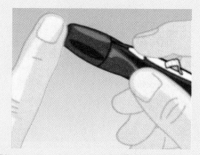

STEP 9c. Pierce skin with lancet. (Courtesy LifeScan, Inc., Milpitas, California.)

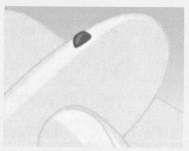

STEP 9d. Transfer droplet to test pad. (Courtesy LifeScan, Inc., Milpitas, California.)

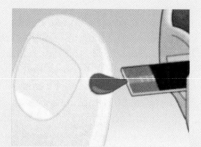

STEP 10a. Wick blood onto test strip. (Courtesy LifeScan, Inc., Milpitas, California.)

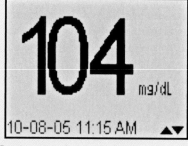

STEP 10b. Read results. (Courtesy LifeScan, Inc., Milpitas, California.)

EVALUATION

1 Observe puncture site for evidence of bleeding or bruising.

2 Compare glucose meter reading with target blood glucose levels and prior test results.

3 Ask client to discuss procedure and test results.

Unexpected Outcomes and Related Interventions

1 Puncture site continues to bleed or is bruised.

a. Apply pressure to site.

b. Notify care provider.

2 Glucose meter malfunctions.

a. Repeat test, following directions.

b. Follow manufacturer's directions for malfunctions.

3 Blood glucose level above or below target range.

a. Continue to monitor client.

b. Follow agency protocol for laboratory confirmation testing of very high or very low results. Laboratory testing is generally considered more accurate.

c. Check medical record to see if there are medication orders for deviations in glucose level; if not, notify physician.

d. Administer insulin or carbohydrate source as ordered (depending on glucose level).

e. Notify physician of client's response.

Recording and Reporting

• Record glucose results on appropriate flow sheet and describe response, including presence or absence of pain or excessive oozing of blood at puncture site.

• Report blood glucose levels out of target range, and take appropriate action for hypoglycemia or hyperglycemia (Table 13-2).

Sample Documentation

(For a client with insulin ordered based on glucose level.)

0730 Blood glucose 110. No sliding-scale insulin administered.

1200 Blood glucose 240. Regular insulin (4 units) administered subcutaneously as prescribed per sliding scale.

Special Considerations

Geriatric Considerations

• Older adults who have difficulty seeing the readings on the meter display screen may use a device with a larger display screen and lighted background or an audio blood glucose meter that gives verbal instructions to guide the client through the procedure.

• Older adults with musculoskeletal alterations may not have the fine motor coordination necessary to manipulate the device and place samples on test strips or insert strips in meter. Some models can be loaded with multiple strips.

• Warming fingertips may facilitate obtaining blood specimen.

Home Care Considerations

• Blood glucose levels are usually assessed before meals, before taking medication, and at bedtime to monitor effectiveness of treatment plan.

• It is generally recommended that one or more family members be able to monitor blood glucose levels in the event that the client is unable to do so independently.

• Some clients with diabetes check blood sugars before driving because they have hypoglycemic unawareness and need to see if their blood sugar is low or getting low before they get behind the wheel of a car.

TABLE 13-2 Signs and Symptoms of Blood Glucose Alterations	
ALTERATION	**ASSESSMENT FINDINGS**
Hyperglycemia (elevated blood glucose)	Thirst, polyuria, polyphagia, weakness, fatigue, headache, blurred vision, nausea, vomiting, abdominal cramps
Hypoglycemia (low blood glucose)	Sweating, tachycardia, palpitations, nervousness, tremors, weakness, headache, mental confusion, fatigue

Skill 13.4 Collecting Blood Specimens—Venipuncture with Syringe, Venipuncture with Vacutainer, and Blood Cultures

Blood tests, one of the most commonly used diagnostic measures, yield valuable information about a client's nutritional, hematological, metabolic, immune, and biochemical status. These tests allow health care providers to screen clients for early signs of physical illness, monitor changes in acute or chronic diseases, and evaluate responses to therapies.

Because veins are major sources of blood for both laboratory tests and routes for intravenous (IV) fluid or blood administration, maintaining their integrity is essential. It is important to use the most distal sites first, and retain one or more appropriate sites for IV access. Do not draw blood from a site proximal to an IV insertion site.

After obtaining a specimen, place it directly into the appropriate blood tube. A color-coding system for the tops of the collection tubes is used to indicate the type of specimen that can be collected within that tube (see agency procedure). Special blood tubes are available, containing anticoagulants, because some tests cannot be performed on clotted or hemolyzed specimens.

Venipuncture is the most common method of obtaining blood specimens. This method involves insertion of a hollow-bore needle into the lumen of a large vein to obtain a specimen using either a needle and syringe or a Vacutainer device that allows the drawing of multiple samples.

Blood cultures aid in the detection of bacteria in the blood. It is important that at least two culture specimens be drawn from two different sites. Because fever and chills may accompany bacteremia, blood cultures may be drawn when symptoms are present (Pagana and Pagana, 2005). If only one culture produces bacteria, the assumption is that the bacteria were skin contaminants rather than the infecting agent. Bacteremia exists when both cultures grow the infectious agent.

ASSESSMENT

1 Determine client's understanding of purpose of test and ability to cooperate with procedure. *Rationale: Some clients may need assistance of another member of the health care team. Procedure can appear threatening to client.*

2 Determine if special conditions need to be met for specimen collection (e.g., client allowed nothing by mouth [NPO], a specific time for collection in relation to time medication is given, need to ice specimen). *Rationale: Conditions may be required for accurate measurement of blood elements (e.g., fasting blood sugar, drug peak and trough, ammonia levels).*

3 Assess client for possible risks of venipuncture, which include anticoagulant therapy, low platelet count, or bleeding disorder. Review medication history. *Rationale: Abnormal clotting caused by low platelet count, hemophilia, or medications increases risk for bleeding and hematoma formation.*

4 Assess client for contraindicated sites for venipuncture: presence of IV infusion, hematoma at potential site, arm on side of mastectomy or axillary surgery, or hemodialysis shunt. *Rationale: Drawing specimens from such sites can result in false test results or may injure client.*

5 Identify latex allergies, tape sensitivity, or betadine allergy. *Rationale: Determines the need for avoiding exposure to these items.*

6 When drawing blood cultures, assess for systemic evidence of bacteremia, including fever and chills. *Rationale: Three blood samples should be drawn at least 1 hour apart beginning at the earliest sign of sepsis (Mermel and others, 2001).*

7 Review physician's order for type of blood tests. *Rationale: Physician's order is required. Type of test determines blood tubes to use and amount of specimen.*

PLANNING

Expected Outcomes focus on the collection of an uncontaminated, appropriate blood specimen by the nurse or trained technician.

1 Client explains purpose of blood collections before collection is attempted.

2 Venipuncture site shows no evidence of continued bleeding or hematoma.

3 Client denies anxiety or discomfort.

4 Laboratory test results are within normal limits (see agency report or appropriate laboratory manual).

Delegation Considerations

The skill of collecting blood specimens by venipuncture may be delegated. In some settings, phlebotomists are available. The nurse directs personnel by:

- Explaining client's condition (e.g., presence of IV therapy, edema that affects extremity or vein for venipuncture selection)
- Instructing personnel to report client's discomfort or signs of excessive bleeding to the nurse

Equipment
All Procedures
- Alcohol or antiseptic swab (check agency policy for specific antiseptic solution)
- Clean gloves
- Small pillow or folded towel
- Sterile gauze pads (2 × 2 inch)
- Tourniquet
- Adhesive bandage or adhesive tape
- Appropriate blood tubes
- Completed identification labels (with appropriate client identifiers)
- Completed laboratory requisition, including appropriate client identification, date, time, name of test, and source of culture
- Small plastic bag for delivery of specimen to laboratory (or container as specified by agency)

Venipuncture with Syringe
- Sterile needles (20- to 21-gauge for adults; 23- to 25-gauge for children)
- Sterile syringe of appropriate size

Venipuncture with Vacutainer
- Vacutainer and safety access device
- Sterile double-ended needles (20- to 21-gauge for adults; 23- to 25-gauge for children)
- Appropriate blood tubes (depending on tests being done)

Blood Cultures
- Antiseptic swabs (check agency policy regarding use of 70% alcohol)
- Two 20-ml syringes
- Sterile needles (20- to 21-gauge for adults; 23- to 25-gauge for children)
- Anaerobic and aerobic culture bottles (check agency policy)

IMPLEMENTATION *for Collecting Blood Specimens—Venipuncture with Syringe, Venipuncture with Vacutainer, and Blood Cultures*

STEPS	RATIONALE

1 See Standard Protocol (inside front cover).

2 Assist client with lying supine or sitting in semi-Fowler's position or in a chair with arm supported and elbow extended. Place small pillow or towel under upper arm. (Option: lower arm briefly so it fills hand and lower arm with blood.)

Helps to stabilize extremity. Supported position in bed reduces chance of injury to client if fainting occurs.

> **COMMUNICATION TIP** "As I begin, you are going to feel a tightness around your arm when I place this rubber tourniquet. The alcohol will feel cool and wet. I will tell you just as I insert the needle; it will feel like an insect sting."

3 Apply tourniquet so that it can be removed by pulling end with single motion.

Tourniquet blocks venous return to heart from extremity, causing veins to dilate for easier visibility.

  a. Position the tourniquet 5 to 10 cm (3 to 4 inches) above venipuncture site selected.

  b. Cross the tourniquet over the client's arm, holding the tourniquet between your fingers close to the arm (see illustration). Tourniquet may be placed over gown sleeve to protect skin.

  c. Tuck a loop between the client's arm and the tourniquet so that the free end can be easily grasped (see illustration).

Free end can be pulled to release tourniquet after venipuncture.

> **NURSE ALERT** Palpate distal pulse (e.g., radial) below tourniquet. If pulse is not palpable, the tourniquet is too tight and is impeding arterial blood flow. If this happens, remove and wait 60 seconds before reapplying tourniquet more loosely or assessing other extremity. Keep tourniquet in place no longer than 1 minute. Minimizes effects of hemoconcentration and hemolysis. Prolonged time may alter test results and cause pain and venous stasis (e.g., falsely elevated serum potassium level) (Malarkey and McMorrow, 2005).

4 Ask the client to *gently* open and close fist several times, finally leaving fist clenched.

5 Quickly inspect extremity for best venipuncture site, looking for straight, prominent vein without swelling or hematoma. Of the three veins located in the antecubital area, the median cubital vein is preferred (see illustration).

This vein is large, well anchored (does not easily move), closer to the surface of the skin, and less painful to puncture. Straight and intact veins are easiest to puncture. The veins of the lower arm and hand are preferred for administering IV fluids.

6 Palpate selected vein with finger (see illustration). Note if vein is firm and rebounds when palpated or if vein feels rigid and cordlike and rolls when palpated.

A healthy vein is elastic and rebounds on palpation. Thrombosed vein is rigid, rolls easily, and is difficult to puncture.

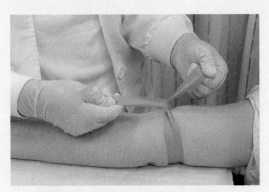

STEP 3b. Cross tourniquet over the arm.

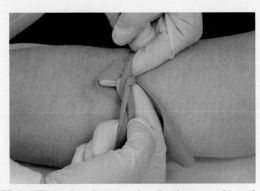

STEP 3c. Tuck a loop between the client's arm and tourniquet.

STEPS	RATIONALE

> **NURSE ALERT** Avoid vigorously slapping veins because this can cause vasospasm.

7 Obtain blood specimen.

a. **Syringe Method:**

    (1) Have syringe with appropriate needle attached.

    (2) Cleanse venipuncture site with antiseptic swabs, moving in a circular motion from site outward for about 5 cm (2 inches) (see illustration). Allow to dry.

> Antimicrobial agent cleans skin surface of resident bacteria so organisms do not enter puncture site. Allowing antiseptic to dry completes its antimicrobial task and reduces "sting" of venipuncture. Alcohol left on skin can cause hemolysis of sample.

       (a) If drawing sample for blood alcohol level or blood cultures, use only antiseptic swab rather than alcohol swab.

> Ensures accurate test results.

    (3) Remove needle cover and inform client of "stick" lasting only a few seconds.

> Prepares client and prevents sudden movement from the needle.

    (4) Place thumb or forefinger of nondominant hand 2.5 cm (1 inch) below site, and gently pull skin taut. Stretch skin steadily until vein is stabilized.

> Stabilizes vein and minimizes rolling during needle insertion.

    (5) Hold syringe and needle at a 15- to 30-degree angle from client's arm with the bevel up.

> Angle and bevel up position facilitate entry of the needle into the vein.

    (6) Slowly insert needle into vein (see illustration), stopping when a "pop" is felt as the needle enters vein.

> Prevents puncture through the opposite side of the vein.

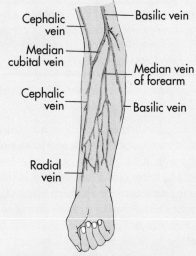

Cephalic vein — Basilic vein
Median cubital vein
Median vein of forearm
Cephalic vein — Basilic vein
Radial vein

STEP 5 Location of antecubital veins.

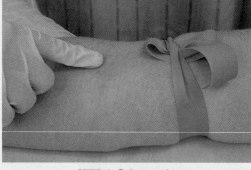

STEP 6 Palpate vein.

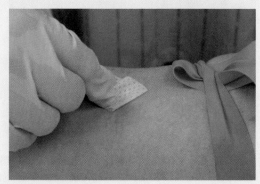

STEP 7a.(2) Cleanse venipuncture site with antiseptic solution.

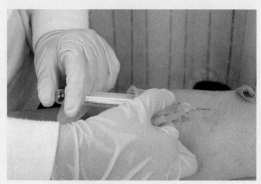

STEP 7a.(6) Perform venipuncture.

STEPS	RATIONALE
(7) Hold syringe securely, and pull back gently on plunger (see illustration).	Creates a vacuum for withdrawal of blood specimen.
(8) Observe for blood return and withdraw until desired amount of blood is obtained.	Verifies placement in the vein.
(9) Release tourniquet before removing needle (see illustration).	Reduces bleeding at site.
(10) Apply 2 × 2 gauze pad or alcohol swab over puncture site without pressure. Quickly, but carefully, withdraw needle and apply pressure after removal of needle (see illustration).	Minimizes discomfort and trauma to vein.
(11) Activate needle safety cover and immediately discard needle in proper receptacle.	Phlebotomy equipment must include needle safety devices. Reduces risk of needlestick injury (OSHA, 2001).

b. Vacutainer System Method:

(1) Attach double-ended needle to Vacutainer tube (see illustration).	
(2) Have proper blood specimen tubes resting inside Vacutainer, but do not puncture rubber stopper.	Tubes are usually color coded to indicate intended use based on size of tube and presence or absence of a chemical additive. Puncture of stopper results in loss of vacuum.
(3) Cleanse venipuncture site with alcohol swab (70% isopropyl alcohol) using a circular motion out from site for approximately 5 cm (2 inches). Allow to dry.	Antimicrobial agent cleans skin surface of resident bacteria so organisms do not enter puncture site. Allowing alcohol to dry reduces "sting" of venipuncture. Alcohol left on skin can cause hemolysis of sample.
(4) Remove needle cover, and inform client that "stick" lasting only a few seconds will be felt.	Client has better control over anxiety when prepared about what to expect.

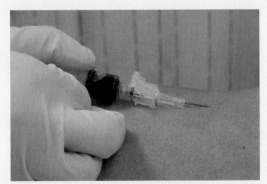

STEP 7a.(7) Pull back on plunger.

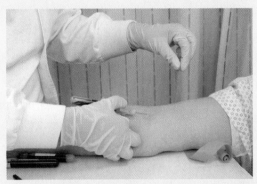

STEP 7a.(9) Release tourniquet before removing needle.

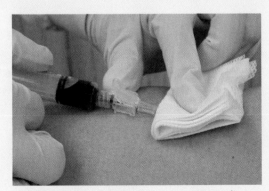

STEP 7a.(10) Apply gauze over puncture site.

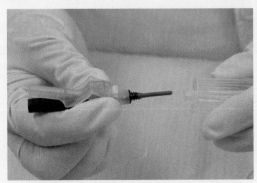

STEP 7b.(1) Attach double-ended needle.

STEPS	RATIONALE
(5) Place thumb or forefinger of nondominant hand 2.5 cm (1 inch) *below* site, and pull skin taut. Stretch skin down until vein is stabilized.	Position of finger below site prevents accidental needle stick. Stretching helps to stabilize vein and prevent rolling during needle insertion.
(6) Hold Vacutainer needle at 15- to 30-degree angle from arm with bevel of needle up.	Reduces chance of penetrating both sides of vein during insertion and is less traumatic to the vein.
(7) Slowly insert needle into vein (see illustration).	Prevents puncture on opposite side.
(8) Grasp Vacutainer securely, and advance specimen tube into needle of holder (Do not advance needle in vein).	Pushing needle through stopper breaks vacuum and causes flow of blood into tube. If needle in vein advances, vein may become punctured on other side.
(9) Note flow of blood into tube, which should be fairly rapid (see illustration).	Failure of blood to appear indicates that vacuum in tube is lost or needle is not in vein.
(10) After specimen tube is filled, grasp Vacutainer firmly and remove tube. Insert additional specimen tubes as needed.	Prevents needle from advancing or dislodging. Tubes with additives should be inverted as soon as possible.

> **NURSE ALERT** When filling tubes with an anticoagulant additive, let tube fill until the vacuum is exhausted. Ratio of blood to additive is important. Gently rotate the tube back and forth 8 to 10 times. Prevents clotting as additives are mixed with blood. Shaking can cause hemolysis of red blood cells (RBCs), producing inaccurate test results.

STEPS	RATIONALE
(11) Release tourniquet and apply gauze; see Steps 7a(9) and 7a(10).	Reduces bleeding at site when needle is withdrawn.
c. Blood Culture:	
(1) Cleanse venipuncture site with antiseptic swab (check agency policy). Allow to dry.	Antimicrobial agent cleans skin surface so organisms do not enter puncture site or contaminate culture. Drying ensures complete antimicrobial action.
(2) Clean bottle tops of Vacutainer tubes or culture bottles. Check agency policy regarding cleaning with 70% alcohol after cleaning with antiseptic solution and air-drying.	Ensures specimen is sterile.
(3) ✋ Collect 10 to 15 ml of venous blood by venipuncture from each venipuncture site.	Cultures must be obtained from two sites to confirm culture growth.
(4) Discard needle on syringe; replace with new sterile needle before injecting blood sample into culture bottles.	Maintains sterile technique and prevents contamination of specimen.
(5) If both aerobic and anaerobic cultures are needed, fill the anaerobic container first (Pagana and Pagana, 2005).	Anaerobic organisms may take longer to grow.
(6) Gently mix blood in the culture bottle.	Mixes medium and blood.
(7) Release tourniquet and apply gauze; see Steps 7a(9) and 7a(10).	

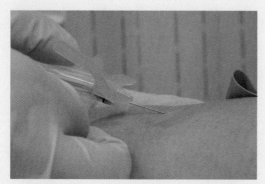

STEP 7b.(7) Insert Vacutainer needle into vein.

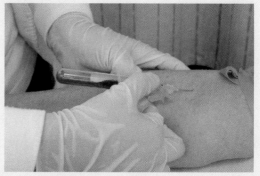

STEP 7b.(9) Note rapid flow of blood into tube.

STEPS	RATIONALE
8 For blood obtained by syringe, transfer specimens to appropriate specimen tubes. Insert needle through stopper of blood collection tube and allow vacuum to fill the tube. Do not force blood into tube.	Forcing blood into tube may cause hemolysis of RBCs.
9 Take blood tubes containing additives; gently rotate back and forth 8 to 10 times.	Additives should be mixed with blood to prevent clotting. Shaking can cause hemolysis of blood cells, producing inaccurate results.
10 Observe for any sign of blood on outside of tube; wipe with 70% alcohol.	
11 Carefully discard uncapped sharps into appropriate container. If needle has built-in safety device, activate (see illustration) and then discard.	One-handed technique helps to avoid needlestick injury (OSHA, 2001).
12 Label the specimen with the client identifiers, date, and time. Affix proper requisition.	Ensures diagnostic information reported on correct client.
13 Place all specimens in appropriate bag for transfer. Transport cultures immediately to laboratory (or at least within 30 minutes).	
14 **See Completion Protocol (inside front cover).**	

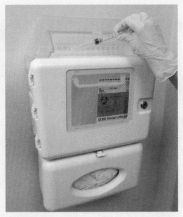

STEP 11 Needle with safety cover.

EVALUATION

1 Ask client to explain purposes of tests.
2 Reinspect venipuncture site for hemostasis.
3 Determine if client is anxious or fearful.
4 Check laboratory report for test results.

Unexpected Outcomes and Related Interventions

1 Hematoma forms at venipuncture site.
a. Apply pressure.
b. Continue to monitor client for pain and discomfort.
2 Bleeding at site continues.
a. Apply pressure and have client help to maintain pressure on site.
b. Monitor client.

3 Laboratory tests reveal significantly abnormal blood results (see laboratory report or laboratory manual for normal limits).
a. Report to physician.

Recording and Reporting

- Record method used to obtain blood specimen, date and time collected, type of test ordered, and laboratory receiving specimen; describe venipuncture site after specimen collection and client's response to procedure.
- Report any stat or abnormal results to physician or charge nurse.

Sample Documentation

1000 Serum chemistry and CBC specimens drawn from L antecubital fossa. 2-cm hematoma noted. Pressure applied using 2 × 2 gauze. Encouraged to elevate arm, continue pressure, and notify nurse if bleeding occurs or hematoma enlarges.

Special Considerations

Pediatric Considerations

- Explain procedure to child using developmentally appropriate language
- Application of EMLA or other local anesthetic cream may be ordered to reduce pain in infants and young children (Hockenberry and others, 2003).
- When performing venipuncture on children, the nurse needs to explore a variety of sources for vein access (e.g., scalp, antecubital fossa, saphenous veins, hand veins).

- Vacutainers are not recommended in children under 2 years of age because of possible vein collapse (Hockenberry and others, 2003).

Geriatric Considerations

- Older adults have fragile skin and veins that are easily traumatized during venipuncture. Sometimes application of warm compresses may help in obtaining samples.
- A small-bore needle/catheter also may be beneficial.

Home Care Considerations

- In the home care setting a blood pressure cuff, rather than a tourniquet, can be used for venipuncture.

SKILL 13.5 Collecting Specimens from the Nose and Throat

When clients have signs and symptoms of upper respiratory or sinus infection, a nose or throat culture is a simple diagnostic tool to identify the presence and type of microorganisms. Cultures should be obtained before antibiotic therapy is started, because the antibiotic may interrupt the organism's growth in the laboratory. If the client is receiving antibiotics, the laboratory needs to be notified and told what specific antibiotics the client is receiving (Pagana and Pagana, 2005).

Collection of a specimen from the nose and throat can cause the client discomfort and gagging because of sensitive mucosal membranes. It is important to collect a throat culture before mealtime or at least 1 hour after eating or drinking to lessen the chance of inducing vomiting. Clients should clearly understand how each specimen is to be collected to minimize anxiety or discomfort.

ASSESSMENT

1 Assess client's understanding of purpose of procedure and ability to cooperate. The nurse may need assistance to obtain throat cultures from confused, combative, or unconscious clients. *Rationale: Provides basis to determine need for health teaching and need for assistance.*
2 Assess condition of and drainage from nasal mucosa and sinuses. *Rationale: Reveals physical signs that may indicate infection or allergic irritation.*
3 Determine if client has experienced postnasal drip, sinus headache or tenderness, nasal congestion, or sore throat. *Rationale: Further clarifies nature of problem.*

4 Assess condition of posterior pharynx (see Chapter 12).
5 Assess for systemic indications of infection, including fever, chills, and malaise.

PLANNING

Expected Outcomes focus on obtaining an uncontaminated specimen in the appropriate amount for diagnosis and appropriate treatment.
1 Client verbalizes understanding of purpose of specimen and how specimen is obtained.
2 Culture specimen is obtained without contamination from adjacent skin or tissues.
3 Client does not experience bleeding of nasal mucosa.

Delegation Considerations

The skills of obtaining specimens from the throat and nose may not be delegated.

Equipment

- Two sterile swabs in sterile culture tubes (flexible wire swab with cotton tip may be used for nose cultures)
- Nasal speculum (optional)
- Tongue blades
- Penlight
- Emesis basin or clean container (optional)
- Facial tissues
- Gauze
- Clean gloves

- Completed identification labels (with appropriate client identifiers)
- Completed laboratory requisition, including appropriate client identification, date, time, name of test, and source of culture
- Small plastic bag for delivery of specimen to laboratory (or container as specified by agency)

IMPLEMENTATION *for Collecting Specimens from the Nose and Throat*

STEPS	RATIONALE

1 See Standard Protocol (inside front cover).

> **COMMUNICATION TIP** Explain that client may have tickling sensation or gag during swabbing of throat. Nasal swab may create urge to sneeze. State that procedures take only a few seconds.

2 Ask client to sit erect in bed or chair facing you. Acutely ill client may lie supported at a 45-degree angle in semi-Fowler's position.	Provides easy access to oral structures.
3 Have swab in tube ready for use. You may want to loosen top so swab can easily be removed.	Most commercially prepared tubes have a top that fits securely over end of swab, which allows nurse to touch outer top without contaminating swab stick.

4   Collect throat culture.

a. Schedule procedure when client's stomach is empty. Instruct client to tilt head backward. For clients in bed, place pillow behind shoulders.	Obtaining specimen on empty stomach reduces risk of vomiting.
b. Ask client to open mouth and say "ah."	Permits exposure of pharynx, relaxes throat muscles, and minimizes gag reflex.
c. Depress tongue with tongue blade if unable to expose pharynx, and note inflamed areas of pharynx or tonsils. Depress anterior third of tongue only, and illuminate with penlight as needed.	Area to be swabbed should be clearly visualized.
d. Insert swab without touching lips, teeth, tongue, or cheeks (see illustration).	
e. Gently but quickly, swab tonsillar area side to side, making contact with inflamed or purulent sites.	Collects microorganisms from the throat tissues without contamination from mouth or tongue.
f. Carefully withdraw without touching oral structures.	

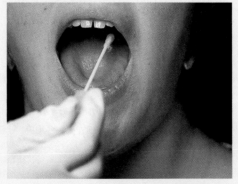

STEP 4d. Obtaining a tonsillar swab.

STEPS	RATIONALE

5 Collect nasal culture.

a. Ask client to blow nose, and then check nostrils for patency with penlight. Select nostril with greatest patency.

Clears nasal passage of mucus that contains resident bacteria.

b. Ask client to tilt head back. Clients in bed should have pillow behind shoulders.

c. Gently insert nasal speculum in one nostril *(optional)*.

d. Carefully pass swab into nostril until it reaches that portion of mucosa that is inflamed or containing exudate. Rotate swab quickly. NOTE: If nasopharyngeal culture is to be obtained, use a special swab on a flexible wire that can be flexed downward to reach nasopharynx.

Swab should remain sterile until it reaches area to be cultured. Rotating swab covers all surfaces where exudate is present.

e. Remove swab without touching sides of speculum or nasal canal.

Prevents contamination by resident bacteria.

f. Carefully remove nasal speculum (if used), and place in basin. Offer client facial tissue.

6 Insert swab into culture tube. Using gauze to protect your fingers, crush ampule at bottom of tube to release culture medium.

Placing tip within culture medium maintains life of bacteria for testing.

7 Push tip of swab into liquid medium.

8 Place top on tube securely.

9 Securely attach properly completed identification label and laboratory requisition to side of specimen container (not lid).

Incorrect identification of specimen could result in diagnostic or therapeutic errors.

10 Enclose specimen in a plastic bag.

11 Send specimen immediately to laboratory, or refrigerate.

12 **See Completion Protocol (inside front cover).**

Reduces transmission of microorganisms.

EVALUATION

1 Ask client to describe purpose of culture.
2 Monitor technique of culture collection process for potential contamination.
3 Inspect specimen for traces of blood, and reinspect mucosa if bleeding is apparent.

Unexpected Outcomes and Related Interventions

1 Cultures reveal heavy bacterial growth.
a. Notify physician of results.
b. Administer antibiotics as ordered.
2 Culture was contaminated by bacteria from adjacent skin or tissues.
a. Notify physician.
b. Repeat collection of cultures.
3 Client experiences minor nasal bleeding.
a. Apply mild pressure and ice pack over bridge of nose.
b. Notify physician of client's condition.

Recording and Reporting

- Record types of specimen obtained, source, and time and date sent to laboratory; describe appearance of site and presence or absence of signs of local or systemic infection; note any unusual client response to procedure.
- Report unusual test results to care provider.

Sample Documentation

0930 C/O sore throat, oral temp 101° F. Pharynx inflamed with green-colored exudate noted on inspection. Obtained throat culture per order. Tolerated without gagging or discomfort. Specimen sent to lab.

Special Considerations
Pediatric Considerations

- Immobilization of child's head and arms is important when obtaining nose or throat culture and should be done in firm, gentle, kind manner. Ask another nurse to assist, if necessary.

- Showing tongue blade and penlight to child and demonstrating how to say "ah" helps to decrease anxiety.
- Throat cultures should not be attempted if acute epiglottitis is suspected, because trauma from swab might cause increase in edema and resulting occlusion of airway (Hockenberry and Wilson, 2007).

SKILL 13.6 Collecting a Sputum Specimen by Suction

Sputum specimens are collected for three purposes:
1 Cytology specimens are used to identify cancer cells.
2 Sputum for C&S can be used to identify specific pathogens and to determine the antibiotics to which they are most sensitive.
3 Sputum for acid-fast bacillus (AFB) is examined to support the diagnosis of pulmonary tuberculosis (TB).

Nasotracheal suctioning is required to collect a sputum specimen when a client cannot expectorate sputum. Suctioning can provoke violent coughing, which can induce vomiting and constriction of pharyngeal, laryngeal, and bronchial muscles. Suctioning can also cause direct stimulation of vagal nerve fibers, resulting in cardiac arrhythmias and increased intracranial pressure (IICP) (Mason and others, 2005). Procedural Guideline 13-3 describes the steps for collecting an expectorated sputum specimen.

ASSESSMENT

1 Check physician's orders for number and type of specimens needed, as well as time and method of collection.
2 Assess client's understanding of procedure and its purpose.
3 Assess client's ability to cough and expectorate sputum. *Rationale: Suction is avoided when an expectorated specimen can be obtained.*
4 Determine when client last ate a meal. *Rationale: It is best to obtain the specimen 1 to 2 hours after or 1 hour before a meal to minimize gagging, which can cause vomiting and aspiration.*
5 Assess client's respiratory status, including respiratory rate, depth, and pattern; lung sounds; and lung color. *Rationale: Changes in respiration may indicate the presence of secretions in tracheobronchial tree and potential need for supplementary oxygenation.*
6 Assess client's anxiety level. *Rationale: Obtain a premedication order (i.e., sedative) if client is extremely anxious. This procedure may be contraindicated in clients who cannot cooperate or remain still during the procedure (Pagana and Pagana, 2005).*

PLANNING

Expected Outcomes focus on collecting an uncontaminated specimen while maintaining a patent airway, adequate oxygenation, and client comfort.
1 Client's respirations are same rate and character as before procedure.
2 Client verbalizes understanding of the purpose and process of specimen collection.
3 Client maintains comfort level and experiences minimal anxiety.
4 Sputum is not contaminated by saliva or oropharyngeal flora.

Delegation Considerations

Collection of a sputum specimen by suction may not be delegated. Collection of expectorated sputum specimens may be delegated. The nurse directs personnel by:
- Instructing to notify nurse if client expectorates bloody sputum

Equipment
- Completed identification labels (with appropriate client identifiers)
- Completed laboratory requisition, including appropriate client identification, date, time, name of test, and source of culture
- Small plastic bag for delivery of specimen to laboratory (or container as specified by agency)
- Suction device (wall or portable)
- Sterile suction catheter (size 13, 16, or 18 Fr [not large enough to cause trauma to nasal mucosa])
- Sterile gloves
- Sterile saline in container
- In-line specimen container (sputum trap)
- Oxygen therapy equipment if indicated
- Protective eyewear (if required)

IMPLEMENTATION *for Collecting a Sputum Specimen by Suction*

STEPS	RATIONALE
1 See Standard Protocol (inside front cover).	
2 Position client in high- or semi-Fowler's position for suctioning.	Promotes full lung expansion and facilitates ability to cough.
3 Explain steps of procedure and purpose. Encourage client to breathe normally to prevent hyperventilation.	
4 Apply glove to nondominant hand. Prepare suction machine or device, and make sure it is functioning properly.	Adequate amount of suction is necessary to aspirate sputum.
5 Connect suction tube to adapter on sputum trap.	
6 Apply sterile glove to dominant hand.	Allows handling of suction catheter without introducing microorganisms into the tracheobronchial tree, which is a sterile body cavity.

> **NURSE ALERT** Preoxygenate for 1 minute with 100% oxygen (if appropriate). Use caution if client has chronic obstructive pulmonary disease (COPD), because 100% oxygen can depress respiratory effort.

STEPS	RATIONALE
7 Using gloved hand, connect sterile suction catheter to rubber tubing on sputum trap.	Aspirated sputum will go directly to trap instead of to suction tubing.
8 Gently insert tip of suction catheter prelubricated with sterile water through nasopharynx, endotracheal (ET) tube, or tracheostomy without applying suction (see Chapter 29).	Minimizes trauma to airway as catheter is inserted. Lubrication allows for easier insertion.
9 Gently and quickly advance catheter into trachea (see illustration).	Triggers cough reflex.

> **COMMUNICATION TIP** Warn client to expect to cough. Entrance of catheter into larynx and trachea triggers cough reflex.

STEPS	RATIONALE
10 As client coughs, apply suction for 5 to 10 seconds, collecting 2 to 10 ml of sputum.	Suctioning longer than 10 seconds can cause hypoxia and mucosal damage.
11 Release suction and remove catheter, then turn off suction.	Releasing suction avoids unnecessary trauma to mucosa as the catheter is withdrawn.
12 Detach catheter from specimen trap, and dispose of catheter into appropriate receptacle.	
13 Connect rubber tubing on sputum trap to plastic adapter (see illustration).	
14 If any sputum is present on outside of container, wipe it off with disinfectant.	Prevents spread of infection to persons handling specimen.

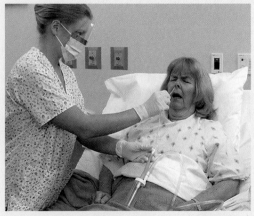

STEP 9 Insert catheter through nasopharynx.

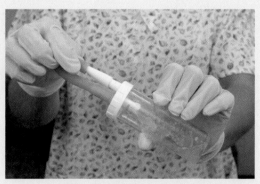

STEP 13 Closing sputum trap.

STEPS	RATIONALE
15 Offer client tissues after suctioning. Dispose of tissues in emesis basin or trash container. Remove and dispose of gloves.	
16 Securely attach properly completed identification label and laboratory requisition to side of specimen container (not lid).	Incorrect client identification could lead to diagnostic or therapeutic error.
17 Enclose specimen in a biohazard plastic bag, attach requisition, and send immediately to laboratory.	Bacteria multiply quickly. Specimen should be analyzed promptly for accurate results.
18 Offer client mouth care.	
19 **See Completion Protocol (inside front cover).**	

EVALUATION

1 Observe respiratory and oxygenation status throughout procedure, especially during suctioning.
2 Note any anxiety or discomfort.
3 Observe character of sputum, color, consistency, odor, volume, viscosity, and/or presence of blood.
4 Refer to laboratory reports for test results.
5 Evaluate client's ability to describe/demonstrate sputum collection process.

Unexpected Outcomes and Related Interventions

1 Client becomes hypoxic with increased respiratory rate and shortness of breath.
a. Discontinue suctioning immediately.
b. Administer oxygen.
c. Monitor vital signs and oxygen saturation.
d. Notify physician if distress is unrelieved.
2 Inadequate amount of sputum is collected, or specimen contains saliva.
a. Repeat collection procedure after client has rested.
b. Encourage client to deep breathe and cough.
3 Client remains anxious or complains of discomfort from suction catheter.
a. Discontinue procedure until client is stable.
b. Provide oxygen as needed (if ordered).
c. Notify physician of client's condition.
d. Continue to monitor client's vital signs. Consider measuring oxygen saturation.

Recording and Reporting

• Record method used to obtain specimen, date and time collected, type of test ordered, and how specimen was transported to the laboratory and describe characteristics of sputum specimen and client's tolerance of procedure.
• Report any unusual findings, such as bloody sputum, or client response, such as increased dyspnea.

Sample Documentation

0730 Suctioned 13 ml thick green sputum; immediately transported to lab for C&S. Reports slightly short of breath. Respirations 26. Rales noted bilaterally in all lung fields.

Special Considerations
Home Care Considerations
• If client is to obtain a sputum specimen at home, instruct client and/or family member regarding proper technique and importance of having sputum (not saliva) specimen sent to laboratory in timely manner.
• Discuss ways to avoid contaminating specimen (e.g., hand washing, using appropriate equipment).

PROCEDURAL GUIDELINE 13-3

Collecting a Sputum Specimen by Expectoration

Delegation Considerations

The skill of collecting a sputum specimen by expectoration may be delegated. The nurse directs AP by:

- Instructing to immediately report the presence of blood in the sputum or changes in client's vital signs.

Equipment

- Completed identification labels (with appropriate client identifiers)
- Completed laboratory requisition, including appropriate client identification, date, time, name of test, and source of culture
- Small plastic bag for delivery of specimen to laboratory (or container as specified by agency)
- Sterile specimen container with cover
- Clean disposable gloves
- Facial tissues
- Emesis basis (optional)
- Toothbrush (optional)

Procedural Steps

1 **See Standard Protocol (inside front cover).**
2 Explain importance that client coughs and expectorates sputum. Client cannot simply clear throat and expectorate saliva.
3 Provide opportunity to cleanse or rinse mouth with water.

NURSE ALERT Client should not use mouthwash or toothpaste. These products may decrease viability of microorganisms and alter culture results.

---

4 Provide sputum cup, and instruct client not to touch the inside of the container.
5 Have client take three to four deep breaths. Instruct client to emphasize slow, full exhalation. Then after a full inhalation ask client to cough forcefully, expectorating sputum directly into specimen container (see illustration).

6 Repeat until 5 to 10 ml (1 to 2 teaspoons) of sputum (not saliva) has been collected.
7 Secure top on specimen container tightly. If any sputum is present on outside of container, wipe it off with disinfectant.
8 Offer client tissues after expectorating, dispose of tissues, and offer mouth care.
9 Remove and dispose of gloves.
10 Securely attach properly completed identification label and laboratory requisition to side of specimen container (not lid).
11 Enclose specimen in a plastic bag.
12 Send specimen immediately to laboratory.
13 **See Completion Protocol (inside front cover).**

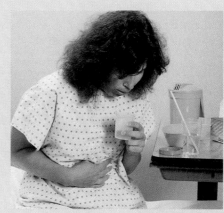

STEP 5 Expectorating sputum. (From Grimes D: *Infectious diseases,* Mosby's clinical nursing series, St Louis, 1991, Mosby.)

SKILL 13.7 Obtaining Wound Drainage Specimens for Culture

- Nursing Skills Online: Specimen Collection, Lesson 5

When caring for a client with a wound, the nurse assesses the wound's condition and observes for the development of infection. Localized inflammation, tenderness, warmth at the wound site, and purulent drainage are signs and symptoms of wound infection. Infection is best treated appropriately with confirmation from a wound culture.

The nurse should collect a wound culture sample from fresh exudate from the center of the wound after removing old drainage. Resident colonies of bacteria on the skin grow in old wound exudate and may not be the true organisms causing infection.

Separate techniques are used to collect specimens for measuring aerobic versus anaerobic microorganism growth.

Aerobic organisms grow in superficial wounds exposed to the air. Anaerobic organisms grow deep within body cavities, where oxygen is not normally present.

ASSESSMENT

1 Assess client's understanding of need for wound culture and ability to cooperate with procedure
2 Assess client for fever, chills, malaise, and elevated white blood cell (WBC) count. *Rationale: Signs and symptoms indicate systemic infection.*
3 Assess severity of pain at wound site (scale of 0 to 10). *Rationale: If client requires analgesic before dressing change or a wound culture, ideally medication is given 30 minutes before dressing change to reach peak effect.*

4 Review physician's order for aerobic or anaerobic culture.

5 Wear clean gloves to remove any soiled dressing. Apply sterile gloves to assess wound. Observe for swelling, opening of wound edges, inflammation, and drainage. Palpate along wound edges and note tenderness or drainage.

6 Determine when dressing change is scheduled. *Rationale: This step may be performed immediately after specimen collection.*

PLANNING

Expected Outcomes focus on obtaining an uncontaminated specimen while maintaining client comfort.

1 Wound culture does not reveal bacterial growth.

2 Culture swab is free of contaminants.

3 Client can discuss purpose and procedure for specimen collection.

Delegation Considerations

The skill of obtaining wound drainage for culture may not be delegated.

Equipment

- Culture tube with swab and transport medium for aerobic culture
- Anaerobic culture tube with swab (tubes contain carbon dioxide or nitrogen gas)
- 5- to 10-ml syringe and 19-gauge needle
- Clean gloves
- Sterile gloves
- Protective eyewear
- Antiseptic swab
- Sterile dressing materials (determined by type of dressing)
- Paper or plastic disposable bag
- Completed identification labels (with appropriate client identifiers)
- Completed laboratory requisition, including appropriate client identification, date, time, name of test, and source of culture
- Small plastic bag for delivery of specimen to laboratory (or container as specified by agency)

IMPLEMENTATION *for Obtaining Wound Drainage Specimens for Culture*

STEPS	RATIONALE
1 See Standard Protocol (inside front cover).	
2 Remove old dressing. Observe drainage. Fold soiled sides of dressing together, and then dispose of in a plastic bag.	
3 Cleanse area around wound edges with antiseptic swab. Remove old exudate.	Removes skin flora, preventing possible contamination of specimen.
4 Discard swab; remove and dispose of soiled gloves in bag.	
5 Open packages containing sterile culture tube and dressing supplies.	Provides sterile field from which nurse can handle supplies.
6 Apply sterile gloves.	
7 Obtain cultures.	
a. Obtain aerobic culture.	
(1) Take swab from culture tube, insert tip into wound in area of drainage, and rotate swab gently. Remove swab from wound, and return to culture tube (wrap outside of ampule with gauze to prevent injury to nurse's fingers). Crush ampule of medium, and push swab into fluid.	Swab should be coated with fresh secretions from within wound. Medium keeps bacteria alive until analysis is complete.
b. Obtain anaerobic culture.	
(1) Take swab from special anaerobic culture tube, swab deeply into draining body cavity, and rotate gently. Remove swab from wound, and return to culture tube.	Specimen is taken from deep cavity where oxygen is not present. Carbon dioxide or nitrogen gas keeps organisms alive until analysis is complete. Air injected into tube would cause organisms to die.
or	
(2) Insert tip of syringe (without needle) into wound, and aspirate 5 to 10 ml of exudate. Attach 19-gauge needle, expel all air, and inject drainage into special culture tube.	

STEPS	RATIONALE
8 Place correct specimen label on each culture tube.	Ensures correct results for correct client.
9 Ask another caregiver to securely attach properly completed labels and laboratory requisition to each tube. NOTE: Indicate on specimen requisition if client is receiving antibiotics. Send specimens to laboratory immediately, within 15 minutes of collection (Parini, 2000).	Bacteria grow rapidly. Cultures should be prepared quickly for accurate results.
10 Clean wound per care provider's orders. Apply new sterile dressing.	Protects wound from further contamination and aids in absorbing drainage and debriding wound.
11 Remove gloves and secure dressings with tape or ties.	
12 **See Completion Protocol (inside front cover).**	

EVALUATION

1 Observe character of wound drainage.
2 Observe edges of wound for redness and bleeding.
3 Ask client to describe purpose of culture.
4 Obtain laboratory report for results of cultures.

Unexpected Outcomes and Related Interventions

1 Wound cultures reveal heavy bacterial growth.
a. Monitor client for fever, chills, and increased WBC count.
b. Inform physician of findings.
2 Laboratory report indicates wound culture is contaminated with superficial skin cells.
a. Monitor client for fever and pain.
b. Inform physician.
c. Repeat collection of specimen as ordered.

Recording and Reporting

• Record type of specimen obtained, source, and time and date specimen sent to laboratory; describe appearance of wound and characteristics of drainage; describe client's tolerance to procedure and response to analgesia.
• Report any evidence of infection to nurse in charge and physician.

Sample Documentation

1320 Complains of pain from surgical site. Dressing change reveals 4-cm wound is separated at top with yellow purulent drainage. Lower half of incision remains well approximated. Aerobic culture obtained from site of drainage, sent to lab as ordered.

Special Considerations

Pediatric Considerations

• If procedure is to be performed on a child and it is anticipated to be painful, some agencies perform procedure in area other than child's room, keeping child's room a safe place (Hockenberry and Wilson, 2007).

Home Care Considerations

• Risks for wound infections are different in the home setting than in the hospital setting because families are less susceptible to infections from microorganisms in their home environment. Careful hand washing and clean technique are usually adequate for performing dressing changes by clients and their families in the home.
• Inform family regarding signs and symptoms of wound infection and under what circumstances to notify the physician for evaluation of the need for a wound culture.

NCLEX® Style Questions

1 A 54-year-old client is seen at the clinic for a possible UTI. Which of the following is an appropriate assessment relating to collecting a urine specimen for C&S?
1. Determine the client's ability to cooperate and level of assistance required.
2. Collect an uncontaminated urine specimen before administration of antibiotics.
3. Notify the physician if the urine has the appearance of blood, cloudiness, or excess sediment.
4. Inform the client that the antiseptic solution will feel cold while wiping from front to back.

2 A 75-year-old man is admitted with severe vomiting and possible GI bleeding. When planning the collection of a gastric specimen for a guaiac test, what should the nurse do prior to the test?
1. Promote a meat-free, high-residue diet for 24 hours.
2. Obtain a nursing history for colon cancer, GI bleeding, ulcers, or diarrhea.
3. Insert an NG tube.
4. Monitor the client's intake and output.

3 Mrs. Murphy is diabetic and performs BGM before each meal and at bedtime. She tells the nurse that she has trouble getting a droplet of blood large enough for testing. Which of the following interventions would be least appropriate?
1. Instruct her to use the lateral side of the finger.
2. Apply pressure to the site for at least 1 minute before puncture.
3. Cleanse site with warm water and allow to dry.
4. Place lancet firmly against the site, to ensure an appropriate depth of puncture.

4 The preferred vein for venipuncture for phlebotomy is:
1. The antecubital vein, which is less painful
2. The basilic vein, which is straight
3. The cephalic vein, which is in the hand and well anchored
4. The median cubital vein, which is larger, well anchored, and closer to the surface

5 One of the unexpected outcomes of collection of a nasal culture is nasal bleeding. Which of the following interventions would be most appropriate if it occurred?
1. Provide analgesia as ordered.
2. Administer antibiotics as ordered.
3. Perform a Hemoccult test.
4. Apply pressure and ice.

6 Place the following steps of obtaining a wound drainage specimen in the correct order:
1. Cleanse around wound with an antiseptic swab and dispose.
2. Apply a fresh dressing.
3. Assess for signs of infection, including redness, tenderness, and drainage.
4. Place culture swab into the container, and attach ID label.
5. Enclose in a biohazard bag and attach a completed lab requisition.
6. Place tip of culture swab into the wound and gently rotate.
7. Remove soiled dressing.

References for all chapters appear in Appendix D.

14

Diagnostic Procedures

MEDIA RESOURCES

- **evolve** http://evolve.elsevier.com/Elkin

Diagnostic procedures may be performed at the client's bedside or in specially equipped rooms for diagnostic purposes. During diagnostic procedures the nurse is responsible for assessing the client's knowledge of the procedure, preparing the client, providing a safe environment throughout the procedure, and providing periprocedural assessment, care, teaching, and documentation. The nurse also supervises any nursing care delegated to assistive personnel (AP).

Invasive procedures involving injection of dye or entrance into a body cavity require informed consent. The physician is responsible for giving an explanation of what is involved with the test, the risks involved, expected benefits, alternative methods of treatment available, and probable outcomes.

EVIDENCE IN PRACTICE

Hoffman and others: Risk reduction in pediatric procedural sedation by application of an American Academy of Pediatrics/American Society of Anesthesiologists process model, *Pediatrics* 109(2):236-243, 2002.

Descriptions of procedural sedation have become more specific as a result of the term "conscious sedation" being misinterpreted. Procedural sedation is now classified as "minimal," "moderate," or "deep" sedation. "Moderate" corresponds to the older term of "conscious" sedation. Objective scales for preassessment are used to help determine client risk for undesirable outcomes. Use of a standard scale such as the American Society of Anesthesiologists (ASA) classification helps reduce the risk of complications by determining when it may be prudent to involve an anesthesiologist in a procedure to help manage the care of a complicated client condition (ASA, 2004a).

NURSING DIAGNOSES

Anxiety is related to anticipating discomfort or pain as a procedure is performed. **Deficient knowledge** regarding purpose and steps of a procedure is common with clients experiencing a procedure for the first time. **Fear** may be related to the unknown test results or the invasive nature of a procedure. Nursing diagnoses to promote oxygenation during diagnostic procedures involving sedation include **risk for impaired gas exchange** and **risk for aspiration. Risk for injury** is appropriate for all of the procedures in this chapter.

SKILL 14.1 Intravenous Moderate Sedation

Certain diagnostic procedures require the client to receive intravenous (IV) moderate sedation (formerly referred to as "conscious sedation"). Moderate sedation helps improve the client's cooperation with the procedure, allows a rapid return to the preprocedure status, and minimizes the risk of injury. In addition, it often raises the pain threshold and provides amnesia concerning the actual procedural events. Use of IV moderate sedation is closely controlled and normally restricted to physicians and nurses who received special training or credentialing. The most common types of drugs used to achieve moderate sedation include benzodiazepines and opiates. Clients are monitored for oversedation using a scoring system that identifies loss of consciousness, which poses the risk of aspiration caused by loss of the protective gag reflex. One such tool is the Modified Ramsay Sedation Scale (Ramsay and others, 1974) (Box 14-1). On this scale, the optimal score is 3. A score higher than 3 suggests oversedation, whereas a score lower than 3 may indicate risk for discomfort or inadequate relaxation. Although the nurse may administer IV moderate sedation when a physician is in attendance, it is the responsibility of the physician to order the appropriate drugs and their dosages. Check agency policy for recommended and maximum doses of medications.

Risks of IV moderate sedation include hypoventilation, airway compromise, hemodynamic instability, and/or altered level of consciousness (LOC), which may include an overly depressed LOC or agitation and combativeness. Emergency equipment and staff prepared to perform emergency medical treatment are immediately accessible in settings where IV sedation is administered. During and after the procedure, clients need continuous monitoring of vital signs and oxygen saturation by pulse oximetry and continual checks for improving LOC.

ASSESSMENT

1 Verify client's identity by using at least two forms of identifiers, neither of which may be the client's room number. Verify the type of procedure to be performed and procedure site with the client. *Rationale: Ensures accurate client identification and improves client safety. Client room number is not an acceptable identifier (JCAHO, 2003, 2006).*

2 If required by the agency, verify the client's ASA Physical Status Classification (Box 14-2). *Rationale: The ASA recommends that clients receiving a classification of 3 or higher have an anesthesia consult before receiving IV sedation (ASA, 2004b).*

BOX 14-1 Assessment of Level of Consciousness for IV Moderate Sedation

Assign the number that best describes the client's response to each category. An optimal score is 4, with acceptable scores ranging from 3 to 5.

Modified Ramsay Sedation Scale

Minimal sedation (anxiolysis)	1	Anxious and agitated, restless, or both.
	2	Cooperative, oriented, and tranquil.
Moderate sedation/ analgesia (conscious sedation)	3	Responds to commands spoken in a normal voice.
Deep sedation/ analgesia	4	Brisk response to a light forehead tap or loud auditory stimulus.
	5	Sluggish response to a light forehead tap or loud auditory stimulus.
	6	No response to a light forehead tap or loud auditory stimulus.

Excerpted from American Society of Anesthesiologists: *Continuum of depth of sedation definition of general anesthesia and levels of sedation/analgesia*, October 2005, p. 37. A copy of the full text can be obtained from ASA, 520 N. Northwest Highway, Park Ridge, IL 60068-2573.

BOX 14-2 ASA Physical Status Classification

1 Healthy client; no organic, physiological, or psychiatric disturbances.
2 Presence of mild systemic disease without functional limitations.
3 Presence of severe systemic disease with significant systemic effects and significant functional limitations.
4 Presence of medical condition that is poorly controlled, associated with significant dysfunction, and is a potential threat to life.
5 Presence of critical medical condition associated with little chance of survival.
6 Presence of brain death.

Based on American Society of Anesthesiologists: *ASA manual for anesthesia department organization and management (MADOM)*, 2005-2006. A copy of the full text can be obtained from ASA, 520 N. Northwest Highway, Park Ridge, IL 60068-2573.

3 Assess the client for a history of substance abuse. *Rationale: A history of substance abuse may require dose adjustment of the sedative.*

4 Verify that the client has not taken food or fluids, except for oral medications, for at least 4 hours. Verify specific agency requirements. *Rationale: Because a risk of moderate sedation is client loss of airway protection, an empty stomach reduces the risk of aspiration.*

5 Determine whether client is allergic to latex, antiseptic, or anesthetic solutions. *Rationale: Common allergic reactions to local anesthetic agents include central nervous system (CNS) depression, respiratory difficulties, and hypotension. Allergic reactions to antiseptic solutions are usually skin irritations. Allergic reactions to latex range from mild skin reaction to anaphylaxis.*

6 Assess baseline heart rate, respiratory rate, blood pressure, LOC, pain level, and oxygen saturation. *Rationale: Establishes a baseline to which the client's status during the procedure may be compared. Physician must be notified of abnormalities.*

7 Determine height and weight. *Rationale: Needed for calculation of drug dosages.*

8 Assess respiratory status, including airway and ability to open mouth wide and hyperextend neck. *Rationale: Factors that influence intubation if needed.*

9 Assess level of anxiety. *Rationale: The higher the anxiety level, the more sedation that is likely to be needed.*

10 Assess and document the client's baseline status via the agency's designated scoring system. *Rationale: Establishes a baseline to which the client's status after the procedure may be compared.*

PLANNING

Expected Outcomes focus on safe, effective, and uncomplicated IV sedation.

1 Client remains relaxed and comfortable (pain less than 4 on a scale of 0 to 10) *and* is responsive to physical and verbal stimuli with protective airway reflexes intact.

2 Client does not experience complications, such as respiratory depression, decreased cardiovascular function, confusion, or diminished reflexes, which are side effects of drugs used for IV sedation.

3 Client explains the purpose and basic steps of the procedure before it begins.

Delegation Considerations

The skill of assisting with IV sedation during the procedure may not be delegated.

Equipment

- Equipment for IV insertion (see Chapter 27)
- Sedatives for IV sedation (diazepam [Valium], midazolam [Versed], and fentanyl [Sublimaze] are commonly used; however, others may be ordered)
- Emergency equipment for resuscitation: oxygen, pulse oximeter (Spo_2, cardiac monitor may be used, depending on the procedure and agency policy)
- Appropriate reversal drugs (naloxone is used for reversal of opioids; flumazenil is used for reversal of benzodiazepines)
- Appropriate pain medication for procedures anticipated to cause postprocedure pain

IMPLEMENTATION *for Intravenous Moderate Sedation*

STEPS	RATIONALE

1 See Standard Protocol (inside front cover).

> **COMMUNICATION TIP** Explain to client that the IV sedation will cause relaxation, but that he or she will be awake during the procedure. If the client will not be able to speak because of the nature of the procedure, teach nonverbal signals for things such as "yes," "no," and "pain." Explain to client that close monitoring of vital signs and frequent checks during the procedure are routine and do not mean that there are problems. Explain to the client briefly the major steps of the procedure.

STEPS	RATIONALE
2 Establish IV access.	Provides route for administration of IV sedation, as well as rapid IV access, should emergency care be needed.
3 Monitor and record vital signs and oxygen saturation (Spo_2) every 5 to 15 minutes.	Vital signs are used to monitor client's ongoing response to sedation. Increasing heart rate and decreasing Spo_2 indicate impaired breathing, possibly caused by position or oversedation.
4 Observe for verbal or nonverbal evidence of pain, facial grimacing, and eye opening.	Physical responses indicate level of sedation.
5 Monitor sedation level (see Box 14-1), and notify physician of unacceptable scores.	Careful monitoring for excessive medication response is essential during IV moderate sedation.

> **NURSE ALERT** A Ramsay sedation level score higher than 3 must be immediately reported to the physician. Ensure the patency of the client's airway.

STEPS	RATIONALE
6 Monitor visually for LOC and responsiveness.	Reduced responsiveness increases risk of airway compromise and aspiration.
7 See Completion Protocol (inside front cover).	

EVALUATION

1 Assess client throughout the procedure using the Ramsay sedation scale.

2 After the procedure, monitor airway patency, respiratory rate, Spo₂, heart rate, pain score, and LOC, every 5 minutes for at least 30 minutes, then every 15 minutes for an hour, then every 30 minutes until client meets discharge criteria on the agency's designated scoring system.

3 Ask client to repeat back what he or she understands to be the steps of the procedure.

Unexpected Outcomes and Related Interventions

1 Client develops respiratory distress evidenced by decreased oxygen saturation, cyanosis, and slow, shallow respirations with periods of apnea.
a. Notify physician immediately.
b. Support client's breathing via positioning and manual bagging.
c. Be prepared to administer reversal agents to counteract the sedative.

2 Client develops cardiac instability as evidenced by irregular heart rate, change in pulse rate, or change in blood pressure.
a. Obtain electrocardiogram (ECG) as ordered.
b. Notify physician immediately.

Recording and Reporting

- Record respiratory rate and sedation level at baseline and each time assessed.
- Record dosage, route, and time of drugs administered during and after the procedure, including the use of reversal agents and significant client reactions during the procedure.
- Report to physician immediately any respiratory distress, cardiac compromise, or altered mental status.

Sample Documentation

1500 Returned to unit after esophagogastroduodenoscopy (EGD) with IV moderate sedation. Alert and awake. BP 120/60, P 92, R 26, O₂ saturation 98%. Respirations deep and regular. Color pale. Morphine 8 mg IV given for pain rating of 6 (0 to 10 scale) in right rib area, worse at 8 with deep breaths.

1530 Resting. Rates pain at 1 (0 to 10 scale). Vital signs unchanged. O₂ saturation 97% to 99% on room air.

Special Considerations
Pediatric Considerations

- A preprocedure medical evaluation is required. One must consider anatomical and physiological variations, preprocedure assessments, and pharmacological techniques to safely administer sedation to the pediatric client (American Academy of Pediatrics, 2002).
- Sedation is used in pediatric clients to attain their cooperation with procedures. Deep sedation is used more often than moderate sedation in children younger than age 6 (American Academy of Pediatrics, 2002).
- Children are more likely than adults to sustain a serious complication resulting from anesthesia. The American Academy of Pediatrics recommends the presence of personnel who are able to manage a child's airway (American Academy of Pediatrics, 2002).

Geriatric Considerations

- Closely monitor the effects of narcotics and hypnotics that may interfere with breathing because older clients may have reduced drug clearance through the kidneys or liver (Phipps and others, 2003).

Home Care Considerations

- Driving is usually restricted for 24 hours after IV sedation has been used.

SKILL 14.2   Contrast Media Studies: Arteriogram (Angiogram), Cardiac Catheterization, Intravenous Pyelogram

Contrast media studies involve visualization of blood vessel structure of the body by the intravascular injection of a contrast medium. An arteriogram (angiogram) permits visualization of the arterial system (Figure 14-1) to help diagnose occlusions, stenosis, emboli, thromboses, aneurysms, tumors, congenital malformations, or trauma anywhere in the body.

Cardiac catheterization is a specialized form of angiography in which a catheter is inserted into either the left or right side of the heart via a peripheral major blood vessel (subclavian or femoral vein). The test studies pressures within the heart, cardiac volumes, valve function, and patency of coronary arteries.

Intravenous pyelography (IVP) is a venographical examination of the flow of radiopaque contrast medium through the kidneys, ureters, and bladder to identify obstruction, hematuria, stones, bladder injury, or renal artery occlusion. Dye is injected into a peripheral vein and serial radiographs are taken over the subsequent 30 minutes.

The diagnostic procedures addressed in this skill are performed in radiology or a special procedures department (Figure 14-2) by a variety of specially trained technicians and physicians. The nurse assists with client preparation, provides support during the procedure, and monitors for complications after the procedure.

ASSESSMENT

1 Verify client's identity by using at least two forms of identifiers, neither of which may be the client's room number. Verify the type of procedure to be performed and procedure site with the client. *Rationale: Ensures accurate client identification and improves client safety. Client room number is not an acceptable identifier (JCAHO, 2003, 2006).*

2 Determine if client is taking anticoagulants. *Rationale: Medication increases risk of bleeding and needs to be stopped before the procedure.*

3 Examine medical record for contraindications.

a. Angiography contraindications: anticoagulant therapy; bleeding disorders; thrombocytopenia; dehydration; uncontrolled hypertension; previous allergy to radiographic dye, iodine, or shellfish; renal insufficiency; and pregnancy (if iodinated contrast media is used, because of radioactive iodine crossing the blood-placental barrier)

b. Cardiac catheterization contraindications: pregnancy (because of radioactive iodine crossing the blood-placental barrier), severe cardiomyopathy, severe arrhythmias, uncontrolled congestive heart failure (CHF)

c. IVP contraindications: dehydration, known renal insufficiency. *Rationale: Anticoagulants and bleeding disorders are contraindications for arterial procedures because of interference with the client's*

FIGURE 14-1 Arteriogram. (From Dougherty DB, Jackson DB: *Gastrointestinal disorders,* Mosby's clinical nursing series, St Louis, 1993, Mosby.)

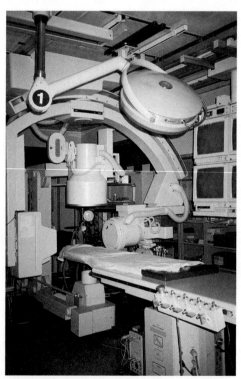

FIGURE 14-2 Cardiac catheterization procedure room. (From Wong and others: *Whaley and Wong's nursing care of infants and children,* ed 7, St Louis, 2003, Mosby.)

blood clotting abilities and risk of too much blood loss. Dehydration and renal insufficiency contraindicate use of radiographic contrast media because the client will have an impaired ability to excrete the contrast media via the kidneys (Chernecky and Berger, 2004).

4 Determine whether client has taken the drug metformin within the past 48 hours. If so, notify the physician immediately. *Rationale: Metformin taken within 48 hours before receiving iodinated contrast media can lead to lactic acidosis. Metformin is contained in the drugs Glucophage and Glucovance (Calabrese and others, 2002).*

5 Assess client's knowledge of the procedure. *Rationale: Determines level of understanding and what teaching may be necessary.*

6 Observe verbal and nonverbal behaviors to determine level of client's anxiety.

7 Assess for allergy to iodine dye, shellfish, or latex; if so, notify cardiologist or radiologist. *Rationale: A hypoallergenic contrast medium can sometimes be used for clients with these allergies. Latex allergies range from moderate (itching) to severe (anaphylaxis).*

8 Obtain vital signs and peripheral pulses. For arterial procedures, mark the client's peripheral pulses before the procedure. For cardiac catheterization, also auscultate heart and lungs. *Rationale: Provides baseline data and locations for comparison with findings during and after procedure.*

9 Determine client's hydration status. *Rationale: Severe dehydration can cause renal shutdown and failure (Pagana and Pagana, 2005).*

10 Assess client's bleeding and coagulation status (e.g., complete blood count [CBC], platelet count, prothrombin time [PT]). *Rationale: Abnormal clotting factors may contraindicate the procedure because of increased risk for bleeding.*

11 Assess client's renal function via electrolyte, urea nitrogen, and creatinine levels. *Rationale: Elevated urea nitrogen or creatinine levels increase the risk for renal failure.*

12 Determine that preprocedure preparation is complete.

a. For cardiac catheterization: Determine whether the site of catheter insertion needs to be shaved and prepped with antiseptic just before the procedure. Antiseptic should be allowed to dry. *Rationale: Reduces risk of site-related infection.*

b. For IVP: Verify that the client has taken the necessary preprocedure orally administered bowel evacuation medication 24 hours before the test or completed an evacuation enema 8 hours before the test. *Rationale: An evacuated lower intestine and bowel improve visualization.*

13 Auscultate heart and lungs (for clients undergoing angiography) to provide baseline data for comparison with findings during and after procedure.

14 Verify that informed consent has been obtained (check agency policy).

15 Determine and document time of last ingested fluid or food. *Rationale: Excessive hydration causes dilution of contrast medium, making structure more difficult to visualize. Iodine dye may cause nausea. Client should be NPO for 6 to 8 hours before the procedure.*

16 Assess client's ability to remain still and cooperate throughout the procedure.

17 Remove metal objects and all of client's jewelry. *Rationale: Eliminates objects that interfere with radiography visualization of the vessels.*

18 Review physician's orders for preprocedure medications and for IV sedation. *Rationale: Increased sedation may be necessary in anxious or confused clients.*

a. Atropine: Decreases salivary secretions and increases heart rate when bradycardia is present.

b. Diphenhydramine (Benadryl): Used to block histamine and decrease allergic response.

c. Preprocedure sedative: Decreases anxiety and promotes relaxation.

d. IV sedation during procedure: See Skill 14.1.

PLANNING

Expected Outcomes focus on prevention of respiratory side effects from sedation and cardiovascular complications from catheter placement.

1 Client assumes the correct position and remains still throughout the entire procedure.

2 Client has pain less than 4 (on a scale of 0 to 10) that is limited to soreness at catheter insertion site and possible backache.

3 Client does not experience postprocedure complications, such as:

a. Flushing, itching, and urticaria, which signify possible allergic reaction to dye

b. Diminished or absent peripheral pulses, signifying thrombosis or embolism

c. Hypotension and tachycardia, signifying hemorrhage or allergic reaction to dye

d. Decreased or absent urine output related to renal failure

4 Client recovers from IV sedation without respiratory complications or reduced LOC.

5 Client tolerates increased fluid intake and voids sufficiently to excrete radiographic dye.

Delegation Considerations

The skill of assisting with angiography and IVP may be delegated if the client is stable and if no IV sedation is used. The nurse directs personnel by:

- Reviewing what to observe and report to the nurse

Equipment

- Protective supplies: mask, goggles, sterile gown, gloves
- Sterile packs containing catheters/equipment for performing the procedures
- Equipment for IV access
- Diazepam, midazolam, or other sedative for IV sedation if indicated
- Emergency equipment: oxygen, pulse oximeter, cardiac monitor, sedative reversal agents

IMPLEMENTATION *for Contrast Media Studies: Arteriogram (Angiogram), Cardiac Catheterization, Intravenous Pyelogram*

STEPS	RATIONALE
1 See Standard Protocol (inside front cover).	
2 Have client empty bladder before procedure.	Ensures that client will not need to void during procedure.
3 Prepare equipment for monitoring client during the procedure, including heart rate and rhythm, oxygen saturation, and blood pressure.	
4 Provide IV access using large-bore cannula. Remove gloves.	Provides access for delivery of IV fluids and/or drugs.
5 Assist client in assuming a comfortable supine position on x-ray table. Clients undergoing IVP may be placed supine or in a slight Trendelenburg position. Immobilize the extremity that will be injected.	For arterial procedures, position may need to be maintained for 1 to 3 hours.
6 Take "Time Out" to verify the client's name, type of procedure to be performed, and procedure site with the client.	"Time Out" verification just before starting the procedure includes the physician and all involved personnel and is a safety precaution to prevent wrong client, wrong site, and wrong procedure errors (JCAHO, 2003, 2006).
7 Physician cleanses site for catheter insertion (femoral, carotid, or brachial) with antiseptic.	
8 All members of the team apply sterile gown and gloves, and the client is draped with sterile drapes, leaving puncture site exposed.	Reduces transmission of infection.
9 The skin at the puncture site is anesthetized with a local anesthetic.	

> **NURSE ALERT**   Be prepared to end the cardiac catheterization procedure early in the event of severe unrelieved chest pain, neurological symptoms of a cerebrovascular accident (CVA), cardiac arrhythmias, or hemodynamic changes (Chernecky and Berger, 2004).

10 Physician inserts needle and guide wire, advances catheter to desired artery or cardiac chamber, and injects contrast medium. During dye injection, specialized machinery takes rapid sequence of x-rays.	Permits radiographic visualization of structures, aneurysms, occlusions, or anomalies.

> **COMMUNICATION TIP**   Tell client that during the injection of the dye, he or she may experience some chest pain and there may be a severe hot flash that is quite uncomfortable but lasts only a few seconds.

11 If iodinated dye is administered, observe client for signs of anaphylaxis, including respiratory distress, palpitations, itching, and diaphoresis.	Allergic reactions can be life threatening.
12 During cardiac catheterization, the nurse assists with measuring cardiac volumes and pressures.	Provides data related to cardiac output, central venous pressure (CVP), ventricular pressures, and pulmonary artery pressure.
13 Nurse administering IV sedation monitors level of sedation and LOC (see Skill 14-1).	IV sedation should not cause loss of consciousness.
14 The physician withdraws catheter and applies pressure to puncture site for 5 to 15 minutes. Alternatively, a vascular closure device may be used.	Pressure on puncture site promotes clotting and prevents bleeding.
15 Remove and discard gown and gloves.	

STEPS	RATIONALE

16 See Completion Protocol (inside front cover).

> **NURSE ALERT** If the client reports any feelings of pain, dyspnea, numbness, tingling, or other untoward symptoms, immediately report these to the physician.

17 For arterial procedures:

a. Keep affected extremity immobilized for 6 to 8 hours after removal of catheter. Use orthopedic bedpan for female client as needed while on bed rest.

Allows time for the body's natural hemostatic mechanisms to form stable initial repair at the insertion site.

b. Emphasize the need to lie flat for 6 to 12 hours (and possibly overnight if the catheters are left in the groin).

Helps prevent disruption of hemostasis.

EVALUATION

1 Assess client's body position and comfort during procedure.

2 Evaluate client's level of comfort on a pain scale of 0 to 10.

3 Monitor for complications:

a. Observe insertion site for bloody drainage or hematoma formation. Assess postprocedure laboratory values (CBC, PT).

b. Palpate peripheral pulses in the affected extremity, as well as skin temperature and color. Changes can indicate altered circulation.

c. Auscultate heart and lungs, and compare findings with preprocedure findings. Monitor ECG recording.

d. Monitor the client for allergic reactions.

(1) Assess client for flushing, itching, and urticaria.

(2) Assess client's respiratory status for sudden, severe shortness of breath.

e. Monitor client's LOC and neurological status.

4 Monitor vital signs compared with baseline every 15 minutes for 1 hour, then every 30 minutes for 2 hours or until vital signs are stable, then every 4 hours (see agency policy) (Ignatavicius and Workman, 2002).

5 Monitor for sedation complications (see Skill 14-1).

a. Measure vital signs as discussed; compare to baseline and subsequent values.

b. Measure Spo2 and compare to baseline.

6 Encourage client to drink 1 to 2 liters of fluid after procedure. Assess client's tolerance of fluids and urinary output.

Unexpected Outcomes and Related Interventions

1 Client experiences vasovagal response (occurs at time of femoral puncture or after procedure with femoral pressure). Symptoms include feeling faint, dizzy, light-headed, and possible loss of consciousness for a few seconds. Bradycardic pulse is caused by stimulation of the vagus nerve via baroreceptors.

a. Support airway.

b. Lower table or head of bed to the Trendelenburg position.

c. Administer IV fluid bolus, if ordered.

2 Client's pedal pulses are nonpalpable bilaterally 2 hours after an angiogram.

a. Assess pulses with a Doppler scope.

b. Notify physician immediately.

3 Client develops hematoma or hemorrhage at catheter insertion site.

a. Maintain direct pressure over insertion site.

b. Contact physician immediately. Follow specific postprocedure orders related to findings.

c. Monitor catheter site every 30 minutes for 2 to 3 hours, then as needed.

4 Oversedation occurs.

a. See Skill 14.1.

5 Retroperitoneal bleeding occurs (when femoral access site is used). A hallmark sign of retroperitoneal bleeding is low back pain radiating to both sides of the body.

a. Prepare client for emergency surgery.

b. Monitor vital signs every 5 to 15 minutes.

c. Monitor distal pulses hourly.

Recording and Reporting

• Record client's condition: vital signs, peripheral pulses for equality and symmetry, blood pressure especially for hypotension, temperature and color of catheterized extremity, condition of IV site, level of comfort and level of client responsiveness, any drainage from puncture site, dressing appearance, and condition of site.

• Report to physician or charge nurse immediately: changes in vital signs and/or oxygen saturation, arrhythmias, excessive bleeding or increasing hematoma at puncture site, decreased or absent peripheral pulses, urine output less than 30 ml per hour, and decreased level of client responsiveness.

Sample Documentation

0800 Returned from angiogram via stretcher awake and alert. Dorsalis pedis and posterior tibial pulses are palpable and equal bilaterally. No bleeding, swelling, or discoloration noted at catheter insertion site in left groin. Sandbag in place over left groin. Left leg extended. Complains of mild discomfort at left groin equal to 2 on a 0 to 10 pain scale, but denies need for analgesics.

Special Considerations

Pediatric Considerations

- Because of their small body size, infants and children are very susceptible to the diuretic effects of radiocontrast dyes and may display complications very quickly. Emphasize the importance of fluid intake with the child and parent(s) (Nagelhout and Zaglaniczny, 2005).
- Blood loss from the procedure occurs from the cutdown site and bleeding into surrounding tissues. Fluid boluses via IV may be required to maintain acceptable circulating plasma volume (Nagelhout and Zaglaniczny, 2005).

Geriatric Considerations

- In the older adult, slight alterations in vital signs or behavior may be precursors to impending problems; therefore skilled observations are critical (Phipps and others, 2003).
- Physical exposure and room temperature may contribute to hypothermia in frail adults who may not be able to communicate that they are cold. Use heated blankets or forced air heat to maintain core temperature at comfortable, safe levels (Negishi and others, 2003).

- Renal insufficiency in older clients may contribute to prolonged sedation.
- The older adult with preexisting dehydration or renal insufficiency in combination with NPO status is at risk for dye-induced renal failure. Carefully monitor intake and output (I&O).

Home Care Considerations

- Instruct client to contact the physician (or affiliated emergency department) if any of the following occur after cardiac catheterization:
  - Bleeding from the catheterization puncture site: Apply gentle pressure with a clean gauze or cloth.
  - Formation of a knot or lump under the skin that increases in size.
  - Worsening of a bruise or its movement down the extremity rather than disappearing.
  - Pain at puncture site or in the extremity used for the catheterization.
  - Extremity where arterial puncture is made becomes pale and cool to touch.
  - Appearance of redness, swelling, or warmth of the affected extremity.
- Although bathing or showering may be allowed the day after the catheterization, the client should be cautioned to avoid slipping because the leg (if this extremity was used) may feel stiff.

SKILL 14.3 | **Assisting with Aspirations: Bone Marrow, Lumbar Puncture, Paracentesis, Thoracentesis**

Aspirations are invasive procedures involving removal of body fluids or tissue for diagnostic purposes. The nurse assists the physician during an aspiration procedure. Informed consent is legally required for these invasive procedures (Table 14-1).

A bone marrow aspiration involves the removal of a small amount of marrow, the liquid material from the bone. The site of aspiration is usually the sternum or the superior iliac crest. In children the proximal tibia may be used. A bone marrow aspiration may be done to diagnose leukemias, certain malignancies, anemias, and thrombocytopenia. The marrow is examined in a laboratory to reveal the number, size, shape, and development of red blood cells (RBCs) and platelet precursors. Culture of bone marrow can help differentiate infectious diseases such as tuberculosis (TB) or histoplasmosis. This test takes about 20 minutes.

A lumbar puncture (LP), also called a spinal puncture or spinal tap, involves the introduction of a needle into the subarachnoid space of the spinal column. The purpose is to measure the pressure in the subarachnoid space; to obtain cerebrospinal fluid (CSF) for visual and laboratory examination; and to inject anesthetic, diagnostic, or therapeutic agents. Laboratory examination of CSF helps diagnose spinal cord tumors, CNS infections, hemorrhage, autoimmune or demyelinating diseases, and degenerative brain disease.

Abdominal paracentesis involves aspiration of peritoneal fluid from the abdomen. The aspirate is then analyzed for cell cytology and the composition of bacteria, blood, glucose, and protein to help diagnose the cause(s) of abdominal effusion. Aspiration paracentesis may also be performed as a palliative measure to provide temporary relief of abdominal and respiratory discomfort caused by severe ascites. Lavage paracentesis, in which a lavage of solution is instilled, then withdrawn, may be done to detect the presence of bleeding, such as in cases of blunt abdominal trauma

TABLE 14-1 Summary of Aspiration Procedures

ASPIRATION PROCEDURE	PREPARATION/ASSESSMENT SPECIFIC TO TEST	POSITION OR SITE PRONE OR SUPINE POSITION	SPECIAL CONSIDERATIONS
Bone marrow aspiration	Assess CBC for abnormalities.	Sternum Superior illiac crest Proximal tibia	Clients with arthritis or orthopnea may have difficulty assuming this position. Pressure is applied to the site after the procedure.
Lumbar puncture	Assess neurological status, including movement, sensation, and muscle strength of legs to provide a baseline for comparison. Assess bladder for distention, and determine last voiding.	Lateral decubitus position L1 L3 L5 L2 L4 Subarachnoid space	*Risk of spinal headache:* Instruct client to remain flat and log roll according to physician orders. Observe for excessive drainage at the site. Fluid loss at the site can predispose client to headache and infection.

(From Ignatavicius DD, Workman ML: *Medical-surgical nursing: critical thinking for collaborative care,* ed 4, Philadelphia, 2002, Saunders.)

Continued

TABLE 14-1 Summary of Aspiration Procedures—cont'd

ASPIRATION PROCEDURE	PREPARATION/ASSESSMENT SPECIFIC TO TEST	POSITION OR SITE SITTING POSITION	SPECIAL CONSIDERATIONS
Paracentesis	Assess bladder for distention, and determine last voiding. Weigh client, assess abdomen, and measure abdominal girth at largest point. Mark location.	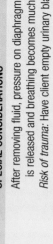	After removing fluid, pressure on diaphragm is released and breathing becomes much easier. *Risk of trauma:* Have client empty urinary bladder before procedure.
Thoracentesis	Assess respiratory rate and depth, symmetry of chest on inspiration and expiration, cough and sputum. Assist client with remaining still during the procedure to prevent trauma to the visceral pleura. Client will need to hold breath and avoid coughing during the procedure.	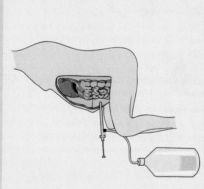 (From Beare P, Myers J: *Adult health nursing,* ed 3, St Louis, 1998, Mosby.) Orthopneic position Area for needle insertion (intercostal space) 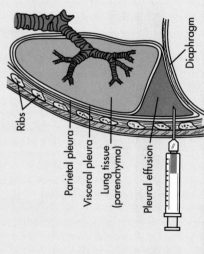 Ribs Parietal pleura Visceral pleura Lung tissue (parenchyma) Pleural effusion Diaphragm	Monitor blood pressure for hypotension if large quantity of fluid is removed. *Risk of pneumothorax:* Observe for sudden shortness of breath, tracheal deviation, anxiety, altered vital signs, and decreased oxygen saturation.

or tumor cells when cancer is suspected. The procedure takes 30 minutes or less.

Thoracentesis is performed to analyze or remove pleural fluid or to instill medications intrapleurally. Specimens are examined for gross appearance and consistency and for protein, glucose, amylase, lactate dehydrogenase (LD), and cellular composition. Cytological specimens are examined for malignancy, differentiated between transudative and exudative characteristics, and cultured for pathogens. Therapeutic thoracentesis is used to relieve pain, dyspnea, and signs of pleural pressure. Diagnostic thoracentesis is used in the presence of pleural effusion of unknown etiology and generally takes 30 minutes or less.

ASSESSMENT

1 Verify client's identity by using at least two forms of identifiers, neither of which may be the client's room number. Verify the type of procedure to be performed and procedure site with the client. *Rationale: Ensures accurate client identification and improves client safety. Client room number is not an acceptable identifier (JCAHO, 2003, 2006).*

2 Review medical record for contraindications:

a. Bone marrow biopsy: Client is unable to maintain positioning or lie still during the procedure.

b. Lumbar puncture: The main contraindication for LP is increased intracranial pressure (IICP). If IICP is present, the sudden release of pressure during an LP may cause herniation of the brain structures through the foramen magnum and subsequent death. Normally a diagnostic computed tomography (CT) scan is done to rule out IICP. However, when the need for diagnostic LP is urgent, such as in clients without brain shift who are comatose and suspected of acute meningitis, prior CT may be omitted (van Crevel, Hijdra, and de Gans, 2002). Other contraindications include spinal degenerative joint disease, spinal deformities, and coagulopathies. In addition, infection near the lumbar site not only risks introduction of infection into the CSF but also affects the accuracy of the resulting CSF cytology (Chernecky and Berger, 2004).

c. Paracentesis: Although not contraindicated, paracentesis should be performed with caution in clients with coagulopathies, intestinal obstruction, or abdominal wall infection with portal hypertension with abdominal collateral circulation, as well as in those who are pregnant.

d. Thoracentesis: Client is unable to maintain positioning or stay motionless during the procedure.

3 Determine client's knowledge of procedure to determine level of teaching required.

4 Observe verbal and nonverbal behaviors to determine client's anxiety.

5 Assess client's ability to follow directions closely, including ability to physically assume and maintain posi-

tion required for procedure and ability to remain still. Bone marrow biopsy requires a prone position. LP requires lateral decubitus position. Paracentesis usually involves a sitting position. Thoracentesis uses an orthopneic position. *Rationale: Client must maintain position, without moving, to avoid complications during needle or trochar insertion.*

6 Determine whether client is allergic to antiseptic, anesthetic solutions, or latex. *Rationale: Common allergic reactions to local anesthetic agents include CNS depression, respiratory difficulties, and hypotension. Allergic reactions to antiseptic solutions are usually skin irritations. Latex allergies range from moderate (itching) to severe (anaphylaxis).*

7 Determine whether informed consent has been obtained. Hold sedatives until this is done. *Rationale: Consent must be given when client is alert and oriented.*

8 Obtain vital signs. *Rationale: Provides baseline data for comparison with postprocedure vital signs. For LP, also carry out a baseline assessment of lower extremity movement, sensation, and muscle strength.*

9 Assess client's use of anticoagulants. *Rationale: Anticoagulants increase risk of bleeding.*

10 For paracentesis, encourage client to void before the procedure. *Rationale: Presence of a distended bladder increases the risk for inadvertent bladder trauma.*

11 For paracentesis, obtain client weight and document measurement of abdominal girth. Use an ink pen to mark the location of the measuring tab on the abdomen. *Rationale: Provides baseline measurements for postprocedure comparison.*

12 Determine need for preprocedure pain medication. *Rationale: Procedure may be painful, and pain control helps client remain still throughout procedure.*

PLANNING

Expected Outcomes focus on proper positioning, client's ability to follow directions, comfort, and absence of complications.

1 Client assumes the correct position and remains still throughout the entire procedure.

2 Puncture site dressing remains clean, dry, and intact.

3 Client is able to explain postprocedure position and activity restrictions.

4 Client maintains respiratory rate, heart rate, and blood pressure within normal limits during and after aspiration procedure.

5 Client verbalizes pain at less than 4 on a scale of 0 to 10 after the procedure.

Delegation Considerations

Assessment of the client's condition cannot be delegated. Monitoring of vital signs after the procedures may be delegated. The nurse directs personnel by:

• Reviewing what to observe and report to the nurse. This information is specific for each client.

Equipment

- Masks, goggles, gowns, and gloves
- Test tubes, laboratory requisitions, and labels
- Aspiration trays: Most institutions provide trays with contents appropriate for the specific aspiration. Contents of trays may differ from one institution to another. Standard aspiration trays may contain:
  - Antiseptic solution (e.g., povidone-iodine)
  - Sterile gauze sponges (4 × 4)
  - Sterile towels
  - Anesthetic agent (e.g., lidocaine 1%)
- Two 3-ml sterile syringes with 16- to 27-gauge needles (NOTE: incidence of postpuncture headache progressively decreases as needle gauge decreases [Evans and others, 2000])
- 2-inch adhesive tape and bandages
- Lumbar puncture: Manometer (to measure spinal fluid pressure)
- Thoracentesis: Vacuum bottles, stopcock with extension tubing, test tubes
- Paracentesis: Sterile specimen containers and bag, vacuum bottles

IMPLEMENTATION *for Assisting with Aspirations: Bone Marrow, Lumbar Puncture, Paracentesis, Thoracentesis*

STEPS	RATIONALE
1 See Standard Protocol (inside front cover).	
2 Explain steps of skin preparation, anesthetic injection, needle insertion, and position required. For bone marrow biopsy, explain to client that pain may occur when the bone marrow is aspirated.	Anticipation of expected sensation reduces anxiety.
3 Set up sterile tray or open supplies to make accessible for physician.	Reduces risk of contamination of sterile field and promotes prompt completion of procedure.
4 Take "Time Out" to verify the client's name, type of procedure to be performed, and procedure site with the client.	"Time Out" verification just before starting the procedure includes the physician and all involved personnel and is a safety precaution to prevent wrong client, wrong site, and wrong procedure errors (JCAHO, 2003, 2006).
5 Obtain a premedication order (i.e., sedative) if client is extremely anxious. Premedicate for pain if a bone marrow biopsy will be done.	Pain occurs when bone marrow is aspirated. Reduces client discomfort and reduces risk of client movement during the procedure.
6 Assist client in maintaining correct position (see Table 14-1). Reassure client while explaining procedure.	Decreases chance of complications during procedure. Explanations increase client comfort and relaxation.
7 Physician cleanses site with antiseptic solution and drapes site with sterile drape.	

COMMUNICATION TIP Tell the client that the local anesthetic needle will cause a mild pinching sensation for a few seconds. This will be followed by a feeling of dull pressure when the trochar is inserted.

STEPS	RATIONALE
8 Physician injects local anesthetic and waits for area to become numb.	Discomfort and pressure may still occur when deep tissues are disrupted.
9 Physician inserts trochar or needle into body cavity involved (see Table 14-1).	
10 To aspirate tissue or body fluid for specimens, a syringe is attached to the trochar or needle and aspirate is placed into appropriate specimen container.	
11 If excess fluid is drained, the physician attaches drainage tubing and container and fluid drains by gravity flow.	
12 Properly label specimens with client information and name of test desired. Transport tubes to the laboratory immediately.	Nurse is responsible for labeling tubes with client's name and tests desired. Test tubes are numbered in sequence of collection (e.g., 1 through 4).
13 Physician removes needle/trochar and applies pressure over insertion site until drainage ceases. Assist with placement of closure device or direct pressure and gauze dressing. Continue to apply pressure for a specific time period if directed.	

STEPS	RATIONALE
14 Note characteristics of fluid/tissue aspirate (e.g., amount, color).	Characteristics are used for observation, reporting, and recording.
15 See Completion Protocol (inside front cover).	

EVALUATION

1 Observe client body position throughout procedure, and assist with maintaining position as necessary.

2 Inspect dressing over puncture site for drainage every hour after the procedure as ordered.

3 Ask client to describe level of comfort using a scale of 0 to 10.

4 Monitor client's respiratory status: rate, rhythm, and depth of respirations, as well as symmetry of chest movement. Compare client's LOC, heart rate, and blood pressure during and after procedure to preprocedure baseline. (Check agency policy; this may be as often as every 15 minutes for 2 hours.)

5 Ask client to describe postprocedure positioning and activity restrictions.

Unexpected Outcomes and Related Interventions

1 Oversedation occurs.
a. Follow Interventions in Skill 14.1.

2 Postdural puncture headache (PDPH) after LP is evidenced by headache, blurred vision, and tinnitus.
a. Medicate for pain as ordered.
b. Notify physician, who may choose to inject a blood patch into the epidural space.
c. IV caffeine sodium benzoate has been used with limited success in relieving PDPH (Yucel and others, 1999).
NOTE: Increasing the fluid intake, a longstanding practice, has not been shown to prevent postpuncture headache.

3 Hematoma develops internally at LP site, evidenced by lower extremity tingling.
a. Compare to baseline assessment.
b. Notify physician.
c. Continue frequent evaluation.

4 LP client develops excessive loss of CSF, evidenced by large amount of CSF drainage from site and reduced LOC, dilated pupils, and increased blood pressure.
a. Maintain airway.
b. Notify physician immediately.
c. Prepare for transfer to intensive care setting.

5 Paracentesis client develops leakage of fluid at the aspiration site as evidenced by continuously saturated dressings.
a. Reinforce dressing. Place collection bag over the site, if needed.
b. Notify physician, who may place a small suture to stop the drainage.

6 Pneumothorax after thoracentesis is evidenced by sudden dyspnea and tachypnea and asymmetrical chest excursion.
a. Administer oxygen (if ordered).
b. Monitor vital signs and respiratory status frequently.
c. Notify physician of findings, and obtain further orders.
d. Anticipate chest x-ray and possible chest tube insertion.

Recording and Reporting

• Record preprocedure and client preparation; name of procedure; location of puncture site (if applicable); amount, consistency and color of fluid drained or specimen obtained; client's tolerance to procedure (e.g., vital signs, comfort); laboratory tests ordered; type of dressing; completion of postprocedure activities, such as chest x-ray; preprocedure, intraprocedure, and postprocedure vital signs; and (if applicable) extremity assessments, abdominal girth, and LOC.

• Immediately report to physician or charge nurse any unexpected drainage or significant changes in vital signs or oxygen saturation status.

Sample Documentation

0930 Voided 300 ml. Abdominal girth measures 42 inches at umbilicus. Assisted with sitting on side of bed. Physician completed abdominal paracentesis with 1100 ml cloudy liquid aspirated. Respirations 18 with moderate depth, pulse 98, and blood pressure 138/86. Rates pain at 6 on scale of 0 to 10. 22-inch gauze dressing applied to puncture site; remains dry and intact.

0940 Morphine sulfate 10 mg given in right vastus lateralis for abdominal pain.

1010 States pain has decreased to 2, which is tolerable. Abdominal girth measures 34 inches at umbilicus. Weight decreased to 158 pounds.

Special Considerations
Pediatric Considerations

• Sedation is recommended for children because of the risk of injury caused by children's movement during LP. Very young children may receive IV moderate sedation or general anesthetic for aspiration procedures. Conscious or unconscious sedation is commonly used. If unconscious sedation is used, an anesthesiologist will be needed for the procedure.

- Prepare child of preschool age before the procedure; make a game out of having child recall the next procedural step, using a doll as a model. This can serve as a distraction mechanism (Haiat, Bar-Mor, and Shochat, 2003).

Geriatric Considerations

- Older adults with arthritis may have difficulty sustaining the position required for the procedure and may need help to sustain the required position.
- Assess closely for nonverbal signs of pain; the older adult may not ask for pain relief.
- During thoracentesis, be aware of ineffective breathing patterns in the older adult because of age-related changes such as reduced elastic lung recoil, declining chest expansion, reduced cough efficiency, and weaker thoracic and diaphragmatic muscles.
- Older adults may exhibit restlessness as an early sign of hypoxia during or after thoracentesis.
- Be aware of need to change positions slowly to minimize risks for postural hypotension.

Home Care Considerations

- Instruct client that some clients experience tenderness at the puncture site for several days, and mild analgesia may be ordered by the physician.
- LP client should seek medical attention immediately if he or she suddenly complains of severe headache or has change in LOC.
- Inform paracentesis client to notify physician of fever or any swelling, pain, or drainage at puncture site. Males should report scrotal edema to the physician.
- Teach the thoracentesis client symptoms of complications related to liver and spleen perforation that may not be present for several days after procedure and to notify the physician. The client should report any new abdominal pain to the physician.

SKILL 14.4 Assisting with Bronchoscopy

Bronchoscopy is the examination of the tracheobronchial tree through a lighted tube containing mirrors (Figure 14-3). The tube, or bronchoscope, most commonly used is a flexible fiberoptic bronchoscope that allows both visualization and simultaneous administration of oxygen. The fiberoptic bronchoscope has lumens for visualization and for obtaining sputum, foreign bodies, and biopsy specimens. Laser ablation of endotracheal (ET) lesions may be performed through the bronchoscope.

Bronchoscopy may be an emergency or scheduled procedure and is performed for both diagnostic and therapeutic reasons. The procedure is usually performed by a pulmonary specialist or surgeon and takes about 30 to 45 minutes. It may be done in a specially equipped room. This is an invasive procedure, and informed consent is required.

ASSESSMENT

1 Verify client's identity by using at least two forms of identifiers, neither of which may be the client's room number. Verify the type of procedure to be performed and procedure site with the client. *Rationale: Ensures accurate client identification and improves client safety. Client room number is not an acceptable identifier (JCAHO, 2003, 2006).*

2 Assess client's history for inability to tolerate interruption of high-flow oxygen, unless intubated. Report this to the physician. *Rationale: Determine need for oxygen administration during procedure.*

3 Assess client's knowledge of procedure to determine level of teaching required.

4 Assess level of anxiety, observing verbal and nonverbal cues.

5 Assess time of last ingested fluid or food. Clients should be NPO 8 hours before bronchoscopy. *Rationale: Excessive hydration causes dilution of contrast medium, making structures more difficult to visualize. NPO decreases chance of aspiration of stomach contents.*

6 Obtain vital signs. *Rationale: Provides baseline data for comparison with findings during and after procedure.*

7 Assess client's allergies. Determine if client previously received topical anesthetic.

8 Assess respiratory status: lung sounds, type of cough, and sputum produced. *Rationale: Provides baseline data for comparison with respiratory status during and after procedure.*

9 Assess need for preprocedure medication (usually atropine and narcotic or sedative). *Rationale: Atropine decreases secretions and inhibits vagally stimulated bradycardia; narcotics or sedatives relieve anxiety and decrease discomfort.*

PLANNING

Expected Outcomes focus on improving client's knowledge of the procedure, reducing anxiety regarding procedure and results, and detecting early detection of potential complications.

1 Client explains what to expect during the procedure before it is begun.

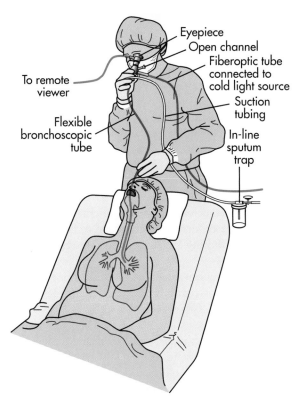

FIGURE 14-3 Flexible fiberoptic bronchoscopy.

2 Client has stable respiratory status without distress.
3 Client has vital signs within normal limits.
4 Client's level of comfort is 4 or less on a pain scale of 0 to 10.

5 Client does not experience complications, including severe shortness of breath resulting from laryngospasm or bronchospasm in response to irritation from bronchoscope or topical anesthetic.

Delegation Considerations

Assessment of the client's condition may not be delegated. Monitoring vital signs may be delegated. The nurse directs personnel by:
- Requesting personnel to report indications of allergic reactions, respiratory distress, or coughing up blood to the nurse immediately
- Instructing how to assist with client positioning

Equipment

- Bronchoscopy tray, which may include gauze sponges (4 × 4); local anesthetic spray (lidocaine); sterile tracheal suction catheters
- Flexible fiberoptic bronchoscope (see Figure 14-3)
- Diazepam, midazolam, or other sedative for IV sedation
- Oxygen, resuscitative equipment, pulse oximeter, cardiac monitor
- Sterile gloves
- Sterile water-soluble lubricating jelly (petroleum-based lubricants should not be used because of the hazard of aspiration and subsequent pneumonia)
- Masks, goggles, and gowns
- Emesis basin
- Tracheal suction equipment

IMPLEMENTATION *for Assisting with Bronchoscopy*

STEPS	RATIONALE
1 See Standard Protocol (inside front cover).	
2 Remove and safely store client's dentures and eyeglasses (if applicable).	
3 Establish IV access using large-bore cannula (see Chapter 27).	Provides access for delivery of IV fluids and/or drugs.
4 Assist client in maintaining position desired by physician, usually semi-Fowler's.	Provides maximal visualization of lower airways and adequate lung expansion.
5 Take "Time Out" to verify the client's name, type of procedure to be performed, and procedure site with the client.	"Time Out" verification just before starting the procedure includes the physician and all involved personnel and is a safety precaution to prevent wrong client, wrong site, and wrong procedure errors (JCAHO, 2003, 2006).

> **COMMUNICATION TIP** Tell the client that the anesthetic spray will make his or her mouth and throat feel numb after a few minutes. Assure client that oral secretions will be removed with suction. Inform the client that while the tube is in place the client will be unable to speak. Agree on hand signals for client to use to indicate the presence of discomfort.

6 Position tip of suction cannula for easy access in the client's mouth.	Drains oral secretions to reduce risk of aspiration.

STEPS	RATIONALE
7 Physician sprays nasopharynx and oropharynx with topical anesthetic. Lidocaine is commonly used for throat spraying, which is done 10 to 15 minutes before the procedure.	
8 Instruct client not to swallow local anesthetic; provide emesis basin.	Swallowed anesthetic may be absorbed systemically and cause CNS and cardiovascular reactions.
9 Physician applies goggles, mask, and sterile gloves and then introduces bronchoscope into mouth to pharynx. The scope is passed through the glottis and then into trachea and bronchi.	
10 Assist the client by giving explanations, verbal reassurance, and support.	Although premedicated and drowsy, clients need to be reminded not to change position and to cooperate.
11 Monitor ECG, pulse, and blood pressure for changes every 5 minutes during procedure.	Establishes monitoring for oversedation (see Skill 14-1).
12 Monitor client's respiratory status every 5 minutes during procedure: observe degree of restlessness and respiratory rate; observe capillary refill and color of nail beds; monitor pulse oximetry (oxygen saturation).	Bronchoscope may cause feelings of suffocation; also, because airway is partially occluded, client may become hypoxic during observations.
13 Note characteristics of suctioned material. A small amount of blood mixed with the aspirate is expected because of tissue trauma.	Information is used to record and report and to make further client observations.
14 Using gloved hand, wipe client's nose to remove lubricant after bronchoscope is removed.	Promotes hygiene and comfort.

> **NURSE ALERT** Do not allow client to eat or drink until the tracheobronchial anesthesia has worn off and gag reflex returns.

15 Instruct client not to try to swallow sputum until gag reflex returns. Provide emesis basis for expectoration of sputum. Assess for return of gag reflex. Gag reflex usually returns in approximately 2 hours.	Helps prevent aspiration pneumonia, which is a risk until gag reflex returns.
16 See Completion Protocol (inside front cover).	

EVALUATION

1 Ask client to explain understanding of the procedure before sedation.

2 Closely monitor client's respiratory status. Assess level of sedation and LOC. Monitor for return of gag reflex, which usually returns within 2 hours. Observe character and amount of sputum. Physician may order serial sputum collection for 24 hours for cytological examination.

3 Monitor vital signs and pulse oximetry.

4 Assess client's level of pain.

5 Monitor for sudden dyspnea indicating laryngospasm or bronchospasm.

Unexpected Outcomes and Related Interventions

1 Laryngospasm and bronchospasm indicated by sudden, severe shortness of breath.

a. Call physician immediately.

b. Prepare emergency resuscitation equipment.

c. Anticipate possible cricothyrotomy.

2 Presence of hypoxemia indicated by gradual shortness of breath and decreasing LOC

a. Maintain airway.

b. Notify physician immediately.

c. Monitor oxygen saturation.

3 Vasovagal response during bronchoscope insertion. Vasovagal response is caused by stimulation of the baroreceptors, causing bradycardia. Symptoms include feeling faint, dizzy, and light-headed and being diaphoretic with a slow, steady pulse. Client may become unconscious for a few seconds.

a. Lower head of table.

b. Support airway.

4 Hemorrhage.

a. Call physician immediately.

b. Emergency resuscitation equipment must be readily available.

c. Follow specific postprocedure orders related to findings.

Recording and Reporting

- Record in nurses' notes name of procedure (include biopsy if performed), duration of procedure, client's tolerance of procedure and complications, and collection and disposition of specimen. Document time gag reflex returns. Include client's response to procedure and level of anxiety.

- Report excessive bleeding or respiratory difficulty after procedure or changes in vital signs beyond client's normal limits to physician immediately.

Sample Documentation

0900 To bronchoscopy via stretcher.

1030 Returned from bronchoscopy. Alert and oriented. Vital signs stable. Oxygen saturation 88%. Resting in semi-Fowler's position. Denies dyspnea. Color pale. Respirations 28; rhonchi noted bilaterally at bases, clears some with cough. Occasional cough noted productive of small amount bright red sputum. No gag reflex present.

1130 Vital signs stable and recorded every 15 min ×4. No change in assessment.

1230 Vital signs stable. Gag reflex present. Taking sips of clear liquids.

Special Considerations

Pediatric Considerations

- In children the procedure is most frequently performed to remove foreign bodies from larynx or trachea and may be done under general anesthesia. Client is placed in the lateral position after the procedure to prevent aspiration.

- Children are at higher risk of hypoxemia than adults because of their smaller bronchus and the bronchoscope decreasing the available breathing space (Pagana and Pagana, 2005).

Geriatric Considerations

- Postprocedure restlessness in the older adult client could indicate either hypoxemia or pain. Thoroughly assess oxygenation status before administration of a narcotic analgesic, which could further deplete the body's oxygen supply.

- Physical exposure and room temperature may contribute to hypothermia in frail older adults, who may not be able to communicate that they are cold. Use heated blankets or forced air heat to maintain core temperature at comfortable, safe levels (Negishi and others, 2003).

- Postprocedure restlessness could indicate hypoxemia, not pain.

- Because of multiple medications the older adult client may be taking, be aware of alterations in administration schedules necessary as a result of the NPO status for the diagnostic test.

Home Care Considerations

- Instruct client to notify the physician if the following symptoms develop: fever, chest pain, dyspnea, wheezing, or hemoptysis.

- Throat discomfort is normal after this procedure. Warm saline gargles or throat lozenges may be helpful.

SKILL 14.5 Assisting with Gastrointestinal Endoscopy

Endoscopy is any study that allows direct visualization of an internal organ or structure by means of a long, flexible fiberoptic scope with a light source attached (Figures 14-4 and 14-5). For visualization of the upper gastrointestinal (GI) tract, esophagoscopy, gastroscopy, gastroduodenojejunoscopy, or duodenoscopy is performed; or more frequently, EGD, which permits visualization of the esophagus, stomach, and duodenum in one examination. Endoscopy enables biopsy of suspicious tissue, polyp removal, and performance of many other procedures, such as direct visual guidance for fine-needle aspiration biopsies and dilation and stenting of strictures. For visualization of the hepatobiliary tree and pancreatic ducts, an endoscopic retrograde cholangiopancreatography (ERCP) is performed. For visual examination of the lower GI tract, a proctoscopy, sigmoidoscopy, or colonoscopy may be performed. Typically, these clients receive IV moderate sedation.

Risks of endoscopic procedures include intestinal perforation, hemorrhage, peritonitis, aspiration, respiratory depression, and myocardial infarction (MI) secondary to vasovagal response. Both upper and lower GI endoscopic examinations are performed in a specially equipped endoscopic unit.

ASSESSMENT

1 Verify client's identity by using at least two forms of identifiers, neither of which may be the client's room

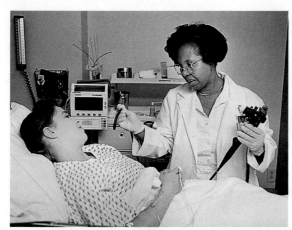

FIGURE 14-4 Physician preparing for endoscopy.

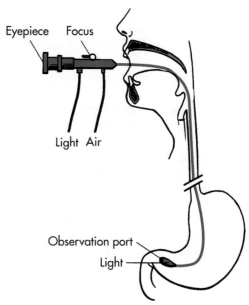

Eyepiece   Focus

Light Air

Observation port

Light

FIGURE 14-5 Flexible endoscope to visualize stomach.

number. Verify the type of procedure to be performed and procedure site with the client. *Rationale: Ensures accurate client identification and improves client safety. Client room number is not an acceptable identifier (JCAHO, 2003, 2006).*

2 Verify that informed consent has been obtained.

3 Assess client's knowledge of the procedure and explain the steps of the procedure. *Rationale: Determines level of teaching required. Answering client questions helps to relieve anxiety.*

4 Observe anxiety level, including verbal and nonverbal behaviors.

5 Determine if signs of GI bleeding are present by observing the character of emesis, stool, and nasogastric (NG) tube drainage for frank blood or black material that looks like coffee grounds. *Rationale: Test is contraindicated in clients with severe upper GI bleeding because viewing lens may get covered with blood clots, preventing visualization (Pagana and Pagana, 2005).*

6 Measure and record baseline vital signs.

7 Verify that client has been NPO for at least 8 hours for upper GI. *Rationale: Promotes adequate visualization; helps prevent aspiration if introduction of the endoscope through the oropharynx stimulates the gag reflex and causes vomiting.*

8 For lower GI studies (proctoscopy, sigmoidoscopy, or colonoscopy), verify that the client has followed a clear liquid diet for 2 days and has completed any ordered bowel cleansing regimen. *Rationale: An empty intestinal tract is necessary to allow the endoscope insertion and good visualization of the interior walls.*

9 Assess client's ability to understand and follow directions. *Rationale: Procedures require client to follow directions closely and assume proper position.*

PLANNING

Expected Outcomes focus on preventing complications, client's ability to follow instructions, and protection of client's airway.

1 Client does not aspirate and has no postprocedure bleeding.

2 Client's level of comfort is equivalent to 4 or less on a pain scale of 0 to 10.

3 Client is without respiratory complications or change in LOC.

Delegation Considerations

The skill of assisting with endoscopy may not be delegated. The nurse directs personnel by:

• Instructing how to assist with client positioning

Equipment

• Endoscopy tray
• Fiberoptic endoscope and camera
• Solutions for biopsy specimens
• Local anesthetic spray
• Tracheal suction equipment
• Blood pressure equipment
• Sterile water-soluble jelly
• Sterile gloves for physician
• Emesis basin
• IV fluid and equipment for IV start (optional)
• Diazepam, midazolam, or other sedative for IV sedation (optional)
• Carbon dioxide source (for lower GI procedures)
• Oxygen, resuscitative equipment, and pulse oximeter
• Protective equipment: mask, gown, gloves, goggles

IMPLEMENTATION *for Assisting with Gastrointestinal Endoscopy*

STEPS	RATIONALE
1 See Standard Protocol (inside front cover).	
2 Administer pain medication or preprocedure medication.	Promotes relaxation and reduces anxiety.
3 ✋ Remove client's dentures and dental appliances.	Prevents dislodgement of dental structures during intubation phase.
4 Take "Time Out" to verify the client's name, type of procedure to be performed, and procedure site with the client.	"Time Out" verification just before starting the procedure includes the physician and all involved personnel and is a safety precaution to prevent wrong client, wrong site, and wrong procedure errors (JCAHO, 2003, 2006).

> **COMMUNICATION TIP** Inform the client that while the tube is in place the client will be unable to speak. Agree on hand signals for client to use to indicate the presence of discomfort.

STEPS	RATIONALE
5 Monitor IV fluids, and administer IV moderate sedation as ordered (see Skill 14.1).	
6 Promote comfort, and keep client informed of what is happening, using a calm and reassuring voice.	Helps to minimize client's anxiety.
7 ✋ Assist physician to spray nasopharynx and oropharynx with local anesthetic (usually Xylocaine).	
8 For upper GI procedures, assist client in maintaining left lateral Sims' position. For lower GI procedures, assist client in maintaining left lateral decubitus position. Drape client for privacy and comfort.	Sims' position allows easy passage of upper or lower endoscope. Provides for airway clearance if client gags and vomits gastric contents. Left lateral decubitus position provides access to lower GI tract.
9 Verify IV line is patent.	Provides route for emergency medications.
10 Administer atropine, if ordered (upper GI studies).	Atropine reduces the quantity of secretions, therefore reducing risk of aspiration for upper GI endoscopic procedures.
11 Position tip of suction cannula for easy access in the client's mouth (upper GI studies).	Drains oral secretions to reduce risk of aspiration.
12 Assist client through procedure.	
a. Anticipate needs and promote comfort.	Client is unable to speak after tube is passed into throat.
b. Tell client what is happening as each portion of the procedure is carried out.	Reassures client about procedure and how long it will last.
13 For upper GI studies, physician slowly passes the endoscope into mouth, esophagus, stomach, or duodenum and advances to desired depth while visualizing the walls. For lower GI studies, a lubricant-coated flexible fiberoptic endoscope is inserted through the anus and slowly advanced through the rectum and colon, while the walls are visualized.	Provides visualization of structures.

> **NURSE ALERT** If client is actively bleeding, physician may order that the stomach be lavaged and aspirated clear of clots before procedure is attempted.

STEPS	RATIONALE
14 Physician insufflates air through endoscope into upper GI tract. For colonoscopies, carbon dioxide is used. Physician examines, photographs, or performs biopsy of structures. Physician slowly removes the endoscope.	Distends GI structures for better visualization. Carbon dioxide insufflation produces less postprocedure abdominal cramping than air insufflation (Chernecky and Berger, 2004).
15 Place tissue specimens in proper laboratory containers. Provide slides and containers for specimens and fix or seal as needed.	Ensures proper labeling and preparation of specimens for microscopic examination.

STEPS	RATIONALE
16 Assist client to comfortable position.	Promotes rest and relaxation.
17 Suction airway if client begins to vomit or accumulate saliva. Remove and discard gloves.	Prevents aspiration of gastric contents or oral secretions.
18 Inform not to eat or drink until after gag reflex returns.	Absence of gag reflex increases risk of aspiration.
19 See Completion Protocol (inside front cover).	

EVALUATION

1 Monitor vital signs for signs of bleeding (tachycardia and hypotension). May be as often as every 15 minutes for 2 hours. Evaluate emesis or aspirate for frank or occult blood

2 Assess level of sedation (see Skill 14.1).

3 Ask client to describe discomfort using a 0 to 10 pain scale.

4 Evaluate any emesis or aspirate for frank or occult blood.

5 If local anesthetic was used to numb the throat, observe for return of gag reflex, usually within 2 to 4 hours. Assess breath sounds, labor of respirations, and oxygen saturation.

6 Ask client to describe purpose and basic steps of the procedure before it begins.

Unexpected Outcomes and Related Interventions

1 For upper GI procedures: Laryngospasm and bronchospasm, as evidenced by sudden, severe shortness of breath.

a. Notify physician immediately. This can be life threatening.

b. Prepare emergency resuscitation equipment.

c. Anticipate possible cricothyrotomy.

2 For upper GI procedures: Hypoxemia caused by aspiration, as evidenced by gradually increasing shortness of breath and decreasing LOC.

a. Support airway.

b. Notify physician immediately.

c. Monitor oxygen saturation.

3 Hemorrhage, as evidenced by hypotension and tachycardia, as well as decreasing LOC with or without visible signs of hemorrhage.

a. Notify physician immediately. This can be life threatening.

b. Follow specific postprocedure orders related to findings.

4 Sharp intense pain in chest, stomach, or abdomen and cool, pale skin.

a. Notify physician immediately. These can be signs of GI perforation.

5 Vasovagal response caused by stimulation of the baroreceptors during bronchoscope insertion, as evidenced by feeling faint, dizzy, and light-headed; diaphoresis with a slow, steady pulse; and/or a few seconds of unconsciousness.

a. Lower head of table.

b. Support airway.

Reporting and Recording

- Record in nurses' notes the procedure, duration, client's tolerance, complications and interventions, and collection and disposition of specimen.

- Report to nurse in charge the duration of procedure, client's tolerance, and changes in vital signs or condition. Report onset of any bleeding, abdominal pain, dyspnea, and vital sign changes to physician.

Sample Documentation

0800 NPO since midnight. Transported to endoscopy department via wheelchair for EGD. Vital signs within normal limits. Consent signed. Reports that physician explained procedure, and he has no questions at present.

1000 Returned from endoscopy. Reports no discomfort. Vital signs at baseline level. No apparent bleeding. Gag reflex present.

Special Considerations
Pediatric Considerations

- Children require deep sedation or general anesthesia (American Academy of Pediatrics, 2002).

- Introduction of the endoscope in infants and small children who have a narrow and collapsible airway may result in respiratory distress.

Geriatric Considerations

- Client is at risk for prolonged sedation because of age-related decreased glomerular filtration rate and decreased hepatic function. Monitor urine output closely.

- Client may have age-related thinning of the gastric mucosa, which increases the incidence of irritation and ulceration (Phipps and others, 2003).

- Physical exposure and room temperature may contribute to hypothermia in frail older adults, who may not be able to communicate that they are cold. Use heated blankets or forced air heat to maintain core temperature at comfortable, safe levels (Negishi and others, 2003).
- Because of multiple medications the older adult client may be taking, be aware of alterations in administration schedules necessary as a result of the NPO status for the diagnostic test.
- The older adult may experience dehydration, electrolyte imbalance, and exhaustion from test preparation combined with NPO status. If the procedure is done on an ambulatory care basis, it may be helpful to have someone stay with the client.

Home Care Considerations

- Ambulatory care clients should be instructed to notify the physician if the following symptoms develop: fever, chest pain or discomfort, dyspnea, wheezing, or hemoptysis.
- Throat discomfort may be managed with throat lozenges.
- After colonoscopy a warm tub bath may be soothing to minimize rectal discomfort.
- Inform client who received sedation not to drive for at least 24 hours after the procedure.

SKILL 14.6 Assisting with Electrocardiogram

An ECG is a graphical representation of the heart's electrical activities, or conduction system. The electrical impulse for each heartbeat originates within the sinoatrial (SA) node, the "pacemaker" of the heart. The SA node is in the right atrium. The rate of impulses initiated at the SA node for an adult at rest is about 75 beats per minute. The electrical impulses are then transmitted through the atria to the atrioventricular (AV) node. The AV node assists with atrial emptying by delaying the impulse before transmitting it through the bundle of His and the ventricular Purkinje network of the ventricles.

The electrical activity of the conduction system is recorded on an ECG. An ECG may be done to determine baseline cardiac function (e.g., preoperative, prediagnostic testing), to help evaluate response to cardiac medications, to help monitor recovery after a MI, or when the client experiences chest discomfort (Chernecky and Berger, 2004). An ECG monitors the regularity and path of the electrical impulse through the conduction system; however, it does not reflect muscular work of the heart. The normal sequence on the ECG is called normal sinus rhythm (NSR), which contains PQRST waves (Figure 14-6). The PR interval represents atrial depolarization during which the atria empty their blood supply into the ventricles. The QRS interval represents ventricular depolarization, during which ventricular contraction occurs. The remainder of the waveform through the end of the T-wave signifies ventricular repolarization. Disturbances in conduction may result when impulses cannot travel through the normal pathways. These rhythm disturbances are called arrhythmias, meaning a deviation from the normal sinus heart rhythm (Table 14-2). Arrhythmias may occur as a response to ischemia, valvular abnormality, anxiety, drug toxicity, or acid-base or electrolyte imbalance. Some common arrhythmias include tachycardia (greater than 100 beats per minute), bradycardia (less than 60 beats per minute), premature ventricular contractions (PVCs) (early beat), or heart block (delayed or absent beat).

A Holter monitor is a small, portable device that records electrical activity of the heart for as long as 24 hours. This

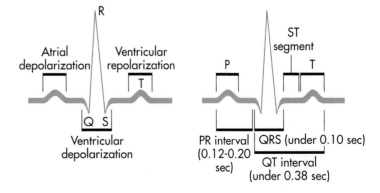

FIGURE 14-6 Normal ECG waves and intervals. (From Pagana KD, Pagana TJ: *Mosby's manual of diagnostic and laboratory tests,* ed 2, St Louis, 2002, Mosby.)

TABLE 14-2 Common Basic Cardiac Dysrhythmias

RHYTHM CHARACTERISTICS	APPEARANCE	CLINICAL SIGNIFICANCE
Sinus tachycardia: Regular rhythm; rate 100-180 beats per minute; normal PQRS complex	(From Wellens HJJ, Conover MB: *The ECG in emergency decision making*, ed 2, Philadelphia, 2006, Saunders.)	Normal response to exercise, emotion, pain, fever, hyperthyroidism, and certain drugs.
Sinus bradycardia: Regular rhythm; rate less than 60 beats per minute; normal P, PR interval; normal QRS complex	(From Potter PA, Perry AG: *Basic nursing: a critical thinking approach*, ed 4, St Louis, 1999, Mosby.)	May be associated with decreased cardiac output, dizziness, syncope, and chest pain.
Premature ventricular contractions (PVCs): Irregular rhythm followed by compensatory pause	(From Potter PA, Perry AG: *Basic nursing: a critical thinking approach*, ed 4, St Louis, 1999, Mosby.)	Caused by irritable focus. If more than six per minute or in pairs, indicates increased ventricular irritability.
Ventricular tachycardia: Rhythm slightly irregular; rate 100-200 beats per minute; P wave absent; PR interval absent; QRS complex wide and bizarre	(From Wellens HJJ, Conover MB: *The ECG in emergency decision making*, ed 2, Philadelphia, 2006, Saunders.)	Often a forerunner of ventricular fibrillation; may cause decreased cardiac output because of decreased ventricular filling time.

makes it possible to monitor the cardiac rhythm for ambulatory clients during activity, rest, and sleep. Clients keep a diary of activity, noting when they experience rapid heartbeats or periods of dizziness. Correlation between activities and abnormal electrical activity can then be determined.

ASSESSMENT

1 Verify client's identity by using at least two forms of identifiers, neither of which may be the client's room number. Verify the type of procedure to be performed and procedure site with the client. *Rationale: Ensures accurate client identification and improves client safety. Client room number is not an acceptable identifier (JCAHO, 2003, 2006).*

2 Determine rationale for obtaining ECG. *Rationale: If the ECG is being done for active chest pain, it should be performed immediately.*

3 Assess client's knowledge of the procedure. *Rationale: Determines level of teaching required.*

4 Assess client's ability to follow directions closely and remain still in a supine position. *Rationale: Provides clear, accurate recording without artifacts.*

PLANNING

Expected Outcomes focus on client's ability to lie still during the procedure and on obtaining an accurate ECG.

1 Client explains purpose and basic steps of the procedure before it begins.

2 Client lays supine and remains still throughout the procedure.

3 A clear recording of the ECG waveform is obtained.

Delegation Considerations
The skill of assisting with the ECG may be delegated to AP.

Equipment
- 12-lead ECG machine
- Electrode gel (optional)
- ECG leads or electrodes (self-stick adhesive)
- Alcohol wipes
- Scissors

IMPLEMENTATION *for Assisting with Electrocardiogram*

STEPS	RATIONALE
1 See Standard Protocol (inside front cover).	
2 Expose client's chest and arms, and cleanse and prepare skin using alcohol wipes.	Alcohol removes oil and fat from the skin and minimizes artifact caused by inadequate contact with the skin (Chernecky and Berger, 2004).
3 If large amounts of hair are present, it may be necessary to clip hair at the placement sites.	Promotes adherence of leads (electrodes) to chest or extremity.
4 Apply self-sticking electrodes, or apply electrode paste and attach leads. For 12-lead ECG (see illustration):	Position of leads promotes proper display of ECG on paper.
a. Chest (precordial leads)	
V_1—Fourth intercostal space (ICS) at right sternal border	
V_2—Fourth ICS at left sternal border	
V_3—Midway between V_2 and V_4	
V_4—Fifth ICS at midclavicular line	
V_5—Left anterior axillary line at level of V_4 horizontally	
V_6—Left midaxillary line at level of V_4 horizontally	
b. Extremities: one on lower portion of each extremity	
aV_r—Right wrist	
aV_l—Left wrist	
aV_f—Left ankle	
5 Turn on machine, enter in any required demographical information, and obtain tracing; 12-lead ECG may be obtained without removing precordial leads.	Transfers electrocardiac conduction on ECG tracing paper for subsequent analysis by cardiologist.

COMMUNICATION TIP Tell client to lie quietly until a reading is obtained.

STEPS	RATIONALE
6 Disconnect leads and wipe excess electrode paste from chest.	Promotes comfort and hygiene.
7 See Completion Protocol (inside front cover).	

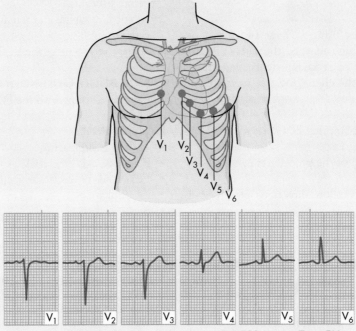

STEP 4 Placement of ECG leads and corresponding ECG waves. (From Phipps WJ and others: *Medical-surgical nursing: health and illness perspectives*, ed 7, St Louis, 2003, Mosby.)

EVALUATION

1 Ask client to explain the procedure.
2 Examine ECG report for artifact.

Unexpected Outcomes and Related Interventions

1 Uninterpretable ECG as evidenced by absence of tracing in one or more leads or the presence of artifact in the ECG tracings.
a. Inspect electrodes for secure placement.
b. Reposition any wires that are moving as a result of client breathing or movement, or vibrations in the environment.
c. Remind client who is moving that lying still is necessary to obtain a good tracing.
d. Manually hold any extremities, if needed.
e. If artifact looks like 60-cycle interference (looks like a very thick-lined waveform), unplug battery-operated equipment in the room, one item at a time, to see if the interference disappears. NOTE: 60-cycle interference is rare.
f. Repeat the tracing.
2 Client experiences chest pain.
a. Continue to monitor.
b. Follow specific postprocedure orders related to findings.

c. Reassess factors contributing to anxiety.
d. Notify physician.

Recording and Reporting

• Record in nurses' notes when ECG was obtained (date and time), where tracing was sent, rationale for obtaining ECG (e.g., pain, discomfort, preoperatively, postoperatively), and baseline vital signs. Include a rhythm strip in the client's chart according to agency policy.
• Report any unexpected outcomes immediately.

Sample Documentation

1030 C/O chest pain at level 4 (0 to 10 scale) for 30 minutes with "heaviness" and "aching" in epigastric region. Pain radiates to L shoulder blade. Very restless. Reports some short episodes of more severe pain at level 7 or 8 (0 to 10 scale) lasting 30 to 60 seconds and somewhat relieved by position changes. BP 160/90, P 110, R 20, O_2 saturation 98%. ECG done; sinus tachycardia noted. (See rhythm strip.) Physician notified.

Special Considerations
Geriatric Considerations

- Many factors can contribute to arrhythmias, including medications such as digitalis and quinidine, hypertrophy of cardiac muscle, alcohol, thyroid dysfunction, coffee, tea, tobacco, electrolyte imbalances, edema, acid-base imbalances, and myocardial ischemia.

- Clients with arrhythmias are at risk for cardiac arrest. The nurse needs to be familiar with crash cart location and be prepared with knowledge of emergency equipment, medications, and cardiopulmonary resuscitation (CPR) skills.

NCLEX® Style Questions

1 You are assessing your client after a cardiac catheterization. What assessments indicate possible internal bleeding?
1. Catheter site pain and loss of distal pulses
2. Anxiety, backache, and heart rate increase from 90 to 105
3. Atrial fibrillation and drowsiness
4. Fever and bradycardia

2 When reviewing your client's history and lab results before preparing him for an IVP, which finding would cause rescheduling of the procedure?
1. Sodium level of 133 mg/dl and potassium level of 3.4 mmol/L
2. Last meal 12 hours ago
3. Age over 85 years
4 History of diabetes; last metformin dose taken yesterday

3 Your pediatric client with leukemia is scheduled for a bone marrow aspiration. What nursing intervention is not appropriate?
1. Apply topical anesthetic to the bone marrow aspiration site 10 minutes before the procedure is scheduled to begin.

2. Verify that parental informed consent has been obtained.
3. Use a doll to demonstrate for the child the steps of the procedure.
4. Check emergency equipment for pediatric sizes.

4 Place the following steps of bronchoscopy preprocedure care in the proper order.
1. Perform the preprocedure "Time Out."
2. Administer IV moderate sedation.
3. Verify that informed consent has been obtained.
4. Position the client on the bronchoscopy table.

5 Your client is unresponsive and febrile, and acute meningitis is suspected. An emergent LP is being done without the normal step of taking a CT first to rule out IICP. Appropriate delegation of care to AP includes:
1. Instructing the nursing assistant to stay with you, the nurse, during the procedure to help maintain the client's side-lying position.
2. Assisting the physician during the procedure and notifying you if the client's vital signs deteriorate.
3. Monitoring the client's airway during the procedure and administering oxygen as needed.
4. Preparing the site and setting up the sterile tray.

References for all chapters appear in Appendix D.

15

Preparation for Medication Administration

Safe and accurate medication administration is one of a nurse's most important responsibilities. As a nurse, you are responsible for having a full understanding of medication therapy and the related nursing implications. The nursing process is a useful framework for administering medications. Assessment and planning involve identifying factors that influence the way you administer medications and provide clients instruction on self-administration. Nursing diagnoses communicate problems related to drug therapy and direct interventions for appropriate nursing care. Implementation includes administering drugs correctly and safely and in many cases teaching clients how to self-administer drugs. Evaluation involves monitoring clients' responses to medications and measuring learning. This chapter includes basic information for preparing to administer medications. Subsequent chapters address administration of nonparenteral medications and injections.

DRUG EFFECTS

When administering medications, know the mechanism of action, the therapeutic effects of the drugs, the purpose for the specific client, and the desired effect. It is also important for you to know possible side effects and adverse reactions.

Mechanism of Action

When giving a drug to a client, you can expect a predictable chemical reaction that changes the physiological activity of the body. This most commonly occurs as the medication bonds chemically at a specific site in the body called a receptor site. The reactions are possible only when the receptor site and the chemical fit together like a key in a lock. When the chemical fits well, the chemical response is good. These drugs are called agonists (Skidmore-Roth, 2006). Some drugs attach at the receptor site but do not produce a new chemical reaction. These drugs are called antagonists. Other drugs attach and produce only a small response or prevent other reactions from occurring. These drugs are called partial agonists.

DRUG ACTIONS

Pharmacokinetics is the study of how drugs enter the body (absorption), reach the site of action (distribution), are metabolized, and are excreted from the body. Absorption describes how a drug enters the body and passes into body fluids and tissues. Absorption influences the route of drug administration. Distribution is the way drugs move to the sites of action in the body. Metabolism refers to the chemical reactions by which a medication is broken down (e.g., in the liver) until it becomes chemically inactive. Excretion is the process of drug elimination from the body through the gastrointestinal (GI) tract, kidneys, or other body secretions (Skidmore-Roth, 2006).

Understanding pharmacokinetics enables you to make the decisions necessary to ensure drugs are given by the appropriate route and to then recognize and act based upon the nature and extent of drug actions, interactions, and adverse actions. In addition, this knowledge helps in planning drug administration schedules. For example, knowing when an analgesic's peak action occurs allows you to administer the drug at a time when you anticipate the client's pain will increase (e.g., during exercise). Most agencies have standard administration schedules (see Appendix B, Abbreviations and Equivalents). Most schedules allow you to administer a drug, for example, one half hour before or after the scheduled time without concern for altering the effectiveness of the medication. Some medications are ordered for administration as needed (prn) within certain parameters prescribed by the physician.

Pharmacokinetics affects how much of a drug dose reaches the site of action. These processes are influenced by factors such as body surface area, body water content, body fat content, and body protein stores. When certain medications, such as antibiotics, are prescribed, the goal is to achieve a constant drug blood level within a safe therapeutic range. The client and nurse must follow regular dosage schedules and administer prescribed doses at correct intervals. Knowledge of the following time intervals of drug action helps you to anticipate a drug's effect:

1 Onset of action: The time interval between when a drug is given and the first sign of its effect.
2 Peak action: The time it takes for a drug to reach its highest effective concentration.
3 Duration of action: The time period from onset of drug action to the time when a response is no longer seen.
4 Plateau: Blood serum concentration reached and maintained after repeated, fixed doses.
5 Therapeutic range: The range of plasma concentration that produces the desired drug effect without toxicity.

The therapeutic levels of drugs, such as antibiotics, are monitored by laboratory blood tests. Test results allow physicians to modify drug dosages to achieve a constant desired blood level. A blood sample is drawn to identify the peak serum level of a drug, which varies according to the specific drug involved. The lowest serum level is known as the trough level. Blood samples for trough levels are usually drawn just before the next scheduled dose of medication. You will coordinate blood sampling with the laboratory to obtain the most accurate peak and trough levels.

Therapeutic Effects

A therapeutic effect is the intended or desired physiological response of a medication. A single medication may have many therapeutic effects. For example, aspirin creates analgesia, reduces inflammation and fever, and slows blood clotting. Other drugs have more specific therapeutic effects. For example, an antihypertensive medication lowers blood pressure.

Side Effects and Adverse Reactions

Medication can react in the body to produce unpredictable and unexplainable responses. A side effect is a predictable and unavoidable secondary effect produced at a usual therapeutic dose. Some side effects may be harmless, whereas others cause injury. A common side effect of codeine phosphate is constipation, which can be managed with a change in diet and fluid intake. If the side effects are serious enough to outweigh the beneficial effects of a drug's therapeutic action, the prescriber may discontinue the drug. Clients often stop taking medications because of side effects such as anorexia, drowsiness, dry mouth, or diarrhea. Report any side effects to a physician or pharmacist so that they are not interpreted as more serious adverse reactions.

Adverse Reactions

Adverse reactions are unintended, undesirable, and often unpredictable drug effects. Some reactions occur immediately, whereas others develop more slowly over time. An example of an adverse reaction is a client becoming comatose after taking a drug. When adverse responses to medications occur, the prescriber discontinues the medication immediately. Adverse reactions can range from mild to toxic effects. Prompt recognition and reporting of adverse reactions can prevent serious injury to clients.

Toxic Effects. Toxic medication effects develop after prolonged intake of high doses of medication, ingestion of drugs intended for external application, or when a drug builds up in the blood because of impaired metabolism or excretion. Toxic effects may be lethal, depending on a drug's action. For example, morphine, an opioid analgesic, relieves pain by depressing the central nervous system (CNS). However, toxic levels of morphine cause severe respiratory depression and death.

Idiosyncratic Reactions. Medications may cause unpredictable effects, such as an idiosyncratic reaction. In this case a client overreacts or underreacts to a drug. Predicting which clients will have an idiosyncratic response is impossible. For example, lorazepam (Ativan), an antianxiety medication, when given to an older adult may worsen anxiety and cause agitation and delirium.

Allergic Reactions. Allergic reactions are also unpredictable responses to medications. Taking a medication the first time may cause an immunological response. The drug acts as an antigen, which causes the production of antibodies. With repeated administration, the client develops an allergic re-

TABLE 15-1 Common Allergic Reactions	
SYMPTOM	DESCRIPTION
Angioedema	An acute, painless, dermal, subcutaneous, or submucosal swelling involving the face, neck, lips, larynx, hands, feet, or genitalia.
Eczema (rash)	Small, raised vesicles that are usually reddened; often distributed over the entire body.
Pruritus	Itching of the skin; accompanies most rashes.
Rhinitis	Inflammation of mucous membranes lining the nose, causing swelling and a clear watery discharge.
Urticaria (hives)	Raised, irregularly shaped skin eruptions with varying sizes and shapes; eruptions have reddened margins and pale centers.
Wheezing	Constriction of smooth muscles surrounding bronchioles that decreases diameter of airways; occurs primarily on inspiration because of severely narrowed airways; development of edema in pharynx and larynx further obstructs airflow.

sponse to the drug, its chemical preservatives, or a metabolite of it.

The antibodies act to create a mild or severe reaction. Allergic symptoms vary, depending on the client and the drug. Among the different classes of drugs, antibiotics cause a high incidence of allergic reactions. Table 15-1 summarizes common allergy symptoms. Severe, or anaphylactic, reactions are characterized by sudden constriction of bronchiolar muscles, edema of the pharynx and larynx, and severe wheezing and shortness of breath. The client may become severely hypotensive, necessitating emergency resuscitation measures.

It is common practice for hospitalized clients with known drug allergies to have their allergy information recorded in a clearly identifiable place. This allows all caregivers to be aware of the client's allergies. In many institutions this information is recorded on the front of the client's medical record on an eye-catching sticker. Clients also wear a wristband that contains the name of the medications to which the client is allergic. Client allergies must be recorded on the client's medication administration record (MAR). Clients cared for in other settings (e.g., home) and who have a known history of an allergy to a medication should wear an identification bracelet or medal that alerts all health care providers to the allergy in case the client is unconscious when receiving medical care.

Medication Interactions

When one medication modifies the action of another, a medication interaction occurs. A medication can enhance or reduce the action of other medications and alter the way in which the body absorbs, metabolizes, or eliminates the drug. When two drugs have a synergistic effect, the effect of the two medications combined is greater than the effect of one drug given separately. Alcohol is a CNS depressant that has a synergistic effect with antihistamines, antidepressants, and opioid analgesics.

A drug interaction may be desirable. Often a physician orders combination drug therapy to create a drug interaction for therapeutic benefit. For example, a client with moderate hypertension may receive several drugs, such as diuretics and vasodilators, which act together to keep blood pressure at a desirable level.

Drug Tolerance and Dependence

Drug tolerance occurs over time. A client receives the same drug for long periods of time and then requires higher doses to produce the same desired effect. Clients taking various pain medications may develop tolerance over time. It may take a month or even longer for tolerance to occur (McCaffery and Robinson, 2002).

Drug tolerance is not the same as drug dependence. Two types of drug dependence exist: psychological (or addiction) and physical. In psychological dependence the client desires the medication for a benefit other than the intended effect. Physical dependence implies that a client will suffer some ill effect if the medication is not given. When clients receive medications for a short term, such as for postoperative pain, dependence is rare (McCaffery and Robinson, 2002).

Nontherapeutic Medication Use

Misuse includes overuse, underuse, erratic use, and contraindicated use of medications. Clients of all ages misuse medications. Older adults are at greatest risk. Some people use medications for purposes other than their intended effect because of peer pressure, curiosity, or the pursuit of pleasure. Problems are not limited to illegal street drugs. The incidence of prescription and over-the-counter (OTC) drug misuse and abuse is also on the rise. The most commonly abused prescriptions medications include opioids, stimulants, tranquilizers, and sedatives.

You are ethically and legally responsible to understand the problems of persons using medications improperly. When caring for clients with suspected medication abuse or dependence, be aware of your values and attitudes about the willful use of harmful substances. Do not let your personal values interfere with understanding the client's needs and concerns.

ADMINISTERING MEDICATIONS

You are not solely responsible for medication administration. The prescriber (e.g., physician or advanced practice nurse [APN]) also help to ensure the right medication gets to the right client. You are accountable for knowing what medications are ordered, understanding their therapeutic effects, and recognizing undesired effects.

Medication Orders

A physician's order is required for all medications to be administered by a nurse (except in states where Nurse Practice Acts allow APNs and nurse practitioners [NPs] to prescribe). A physician's order sheet is a written or electronic form on which the physician writes the date, time, and drug order, including:

1 The name of the drug, which may be either the trade name (e.g., Percocet) or the generic name (e.g., oxycodone)
2 The dose (e.g., 5 mg)
3 The route (e.g., by mouth [PO])
4 The frequency (e.g., every 4 hours [q4h])
5 Orders for drugs to be given prn also include the reason they are to be given (e.g., for pain)
6 The signature of the prescriber

Verbal and telephone orders are optional forms of orders when written or electronic communication between the prescriber and nurse is not possible. When you receive a verbal or telephone order you enter the order on the physician's order sheet (Figure 15-1). The name of the prescriber and your signature are included. The prescriber will countersign the order at a later time, usually within 24 hours after making the order (see agency policy). Box 15-1 provides guidelines for safely taking verbal or telephone orders for medications.

There are five common types of medication orders. The type of order is based on the frequency and/or urgency of medication administration. Types of medication orders include standing orders; prn orders; and single (one-time) orders, which also include stat orders and now orders.

You carry out a standing order until the physician cancels it by another order or until a prescribed number of days elapse. A standing order sometimes indicates a final date or number of doses. Many institutions have a policy for automatically discontinuing standard orders.

The physician sometimes orders a medication to be given only when a client requires or requests it. This is a prn order. You must assess a client thoroughly to determine whether the client needs the medication. Sometimes a different type of therapy is more appropriate. A prn order usually has minimum intervals set for the time of administration. This means you cannot give the drug any more frequently than what is prescribed.

Single (one-time) orders are common for preoperative medications or medications given before diagnostic examinations. A physician will order the medication to be given only once at a specified time. A stat order means that you give a single dose of a medication immediately and only once. Physicians usually write stat orders for emergencies when the client's condition changes suddenly. A now order is more specific than a one-time order. It is used when a client needs a medication quickly but not as soon as a stat order. When you receive a now order, you have as long as 90 minutes to give the drug. Nursing students cannot take medication orders.

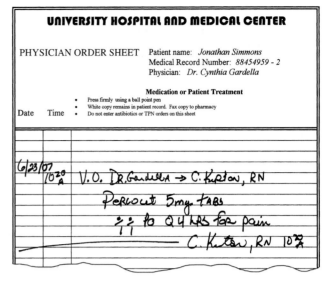

FIGURE 15-1 Example of a verbal physician's order.

BOX 15-1 Guidelines for Telephone Orders and Verbal Orders

- Clearly identify client's name, room number, and diagnosis. Read back all orders to physician or health care provider (JCAHO, 2005).
- Use clarification questions to avoid misunderstandings.
- Write "TO" (telephone order) or "VO" (verbal order), including date and time, name of client, and complete order; sign the name of the physician or health care provider and nurse.
- Follow agency policies; some institutions require documentation of the "read-back" or require two nurses to review and sign telephone or verbal orders.
- Physician or health care provider co-signs the order within the time frame required by the institution (usually 24 hours; verify agency policy).

Communication and Transcription of Orders

After new medication orders are written, the drugs must be obtained from the pharmacy. Usually the copy of the physician's order sheet is sent to the pharmacy. The pharmacist is responsible for preparing the correct medications and delivering them to the nursing unit. Pharmacists also assess the medication plan and ensure that orders are valid.

Drug Distribution Systems

Systems for storing and distributing medications vary. Institutions providing nursing care have special areas for stocking and dispensing medications. Medication storage areas must be locked when unattended.

Unit-Dose System

The unit-dose system uses portable carts containing a drawer with a 24-hour supply of medications for each client. The unit dose is the ordered dose of medication the client receives at one time. Each medication form is wrapped

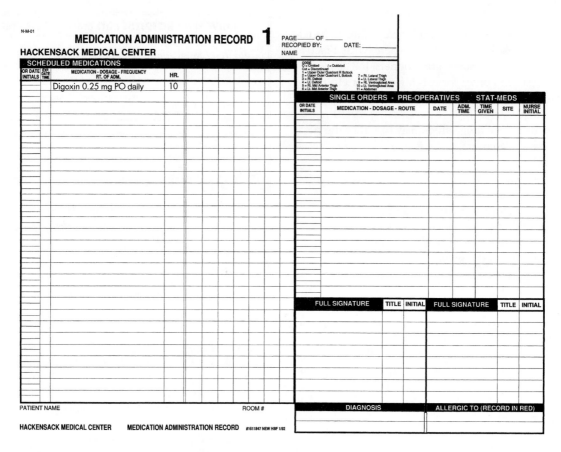

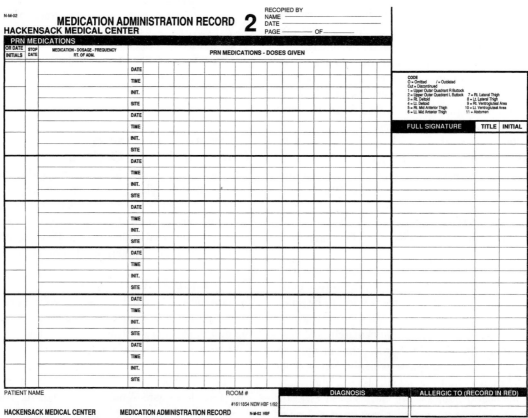

FIGURE 15-2 Examples of medication administration records. (Courtesy Hackensack University Medical Center, Hackensack, NJ.)

separately. The cart also contains limited amounts of prn and stock medications for special situations. The medication cart can be pushed from room to room to facilitate administration of medications at routine times. The cart is kept locked when not attended. In some settings the medications are kept in a locked cabinet in the client's room.

Computer-Controlled Dispensing Systems

Computer-controlled dispensing systems are variations of unit-dose and floor stock systems. For example, the Pyxis Corporation designs the MedStation. This system can carry a variety of medications, housed in individual compartments that a nurse accesses after requesting the medication from a computerized screen. Each nurse has a security code

for access to only those medications specifically ordered for a client. All medications retrieved from the MedStation are recorded in the system's computer and can be automatically charged to the client.

Medication Administration Record

An MAR is a form used to verify that the right medications are being administered at the correct times. Examples of MAR forms are given in Figures 15-2 and 15-3. Every 24 hours an MAR is distributed for each client for that day. As the nurse you are responsible for verifying that the MAR is accurate and up-to-date by comparing each medication to the original order, including the client's name, drug name, dose, route of administration, and times to be given. If a

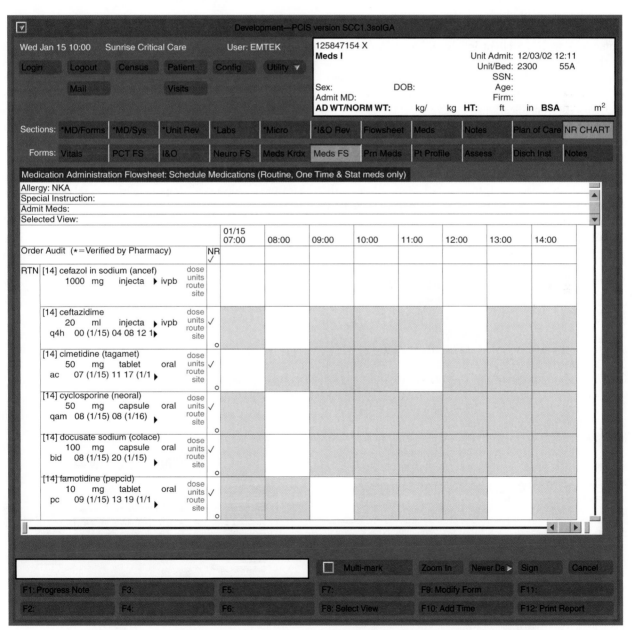

FIGURE 15-3 Computer list of ordered medications. (Courtesy Barnes-Jewish Hospital, St Louis, Mo.)

medication is to be given before the computer printout is available, you or the unit secretary writes the complete order on the MAR. The nurse who checks all transcribed orders is responsible for accuracy. If an order seems incorrect or inappropriate, the nurse consults the prescriber.

The Six Rights of Medication Administration

Preparing and administering medications requires accuracy and your full attention. The six rights is a traditional checklist to promote accuracy in drug administration.

Right Medication

The Joint Commission on Accreditation of Healthcare Organizations (JCAHO) included medication reconciliation as a national patient safety goal for 2006 (JCAHO, 2006). When a client enters a hospital setting, a complete list of the client's current medications must be reviewed and documented, with the client involved. You will also compare the medications the hospital provides to those on the client's list. When the client is transferred to another service or health care setting, you once again must reconcile the client's list of medications.

The JCAHO (2005) published a list of unacceptable abbreviations that were found to increase the incidence of error in medication administration (Table 15-2). You are responsible for using correct abbreviations and verifying that the order was accurately transcribed. Many institutions have a policy that requires that registered nurses (RNs) on a specific shift verify the accuracy of MAR forms printed for each client each day. Whenever new orders are handwritten on the MAR, the RN adding the orders must verify that

they are accurately added to the MAR. When verification is done, you initial and sign the order.

During drug administration, you compare the label of the drug (Figure 15-4) with the MAR three times: (1) when removing the drug from the storage bin; (2) before placing the drug in the medicine cup or before taking the drug to the client's room; and (3) again before giving the drug to the client. If the drug is ordered by trade name and dispensed from the pharmacy by generic name, you must verify that there is no discrepancy.

If a client questions the medication, stop and recheck to be certain there is no mistake. In most cases the drug order has been changed or is manufactured by a different company than the client has been using at home. Sometimes, however, attention to a client's question is how errors are identified and prevented.

Right Dose

When a medication is prepared from a dose other than what is ordered, the chance of errors increases. After calculating the dose, compare the calculation with a calculation done independently by a second nurse. This is especially important if it is an unusual calculation or involves a potentially toxic drug, such as Coumadin (an anticoagulant preparation that can be life threatening if an incorrect dose is given).

After calculating dosages, use appropriate measuring devices to prepare medications. Liquid preparations can be measured using a medicine cup marked in ml or a syringe for oral use. Some pediatric medications come with a scaled dropper (Figure 15-5).

The JCAHO now discourages the use of range orders for prn medications. An example of a range order is morphine sulfate 2 to 6 mg IV push q2-4h prn for pain. Range orders are often unclear and a source of medication errors. The JCAHO recommends that organizations develop practice guidelines to define how range orders can be implemented (Rich, 2002).

Right Client

Clients must be identified by using two client identifiers, neither of which is the client's room number (JCAHO, 2006). Check the MAR against the client's identification bracelet and ask the client to state his or her full name. In

TABLE 15-2 Prohibited and Error-Prone Abbreviations*	
ABBREVIATION	**PREFERRED TERM**
U (unit)	Write "unit"
IU (international unit)	Write "international unit"
Q.D., QD, q.d., qd (daily)	Write "daily"
Q.O.D., QOD, q.o.d., qod (every other day)	Write "every other day"
Trailing zero (X.0 mg)[†]	Write X mg
Lack of leading zero (.X)	Write 0.X
MS, MSO$_4$, and MgSO$_4$	Write "morphine sulfate" or write "magnesium sulfate"
HS (half-strength); hs (bedtime)	Write "half strength" or "bedtime"
SC, SQ (subcutaneous)	Write "subcutaneous" or "sub Q"
D/C (discharge or discontinue)	Write "discharge" or "discontinue"
cc (cubic centimeters)	Write "ml"

Data from JCAHO: The official "Do Not Use" list, 2005, http://www.jcaho.org/accredited+organizations/patient+safety/dnu.htm.
*Applies to all orders and all medication-related documentation that is handwritten (inlcuding free-text computer entry or on preprinted forms).
[†]Exception: A "trailing zero" is used only when needed to show precision of a reported value (e.g., laboratory test results), studies that report the size of lesions, or catheter and tube sizes. A "trailing zero" cannot be used in medication orders or medication-related documentation.
© Joint Commission on Accreditation of Healthcare Organizations, 2006. Reprinted with permission.

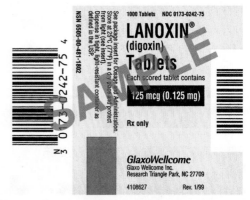

FIGURE 15-4 Sample drug label. (Reproduced with permission of Glaxo Wellcome, Inc., Research Triangle Park, NC.)

some agencies a nurse also compares the medical record number on the MAR with the identification bracelet. When nursing students are caring for one client, this process may seem awkward. However, when a nurse is giving medications to many clients, this practice is invaluable. This is essential even after caring for the same client for several days. Performing this identification routine systematically every time is a good habit that can prevent serious medication errors. If the client questions the practice, explain that this is the routine practice for making sure the client is getting the correct medication.

Right Route

The prescriber's order must designate a route of administration (Table 15-3). If the route of administration is missing, or if the specified route is not the recommended route, you must consult the prescriber immediately. When injections are administered, use only preparations intended for parenteral use. Injection of a liquid intended for oral use can produce local complications, such as sterile abscess, or fatal systemic effects. Medication companies label parenteral medications "for injectable use only."

Right Time

Each agency has routine time schedules for medications ordered at standard intervals. For example, medications to be given three times a day (tid) may be routinely scheduled for 0800, 1400, and 2000; or 0900, 1300, and 1900, depending on the agency policy. A drug may also be ordered every 8 hours (q8h), which is also three times a day. The medication ordered q8h needs to be given around the clock (ATC) to maintain adequate therapeutic levels and would, for example, be given at 0800, 1600, and 2400. Generally, the standard is for all routinely ordered medications to be given within 30 minutes before or after the scheduled time. Nursing judgment may allow some variance depending on the medication involved. There are institutions now allowing administration 60 minutes before and after the scheduled time.

A medication may also be ordered for special circumstances. A preoperative medication may be ordered "stat" (to be given immediately); "now," which means as soon as available, usually within an hour; or "on call," which means the operating or procedure room personnel will notify the nurse when it is the appropriate time. A drug may be ordered before meals ("ac") or after meals ("pc").

Right Documentation

To ensure the right documentation, first make sure that the information on your client's MAR corresponds exactly with the prescriber's order and the label on the medication container. Do not give medications that have illegible or incomplete orders. Verify inaccurate documentation before giving medications. It is better to give the correct medication at a later time than to give your client the wrong drug. Record the administration of each medication on the MAR as soon as you give it. Never document that you have given a medication until you have actually given it. Document the name of the medication, the dose, the time of administration, and the route. Also document the site of any injections you give. Also document the client's response to the medication in the nurses' notes. Accurate documentation prevents medical errors.

Medication Preparation

It is legally advisable to administer only the medications you prepare. Administering a drug prepared by another nurse increases the opportunity for error. The nurse who gives the wrong medication or an incorrect dose is legally responsible for the error. The importance of checking similar names and verifying for the correct drug cannot be overemphasized.

Interpreting Drug Labels

Drug labels include several basic pieces of information: the trade name of the drug in large letters, the generic name in smaller letters, the form of the drug, the dosage, the expiration date, the lot number, and the name of the manufacturer. The trade name given by the manufacturer often suggests the action of the drug, and the generic name is the chemical name (Figure 15-6).

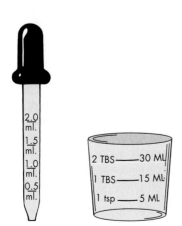

FIGURE 15-5 Scaled dropper for pediatric use and cup to measure oral liquids. (From Clayton BD, Stock YN: *Basic pharmacology for nurses,* ed 13, St Louis, 2004, Mosby.)

TABLE 15-3 Routes of Drug Administration	
ROUTE	**DESCRIPTION**
Nonparenteral	
Oral	By mouth
Sublingual	Under the tongue
Topical	On the skin (as a cream or patch), and eye/ear drops
Suppository	Into rectum or vagina
Parenteral	
Intradermal (ID)	Into the dermis
Intramuscular (IM)	Into the muscle
Intravenous (IV)	Into the vein
Subcutaneous (Sub-Q)	Into the subcutaneous tissue

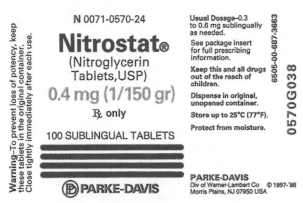

FIGURE 15-6 Interpreting a drug label. (Reproduced with permission of Warner-Lambert Company.)

Conversions

Drugs are not always dispensed in the unit of measure in which they are ordered. Drug companies package and bottle certain standard equivalents. You must convert available units of volume and weight to desired dosages or vice versa. You must know approximate equivalents in all of the measurement systems or make use of conversion tables. An example follows:

The order reads: vancomycin 1 g IV.

The pharmacy supplies vancomycin in 500-mg vials.

Because the drug dose on the drug label is in milligrams, conversion should be from grams to milligrams; 1 gm = 1000 mg.

SYSTEMS OF DRUG MEASUREMENT

The proper administration of medication depends on your ability to compute drug dosages accurately and measure medications correctly. A careless mistake in placing a decimal point or adding a zero to a dosage can lead to a fatal error. The prescriber and client depend on you to check the dosage before giving a drug. The metric system is the most common system used in the measurement of medications.

Metric System

As a decimal system, the metric system is the most logically organized of the measurement systems. Each basic unit of measure is organized into units of 10. Multiplying or dividing by 10 forms secondary units. In multiplication, the decimal point moves to the right; in division, the decimal moves to the left. To convert grams to milligrams you multiply by 1000 or move the decimal point three places to the right (0.5 g = 500 mg). Conversely, to convert milligrams to grams you divide by 1000 or move the decimal point three places to the left (500 mg = 0.5 g).

The basic units of measure in the metric system are the meter (length), liter (volume), and gram (weight). For drug calculations you will use primarily volume and weight units. In the metric system small or large letters designate the basic units:

Gram: g or Gm

Liter: l or L

Small letters are abbreviations for subdivisions of major units:

Milligram: mg

Milliliter: ml

Household Measurements

Household measures are familiar to most people, but these measures are not recommended for medication administration because of the variability in the size of household utensils. Included in household measures are drops, teaspoons, tablespoons, and cups for volume and ounces and pounds for weight. Before the actual administration of medication, you may need to convert units within a system or between systems and calculate drug dosages (Box 15-2).

> **NURSE ALERT** Drugs ordered in units and milliequivalents are not convertible to metric, apothecary, or household measurements.

Solutions

Solutions are used for injections, irrigations, and infusions. A solution is a given mass of solid substance dissolved in a known volume of fluid, or a given volume of liquid dissolved in a known volume of another fluid. Solutions are available in units of mass per units of volume (e.g., g/ml, g/L). You can also express a concentration of a solution as a percentage. A 10% solution is 10 g of solid dissolved in 100 ml of solution.

Dosage Calculations

Dosage calculations are necessary when the dose on the drug label differs from the dosage ordered. There are several dosage calculation methods. The most common methods are ratio-proportion or use of a formula (Box 15-3). Dimensional analysis is a method for dosage calculation that involves simple multiplication and division and not algebra (Box 15-4).

BOX 15-2 Approximate Equivalents

1 g* = 60 mcg	5 ml = 1 tsp†
1 g = 1000 mg	3 tsp† = 1 Tbsp†
1000 mcg(μg) = 1 mg	30 ml = 1 oz†
1 kg = 2.2 lb	1000 ml = 1 L
1 ml or mL = 15-16 minims*	

*Apothecary measure.
†Household measure.

BOX 15-3 Formula Method

$$\frac{D}{H} \times V = \text{amount to give}$$

D is the desired dose or the dose ordered by the physician for the client (e.g., 250 mg of penicillin PO 4 times daily).

H is the drug dose on hand or available for use. The dose is on the drug label (e.g., penicillin tablets of 250 mg each).

V is the volume (liquid) or vehicle (tablets, capsules) that delivers the available dose.

NOTE: The desired dose **(D)** and the on-hand dose **(H)** must be in the same unit of measurement. If they are in different units, you must perform conversions before completing the formula.

BOX 15-4 Dimensional Analysis

Step 1: Identify the starting factor (amount ordered), which is the first item of the equation, and the answer label (tablets, capsules, or ml), which is the last item.

Step 2: Identify appropriate equivalents with a 1:1 ratio (e.g., 1 g = 1000 mg). Set up the equation so that labels can be canceled; for example, if mg is in the numerator, mg must be in the denominator to cancel.

Step 3: Solve the equation.
  a. Cancel labels first; the answer label should not cancel.
  b. Reduce numbers to lowest terms.
  c. Multiply/divide to solve equation.
  d. Reduce answer to lowest terms, convert to decimal, and round to a measurable quantity.

$$\text{Starting factor} \times \frac{\text{Equivalent}}{\text{Equivalent}} = \text{Answer label}$$

Example 1

When the dose ordered has the same label as the dose available:

  Dose ordered: 0.5 g
  Tablets available: 0.25 g per tablet

Step 1. The starting factor is 0.5 g.

  The answer label is tablets; that is, how many tablets should be given?

Step 2. Formulate the conversion equation:

  The equivalent needed is 1 tablet = 0.25 g.

$$\frac{0.5 \text{ g}}{1} \times \frac{1 \text{ tab}}{0.25\text{g}} = \text{tabs}$$

  Cancel labels (g).

  NOTE: If properly written, all labels except the answer label will cancel.

Step 3. Solve the equation:

  Reduce the numerical values, and multiply the numerators and the denominators.

$$\frac{\overset{2}{\cancel{0.5 \text{ g}}}}{1} \times \frac{1 \text{ tab}}{\cancel{0.25\text{g}}} = 2 \text{ tabs}$$

Example 2

When the dose ordered has a different label than the dose available:

  Dose ordered: 0.5 g
  Tablets available: 250 mg per tablet

Step 1. The starting factor is 0.5 g.

  The answer label is tablets; that is, how many tablets should be given?

Step 2. Formulate the conversion equation:

  The equivalents needed are 1 g = 1000 mg and 1 tab = 250 mg.

$$\frac{0.5 \text{ g}}{1} \times \frac{1000 \text{ mg}}{1 \text{ g}} \times \frac{1 \text{ tab}}{250 \text{ mg}} = \text{tabs}$$

Cancel labels (g, mg).

Step 3. Solve the equation:

  Reduce the values, and multiply the numerators and the denominators.

$$\cancel{0.5 \text{ g}} \times \frac{\overset{4}{\cancel{1000 \text{ mg}}}}{\cancel{1 \text{ g}} \, 2} \times \frac{1 \text{ tab}}{\cancel{250 \text{ mg}}} = \frac{4}{2} = 2 \text{ tabs}$$

Example 3

When the dose ordered is available in a liquid form:

  Dose ordered: Keflex 250 mg PO
  Available: 125 mg per 5 ml

Step 1. The starting factor is 250 mg.

  The answer label is ml.

Step 2. Formulate the conversion equation:

  The equivalent needed is 125 mg = 5 ml.

$$\frac{250 \text{ mg}}{1} \times \frac{5 \text{ ml}}{125 \text{ mg}} = \text{ml}$$

Cancel labels (mg).

Step 3. Solve the equation:

  Reduce and multiply.

$$\frac{\overset{2}{\cancel{250 \text{ mg}}}}{1} \times \frac{5 \text{ ml}}{\cancel{125 \text{ mg}}} = 10 \text{ ml}$$

Example 4

When dosage is ordered based on body surface area (commonly done for pediatric dosages), the body surface area is estimated on the basis of weight, using standard charts or a nomogram. The formula is a ratio of the child's body surface area compared with the body surface area of an average adult (1.7 square meters, or 1.7 m²).

$$\text{Child's dose} = \frac{\text{Surface area of child}}{1.7 \text{ m}^2} \times \text{Normal adult dose}$$

  The physician orders ampicillin for a child weighing 12 kg, and the nomogram chart shows that the body surface area for this child is 0.54 m². The normal single adult dose is 250 mg.

  1 Child's dose $= \dfrac{0.54 \text{ m}^2}{1.7 \text{ m}^2} \times 250 \text{ mg}$

  2 The m² units cancel out and can be ignored.

3 Child's dose $= \dfrac{0.54}{1.7} \times 250$ mg

4 0.3×250 mg $= 75$ mg

5 Child's dose $= 75$ mg

NURSING PROCESS

Nurses use the nursing process to integrate drug therapy into client care. As a nurse, your role extends beyond simply giving drugs to a client. You are responsible for monitoring clients' responses to medications, providing education to the client and family about the medication regimen, and informing the physician when medications are effective, ineffective, or no longer necessary.

ASSESSMENT

Begin your assessment with the client's medical history, which provides any indications or contraindications for medication therapy. Certain diseases or illnesses place clients at risk for adverse medication effects. For example, if a client has a gastric ulcer, forms of aspirin will increase the chance of bleeding. Long-term health problems require specific medications. This knowledge helps you anticipate the medications your client requires.

Include an assessment of client allergies. Many medications have ingredients found in food sources. For example, if your client is allergic to shellfish, he or she may be sensitive to products containing iodine, such as Betadine or dyes used in radiological testing. When assessing for drug allergies, you must differentiate between actual allergic reactions, which can be life threatening, and drug intolerances, which are uncomfortable side effects.

Your assessment also involves identifying drugs the client takes every day at home, including prescriptions, OTC preparations, and herbal supplements. Determine how long the client has taken each drug, current dosage schedule, and whether the client has had any adverse effects to any of the medications. The client should know the name, purpose, dosage, route, and side effects of medications and supplements that are being taken. Often clients take many drugs and carry a list that includes this information. Clients have different levels of understanding. One client may describe a diuretic as a "water pill," whereas another describes it as a drug to minimize swelling and lower blood pressure. Still another may describe it as "the little white pill I take in the morning." By assessing the client's level of knowledge, you determine the need for teaching. If a client is unable to understand or remember pertinent information, it may be necessary to involve a family member.

NURSING DIAGNOSES

Ineffective therapeutic regimen management may be related to a knowledge deficit about prescribed medications, the complexity of a drug schedule, or unpleasant side effects. **Health-seeking behaviors (medications)** may apply when clients have a knowledge deficit and want to learn how to provide self-medication. **Noncompliance** involves a person's informed decision not to adhere to a therapeutic regimen of medication administration, which may be related to economical, cultural, or spiritual beliefs. Certain medications, such as chemotherapeutic agents, steroids, and anticoagulants, may contribute to **ineffective protection,** in which therapy alters the client's ability to respond normally to infection or bleeding. **Disturbed sensory perception (visual or auditory)** is appropriate in clients receiving eye or ear medications.

PLANNING

When you administer medications, the following general goals are met:
1 Client achieves therapeutic effect of the prescribed medication
2 Absence of client complications related to the prescribed medication
3 Client and/or family understand drug therapy
4 Client and family self-administer medication safely (when appropriate)

IMPLEMENTATION

Nursing interventions focus on safe and effective drug administration. This includes careful drug preparation, accurate and timely administration, and client education.

Preadministration Activities
1 Identify the drug action, purpose, side effects, and nursing implications for administering and monitoring. Ensure that the medication order has not expired.
2 Complete appropriate assessments, which may include, but are not limited to, vital signs, laboratory data, or nature and severity of symptoms. If data contraindicates medication administration, hold the drug and notify the prescriber.
3 Calculate drug doses accurately and use appropriate measuring devices. Verify that the dose prescribed is appropriate for the client situation.
4 Give medications within 30 minutes before or after the scheduled time to maintain a therapeutic level. NOTE: Medications ordered stat should be given immediately. Preoperative medications may be ordered "on call" and are given when the operating or procedure room personnel notify the nurse of the appropriate time. Certain drugs, such as insulin, should be given at a precise interval before a meal. Others should be given with meals or on an empty stomach.
5 Use good hand-hygiene technique for nonparenteral medications. Avoid touching tablets and capsules. Use sterile technique for parenteral medications. Wear clean gloves when administering parenteral medications.

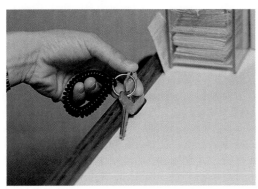

FIGURE 15-7 Medication carts must be kept locked when unattended and the key kept by an authorized person.

6 Administer only those medications you personally prepare. Do not ask another person to administer drugs you prepare. Keep drugs secure (Figure 15-7). Do not administer medications prepared by someone else.

7 When preparing medications, be sure the label is clear and legible and the drug is properly mixed; has not changed in color, clarity, or consistency; and has not expired.

8 Keep tablets and capsules in their wrappers and open them at the client's bedside. This allows you to review each drug with the client. If a client refuses medication, there is no question about which one is withheld.

Drug Administration

1 Follow the six rights for medication administration.

2 Inform the client of each drug's name, purpose, action, and common side effects. Evaluate the client's knowledge of the drug, and provide appropriate teaching.

3 Stay with the client until the medication is taken. Provide assistance as necessary. Do not leave medication at the bedside without a prescriber's order to do so. For example, some clients may take their own vitamins or birth control pills while in the hospital.

4 Respect the client's right to refuse medication. If the medication wrapper is intact, the medication may be returned to the client's storage bin. When medication is refused, determine the reason for this, and take action accordingly. If, for example, the client has unpleasant side effects, it may be possible to eliminate them by giving the pills with food or using a different time schedule.

Postadministration Activities

1 Record medications immediately according to agency policy. Include the drug name, dose, route, time, and your signature.

2 Document data pertinent to the client's response. This is especially important when giving drugs ordered prn.

3 If a drug is refused, document that it was not given, the reason for the refusal, and when the physician was notified.

EVALUATION

1 Monitor for evidence of therapeutic effects, side effects, and adverse reactions. This includes monitoring physical response (e.g., heart rhythm, blood pressure, urine output, or laboratory results).

2 When a drug is given for relief of symptoms, ask the client to report if symptoms have diminished or been relieved.

3 Observe injection sites for bruises, inflammation, localized pain, numbness, or bleeding.

4 Evaluate client's understanding of drug therapy and ability to self-administer medication.

CLIENT AND FAMILY TEACHING

A well-informed client is more likely to take medications correctly. However, many clients have limited health literacy, meaning they do not understand how to read medication labels or calculate doses. Provide an individualized approach to teaching, using visual aids, instructional booklets, or even video tapes. When teaching clients about their medications include persons identified as being significant to the client's recovery. This may include family members, partners, or home care providers. There are specific nursing interventions that are appropriate in the home setting (Box 15-5).

Teaching Clients About Side Effects

All medications have side effects. You are responsible for teaching the client and family members about side effects associated with each medication prescribed. Because medications can have many side effects, teaching the client about all of them can overwhelm the client and impede learning. Remember, client learning is a continual process. When beginning to teach a client about a new medication, evaluate each of the side effects. Then teach the client about the ones that are the most likely to occur and occur early after administration. For example, some antibiotics cause hypersensitivity reactions, hepatotoxicity, nephrotoxicity, and platelet dysfunction. Hypersensitivity reactions are likely to occur shortly after taking a few doses of an antibiotic. The other side effects tend to occur after long-term antibiotic administration. Teach clients about side effects in terms of things that they can see, feel, touch, or hear. For example, thrombocytopenia, a reduction in the number of platelets in the blood, can be a side effect of a drug. The client cannot see, feel, touch, or hear thrombocytopenia. However, thrombocytopenia can cause bleeding. Teach the client how to look for evidence of bleeding. Be sure to teach the client what to do about side effects when they are discovered.

Medications and the Client's Activities of Daily Living

Evaluate the client's activities of daily living (ADLs) and the effect they will have on the client's ability to comply

---

BOX 15-5 Home Care

1 During each home visit, assess all prescription and nonprescription medications being taken by the client.

2 Document and notify the primary health care provider of the client's medication regimen and of multiple physician sources for medications.

3 Teach the complications and interactions of all OTC medications to clients and their caregivers.

4 Collaborate with social workers to identify community resources for financial assistance with pharmaceutical needs.

5 Use laboratory parameters to monitor overuse and underuse of medications, as well as interactive states of medications.

6 Monitor urinary output status of clients, because changes in renal excretion may require a decrease or increase in drug dosage.

7 Teach the homebound older client to set up a daily or weekly schedule of medications using a method or tool that fosters safe, independent administration.

8 Reduce the chance of medication error by labeling or color-coding medication bottles.

9 Keep an accurate record of the homebound client's weight, especially the older adult, because many medication dosages are calculated by body weight.

10 Teach drug safety in the home environment by instructing clients to do the following:
   a. Keep drugs in original, labeled containers.
   b. Dispose of outdated medications in a sink or toilet only; never dispose of them in the trash within reach of children.
   c. Never "share" drugs with friends or family members.
   d. Always finish a prescribed medication; do not save it for a future illness.
   e. Read labels carefully and follow all instructions.

11 Instruct clients with muscle weakness and older adults who have difficulty opening child-proof containers to request health care providers ask for non–child-proof containers when writing prescriptions.

Data from Meiner SE, Lueckenotte AA: *Gerontologic nursing,* ed 3, St Louis, 2006, Mosby.

---

with medication schedules. When medications are initiated in the acute care setting, they are often given ATC. In the community it may not be reasonable to think clients can administer medications according to this schedule. In collaboration with the prescriber or the pharmacist, teach the client and family members how to adjust medication schedules that are consistent with the client's lifestyle. Include what to do if doses are missed.

Evaluating the effectiveness of teaching ensures that the client can administer drugs in a safe manner. One method of evaluating client understanding is to create medication cards with the generic and trade names of the drug on the front of the card and all pertinent drug information on the back of the card. You can flash the card in front of the client, and ask the client to read the names of the medication. Another method is to have clients read labels on prepared medications. Remember, drug bottles often have fine print and are difficult to read by the client with impaired vision.

If the client correctly identifies the name of the medication, ask the client the following questions:
- Why are you taking this medication?
- How often do you take this medication?
- What side effects can occur with this medication?
- If this side effect occurs, what are you going to do about it?

For clients who are unable to identify drug names, consider further assessment for a possible literacy problem. Be sure to also assess the client's sensory, motor, and cognitive functions. Impairments may affect the client's ability to safely self-administer medications, and family members, friends, or home health aides may need to assist with medication administration. Many self-help devices are also available for purchase (e.g., pill boxes with times displayed and electronic dispensers).

SPECIAL HANDLING OF CONTROLLED SUBSTANCES

As a nurse, you are responsible for following legal regulations when administering controlled substances (drugs with potential for abuse). Violations of the Controlled Substances Act may result in fines, imprisonment, and loss of license. Health care institutions have policies for the proper storage and distribution of controlled substances, including opioids (Box 15-6). Many agencies use computerized systems for medication access and distribution (Figure 15-8).

EVIDENCE IN PRACTICE

Sullivan C and others: Medication reconciliation in the acute care setting, *J Nurs Care Qual* 20(2):95, 2005.

In 1999 the Institute of Medicine (IOM) reported that medical errors in hospitals possibly caused between 44,000 and 98,000 deaths in the United States (Kohn, Corrigan, and Donaldson, 1999). This report sparked a movement to develop strategies to prevent medical errors and specifically reduce medication errors (Box 15-7). Sullivan and others (2005) noted that nurses have a vital part in any effort to reduce medication errors. This study concluded that medication errors can be decreased and avoided by having nurses consistently perform medication reconciliation, which was defined as systematic validation and verification of a client's medication history and medication orders. Medication reconciliation occurs when clients transfer to new units or are discharged to other facilities.

MEDICATION ERRORS

The JCAHO (2005) defines a medication error as any preventable event that may cause inappropriate medication use or jeopardize client safety. Medication errors can be made by anyone involved in the prescribing, transcribing, preparation, dispensing, and administration of medications (Smetzer, 2001). Hospital delivery systems have a system of (see Figure 15-8).

BOX 15-6 Storage and Accountability for Controlled Substances

- All controlled substances are stored in a locked cabinet or container (see Figure 15-8).
- Authorized nurses carry a set of keys or computer entry code for the cabinet.
- An inventory record is kept to record all controlled substances used, including client's name, date, name of drug, and time of drug administration.
- Before any drug is removed from the cabinet, the number actually available is compared with the number indicated on the controlled substance record. If incorrect, the discrepancy must be rectified before proceeding.
- If any part of a dose of a controlled substance is discarded, a second nurse witnesses disposal of the unused portion, and the record is signed by both nurses.
- At change of shift one nurse going off duty counts all controlled substances with a nurse coming on duty. Both nurses sign the record to indicate the count is correct. (Computerized storage has eliminated this process.)
- Discrepancies in controlled substance counts are reported immediately.

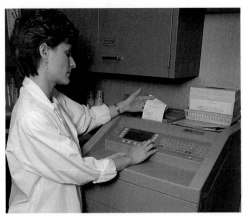

FIGURE 15-8 Computerized system for medication distribution.

Box 15-7 Steps to Take in Preventing Medication Errors

- Follow the six rights of medication administration.
- Be sure to read labels at least three times (comparing MAR with label): when removing drug from storage, before taking to client's room, before giving drug.
- Use at least two client identifiers (e.g., name band, client pronouncing name) whenever administering a medication.
- Do not allow any other activity to interrupt your administration of medication to a client.
- Double-check all calculations, and verify with another nurse.
- Do not interpret illegible handwriting; clarify with prescriber.
- Question unusually large or small doses.
- Document all medications as soon as they are given.
- When you have made an error, reflect on what went wrong, and ask how you could have prevented the error.
- Evaluate the context or situation in which a medication error occurred. This helps to determine if nurses have the necessary resources for safe medication administration.
- When repeated medication errors occur within a work area, identify and analyze the factors that may have caused the errors, and take corrective action.
- Attend in-service programs on the medications you commonly administer.

checks that help prevent medication errors. *Conscientious adherence to the six rights of medication administration is your best way to prevent errors.*

When an error occurs, acknowledge it immediately, and then assess the client. You have an ethical and professional obligation to report the error to the client's physician, the nurse manager, and any other persons as indicated by the institution's policy regarding errors. Appropriate follow-up may include administering an antidote, withholding a subsequent dose, and monitoring the effects of the drug. The client's record should include a notation that indicates what was given, who was notified, the observed effects of the drug, and follow-up measures taken.

You are also responsible for completing a report describing the incident. Most institutions have a policy or protocol for reporting adverse events. This report provides an objective analysis of what went wrong. It provides information for the risk management team to identify factors contributing to errors and develop ways to avoid similar errors in the future (Benner, 2001).

SPECIAL CONSIDERATIONS FOR SPECIFIC AGE-GROUPS

Pediatric Considerations

Children vary in age, weight, and ability to absorb, metabolize, and excrete medications. Children's dosages are lower than those of adults, and caution is needed in preparing medications. Drugs may or may not be prepared and packaged in doses appropriate for children. Preparing appropriate doses often requires calculation based on body weight

(Hockenberry, 2004). A child's parents may be helpful in determining the best way to give a child medication. Sometimes it is more effective to have the parent give the drug as you stand by.

Geriatric Considerations

Individuals older than age 65 are the largest users of drugs (Meiner and Lueckenotte, 2006). Because of physiological changes associated with the aging process, special nursing interventions are needed to promote safe and effective medication administration (Table 15-4). Be aware of the following patterns related to drug use:

- *Polypharmacy.* The client takes two or more medications to treat the same illness, takes two or more medications from the same chemical class, or takes

TABLE 15-4 Drug Effects in Older Adults

DRUG EFFECT	RELATED INTERVENTIONS
Difficulty swallowing large tablets or capsules; tissue damage related to uncoated medications such as aspirin and potassium chloride	Position client sitting upright. Give full glass of liquid (if unrestricted). Crush tablets and mix with food, or give liquid form if available.
Slowing of drug excretion; overuse and abuse of laxatives by client	Instruct client to increase fluid intake, eat high-fiber foods, and avoid daily use of laxatives.
Longer biotransformation of drugs by the liver with greater risk for drug sensitivity and toxicity	Monitor for signs of liver dysfunction (laboratory tests, jaundice, and dark urine). Monitor for contraindications in clients with known liver disease.
Risk of drug accumulation and toxicity related to altered kidney function or renal blood flow	Monitor for renal impairment (decreased urine output) and for contraindications to medications (e.g., gentamycin) in clients with known renal disease.

two or more medications with the same or similar actions to treat different illnesses (Brager and Sloan, 2005). This increases the risk of drug interactions with other drugs or with foods.

* *Self-prescribing.* Older adults often attempt to seek relief from a variety of problems with OTC preparations, folk medicines, and herbs.

* *Misuse of drugs.* Misuse by older adults includes overuse, underuse, erratic use, and contraindicated use.
* *Noncompliance.* Deliberate misuse of medication is considered to be noncompliance. Older adults alter doses because of ineffectiveness, unpleasant side effects, and lack of financial resources.

NCLEX® Style Questions

1 The nurse uses a current drug index to look up a pain medication and finds that the drug's onset of action is 30 minutes, it peaks in 60 minutes, and the duration of action is 3 hours. The client asks the nurse to administer this medication so it will be most effective when the client participates in a strenuous hour-long physical therapy session later in the day. When should the nurse give this medication to the client?
1. Now
2. Fifteen minutes before the physical therapy session
3. An hour before the physical therapy session
4. Just before the client begins the physical therapy session

2 The nurse finds the following new medication order written in a client's hospital chart: "3/17/06 0815 Furosemide 40 mg twice a day. Dr. Eagleton" What should the nurse do?
1. Enter the order in the hospital computer.
2. Administer the medication.
3. Contact Dr. Eagleton.
4. Review the order with a pharmacist.

3 List the six rights of medication administration.

4 A client is to receive 500 mg of a medication that is available in scored tablets of 1 gram. How many tablets should the client receive?

5 A client is to receive 500 mg of a liquid medication that is available as 1 gram in 10 ml. How much should the client receive?

References for all chapters appear in Appendix D.

Administration of Nonparenteral Medications

MEDIA RESOURCES

- **evolve** http://evolve.elsevier.com/Elkin

- **View Video!** **Video Clips**

- **Nursing Skills Online**

Nurses administer nonparenteral medications by several routes that do not invade the skin, including oral, topical, inhalation, or instilled into the eye, ear, rectum, or vagina. The route chosen depends on the properties and desired effects of the medication, as well as the physical and mental condition of the client. Each route has advantages and disadvantages (Table 16-1). There are many reasons you may find it necessary to recommend a change from one route to another. When this occurs, you are responsible for consulting with the physician or health care provider for an order or conferring with a pharmacist to safely meet the client's needs.

The easiest and most desirable way to administer medications is orally (by mouth). Clients usually are able to ingest or self-administer oral drugs with few problems. However, situations may arise that contraindicate clients receiving medications by mouth, including the presence of gastrointestinal (GI) alterations, the inability of a client to swallow food or fluids, and the use of gastric suction. An important precaution to take when administering any oral preparation is to protect clients from aspiration. Aspiration is a life-threatening condition that occurs when food, fluid, or medication intended for GI administration accidentally enters the respiratory tract. You can protect clients from aspiration by evaluating their ability to safely swallow (Box 16-1). Properly positioning the client is also essential in preventing aspiration. Unless contraindicated, position the client in a seated high-Fowler's position when administering oral medications. The lateral position is also used when the client's swallow, gag, and cough reflexes are intact. A client who has difficulty swallowing should be evaluated by appropriate personnel (e.g., speech therapist) before receiving oral preparations. In addition, the physician should be notified. When a feeding tube is present, it is imperative to verify

Table 16-1 Nonparenteral Routes of Administration

ROUTE	ADVANTAGES	DISADVANTAGES
Inhalation	Provides direct effects on lung tissues and rapid relief of respiratory distress.	Difficult for some clients to administer correctly. Clients must be taught how to use equipment.
Mucous membranes: eyes, ears, nose; vaginal, rectal, buccal, sublingual	Local application to involved site; limited side effects. Buccal and sublingual rapidly absorbed. Rectal route an alternative when oral route not available.	Insertion of vaginal or rectal products may cause embarrassment. Rectal suppositories are contraindicated with rectal surgery or active rectal bleeding.
Oral (swallowed)	Easy, comfortable, economical; may produce local or systemic effects.	Some drugs are destroyed by gastric secretions. Cannot be given if client is NPO, unable to swallow, is nauseated, has gastric suction, or is unconscious or confused and unwilling to cooperate. May irritate lining of gastrointestinal (GI) tract, discolor teeth, or have unpleasant taste.
Skin: topical application or transdermal patches	Provides primarily local effect; painless; limited side effects. Transdermal application provides systemic effects and bypasses the liver and its first-pass effects.	Extensive topical applications may be bulky or cause difficulty in maneuvering. May leave oily or pasty substance on skin; may soil clothing. Systemic absorption can be unreliable. Allergies to the adhesive in transdermal patches may develop.

Modified from Lilley LL, Harrington S, Snyder JS: *Pharmacology and the nursing process,* ed 4, St Louis, 2004, Mosby.

BOX 16-1 Dysphagia

Dysphagia, or difficulty in swallowing, may lead to aspiration of food or fluid into the lungs. Signs and symptoms associated with dysphagia include:

- Choking while eating or drinking
- Frequent need to clear the throat
- Drooling or leakage of food from the mouth
- Coughing during or after meals
- Holding pockets of food in the cheeks
- Unusually intense chewing, or repeated attempts to swallow just one bite of food
- Gurgled voice after eating (have the client say "Ah" to assess)
- Increased congestion or secretions after eating or drinking

Assess the client's swallow, cough, and gag reflexes carefully. Assess swallowing by placing the thumb and index finger on both sides of the client's Adam's apple and feel for elevation of the larynx when the client tries to swallow. The elevation should be the same on both sides. Next, have client demonstrate a cough, by taking a slow deep breath and holding it for 2 seconds, contracting expiratory muscles and coughing through an open mouth. Determine presence or absence of gag reflex by gently stroking the back of the throat with a tongue blade. Also observe how the client places food and liquid in his or her mouth, how the food bolus is chewed or moved before it is swallowed, and how well the tongue moves the food bolus to the back of the throat. Look for food residue in the mouth after swallowing.

If swallowing difficulties are suspected or detected, a referral to a speech pathologist is needed for definitive diagnosis. Dysphagia that is not recognized or managed may lead to aspiration pneumonia.

Modified from Galvan TJ: Dysphagia: going down and staying down, *Am J Nurs* 101(1):37-43, 2001; Mahan LK, Escott-Stump S: *Krause's food, nutrition, and diet therapy,* ed 11, Philadelphia, 2004, Saunders; and Terrado M, Russell C, Bowman JB: Dysphagia: an overview, *Medsurg Nurs* 10(5):233-247, 2001.

correct tube placement prior to giving medications in order to prevent aspiration.

Topical administration of medications involves applying drugs directly to skin, mucous membranes, or tissue membranes. You apply medications to the skin by painting, spraying, or spreading medication over a localized area. Transdermal patches (adhesive-backed medicated disks) applied to the skin provide a continuous release of medication over several hours or days. Systemic effects from topical agents can occur if the skin is thin, if the drug concentration is high, or if contact with the skin is prolonged. Topical administration avoids puncturing the skin and lessens tissue injury and risk of infection that may occur with injections. The risk of serious side effects is generally low, but they can occur. You will need to wear gloves while applying these preparations to avoid the effects of the topical medications.

Drugs applied to membranes such as the cornea of the eye or rectal mucosa are absorbed quickly because of the membrane's vascularity. When drug concentrations are high, systemic effects can occur. For example, bradycardia and hypotension may occur after instillation of ophthalmic beta blockers such as timolol (Timoptic). Mucous and other tissue membranes differ in their sensitivity to medications. The cornea of the eye, for example, is extremely sensitive to chemicals. Clients commonly experience burning sensations during administration of eye and nose drops. Medications are generally less irritating to vaginal or rectal mucosa.

Medications for topical use can be administered in the following ways:

1 Direct application to skin or mucosa (lotion, creams, patches, disks, ointments, gargling, swabbing throat) or membrane of eye (eye drops)

2 Insertion of a drug into body cavity: suppository into rectum or vagina; creams and foams into the vagina

3 Instillation of fluid into body cavity (fluid is retained): ear drops, nose drops, bladder and rectal instillation

4 Irrigation of body cavity (fluid is not retained): flushing eye, ear, vagina, bladder, or rectum with medicated fluid

5 Spray: instillation into nose or throat, or sublingually

6 Inhalation of medicated aerosol spray (via nebulizer or metered-dose inhaler [MDI]) or dry powder (through an inhaler): distributes medication throughout the nasal passages and tracheobronchial airway

NURSING DIAGNOSES

Nursing diagnoses affecting the client's ability to self-administer drugs include **ineffective therapeutic regimen management,** which may be related to a knowledge deficit of the purpose of prescribed medications, the complexity of a drug schedule, or unpleasant side effects. **Health-seeking behaviors** applies when clients want to learn how to provide self-medication. You may identify nursing diagnoses based on therapeutic effects or side effects of specific prescribed medications. For example, **impaired skin integrity** applies when you use topical medications to treat rashes and skin injury, and **impaired gas exchange** is appropriate when you give medications by inhalation. Certain medications such as chemotherapeutic agents, steroids, and anticoagulants may contribute to **ineffective protection,** in which the client's ability to respond normally to infection or bleeding is decreased. Clients who receive medications through a feeding tube may have **risk for aspiration.**

SKILL 16.1 Administering Oral Medications

- **Nursing Skills Online: Non–Parenteral Medication Administration, Lesson 1**

The majority of medications you administer in many health care settings are given by mouth. You typically prepare the oral medications for the client to self-administer in an area designed for medication preparation or at the unit-dose cart.

Absorption of an oral medication after it is ingested depends largely on its form or preparation. Solutions and suspensions that are already in a liquid state (Figure 16-1) are absorbed more readily than tablets or capsules. Oral medications are absorbed more easily when administered between meals and when the stomach is not filled with food, which slows the absorption process. When effective absorption in the stomach is required, give those drugs at least 1 hour before or 2 hours after meals or antacids. Acidic drugs are absorbed quickly in the stomach.

Some drugs are not absorbed until reaching the small intestine. Enteric coatings on some tablets resist being dissolved by gastric juices and prevent digestion in the upper GI tract. The coating protects the stomach lining from irritation by the medication. Eventually the drug is absorbed in the intestine. Do *not* crush or dissolve enteric-coated medications before administration.

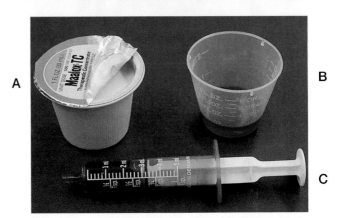

FIGURE 16-1 A, Liquid medication in a single-dose package. **B,** Liquid measured in a medicine cup. **C,** Oral medicine in syringe.

ASSESSMENT

1 Identify the drug(s) ordered: action, purpose, normal dosage and route, common side effects, time of onset and peak action, and nursing implications. *Rationale: This allows you to anticipate effects of drugs and to observe client's response.*

2 Assess for any contraindications to oral medication, including inability to swallow, nausea/vomiting, bowel in-

flammation, reduced peristalsis, GI surgery, gastric suction, and decreased level of consciousness (LOC). Notify the prescriber if any contraindications are discovered. *Rationale: Alterations in GI function can interfere with drug absorption, distribution, and excretion. Giving oral medication to clients with impaired swallowing or decreased LOC increases their risk of aspiration.*

3 Check for a history of allergies and related response (e.g., rash, anaphylactic shock). Notify prescriber.

4 Assess client's knowledge regarding each medication. *Rationale: Determines need for drug education and assists in preparing for drug therapy at home.*

5 Assess client's preferences for fluids. Maintain fluid restrictions as prescribed. *Rationale: Offering fluids during drug administration is an excellent way to increase client's fluid intake. Fluids ease swallowing and facilitate absorption from the GI tract. However, fluid restrictions must be maintained.*

PLANNING

Expected Outcomes focus on safe, accurate, and effective drug therapy.

1 Client takes medications as prescribed, with evidence of improvement in condition (e.g., relief of pain, regular heart rate, stable blood pressure).

2 Client explains purpose of medication and drug dose schedule.

Delegation Considerations

In acute care settings, administration of oral medication cannot be delegated. The nurse directs personnel by:

• Instructing about potential side effects of medications and to report their occurrence.

• In some long-term care settings, trained and certified assistive personnel (AP) administer certain nonopioid, nonparenteral medications to stable clients. However, knowledge of desired effects and adverse reactions is very limited; therefore, assessment and evaluation of medication effects remains primarily the responsibility of the nurse.

Equipment

• Medication administration record (MAR)
• Automated, computer-controlled drug dispensing system (Figure 16-2), or medication cart (Figure 16-3)
• Disposable medication cups
• Glass of water, juice, or preferred liquid and drinking straw
• Device for crushing or splitting tablets (optional)

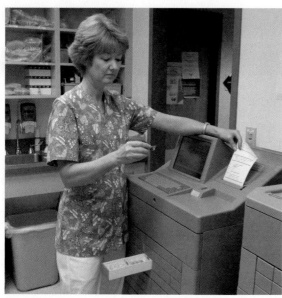

FIGURE 16-2 The nurse removes medications from an automated, computer-controlled drug dispensing system. (From Lilley LL, Harrington S, Snyder JS: *Pharmacology and the nursing process,* ed 4, St Louis, 2004, Mosby.)

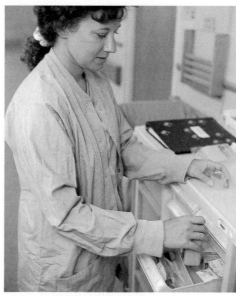

FIGURE 16-3 The nurse removes medications from a drawer in a medication cart, which is kept locked when not in use.

IMPLEMENTATION *for Administering Oral Medications*

STEPS	RATIONALE
1 See Standard Protocol (inside front cover).	
2 Prepare medications.	
a. Compare MAR with scheduled medication list or physician's orders. Check the client's name and the drug name, dosage, route, and time of administration. If discrepancies exist, check against original physician orders.	Physician's order is most reliable source and only legal record of drugs client is to receive. Check orders at least every 24 hours and when client questions a drug order (Lilley, Harrington, and Snyder, 2004).

> **NURSE ALERT** Clarify incomplete or unclear orders with the prescriber before implementation.

| b. Arrange medication tray and cups in medication preparation area, or move medication cart to position outside client's room. | Organization of equipment saves time and reduces error. |

STEPS	RATIONALE
c. Unlock medicine drawer or cart if applicable.	Unauthorized access to medications is prevented when cabinet or cart is locked.
d. Prepare medications for one client at a time. Follow the six rights of medication administration. Keep all pages of MARs or computer printouts for one client together.	Prevents preparation errors.
e. Select correct drug from stock supply, unit-dose drawer, or automated dispensing system. Compare name of medication on the label with MAR or computer printout (see illustration).	Reading label and comparing it against transcribed order reduces errors. *This is the first check for accuracy.*
f. Check drug dose. If dose printed on the package differs from ordered dose, calculate correct amount to give.	Double-checking pharmacy calculations reduces risk of error. Some agencies require nurses to check calculations of certain medications, such as insulin, with another nurse.
g. Check expiration date on medication. Return all outdated drugs to pharmacy.	Medications used past expiration date may be inactive or harmful to client.
h. To prepare unit-dose tablets or capsules, place prepackaged tablet or capsule directly into medicine cup without removing wrapper (see illustration). Give medications only from containers with labels that are clearly marked and legible.	Wrapper identifies drug name and dosage, which can facilitate teaching.
i. To prepare tablets or capsules from a floor stock bottle, pour required number into bottle cap and transfer medication to medication cup. Do not touch medication with fingers. Extra tablets or capsules may be returned to bottle.	Floor stock bottles are often used in long-term care settings for common over-the-counter (OTC) drugs such as laxatives and nonopioid analgesics.
j. Place all tablets or capsules requiring preadministration assessments (e.g., pulse rate, blood pressure) in a separate cup.	Serves as a reminder to complete appropriate assessment and facilitates withholding drugs (if necessary).
k. Medications that must be broken in order to administer half the dose can be broken using a gloved hand or cut with a cutting device. Tablets that are broken in half should be scored, as identified by a manufactured line across the center of the tablet. Unused portions of divided tablets or capsules may be discarded or returned to the original container, depending on agency policy.	Discarding prevents mislabeling by placement in the incorrect container. Returning unused portion is more cost-effective.

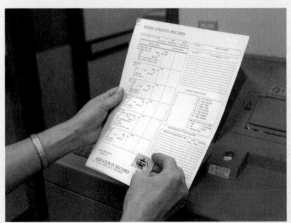

STEP 2e. The nurse compares the MAR to the medication label. (From Lilley LL, Harrington S, Snyder JS: *Pharmacology and the nursing process,* ed 4, St Louis, 2004, Mosby.)

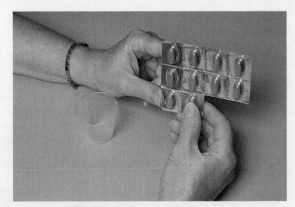

STEP 2h. Place tablet into medicine cup without removing wrapper.

STEPS	RATIONALE
l. If client has difficulty swallowing, use a mortar and pestle or a pill-crushing device (see illustrations). Mix ground tablet in small amount of soft food (custard or applesauce).	Ground tablet mixed with palatable soft food is usually easier to swallow.

> **NURSE ALERT** Not all drugs can be crushed (e.g., capsules, enteric-coated, long-acting/slow-release drugs). The coating of these drugs is designed to protect the stomach from irritation, protect the drug from destruction from stomach acids, or control the rate of release of medication. If a medication has the notation of "extended release," "sustained release," or abbreviations such as "XL," "SR," or "CD," it should not be crushed. Consult with the pharmacist when in doubt or to determine if the medication is available in a liquid, injection, or suppository form that would be more appropriate (Miller and Miller, 2000).

STEPS	RATIONALE
m. When using a blister pack, "pop" medications through foil or paper backing into a medication cup.	Many long-term care agencies use blister packs, which provide about 1 month's supply of prescription drugs for an individual client. Each "blister" usually contains a single dose. Blister packs are prepared by a pharmacist or pharmaceutical company.
n. When preparing liquids, thoroughly mix by shaking gently before administering. Check and discard medications that are cloudy or have changed color.	Liquid medications packaged in single-dose cups need not be poured into medicine cups. Mix liquid suspensions thoroughly just before pouring to ensure that the correct amount of medication, and not just the solvent, is measured for the dose.
(1) Remove bottle cap from container, and place cap upside down.	
(2) Hold bottle with label against palm of hand while pouring.	Spilled liquid will not soil or obscure label.
(3) Place medication cup at eye level on countertop, or when necessary, in hand, and fill to desired level (see illustration).	Ensures accurate measurement.
(4) Wipe lip of bottle with paper towel.	Prevents contamination of bottle's contents and prevents bottle cap from sticking.
(5) If giving less than 5 ml of liquids, prepare medication in an oral dosing syringe (see Figure 16-1). Do not use a hypodermic syringe or a syringe with a needle or syringe cap.	Allows more accurate measurement of small amounts. If hypodermic syringes are used, the medication may accidentally be given parenterally. If the needle or syringe cap is not removed, it may dislodge and become aspirated during administration of oral drugs (ISMP, 2001).
o. When administering controlled drugs such as opioids, check the controlled drug record for previous drug count and compare with supply available. Controlled drugs may be stored in a computerized locked cart (see Chapter 15).	Controlled substance laws require careful monitoring of dispensed opioids. In most facilities, co-signature by a registered nurse (RN) is required when students administer controlled drugs.

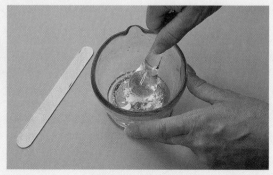 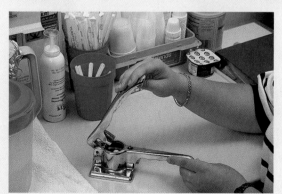

STEP 2l. A, Using a mortar and pestle to grind pills. **B,** Using a pill-crushing device.

STEPS	RATIONALE
p. Before going to client's room, compare MAR with prepared drugs and continue.	Reading labels a second time reduces errors. *This is the second check for accuracy.*
3 Administer medications.	
a. Take medications to client within 30 minutes before or after scheduled time. Stat and single-order medications are given at the exact time ordered.	Promotes intended therapeutic effect.

> **NURSE ALERT** Apply the six rights of medication administration (see Chapter 15).

STEPS	RATIONALE
b. Before going to client's room, compare the MAR or computer printout with the names of medications on the medication labels.	*This is the third check for accuracy and ensures the client receives the correct medication.*
c. Identify client by checking identification bracelet and asking client's name. Compare with MAR. In long-term care settings, client photographs may also be used. Replace any missing, outdated, or faded identification tools.	Ensures correct client receives medication. At least two client identifiers (neither to be the client's room number) are to be used whenever administering medications (JCAHO, 2006).

> **COMMUNICATION TIP** Asking client to state name may elicit a surprised reaction, especially when you have previously established a relationship; however, it is a routine practice that has prevented identification errors. Explain to client why you are asking for his or her name.

STEPS	RATIONALE
d. Perform necessary preadministration assessment (e.g., blood pressure, pulse) for specific medications.	Determines whether specific medications should be withheld at that time.
e. Discuss the purpose of each medication and its action with client. Allow client to ask any questions about drugs.	Client has the right to be informed, and client's understanding of purpose of each medication improves compliance with drug therapy.
f. Assist client to sitting or side-lying position.	Position prevents aspiration during swallowing.

> **NURSE ALERT** If in doubt about client's ability to swallow, check swallow, cough, and gag reflexes (see Box 16-1). If these reflexes are impaired, or if the client is unable to swallow pills without choking, withhold the medication, keep the client NPO, and notify the prescriber. It may be necessary to ask the prescriber to consider administering the drug in another form (crushed, oral liquid, suppository, or by injection).

STEPS	RATIONALE
g. Client may wish to hold solid medications in hand or cup before placing in mouth.	Client becomes familiar with medications by seeing each drug.

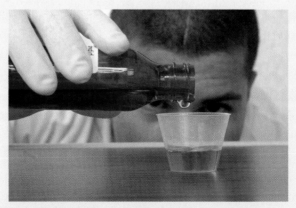

STEP 2n.(3) Measuring liquid medication. Look at meniscus at eye level. (From Lilley LL, Harrington S, Snyder JS: *Pharmacology and the nursing process,* ed 4, St Louis, 2004, Mosby.)

STEPS	RATIONALE
h. If client is unable to hold medications, place medication cup to the lips and gently introduce each drug into the mouth, one at a time. A spoon can also be used to place the pill in the client's mouth. Do not rush or force medications.	Administering single tablet or capsule eases swallowing and decreases risk of aspiration.
i. Offer water or juice to help client swallow medications.	Choice of fluid promotes client's comfort and can improve fluid intake.

> **NURSE ALERT** Be sure there are no interactions between the medications given and the juice used. For example, grapefruit juice interacts with several drugs, such as some calcium channel blockers (Lilley, Harrington, and Snyder, 2004; McKenry, Tessier, and Hogan, 2006).

STEPS	RATIONALE
j. For sublingual-administered drugs, have client place medication under tongue and allow it to dissolve completely. Caution client against swallowing tablet.	Drug is absorbed through blood vessels of undersurface of tongue. If swallowed, drug is destroyed by gastric juices or so rapidly detoxified by liver that therapeutic blood levels are not attained.
k. For buccal-administered drugs, have client place medication in mouth against mucous membranes of the cheek until it dissolves.	Buccal medications act locally on mucosa or systemically as they are swallowed in saliva.

> **NURSE ALERT** If client is to receive a combination of oral tablets, capsules, and sublingual or buccal drugs, administer tablets/capsules first and have client take sublingual and buccal medications last. Do not give liquids until buccal medication has dissolved.

STEPS	RATIONALE
l. Mix powdered medications with liquids at bedside, and give to client to drink.	When prepared in advance, powdered drugs may thicken and even harden, making swallowing difficult.
m. Caution client against chewing or swallowing lozenges.	Drug acts through slow absorption through oral mucosa, not gastric mucosa.
n. Give effervescent powders and tablets immediately after dissolving.	Effervescence improves unpleasant taste of drug and often relieves GI problems.
o. Stay until client has completely swallowed each medication. If concerned about ability or willingness to swallow, ask client to open mouth and inspect for presence of medication.	Nurse is responsible for ensuring that client receives ordered dosage. If left unattended, client may forget to take it, drop it, or intentionally not take dose.
p. For certain medications that should not be given on an empty stomach (e.g., aspirin), offer client nonfat snack (e.g., crackers) if not contraindicated by client's condition.	Reduces gastric irritation. The fat content of foods may delay absorption of the medication.
4 Replenish stock such as cups and straws, return cart to medicine room, and clean work area.	Well-stocked, clean working space assists other staff in completing duties efficiently.
5 See Completion Protocol (inside front cover).	

EVALUATION

1 Return within appropriate time to determine client's response to medications, including therapeutic effects, side effects or allergy, and adverse reactions. Sublingual/buccal medications act in 15 minutes; most oral medications act in 30 to 60 minutes.

2 Ask client or family member to identify drug name and explain purpose, action, dosage schedule, and potential side effects of drug.

Unexpected Outcomes and Related Interventions

1 Client exhibits allergic effects related to the medication (symptoms include urticaria, pruritus, rhinitis, and wheezing) or toxic effects as a result of prolonged high doses or altered excretion.

a. Notify the physician. If symptoms are severe, other drugs may be prescribed to counteract adverse effects.

b. Withhold further doses, notify physician, and provide supportive therapy as prescribed.

2 Tablet or capsule falls to the floor.

a. Discard it and repeat preparation.

3 Client exhibits side effects common to medication.

a. Identify comfort measures that relieve symptoms.

b. Report severe or intolerable side effects to physician. Dosage or form of medication may be changed.

4 Client refuses medication or questions a drug order.

a. Assess reasons the client is refusing the medication. Do not force the client to take the medication; always listen when a client questions an order.

b. Explain the purpose of the medication.

c. Notify the prescriber and document refused medication and client's rationale.

5 Client is unable to explain drug information and is unable or unwilling to remember information about purpose, schedule, or adverse effects.

a. Reassess client's ability to read. Identify family member willing to assume responsibility.

b. Refer to home health agency for discharge follow-up.

c. Utilize appropriate aids to facilitate accurate self-administration, which may include homemade calendars for each week with plastic bags containing medications to take at specific times, egg cartons divided into color-coded sections with medications for each day, clock faces for clients who cannot read or see clearly, or color coding for drug types (e.g., blue for sedative, red for pain pill).

6 Administration error is made (wrong drug, dose, client, route, or time).

a. Acknowledge it immediately.

b. Take measures to counteract the effects of the error if necessary (e.g., keep client on bed rest, administer ordered antidotes, hold other medications if ordered).

c. Monitor client for untoward effects according to the drug action and side effects.

d. Notify physician.

e. Complete medication error form as required by the agency. These reports can assist in preventing similar errors in the future.

Recording and Reporting

- Record actual time each drug was administered on the MAR or computer printout. Do not chart medication administration until *after* it is given to the client. Include initials or signature.

- If drug is withheld, record reason in nurses' notes. Follow facility policy for marking held medications on the MAR. Many facilities require that the nurse circle the time the drug normally would have been given on the MAR or computer printout.

- Report adverse effects/client response and/or withheld drugs to nurse in charge or physician.

Sample Documentation

0900 Apical pulse 50 regular; complains of nausea. Digoxin held and Dr. Jay notified.

Special Considerations

Pediatric Considerations

- Oral liquids available in colorful and palatable forms are preferred for administration of medications to children. Small pills may be aspirated.

- Pediatric doses are usually calculated based on body weight. Nurses are responsible for verifying that the prescribed dose is safe.

- Bitter or distasteful oral preparations will be rejected by the child. Mix the drug with a small amount (about 1 teaspoon) of a sweet-tasting substance, such as jam, applesauce, or fruit puree. Do not use honey in infants because of the risk of botulism. Offer the child juice or an ice pop after medication administration. Do not place medication in an essential food item, such as milk or formula; the child may refuse the food at a later time. Offer a "chaser" of water, juice, or a flavored ice pop after the drug.

- Measure small amount of liquid medications using a plastic calibrated syringe. Amounts less than a teaspoon are impossible to measure accurately with a molded medicine cup. (Hockenberry and Wilson, 2007).

Geriatric Considerations

- Physiological changes of aging may influence how oral medications affect the client. Common changes include reduction in parotid gland secretion, causing dry mouth; delayed esophageal clearance, impairing swallowing; reduction in gastric acidity and stomach peristalsis; reduced liver function, resulting in altered drug metabolism; and reduced renal function and colon motility, slowing drug excretion.

- Administer with a full glass of water (unless restricted) to aid passage of the drug. Give client time to swallow.

- Clients may have several health problems or chronic conditions that require the use of multiple drugs, often prescribed by different health care providers. Polypharmacy creates a high risk for drug interactions and adverse reactions. Assess for potential drug interactions.

- The most common adverse reactions that may occur in older adults are lethargy, sedation, falls, confusion, GI upset, and constipation.

- When instructing clients about their medication regimen, include the client's spouse or another family member.

- If possible, provide a written medication schedule for client to follow at home. Use large print in written materials if vision is impaired (Ebersole and Hess, 2004).

Home Care Considerations

- Instruct client about specific drug regimen (purpose, action, dose, dosage intervals, side effects, food to avoid or take with drugs).

- When measuring liquid medications at home, clients should use kitchen measuring spoons or measuring spoons designed for medications, not eating utensil spoons that may vary in volume.

SKILL 16.2 Administering Medications Through a Feeding Tube

This skill involves the safe administration of oral medications through a feeding tube, which can be either nasogastric (NG) or nasojejunal. Pay specific attention to proper placement of the tube (see Chapter 31) and whether the medication can be safely crushed for administration through the tube. Liquid medications and elixirs are the best choice to administer through a feeding tube, but some medicines come only in tablet form. Most tablets may be crushed; however, those that are sublingual, enteric coated, or sustained release should not be given by tube, because their absorption, metabolism, and effectiveness will be unpredictable. Consult a pharmacist before you crush pills or before you open and dissolve capsules for tube feeding administration.

Do not mix medications in with tube feedings because of potential interruptions in tube feeding flow (e.g., turning feeding off while client is in radiology department), spillage, delayed absorption of the medication, or possible drug precipitation. If a medication is to be administered through an NG tube inserted for decompression, consult the physician because the tube must be clamped for 30 minutes to an hour after instillation of the medication. In most cases, do not administer medications into NG/intestinal tubes that are inserted for decompression of the stomach.

ASSESSMENT

1 Identify the drug(s) ordered: action, purpose, normal dosage and route, common side effects, time of onset and peak action, and nursing implications. *Rationale: This allows you to anticipate effects of drugs and to observe client's response.*

2 Assess for any contraindications to client receiving oral medication: Has the client been diagnosed as having bowel inflammation or reduced peristalsis? Has client had recent GI surgery? Does client have gastric suction? *Rationale: Alterations in GI function interfere with drug distribution, absorption, and excretion. Clients with GI suction might not receive benefit from the medication because it may be suctioned from GI tract before it can be absorbed.*

3 Assess medical history: history of allergies, previous drug regimen, and diet history. *Rationale: These factors can influence how certain drugs act. Information also reflects client's need for medications.*

4 Gather and review assessment data (e.g., bowel sounds, abdominal distention or pain, laboratory data that may influence drug administration). *Rationale: Physical examination findings or laboratory data may contraindicate drug administration.*

5 Assess for potential drug-food interactions if you must administer drugs through a feeding tube. Some drugs, such as phenytoin, warfarin, and fluoroquinolone antimicrobials may require the feeding be stopped for an hour before and 2 hours after the dose (McKenry, Tessier, and Hogan, 2006).

6 Check with the pharmacy for availability of liquid preparations for client's medications. An order from the prescriber may be needed to change the dosage form. *Rationale: Liquid preparations are always preferable to crushing tablets.*

PLANNING

Expected Outcomes focus on administration of appropriate medication via the feeding tube route and avoidance of tube clogging from medication administration as well as safe, accurate, and effective drug therapy.

1 Client experiences desired medication effect within period of onset of medication.

2 Client's feeding tube remains patent after medication administration.

3 Client does not aspirate during or after medication administration.

Delegation Considerations

The skill of administering medications through a feeding tube cannot be delegated. The nurse directs personnel by:

• Instructing about potential side effects of medications and to report their occurrence.

Equipment

• 50- to 60-ml syringe, catheter tip for large-bore tubes, Luer-Lok tip for small-bore tubes
• pH test strip (scale 0.0 to 14.0)
• Graduate container
• Medication to be administered
• Pill crusher if medication in tablet form
• Syringe with needle if medication in gelatin form
• Water
• Tongue blade or straw to stir dissolved medication
• MAR
• Clean gloves (required if handling medications)

IMPLEMENTATION *for Administering Medications Through a Feeding Tube*

STEPS	RATIONALE
1 See Standard Protocol (inside front cover).	
2 Compare MAR with scheduled medication list or physician's orders. Check client's name, drug name, dosage, route, and time of administration. If discrepancies exist, check original physician orders.	Physician's order is most reliable source and only legal record of drugs client is to receive. Check orders at least every 24 hours and when client questions a drug order (Lilley, Harrington, and Snyder, 2004).

STEPS	RATIONALE
3 Select correct drug from stock supply, unit-dose drawer, or automated dispensing system. Compare name of medication on the label with MAR or computer printout.	Reading label and comparing it against transcribed order reduces errors. *This is the first check for accuracy.*
4 Prepare medication for instillation in feeding tube (see Skill 16-1).	Adequate preparation saves nursing time.
a. Check expiration date on medication.	Medications used past expiration date may be inactive or harmful to client.
b. Check drug dose. If dose printed on package differs from ordered dose, calculate correct amount to give.	Double-checking pharmacy calculations reduces risk of error.

> **NURSE ALERT** Apply the six rights of medication administration (see Chapter 15).

STEPS	RATIONALE
c. Verify that medications to be administered do not include any sublingual, enteric-coated, or sustained-release medications.	Crushing these medication forms will alter their absorption and effectiveness (Miller and Miller, 2000).
d. **Tablets:** Crush pill (in its package if possible) with pill crusher (see Skill 16.1). Dissolve the powder in 15 to 30 ml warm water.	Crushing medication in its package prevents some from being lost.
e. **Capsules:** Ensure that contents of capsule (granules or gelatin) can be expressed from the covering (check with pharmacist). Open capsule or pierce gelcap with sterile needle and empty contents into 15 to 30 ml of warm water. Gelcaps can also be dissolved in warm water, but this may take 15 to 20 minutes to occur.	Medication must be prepared properly for administration through the feeding tube.
f. Before going to client's room, compare MAR with labels of prepared drugs and continue.	Reading labels a second time reduces errors. *This is the second check for accuracy.*
5 Take medications to client within 30 minutes before or after scheduled time. Give stat and single-order medications at exact time ordered.	Promotes intended therapeutic effect.
6 At the bedside, again compare the MAR or computer printout with the names of medications on the medication labels.	*This is the third check for accuracy, and ensures the client receives correct medication.*
7 Identify client by checking identification bracelet and asking client's name. Compare with MAR. Replace any missing, outdated, or faded identification tools.	Ensures correct client receives medication. At least two client identifiers (neither to be the client's room number) are to be used whenever administering medications (JCAHO, 2006).
8 Elevate the head of bed to high-Fowler's position (45 to 90 degrees) or reverse Trendelenburg's position if spinal injury is present.	Reduces risk of aspiration, keeping head above stomach.
9 Check placement of feeding tube (see Chapter 31).	Ensures proper tube placement and reduces the risk of introducing fluids into the respiratory tract (Metheny and others, 2005).
10 Check for residual by aspirating stomach contents (see illustration) (see Chapter 31), determine volume with graduate container if necessary, and reinstill to client. If residual volume is greater than 100 ml (or as defined by agency policy), hold the medication and contact the prescriber for orders.	Excess residual volume indicates that gastric emptying is delayed. Administering more fluids may lead to aspiration of gastric contents into the lungs (Ignatavicius and Workman, 2006).
11 Clamp feeding tube by pinching it, and remove the syringe. Draw up 30 ml of water into the syringe, reinsert tip of syringe into the feeding tube, and flush tubing. Clamp feeding tube again, then remove bulb or plunger of syringe, keeping syringe attached to tube.	Clamping the tubing prevents leakage or spillage of stomach contents. Flushing ensures that the tube is patent.

STEPS	RATIONALE

12 Administer medication.

a. Pour first dissolved medication into syringe, and allow to flow by gravity into feeding tube (see illustration).

b. If only one dose of medication is given, flush with 30 to 60 ml of water.

   Ensures medication passes through tube to stomach.

c. To administer more than one medication, give each separately and flush between medications with 15 to 30 ml of water.

   Giving the medications separately allows for accurate identification of medication if a dose is spilled. Also, some medications may be incompatible (Lilley, Harrington, and Snyder, 2004).

d. Follow last medication with 30 to 60 ml of water.

   Avoids tube clogging with medication and ensures medication enters stomach.

13 Clamp the tubing if a tube feeding is not being administered.

   Prevents air from entering the stomach.

14 Assist the client to a comfortable position, and keep the head of the bed elevated for at least 1 hour (per facility policy).

   Promotes adequate passage of the medication through the stomach and reduces risk of aspiration (Ignatavicius and Workman, 2006).

15 **See Completion Protocol (inside front cover).**

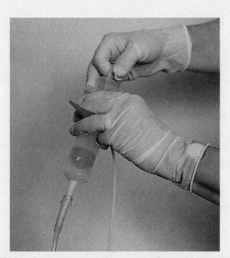

STEP 10 Aspirate stomach contents for residual volume.

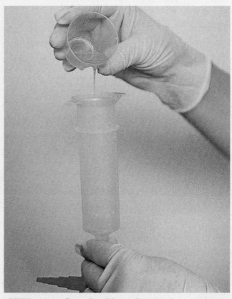

STEP 12a. Pour liquid medication into syringe.

EVALUATION

1 Observe for desired effects within appropriate time frame depending on medication administered.

2 Observe tube patency before and after medication administration.

3 Monitor client for signs of aspiration, such as dyspnea, choking, gurgling speech, or congested breath sounds, during and after medication administration.

Unexpected Outcomes and Related Interventions

1 Client is unable to receive medication because of blockage in tube.

a. For newly inserted tube, notify physician and obtain x-ray confirmation of positioning.

b. Attempt to flush tube with large-bore syringe and warm water to clear clog. (Avoid using a small-bore syringe because this exerts large amounts of pressure and may rupture tube.)

c. If unable to flush clog, contact physician for replacement of tube and potential need to reroute medication if dose cannot be skipped or delayed until a new feeding tube is placed.

2 Client exhibits signs of aspiration, such as respiratory distress, changes in vital signs, and decreased oxygen saturation.

a. Stop the administration of all fluids/medications through the feeding tube.

b. Elevate the head of the bed and stay with the client. Have another staff member notify the client's physician.

c. Assess vital signs, oxygen saturation, and breath sounds.

Recording and Reporting

- Record in nurses' notes the method used to check tube placement (see Chapter 31) and volume of aspirate.
- Record time each drug was administered on the MAR or computer printout. Include initials and signature (check agency policy).
- Report adverse effects, client response, and/or withheld drugs to nurse in charge or physician.

Sample Documentation

NOTE: Documentation for medications via feeding tube is usually done on the MAR, the same as for any other medication. Fluids given without medications must be recorded as intake or I&O. Other documentation occurs only if a problem is noted.

1300 Unable to administer medication because of clogged feeding tube, despite attempts to irrigate. Dr. James notified; medications and tube feeding held pending placement of new tube.

Special Considerations
Geriatric Considerations

- Assess the client for use of medications that may affect the pH of gastric secretions, such as H_2-receptor antagonists or antacids.

Home Care Considerations

- Teach the client or primary caregiver to check placement of tube before administering any medication.
- Instruct the client or primary caregiver not to administer medication and to notify the physician if there is any doubt concerning the placement of the tube.
- Provide the client or primary caregiver with resources to determine which medications can be crushed, which medications should not be crushed, and how to obtain liquid formulations of the medications.
- Instruct the client or primary caregiver about the importance of consistent irrigation of feeding tubes before, during, and after medication administration.

SKILL 16.3 Applying Topical Medications to the Skin

- Nursing Skills Online: Non–Parenteral Medication Administration, Lesson 2

Topical administration of medications involves applying drugs locally to skin, mucous membranes, or tissue membranes. Many topically applied drugs such as lotions, patches, pastes, and ointments can create systemic and local effects if absorbed through the skin. Adhesive-backed medicated patches applied to the skin provide sustained, continuous release of medication over several hours or days. Systemic effects from topical agents can occur if the skin is thin, if drug concentration is high, if contact with the skin is prolonged, or if the drug is applied to broken skin.

Use gloves and applicators to protect yourself from accidental exposure to topical medications. Clean the client's skin gently and thoroughly with soap and water before applying topical medications. When applied over skin encrustations, the dead tissues harbor microorganisms and block contact of medications with the tissues to be treated. Simply applying new medications without cleansing does not offer maximum therapeutic benefit. Follow the correct application procedure for each medication form, such as lotion, powder, or patch, to ensure proper absorption.

2 Assess condition of client's skin (see Chapter 12). Cleanse skin if necessary to visualize adequately. Note if client has symptoms of skin irritation, such as pruritus or burning. Do not administer topical medications to skin where the integrity is altered unless indicated. *Rationale: Assessment provides baseline to determine change in condition of skin after therapy. Topical agents can lessen or aggravate these symptoms.*

3 Determine whether client has a known allergy to latex or the topical agent. Ask if client has had a reaction to a cream or lotion applied to the skin. *Rationale: Allergic contact dermatitis is relatively common and can intensify existing dermatological condition.*

4 Determine amount of topical agent required for application by assessing skin site, reviewing physician's order, and reading application directions carefully (a thin, even layer is usually adequate). *Rationale: An excessive amount of topical agent can cause chemical irritation of skin, negate drug's effectiveness, and/or cause adverse systemic effects, such as decreased white blood cell (WBC) counts.*

5 Determine if client is physically able to apply medication by assessing grasp, hand strength, reach, and coordination. *Rationale: This is necessary if client is to self-administer drug in the home.*

ASSESSMENT

1 Identify the drug(s) ordered: action, purpose, normal dosage and route, common side effects, time of onset and peak action, and nursing implications. *Rationale: Allows you to anticipate effects of drug and to observe client's response.*

PLANNING

Expected Outcomes focus on safe, accurate, and effective drug therapy.

1 Client's condition improves (e.g., relief of pain, inflammation, or itching).

2 Client self-administers topical medication or patch correctly.

3 Client explains purpose of medication, dosage schedule, and possible side effects.

Delegation Considerations

The skill of administering most topical preparations, including patches, cannot be delegated. *Some* lotions and ointments applied to irritated skin or for protection of the perineum may be delegated (check agency policy). Periodic assessment of the affected areas may not be delegated.

Equipment

- Clean gloves (for intact skin) or sterile gloves (for nonintact skin)
- Cotton-tipped applicators or tongue blades
- Ordered medication (powder, cream, ointment, spray, patch)
- Basin of warm water, washcloth, towel, nondrying soap
- Sterile dressing, tape (if needed)
- MAR

IMPLEMENTATION *for Applying Topical Medications to the Skin*

STEPS	RATIONALE
1 See Standard Protocol (inside front cover).	
2 Compare MAR with scheduled medication list or physician's orders. Check the client's name, drug name, dosage, route, and time of administration. If discrepancies exist, check against original physician orders.	Physician's order is most reliable source and only legal record of drugs client is to receive. Check orders at least every 24 hours and when client questions a drug order (Lilley, Harrington, and Snyder, 2004).
3 Select correct drug from stock supply, unit-dose drawer, or automated dispensing system. Compare name of medication on the label with MAR or computer printout.	Reading label and comparing it against transcribed order reduces errors. *This is the first check for accuracy.*
4 Prepare medication for administration.	
a. Check expiration date on medication.	Medications used past expiration date may be inactive or harmful to client.
b. Check drug dose. If dose printed on package differs from ordered dose, calculate correct amount to give.	Double-checking pharmacy calculations reduces risk of error.
c. Before going to client's room, compare name of medication on the label with MAR or computer printout.	Reading label and comparing it against transcribed order reduces errors. *This is the second check for accuracy.*

> NURSE ALERT Apply the six rights of medication administration (see Chapter 15).

5 Take medications to client within 30 minutes before or after scheduled time. Give stat and single-order medications at the exact time ordered.	Promotes intended therapeutic effect.
6 At the bedside, again compare the MAR or computer printout with the names of medications on the medication labels.	*This is the third check for accuracy and ensures the client receives correct medication.*
7 Identify client by checking identification bracelet and asking client's name. Compare with MAR. Replace any missing, outdated, or faded identification tools.	Ensures correct client receives medication. At least two client identifiers (neither to be the client's room number) are to be used whenever administering medications (JCAHO, 2006).
8 Apply topical creams, ointments, and oil-based lotions.	
a. Expose affected area while keeping unaffected areas covered.	Adequate visualization is necessary for evaluation of the effectiveness of treatment.
b. Wash affected area, removing all debris, encrustations, and previous medication.	Removal of debris enhances penetration of topical drug through skin. Cleansing removes microorganisms resident in remaining debris.
c. In some cases, soaking in plain warm water and rinsing without soap are needed to remove crusted tissues.	Minimizes inflammation and irritation of underlying tissue.

STEPS	**RATIONALE**
d. Pat skin dry, or allow area to air-dry.	Excess moisture can interfere with even application of topical agent.
e. If skin is excessively dry and flaking, apply topical agent while skin is still damp.	Retains moisture within skin layers.
f. Remove gloves, and apply new clean or sterile gloves.	Sterile gloves and sterile procedure are used when applying agents to open, noninfectious skin lesions. Changing gloves prevents cross contamination of infected or contagious lesions. Gloves also protect the nurse from drug effects.

> **COMMUNICATION TIP** Tell client what to expect (e.g., "Your skin will feel soothed after the topical application" or "This might feel cold").

STEPS	**RATIONALE**
g. Place required amount of medication in palm of gloved hand and soften by rubbing briskly between hands.	Softening of topical agent makes it easier to apply to skin.
h. After medication is thin and smooth, smear it evenly over skin surface, using long, even strokes that follow direction of hair growth. Apply to thickness as directed by manufacturer's instructions.	Ensures even distribution of medication. Technique prevents irritation of hair follicles.
i. Explain to client that skin may feel greasy after application.	Applications often contain oil.
9 　 Apply antianginal (nitroglycerin) ointment.	
a. Remove previous dosage paper, and wipe off residual medication with a tissue.	Prevents overdose that can occur with multiple dosage papers or excess medication left in place. Wearing gloves protects the nurse from exposure to the medication.
b. Antianginal (nitroglycerin) ointments are usually ordered in inches and can be measured on small sheets of paper marked off in ½-inch markings (McConnell, 2001). Apply desired number of inches of ointment over paper measuring guide (see illustration).	Ensures correct dose of medication.

> **NURSE ALERT** Unit-dose packages are available. (WARNING: One package equals 1 inch; smaller amount should not be measured from this package.)

STEPS	**RATIONALE**
c. Apply nitroglycerin ointment to the chest area, back, upper arm, or legs. Do not apply on hairy surfaces or over scar tissue.	Application on hairy surfaces or scar tissue may interfere with absorption.
d. Be sure to rotate application sites.	Minimizes skin irritation.

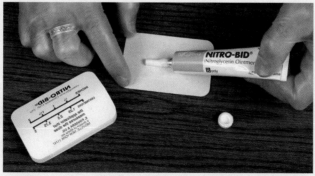

STEP 9b. Antianginal ointment is spread in inches over the measuring guide paper.

STEPS	RATIONALE
e. Apply ointment to skin surface by holding edge or back of the paper wrapper and placing ointment and wrapper directly on the skin (see illustration).	Minimizes chance of ointment covering gloves and later touching nurse's hands.
f. Do not rub or massage ointment into skin.	Medication is designed to absorb slowly over several hours; massaging may increase absorption.
g. Write date, time, and nurse's initials on application paper.	Promotes accuracy.
h. Cover ointment and paper with plastic wrap and tape securely, or follow manufacturer's directions	Prevents staining of clothes or accidental removal of the medication (McConnell, 2001).
10 Apply transdermal patches (e.g., analgesic, nitroglycerin, nicotine, estrogen).	
a. If a patch is present, remove the old patch and wipe the skin clean.	Failure to remove old patches may result in overdose (Schulmeister, 2005).
b. Dispose of old patch carefully (per facility policy).	Proper disposal prevents accidental exposure to medication.
c. Choose a clean, dry area of the body that is free of hair. Do not apply the patch on skin that is oily, burned, cut, or irritated in any way.	Ensures complete medication absorption.

NURSE ALERT Estrogen patches should never be applied to the breast tissue or waistline.

STEPS	RATIONALE
d. Carefully remove the patch from its protective covering (see illustration). Hold the patch by the edge without touching the adhesive edges.	Touching only the edges ensures that the patch will adhere and that the medication dosage has not been changed.
e. Immediately apply the patch, pressing firmly with the palm of one hand for 10 seconds. Make sure it sticks well, especially around the edges. Date and initial patch, and note time.	Adequate adhesion prevents loss of the patch, which results in decreased dosage and effectiveness. Visual reminders of dose applications prevent missing doses.
f. Advise clients not to use heating pads anywhere near the site.	Heat increases circulation and the rate of absorption.
g. Instruct client that transdermal patches are never to be cut in half; a change in dosage would require a prescription for a new strength of transdermal medication.	Cutting a transdermal patch in half would alter the intended medication delivery of the transdermal system, resulting in inadequate or altered drug levels.

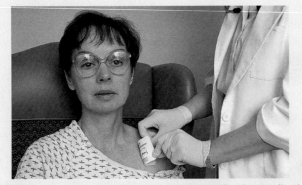

STEP 9e. Nurse applies dosage paper with medication to client's skin.

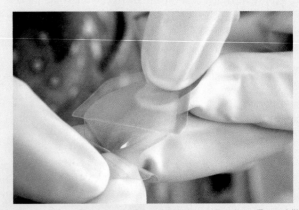

STEP 10d. Opening a transdermal patch medication. (From Lilley LL, Harrington S, Snyder JS: *Pharmacology and the nursing process*, ed 4, St Louis, 2004, Mosby.)

STEPS	RATIONALE

> **NURSE ALERT** It is recommended that nitroglycerin transdermal patches be removed after 10 to 12 hours to allow for a nitrate-free interval and reduce the chance of tolerance to the medication. Check with the client's prescriber (Lilley, Harrington, and Snyder, 2004).

STEPS	RATIONALE
h. Avoid previously used sites for at least 1 week.	Minimizes skin irritation.
i. Caution clients to not use alternative forms of medications or drugs when using patches. For example, clients should not smoke while using a nicotine patch. Clients should not apply nitroglycerin ointment in addition to the patch unless specifically ordered to do so by their physician.	Use of patch with an additional/alternative preparation of drug can result in toxicity and other side effects.
11 Administer aerosol sprays (e.g., local anesthetic sprays).	
a. Shake container vigorously.	Mixes contents and propellant to ensure distribution of a fine, even spray.
b. Read container's label for distance recommended to hold spray away from area, usually 6 to 12 inches (15 to 30 cm).	Proper distance ensures fine spray hits skin surface. Holding container too close results in thin, watery distribution.
c. If neck or upper chest is to be sprayed, ask client to turn face away from spray or briefly cover face with towel.	Prevents inhalation of spray.
d. Spray medication evenly over affected site (in some cases, spray is timed for period of seconds).	Entire affected area of skin should be covered with thin spray.
12 Apply suspension-based lotion.	
a. Shake container vigorously.	Mixes powder throughout liquid to form well-mixed suspension.
b. Apply small amount of lotion to small gauze dressing or pad, and apply to skin by stroking evenly in direction of hair growth.	Method of application leaves protective film of powder on skin after water base of suspension dries. Technique prevents irritation of hair follicles.
c. Explain to client that area will feel cool and dry.	Water evaporates to leave thin layer of powder.
13 See Completion Protocol (inside front cover).	

EVALUATION

1 Inspect condition of skin between applications to determine if skin condition improves.
2 Observe client applying topical medication or patch.
3 Ask the client or significant other to name the medication and its purpose, dosage, schedule, and side effects.

Unexpected Outcomes and Related Interventions

1 Skin site may appear inflamed and edematous with blistering and oozing of fluid from lesions, or client continues to complain of pruritus and tenderness.
a. Notify prescriber; additional or alternative therapies may be needed.
2 Client is unable to explain information about topical application or does not administer as prescribed.
a. Identify possible reasons for noncompliance and explore alternative approaches or options.

Recording and Reporting

- Describe objective data (appearance of abnormal skin, including size, shape, and characteristics of lesions) and subjective data (such as complaints of pain and itching) in nurses' notes.
- Report and record changes in appearance and condition of skin lesions.

Sample Documentation

0930 Skin on the back of both hands and wrists is dry, red, and flaky. Complains of itching. Hydrocortisone cream 1% applied sparingly to affected areas as prescribed.

1000 Reported itching is relieved.

Special Considerations
Geriatric Considerations
- Handle older persons gently, and observe for changes that may occur in the skin of the older client, including (Lewis, Heitkemper, and Dirksen, 2004):
  - Increased wrinkling
  - Slowness of skin to flatten when pinched together (tenting)
  - Dry, flaking skin with possible signs of excoriation caused by pruritus
  - Increased tendency to bruise
  - Increased tendency for skin to tear, especially if adhesive tape is applied

- Diminished awareness of pain, touch, temperature
- Diminished rate of wound healing

Home Care Considerations
- Instruct client on safe disposal techniques at home. Used patches should be folded with medication sides together and wrapped in newspaper before discarding. Used applicators or patches are placed into cardboard or plastic disposable containers. Children and pets may become ill if they ingest or handle used patches; careful disposal is necessary to ensure safety in the home.

SKILL 16.4   Instilling Eye and Ear Medications

- Nursing Skills Online: Non–Parenteral Medication Administration, Lessons 3 and 4

Eye (ophthalmic) medications commonly used by clients include both topical drops and ointments. Intraocular disks are a third type of medication delivery option. Medications resemble a contact lens. The disk is placed into the conjunctival sac, not the cornea, where it remains in place for as long as 1 week.

Many clients receive prescribed ophthalmic drugs after cataract extraction and for eye conditions such as glaucoma. Eye medications come in a variety of concentrations. Instilling the wrong concentration may cause local irritation to eyes, as well as systemic effects. Certain eye medications that dilate or constrict the pupil, such as mydriatics and cycloplegics, temporarily blur a client's vision. Use of the wrong drug concentration can prolong these undesirable effects. Orders for eye medications must indicate administration to one or both eyes.

The eye is extremely sensitive because the cornea is richly supplied with sensitive nerve fibers to protect the eye. The conjunctival sac is much less sensitive and thus a more appropriate site for medication instillation. Care is taken to prevent instilling medication directly onto the sensitive cornea.

Clients receiving topical eye medication should learn correct self-administration of the medication. Clients with glaucoma, for example, usually require lifelong eye drops for control of their disease. At times it may become necessary for family members to learn how to administer eye drops or ointment, particularly immediately after eye surgery, when clients' vision is so impaired that it is difficult for them to assemble needed supplies and handle applicators correctly.

Medications used in the ear are usually in a solution and instilled by drops. Internal ear structures are very sensitive to temperature extremes, and therefore solutions are administered at room temperature. When drops are instilled cold from a refrigerator, the client may experience vertigo (severe dizziness) or nausea.

Although structures of the outer ear are not sterile, it is wise to use sterile drops and solutions because the eardrum can rupture without the awareness of the client or nurse. Introduction of nonsterile solutions into the middle ear can cause serious infection. Avoid forcing solution into the ear or occluding the ear canal with a medicine dropper, because medication administered under pressure within the canal can injure the eardrum.

ASSESSMENT

1   Identify the drug(s) ordered: action, purpose, normal dosage and route, common side effects, time of onset and peak action, and nursing implications. *Rationale: This allows you to anticipate effects of drugs and to observe client's response.*

2   Assess condition of external eye or ear structures (see Chapter 12). *Rationale: This may also be done just before drug instillation to provide a baseline to determine later if local response to medications occurs. This also indicates the need to clean the area before drug application.*

3   Determine whether client has symptoms of discomfort or hearing or visual impairment. *Rationale: Certain eye medications can act to either lessen or increase symptoms. Occlusion of external ear canal by swelling, drainage, or cerumen can impair hearing acuity and is painful.*

4   Determine whether client has any known allergies to medications. Also, ask if client has allergies to latex, if using latex gloves.

5   Assess client's LOC and ability to follow instructions. *Rationale: Client must lie still during drug administration. Sudden movements can cause injury from eye or ear dropper.*

6   Assess client's knowledge regarding drug therapy and desire to self-administer medication. Assess client's ability

to manipulate and hold dropper. *Rationale: Client's level of under-standing may indicate need for health teaching. Motivation influences teaching approach. Reflects client's ability to learn to self-administer medication.*

7 Assess client's ability to manipulate and hold dropper or ocular disks. *Rationale: Reflects client's ability to self-administer drug.*

PLANNING

Expected Outcomes focus on relief of symptoms without unpleasant adverse reactions and safe, accurate, and effective drug therapy.

1 Client states that symptoms (e.g., irritation, dryness) are relieved.

2 Client denies unpleasant side effects or adverse reactions.

3 Client describes medication effects and technique of application.

4 Client correctly demonstrates self-instillation of eye drops or ear drops.

Delegation Considerations

The skills of administering eye/ear drops may not be delegated. The nurse directs personnel by:

- Instructing about potential side effects of medications and to report their occurrence, including vision impairment.

Equipment

- Appropriate medication (eye drops with sterile dropper, ointment tube, medicated intraocular disk, or ear drops)
- Cotton-tipped applicator, cotton balls, or tissue
- Warm water and washcloth
- Clean gloves
- Eye patch and tape (optional)
- MAR

IMPLEMENTATION *for Instilling Eye and Ear Medications*

STEPS	RATIONALE
1 See Standard Protocol (inside front cover).	
2 Compare MAR with scheduled medication list or physician's orders. Check the client's name, drug name, dosage, route, and time of administration. If discrepancies exist, check against original physician orders.	Physician's order is most reliable source and only legal record of drugs client is to receive. Check orders at least every 24 hours and when client questions a drug order (Lilley, Harrington, and Snyder, 2004).
3 Select correct drug from stock supply, unit-dose drawer, or automated dispensing system. Compare name of medication on the label with MAR or computer printout.	Reading label and comparing it against transcribed order reduces errors. *This is the first check for accuracy.*
4 Prepare medication for administration.	
a. Check expiration date on medication.	Medications used past expiration date may be inactive or harmful to client.
b. Check drug dose/concentration. If dose/concentration printed on package differs from what is ordered, calculate correct amount to give.	Double-checking pharmacy calculations reduces risk of error.
c. Before going to client's room, compare name of medication on the label with MAR or computer printout.	Reading label and comparing it against transcribed order reduces errors. *This is the second check for accuracy.*

> **NURSE ALERT** Review the six rights of medication administration (see Chapter 15).

STEPS	RATIONALE
5 At the bedside, again compare the MAR or computer printout with the names of medications on the medication labels.	*This is the third check for accuracy and ensures the client receives correct medication.*
6 Identify client by checking identification bracelet and asking client's name. Compare with MAR. Replace any missing, outdated, or faded identification tools.	Ensures correct client receives medication. At least two client identifiers (neither to be the client's room number) are to be used whenever administering medications (JCAHO, 2006).
7 Explain procedure to client. Clients experienced in self-instillation may be allowed to give drops under nurse's supervision (check agency policy).	Clients often become anxious about medication being instilled into eye because of potential discomfort.

STEPS	RATIONALE

COMMUNICATION TIP Tell clients receiving mydriatics or cycloplegics that vision will be temporarily blurred, and that photophobia (sensitivity to light) may occur. They should not drive or attempt to perform any activity that requires acute vision or sensitivity to light until vision returns to normal.

8 Instill eye drops.

a. Ask client to lie supine or sit back in chair with neck slightly hyperextended.

Position provides easy access to eye/ear for medication instillation. Correct positioning minimizes drainage of eye medication into tear duct.

b. If crusting or drainage is present along eyelid margins or inner canthus, gently wash away from inner to outer canthus. If indicated, soak any crusting with a warm, damp washcloth for several minutes.

Cleansing eye from inner to outer canthus avoids introducing microorganisms into lacrimal ducts. Soaking allows easy removal of crusts that harbor microorganisms.

NURSE ALERT Do not hyperextend the neck of a client with a cervical neck injury.

c. Instill drops by holding clean tissue in nondominant hand on client's cheekbone just below lower eyelid.

Tissue absorbs medication that escapes eye. Avoid cotton balls, which may leave fibers that may get into the eyes.

d. With tissue resting below lower lid, gently press downward with thumb or forefinger against bony orbit, exposing conjunctival sac (see illustration).

Prevents pressure and trauma to eyeball and prevents fingers from touching eye.

e. Ask client to look at ceiling.

Moves the sensitive cornea up and away from conjunctival sac and reduces stimulation of blink reflex.

f. Rest dominant hand gently on client's forehead, and hold filled medication eyedropper approximately 1 to 2 cm (½ to ¾ inch) above conjunctival sac.

Resting hand helps prevent accidental contact of eyedropper with eye and reduces risk of injury and transfer of microorganisms to dropper. Contact of eyedropper with eye contaminates the container (ophthalmic medications are sterile).

g. Drop prescribed number of medication drops into conjunctival sac.

Conjunctival sac normally holds 1 or 2 drops. Applying drops to sac provides even distribution of medication across eye.

h. If client blinks or closes eye, causing drops to land on outer lid margins, repeat procedure.

Therapeutic effect of drug is obtained only when drops enter conjunctival sac.

i. When administering drugs that may cause systemic effects, apply gentle pressure to client's nasolacrimal duct with a tissue for 30 to 60 seconds. Avoid pressure directly against client's eyeball.

Prevents overflow of medication into nasal and pharyngeal passages. Minimizes absorption into systemic circulation.

j. After instilling drops, ask client to close eyes gently.

Helps to distribute medication. Squinting or squeezing of eyelids forces medication from conjunctival sac. Distributes medication evenly across eye and lid margin.

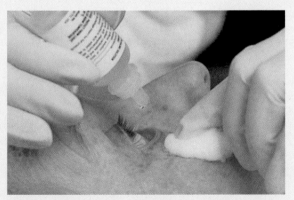

STEP 8d. Instilling eye drops into the nonjunctival sac.

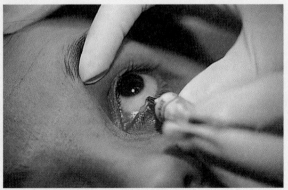

STEP 9b. Applying eye ointment along the inside edge of the lower eyelid on the conjunctiva from the inner to outer canthus.

STEPS	RATIONALE

9 Instill eye ointment.

a. Ask client to look up.
    Moves the sensitive cornea up and away from the conjunctival sac and reduces stimulation of the blink reflex during ointment application.

b. Holding ointment applicator above lower lid margin, apply thin ribbon of ointment evenly along inner edge of lower eyelid on conjunctiva (see illustration) from the inner canthus to the outer canthus.
    Distributes medication evenly across eye and lid margin.

c. Have client close eye, and rub lid lightly in circular motion with a tissue, if rubbing is not contraindicated.
    Further distributes medication without traumatizing eye. Avoid pressure directly against client's eyeball.

d. If excess medication is on eyelid, gently wipe it from inner to outer canthus.
    Promotes comfort and prevents trauma to eye.

10 If client needs an eye patch, apply clean one by placing it over affected eye so entire eye is covered. Tape securely without applying pressure to eye.
    Clean eye patch reduces chance of infection.

11 Apply intraocular disk.

a. Open package containing the disk. Gently press your fingertip against the disk so that it adheres to your finger. Position the convex side of the disk on your fingertip. It may be necessary to moisten gloved finger with sterile saline.
    Allows you to inspect disk for damage or deformity.

b. With your other hand, gently pull the client's lower eyelid away from the eye. Ask client to look up.
    Prepares conjunctival sac for receiving medicated disk and moves sensitive cornea away.

c. Place the disk in the conjunctival sac, so that it floats on the sclera between the iris and lower eyelid (see illustration).
    Ensures delivery of medication.

d. Pull the client's lower eyelid out and over the disk. You should not be able to see the disk at this time. Repeat if you can see the disk (see illustration).
    Ensures accurate medication delivery.

12 Remove intraocular disk.

a. Gently pull downward on the lower eyelid.
    Exposes the disk.

b. Using your forefinger and thumb of your opposite hand, pinch the disk and lift it out of the client's eye (see illustration).

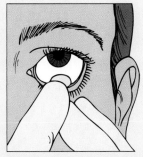

STEP 11c. Place disk in the conjunctival sac between the iris and lower eyelid.

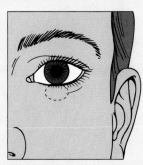

STEP 11d. Gently pull lower eyelid over the disk.

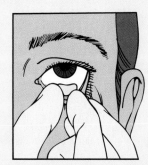

STEP 12b. Carefully pinch the disk to remove it from client's eye.

STEPS	RATIONALE
c. If excess medication is on eyelid, gently wipe it from inner to outer canthus.	Promotes comfort and prevents trauma to eye.
d. If client had eye patch, apply clean one by placing it over affected eye so entire eye is covered. Tape securely without applying pressure to eye.	Clean eye patch reduces chance of infection.

13 Instill ear drops.

STEPS	RATIONALE
a. Apply gloves if drainage is present.	
b. Warm medication to room temperature by running warm water over the bottle (making sure not to damage the label or allow water to enter the bottle).	Ear structures are very sensitive to temperature extremes. Cold may cause vertigo and nausea.
c. Position client on side or sitting in a chair with affected ear facing up. Stabilize the client's head with his or her hand.	Facilitates distribution of medication into ear.
d. Straighten ear canal by pulling auricle upward and outward (adult or child older than age 3) or down and back (child) (see illustrations).	Straightening of ear canal provides direct access to deeper external ear structures. Anatomical differences in younger children and infants require different methods of doing this (Lilley, Harrington, and Snyder, 2004).
e. If cerumen or drainage occludes outermost portion of ear canal, wipe out gently with cotton-tipped applicator, taking care not to force wax inward.	Cerumen and drainage harbor microorganisms and can block distribution of medication into canal. Occlusion blocks sound transmission.
f. Instill prescribed drops, holding dropper 1 cm (½ inch) above ear canal.	Avoiding contact prevents contamination of the dropper, which could contaminate the medication in the container.
g. Ask client to remain in side-lying position 5 to 10 minutes, and apply gentle massage or pressure to tragus of ear with finger (see illustration).	Allows complete distribution of medication. Pressure and massage move medication inward.
h. If ordered, gently insert a portion of cotton ball into outermost part of canal. Do not press cotton into canal.	Prevents escape of medication when client sits or stands.
i. Remove cotton after 15 minutes. Assist client to comfortable position after drops are absorbed.	Allows adequate time for drug distribution and absorption.

14 See Completion Protocol (inside front cover).

STEPS	RATIONALE

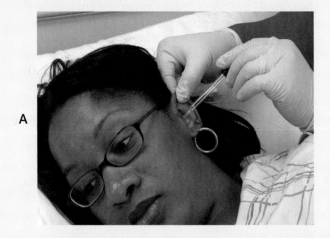

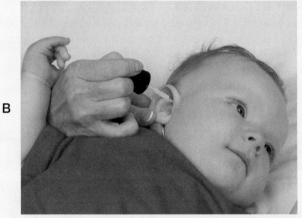

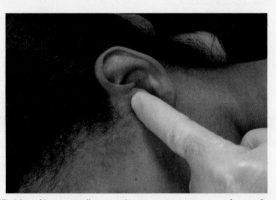

STEP 13d. A, Pull the pinna *up* and *outward* for adults and children older than age 3. **B,** Pull the pinna *down* and *back* for children age 3 or younger. (From Lilley LL, Harrington S, Snyder JS: *Pharmacology and the nursing process,* ed 4, St Louis, 2004, Mosby.)

STEP 13g. Nurse applies gentle pressure to tragus of ear after instilling drops.

EVALUATION

1 Observe effects of medication by evaluating desired changes.
2 Note client's response to instillation, observe for side effects, and ask if any discomfort was felt.
3 Ask client to discuss drug's purpose, action, side effects, and technique of administration.
4 Observe client demonstrate self-administration of next dose.

Unexpected Outcomes and Related Interventions

1 Client complains of burning or pain after administration of eye drops.
a. Use greater caution during next instillation to instill drops into conjunctival sac and not onto the cornea.

2 Client experiences local side effects, for example, headache, bloodshot eyes, and local eye irritation.
a. Monitor closely and notify prescriber if needed.
3 Client experiences systemic effects from eye drops, for example, increased heart rate and blood pressure from epinephrine or decreased heart rate and blood pressure from timolol. Local anesthetics and antibiotics can cause anaphylaxis.
a. Systemic absorption through tear duct can cause potentially dangerous effects. Monitor client and notify prescriber.
4 Client experienced increased ear pain. Rupture of eardrum may have occurred.
a. Notify prescriber immediately.
5 Ear canal remains occluded with cerumen.
a. Irrigation may be required.

6 Client lacks confidence or ability to instill medication without supervision.

a. If client is unable to manipulate the dropper or is unable to see, instruct a family member in the technique.

Recording and Reporting

- Include objective data related to condition of tissues involved (redness, drainage, irritation) and subjective data (discomfort, itching, altered vision or hearing).
- Include evaluation related to desired effects of medications instilled and evidence of any side effects experienced.

Sample Documentation

1300 Complaining of dry and irritated eyes. Redness noted on both sclerae. Artificial Tears 2 drops instilled into each eye after eyes cleansed.

Special Considerations

Pediatric Considerations

- When instilling drops in an infant or young child, have another nurse gently restrain child's head with child in parent's lap. Be sure that the child's hands do not interfere with instillation.

- Infants often clench the eyes tightly to avoid eye drops. To administer drops in an uncooperative infant, with the head gently restrained, place the drops at the nasal corner where the lids meet. When the infant opens the eye, the medication will flow into the eye.
- Use cotton pledgets to prevent medication from flowing out of external canal. They should be inserted loosely enough to allow any discharge to exit from ear. To prevent cotton from absorbing medication in ear, premoisten cotton with a few drops of medication (Hockenberry and others, 2003).

Geriatric Considerations

- Many older adults experience excessive accumulation of cerumen in the ear. This should be removed before administration of medication.

Home Care Considerations

- Have clients with chronic health problems consult their health care provider before using over-the-counter (OTC) eye medications.
- Clients should not share eye drops with other family members. Risk of infection transmission is high.

SKILL 16.5 Using Metered-Dose Inhalers (MDI)

- **Nursing Skills Online: Non–Parenteral Medication Administration, Lesson 5**

MDIs are handheld inhalers that dispense a measured dose of aerosol spray, mist, or fine powder to penetrate lung airways. The deeper passages of the respiratory tract provide a large surface area for drug absorption. The alveolar-capillary network absorbs medication rapidly.

Inhaled medications are designed to produce local effects; for example, bronchodilators open narrowed bronchioles, and mucolytic agents liquefy thick mucous secretions. However, because these medications are absorbed rapidly through the pulmonary circulation, most create systemic side effects. For example, albuterol dilates bronchioles and can also cause nervousness and tremors.

Clients who receive drugs by inhalation frequently have chronic respiratory disease. Because clients depend on medications for airway management, they need to know how to administer them safely. It is *not* appropriate to try to teach a client how to use an inhaler during an episode of shortness of breath, because the client's ability to learn is greatly diminished.

Drugs can be delivered by MDIs, which deliver a measured dose of drug with each push of a canister. Because use of an MDI requires coordination during the breathing cycle, clients may spray only the back of their throats thus not receive a full dose. The inhaler must be depressed to expel medication just as the client inhales. This ensures the medication reaches the lower airways. Difficulty with coordination can be resolved by the use of spacer devices, breath-activated inhalers, or dry powder inhalers (DPIs) (Figure 16-4).

EVIDENCE IN PRACTICE

Rubin DK, Durotoye L: How do clients determine that their metered dose inhaler is empty? *Chest* 126(4):1134-1137, 2005.

Clients who use MDIs need to know how to determine whether the medication is depleted. For years, clients were taught to measure the amount of medication remaining in a canister of an MDI by floating it in a container of water. The angle of flotation, or the degree of sinking, was thought to indicate whether the canister was full, half-full, or empty. However, this method is not reliable because of differences in canister sizes and designs. In addition, exposing the neck of the actuation valve to water may cause damage. Recent research by Rubin and Durotoye (2005) found that clients used a variety of methods to determine if a canister was empty, but none of the methods were found to be reliable. Consequently, the medication canister is used long past its intended duration. The researchers recommended that when MDIs do not have built-in dose counters, instruction

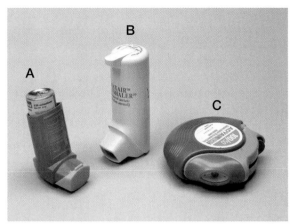

FIGURE 16-4 Types of inhalers. **A,** Metered-dose inhaler (MDI). **B,** Breath-activated inhaler. **C,** Dry powder inhaler (DPI). (From Lilley LL, Harrington S, Snyder JS: *Pharmacology and the nursing process,* ed 4, St Louis, 2004, Mosby.)

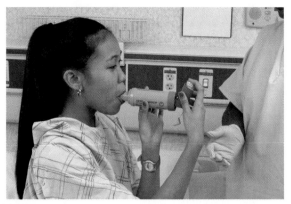

FIGURE 16-5 Using a spacer device with an MDI. (From Lilley LL, Harrington S, Snyder JS: *Pharmacology and the nursing process,* ed 4, St Louis, 2004, Mosby.)

in dose counting (calculating the number of puffs used per day and calculating how many days the inhaler should last) is vital to correct MDI use.

ASSESSMENT

1 Identify the drug(s) ordered: action, purpose, concentration, route, common side effects, time of onset and peak action, and nursing implications. *Rationale: This allows you to anticipate effects of drugs and to observe client's response.*

2 Assess respiratory pattern and auscultate breath sounds. *Rationale: Establishes baseline of airway status for comparison during and after treatment.*

3 Assess client's ability to hold, manipulate, and depress canister and inhaler. *Rationale: Impairment of grasp or presence of tremors of hands interferes with client's ability to depress canister within inhaler.*

4 Assess client's readiness to learn: Client asks questions about medication, disease, or complications; requests education in use of inhaler; is mentally alert; and participates in own care.

5 Assess client's ability to learn: Client should not be fatigued, in pain, or in respiratory distress; assess level of understanding of terms.

6 Assess client's knowledge and understanding of disease and purpose and action of prescribed medications. *Rationale: May assist in assessing client's potential for compliance with self-administration.*

NURSE ALERT If the client is to receive inhaled bronchodilators and inhaled corticosteroids at the same time, the bronchodilators should be given first to promote opening of the airways. After 5 minutes, administer the second drug (McKenry, Tessier, and Hogan, 2006).

PLANNING

Expected Outcomes focus on relief of symptoms; promoting knowledge for self-administration of inhalers; and safe, accurate, and effective drug therapy.

1 Client manipulates mouthpiece, canister, and inhaler correctly and cleans inhaler after use.

2 Client describes proper time during respiratory cycle to inhale spray and number of inhalations for each administration.

3 Client's breathing pattern improves, and airways become less restrictive, with adequate gas exchange.

4 Client lists side effects of medications and criteria for calling health care professional if dyspnea develops.

Delegation Considerations

The skill of administering MDIs should not be delegated. The nurse directs personnel by:

• Instructing about potential side effects of medications and to report their occurrence.

Equipment

• Inhaler device with medication canister (MDI or DPI) (see Figure 16-4)
• Spacer device, such as AeroChamber or InspirEase (optional) (Figure 16-5)
• Facial tissues (optional)
• MAR
• Stethoscope
• Pulse oximeter (optional)

IMPLEMENTATION *for Using Metered-Dose Inhalers (MDI)*

STEPS	RATIONALE
1 See Standard Protocol (inside front cover).	
2 Compare MAR with scheduled medication list or physician's orders. Check the client's name, drug name, number of inhalations prescribed, concentration, route, and time of administration. If discrepancies exist, check against original physician orders.	Physician's order is most reliable source and only legal record of drugs client is to receive. Check orders at least every 24 hours and when client questions a drug order (Lilley, Harrington, and Snyder, 2004).
3 Select correct drug from stock supply, unit-dose drawer, or automated dispensing system. Compare name of medication on the label with MAR or computer printout.	Reading label and comparing it against transcribed order reduces errors. *This is the first check for accuracy.*
4 Prepare medication for administration.	
a. Check expiration date on medication.	Medications used past expiration date may be inactive or harmful to client.
b. Check drug dose/concentration. If dose/concentration printed on package differs from what is ordered, calculate correct amount to give.	Double-checking pharmacy calculations reduces risk of error.
c. Before going to client's room, compare name of medication on the label with MAR or computer printout.	Reading label and comparing it against transcribed order reduces errors. *This is the second check for accuracy.*

> **NURSE ALERT** Review the six rights of medication administration (see Chapter 15).

5 At the bedside, again compare the MAR or computer printout with the names of medications on the medication labels.	*This is the third check for accuracy and ensures the client receives correct medication.*
6 Identify client by checking identification bracelet and asking client's name. Compare with MAR. Replace any missing, outdated, or faded identification tools.	Ensures correct client receives medication. At least two client identifiers (neither to be the client's room number) are to be used whenever administering medications (JCAHO, 2006).
7 Allow client opportunity to manipulate inhaler, canister, and spacer device (if provided). Explain and demonstrate how canister fits into inhaler.	Client must be familiar with how to assemble and use equipment.
8 Explain what metered dose is, and warn client about overuse of inhaler, including drug side effects.	Client needs to know the dangers of excessive inhalations because of risk of serious side effects. If drug is given in recommended doses, side effects are minimal.
9 Remove mouthpiece cover from inhaler. Shake inhaler well, three or four times.	Ensures mixing of medication in canister.

> **NURSE ALERT** If using an MDI that is new or has not been used for several days, push a "test spray" into the air once or twice to prime the device before using. This ensures that the MDI is patent and that the metal canister is positioned properly (Togger and Brenner, 2001).

10 Without spacer device:	
a. Have client take a deep breath and exhale completely. Place lips around the mouthpiece, inhale slowly through the mouth, and simultaneously depress the top of the inhaler canister (see illustration).	Directs aerosol spray toward the airway. Correct coordination of breathing with inhaler activation ensures adequate absorption of medication (Capriotti, 2005).
b. An alternative technique is to position the mouthpiece 2 to 4 cm (1 to 2 inches) from the widely open mouth, with the opening of the inhaler toward the back of the throat. Lips should not be touching the inhaler (see illustration).	Directs aerosol spray toward the airway.

STEPS	RATIONALE

> **NURSE ALERT** A spacer device may be used with MDIs to facilitate medication inhalation when clients have trouble coordinating breathing and depressing the canister. Releasing the medication into the chamber allows the client extra time to inhale the medication and increases the amount of medication that reaches the lungs. Puffs are administered one at a time, and the client should breathe slowly after depressing the inhaler. The nurse should assess whether a spacer would improve MDI administration (see Figure 16-4) (Capriotti, 2005).

11 Instruct client to tilt head back slightly, inhale slowly and deeply through mouth, and depress medication canister fully.

Medication is distributed to airways during inhalation.

12 Instruct client to breathe in slowly for 2 to 3 seconds. Hold breath for approximately 10 seconds.

As client inhales, particles of medication are delivered to airway. Holding breath allows tiny drops of aerosol spray to reach deeper branches of airways (Capriotti, 2005).

13 Instruct client to exhale slowly through pursed lips.

Pursed-lip breathing keeps small airways open during exhalation.

14 After 30 seconds, these steps may be repeated if more than one puff is prescribed (Capriotti, 2005).

First inhalation opens airways. Second or third inhalations penetrate deeper airways.

15 If more than one type of inhaled medications is prescribed, wait 5 to 10 minutes between inhalations or as ordered by physician.

Drugs are prescribed at intervals during day to promote bronchodilation and minimize side effects.

> **COMMUNICATION TIP** Explain that there should not be a gagging sensation in the throat. These sensations occur when inhalers are used incorrectly.

16 If steroid medications are administered via MDI, instruct client to rinse mouth.

Removing medication residue from oral cavity area reduces risk of oral yeast infection (oral candidiasis) (Lilley, Harrington, and Snyder, 2004).

17 Instruct client to remove medication canister and clean inhaler in warm water after each use.

Accumulation of spray around the mouthpiece can interfere with proper distribution during use.

18 Instruct client against repeating inhalations before next scheduled dose.

Drugs are prescribed at intervals during the day to provide constant drug levels and minimize side effects.

19 Teach client to keep track of doses used by noting the first day of use on the canister and calculating doses that will be used. For example, if 2 puffs are taken 3 times a day, and an inhaler has a capacity for 200 inhalations, then 2 puffs times 3 times a day equals 6 inhalations per day. Six divided into 200 indicates that the inhaler will last approximately 33 days, assuming that the client does not use extra doses.

This technique will help clients keep track of doses remaining in the inhaler canister (Capriotti, 2005). Floating the inhaler canister in water is not a reliable method for determining the amount of medication remaining (Rubin and others, 2005).

20 **See Completion Protocol (inside front cover).**

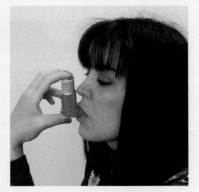

STEP 10a. Using an MDI.

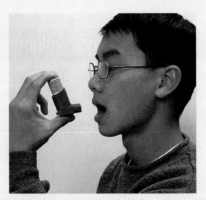

STEP 10b. Alternative technique for using an MDI.

EVALUATION

1 Have client explain and demonstrate steps in use and cleaning of inhaler.
2 Ask client to explain drug schedule and dose of medication.
3 After medication instillation, assess client's respirations, breath sounds, and SpO_2 (with pulse oximeter).
4 Ask client to list side effects and criteria for calling physician.

Unexpected Outcomes and Related Interventions

1 Client's breathing pattern is ineffective; respirations are rapid and shallow, and gas exchange is inadequate. Client's need for a bronchodilator more than every 4 hours can signal respiratory problems. Notify the physician.
a. Reassess type of medication or delivery method. Make sure client shakes canister before administration.
b. Determine fullness of canister.
c. Wait adequate time between puffs to allow deeper penetration into the lungs.
d. Observe whether the canister is releasing a spray. If not, the valve may need to be cleaned.
2 Client experiences gags or paroxysms of coughing from inability to inhale.
a. Reinstruct on proper way to inhale.
3 Client is experiencing cardiac arrhythmias. Signs and symptoms of overuse of sympathomimetic drugs include tachycardia, palpitations, headache, restlessness, and insomnia.
a. Notify physician; monitor heart rate and rhythm.
4 Client is unable to depress medication canister because of weakened grasp or presses the canister before or after taking a breath.
a. Client may need practice with assistance for several different steps of procedure before being able to perform each skill independently.
b. Alternative delivery routes or methods may need to be explored. Assess potential benefits of a spacer device.

Recording and Reporting

- Include objective data related to the desired effects of the MDI (e.g., respiratory rate and pattern, breath sounds).
- Include evidence of side effects (e.g., heart rate, client's description of feelings experienced [anxiety and others]).
- Include ability to demonstrate correct use of the MDI.

Sample Documentation

0900 Coughing violently and reports difficulty breathing. Wheezing noted throughout all lung fields. R 32, P 98. Self-administered MDI (2 puffs) correctly with no verbal coaching. Reported relief from shortness of breath within 1 minute.

0915 Reports breathing more at ease, R 24, P 94.

Special Considerations
Pediatric Considerations

- Because of difficulty with coordination of activating inhaler and inhaling, the use of a spacer device is recommended for young children (Hockenberry and Wilson, 2007).
- Educate child and parent about the need to use inhaler during school hours. Help family find resources within the school or day care facility. Keep in mind that many school systems do not permit self-administration of MDIs. Follow the school's policy regarding having the MDI available for use during school hours. A physician's order is required.

Geriatric Considerations

- Older adult client may be unable to depress medication canister because of weakened grasp. If there is difficulty with coordinating activation of the inhaler and inhalation, the use of a spacer device may be helpful.

Home Care Considerations

- Remind clients to carry prescribed inhalers with them at all times to use as immediate treatment in case of an acute asthma attack.

SKILL 16.6 Using Small-Volume Nebulizers

Nebulization is a process of adding medications or moisture to inspired air by mixing particles of various sizes with air. Adding moisture to the respiratory system through nebulization may improve clearance of pulmonary secretions. Medications such as bronchodilators, mucolytics, and corticosteroids are often administered by nebulization. Nebulizers provide medications in an aerosolized form that can be inhaled by the client into the tracheobronchial tree and possibly into the bloodstream through the alveoli. As a result, systemic effects from the medications may occur. In the hospital setting, medications may be given with nebulization bottles and tubing that are attached to an air compressor in the wall. In some facilities, and in the home setting, a small-volume nebulizer provides a portable way to receive these medications.

Clients who receive drugs by nebulization frequently suffer from chronic lung disease characterized by airway hyperreactivity or constriction. Because clients depend on these medications for adequate oxygenation, they must learn how they work and how to administer them safely.

ASSESSMENT

1 Identify the drug(s) ordered: action, purpose, normal dosage and route, common side effects, time of onset and peak action, and nursing implications. *Rationale: This allows you to anticipate effects of drugs and to observe client's response.*

2 Assess client's medical history, history of allergies, and medication history. *Rationale: These factors can influence how certain drugs act. Information also reflects client's need for medications.*

3 Assess client's ability to assemble, hold, and manipulate the nebulizer equipment. *Rationale: Impaired grasp or presence of hand tremors interferes with client's ability to use the equipment.*

4 Assess pulse, respirations, and breath sounds before beginning treatment. *Rationale: Establishes a baseline for comparison during and after treatment.*

PLANNING

Expected Outcomes focus on safe, accurate, and effective drug therapy; relief of symptoms; and promoting knowledge for self-administration of small-volume nebulizers.

1 Client's breathing patterns are effective and gas exchange is adequate.

2 Client describes techniques for use of small-volume nebulizers.

3 Client correctly self-administers medication using small-volume nebulizer.

4 Client correctly describes care of and cleaning of small-volume nebulizer and equipment.

5 Client lists side effects of medications and criteria for calling health care professional if dyspnea develops.

Delegation Considerations

The skill of administering medications by nebulizer cannot be delegated; however, in many institutions, respiratory therapists may also perform administration of nebulizer medications. The nurse directs personnel by:

- Instructing personnel on the side effects to report, should they develop.

Equipment

- Medication ordered
- Diluent (if needed)
- Nebulizer bottle and tubing assembly
- Small-volume nebulizer machine (often called handheld nebulizer or, simply, nebulizer) or access to wall compressed air mechanism
- Stethoscope
- MAR
- Pulse oximeter (optional)

IMPLEMENTATION *for Using Small-Volume Nebulizers*

STEPS	RATIONALE
1 See Standard Protocol (inside front cover).	
2 Compare MAR with scheduled medication list or physician's orders. Check the client's name, drug name, dosage/concentration, route, and frequency of administration. If discrepancies exist, check against original physician orders.	Physician's order is most reliable source and only legal record of drugs client is to receive. Check orders at least every 24 hours and when client questions a drug order (Lilley, Harrington, and Snyder, 2004).
3 Select correct drug from stock supply, unit-dose drawer, or automated dispensing system. Compare name of medication on the label with MAR or computer printout.	Reading label and comparing it against transcribed order reduces errors. *This is the first check for accuracy.*
4 Prepare medication for administration.	
a. Check expiration date on medication.	Medications used past expiration date may be inactive or harmful to client.
b. Check drug dose/concentration. If dose/concentration printed on package differs from what is ordered, calculate correct amount to give.	Double-checking pharmacy calculations reduces risk of error.
c. Check amount and type of diluent (if unit dose is not available).	Unit-dose medications do not require dilution; however, a diluent may be used along with a unit-dose medication if a different concentration of drug is desired.
d. Before going to client's room, compare MAR with selected drugs and continue.	Reading labels a second time reduces errors. *This is the second check for accuracy.*
5 Take medications to client within 30 minutes before or after scheduled time. Stat and single-order medications are given at the exact time ordered.	Promotes intended therapeutic effect.

STEPS	RATIONALE
6 At the bedside, again compare the MAR or computer printout with the names of medications on the medication labels.	*This is the third check for accuracy and ensures the client receives correct medication.*
7 Identify client by checking identification bracelet and asking client's name. Compare with MAR. Replace any missing, outdated, or faded identification tools.	Ensures correct client receives medication. At least two client identifiers (neither to be the client's room number) are to be used whenever administering medications (JCAHO, 2006).

> **NURSE ALERT** Review the six rights of medication administration (see Chapter 15).

8 Explain the use of the nebulizer, and describe possible drug side effects.	Helps to make the client more knowledgeable about the treatment and the medication.

> **NURSE ALERT** Some respiratory medications cause systemic effects such as restlessness, nervousness, and palpitations. Administer these medications with caution to clients with cardiac disease because of the possibility of hypertension, arrhythmias, or coronary insufficiency. If severe bronchospasm occurs during treatment, discontinue drug immediately, and notify physician. Monitor client closely.

> **COMMUNICATION TIP** Do not try to teach client how to use a nebulizer during an episode of shortness of breath.

9 Assemble the nebulizer equipment per manufacturer's directions.	Assembly may vary slightly with different manufacturers. Proper assembly ensures safe delivery of medication.
10 Add the prescribed medication and diluent (if needed) to the nebulizer.	Ensures proper dosage and delivery of ordered medication.
11 Have client hold the mouthpiece between the lips with gentle pressure (see illustration).	
a. Use a face mask for a child; an infant; or an adult who is fatigued, who cannot follow instructions, or who is unable to follow instructions.	Use of a face mask does not require the client to remember to hold mouthpiece correctly. Correct delivery ensures sufficient deposition of medication.
b. Use special adaptors for clients with a tracheostomy.	
12 Have client take a deep breath, slowly, to a volume slightly greater than normal. After inspiration have the client pause briefly, then have the client exhale passively.	Promotes greater deposition of medication in the airways.
a. If client is dyspneic, encourage client to hold every fourth or fifth breath for 5 to 10 seconds.	Improves effectiveness of medication.
13 Turn on the small-volume nebulizer machine, and ensure that a sufficient mist is formed.	Verifies that the equipment is working properly during delivery of medication.
a. Tap the nebulizer cup occasionally during treatment and toward the end of the treatment.	Releases droplets that may be clinging to the side of the cup, thus allowing for renebulization of the solution.

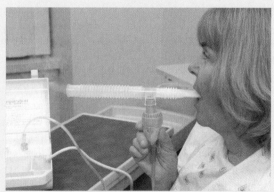

STEP 11 Nebulizer mouthpiece placed between client's lips during treatment.

STEPS	RATIONALE
b. Remind client to repeat the breathing pattern described in Step 12 until the drug is completely nebulized. Some practitioners prefer to set a time limit as the length of the treatment (e.g., 20 minutes) rather than waiting for the medication to completely nebulize.	Maximizes effectiveness of medication.
c. Monitor client's pulse for tachycardia during procedure, especially if beta-adrenergics are used. If tachycardia occurs, stop the procedure and notify the physician.	Helps observe for potential side effects of medications. Stopping the treatment helps to reduce the adverse effects (Lilley, Harrington, and Snyder, 2004).
14 When medication is completely nebulized and liquid is gone, turn off machine and store tubing assembly per agency policy.	Proper storage reduces transfer of microorganisms.
a. Shake the nebulizer bottle, attempting to remove all remaining solution.	
b. Teach client not to store medication in nebulizer for later use.	Stored medication may contain microorganisms, and medication may lose effectiveness.
15 If steroids are nebulized, have client rinse mouth and gargle with warm water after nebulizer treatment.	Removes medication residue from oral cavity and helps to prevent thrush, a possible side effect of therapy with these drugs (Lilley, Harrington, and Snyder, 2004).
16 See Completion Protocol (inside front cover).	

EVALUATION

1 Measure client's pulse, respiratory rate, breath sounds, and SpO_2 (if indicated) after procedure.
2 Have client describe techniques for use of small-volume nebulizer.
3 Observe while client self-administers medication using small-volume nebulizer.
4 Ask client to explain and demonstrate care of and cleaning of small-volume nebulizer and equipment.
5 Ask client to describe side effects of medications and criteria for calling physician.

Unexpected Outcomes and Related Interventions

1 Client's breathing pattern is ineffective; respirations are rapid and shallow; SpO_2 is less than 90%.
a. Reassess type of medication or delivery method. Notify physician.
2 Client experiences paroxysms of coughing. Aerosolized particles irritate posterior pharynx.
a. Notify prescriber; may need to reassess type of medication or delivery method.
3 Client experiences cardiac arrhythmias as a side effect of medication.
a. Notify prescriber; monitor heart rate and rhythm.
4 Client is unable to self-administer medication properly.
a. Alternative delivery routes or methods may need to be explored.

5 Client is unable to explain technique and risks of drug therapy.
a. Further teaching may be required.
b. Include family in any instruction; they can serve as coaches.

Recording and Reporting

• Record the drug used, dosage and concentration, and time and date of administration on the MAR or computer printout immediately after administration.
• Record the client's baseline pulse, respirations, and breath sounds.
• Record the client's response to the medication, including pulse, respirations, and breath sounds assessed.
• Document skills taught and client's ability to perform them.

Sample Documentation

0900 Reports that he "cannot catch his breath" after getting up to the bathroom. Dyspnea noted, with R 32, P 95, and scattered wheezes throughout lung fields bilaterally. Albuterol 2.5 mg given by nebulizer over 20 minutes. Postnebulizer R 26, P 102; wheezes decreased. States he is "breathing easier now."

Special Considerations
Pediatric Considerations
- Use a mask for the nebulizer treatment if the child is too young to hold the mouthpiece correctly for the duration of the treatment.
- Instruct the child to breathe normally with the mouth open to provide a direct route to the airways for the medication (Hockenberry and Wilson, 2007).
- Use a peak flow meter before and after the treatment to monitor the child's airway status (McKenry, Tessier, and Hogan, 2006).
- Educate child and parent about the need to use nebulizer during school or day care hours. Help family find resources within the school or day care facility. Follow the school's policy regarding having the nebulizer and medication available for use during school hours. A physician's order may be necessary.

Home Care Considerations
- When used at home, the nebulizer parts should be rinsed after each use with clear water and air-dried. In addition, the parts should be cleaned daily with warm, soapy water, rinsed, and allowed to dry.
- Once a week the nebulizer parts should be soaked in a solution of vinegar and water (one part white vinegar to four parts water) for 30 minutes, rinsed thoroughly with clean water, and air-dried. Nebulizer parts should never be stored until totally dried. Wet equipment encourages the growth of bacteria and mold (Lilley, Harrington, and Snyder, 2004).
- Follow manufacturer's recommendations for maintenance of small-volume nebulizer machine, including changing the filters when they become discolored (grayish).
- Advise clients taking long-acting beta-agonists, which are used for long-term control of symptoms, about possible adverse effects: nervousness, restlessness, tremor, headache, nausea, rapid or pounding heart rate, and dizziness. Emphasize that the drug should be taken only as ordered so that a tolerance to the drug is not developed.

SKILL 16.7 Inserting Rectal and Vaginal Medications

- Nursing Skills Online: Non–Parenteral Medication Administration, Lesson 6

Drugs administered rectally exert either a local effect on GI mucosa, such as promoting defecation, or systemic effects, such as relieving nausea or providing analgesia. The rectal route is not as reliable as oral or parenteral routes in terms of drug absorption and distribution. However, the medications are relatively safe and rarely cause local irritation or side effects. Rectal medications are contraindicated in clients who have had rectal surgery or have active rectal bleeding.

Vaginal medications also exert local or systemic effects. Female clients who develop vaginal infections require topical application of antiinfective agents. Estrogens are available in vaginal creams. Vaginal medications are also available in foam, gel, or suppository form. Medicated irrigations or douches may also be ordered for cleansing. However, their excessive use can lead to vaginal irritation.

Suppositories come individually packaged in foil wrappers and are usually stored in a refrigerator to prevent melting. *Caution:* Rectal and vaginal suppositories may be stored together in a refrigerator. Rectal suppositories are thinner than vaginal suppositories and bullet shaped (Figure 16-6). The rounded end prevents anal trauma during insertion. To administer a suppository, place it past the internal sphincter and against the rectal mucosa. Avoid placing a rectal suppository into a mass of fecal material.

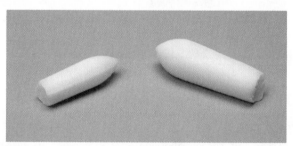

FIGURE 16-6 Vaginal suppositories *(right)* are larger and more oval than rectal suppositories *(left)*. (From Lilley LL, Harrington S, Snyder JS: *Pharmacology and the nursing process,* ed 4, St Louis, 2004, Mosby.)

After a suppository is inserted into either the rectum or vagina, body temperature melts the suppository so the medication can be distributed. Clients may prefer self-administering suppositories. If possible, allow privacy when the client is capable of self-administering without difficulty. Proper placement is important to promote retention of the medication until it dissolves and is absorbed into the mucosa. If necessary, obtain a physician's order to administer a small cleansing enema to evacuate the lower bowel before inserting the suppository.

ASSESSMENT

1 Identify the drug(s) ordered: action, purpose, normal dosage and route, common side effects, time of onset and peak action, and nursing implications. *Rationale: This allows you to anticipate effects of drugs and to observe client's response.*

2 Inspect condition of external genitalia and anal area (may be done just before insertion). *Rationale: Provides a baseline to determine later if local response to medication occurs.*

3 Ask if client is experiencing any symptoms of pruritus, burning, rectal bleeding, or discomfort. *Rationale: May indicate adverse effects.*

4 Review client's knowledge of purpose of drug therapy, as well as ability and willingness to self-administer medication.

5 Review medical record for history of rectal surgery or bleeding. *Rationale: May alter tissue integrity and level of discomfort. May contraindicate use of suppository.*

PLANNING

Expected Outcomes focus on relief of symptoms without unpleasant side effects and on safe, accurate, and effective drug therapy.

1 Client reports relief of symptoms (e.g., discomfort, itching, constipation).

2 Client is able to self-administer suppository correctly.

3 Client explains purpose of medication, side effects, and steps to use for proper suppository insertion.

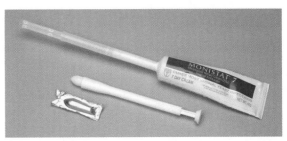

FIGURE 16-7 *From top:* Vaginal cream with applicator, applicator, and vaginal suppository. (From Lilley LL, Harrington S, Snyder JS: *Pharmacology and the nursing process,* ed 4, St Louis, 2004, Mosby.)

Delegation Considerations

The skills of administering rectal and vaginal medications cannot be delegated. Judgment must be used regarding allowing the client to self-administer rectal or vaginal medications. The nurse directs personnel by:

- Instructing about potential side effects of medications and to report their occurrence.

Equipment

- Clean gloves
- Suppository
- Lubricant (water soluble)
- Suppository inserter (vaginal only)
- Vaginal creams or foam instillation (Figure 16-7)
- Vaginal cream or foam in plastic tube or can
- Perineal pad (optional)
- MAR

IMPLEMENTATION *for Inserting Rectal and Vaginal Medications*

STEPS	RATIONALE
1 See Standard Protocol (inside front cover).	
2 Compare MAR with scheduled medication list or physician's orders. Check the client's name, drug name, dosage, route, and time of administration. If discrepancies exist, check against original physician orders.	Physician's order is most reliable source and only legal record of drugs client is to receive. Check orders at least every 24 hours and when client questions a drug order (Lilley, Harrington, and Snyder, 2004).
3 Select correct drug from stock supply, unit-dose drawer, or automated dispensing system. Compare name of medication on the label with MAR or computer printout.	Reading label and comparing it against transcribed order reduces errors. *This is the first check for accuracy.*
4 Prepare medication for administration.	
a. Check expiration date on medication.	Medications used past expiration date may be inactive or harmful to client.
b. Check drug dose. If dose printed on package differs from what is ordered, calculate correct amount to give.	Double-checking pharmacy calculations reduces risk of error.
c. Before going to client's room, compare name of medication on the label with MAR or computer printout.	Reading label and comparing it against transcribed order reduces errors. *This is the second check for accuracy.*
5 Take medications to client within 30 minutes before or after scheduled time. Stat and single-order medications are given at the exact time ordered.	Promotes intended therapeutic effect.

STEPS	RATIONALE
6 At the bedside, again compare the MAR or computer printout with the names of medications on the medication labels.	*This is the third check for accuracy and ensures the client receives correct medication.*
7 Identify client by checking identification bracelet and asking client's name. Compare with MAR. Replace any missing, outdated, or faded identification tools.	Ensures correct client receives medication. At least two client identifiers (neither to be the client's room number) are to be used whenever administering medications (JCAHO, 2006).

> **NURSE ALERT** Review the six rights of medication administration (see Chapter 15).

8 Administer rectal suppository.

a. Assist client in assuming a left side-lying Sims' position with upper leg flexed upward.	Position exposes anus and helps client to relax external anal sphincter. Left side lessens the likelihood of the suppository or feces being expelled.
b. Keep client covered with only anal area exposed.	Maintains privacy and facilitates relaxation.
c. Examine condition of anus externally, and palpate rectal walls as needed (see Chapter 12).	Determines presence of active rectal bleeding. Palpation determines whether rectum is filled with feces, which may interfere with suppository placement.

> **NURSE ALERT** Do not palpate a client's rectum after rectal surgery. For clients with hemorrhoids, use a liberal amount of lubricant and gently manipulate the tissues to visualize the anus. Generally, rectal suppositories are contraindicated in the presence of active rectal bleeding and diarrhea (McKenry, Tessier, and Hogan, 2006).

d. Discard soiled gloves.	Minimizes contact with fecal material to reduce transmission of infection.
e. Remove suppository from foil wrapper, and lubricate rounded end with water-soluble lubricant.	Lubrication reduces friction as suppository enters rectal canal. Leaving the wrapper in place may cause damage to the rectal wall (ISMP, 2006).
f. Retract client's upper buttock with nondominant hand. Ask client to take slow, deep breaths through mouth and to relax anal sphincter.	Forcing suppository through constricted sphincter causes discomfort.
g. With gloved index finger of dominant hand, insert suppository, rounded end first gently through anus, past internal sphincter, and against rectal wall, 10 cm (4 inches) in adults (see illustration).	Inserting the suppository against the rectal wall enhances the effectiveness of the medication; inserting the suppository into a mass of fecal material reduces the medication's effectiveness.
h. Wipe client's anal area, and discard gloves by turning them inside out and disposing of them in appropriate receptacle.	Inverting the gloves contains the microorganisms and prevents contamination of other articles.
i. Ask client to remain on side for 5 to 10 minutes or until urge to eliminate is strong.	Prevents expulsion of suppository. Provides sufficient time for suppository to reach maximum effectiveness.

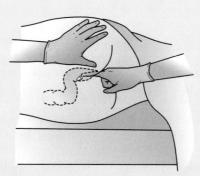

STEP 8g. Inserting a rectal suppository.

STEPS	RATIONALE

j. If client has difficulty retaining the suppository, hold client's buttocks together for 30 seconds.

Helps the suppository to stay in place, especially in clients who have poor sphincter control.

k. If suppository contains laxative or fecal softener, place call light within reach so client can obtain assistance to reach bedpan or toilet.

Ability to call for assistance provides client with sense of control over elimination.

9   Administer vaginal suppository.

a. Assist client with lying in dorsal recumbent position with abdomen and lower extremities covered.

Provides easy access to vaginal canal and allows suppository to dissolve in vagina without leaking out.

b. Be sure vaginal orifice is well illuminated. If needed, cleanse perineal area.

Proper insertion requires visualization of external genitalia if not self-administered.

c. Remove suppository from foil wrapper, and apply liberal amount of water-soluble lubricant. Lubricate gloved index finger of dominant hand.

Lubrication reduces friction against mucosal surfaces during insertion. Use of petroleum jelly may leave a residue that harbors bacteria and fungi.

d. With nondominant gloved hand, gently retract labial folds to expose vaginal orifice.

e. Insert rounded end of suppository along posterior wall of vaginal canal entire length of finger (7.5 to 10 cm, or 3 to 4 inches) (see illustration).

Proper placement of suppository ensures equal distribution of medication along walls of vaginal cavity.

f. Wipe away remaining lubricant from around orifice and labia. Wipe the applicator clean (if used), rinse with warm water, and dry before storing. Remove and discard gloves.

Cleansing the area promotes comfort. Cleansing applicator prepares it for use with the next dose.

g. Tell client there may be a small amount of discharge that is the color of medication exiting from vaginal canal. Instruct client to remain supine for at least 10 minutes. Client may wish to use disposable panty liners.

As the medication liquefies at body temperature, it is absorbed; however, small amounts may ooze from the vaginal canal.

10   Administer vaginal cream or foam.

a. Fill cream or foam applicator following package directions.

Dose is instilled based on volume in applicator.

b. With nondominant gloved hand, gently retract labial folds to expose vaginal orifice.

c. With dominant gloved hand, insert applicator approximately 5 to 7.5 cm (2 to 3 inches). Push applicator plunger to deposit medication into vagina (see illustration).

d. Withdraw applicator, and place on paper towel. Wipe off residual cream from labia or vaginal orifice. Wipe the applicator clean, rinse with warm water, and dry before storing.

Residual cream on applicator may contain microorganisms.

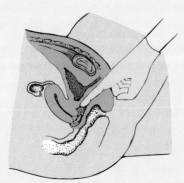

STEP 9e. Vaginal suppository insertion.

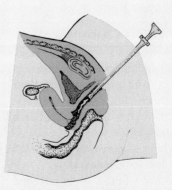

STEP 10c. Applicator inserted into vaginal canal.

STEPS	RATIONALE
e. Instruct client to remain supine for at least 10 minutes. f. Offer disposable panty liners for use during ambulation.	Medication will be distributed and absorbed more evenly. Small amounts of medication may ooze from the vaginal orifice.

11 **See Completion Protocol (inside front cover).**

EVALUATION

1 Ask client about relief of symptoms for which medication was prescribed.

2 Inspect condition of vagina or rectum, external genitalia, and anal area between applications. Ask about the presence of itching, burning, or discomfort.

3 Ask client to discuss purpose, side effects, and method of administration of medication.

Unexpected Outcomes and Related Interventions

1 Vaginal yeast infections may develop, characterized by thick, white, patchy, curdlike discharge.

a. Report findings to physician; vaginal infections often are treated with topical application of antiinfective agents.

2 Client reports localized pruritus and burning, which may indicate infection or inflammation.

a. Report symptoms to physician. Antiinfective agent may be ordered.

3 Client reports rectal pain during insertion of a rectal suppository.

a. Use more lubrication before inserting suppository.

b. The rectal route may be contraindicated; consult with physician.

Recording and Reporting

- Record appearance of external genitalia and anal area in nurses' notes, and report any unusual findings.
- Record drug name, dosage, time administered, and route on MAR.
- Record and report client's ability to self-administer, as well as response to medication.

Sample Documentation

0800 Complains of constipation. Has not had bowel movement for 3 days. Dulcolax suppository given per rectum as ordered. Expelled large, hard, dark-brown stool. States feeling much relieved. Encouraged to drink more fluids, to choose high-fiber foods from menu, and to ambulate as much as possible to prevent further problems. Verbalized understanding and willingness to comply.

Special Considerations
Pediatric Considerations

- With children it may be necessary to gently hold the buttocks together for 5 to 10 minutes to relieve pressure on the anal sphincter until the urge to expel the suppository is gone (Hockenberry and Wilson, 2003).

Geriatric Considerations

- Older adult clients with loss of sphincter control may have difficulty retaining suppository.
- Older female clients may experience vaginal atrophy and dryness and may require very generous lubrication of suppositories and applicators.

Home Care Considerations

- If the client will be self-administering suppositories at home, be sure to provide thorough instructions. Clients have been known to insert suppositories without removing wrappers, and even have swallowed them orally. Always give specific instructions (ISMP, 2006).

NCLEX® Style Questions

1 The nurse should include which instruction when teaching the client about using transdermal patches for chronic pain management?

1. Apply the patch to the same spot each day for consistent dosing.
2. If the client experiences severe sedation, cut the patch in half for the next dose.
3. If pain is not relieved, apply a second patch without removing the first one.
4. Remove the old patch and cleanse the area before applying a new patch.

2 Prior to giving a rectal suppository, the nurse assesses for which contraindication?

1. Rectal hemorrhoids
2. Diarrhea
3. Constipation
4. Stool in the rectum

3 Which nursing action is correct when giving an MDI medication to a client?

1. Administer the corticosteroid first, then the bronchodilator, if two different medications are due at the same time.
2. Give two puffs in rapid succession if the client is experiencing severe dyspnea.
3. Rinse the mouth with water thoroughly after taking inhaled corticosteroids.
4. Determine whether the inhaler is empty by shaking it or performing a test spray.

4 When administering ear drops to a 2-year-old child, how should the nurse hold the child's ear?

1. Pull the pinna down and back before administering the ear drops.
2. Pull the pinna up and outward before administering the ear drops.
3. Retract the tragus out from ear canal.
4. Have infant sit up and pull pinna forward.

5 Arrange the steps in the correct order to follow when giving medications through a feeding tube.

1. Administer each medication, flushing with 15-30 ml of water after each medication.
2. After last medication, flush tubing with 30 to 60 ml of water.
3. Prepare medication for administration through the feeding tube (e.g., crushing tablets as appropriate, pouring liquid medications).
4. Aspirate contents to measure residual volume, and reinstill residual to client.
5. Flush tubing with 30 ml of water.
6. Check for correct placement of feeding tube.

References for all chapters appear in Appendix D.

Administration of Injections

MEDIA RESOURCES

- **evolve** http://evolve.elsevier.com/Elkin
- **Video Clips**
- **Nursing Skills Online**

Injections instill medications into body tissues for systemic absorption. Injected drugs are more quickly absorbed than oral medications, and these routes may be used when clients are vomiting, cannot swallow, and/or are restricted from taking oral fluids. Injections are administered through three routes:

- *Subcutaneous:* injection into tissues just below the dermis of the skin
- *Intramuscular (IM):* injection into the body of a muscle
- *Intradermal:* injection into the dermis just under the epidermis

Injections are invasive. Use strict aseptic technique during preparation and administration to minimize the risk of infection. Injections involve some discomfort. Because risk of tissue or nerve damage exists, site selection is an important nursing concern. You must monitor the client's response closely and know potential side effects or allergic reactions.

SYRINGES

Syringes are single dose and disposable. They are packaged separately, in a paper wrapper or rigid plastic container. Syringes come with or without a sterile needle or with a needleless device. The parts of a syringe are shown in Figure 17-1. Syringes are classified as either Luer-Lok or non–Luer-Lok. Non–Luer-Lok syringes use needles that slip onto the tip. Luer-Lok syringes (Figure 17-2, A) use standard needles or needleless devices that are twisted onto the tip and lock themselves in place. The Luer-Lok design prevents the accidental removal of the needle from the syringe.

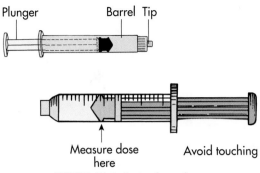

FIGURE 17-1 Parts of a syringe.

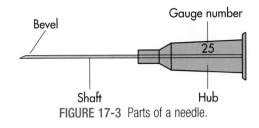

FIGURE 17-3 Parts of a needle.

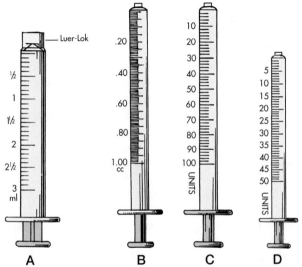

FIGURE 17-2 Types of syringes. **A,** 3-ml Luer-Lok syringe marked in 0.1 (tenths). **B,** Tuberculin syringe marked in 0.01 (hundredths) for doses of less than 1 ml. **C,** Insulin syringe marked in units (100). **D,** Insulin syringe marked in units (50) for low dose.

Syringes come in a variety of sizes, ranging in capacity from 0.3 to 60 ml (see Figure 17-2). When you select a syringe, choose the smallest syringe size possible to improve accuracy of medication preparation. In addition, you must avoid injecting a large volume of fluid into tissues. It is unusual to use a syringe larger than 5 ml for IM injections. A larger volume creates discomfort. Syringes are most commonly marked in a scale by tenths of a milliliter (Figure 17-2, A). Tuberculin (TB) syringes, which are marked in hundredths, are used to measure very small dosages (Figure 17-2, B).

Insulin syringes (Figure 17-2, C and D) hold 0.3 to 1 ml, come with preattached needles, and are calibrated in units. Insulin syringes that hold 30 units and 50 units are known as low-dose syringes and are easier to read. Clients with visual problems and children with diabetes mellitus often use these syringes. Some insulin syringes have a single scale in increments of 2 units, and others have a dual scale that allows for odd and even-numbered doses. Insulin syringes in the United States and Canada are U-100s, designed for use with U-100 strength insulin. Each milliliter of solution contains 100 units of insulin. Before use, examine the syringe to determine which measurement scale is marked on the syringe to ensure that the correct syringe is being used to prepare the ordered medication.

NEEDLES

Needles come packaged in individual sheaths to allow flexibility in choosing the right needle for a client. Some needles are preattached to standard-size syringes. A needle has three parts: the hub, which fits onto the tip of the syringe; the shaft, which connects to the hub; and the bevel, or slanted tip (Figure 17-3). The needle hub, shaft, and bevel must remain sterile at all times. To prevent contamination, place the needle onto the syringe with the cap intact using gentle force.

The tip of a needle, or the bevel, is always slanted. The bevel creates a narrow slit when injected into tissue that quickly closes as the needle is removed, to prevent leakage of medication, blood, or serum. Longer beveled tips are sharper and narrower, which minimizes discomfort from a subcutaneous or IM injection.

Needles vary in length from ¼ to 3 inches (Figure 17-4). Often they are color-coded for ease of selection. Use longer needles (1 to 1½ inches) for IM injections and shorter needles (⅜ to ⅝ inch) for subcutaneous injections. Choose the needle length according to the client's size and weight and the type of tissue into which the drug is to be injected. Children and very small, thin adults generally require a shorter needle. The smaller the needle gauge is, the larger the needle diameter. The selection of a gauge depends on the viscosity of fluid to be injected. For example, a larger 22-gauge 1½-inch needle is typically used for IM injections. A smaller 25-gauge ⅝-inch needle is used for subcutaneous injections.

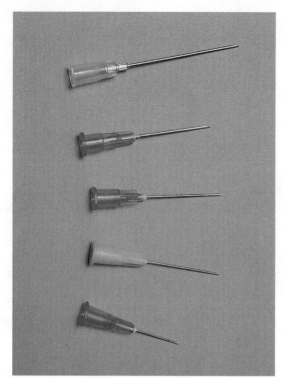

FIGURE 17-4 Needles *(top to bottom):* 19-gauge, 1-½ inch length; 20-gauge, 1-inch length; 21-gauge, 1-inch length; 23-gauge, 1-inch length; and 25-gauge, ⅝-inch length.

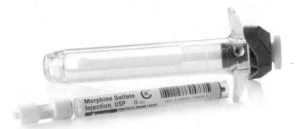

FIGURE 17-5 Carpuject syringe holder and needleless, prefilled, sterile cartridge. (2006 Hospira, used with permission.)

DISPOSABLE INJECTION UNITS

Single-dose, prefilled, disposable syringes are available for some medications. You do not need to prepare medication doses, except perhaps to expel portions of unneeded medication. However, it is important to carefully check the medication and concentration, because prefilled syringes appear very similar.

One example of a disposable injection system is Carpuject. The Carpuject syringe system includes reusable plastic syringe holders and disposable, prefilled, sterile cartridge units (Figure 17-5). To assemble, place the cartridge, Luer tip first, into the plastic syringe holder. Following manufacturer's instructions, turn the plunger rod to the left (counterclockwise) and the lock to the right (clockwise) until it "clicks." Finally, remove the needle guard and advance the plunger to expel air and excess medication, as with a regular syringe. The cartridge may be used with needleless systems or safety needles. After you administer the medication, you can safely dispose of the cartridge in a puncture-proof and leak-proof receptacle. This design reduces the risk of needlestick injury.

NEEDLESTICK PREVENTION

The most frequent route of exposure to blood-borne disease is from needlestick injuries (ANA, 2002; Perry, Parker, and Jagger, 2003). It is estimated that 80% of needle sticks can be prevented by the use of safer needle devices and proper education about needle safety (Foley, 2004). The Needlestick Safety and Prevention Act is a federal law that mandates health care facilities to use safe needle devices to reduce the frequency of needlestick injury. In addition, employers must update their exposure control plans and seek employees' input when evaluating and selecting safer medical devices (OSHA, 2001). It is estimated that these devices reduce the occurrence of needlestick injuries by 62% to 88% (Wilburn, 2004).

One type of safe needle device is the safety syringe, which is equipped with a plastic guard or sheath that slips over as it is withdrawn from the skin (Figure 17-6, A and B). Another type of safety device is found in needleless intravenous (IV) line connection systems (Figure 17-6, C, D, and E). Box 17-1 lists recommendations for health care workers to use to reduce their risk of needlestick injuries.

Special puncture-proof and leak-proof containers are available in health care agencies for the disposal of sharps. Containers are made so that only one hand needs to be used when disposing of uncapped needles. Keeping the other hand well away from the container prevents accidental injury (Figure 17-7). Never force a needle into a full needle-disposal receptacle. You should dispose of used needles and syringes immediately in the appropriate container.

EVIDENCE IN PRACTICE

Nicoll LH, Hesby A: Intramuscular injection: an integrative research review and guideline for evidence-based practice, *Appl Nurs Res* 16(2):149, 2002.

The injection site used for IM injections is the one factor most predictive of complications such as nerve injury or hematoma. To avoid these complications, assess the client's age and the medication type and volume when selecting an injection site. The dorsogluteal site should *not* be used as a site for IM injections. Although the dorsogluteal was formerly the traditional site for IM injections, studies have demonstrated the exact location of the sciatic nerve varies from one person to another. When a needle hits the sciatic nerve, the client may experience permanent or partial paralysis of the involved leg.

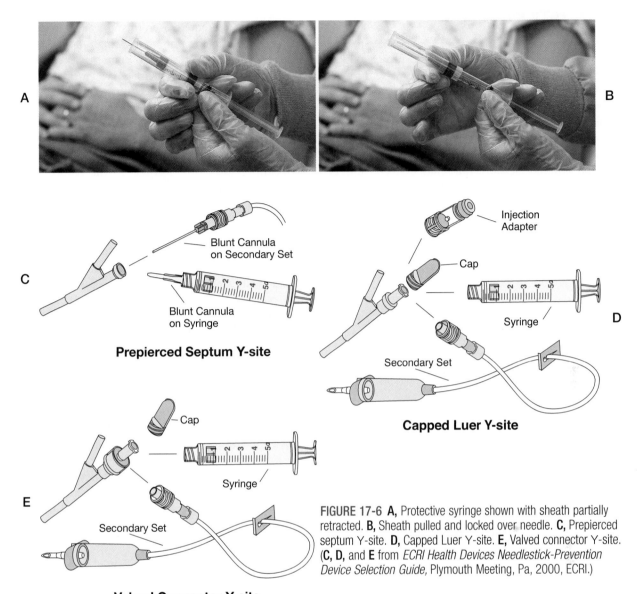

FIGURE 17-6 **A,** Protective syringe shown with sheath partially retracted. **B,** Sheath pulled and locked over needle. **C,** Prepierced septum Y-site. **D,** Capped Luer Y-site. **E,** Valved connector Y-site. (**C, D,** and **E** from *ECRI Health Devices Needlestick-Prevention Device Selection Guide,* Plymouth Meeting, Pa, 2000, ECRI.)

BOX 17-1 Recommendations for the Prevention of Needlestick Injuries

1 Avoid using needles when effective needleless systems or sharps with engineered sharps injury protection (SESIP) safety devices are available.

2 Do not recap needles after medication administration.

3 Plan safe handling and disposal of needles before beginning a procedure that requires the use of a needle.

4 Immediately dispose of used needles, needleless systems, and SESIP into puncture-proof and leak-proof sharps disposal containers.

5 Maintain a sharps injury log (see agency policy).

6 Attend educational offerings regarding blood-borne pathogens, and follow recommendations for infection prevention, including receiving the hepatitis B vaccine.

7 Report all needlestick and sharps-related injuries immediately, according to institutional policies, to ensure the receipt of appropriate follow-up care.

8 Participate in the selection and evaluation of needleless systems and devices with safety features within your place of employment whenever possible.

9 Support legislation that promotes the safe use of needles and sharps.

Data from Occupational Safety and Health Administration (OSHA): Occupational exposure to bloodborne pathogens; needlestick and other sharps injuries; final rule, *Fed Regist* 66:5317, January 18, 2001; available at http://needlestick.org.

PREPARATION OF INJECTABLE MEDICATIONS

Ampules contain single doses of injectable medication in a liquid form. They are available in several sizes, from 1 to 10 ml or more. An ampule is made of glass with a constricted neck that is snapped off to allow access to the medication (Figure 17-8, A). A colored ring around the neck indicates where the ampule is prescored to be broken easily. Medication is easily withdrawn from the ampule by aspirating the fluid with a filter needle and syringe. Filter needles must be used when preparing medication from a glass ampule to prevent glass particles from being drawn into the syringe (Nicoll and Hesby, 2002). *Do not* use a filter needle to administer the medication.

A vial is a single-dose or multidose plastic or glass container with a rubber seal at the top (Figure 17-8, B). A single-dose vial is entered and then discarded, regardless of the amount of medication used. A multi-dose vial can be entered into several times and contains several doses of medication. When using a multidose vial, write the date the vial is opened on the vial label. Verify with the institution how long an opened multidose vial may be used. Vials that exceed the time allowed by the institutional policy must be properly discarded.

A metal or plastic cap protects the vial's rubber seal. Remove the cap when you first prepare the vial for use. Vials may contain liquid or dry forms of medications; drugs that are unstable in solution are packaged in dry form. The vial label specifies the liquid to use to dissolve the dry drug and the amount needed to prepare a desired drug concentration. Some vials contain a diluent solution in one chamber and a powdered substance in another chamber. A rubber stopper separates the two chambers. Before preparing the medication, push on the upper chamber to dislodge the rubber stopper and allow the powder and the diluent to be mixed. Unlike an ampule a vial is a closed system. You must inject air into the vial to permit easy withdrawal of the solution. Some medications, even when in a vial, may need to be drawn up with a filter needle because of the nature of the drug. Institutional policies and package inserts from the manufacturer indicate drugs that should be prepared with a filter needle.

Tables 17-1 and 17-2 describe the steps and rationales for drawing up medications from ampules and vials.

Occasionally the prescriber will order an injectable medication that must be reconstituted. This frequently occurs for time-sensitive injectable medication, which must be administered within a specific time period in order to guarantee full drug effectiveness. Procedural Guideline 17-1 describes the steps for reconstituting medication from a powder.

Text continued on p. 424

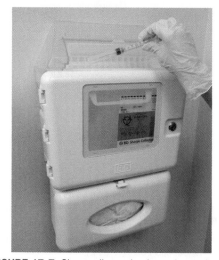

FIGURE 17-7 Sharps disposal using only one hand.

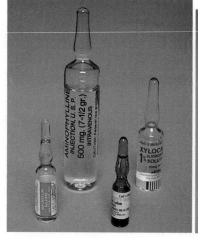
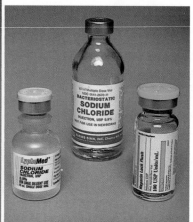

FIGURE 17-8 A, Medication in ampules. **B,** Medication in vials.

TABLE 17-1 Drawing up Medication from an Ampule

STEPS	RATIONALE
1 Compare medication administration record (MAR) with scheduled medication list or physician's orders. Check the client's name, drug name, dosage, route, and time of administration. If discrepancies exist, check against original physician orders.	Physician's order is most reliable source and only legal record of drugs client is to receive. Check orders at least every 24 hours and when client questions a drug order (Lilley, Harrington, and Snyder, 2004).
2 Perform hand hygiene and prepare supplies, including syringe, filter needle, needle or needleless system device, small gauze pad or unopened alcohol swab, and MAR.	Ensures organized, uninterrupted procedure.
3 Prepare medications for one client at a time. Follow the six rights of medication administration. Keep all pages of MARs or computer printouts for one client together.	Prevents preparation errors.
4 Select ampule from stock supply, unit-dose drawer, or automated dispensing system. Compare name of medication on the label with MAR or computer printout.	Reading label and comparing it against transcribed order reduces errors. *This is the first check for accuracy.*
5 Check expiration date on ampule.	Medications used past expiration date may be inactive or harmful to client.
6 Check drug dose. If dose printed on the ampule differs from ordered dose, calculate correct amount to give.	Calculation reduces risk of error.
7 Tap top of ampule lightly and quickly with finger until fluid moves from neck of ampule (see illustration).	Dislodges fluid that collects above neck of ampule and all solution moves into the lower chamber.
8 Place small gauze pad or unopened alcohol pad around neck of ampule (see illustration).	Placing pad around neck of ampule protects fingers from trauma as glass tip is broken off. Do not use opened alcohol swab to wrap around top of ampule because alcohol may leak into ampule.
9 Snap neck of ampule quickly and firmly away from hands (see illustration).	Protects fingers and face from being cut by glass.
10 Draw up medication quickly, using a filter needle long enough to reach the bottom of ampule.	System is open to airborne contamination. Proper length needle makes sure needle accesses medication. Filter needle prevents withdrawal of glass fragments (Nicoll and Hesby, 2002).
11 Hold ampule upside down, or set it on a flat surface. Insert filter needle into center of ampule. Do not allow needle tip or shaft to touch rim of ampule.	Broken rim of ampule is considered contaminated. When ampule is inverted, solution dribbles out of ampule if needle tip or shaft touches rim of ampule.
12 Aspirate medication into syringe, by gently pulling back on plunger (see illustrations).	Withdrawal of plunger creates negative pressure within syringe barrel, which pulls fluid into the syringe.
13 Keep needle tip under surface of liquid. Tip ampule to bring all of fluid within reach of the needle. If air bubbles are aspirated, do not expel air into ampule.	Expelling air creates pressure that may force fluid out of ampule and medication will be lost.
14 To expel excess air bubbles, remove needle from ampule. Hold syringe with needle pointing up. Tap side of syringe to cause bubbles to rise toward needle (see illustration). Draw back slightly on plunger, and then push the plunger upward to eject air. *Do not eject fluid.*	Withdrawing plunger too far will remove it from barrel. Holding syringe vertically allows air bubbles to rise to top of barrel and fluid to settle in bottom of barrel. Pulling back on plunger allows fluid within needle to enter barrel so fluid is not expelled. Air at tip of barrel and within needle is then expelled.

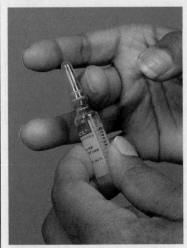

STEP 7 Tapping ampule moves fluid down neck.

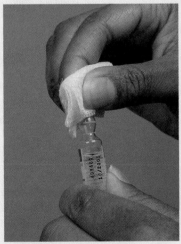

STEP 8 Gauze pad placed around neck of ampule.

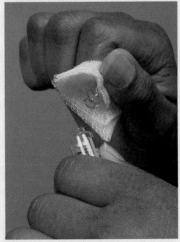

STEP 9 Neck snapped away from hands.

Continued

TABLE 17-1 Drawing up Medication from an Ampule—cont'd

STEPS	RATIONALE
15 If syringe contains excess fluid, use sink for disposal. Hold syringe vertically with needle tip up and slanted slightly toward sink. Slowly eject excess fluid into sink. Recheck fluid level in syringe by holding it vertically at eye level at a 90-degree angle to measure accurately.	Safely disperses medication into sink. Position of needle allows medication to be expelled without it flowing down needle shaft. Rechecking fluid level ensures proper dose.
16 Cover needle with its safety cap. Replace filter needle with proper needle length and gauge for injection (see Skills 17.1, 17.2, and 17.3). Dispose of filter needle properly.	Reduces needlestick injuries and prevents contamination of needle. Filter needles cannot be used for injection (Nicoll and Hesby, 2002).
17 Compare MAR with label of prepared drug.	Reading labels a second time reduces errors.
18 Perform Completion Protocol (inside front cover) and take medication to client's bedside for administration.	

A   B

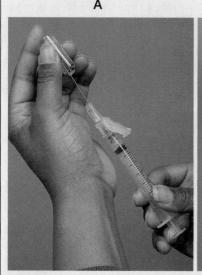 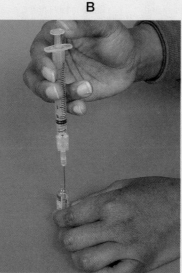

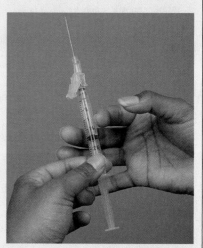

STEP 12 A, Medication aspirated with ampule inverted. **B,** Medication aspirated with ampule on flat surface.

STEP 14 Hold syringe upright; tap barrel to dislodge air bubbles from syringe.

TABLE 17-2 Drawing up Medication from a Vial

STEPS	RATIONALE
1 Compare MAR with scheduled medication list or physician's orders. Check the client's name, drug name, dosage, route, and time of administration. If discrepancies exist, check against original physician orders.	Physician's order is most reliable source and only legal record of drugs client is to receive. Check orders at least every 24 hours and when client questions a drug order (Lilley, Harrington, and Snyder, 2004).
2 Perform hand hygiene and prepare supplies, including syringe, needles (blunt tip vial access cannula, filter needle if indicated, and needle for injection), small gauze pad or alcohol swab, diluent (e.g., normal saline or sterile water) if indicated, and MAR.	Ensures organized, uninterrupted procedure.
3 Prepare medications for one client at a time. Follow the six rights of medication administration. Keep all pages of MARs or computer printouts for one client together.	Prevents preparation errors.
4 Select vial from stock supply, unit-dose drawer, or automated dispensing system. Compare name of medication on the label with MAR or computer printout.	Reading label and comparing it against transcribed order reduces errors. *This is the first check for accuracy.*
5 Check expiration date on vial.	
6 Check drug dose. If dose printed on the vial differs from ordered dose, calculate correct amount to give.	Medications used past expiration date may be inactive or harmful to client. Double-checking pharmacy calculations reduces risk of error.
7 Remove cap covering top of unused vial. If using a multidose vial that has been opened, cap is already removed. Firmly and briskly wipe surface of rubber seal with alcohol swab, and allow it to dry.	Vial comes packaged with cap that cannot be replaced after removal. Not all drug manufacturers guarantee that seals of unused vials are sterile. Therefore seals must be swabbed before drawing up medication. Allowing alcohol to dry prevents alcohol from coating needle and mixing with medication.

TABLE 17-2 Drawing up Medication from a Vial—cont'd

STEPS	RATIONALE
8 Pick up syringe and remove cap covering needleless vial adapter (see illustration). Pull back on plunger to draw amount of air into syringe equivalent to volume of medication to be aspirated from vial.	Injecting air into the vial prevents buildup of negative pressure in vial when aspirating medication.
9 With vial on flat surface, insert tip of needle or needleless access device through center of rubber seal (see illustration). Apply pressure to tip of needle during insertion.	Center of seal is thinner and easier to penetrate. Inserting the needle with the bevel up prevents coring of rubber seal, which could cause the rubber to enter vial or needle (Nicoll and Hesby, 2002).
10 Inject air into vial's airspace, holding on to plunger with firm pressure. Hold plunger with firm pressure; plunger sometimes is forced backward by air pressure in vial.	Air must be injected before aspirating fluid to create vacuum needed to get medication to flow into syringe. Injecting into vial's airspace prevents formation of bubbles and inaccuracy in dose.
11 Invert vial while keeping firm hold on syringe and plunger (see illustration). Hold vial between thumb and middle fingers of nondominant hand. Grasp end of syringe barrel and plunger with thumb and forefinger of dominant hand to counteract pressure in vial.	Inverting vial allows fluid to settle in lower half of container. Position of hands prevents forceful movement of plunger and permits easy manipulation of syringe.
12 Keep tip of needleless adapter below fluid level.	Prevents aspiration of air.
13 Allow air pressure to fill syringe gradually with medication. If necessary, pull back slightly on plunger to obtain correct amount of solution.	Positive pressure within vial forces fluid into syringe. Pulling back too quickly or forcefully on the plunger will pull unwanted air into the syringe.
14 When desired volume has been obtained, position tip of needleless adapter into vial's airspace; tap side of syringe barrel carefully to dislodge any air bubbles. Eject any air remaining at top of syringe into vial.	Forcefully striking barrel while needle is inserted in vial may bend needle. Accumulation of air displaces medication and may cause dosage errors.
15 Remove needleless vial access device from vial by pulling on barrel of syringe.	Pulling plunger rather than barrel causes plunger to separate from barrel, resulting in loss of medication.
16 Hold syringe at eye level at a 90-degree angle to ensure correct volume and absence of air bubbles. Draw back slightly on plunger; then push plunger upward to eject air. Do not eject fluid. Recheck volume of medication.	Holding syringe vertically allows fluid to settle in bottom of barrel. Pulling back on plunger allows fluid within needle to enter barrel so fluid is not expelled. Air at top of barrel and within needle is then expelled.
17 If medication is to be injected into a client's tissue, change adapter for a needle of appropriate gauge and length according to route of administration (see Skills 17.1, 17.2, and 17.3).	A needleless vial access device must be changed because it cannot pierce the skin. Filter needles cannot be used for injections (Nicoll and Hesby, 2002).
18 Compare MAR with label of prepared drug.	*Reading labels a second time reduces errors.*
19 For multidose vial, make a label that includes date of opening, mixing (if necessary), concentration of drug per milliliter, and nurse's initials.	Ensures that future doses will be prepared correctly. Some drugs must be discarded after a certain number of days after opening or mixing.
20 Perform Completion Protocol (inside front cover) and take medication to client's bedside for administration.	Proper disposal of glass and needle prevents accidental injury to staff (OSHA, 2001). Controls transmission of infection.

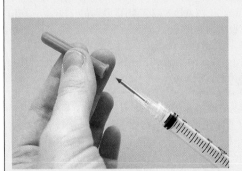

STEP 8 Syringe with needleless vial adapter.

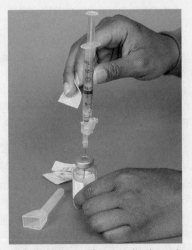

STEP 9 Insert safety needle through center of vial diaphragm (with vial flat on table).

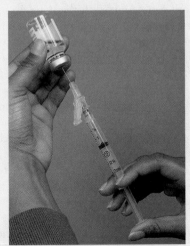

STEP 11 Insert safety needle through center of vial diaphragm.

PROCEDURAL GUIDELINE 17-1
Reconstituting Medications from a Powder

Delegation Considerations

The skill of reconstituting medications from a powder may not be delegated.

Equipment
- Vial with medication
- Vial with diluent solution
- Blunt-tip vial adapter
- Filter needle if indicated (see agency policy)
- Syringe
- Appropriate size needle for injection
- Alcohol swab
- Medication administration record (MAR) or computer printout

Procedural Steps
1. Compare MAR with scheduled medication list or physician's orders. Check the client's name, drug name, dosage, route, and time of administration. If discrepancies exist, check against original physician orders.
2. Perform hand hygiene and prepare supplies.
3. Prepare medications for one client at a time. Follow the six rights of medication administration.
4. Select vial from stock supply, unit-dose cart, or automated dispensing system. Compare name of medication on the label with MAR or computer printout.
5. Check drug dose. If dose printed on the vial differs from ordered dose, calculate correct amount to give.
6. Check expiration date on vial.
7. Remove cap covering vial containing powdered medication and vial containing proper diluent. (Label may specify use of sterile water, normal saline, or special diluent provided with the medication.) Firmly cleanse both rubber seals with alcohol swab and allow alcohol to dry.
8. Draw up diluent into syringe with vial adapter (see Table 17-2, Steps 8 to 14).
9. Insert tip of needleless vial adapter through center of rubber seal of vial of powdered medication. Inject diluent into vial. Remove adapter.
10. Mix medication by gently rolling vial between hands until completely dissolved. Do not shake.
11. Reconstituted medication in vial is ready to be drawn into syringe. Read label and compare with MAR carefully to determine concentration after reconstitution.
12. Draw up reconstituted medication into syringe using adapter (see Table 17-2, Steps 8 to 16).
13. If medication is to be injected into a client's tissue, change adapter for a needle of appropriate gauge and length according to route of administration (see Skills 17.1, 17.2, and 17.3).
14. Compare MAR with label of prepared drug.
15. **Perform Completion Protocol (inside front cover)** and take medication to client's bedside.

MIXING MEDICATIONS IN ONE SYRINGE

To avoid giving two injections at one time, some medications can be mixed in the same syringe. It is essential that any medications mixed be compatible. You can determine medication compatibility by referring to a compatibility chart. Compatibility charts are available in various drug reference guides or are posted within client care areas. Consult a pharmacist, compatibility chart, or drug handbook when you are unsure about the compatibility of medications. When mixing medications, observe for changes in the appearance of the solution, which suggests incompatibility. Whenever two medications are mixed in one syringe, it is essential to remember how to correctly aspirate fluid from each type of container. When using multidose vials, do not contaminate the vial's contents with medication from another vial or ampule.

Mixing medications from a vial and an ampule is simple because adding air to withdraw medication from an ampule is unnecessary. Prepare medications from the vial first and then, using the same syringe and a safety filter needle, withdraw medication from the ampule. Mixing medications from two vials is somewhat more complicated because air must be added to both vials.

Give special consideration to the proper preparation of insulin, which comes in vials. Insulin is the hormone used to treat high blood glucose levels most frequently associated with diabetes. Often clients with diabetes receive a combination of different types of insulin to control their blood glucose levels. Before preparing insulin doses, gently roll all cloudy insulin preparations (*not* rapid- and short-acting insulin and insulin glargine) between palms of the hands to resuspend the insulin (ADA, 2004b). Do not shake insulin vials. Shaking causes bubbles to form. Bubbles take up space in a syringe and alter the dosage.

Some insulins can be mixed in the same syringe. When insulins are mixed, chemical changes may occur either immediately or over time. This can result in a client response to insulin that is different than the response that would occur if the insulins had been given separately. Always prepare the short- or rapid-acting insulin first to prevent it from becoming contaminated with the longer-acting insulin (ADA, 2004b). In some settings insulin is not mixed. Box 17-2 lists recommendations from the American Diabetes Association (ADA) for mixing insulins. Procedural Guideline 17-2 describes the steps for mixing mediations, including two types of insulin, in the same syringe.

BOX 17-2 Recommendations for Mixing Insulins

- Clients whose blood sugar glucose is well controlled on a mixed insulin dose should maintain their individual routine when preparing and administering their insulin.
- Insulin should not be mixed with any other medications or diluent unless approved by the prescribing physician or advanced practice nurse (APN).
- Insulin glargine should not be mixed with any other forms of insulin.
- Commercially available premixed insulins may be used if the ratio of the insulins within the vial matches the client's current insulin requirements.
- Injections that mix NPH and short-acting insulins may be administered immediately or they may be stored for future use.

- Rapid-acting insulin may be mixed with NPH, lente, and ultralente.
- Mixtures of rapid-acting insulin with either an intermediate- or long-acting insulin should be injected within 15 minutes before a meal.
- Short-acting and lente insulins should not be mixed unless the client's blood sugar levels are currently under control with this mixture.
- Phosphate-buffered insulins (e.g., NPH) should not be mixed with lente insulins. If they are mixed, a precipitate may form and the time of onset and peak action of the insulins will change.
- Insulin formulations may change. Always follow manufacturer's guidelines regarding mixing.

Copyright © 2004 American Diabetes Association. From *Diabetes Care* 27:S106-S107, 2004. Reprinted with permission from the American Diabetes Association.

PROCEDURAL GUIDELINE 17-2
Mixing Medications from Vials

Delegation Considerations
The skill of mixing medications from two vials may not be delegated.

Equipment
- Single-dose or multidose vials or ampules containing medications
- Syringe with needleless vial adapter or filter needle and syringe
- Extra needle for injection
- Alcohol swab
- Puncture-proof container for disposing of syringes, needles, and glass
- MAR or computer printout

Procedural Steps
1. Compare MAR with scheduled medication list or physician's orders. Check the client's name, drug name, dosage, route, and time of administration. If discrepancies exist, check against original physician orders.
2. Perform hand hygiene and prepare supplies.
3. Prepare medications for one client at a time. Follow the six rights of medication administration.
4. Select vials from stock supply, unit-dose cart, or automated dispensing system. Compare name of medication on the label with MAR or computer printout.

5. Check drug dose. If dose printed on a vial differs from ordered dose, calculate correct amount to give.
6. Check expiration date on vials.
7. **Mixing medications from two vials:**
   a. Remove protective caps from top of vials, and cleanse seals of both vials with alcohol swab.
   b. Take syringe with needleless vial adapter or filter needle, and aspirate volume of air equivalent to first medication's dose (vial A) into syringe.
   c. Inject air into vial A, making sure needleless adapter or filter needle does not touch solution (see illustration).
   d. Withdraw needle or needleless adapter from vial A. Aspirate air equivalent to second medication's dose (vial B) into the syringe.
   e. Inject the volume of air into vial B, and immediately withdraw the medication in vial B into the syringe (see illustration). Check dose for accuracy.
   f. Insert needle or needleless adapter into vial A, being careful not to push plunger and expel medication into vial. Withdraw the correct amount of medication from vial A into syringe (see illustration).
   g. After preparing the correct combined dose, withdraw adapter or needleless access device from vial A and apply needle suitable for injection.

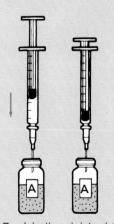

STEP 7c. Injecting air into vial A.

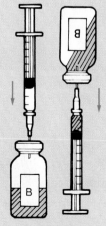

STEP 7e. Injecting air into vial B and withdrawing dose.

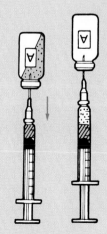

STEP 7f. Withdrawing medication from vial A.

Continued

PROCEDURAL GUIDELINE 17-2—cont'd

8 Mixing insulins:

> **NURSE ALERT** In some institutions insulin doses must be verified by another nurse for accuracy. Have dose of clear insulin verified with needle in vial before proceeding with mixing of insulin. Also verify dose after mixing the medications.

a. If mixing rapid- or short-acting insulin with intermediate- or long-acting insulin, take insulin syringe and aspirate volume of air equivalent to dose to be withdrawn from intermediate- or long-acting insulin first (see illustration). If mixing two intermediate- or long-acting insulins, it makes no difference which you prepare first.

b. Insert needle, and inject air into vial of intermediate- or long-acting insulin. Do not let the tip of the needle touch the insulin.

c. Withdraw needle and syringe from vial without aspirating medication.

d. With the same syringe, inject air, equal to the dose of the rapid- or short-acting insulin, into the vial and withdraw the correct dose into the syringe (see illustration).

e. Remove the syringe from the rapid- or short-acting insulin and remove air bubbles to ensure correct dose.

f. After verifying insulin doses with the MAR again, determine which point on syringe scale correctly combines units of insulin measure by adding the number of units of both insulin preparations (e.g., 5 units of regular insulin + 10 units of NPH insulin = 15 units total).

g. Insert needle into vial of intermediate- or long-acting insulin. Be careful not to push plunger and expel medication into vial. Invert vial and carefully withdraw desired amount of insulin into syringe (see illustration).

h. Withdraw needle and check fluid level in syringe. Keep needle of prepared syringe sheathed or capped until administering medication.

> **NURSE ALERT** Administer mixture of insulins within 5 minutes of preparation. Rapid- or short-acting insulin can bind with intermediate- or long-acting insulin, thus reducing the action of the more rapid-acting insulin (Strowig, 2001).

9 Check syringe carefully for total combined dose of medications.

10 Compare MAR with label of prepared drug a second time.

11 Because combined insulins are injected into a client's tissue, change adapter for a subcutaneous needle of appropriate gauge and length (see Skills 17.1, 17.2, and 17.3).

12 Perform Completion Protocol (inside front cover) and take medication to client's bedside.

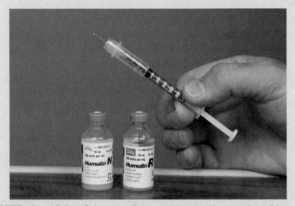

STEP 8a. Vials of intermediate- or long-acting and rapid- or short-acting insulin and syringe with air aspirated.

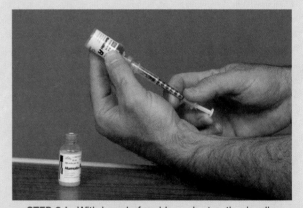

STEP 8d. Withdrawal of rapid- or short-acting insulin.

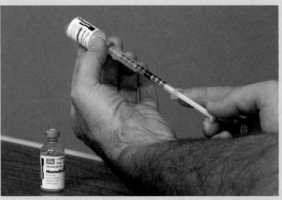

STEP 8g. Withdrawal of intermediate- or long-acting insulin.

NURSING DIAGNOSES

Nursing diagnoses may be identified based on therapeutic effects or side effects of specific prescribed medications and effect of injection into tissues. **Acute pain** is a diagnosis that may apply when clients are receiving medications to help control pain. **Anxiety** is a common diagnosis for clients who are uncomfortable with having injections. **Deficient knowledge** regarding self-administration of medications is appropriate for clients who need to learn or review injection techniques. **Ineffective therapeutic regimen management** is appropriate when the client is having difficulties complying with prescribed medication schedules.

SKILL 17.1   Subcutaneous Injections—Including Insulin

- **Nursing Skills Online: Injections, Lesson 3**

A subcutaneous injection deposits medication into the loose connective tissue underlying the dermis. Subcutaneous tissue is not as richly supplied with blood vessels as muscles; thus drugs are not absorbed as quickly as those given intramuscularly. Anything affecting local blood flow to tissues influences the rate of drug absorption. This includes physical exercise or the local application of hot or cold compresses. Conditions such as circulatory shock or occlusive vascular disease impair a client's blood flow and thus contraindicate subcutaneous injections.

Drugs given subcutaneously are isotonic, nonirritating, nonviscous, and water-soluble. Examples include epinephrine, insulin, allergy medications, narcotics, and heparin. To avoid tissue irritation, give only small doses of medications (0.5 to 1 ml) subcutaneously. Avoid irritating medications that collect within the tissues and can cause sterile abscesses, which appear as hardened, painful lumps.

The best sites for subcutaneous injections include the outer posterior aspect of the upper arms, the abdomen from below the costal margins to the iliac crests, and the anterior aspects of the thighs (Figure 17-9). These areas are easily accessible, especially for clients who must self-administer subcutaneous injections such as insulin. They also are large enough areas so that multiple injections may be rotated within each anatomical location.

Injection sites must be free of infection, skin lesions, scars, bony prominences, and large underlying muscles or nerves. Body weight and the amount of adipose tissue influence the choice of needle length and angle of needle insertion. Generally a 25-gauge ⅜- to ⅝-inch needle with a medium bevel inserted at a 45- to 90-degree angle (Figure 17-10) deposits medication into the subcutaneous tissue of a normal-size client. If a client is obese, you need to gently pinch or elevate the tissue and use a needle long enough to insert through the fatty tissue at the base of the skinfold; the angle of injection is 90 degrees. Thin or cachectic clients may have insufficient tissue for subcutaneous injections. The upper abdomen is the best injection site for clients with little peripheral subcutaneous tissue. The preferred needle length is one half the width of the skinfold. To ensure that the medication reaches subcutaneous tissue, gently pinch or elevate the subcutaneous tissue to prevent injecting the medication into the muscle. Insert the syringe at a 45- to 90-degree angle depending on how much subcutaneous tissue is pinched (Pope, 2002).

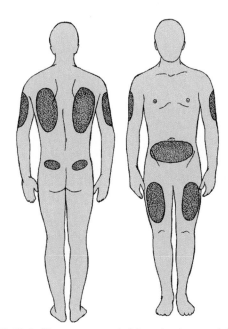

FIGURE 17-9 Sites recommended for subcutaneous injections.

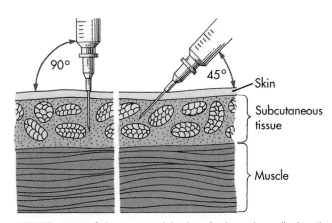

FIGURE 17-10 Subcutaneous injection. Angle and needle length depend on thickness of skinfold.

Aspiration is unnecessary with a subcutaneous injection. Piercing a blood vessel in a subcutaneous injection is very rare and with heparin may cause hematoma formation (ADA, 2004b; McConnell, 2000).

SPECIAL CONSIDERATIONS FOR ADMINISTRATION OF INSULIN

Insulin is the hormone used to treat diabetes mellitus. Clients' blood sugars may also elevate whenever they experience unusual stress (e.g., hospitalization, trauma). Insulin may be used in these situations as well. Clients may receive a combination of different types of insulin to control blood glucose levels. Clients can choose one anatomical area (e.g., the abdomen) and systematically rotate sites within that region. This helps maintain consistency in insulin absorption from day to day. After all potential sites within that area are used, the client may choose either to move to another anatomical site (e.g., the thigh) or to start the rotation pattern over in the same anatomical area (ADA, 2004b). Absorption rates of insulin vary based on the injection site. Insulin is absorbed the quickest in the abdomen, followed by the arms, thighs, and buttocks (Caffery, 2003). Rotation of injection from major site to major site (e.g., rotating from abdomen to upper arms to thighs from one injection to the next), once a common practice for clients who use insulin, is no longer necessary for clients who take

human insulin because human insulins carry a much lower risk for hypertrophy.

When planning insulin injection times, determine when the client will eat or be fed next and know the client's current blood glucose level. Also, check pharmacology resources for the peak action and duration of the client's insulin. Table 17-3 compares the onsets, peaks, and durations of various insulin preparations. Box 17-3 provides general guidelines for insulin administration.

SPECIAL CONSIDERATIONS FOR ADMINISTRATION OF HEPARIN

Heparin therapy provides therapeutic anticoagulation to reduce the risk of thrombus formation. The drug is administered subcutaneously or intravenously. Heparin suppresses clot formation. Therefore, clients receiving heparin are at risk for bleeding. When giving clients long-term anticoagulation, be alert for signs of bleeding (e.g., bleeding gums, hematemesis, hematuria, melena). Results from coagulation blood tests (e.g., aPTT [activated partial thromboplastin time], PTT [partial thromboplastin time]) allow you to monitor the desired therapeutic range for IV heparin therapy.

Before administering heparin, assess for preexisting conditions that may contraindicate the use of heparin, including threatened abortion, cerebral or aortic aneurysm, cerebrovascular hemorrhage, severe hypertension, blood dyscrasias,

TABLE 17-3 Comparison of Insulin Preparations

INSULIN TYPE*	ONSET (HOURS)	PEAK EFFECT (HOURS)	DURATION OF ACTION (HOURS)
Rapid-Acting			
Insulin lispro (Humalog)	¼	1	4
Regular insulin[†]	½-1	2-4	5-7
Prompt insulin zinc suspension (semilente)	1-3	2-8	12-16
Intermediate-Acting			
Insulin zinc suspension (lente)	1-3	8-12	18-28
Isophane insulin suspension (NPH)	3-4	6-12	18-28
Combination insulins			
Humulin 70/30 or Novolin 70/30 (70% NPH; 30% regular insulin)	½	4-8	24
Humulin 50/50 (50% NPH; 50% regular insulin)	½	3	22-24
Humalog Mix 75/25 (75% lispro protamine suspension; 25% lispro insulin)	¼	½-1½ and 2-4	6-12
NovoLog Mix 70/30 (70% insulin aspart protamine; 30% insulin aspart)	¼	1-4	12-24
Long-Acting			
Extended insulin zinc suspension (ultralente)	4-6	18-24	36
Protamine zinc insulin suspension (PZI)	4-6	14-24	36
Insulin glargine (Lantus)[‡]	1	None	24

Modified from McKenry LM, Salerno E: *Pharmacology in nursing,* ed 21, St Louis, 2003, Mosby.
*All of the above insulins are available in 100-unit strengths. Beef, pork, beef-pork, and human insulins are available in rapid-acting insulins and in lente and NPH intermediate insulins.
[†]This is the only insulin for IV use. Intravenously, the onset of action is within 10 to 30 minutes, peak effect within 15 to 30 minutes, and duration of action within 30 minutes to 1 hour.
[‡]Cannot be mixed with other insulins.

and recent ophthalmic surgery or neurosurgery. In addition, assess for conditions in which increased risk of hemorrhage is present: recent childbirth, severe diabetes, severe renal disease, liver disease, severe trauma, vasculitis, and active ulcers or lesions of the gastrointestinal (GI), genitourinary (GU), or respiratory tract. Obtain information about the client's current medication regimen, including over-the-counter (OTC) and herbal medications, for possible drug interactions with heparin. Drugs that interact with heparin include aspirin, nonsteroidal antiinflammatory drugs (NSAIDs), cephalosporins, antithyroid agents, probenecid, and thrombolytics (McKenry and Salerno, 2003).

Low molecular weight (LMW) heparins (e.g., enoxaparin) are more effective than heparin in some clients. The anticoagulant effects are more predictable (McKenry and others, 2006). LMW heparins have a longer half-life, requiring less laboratory monitoring. These medications often come from the manufacturer in a prepared syringe (see manufacturer's guidelines). To minimize the pain and bruising associated with LMW heparin, it is given subcutaneously on the right or left side of the abdomen, at least 2 inches away from the umbilicus (Aventis, 2006). LMW

heparin has slightly fewer hemorrhagic complications than standard heparin (Bick and others, 2005).

ASSESSMENT

1 Identify the drug(s) ordered: action, purpose, normal dosage and route, common side effects, time of onset and peak action, and nursing implications. *Rationale: This allows you to anticipate effects of drugs and to observe client's response.*
2 Assess client's medical history, history of allergies, and medication history.
3 Observe client's verbal and nonverbal response to injection. *Rationale: Injections can cause anxiety, which may increase pain.*
4 Assess for factors that may contraindicate subcutaneous injections, such as circulatory shock or reduced local tissue perfusion. *Rationale: Reduced tissue perfusion interferes with drug absorption and distribution. Physiological changes of aging or repeated injections may create changes in subcutaneous tissue affecting absorption.*
5 Assess client's knowledge regarding medication and dosage schedule. *Rationale: Information may pose implications for client education.*

PLANNING

Expected Outcomes focus on safe, effective administration of injections with minimal anxiety and discomfort.
1 Client experiences no pain or mild burning at injection site.
2 Desired effect of medication achieved with no signs of allergies or undesired effects.
3 Client explains purpose, dosage, and effects of medication.

Delegation Considerations
The skill of administering subcutaneous medications may not be delegated. The nurse directs personnel by:
- Having personnel immediately notify nurse for medication side effects, client reports of pain at injection site, and changes in client's physical status, vital signs, or level of consciousness (LOC)
- Instructing personnel in the care of diabetic clients to immediately notify nurse if client suddenly appears disoriented or confused

Equipment
- Proper size syringe
- Appropriate syringe (1 to 3 ml) and needle (25 to 27 gauge, ⅜ to ⅝ inch)
- U-100 insulin syringe (0.3, 0.5, or 1 ml) with preattached needle (28 to 31 gauge, ⁵⁄₁₆ to ½ inch (ADA, 2005)
- Small gauze pad (optional)
- Alcohol swab
- Medication ampule or vial
- Clean gloves
- MAR or computer printout

BOX 17-3 General Guidelines for Insulin Administration

- Store vials of insulin in the refrigerator. Vials of insulin currently in use may be kept at room temperature to reduce irritation at the injection site. Do not inject cold insulin.
- Inspect insulin vials before each use for changes in appearance (e.g., clumping, frosting, precipitation, change in clarity or color) that may indicate a loss in potency.
- Do not interchange insulin types unless approved by the client's prescriber.
- The usual recommended interval between injection of short-acting insulin and a meal is 30 minutes.
- Preferred injection sites include the upper arm, anterior and lateral aspects of the thigh, buttocks, and abdomen, avoiding a 2-inch radius around the navel. Site selection should be based on anticipated rate of absorption. Insulin absorbs quickest in the abdomen, followed by the arms, thighs, and buttocks.
- Have the client self-administer insulin whenever possible. Consider a child's developmental level when determining the appropriate age for self-administration. Generally, self-administration of insulin should begin by adolescence.
- Clients who use insulin should self-monitor their blood sugars whenever possible.
- Various changes in a client's status may require a different insulin dose. Information about blood glucose values helps clients adjust their insulin dosage during times of illness or stress.
- All clients who take insulin should carry at least 15 g carbohydrate (e.g., 4 oz juice, 8 oz milk) to be eaten or taken in liquid form in the event of a hypoglycemic reaction. Monitor blood glucose levels.
- Teach significant others how to administer insulin and glucagon for situations in which the client is unable to self-administer insulin or is unable to ingest oral carbohydrates during hypoglycemia.

Modified from American Diabetes Association: Insulin administration: position statement, *Diabetes Care* 27(suppl 1):S106, 2004b.

IMPLEMENTATION *for Subcutaneous Injections—Including Insulin*

STEPS	RATIONALE
1 See Standard Protocol (inside front cover).	
2 Prepare medication in syringe (see Tables 17-1 and 17-2 and Procedural Guidelines 17-1 and 17-2). Be sure syringe has needle of appropriate length and gauge.	Ensures that medication is sterile and the dose is correct.
3 Take medication to client at right time, and perform hand hygiene.	Ensures correct timing for therapeutic benefit.
4 Identify client by checking identification bracelet and asking client's name. Compare with MAR. In some settings, client photographs may also be used. Replace any missing, outdated, or faded identification tools.	Ensures correct client receives medication. At least two client identifiers (neither to be the client's room number) are to be used whenever administering medications (JCAHO, 2006). In many long-term care settings pictures may be used along with identification bands.
5 Compare the label of the medication with the MAR one more time at the client's bedside.	Third comparison of medication label with the MAR decreases risk of medication administration errors.
6 Explain steps of procedure, and tell client injection will cause a slight burning or stinging.	Helps minimize anxiety.
7 Select appropriate injection site. Inspect surface of skin over sites for bruises, inflammation, or edema. Palpate site for masses, edema, or tenderness.	Injection site should be free of lesions that might interfere with drug absorption.
a. When administering LMW heparin subcutaneously, choose a site on the right or left side of the abdomen, at least 2 inches away from the umbilicus.	Anticoagulant may cause local bleeding and bruising when injected into areas such as arms and legs, which are involved in muscular activity. Injecting LMW heparin on the side of the abdomen will help decrease pain and bruising at the injection site (Aventis, 2006).
b. When administering insulin, rotate the injection site within the same anatomical area (e.g., abdomen), and systematically rotate sites within that area. After all potential sites within that area are used, the client may choose either to move to another anatomical site (e.g., thigh) or to start the rotation pattern over in the same anatomical area.	Rotating insulin sites within the same anatomical area helps maintain consistency in insulin absorption from day to day (ADA, 2004b).
8 Be sure needle size is correct by grasping skinfold at site with thumb and forefinger. Measure skinfold from top to bottom, and be sure needle is approximately half this length.	Subcutaneous injections can be inadvertently given in the muscle, especially in the abdomen and thigh sites. Appropriate needle size ensures that needle will be injected into subcutaneous tissue.
9 Assist client to comfortable position, and ask client to relax arm, leg, or abdomen depending on site chosen for injection. Talk with client about subject of interest.	Relaxation of area minimizes discomfort during injection. Promoting client's comfort through positioning and distraction helps reduce anxiety.
10 Relocate site using anatomical landmarks (see Figure 17-9).	Accurate injection of medication requires insertion in correct site to avoid injury to underlying nerves, bone, or blood vessels.
11 Cleanse site with an antiseptic swab. Apply swab at center of site and rotate outward in circular direction for about 5 cm (2 inches) (see illustration).	Mechanical action removes secretions containing microorganisms.
12 Hold swab or square of gauze between third and fourth fingers of nondominant hand.	Swab or gauze remains readily accessible for when needle is withdrawn.
13 Remove needle cap or sheath from needle by pulling it straight off.	Preventing needle from touching sides of cap prevents contamination of needle.
14 Hold syringe between thumb and forefinger of dominant hand as if grasping dart, holding syringe across tops of fingertips (see illustration).	Quick, smooth injection requires proper manipulation of syringe parts.

STEPS	RATIONALE

15 Prepare site for injection.

a. *Average-size client:* Spread skin tightly across injection site or elevate skin with nondominant hand.

Needle penetrates tight skin easier than loose skin. Elevating skin raises subcutaneous tissue.

b. *Obese client:* Elevate skin at site.

Obese clients have fatty layer of tissue above subcutaneous layer. Elevating raises subcutaneous tissue.

16 Administer injection.

a. *Average-size client:* Inject needle quickly and firmly at 45- to 90-degree angle (then release skin, if pinched).

Quick, firm insertion minimizes discomfort. Angle ensures that medication reaches subcutaneous tissue rather than muscle. (Injecting medication into compressed tissues irritates nerve fibers.)

b. *Obese client:* Inject at 90-degree angle below tissue fold.

c. After needle enters site, grasp lower end of syringe barrel with nondominant hand to stabilize it. Move dominant hand to end of plunger and slowly inject medication (see illustration). Avoid moving syringe.

Movement of syringe may displace needle and cause discomfort. Slow injection minimizes discomfort.

> **NURSE ALERT** Aspiration after injecting a subcutaneous medication is not necessary. Piercing a blood vessel in a subcutaneous injection is very rare (Stephens, 2003). Aspiration after injecting heparin or insulin is not recommended (ADA, 2004b; McConnell, 2000).

d. Withdraw needle quickly while placing antiseptic swab or sterile gauze gently above or over site.

Supporting tissues around injection site minimizes discomfort during needle withdrawal. Dry gauze may lessen discomfort associated with alcohol on nonintact skin.

> **NURSE ALERT** Applying ice to the injection site for 5 minutes before and after the injection may decrease the client's perception of pain (Kuzu and Ucar, 2001).

17 Apply gentle pressure to site. Do *not* massage site. (If heparin is given, hold alcohol swab or gauze to site for 30 to 60 seconds.)

Aids absorption. Massage can injure underlying tissue.

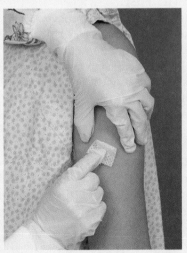
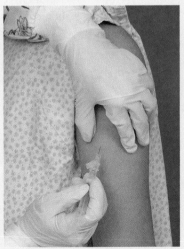
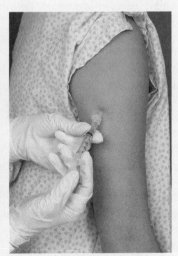

STEP 11 Cleansing site with circular motion.

STEP 14 Holding syringe as if grasping a dart.

STEP 16c. Inject medication slowly.

STEPS	RATIONALE
18 Discard sheathed or uncapped needle or needle enclosed in safety shield (see illustrations) in appropriately labeled receptacle. **19 See Completion Protocol (inside front cover).**	Prevents injury to client and health care personnel. Recapping needles increases risk of needlestick injury (OSHA, 2001).

> **COMMUNICATION TIP** Use this time with client to ask if client has questions regarding medication and its effects. Explain what to expect from a medication. If caring for client who has self-administered injection, give immediate feedback regarding how well the injection was performed.

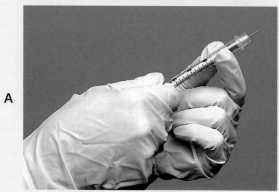 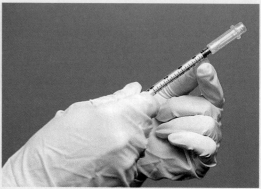

STEP 18 Needle with plastic guard to prevent needle sticks. **A,** Position of guard before injection. **B,** After injection the guard locks in place, covering the needle.

EVALUATION

1 Observe client's response to medication at times that correlate with the medication's onset, peak, and duration to determine effectiveness of drug and observe for adverse reactions.
2 Ask if client feels any acute pain, burning, numbness, or tingling at injection site.
3 Inspect and palpate injection site for lumps, tenderness, or swelling.
4 Have client describe purpose, dosage, intended effects, and side effects of medication.

Unexpected Outcomes and Related Interventions

1 Client complains of localized pain or continued burning at injection site, possibly indicating potential injury to nerves or vessels.
a. Assess injection site for abscess formation. Warm or cool compresses may be provided for comfort.
b. Monitor client's heart rate, respirations, blood pressure, and temperature.
c. Notify client's health care provider and do not reuse site.
2 Client displays signs of urticaria, eczema, pruritus, wheezing, and dyspnea.
a. Monitor client's heart rate, respirations, and blood pressure.

b. Follow institutional policy or guidelines for appropriate response to allergic reactions, and notify client's health care provider immediately.

Recording and Reporting
- Immediately after administration, record medication dose, route, site, time, and date given on MAR to record care provided and future medication administration errors. Correctly sign MAR according to institutional policy.
- Record client's response to medication.
- Report any undesirable effects from medication to client's health care provider, and document any adverse effects according to institutional policy.

Sample Documentation
0900 Heparin injection given in RLQ of abdomen. Bruise (4 cm in diameter) noted on LLQ of abdomen, deep purple, soft, and nontender. Urine clear; stool negative for occult blood.

Special Considerations
Pediatric Considerations
- Only amounts up to 0.5 ml may be administered subcutaneously to small children (Hockenberry and Wilson, 2007).

Geriatric Considerations

- Aging clients have reduced subcutaneous skinfold thickness, and skin is less elastic than that of younger clients. The upper abdominal site is the best site to use when the client has little subcutaneous tissue.

Home Care Considerations

- Clients should always have a spare bottle of each type of insulin used. A slight loss in potency may occur after the bottle has been in use for more than 30 days (ADA, 2004b).
- Pain during insulin injections may be decreased by injecting insulin at room temperature, waiting for alcohol to dry before injecting insulin, relaxing muscles around the injection site, and injecting needle quickly (ADA, 2004b).

- Injections may be given by the client or family members/friends. Instruction will be necessary in proper injection preparation and administration and disposal of syringes and needles (see Procedural Guideline 38-1).
- Properly discarding used needles and sharps in the home setting is essential to reduce health risks to the sanitation workers and the public. Consult local trash or disposal authorities or local fire stations to determine appropriate disposition of containers. In addition, pamphlets for safe home disposal of needles and sharps can be found on the Environmental Protection Agency (EPA, 2005) website: http://www.epa.gov/epaoswer/other/medical/sharps.htm.

SKILL 17.2   Intramuscular Injections

- **Nursing Skills Online: Injections, Lesson 5**

The intramuscular (IM) route deposits medication into deep muscle tissue and provides faster medication absorption than the subcutaneous route because of the muscle's greater vascularity. However, an increased risk of injecting drugs directly into blood vessels exists. Any factor that interferes with local tissue blood flow affects the rate and extent of drug absorption.

An IM injection requires use of a longer and larger-gauge needle to penetrate deep muscle tissue. The viscosity of the medication, the injection site, and the client's weight and amount of adipose tissue influence needle size selection. The needle gauge is often determined by the length of the needle. Most immunizations and parenteral medications mixed in aqueous solutions can be administered to adults using a 22- to 27-gauge needle. However, medications that are in an oil-based solution or medications that are more viscous are administered with an 18- to 25-gauge needle (Nicoll and Hesby, 2002). A 22- to 25-gauge needle is recommended for children (Hockenberry and Wilson, 2007).

An older adult, thin, or cachectic client may require a shorter, smaller-gauge needle because of muscle atrophy. Infants younger than 4 months of age require a ⅝-inch needle. For infants older than 4 months, a 1-inch needle is acceptable. The vastus lateralis or ventrogluteal sites are preferred in all infants and children (Hockenberry and Wilson, 2007). For well-developed children through adolescence, use a ⅝-inch needle for deltoid injections and a 1-inch needle for ventrogluteal injections (Hockenberry and Wilson, 2007).

Administer IM injections so that the needle is perpendicular to the client's body and as close to a 90-degree angle as possible (Nicoll and Hesby, 2002; Katsma and Katsma,

2000). Also, be sure to rotate IM injection sites to decrease the risk of hypertrophy. Emaciated muscles absorb medication poorly, so avoid them whenever possible.

Muscle is less sensitive to irritating and viscous drugs. A normal, well-developed adult client can safely tolerate as much as 5 ml of medication in larger muscles such as the ventrogluteal (Nicoll and Hesby, 2002). However, in most clinical situations it is unusual to administer more than 3 ml in a single injection. Older adults and thin clients tolerate only 2 ml of an injection. Children can tolerate 0.5 ml (infant) to 2 ml (child) for IM injections into the ventrogluteal and vastus lateralis muscles (Hockenberry and Wilson, 2007). In the deltoid muscle, children can tolerate 0.5 ml to 1 ml of drug.

The Z-track method is recommended for IM injections. The Z-track technique, pulling the skin laterally before injection, minimizes irritation by sealing the medication in the muscle tissues (Nicoll and Hesby, 2002). To use the Z-track method, apply a new needle to the syringe after preparing the medication so that no solution remains on the outside of the needle shaft. Select an IM site, preferably in a large, deep muscle, such as the ventrogluteal. Pull the overlying skin and subcutaneous tissues approximately 2.5 to 3.5 cm (1 to 1½ inches) laterally to the side with the ulnar side of the nondominant hand. Hold the skin in this position until the injection has been administered. After cleaning the site, inject the needle deep into the muscle. Slowly inject the medication if there is no blood return on aspiration. Keep the needle inserted for 10 seconds to allow the medication to disperse evenly. Then release the skin after withdrawing the needle. This leaves a zigzag path that seals the needle track wherever tissue planes slide across each other (Figure 17-11). The medication cannot escape from the muscle tissue.

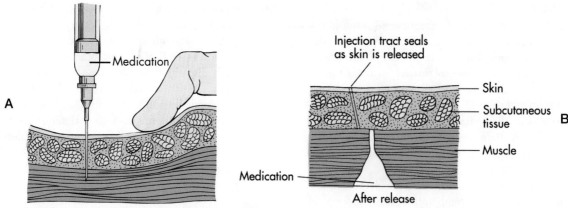

FIGURE 17-11 A, Pulling on overlying skin during IM injection moves tissue to prevent later tracking. **B,** The Z-track left after injection prevents the deposit of medication through sensitive tissue.

INTRAMUSCULAR SITE SELECTION

When selecting an IM site, you must determine if the area is free of pain, infection, necrosis, bruising, and abrasions. Also consider the location of underlying bones, nerves, and major blood vessels and the volume of medication to be given. Each site has certain advantages and disadvantages (Box 17-4). Because the sciatic nerve is near the dorsogluteal muscle, this muscle is no longer recommended as an injection site. If a needle hits the sciatic nerve, the client may experience permanent or partial paralysis of the involved leg (Beyea and Nicoll, 1995; Nicoll and Hesby, 2002). The preferred site for an IM injection for adults and children older than 7 months is the ventrogluteal site (Beyea and Nicoll, 1995). This site provides the greatest thickness of gluteal muscle, does not have nerves and blood vessels penetrating it, has the most consistent and thin layer of fat covering it, and has very few documented injuries associated with it (Rodger and King, 2000).

Location of an appropriate site for IM injection involves the ability to palpate anatomical landmarks accurately with knowledge of the location of underlying nerves and major blood vessels. Presence of excessive fatty tissue may make location of bony structures difficult; however, with experience you can achieve accurate site location. Table 17-4 describes correct techniques for locating standard IM sites for injection.

ASSESSMENT

1 Identify the drug(s) ordered: action, purpose, normal dosage and route, common side effects, time of onset and peak action, and nursing implications. *Rationale: This allows you to anticipate effects of drugs and to observe client's response.*

2 Assess client's medical history, history of allergies, and medication history.

3 Observe client's verbal and nonverbal response to injection. *Rationale: Injections can cause anxiety, which may increase pain.*

4 Review medical record or assess for factors that may contraindicate IM injection, for example, muscle atrophy, reduced blood flow, and circulatory shock. If these

---

BOX 17-4 Advantages and Disadvantages of Intramuscular Injection Sites

- *Ventrogluteal:* The ventrogluteal muscle involves the gluteus medius and minimus. It is situated deep and away from major nerves and blood vessels and is a safe site for all clients. Research has shown that injuries such as fibrosis, nerve damage, abscess, tissue necrosis, muscle contraction, gangrene, and pain have been associated with all the common IM sites except the ventrogluteal site (Nicoll and Hesby, 2002). Therefore, the ventrogluteal site is the preferred injection site for infants, children, and adults (Hockenberry and Wilson, 2007; Nicoll and Hesby, 2002).
- *Vastus lateralis:* The vastus lateralis muscle is another injection site used in the adult client and is the preferred site for administration of biologicals (e.g., immunizations) to infants younger than 12 months of age (Nicoll and Hesby, 2002). Has small nerve endings resulting in discomfort after injection.
- *Deltoid:* Easily accessible muscle. Use this site only for small medication volumes (0.5 to 1 ml), and for administration of routine immunizations in toddlers, older children, and adults (Nicoll and Hesby, 2002). Give hepatitis B vaccine only in the deltoid (Beyea and Nicoll, 1995).

---

conditions are present, call prescriber for an alternative route of administration. *Rationale: Atrophied muscle absorbs medication poorly. Factors interfering with blood flow to muscles impair drug absorption (McKenry and Salerno, 2003).*

5 Assess client's knowledge regarding medication and dosage schedule. *Rationale: Information may pose implications for client education.*

PLANNING

Expected Outcomes focus on safe, effective administration of injection with minimal anxiety and discomfort.

1 Client demonstrates desired effect of medication without evidence of adverse effects.

TABLE 17-4 Locating Sites for Intramuscular Injections

SITE/STEPS	FIGURE
Ventrogluteal Site	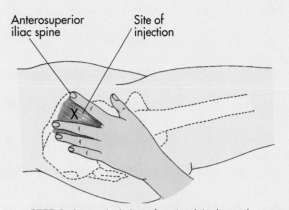

Ventrogluteal Site

1. Position client on either side, with knee bent and upper leg slightly ahead of the bottom leg. Client may also remain supine or may be lying on abdomen. Instruct client to relax muscles to be injected.
2. Palpate the greater trochanter at the head of the femur and the anterior superior iliac spine. To locate the proper site, use the left hand when the client lies on the left side and the right hand when the client lies on the right side.
3. Using the right hand for the left hip and the left hand for the right hip, place the heel of the hand over the greater trochanter of client's hip. Point thumb toward the client's groin and point index finger toward the anterior superior iliac spine and extend the middle finger back along the iliac crest toward the buttock as far as possible (note: a "V" is formed between the index and middle finger) (see illustration).
4. The injection site is the center of the triangle formed by the index and middle fingers.
5. Spread skin taut to give injection. Use dominant hand to give injection (see illustration).

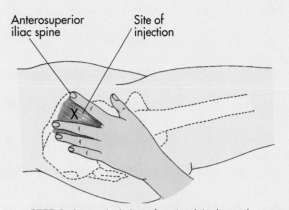

STEP 3 Anatomical view of ventrogluteal muscle.

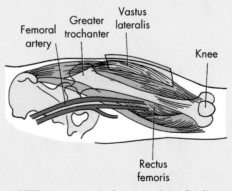

STEP 5 Injection site for ventroglueteal muscle avoids major nerves and blood vessels.

Vastus Lateralis Site

1. Position client lying supine or sitting with site well exposed. If supine, have client flex knee on side where medication will be given.
2. Use the greater trochanter and the knee as landmarks for injection site (see illustration). Place one hand above the knee and one hand below the greater trochanter of the femur.
3. Locate the middle third of the muscle and the midline of the anterior thigh and the midline of the thigh's lateral (outer) side.

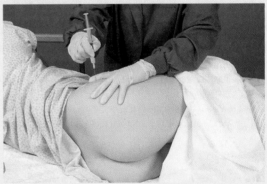
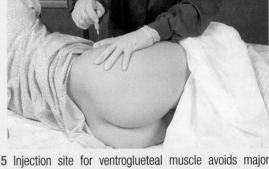

STEP 2 Landmarks for vastus lateralis site.

Continued

TABLE 17-4 Locating Sites for Intramuscular Injections—cont'd

SITE/STEPS	FIGURE

Vastus Lateralis Site—cont'd

4 The injection site is located within a rectangle formed by these boundaries (see illustration).

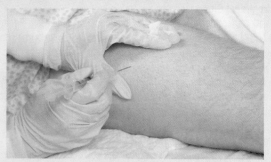

STEP 4 Administering IM injection in vastus lateralis site.

Deltoid Site

1 Position client sitting or lying down, exposing the upper arm and shoulder. Remove any tight-fitting sleeves rather than rolling up.
2 Ask client to relax the arm at the side with the elbow flexed. Instruct client to place the lower arm across the abdomen or chest.
3 Palpate the lower edge of the acromion process, which forms the base of a triangle in line with the midpoint of the lateral aspect of the upper arm (see illustration).
4 Place four fingers across the deltoid muscle, with the top finger along the acromion process.
5 The injection site is in the center of the triangle, about 3 to 5 cm (1 to 2 inches) below the acromion process (see illustration).

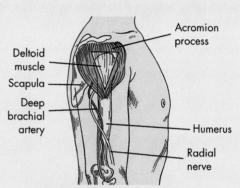

STEP 3 Anatomical view of deltoid muscle.

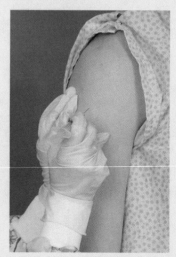

STEP 5 Administering IM injection in deltoid site.

2 Client experiences minimal pain or burning at the injection site.

3 Client understands purpose and desired effects of medication.

Delegation Considerations

The skill of administering IM injections may not be delegated. The nurse directs personnel by:

- Reviewing what to immediately report back to the nurse (e.g., specific medication side effects; reports of pain at injection site; changes in client's physical status, vital signs, or LOC).

Equipment

- IM syringe with needleless vial adapter or filter needle: 2 to 3 ml for adult; 0.5 to 1 ml for infants and small children
- Needle, length, and gauge corresponding to site of injection and age of client according to the following guidelines (Nicoll and Hesby, 2002):
  - Infants and children: ⅝ to 1 inch (based on size of child); 22 to 25 gauge
  - Adults: 1 to 1½ inch; 22 to 27 gauge (aqueous solution); 18 to 25 gauge (oil based)
- Small gauze pad
- Alcohol swab
- Medication ampule or vial
- Clean gloves
- MAR or computer printout

IMPLEMENTATION *for Intramuscular Injections*

STEPS	RATIONALE
1 See Standard Protocol (inside front cover).	
2 Prepare medication in syringe (see Tables 17-1 and 17-2 and Procedural Guidelines 17-1 and 17-2). Be sure syringe has needle of appropriate length and gauge.	Ensures that medication is sterile and the dose is correct.
3 Take medication to client at right time, and perform hand hygiene.	Ensures correct timing for therapeutic benefit.
4 Identify client by checking identification bracelet and asking client's name. Compare with MAR. In some settings, client photographs may also be used. Replace any missing, outdated, or faded identification tools.	Ensures correct client receives medication. At least two client identifiers (neither to be the client's room number) are to be used whenever administering medications (JCAHO, 2006). In many long-term care settings pictures may be used along with identification bands.
5 Compare the label of the mediation with the MAR one more time at the client's bedside.	Third comparison of medication label with the MAR decreases risk of medication administration errors.
6 Explain steps of procedure, and tell client injection will cause a slight burning or stinging.	Helps minimize anxiety.
7 Explain procedure, location of injection site, and how positioning reduces discomfort. Proceed in calm manner.	Allows client to anticipate injection so as to lessen anxiety.
8 Select appropriate IM injection site by assessing size and integrity of muscle. Palpate for areas of tenderness or hardness. Note presence of bruising or area of infection.	The ventrogluteal site is the preferred site for infants, children, and adults unless there are contraindications (e.g., the hepatitis B vaccine should be administered in the deltoid muscle in all clients older than 12 months of age).

> **NURSE ALERT** When choosing an injection site, do not use an area that is bruised, has indurations, has muscular atrophy, has decreased circulation, or has signs associated with infection.

9 Assist client to comfortable position, depending on site (see Table 17-4). Ensure position to relax muscles.	Minimizes discomfort of injection.
10 Relocate site using anatomical landmarks.	Injection into correct anatomical site prevents injury to nerves, bones, and blood vessels.
11 Cleanse site with antiseptic swab. Apply swab to center of site, and rotate outward in circular direction for about 5 cm (2 inches).	Mechanical action of swab removes secretions containing microorganisms.
12 Hold swab or square of sterile gauze between third and fourth fingers of nondominant hand.	Swab or gauze remains readily accessible for when needle is withdrawn.

STEPS	RATIONALE
13 Remove needle cap or sheath from needle by pulling it straight off.	
14 Position the nondominant hand just below site, and pull skin approximately 2.5 to 3.5 cm down or laterally with ulnar side of hand to administer in a Z-track (see Figure 17-12). Hold this position until medication is injected.	Reduces discomfort and incidence of lesions. Z-track technique reduces discomfort and leakage of medication into subcutaneous tissues (McConnell, 2000).

> **NURSE ALERT** If the client's muscle mass is small, grasp the body of the muscle between the thumb and fingers. This ensures that the medication reaches the muscle mass (Hockenberry and Wilson, 2007; Nicoll and Hesby, 2000).

STEPS	RATIONALE
15 Hold syringe between thumb and forefinger of dominant hand as if holding a dart. Hold it with palm down with needle perpendicular to the client's body.	Quick, smooth injection requires proper manipulation of syringe.
16 Administer injection.	
a. Inject needle quickly perpendicular to the client's body, as close to a 90-degree angle as possible.	Smooth, quick injection lessens pain. Angle ensures that the medication reaches muscle mass (Katsma and Katsma, 2000; Nicoll and Hesby, 2002).
b. After needle enters site, grasp lower end of syringe barrel with nondominant hand (while still holding skin back) to stabilize syringe. Continue to hold skin tight with nondominant hand. Move dominant hand to end of plunger. Avoid moving syringe.	Smooth manipulation of syringe parts reduces discomfort from needle movement. Skin must remain pulled until after drug is injected to ensure Z-track administration.
c. Pull back on plunger 5 to 10 seconds. If no blood appears, inject medication slowly at a rate of 1 ml per 10 sec.	Aspiration of blood into syringe indicates accidental IV placement of needle. IM medications are not for IV use. Slow injection allows the muscle fibers to stretch and accommodate the injected volume, which reduces pain and tissue trauma (Nicoll and Hesby, 2002).

> **NURSE ALERT** If blood appears in syringe, remove needle, and dispose of medication and syringe properly. Repeat preparation procedure.

STEPS	RATIONALE
d. Wait 10 seconds, then smoothly and steadily withdraw needle and release skin while placing antiseptic swab or dry gauze gently over injection.	Support of tissues around injection site minimizes discomfort during needle withdrawal. Dry gauze may minimize client discomfort from alcohol on nonintact skin.
17 Apply gentle pressure at site with dry sponge or swab. *Do not massage*.	Minimizes tissue injury. Leaves a zigzag path that seals the needle track where tissue planes slide across each other. Massaging site can cause tissue irritation (Beyea and Nicoll, 1995).
18 For ventrogluteal and vastus lateralis sites, encourage leg exercises. For deltoid site, have client move arm several times.	Promotes drug absorption.
19 Discard sheathed or uncapped needle or needle enclosed in safety shield in appropriately labeled receptacle.	Prevents injury to client and health care personnel. Recapping needles increases risk of needlestick injury (OSHA, 2001).
20 See Completion Protocol (inside front cover).	

EVALUATION

1 Observe and ask about client's response to medication at times that correlate with the medication's onset, peak, and duration to determine effectiveness of drug and observe for adverse reactions.
2 Inspect injection site for bruising, irritation, or induration.
3 Ask client to explain purpose and effects of medication.

Unexpected Outcomes and Related Interventions

1 While administering injection, it feels as though the needle has hit a bone.
a. Pull back on the syringe about ¼ inch, being careful not to pull needle out of skin. Continue with medication administration (Gilsenan, 2000).
2 During injection, nurse aspirates blood.
a. Stop injection and remove needle.
b. Prepare new syringe for administration.
3 Client develops signs and symptoms of allergy or side effects.
a. Follow institutional guidelines for the appropriate response and reporting of adverse drug reactions, and notify client's health care provider immediately.
4 Client complains of localized pain, numbness, or tingling, indicating potential injury to nerves or tissues.
a. Assess injection site and other involved areas, and notify client's health care provider.

Recording and Reporting

• Immediately after administration, record medication dose, route, site, time, and date given on MAR. Correctly sign MAR according to institutional policy.
• Record client's response to medication in nurses' notes.
• Report any undesirable effects from medication to client's health care provider, and document any adverse effects according to institutional policy.

Sample Documentation

1826 Rates incision pain as an 8 on 0 to 10 pain scale. 10 mg morphine sulfate IM given as ordered in right ventrogluteal site.

1900 Rates incision pain as a 4 on 0 to 10 pain scale. Injection site clean, intact, no erythema.

Special Considerations
Pediatric Considerations

• Children can be very anxious or fearful of needles. Assistance with proper positioning and holding of the child may be necessary. Distraction, such as bubble blowing and touch, can help reduce the child's anxiety and pain perception (Sparks, 2001).
• If possible, apply EMLA on site 2½ hours before IM injection or use a vapocoolant spray (e.g., Flouri-Methane) just before injection to decrease pain (Hockenberry and Wilson, 2007).

Geriatric Considerations

• Older adults are prone to muscle atrophy, requiring careful assessment and selection of injection sites. The muscle may have to be grasped between the thumb and fingers for injection.

Home Care Considerations

• Clients requiring regular injections (e.g., vitamin B_{12}) should learn the importance of rotating sites. Injections may be given by family members or client. Instruction will be necessary in proper injection preparation and administration and disposal of syringes and needles (see Procedural Guideline 38-1).
• Consult local agencies for guidelines on properly discarding used needles and sharps in the home setting.

SKILL 17.3 Intradermal Injections

• Nursing Skills Online: Injections, Lesson 4

Nurses administer intradermal injections for small amounts of local anesthetic and skin testing, such as in tuberculosis (TB) screening and allergy testing. Because these medications are potent, they are injected in small amounts into the dermis, where blood supply is reduced and drug absorption occurs slowly. A client may have an anaphylactic reaction if the medication enters the circulation too rapidly. For clients with a history of numerous allergies, the physician may perform skin testing.

Skin testing requires the identification of changes in color and tissue integrity. Therefore choose an intradermal site that is lightly pigmented, free of lesions, and relatively hairless. The inner forearm and upper back are ideal locations.

To administer an injection intradermally, use a TB or small 1-ml syringe with a short (⅜- to ⅝-inch), fine-gauge (25 or 27) needle. The angle of insertion for an intradermal injection is 5 to 15 degrees. Inject only very small amounts of medication (0.01 to 0.1 ml) intradermally. If a bleb does not appear, or if the site bleeds after needle withdrawal, the medication may have entered subcutaneous tissues. In this situation skin test results will not be valid.

ASSESSMENT

1 Identify the drug(s) ordered: action, purpose, normal dosage and route, common side effects, time of onset and peak action, and nursing implications. *Rationale: This allows you to anticipate effects of drugs and to observe client's response.*

2 Assess client's medical history, history of allergies, and medication history.

3 Observe client's verbal and nonverbal response to injection. *Rationale: Injections can cause anxiety, which may increase pain.*

4 Assess for factors that may contraindicate intradermal injections, such as skin infection or lesions. *Rationale: Impedes ability to correctly assess site for skin reaction.*

5 Determine if client had a previous reaction to skin testing. *Rationale: Can prevent a major allergic response.*

6 Assess client's knowledge regarding medication dosage schedule. *Rationale: Information may pose implications for client education.*

PLANNING

Expected Outcomes focus on safe administration and the identification of allergies or exposure to TB.

1 Client experiences very mild burning sensation during injection but no discomfort or adverse effects from the medication after the injection.

2 Small, light-colored bleb, approximately 6 mm (¼ inch) in diameter, forms at site and gradually disappears. Minimal bruising may be present.

3 Client is able to identify signs of a skin reaction and their significance.

Delegation Considerations

The skill of administering intradermal injections may not be delegated. The nurse directs personnel by:

• Reviewing what to immediately report back to the nurse, including signs of possible allergic reactions (e.g., flushing, shortness of breath, anxiety, rapid heart rate, decreased blood pressure).

Equipment

• 1-ml TB syringe with preattached 25- or 27-gauge needle
• Small gauze pad
• Alcohol swab
• Vial or ampule of skin test solution
• Disposable gloves
• Skin pencil (optional)
• MAR or computer printout

IMPLEMENTATION *for Intradermal Injections*

STEPS	RATIONALE
1 See Standard Protocol (inside front cover).	
2 Prepare medication or test solution in syringe (see Tables 17-1 and 17-2). Check dose carefully.	Ensures that medication is sterile and the correct dose.
3 Take medication to client at right time, and perform hand hygiene.	Ensures correct timing for therapeutic benefit.
4 Identify client by checking identification bracelet and asking client's name. Compare with MAR. In some settings, client photographs may also be used. Replace any missing, outdated, or faded identification tools.	Ensures correct client receives medication. At least two client identifiers (neither to be the client's room number) are to be used whenever administering medications (JCAHO, 2006). In many long-term care settings pictures may be used along with identification bands.
5 Compare the label of the medication with the MAR one more time at the client's bedside.	Third comparison of medication label with the MAR decreases risk of medication administration errors.
6 Explain steps of procedure, and tell client injection will cause a slight burning or stinging.	Helps minimize anxiety.
7 Select appropriate injection site. Inspect skin surface for bruises, inflammation, or edema. If possible, select site three to four fingerwidths below antecubital space and one handwidth above wrist (CDC, 2006). If forearm cannot be used, inspect the upper back. NOTE: If necessary, use sites appropriate for subcutaneous injections (see Figure 17-10).	Injection sites should be free of abnormalities that may interfere with drug absorption. An intradermal site should be clear so results of skin test can be seen and interpreted correctly.
8 Assist client to comfortable position with elbow and forearm extended and supported on flat surface.	Stabilizes injection site for easiest accessibility.

STEPS	RATIONALE

9 Cleanse site with an antiseptic swab, beginning at center of the site and rotating outward in a circular direction for about 5 cm (2 inches). Allow to dry.

Mechanical action of swab removes secretions containing microorganisms. Drying prevents antiseptic from affecting test results.

10 Hold swab or square of sterile gauze between third and fourth fingers of nondominant hand or lay aside.

Gauze or swab remains readily accessible when needle is withdrawn.

11 Remove needle cap or sheath from needle by pulling it straight off.

Preventing needle from touching sides of cap prevents contamination.

12 Hold syringe between thumb and forefinger of dominant hand with bevel of needle pointing up.

Smooth injection requires proper manipulation of syringe parts. With bevel up, medication is less likely to be deposited into tissues below dermis.

13 With nondominant hand, stretch skin over site with forefinger or thumb.

Needle pierces tight skin more easily.

14 With needle almost against client's skin, insert it carefully bevel up at a 5- to 15-degree angle until resistance is felt (see illustration). Then advance needle through epidermis to approximately 3 mm (⅛ inch) below skin surface. Needle tip can be seen through skin.

Ensures needle tip is in dermis. Results will be inaccurate if needle is not injected at correct angle and depth (CDC, 2006).

15 Inject medication slowly. Normally resistance is felt. If not, needle is too deep; remove and begin again.

Slow injection minimizes discomfort at site. Dermal layer is tight and does not expand easily when solution is injected.

> **NURSE ALERT** It is not necessary to aspirate, because dermis is relatively avascular.

16 While injecting medication, a bleb resembling a mosquito bite approximately 6 mm (¼ inch) in diameter forms at site (see illustration).

Bleb indicates medication is in dermis.

> **COMMUNICATION TIP** During this time, explain to client that the skin at the site of injection will be marked and not to wash off marking. Tell the client that redness and a lump at the site indicate a positive response to the skin test.

17 Withdraw needle while applying dry gauze gently over site.

Support of tissue around injection site minimizes discomfort during needle withdrawal.

18 *Do not massage* site or apply bandage.

Massage or pressure from a bandage may disperse medication into underlying tissue layers and alter test results.

19 Assist client to comfortable position.

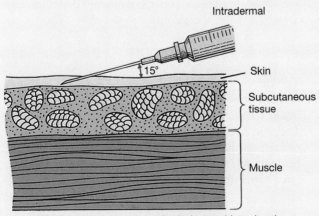

STEP 14 Intradermal needle tip inserted into dermis.

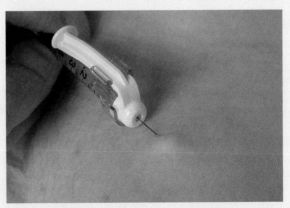

STEP 16 Injection creates a small bleb.

STEPS	RATIONALE
20 Discard sheathed or uncapped needle or needle enclosed in safety shield in appropriately labeled receptacle.	Prevents injury to client and health care personnel. Recapping needles increases risk of needlestick injury (OSHA, 2001).
21 Use skin pencil, and draw circle around perimeter of injection site. Read site within appropriate amount of time, designated by type of medication or skin test given. If client is tested in a clinic or other outpatient setting, have client return to health care provider's office.	The results of skin testing are determined at various times based on the type of medication used or the type of skin testing (see manufacturer's directions).

> **NURSE ALERT** Read TB test at 48 to 72 hours. Positive TB reaction is indicated by induration (hardened raised area) of skin around injection site of:
>
> 15 mm or more in clients with no known risk factors for TB
>
> 10 mm or more in clients who are recent immigrants; injection drug users; residents and employees of high-risk settings; clients with certain chronic illnesses; children younger than 4 years of age; and infants, children, and adolescents exposed to high-risk adults
>
> 5 mm or more in clients who are human immunodeficiency virus (HIV) positive, immunocompromised clients (e.g., clients who have organ transplants or are receiving cancer chemotherapy), or clients recently exposed to TB (CDC, 2006)

22 See Completion Protocol (inside front cover).

EVALUATION

1 Remain with client and observe for any allergic reactions NOTE: Severe anaphylactic reaction is characterized by dyspnea, wheezing, and circulatory collapse and requires immediate attention.

2 Inspect bleb. *Optional:* Use skin pencil and draw circle around perimeter of injection site. Tell client not to wash off markings around injection site.

3 Ask client to describe implications of skin testing and signs of expected skin reaction or hypersensitivity.

Unexpected Outcomes and Related Interventions

1 Raised, reddened, or hard zone (induration) appears at injection site, indicating sensitivity to injected allergen or positive test for TB skin testing.

a. Document results, and notify client's health care provider.

b. Positive TB reaction is indicated by induration 5 mm or more at injection site. (See Skill 17.3, Step 21 Nurse Alert.)

2 Onset of allergic reaction occurs within minutes.

a. Follow institutional policy or guidelines for appropriate response to allergic reactions.

b. Notify client's health care provider immediately.

3 Client is unable to explain purpose or reading of skin testing.

a. Provide further instruction, or make alternative plans for reading of skin site if client is unable to learn at this time.

Recording and Reporting

- Record amount, type of medication, site of injection, and date and time on medication record.
- Record area of injection and appearance of skin in nurses' notes.
- Report any undesirable effects from medication to client's health care provider, and document adverse effects according to institutional policy.

Sample Documentation

1000 PPD injection site in left lower forearm; approximate 6-mm diameter bleb formed at injection site marked with skin pencil. Client instructed not to wash the skin pencil off and to return to clinic in 48 hours to read results. Client remained in clinic waiting room for 20 minutes and discharged after no allergic response noted.

Special Considerations
Geriatric Considerations

- TB skin testing in older adults is an unreliable indicator of TB. Older adults often display a false-negative skin test as a result of reduced immune system activity.
- The skin becomes less elastic because of physiological changes in the older adult. Therefore the skin must be held taut to ensure the intradermal injection is administered correctly.

SKILL 17.4 Continuous Subcutaneous Medications

The continuous subcutaneous infusion (CSQI or CSCI) route of medication administration is an alternative to IV, IM, or subcutaneous injections of medication. The CSQI route is appropriate for continuous administration of medications for pain management (e.g., opioids) and for insulin administration. It has also been used with medications (e.g., terbutaline) to stop preterm labor. One factor that determines the infusion rate of CSQI medications is the rate of medication absorption. As the rate of infusion increases, absorption of the medication decreases. Most clients can absorb 2 to 3 ml of medication per hour (Pasero, 2002).

CSQI is used in many settings, including the home, because it enables clients to manage their illness or pain without the risks and expenses involved with IV medication administration. When used for pain management, this route provides better pain control and less sleep disturbance related to pain when compared with IV pain medications (Pasero, 2002). Box 17-5 summarizes benefits for the use of CSQI in clients requiring pain management.

Diabetics who use CSQI for blood glucose management must have intense diabetes self-management education. Newer insulin pumps provide simultaneous glucose monitoring as well as insulin delivery (Medtronic MiniMed, 2006). Selection criteria for clients' use of an insulin pump are listed in Box 17-6.

The procedure to start and discontinue CSQI therapy is similar regardless of the type of medication being delivered. However, nursing assessment and interventions vary depending on the type of medication. For example, if the medication is used for pain management, you evaluate the effectiveness of the medication by measuring the client's pain severity. Alternatively, if the client is receiving insulin, you monitor and evaluate the client's blood glucose levels, weight gain, and occurrences of hypoglycemia and hyperglycemia (Weissberg-Benchell and others, 2003).

Use a small-gauge (25 to 27) winged butterfly IV needle to deliver medications through CSQI. Alternatively, you may use a special commercially prepared Teflon cannula. Although Teflon cannulas are generally more expensive,

they tend to be more comfortable for the client, have lower rates of complications when compared with winged IV needles, and are associated with fewer needlestick injuries (Dawkins and others, 2000; Torre, 2002). The choice of needle type is based on institutional guideline or client preference. Use the needle that has the shortest length and the smallest gauge necessary to establish and maintain the infusion.

Use the same anatomical sites for subcutaneous injections (see Figure 17-10) and the upper chest. Site selection depends on the client's activity level and the type of medication delivered. For example, insulin is absorbed most consistently in the abdomen; thus a site in the abdomen, away from the waistline, is the preferred administration site. Sites should avoid scar tissue and areas of hardened tissues. Always try to avoid sites where clothing could rub or constrict the pump's tubing. Sites should be free from irritation and away from bony prominences and the waistline. Rotate sites at least every 72 hours or whenever complications, such as leaking or infection, occur (Medtronic MiniMed, 2006).

This route requires the use of a computerized pump with safety features, including lockout intervals and warning alarms. A variety of medication pumps are currently available (Figure 17-12). Ideally, medication pumps should be chosen for each individual, based on the medication being delivered and the client's needs. The availability and cost of the pump and its supplies should also be considered. When possible, have clients select the pump that fits their needs the best and that is the easiest to use.

Box 17-6 Selection Criteria for Clients Using Insulin Pumps

- Possesses strong motivation and commitment to use diabetes management skills.
- Requires or desires improved control of blood glucose levels.
- Requires greater flexibility than allowed by traditional insulin injection schedules.
- Is willing to participate in formal diabetes education program.
- Possesses strong critical-thinking and problem-solving skills.
- Accepts responsibilities associated with the self-management of diabetes.
- Able to perform self–blood glucose monitoring and to operate the insulin pump.
- Displays evidence of effective coping patterns.
- Has support systems available.
- Secures financial resources to cover costs associated with CSQI.

Modified from American Diabetes Association: Continuous subcutaneous insulin infusion, *Diabetes Care* 27(suppl 1):S110, 2004a; Lenhard MJ, Reeves GD: Continuous subcutaneous insulin infusion: a comprehensive review of insulin pump therapy, *Arch Intern Med* 161(19):2293, 2001.

BOX 17-5 Benefits Associated with Pain Management Delivered by Continuous Subcutaneous Infusion

- Can be used in clients with poor venous access.
- Provides pain relief to clients who are unable to tolerate oral pain medications.
- Allows clients greater mobility.
- Onset of action takes about 20 minutes.
- Provides better pain control than IM injections.
- Costs are almost half of costs associated with IV infusion.

Modified from Pasero C: Subcutaneous opioid infusion, *Am J Nurse* 102(7)61: 2002.

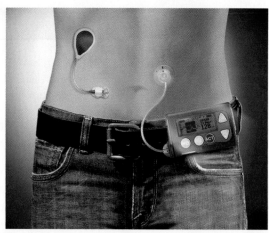

FIGURE 17-12 MiniMed Paradigm REAL-Time Insulin Pump and Continuous Glucose Monitoring System. (Courtesy Medtronic MiniMed, Northridge, Calif.)

ASSESSMENT

1 Identify the drug(s) ordered: action, purpose, normal dosage and route, common side effects, time of onset and peak action, and nursing implications. *Rationale: This allows you to anticipate effects of drugs and to observe client's response.*

2 Assess client's medical history, history of allergies, and medication history.

3 Observe client's verbal and nonverbal response to needle insertion. *Rationale: Injections can cause anxiety, which may increase pain.*

4 Assess adequacy of client's adipose tissue. *Rationale: Physiological changes associated with aging or client illness influence the amount of subcutaneous tissue, which affects choice of catheter insertion site.*

5 Assess client's knowledge regarding medication to be received and use of the medication pump. *Rationale: Determines client's ability to problem-solve and manage pump.*

6 Assess client's symptoms before initiation of medication therapy. Determine client's severity of pain (if using analgesia) or measure blood glucose level (if using insulin). *Rationale: Provides data to evaluate desired effects of CSQI medication.*

PLANNING

Expected Outcomes focus on effective pain management or blood glucose control with minimal anxiety and discomfort.

1 Needle insertion site remains free from infection.

2 Desired effect of medication is achieved with no signs of adverse reactions.

3 Client explains purpose, dosage, and effects of medication and verbalizes understanding of CSQI therapy.

Delegation Considerations

The skill of administering continuous subcutaneous medications may not be delegated. The nurse directs personnel by:

• Explaining how to adapt hygiene techniques so as not to damage the cannula or needle insertion site

• Reviewing what to immediately report back to the nurse (e.g., symptoms of poor glucose control, skin irritation, changes in client status)

Equipment
Initiation of CSQI

• Clean gloves
• Alcohol swab
• Antibacterial skin prep, such as chlorhexidine
• Small-gauge (25 to 27) winged IV needle with attached tubing or cannula especially for CSQI (e.g., Sof-Set)
• Infusion pump
• Occlusive, transparent dressing
• Tape
• Medication in appropriate syringe or container

Discontinuation of CSQI

• Clean, nonsterile gloves
• Small, sterile gauze dressing and tape or adhesive bandage
• Alcohol swab and chlorhexidine (optional)

IMPLEMENTATION *for Continuous Subcutaneous Medications*

STEPS	RATIONALE
1 See Standard Protocol (inside front cover).	
2 Review manufacturer's directions.	Ensures proper use of equipment, as there may be differences from one manufacturer to another.
3 Prepare medication from vial or ampule (see Tables 17-1 and 17-2), or check dose on prefilled syringe and prime tubing with medication.	Ensures that medication is sterile and the correct dose.
4 Obtain and program medication administration pump.	Ensures that dose is accurate and medication is sterile.
5 Take medication to client at right time, and perform hand hygiene.	Ensures correct timing for therapeutic benefit.

STEPS	RATIONALE
6 Identify client by checking identification bracelet and asking client's name. Compare with MAR. In some settings, client photographs may also be used. Replace any missing, outdated, or faded identification tools.	Ensures correct client receives medication. At least two client identifiers (neither to be the client's room number) are to be used whenever administering medications (JCAHO, 2006). In many long-term care settings pictures may be used along with identification bands.
7 Compare the label of the mediation with the MAR one more time at the client's bedside.	Third comparison of medication label with the MAR decreases risk of medication administration errors.
8 Explain steps of procedure and tell client that needle insertion will cause a slight burning or stinging.	Provides opportunity to demonstrate use of CSQI.
9 Initiate CSQI.	
a. Select appropriate injection site. Most common sites used are subclavicular, abdominal, upper arms, and thighs.	Site must be free from irritation and not over bony prominences.
b. Assist client to comfortable position.	Eases pain associated with insertion of needle.
c. ✋ Cleanse injection site with alcohol using a circular motion, followed by skin prep agent, such as chlorhexidine, using straight cleansing strokes. Allow both agents to dry.	Reduces risk of infection at insertion site.

> **NURSE ALERT** Clients managing CSQI at home may use an antibacterial soap (e.g., Hibiclens, pHisoHex) instead of alcohol and chlorhexidine to cleanse insertion site.

STEPS	RATIONALE
d. Hold needle in dominant hand, and remove needle guard.	Prepares needle for insertion.
e. Gently pinch or lift up skin with nondominant hand.	Ensures needle will enter subcutaneous tissue.
f. Gently and firmly insert needle at 45- to 90-degree angle (see illustration).	Decreases pain related to insertion of needle.

> **NURSE ALERT** Some prepackaged needles (e.g., Sof-Set, Sub-Q-Set) are inserted at a 90-degree angle. These needles are shorter than butterfly needles. Refer to manufacturer's directions.

STEPS	RATIONALE
g. Release skinfold, and apply tape over "wings" of needle.	Secures needle.
h. Place occlusive, transparent dressing over insertion site (see illustration).	Protects site from infection and allows nurse to assess site during medication infusion.
i. Attach tubing from needle to tubing from infusion pump, and turn pump on.	Allows medication to be administered.

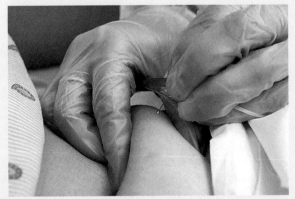

STEP 9f. Insertion of butterfly needle into subcutaneous tissue of abdomen.

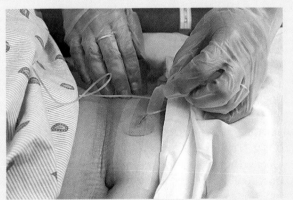

STEP 9h. Securing injection site.

STEPS	RATIONALE

> **NURSE ALERT** Some cannulas have a sharp needle with a plastic catheter covering the needle. In this case, remove the needle and leave the plastic catheter in the skin.

j. Dispose of any sharps into appropriate leak-proof, puncture-resistant container.	Prevents injury to clients and health care personnel (OSHA, 2001).
k. Assess site before leaving client, and instruct client to inform nurse if site becomes red or begins to leak.	A new site with a new needle must be initiated whenever erythema or leaking occurs (Pasero, 2002).

> **COMMUNICATION TIP** Some medications (e.g., fentanyl) burn with initiation of medication pump. Tell client, "You may feel some burning with this medication, but it should go away as the medication infuses for a while. Please let me know if this medication makes you uncomfortable."

10 Discontinue CSQI.	
a. Verify order, and establish alternative method for medication administration if applicable.	If medication will be required after discontinuing CSQI, a different medication and/or route may be necessary to continue to manage client's illness or pain.
b. Stop infusion pump.	Prevents spillage of medication.
c. Perform hand hygiene.	Follows Centers for Disease Control and Prevention (CDC) recommendations to prevent accidental exposure to blood and body fluids (OSHA, 2001).
d. Remove dressing without dislodging or removing needle.	Exposes needle.

> **NURSE ALERT** If site is infected or if included in institutional guidelines, cleanse site with alcohol and skin prep agent such as chlorhexidine. Apply triple antibiotic cream to site if it is excoriated (Pasero, 2002).

e. Remove tape from wings of needle, and pull needle out at the same angle it was inserted.	Minimizes discomfort to client.
f. Apply gentle pressure at site until no fluid leaks out of skin.	Dressing will adhere to site if the skin remains dry.
g. Apply small sterile gauze dressing or adhesive bandage to site.	Prevents bacterial entry into puncture site.
11 See Completion Protocol (inside front cover).	

EVALUATION

1 Evaluate client's response to medication.
2 Assess site at least every 4 hours for redness, pain, drainage, or swelling.
3 Ask client to verbalize understanding of medication and CSQI therapy.

Unexpected Outcomes and Related Interventions

1 Client complains of localized pain or burning at needle's insertion site, or site appears red, swollen, or is leaking, indicating potential infection or dislodgement of needle.
a. Remove needle, and place new needle in different site.
b. Continue to monitor old site for signs of infection, and notify health care provider if infection is suspected.

2 Client displays allergic symptoms to medication.
a. Follow institutional policy or guidelines for appropriate response to allergic reactions, and notify client's health care provider immediately.
3 CSQI becomes dislodged.
a. Stop the infusion, apply pressure at the site until no fluid leaks from skin, cover site with gauze dressing or adhesive bandage, and initiate a new site.
b. Assess client to determine effects of not receiving medication (e.g., assess client's level of comfort using a pain scale, obtain blood glucose levels if receiving insulin).

Recording and Reporting

- Immediately after initiating CSQI, chart medication, dose, route, site, time, date, and type of medication pump in client's medical record.
- Record client's response to medication and appearance of site every 4 hours or according to institutional policy in nurses' notes.
- Report any adverse effects from medication or infection at insertion site to client's health care provider, and document according to institutional policy. Client's condition may indicate need for additional or different medical therapy.

Sample Documentation

2210 Initiated CSQI in left middle abdominal site. Current pain status 8 on a 0 to 10 scale. Instructed client regarding need to call if pain persists or if site becomes red or begins to drain.

2250 Infusion running; pain rating at 4 on a 0 to 10 scale.

Special Considerations

Pediatric Considerations

- Insulin pump therapy has been successfully used in toddlers and preschoolers. Toddlers have better glycemic control with fewer episodes of hypoglycemia (Litton and others, 2002).

- Insulin pumps are effective with adolescents. Use of these pumps offers the child greater flexibility and transfers responsibility of diabetes management from parent to child. Extensive education is needed for both the adolescent and the parent to ensure effective diabetes management (Hockenberry and Wilson, 2007).

Geriatric Considerations

- CSQI can deliver isotonic IV solutions to dehydrated older adults. This is called hypodermoclysis therapy. This method of providing hydration avoids the need to transfer the client from home or long-term care facility to an acute care hospital. Fluids should infuse slowly (e.g., 30 ml/hr) during the first hour of therapy.

Home Care Considerations

- Clients at home with CSQI must identify an additional caregiver if possible.
- Educate the client and the caregiver about the desired effect of the medication, side effects and adverse effects of the medication, operation of the pump, when and how to assess and rotate injection sites, and when to call a health care provider for problems.

NCLEX® Style Questions

1 To prepare a medication from an ampule, the nurse:
1. Wipes the top of the ampule with alcohol
2. Uses a filter needle
3. Injects air into the ampule before withdrawing the dose
4. Breaks off the top of the ampule toward the hands

2 When mixing two medications in one syringe when one medication is in a vial and the other is in an ampule, the nurse prepares the medication in the ampule first.
1. True
2. False

3 Which of the following assessment findings indicates a positive TB reaction in a client with no known risk factors for TB?
1. A large area of redness and swelling at the injection site
2. An induration of 18 mm
3. Frequent, productive cough accompanied by a fever
4. Sudden onset of shortness of breath and wheezing

4 Which of the following symptoms may indicate that a client has sustained an injury to a nerve after an IM injection?
1. Pain, numbness, and tingling at the injection site 2 hours after the injection
2. Pain experienced during the injection
3. Urticaria, eczema, wheezing, and dyspnea
4. Nausea, vomiting, and diarrhea

5 Match the best needle size to use when administering an IM injection, in each situation listed.
1. 25-gauge, ⅝- to 1-inch _____
2. 22-gauge, 1½-inch _____
3. 18-gauge, 1½-inch _____
   a. Viscous or oil-based solution
   b. Children older than 1 year
   c. Average size 30-year-old female

References for all chapters appear in Appendix D.

18

Preparing the Client for Surgery

MEDIA RESOURCES

- **evolve** http://evolve.elsevier.com/Elkin

- **View Video!** Video Clips

Surgery is a stressful experience for the client, both psychologically and physiologically. The client has little control over the situation or the outcome, resulting in feelings of anxiety, fear, and powerlessness. As with trauma, surgery is a physiological stressor affecting the major body systems. Preoperative care can reduce this stress and place the client in the best condition possible to undergo the surgery. The nurse thoroughly assesses the client's condition, teaches the client and family what to expect, and prepares the client physically and psychologically for surgery.

For any surgical procedure, it is important to complete a thorough preoperative assessment. For clients who are already hospitalized, this may occur the day before surgery. For clients having surgery in an ambulatory surgery unit, the preoperative assessment may begin several days before surgery and be completed the morning of surgery. Regardless of the setting, the preoperative assessment forms the basis for a plan of care for the client during and after surgery.

Often the client is unsure of what to expect and has concerns about the amount of pain, disfigurement involved with surgery, and length of recovery. Many clients return home the same day, and family members may be unsure about their role in the client's care and recovery. Before the client undergoes surgery, and again before discharge, teach the client and family what to expect and what they can do to assist in the recovery process.

Physically preparing the client to undergo surgery and anesthesia involves important skills. Regardless of the surgery, safety measures, such as verifying the procedure and surgical site, and consent, are critical. Other steps, such as urinary catheterization or special laboratory tests, are completed only for specific surgical procedures. Physical preparation focuses on minimizing the risks involved with surgery and anesthesia, while optimizing the client's condition.

EVIDENCE IN PRACTICE

Crowther M, McCourt K: Get the edge on deep vein thrombosis: head off progression of this deadly condition by knowing when to assess and what to look for during patient screening, *Nurs Manage* 35(1):21, 2004.

Deep vein thrombosis (DVT) is a common complication of surgery. According to Crowther and McCourt (2004), more than 50% of clients undergoing orthopedic surgeries (hip and knee replacements in particular) and between 10% and 40% of clients undergoing abdominal or thoracic surgeries develop DVT. Nurses play an important role in DVT prevention through client education regarding leg exercises, early ambulation, avoidance of prolonged inactivity and constrictive clothing, hydration maintenance, and use of graduated compression stockings. Use of low-dose unfractionated heparin or low molecular weight (LMW) heparin is highly successful in preventing DVT. The subcutaneous administration of these medications just before surgery is recommended.

NURSING DIAGNOSES

Nursing diagnoses associated with the surgical experience include **risk for infection** related to the surgical incision, urinary catheter, and invasive lines, **risk for injury** related to inadequate identification and communication of risks, and **risk for perioperative positioning injury** related to surgical positioning and placement of electrical equipment used in the operating room (OR). Psychological states such as **deficient knowledge, anxiety,** and **fear** often result when a client is unsure what to expect during the surgical experience. The inability to control the situation often results in **powerlessness,** and the inability to accept the situation may result in **ineffective coping.** During and after surgery using general anesthesia, the client's cough and gag reflexes are suppressed. In addition, inhaled anesthesia may cause increased mucus production. This results in a risk for **ineffective airway clearance** related to retention of secretions.

SKILL 18.1 Preoperative Assessment

To identify risks and plan for the client's care during and after surgery, perform a thorough preoperative assessment of the client's physiological and psychological condition. Many health care facilities have a designated department devoted to completing thorough preoperative screening and testing. Laboratory tests, electrocardiograms (ECGs), chest x-rays, and other tests are often obtained in these facilities 1 to 2 weeks in advance of the scheduled surgical procedure. Perioperative staff perform a thorough assessment and review the test results to identify any potential abnormalities that may need further evaluation and treatment before surgery. Clients are assessed again 1 to 2 hours before the scheduled time of surgery to ensure there are no changes to their medical condition. Advanced planning allows time for nurses to follow up on any unexpected outcomes. Before beginning this assessment, establish a trusting relationship with the client. It is not unusual for the client to remember and report at this time facts that were not told to the physician earlier. Provide the client privacy and a location free of interruption to encourage open communication.

PLANNING

Expected Outcomes focus on obtaining accurate information and identifying risk factors related to the intended surgery.
- Client provides the information required to establish a plan of care.
- Client remains alert and appropriately responsive to nurse's assessment questions.

Delegation Considerations
The skills of preoperative assessment may not be delegated. However, in stable clients the nurse directs personnel by:
- Instructing when to obtain vital signs and weight and height measurements.
- Reporting any abnormal assessment findings to the nurse.

Equipment
- Stethoscope
- Blood pressure cuff
- Pulse oximeter
- Thermometer
- Watch or clock with a second hand
- Scale
- Preoperative assessment form (Figure 18-1)

A-1c4 NURSE'S DETAILED PERIOPERATIVE NOTE

DATE

HOSP. #

NAME

BIRTH DATE

ADDRESS

SS#

1. Place initials in the space preceding the appropriate response (YES/NO, MET/NOT MET, NOT APPLICABLE)
2. Explain any "NO" or "NOT MET" in the space provided adjacent to the item or in the comment section provided, except for * items.
3. Record additional information in the comment section.
4. Record initials immediately following narrative entry.

IF NOT IMPRINTED, PLEASE PRINT DATE, HOSP. #, NAME AND LOCATION

PERIOPERATIVE TRANSPORT BY:	METHOD:	PREOPERATIVE UNIT/AREA:
TIME RECEIVED IN PRESURGICAL CARE UNIT:	TIME RECEIVED IN OR:	

PATIENT ASSESSMENT/PREPARATION	YES	NO	COMMENT	
PATIENT IDENTIFIED			ID Band Location	
BLOOD BAND PRESENT*			#/Location	
ALLERGIES* (If yes, please list)				
LATEX PRECAUTIONS INDICATED*				
CONSENT				
NPO				
HEALTH CHANGED SINCE LAST APPT			If Yes, Specify:	Physician Notified:
INFECTIONS, PROBLEMS WITH HEART OR LUNGS			If Yes, Specify:	Physician Notified:
TAKING ANY NEW MEDICATIONS			If Yes, Specify:	Physician Notified:
PREOPERATIVE ORDERS COMPLETED				
SKIN ASSESSMENT COMPLETED				
VITALS OBTAINED DAY OF SURGERY				
HISTORY AND PHYSICAL PRESENT				
LAB VALUES REVIEWED				
LEVEL OF CONSCIOUSNESS—Answers questions/responds appropriately for age				
IMPLANTS/PROSTHESIS* (If yes, please list)				

Preoperative pain score (0–10) _____
Surgical site verified and marked with patient ☐ _____
Patient voided @ _____ Belongings: _____
Nursing comments _____

NURSING DIAGNOSIS	NURSING ORDERS/INTERVENTIONS	EXPECTED PATIENT OUTCOMES
ANXIETY—Risk of, Related to Surgical Intervention and Outcomes	1. Psychologic & physiologic comfort measures are provided. ___ Yes ___ No	The patient reports and/or demonstrates a reduction in anxiety. ___ MET ___ NOT MET
KNOWLEDGE DEFICIT—Risk of, Related to Surgical Intervention	1. The patient's understanding is assessed and questions/concerns are addressed by the appropriate individuals. ___ Yes ___No	The patient's (guardian's) description of surgery corresponds with the Operative Consent (G-2d). ___ MET ___ NOT MET
INJURY—Risk for, Related to Tubes, Catheters, Lines ___ Not Applicable	1. Integrity of tubes, catheters, and lines is maintained. ___ Yes ___ No Catheters/Tubes/Drains/Lines: _____	The patient's risk for injury related to care and management of tubes, catheters, and lines is minimized. ___ MET ___ NOT MET

Initials	Standards Implemented By:	Initials	Standards Implemented By:

26304/9-01/MH05859

UNIVERSITY OF IOWA HOSPITALS AND CLINICS

Side tabs: A -1c4 / B CLIN. NOTES / C LABORATORY / D X-RAY EXAM / E CONSULTATION / F SPEC. EXAM / G THERAPY / H PATHOLOGY / I PT. QUES.

FIGURE 18-1 Preoperative assessment form. (Courtesy University of Iowa Hospitals and Clinics.)

IMPLEMENTATION *for Preoperative Assessment*

STEPS	RATIONALE
1 See Standard Protocol (inside front cover).	
2 Determine if the client has any communication impairment (e.g., blindness, hearing loss), is able to read and understand English, and is mentally competent. For example, give client an informational brochure and have him or her explain a portion of the contents.	Allows you to determine whether your assessment approach needs to be adapted. Clients with reading difficulties may take the opportunity to open up and discuss the issue (Weiss, 2003).
3 Assess the client's understanding of the intended surgery and anesthesia. Have the client describe in his or her own words.	Asking client to offer a description rather than asking a simple yes or no question (e.g., "Do you understand your surgery?") provides a better determination of level of understanding.
4 Ask if client has an advance directive (see Chapter 37).	Advance directives protect the client's rights by communicating client's treatment preferences if he or she is unable to communicate.
5 Obtain a nursing history.	
a. Condition leading to surgery.	Allows you to anticipate postoperative needs and complications.
b. Chronic illnesses and associated risks (e.g., hypertension—bleeding and stroke; asthma—impaired ventilation; hiatal hernia—aspiration; diabetes—poor wound healing; MRSA—impaired wound healing and sepsis).	Some chronic conditions increase the risk of complications from surgery and anesthesia.
c. Last menstrual period (for female clients in childbearing years).	Anesthetic agents and other medications could injure the fetus.
d. Previous hospitalizations.	Determines if client is familiar with hospital procedures.
e. Medication history, including prescription, over-the-counter (OTC), and herbal remedies and date/time of last doses.	Client may not report OTC medications and herbal remedies unless specifically asked. All may interact with anesthetic agents or other medications given during surgery. The client may be instructed to take any routine blood pressure, cardiac, or seizure medications. Changes in dosages of oral diabetic agents or insulin may be ordered.
f. Previous experience with surgery and anesthesia. Have client clarify if any undesirable outcomes occurred.	Information will assist in preventing recurrent problems with the planned surgery.
g. Family history of complications from surgery or anesthesia.	A family history of reactions to anesthetic agents may indicate a familial condition such as malignant hyperthermia, which is life threatening.
h. Allergies to medications, food, or tape, including specific questions about natural rubber latex (see Chapter 5). Ask clients if they have had any problem with medication or anything placed on their skin.	Reactions to latex can be life threatening, and prevention in sensitized clients requires specific precautions. Often clients with latex allergies are scheduled as first case of the day. Also, many clients do not understand that rubber and latex are the same. Using both words will help obtain accurate information.

> **COMMUNICATION TIP** When asking the client about allergies, ask a specific question about reactions or problems the client might have had to natural rubber latex. Most clients do not know that rubber is latex. Using both words with the examples of balloons and gloves helps to obtain otherwise missed information.

STEPS	RATIONALE
i. Physical impairment.	Physical impairments may cause limited mobility and situations that could lead to problems with positioning during surgery. Communicate this information to the OR nurse because these clients may need special positioning or considerations (Heizenroth, 2003).

STEPS	RATIONALE
j. Prostheses and implants (e.g., implantable medication delivery pump, dentures, hearing aid, pacemaker, internal defibrillator, hip prosthesis).	These devices could become damaged or malfunction from electrical equipment used during surgery. Report this information to the OR nurse.
k. Smoking, alcohol, and drug use.	Increases risk of intraoperative and postoperative complications.
l. Occupation.	Anticipates how postoperative restrictions affect a client's return to work.
6 Assess client's weight (see Procedural Guideline 8-1), height, and vital signs (see Skill 11.1).	Height and weight are used to calculate drug dosages. Vital signs provide a baseline for postoperative comparison.
7 Assess client's respiratory status, including character and rate of respirations, oxygen saturation, ability to breathe lying flat, use of oxygen or continuous positive airway pressure (CPAP) at home, and chest x-ray report.	Poor respiratory condition can affect the client's response to general anesthesia. Use of CPAP may indicate client has obstructive sleep apnea, a condition that poses risks postoperatively.
8 Evaluate client's circulatory status, including apical pulse, ECG report, and peripheral pulses (see Skill 12.4).	Circulation may be a factor in positioning the client on the OR table.
9 Determine client's neurological status, including level of consciousness (LOC) (see Skill 12.1).	Client's neurological status affects attentiveness to instruction. Offers important baseline for postoperative evaluation.
10 Evaluate client's musculoskeletal system, including range of motion (ROM) of joints (see Skill 12.6).	If the ROM is limited, extra care will be needed to prevent injury related to positioning in surgery.
11 Examine client's skin; identify any breaks in skin integrity and determine level of hydration (see Skill 12.1). Pay particular attention to area of body in which client will be positioned.	If skin is thin, broken, or bruised, extra padding will be needed in surgery. Hydration may affect skin integrity.
12 Evaluate client's emotional status, including level of anxiety, coping ability, and family support.	If client has high level of anxiety or fear, consultation with a social worker, pastoral care, or advanced practice nurse (APN) might be useful.
13 Review the results of laboratory tests, including complete blood count (CBC), electrolytes, urinalysis, and other diagnostic tests.	Laboratory work provides an assessment of major body systems.
14 Identify the time of client's last intake of food or drink.	With client under general anesthesia, the esophageal sphincter relaxes and the stomach contents can be aspirated.
15 See Completion Protocol (inside front cover).	

EVALUATION

1 Determine if client information is complete so plan of care can be established. Validate unclear information with family.

2 Evaluate client's ability to cooperate (e.g., makes eye contact, answers appropriately).

Unexpected Outcomes and Related Interventions

1 The client does not understand English.

a. Obtain a professional medical interpreter.

2 The client is not mentally competent.

a. Determine who is legally authorized to consent to surgery (see agency policy).

b. Determine who can provide health history.

3 Client does not understand what surgery will be performed.

a. Notify the surgeon.

4 The client reports a condition that is a risk factor for surgery or postoperatively, such as hiatal hernia, pregnancy, family history of complications with anesthesia, cold or upper respiratory infection, recent chest pain, or sleep apnea.

a. Notify the surgeon and anesthesia provider.

5 The client has been taking anticoagulants.

a. Notify the surgeon.

6 Client reports an allergy to latex.

a. Remove all supplies containing latex from client's room.

b. Post a latex precautions sign on the door or stretcher.

c. Notify surgeon, anesthesia provider, and OR nurse.

7 Appropriate laboratory tests were not ordered or completed.

a. Notify surgeon and anesthesia provider, and make arrangements for tests to be completed.

8 Chest x-ray report, ECG, or laboratory tests show abnormal findings.

a. Notify surgeon and anesthesia provider.

9 Client has a blister, abrasion, or boil near the incision site.

a. Notify surgeon.

Recording and Reporting

- Document findings on the preoperative portion of the nurses' detailed preoperative notes (see Figure 18-1) or other designated agency form.
- Report abnormal laboratory values or other concerns to the surgeon or anesthesiologist.

Sample Documentation

0830 Nursing history completed. States that after knee surgery last year she "vomited for 6 hours." Anesthesiologist notified of client history of vomiting after surgery.

Special Considerations
Pediatric Considerations

- Consider a child's developmental level when performing preoperative preparation; for example, use toys and games to demonstrate preoperative procedures (Hockenberry, 2005).
- Allow the parents to wait with the child until initial sedation begins to take effect. The child does not remember the parents leaving. Reunite parents with child postoperatively as soon as the child is waking in recovery.

Geriatric Considerations

- Age-related changes may result in diminished short-term memory. Additional assessment and teaching may be necessary in this area.
- An older adult may have some limitation in ROM. If this limitation is significant, notify the OR nurse so that surgical position can be modified.

SKILL 18.2 Preoperative Teaching

Preoperative client teaching involves assisting a client with understanding and mentally preparing for the surgical experience (Iowa Intervention Project, 2000). Research shows that preoperative teaching decreases complications, increases client satisfaction, decreases length of stay, and promotes psychological well-being (Oetker-Black and others, 2003). Plan your teaching based on the preoperative assessment. Make every attempt to ensure the client's privacy. Select the best learning method for the client. In many settings, videotape and written materials are available to assist you. Whenever possible, have the family members responsible for the client's care after surgery present. Later they serve as coaches and assist the client in performing exercises. Plan to have the client demonstrate expected postoperative skills to allow for practice and facilitate understanding.

Clients and their families are often anxious about impending surgery. Learning is impaired by anxiety. Speak in a clear, slow voice to reduce the client's anxiety and promote understanding. You may need extra time for teaching and reinforcement to ensure client understanding. Postoperatively, high anxiety can lead to negative psychological and physiological outcomes. Preoperative information about expected perioperative sensations decreases the distress associated with surgery. By teaching the client preoperatively, the nurse can make a significant contribution to the success of surgery and to the client's postoperative recovery (Oetker-Black and others, 2003).

ASSESSMENT

1 Ask about client's previous experiences with surgery and anesthesia. *Rationale: This allows you to individualize teaching and address specific concerns of the client.*

2 Determine client and family's understanding of surgery. *Rationale: This information determines if correction of misunderstanding is necessary.*

3 Identify the client's cognitive level, language, and culture. *Rationale: These factors may alter the client's ability to understand the meaning of surgery and can affect the postoperative healing course if there are mixed messages or misunderstanding.*

4 Assess client's anxiety related to surgery. *Rationale: Directs you to provide additional emotional support and indicates the client's readiness to learn.*

PLANNING

Expected Outcomes focus on reducing the anxiety level of the client and family and having the client demonstrate understanding of key information and specific skills necessary to prevent complications.

- Client demonstrates eye contact and asks and answers questions appropriately.
- Client correctly performs splinting, turning and sitting, breathing exercises, and leg exercises.
- Family identifies the location of the waiting room.
- Family verbalizes the ability to care for client at home.

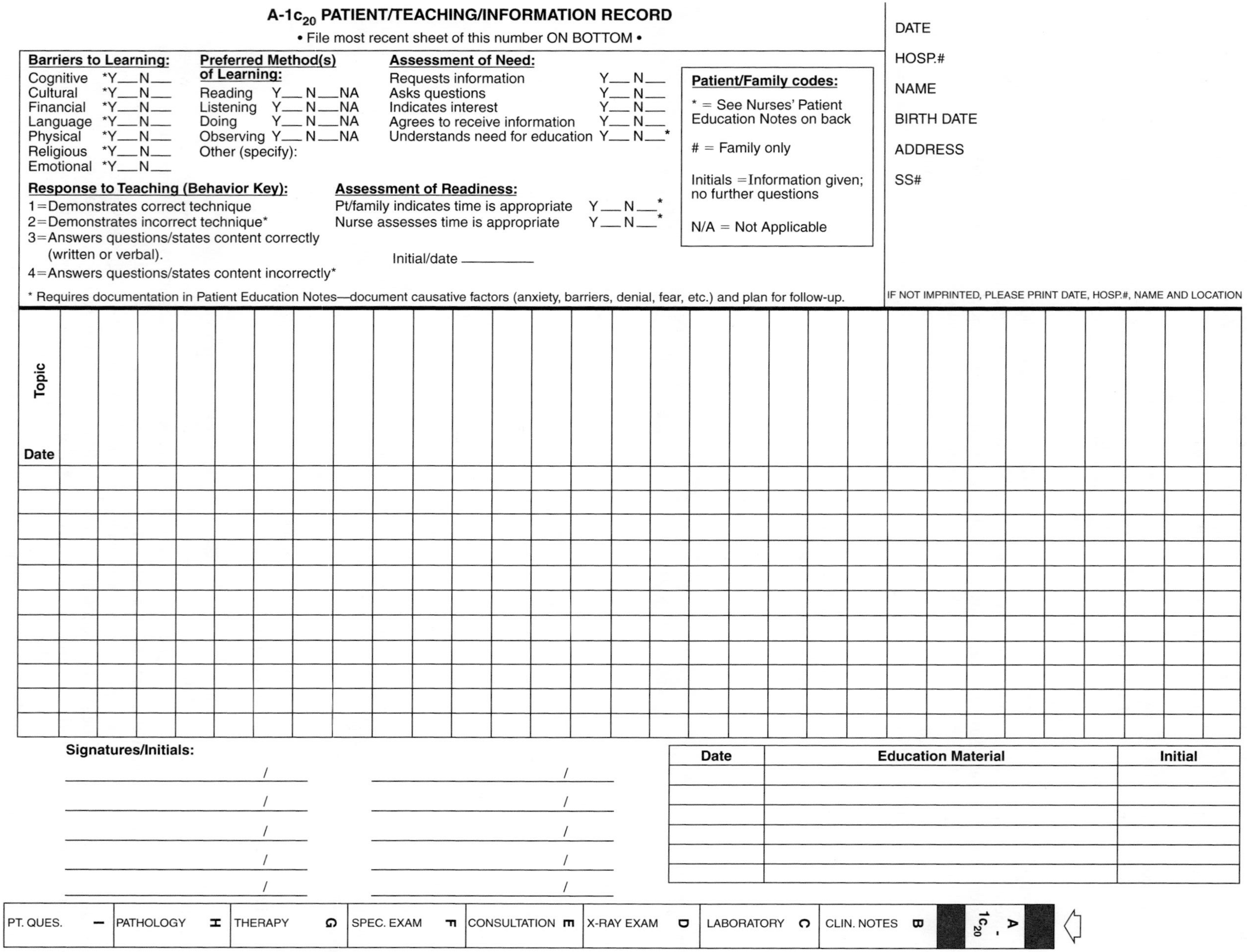

A-1c₂₀ PATIENT/TEACHING/INFORMATION RECORD

• File most recent sheet of this number ON BOTTOM •

Barriers to Learning:

Cognitive *Y___ N___
Cultural *Y___ N___
Financial *Y___ N___
Language *Y___ N___
Physical *Y___ N___
Religious *Y___ N___
Emotional *Y___ N___

Preferred Method(s) of Learning:

Reading Y___ N___ NA
Listening Y___ N___ NA
Doing Y___ N___ NA
Observing Y___ N___ NA
Other (specify):

Assessment of Need:

Requests information Y___ N___
Asks questions Y___ N___
Indicates interest Y___ N___
Agrees to receive information Y___ N___
Understands need for education Y___ N___*

Assessment of Readiness:

Pt/family indicates time is appropriate Y___ N___*
Nurse assesses time is appropriate Y___ N___*

Initial/date ___

Response to Teaching (Behavior Key):

1 = Demonstrates correct technique
2 = Demonstrates incorrect technique*
3 = Answers questions/states content correctly (written or verbal)
4 = Answers questions/states content incorrectly*

* Requires documentation in Patient Education Notes—document causative factors (anxiety, barriers, denial, fear, etc.) and plan for follow-up.

Patient/Family codes:

* = See Nurses' Patient Education Notes on back

= Family only

Initials = Information given; no further questions

N/A = Not Applicable

DATE

HOSP.#

NAME

BIRTH DATE

ADDRESS

SS#

IF NOT IMPRINTED, PLEASE PRINT DATE, HOSP.#, NAME AND LOCATION

Topic

Date

Signatures/Initials:

Date	Education Material	Initial

A - 1c₂₀	B	C	D	E	F	G	H	I
	CLIN. NOTES	LABORATORY	X-RAY EXAM	CONSULTATION	SPEC. EXAM	THERAPY	PATHOLOGY	PT. QUES.

FIGURE 18-2 Preoperative education flow sheet. (Courtesy University of Iowa Hospitals and Clinics.)

- Family provides emotional support for client preoperatively.
- Client and family demonstrate appropriate coping skills.

Delegation Considerations

The skills of preoperative teaching may not be delegated. Assistive Personnel (AP) can reinforce and assist clients in performing postoperative exercises. The nurse directs personnel by:

- Reviewing any precautions for turning a particular client.
- Instructing staff to inform the registered nurse (RN) if the client is unable to perform the exercises correctly

Equipment
- Stretcher or bed
- Pillow
- Incentive spirometer
- Preoperative education flow sheet (Figure 18-2)

IMPLEMENTATION *for Preoperative Teaching*

STEPS	RATIONALE
1 See Standard Protocol (inside front cover).	
2 Inform client and family of date, time, and location of surgery; anticipated length of surgery; additional time in the postanesthesia recovery area; and where to wait.	Accurate information helps reduce the stress associated with surgery.
3 Answer questions client and family ask.	Responding to client and family questions helps to decrease anxiety and demonstrates your concern for them.
4 Instruct client on extent and purpose of food and fluid restrictions for period specified before surgery. (No oral intake for 2 hours before surgery; no meat or fried foods 8 hours before surgery, unless otherwise specified by surgeon or anesthesiologist [ASA, 1999]).	During use of general anesthesia, muscles relax and gastric contents can reflux into esophagus, leading to aspiration. Anesthetic eliminates client's ability to gag.
5 Describe perioperative routines (e.g., time out, site marking, intravenous [IV] therapy, urinary catheterization, enema, hair clipping/removal, laboratory tests, transport to OR).	Allows client to anticipate and recognize routine procedures, reducing anxiety.
6 Describe planned effect of preoperative medications.	Provides information about what to expect, thereby decreasing anxiety.
7 Review which routine medications are to be discontinued before surgery.	Some medications are discontinued before surgery to minimize effects that can cause surgical risks. For example, anticoagulants may increase bleeding and are usually discontinued several days before surgery. Insulin dosages are usually adjusted because of the reduced intake of food preoperatively.
8 Describe perioperative sensations (e.g., blood pressure cuff tightening, ECG leads, cool room, beep of monitor).	Sensation/discomfort information was ranked high among valued information by both inpatients and outpatients (Bernier and others, 2003).
9 Describe pain-control methods. Many clients have a patient-controlled analgesia (PCA) pump (see Chapter 10).	Clients are fearful of postoperative pain. Explaining pain-management techniques will reduce this fear.
10 Describe what client will experience postoperatively (e.g., frequent vital signs, turning, catheters, drains, tubes, alternating pressure from sequential compression device [SCD]).	Provides a concrete description of what the client can expect after surgery so that the client is prepared.
11 If surgical incision is to be either thoracic or abdominal, teach client to place either hands or a pillow over incisional area and to splint incision. Hold pillow to abdomen for support while sitting up or coughing (see illustration).	Splinting the incisional area protects the abdominal incision and provides support for weakened muscles (Lewis and others, 2004).

STEPS	RATIONALE

12 Instruct client on turning and sitting up (especially suited for abdominal and thoracic surgery).

a. Turn onto right side: Instruct client to flex knees while lying supine and move toward left side of bed.

Promotes circulation and ventilation.

b. Have client splint incision with right arm and pillow. Have client keep right leg straight and flex left knee up. Have client grab right side rail with left hand, pull toward right, and roll onto right side. Reverse process to turn to left side.

Supports incision and decreases discomfort while turning.

c. Instruct client to turn every 2 hours from side to side while awake.

Reduces risk of vascular and pulmonary complications.

d. Sit up on right side of bed: Elevate head of bed and have client turn onto right side. While lying on the right side, client pushes on the mattress with right arm and swings feet over the edge of the bed (see illustration), with nurse's assistance. To sit up on the left side of the bed, reverse this process.

Sitting position lowers diaphragm to permit fuller lung expansion.

13 Instruct client in deep breathing and coughing (see illustration).

Client may be unable or reluctant to deep breathe because of weakness or pain, resulting in secretions remaining in the base of the lungs. Collection of secretions increases the risk of pulmonary atelectasis and pneumonia.

a. Assist client to high-Fowler's position in bed with knees flexed or sitting on side of bed or chair in upright position.

Sitting position facilitates diaphragmatic expansion.

b. Instruct client to place palms of hands across from each other along the lower border of the rib cage with tips of third fingers lightly touching.

This allows the client to feel the rise and fall of the abdomen during deep breathing (Lewis and others, 2004).

c. Have client take slow, deep breaths, inhaling through the nose, and pushing abdomen against hands. Client will feel fingers separate during inhalation. Explain that client will feel normal downward movement of diaphragm during inspiration. Demonstrate as needed.

This will help prevent hyperventilation or panting. Slow deep breath allows for more complete lung expansion.

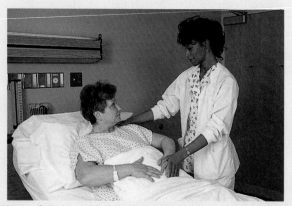

STEP 11 Splinting the incision for coughing after abdominal surgery.

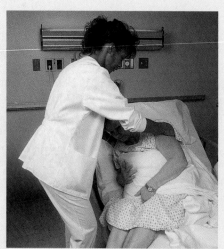

STEP 12d. Splinting the incision while sitting up after abdominal surgery.

STEPS	RATIONALE
d. Have client avoid using chest and shoulder muscles while inhaling.	Increases unnecessary energy expenditure and does not promote full lung expansion.
e. Have client take slow, deep breath and hold for count of 3 seconds, then slowly exhale through the mouth as if blowing out a candle (pursed lips).	Resistance during exhalation helps to prevent alveolar collapse.
f. Have client repeat breathing exercise three to five times.	Repetition reinforces learning.
g. Have client take two slow, deep breaths, inhaling through nose and exhaling through pursed lips.	Deep breaths expand lungs fully so that air moves behind mucus to facilitate coughing.
h. Have client inhale deeply a third time, and hold breath to count of 3. Cough fully for two to three consecutive coughs without inhaling between coughs.	Deep breathing moves up secretions in the respiratory tract to stimulate the cough reflex without voluntary effort on the part of the client (Lewis and others, 2004).
g. Caution client against just clearing throat.	Clearing throat does not remove mucus from deeper airways.
h. Have the client practice several times. Instruct client to perform turn, cough, and deep breathing every 2 hours.	Ensures mastery of technique. Frequent pulmonary exercises and movement will decrease risk of postoperative pneumonia (Lewis and others, 2004).
14 Instruct client in use of an incentive spirometer (see illustration).	Encourages deep breathing and loosens secretions in lung bases.
a. Position in a sitting or reclining position.	Facilitates diaphragm lowering and lung expansion.
b. Instruct client to exhale completely, then place mouthpiece so that lips completely cover it and inhale slowly, maintaining constant flow through unit.	Promotes complete inflation of lungs and minimizes atelectasis.
c. After maximum inspiration, client should hold breath for 2 to 3 seconds and then exhale slowly.	Promotes alveolar inflation.
d. Set marker on spirometer at maximum inspiration point to establish postoperative target.	Establishes measure of normal maximum breath for client. Provides outcome measure to determine postoperative return to the preoperative volumes.
e. Instruct client to breathe normally for a short period, and then repeat process.	Prevents hyperventilation and fatigue.
15 Instruct client in leg exercises: ankle rotation, dorsiflexion and plantar flexion, leg extension and flexion, straight leg raises.	Leg exercises promote circulation in the lower extremities and reduce the risk of circulatory complications such as a venous thrombus.
a. Position client supine.	
b. Instruct client to rotate each ankle in a complete circle and draw imaginary circles with the big toe five times.	Promotes joint mobility.

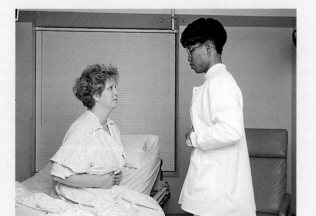

STEP 13 Position for coughing and deep breathing after abdominal surgery.

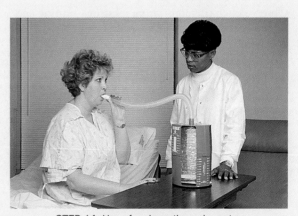

STEP 14 Use of an incentive spirometer.

STEPS	RATIONALE
c. Alternate dorsiflexion and plantar flexion while instructing client to feel calf muscles tighten and relax. Repeat five times (see illustration).	Helps maintain joint mobility and promote venous return to prevent thrombus formation.
d. Instruct client to alternate flexing and extending knees one leg at a time. Repeat five times (see illustration).	Maintains knee joint mobility and contracts muscles of upper leg.
e. Instruct client to alternate raising leg straight up from bed surface. Leg should be kept straight. Repeat five times.	Causes quadriceps muscle contraction and relaxation that helps promote venous return (Lewis and others, 2004).
f. Instruct client to perform these four leg exercises 10 to 12 times every 1 to 2 hours while awake.	Leg exercises lessen venous stasis and help prevent formation of DVT (Crowther and McCourt, 2004).
16 Verify that client's expectations of surgery are realistic. Correct expectations as needed.	Can prevent postoperative anxiety or anger.
17 Reinforce therapeutic coping strategies. If ineffective, encourage alternatives.	Therapeutic coping strategies will promote postoperative compliance and recovery.
18 See Completion Protocol (inside front cover).	

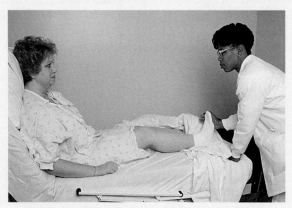

STEP 15c. Dorsiflexion and plantar flexion of foot.

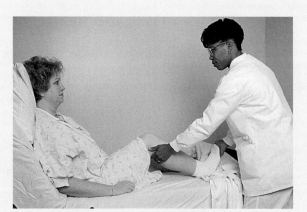

STEP 15d. Flexion and extension of knees.

EVALUATION

1 Ask client to repeat key information (e.g., rationale for withholding food and fluids).
2 Observe client demonstrating splinting, turning and sitting, deep breathing, and leg exercises.
3 Ask family to identify location of the waiting room.
4 Ask family if they are able to care for client at home after discharge.
5 Observe the level of emotional support family provides client.
6 Observe client and family coping strategies.

Unexpected Outcomes and Related Interventions

1 Client identifies an incorrect procedure, site, date, or time of surgery.
a. Provide the correct information verbally and in writing for client and family.

2 Client questions the importance of not drinking the morning of surgery.
a. Explain that under anesthesia, the fluid can come up from the stomach and go into the lungs.
3 Client incorrectly performs breathing exercises.
a. Explain and demonstrate the correct breathing technique.
b. Explain the importance of postoperative breathing.
c. Instruct client to repeat the demonstration.
4 Family verbalizes anxiety about caring for client at home.
a. Explain that these feelings are normal.
b. Provide written instructions and a telephone number for contact if there are further questions.

5 Family indicates that they are unable to care for client at home.

a. Contact physician and discuss the alternative of a home health care referral.

Recording and Reporting

- Record preoperative teaching on the preoperative education flow sheet (see Figure 18-2) or designated agency form.

Sample Documentation

0940 Preoperative teaching completed. Instructed on continued need to be NPO; routine events to expect in OR and recovery room; presence of oxygen; IVF; postoperative drains; and postoperative activities including TCDB, use of IS, and leg exercises. Daughter expressed concern about her mother being able to care for herself at home after surgery. Home health nurse contacted to see client before discharge.

Special Considerations

Pediatric Considerations

- Use an age-appropriate level of communication and provide simple explanations using familiar terms.

- The use of pictures, models, equipment, and play rather than verbal explanations increases preschool and school-age children's learning.

Geriatric Considerations

- Age-related changes in the central nervous system (CNS) may diminish short-term memory. Additional time and reinforcement may be necessary for older adult clients to learn and comprehend information (Spry, 2003). The greater the number of different exposures to new material, the higher the probability that the material will be learned (Eliopoulos, 2005).
- Reinforce teaching with verbal explanations, audiovisual resources, pamphlets, and demonstrations (Eliopoulos, 2005). Sight and hearing deficits should be considered when providing both written and verbal instructions (Spry, 2003).

Home Care Considerations

- Review coughing, deep breathing, abdominal splinting, relaxation, leg exercises, and ambulation before admission to hospital or surgical clinic and after discharge.

SKILL 18.3 Physical Preparation for Surgery

Physical preparation of the client for surgery involves providing nursing care immediately before surgery, verifying required procedures and tests, and documenting care in the client's record (Iowa Intervention Project, 2000). You will follow specific steps to prepare every client. These steps depend on the type of surgery being performed and the risks involved. For example, you will use antiembolism stockings, sequential compression stockings, and the venous foot pump for adult clients undergoing surgery that will last several hours and require a long period of immobilization afterward (Bartley, 2005). You will provide a bowel preparation, administering an enema, laxative, or cathartic (this may be done at home by clients admitted the morning of surgery) for abdominal surgery on or near the intestine. You may need to clip hair near the incision site. Always check the physician's orders to determine what procedures are needed for the surgical client. Regardless of the type of surgery, the goal of physical preparation is to place the client in the best condition possible to minimize the risks of the surgery that is planned.

ASSESSMENT

1 The preoperative assessment forms the basis for physical preparation of the client for surgery (see Skill 18.1).

PLANNING

Expected Outcomes focus on the proper physical preparation of the client for surgery.

- Client cooperates during preparatory measures (e.g., starting an IV, undergoing an enema).
- Client undergoes measures to reduce the risk of infection (e.g., preoperative antibiotic, skin preparation).

Delegation Considerations

Coordinating the client's preparation for surgery may not be delegated. However, AP may administer an enema or a douche, obtain vital signs in stable clients, apply antiembolic stockings, and assist clients in removing clothing, jewelry, and prostheses. The nurse directs personnel by:

- Instructing personnel in proper precautions when preparing a client for surgery
- Reviewing observations and precautions if the client has an IV catheter in place

Equipment

NOTE: Equipment varies by procedure ordered.

- Hospital gown
- IV solution and equipment (see Chapter 27)
- Skin cleansing solution

- Antiembolism stockings
- SCD
- Venous foot pump
- Urinary catheterization kit (see Chapter 33)

- Preoperative checklist
- Medications (e.g., sedative)
- Enema set and prescribed solution (see Chapter 9)
- Douche set and prescribed solution

IMPLEMENTATION *for Physical Preparation for Surgery*

STEPS	RATIONALE
1 See Standard Protocol (inside front cover).	
2 Assist client with putting on hospital gown and removing personal items.	
3 Instruct client to remove makeup, nail polish, hairpins, and jewelry.	During and after surgery, anesthesiologist and nurse must assess the skin and nails to determine tissue perfusion. (In some settings, clients are allowed to have a ring taped and to remove polish from only one nail.)
4 Ensure that money and valuables have been locked up or given to a family member.	Client may not return to same location postoperatively. Prevents valuables from being misplaced or lost.
5 Verify that client's identification and blood band are correct and legible.	Correct client identification ensures right client undergoes right procedure and receives correct blood product.

> **NURSE ALERT** Before placing identification and blood band, have client state name (if able); also check a second identifier (e.g., date of birth, client's registration number). Verify agency policy regarding identifiers to use (JCAHO, 2006).

6 Ensure that client has followed appropriate fluid and food restrictions per surgeon or anesthesiologist order (see Skill 18.2).	Extent and type of restriction will vary by institution and practitioner. Under general anesthesia, the sphincters in the stomach relax, and contents can reflux into the esophagus and trachea.
7 Verify that client has followed request for omission or ingestion of medications as instructed.	Missed or inaccurate dosage could precipitate complications.
8 Verify that a bowel preparation (e.g., laxative, cathartic, enema) is completed if ordered.	For clients admitted the morning of surgery, this may have been performed at home.
9 Ensure that a medical history and physical examination results are in client's record.	Establishes database for future comparison.
10 Verify that surgical consent is complete. The name of the procedure, name of surgeon, date, name of person authorized to obtain consent, and client's signature should all be present.	Ensures client's agreement to undergo intended procedure. In most settings the surgeon obtains the consent and the RN verifies that it is complete and consistent with the client's understanding (refer to agency policy).
11 Ensure that necessary laboratory work, ECG, and chest x-ray studies are completed and results are on the chart.	Diagnostic test results may indicate a medical problem as well as provide data for postoperative comparison.
12 Verify that blood type and crossmatch are completed if ordered by the physician and that blood transfusions are available as needed.	In many cases, surgery cannot begin without availability of blood units.
13 Ask if client has an advance directive. If so, place it in client's record.	Document conveys client's wishes if life support measures are necessary.

> **NURSE ALERT** Some inpatient clients with "do not resuscitate" (DNR) orders may require surgery for palliative care. DNR orders should not routinely be upheld nor should they be routinely suspended during anesthesia and surgery. The client's physicians are responsible for discussing and documenting issues with the client and/or family to determine whether the DNR order is to be maintained or whether it is to be partially or completely suspended during surgery (AORN, 2005).

14 Assess and record client's heart rate, blood pressure, respiratory rate, oxygen saturation, and temperature.	Provides a baseline for client's preoperative status.

STEPS	RATIONALE

15 Administer cathartics or enemas if ordered (see Skill 9.5).

Emptying the bowel is necessary for bowel surgery and the procedure to decrease the risk of postoperative ileus. Enemas are used when surgery is near the lower intestine.

16 Instruct client to void.

Prevents risk of bladder distention or rupture during surgery.

17 Start an IV line; refer to unit standards or physician's orders (see Chapter 27).

IV provides access for fluids and medications administered in OR.

18 Administer preoperative medications as ordered.

Preoperative medication may be used for a variety of reasons and should be administered as ordered for maximum effectiveness.

> **NURSE ALERT** To be most effective, most preoperative prophylactic antibiotics require administration to be as close to the time of incision as possible (30 to 60 minutes) and not be given for longer than 24 hours postoperatively (CDC, 2003). However, prophylactic antibiotics following cardiothoracic surgery may be given for as long as 48 hours postoperatively.

> **COMMUNICATION TIP** Clients are often anxious before surgery. Explaining how equipment or skin preparation will feel (e.g., cold, tight) before it touches the client reduces anxiety.

19 Apply antiembolism stockings (see illustrations) (see Procedural Guideline 6-1).

Antiembolism stockings promote circulation during periods of immobilization, reducing the risk of an embolism.

20 Apply sequential compression stockings if ordered (see illustrations) (see Procedural Guideline 6-1).

Sequential compression stockings promote circulation by sequentially compressing the legs from the ankle upward. This will improve venous flow and reduce swelling (Day, 2003).

21 Apply venous plexus foot pump if ordered. Apply foot cover. Attach cover to the device and verify correct settings (see illustration).

Venous plexus foot pumps promote circulation by mimicking the natural action of walking by intermittently compressing the sole of the foot and then relaxing it, so the venous plexus can fill with blood.

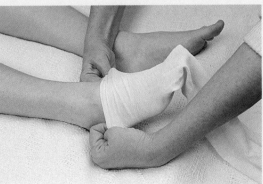

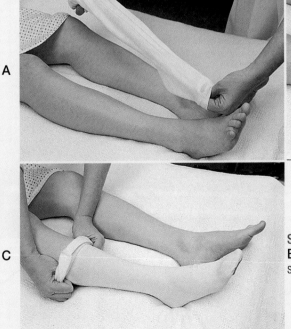

STEP 19 **A,** Turn stocking inside out; hold toe and pull through. **B,** Slip antiembolism stockings over foot. **C,** Ease antiembolism stockings over the leg.

STEPS	RATIONALE
22 Cleanse and prepare the surgical site if ordered.	Cleansing with an antimicrobial soap decreases bacterial flora on the skin.
23 Insert a urinary catheter if ordered (see Chapter 33). Maintains bladder decompression and provides for monitoring output during surgery.	
24 Administer an enema if ordered (see Chapter 9).	Cleansing of the bowel may need to be done before surgery to reduce the risk of fecal contamination during surgery.

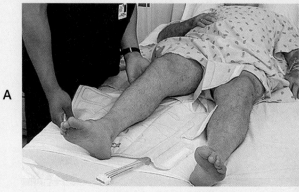

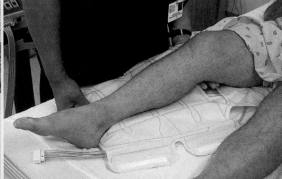

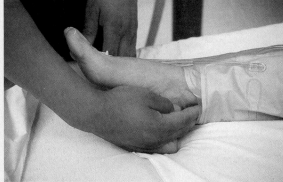

STEP 20 **A,** Correct leg position on inner lining. **B,** Position back of client's knee with popliteal opening. **C,** Check fit of SCD sleeve.

STEP 21 Venous plexus foot pump with bedside controls. (Courtesy Tyco Healthcare Group LP.)

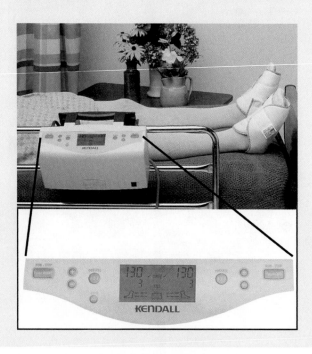

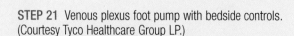

STEPS	RATIONALE
25 Remove gloves, and perform hand hygiene.	
26 Allow the client to wear eyeglasses, dentures, or hearing aid as long as possible before surgery. Remove contact lenses, eyeglasses, hairpieces, and dentures just before surgery.	These aids facilitate client cooperation by ensuring that the client has clear vision and maximal auditory perception throughout the preoperative phase. In some settings, dentures are left in place.
27 Place a cap on client's head.	The cap contains the hair and minimizes OR contamination during surgery. Plastic or reflective caps reduce heat loss during surgery.
28 Assist client onto stretcher for transport to OR.	Some ambulatory surgery clients walk to OR.
29 See Completion Protocol (inside front cover).	

EVALUATION

1 Observe client's level of cooperation during preparation.
2 Ask client to assist with measures to reduce the risk of infection (preoperative antibiotics, skin preparation).

Unexpected Outcomes and Related Interventions

1 Client reports having eaten breakfast or drinking fluids.
a. Notify surgeon and anesthesia provider.
2 Client refuses to go to surgery until contacting a family member.
a. Notify surgeon.
b. Assist client with contacting family member.
3 Consent is incomplete or incorrect.
a. Notify surgeon and anesthesia provider.
4 Client did not follow instructions regarding medications.
a. Notify surgeon.
5 Client has a reaction to a preoperative medication.
a. Discontinue the medication.
b. Treat the reaction as per institutional policy.
c. Notify surgeon.

Recording and Reporting

• Document preoperative physical preparation on preoperative checklist (Figure 18-3).

Sample Documentation

0850 Verified client has been NPO since midnight. Dentures, gold wedding band, and wallet given to client's wife. Fleets enema given with results of large amount soft brown stool. Antiembolism stockings applied. Stated he did not take his morning dose of 20 units of NPH insulin. Bedside blood sugar 110. Dr. Thompson notified. 10 units of NPH insulin administered subcutaneously per order. IV of 5% dextrose and ½ normal saline started in right hand per order. Voided and taken to OR by stretcher per transporter.

Special Considerations
Pediatric Considerations

• Give the child as many choices related to procedures as possible.
• Keep parent-child separation to the minimum time possible. When a parent cannot be present, it is important to leave a favorite possession with the child.

Geriatric Considerations

• Because of cognitive, sensory, or physical impairments, it may take the older client increased time to dress for surgery and complete needed physical preparation.

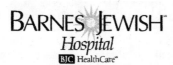

SURGICAL/PROCEDURE CHECKLIST
Complete this side for inpatients & outpatients
having any invasive procedure

Please check (✔) the appropriate box (□) and fill in the blank(s) as needed.

ADDRESSOGRAPH

Date of Procedure: _____ Type of Procedure: _____

Off Floor Reports printed and placed in chart: □ Yes □ No □ N/A: _____

ITEM	Yes/Initials	NA	COMMENT	Date
Face sheet in chart				
Consent to Surgery or Other Procedure signed			□ To be signed in treatment area.	
SPECIALTY Consent signed			□ To be signed in treatment area. (Specify)	
Transfusion consent signed				
ID Band on				
Allergies Noted: □ Armband □ Medication Record □ Allergies/Sensitivities Record/Override Order Form				
Height & Weight documented				
Dentures, eyeglasses, contact lenses, nail polish, hairpins, prosthesis, jewelry removed				
Surgical/Procedural skin prep done				
Patient in hospital gown/pajamas				
Patient has been NPO since: _____				
Voided or catheterized				
Vital Signs taken and documented				
Patient is on Isolation			(Specify)	
History & physical in chart				
Lab work in chart (Printed Off Floor reports)				
Urinalysis in chart				
EKG in chart				
Chest X-ray (done if ordered)				
Change in condition/VS reported to:				
Valuables/Inventory checklist done				
Pre-Operative meds given:				
Addressograph plate in chart				
Patient transferred to Surgical/Procedure area in HIS				
Mode of travel: □ Amb □ W/C □ Stretcher □ Bed				
Operative Site Marked			□ Site to be marked in holding area	
Case Cancelled				

Family contact during surgery:

Name: _____ Location: _____ Phone: _____

INITIALS	SIGNATURES	INITIALS	SIGNATURES

BJ 2-3343-465 V1 (08/01/05) Page 1 of 2 TAB: TREATMENT   **DO NOT WRITE BELOW THIS LINE**

BJ 2-3343-465

FIGURE 18-3 Preoperative checklist. (Courtesy Barnes-Jewish Hospital, St Louis, Mo.)

- Incorporate play into the time the child is required to soak. Placing items in the basin for the child to play with may be helpful. Continuous adult supervision is necessary.
- Perform frequent neurovascular evaluations to ensure adequate blood flow before and after treatment.

Geriatric Considerations
- Older clients, especially those undergoing long-term steroid therapy, may have thinner, more fragile skin.
- Older clients may have impaired circulation or diminished subcutaneous fat leading to alterations in thermoregulation (Meiner and Lueckenotte, 2006).

- In some cases, such as with clients who have cardiac conditions, it may be necessary to monitor vital signs throughout the procedure.

Home Care Considerations
- When necessary, assess availability of primary caregiver to assist client in application of moist heat. Assess the caregiver's understanding of purpose of procedure and willingness to comply with procedure and not leave client.
- Assess physical environment to determine adequacy of facilities for use by client. Contact medical equipment companies for assistance in determining best product for client.

SKILL 24.2 | Dry Heat

Dry heat can be applied directly to the skin with an aquathermia pad, electric heating pad, or commercial heat pack. Dry heat treatments penetrate superficially but maintain temperature changes longer than moist heat treatments. This superficial heating is not effective in penetrating deep joints such as the knee or hip. The temperature and duration of these treatments must be controlled carefully. It is important to protect the client from burns, skin dryness, and loss of body fluids through diaphoresis. Because of the constant temperature control, aquathermia pads tend to be safer than electric heating pads. Special consideration must be given to clients returning home with this therapy.

ASSESSMENT

1 Assess client's skin for integrity, color, temperature, sensitivity to touch, blistering, and excessive dryness. *Rationale: Establishes baseline for condition of skin.*
2 Ask the client to report pain on scale of 0 to 10 or other appropriate scale. *Rationale: Provides baseline to determine if pain relief is achieved.*
3 Assess ROM of body part. *Rationale: Provides baseline to determine changes in joint mobility.*
4 Check electrical plugs and cords for obvious fraying or cracking.
5 Determine client's or family members' knowledge of procedure and related safety factors. *Rationale: Heating pads are frequently used in homes; assessment determines client's health teaching needs.*

PLANNING

Expected Outcomes focus on decreasing pain and improving mobility while preventing burns and dehydration.
1 Client reports decreased level of pain.
2 Client's ROM increases.
3 Client's skin remains intact, pink, warm, and sensitive to touch, with no excessive dryness and no blisters. Immediately after treatment, skin may be pink to red and warm.
4 Client correctly applies pad.

Delegation Considerations
Assessment of the client's condition may not be delegated; however, the skill of applying dry heat may be delegated. The nurse directs personnel by:
- Explaining specific positioning requirements for the client
- Reviewing what to observe, such as excessive redness, and report back to the nurse

Equipment
- Aquathermia pad, electric heating pad, or commercial chemical heat pack
- Electrical control unit
- Distilled water (for aquathermia pad)
- Bath towel or pillow case
- Ties or tape

IMPLEMENTATION *for Dry Heat*

STEPS	RATIONALE

1 See Standard Protocol (inside front cover).

> **COMMUNICATION TIP** Tell client that it is normal for treatment to feel warm, but that if it feels uncomfortably so, the nurse should be notified so the treatment can be evaluated.

STEPS	RATIONALE
2 For aquathermia pad or uncovered heating pad, cover or wrap affected area with bath towel, or enclose pad in pillowcase.	Prevents the heated surface from touching the client's skin directly and increasing risk for injury to client's skin.
3 Place pad over affected area (see Figure 24-1) and secure with tape or ties as needed.	

NURSE ALERT Never position client so that client is lying directly on pad. Lying directly on pad prevents dissipation of heat and increases risk of burns.

4 Turn heating pad on low or medium setting. Check temperature on aquathermia unit. Most units are preset to 105° F, or 40.5° C to 43° C.	To determine correct function of equipment and check for proper temperature. Prevents exposure of client to temperature extremes.
5 If using a commercially prepared heat pack, break pouch inside larger packet (follow manufacturer's instructions for use).	

NURSE ALERT Do not puncture outer pack. Do not allow chemicals to come in contact with the skin or eyes.

6 Monitor condition of site every 5 minutes, and ask client about sensation of burning.	Determines if heat exposure is resulting in burn.
7 Remove treatment after 20 to 30 minutes (or time ordered by physician).	Local application of heat longer than 20 minutes without interruption may result in burn or changes to the microcirculation, such as vasoconstriction (Stitik and Nadler, 1999).
8 See Completion Protocol (inside front cover).	

EVALUATION

1 Assess client's skin for integrity, color, temperature, dryness, and blistering. Evaluate again after 30 minutes.
2 Ask client to rate pain level on scale of 0 to 10 or other appropriate scale.
3 Measure client's ROM.

Unexpected Outcomes and Related Interventions

1 See Unexpected Outcomes, Skill 24.1.
2 Body part is painful to move.
a. Discontinue treatment.
b. Assess for edema or increased swelling.
c. Notify health care provider.

Recording and Reporting

• Record pain level; ROM of body part; skin integrity, color, temperature, sensitivity to touch, dryness, and blistering; temperature and duration of treatment; and client response to treatment.
• Report any unusual findings such as blistering, decreased ROM, or increased pain.

Sample Documentation

1000 Heating pad on low setting applied to right bicep for pain with motion. Pain severity 6 on 0 to 10 scale. Flexion 140 degrees and extension 20 degrees. Skin intact, pink, and warm; turgor elastic.

1020 Heating pad removed. Right bicep pink to red and warm. No blisters; turgor elastic. States feels light touch to affected area. States pain is 2 on 0 to 10 scale. Flexion 145 degrees, extension 20 degrees.

Special Consideraions
Pediatric Considerations

• Because of the risk of injury from heating pads, this treatment is used infrequently in children. If prescribed, remain with the client to ensure safety and effectiveness.

Geriatric Considerations

• Older clients have thinner, more fragile skin that is more susceptible to burns. Use extreme caution with electric heating pads in older clients.
• Older clients have an increased risk of burns because of diminished heat sensation.

Home Care Considerations

• Assess client's use of alternative treatments at home (e.g., use of rice socks or herb packs). Evaluate for proper use of such treatments.
• Assess the home environment for facilities to adhere to implementation of the procedure.

SKILL 24.3 Cold Applications

Cold is applied in many different ways, such as ice bags, moist cold compresses, commercial cold packs or compresses, and electromechanical devices. Cold exerts a profound physiological effect on the body, reducing inflammation, pain, and swelling caused by injuries to the soft tissues of the musculoskeletal system (Airaksinen and others, 2003: Poddar, 2003). Because reduction of inflammation is the primary goal, application of cold (cryotherapy) is the treatment of choice for the first 24 to 48 hours after a soft tissue injury. Cold is also indicated as an analgesic for chronic pain and spasticity control and after orthoscopic surgical procedures.

Cold applications cause vasoconstriction and reduces blood flow to the injured part; as a result, fluid accumulation, bleeding, and hematoma formation associated with trauma are decreased. The lower temperature also reduces muscle spasm and produces a local anesthetic response.

There are electronically controlled cooling devices that work much like aquathermia pads. The cooling pads deliver a constant cool temperature. Cold devices that simultaneously provide compression are effective in treating acute musculoskeletal injury with soft tissue swelling (Arnold and Shelbourne, 2000). Whether using one of these devices or a cold compress, use the acronym RICE: **R**est, **I**ce, Compression bandages (such as snug elastic wraps), and **E**levation of the injured area to effectively manage musculoskeletal injuries (Stitik and Nadler, 1998).

ASSESSMENT

1 Assess area of injury for edema and bleeding. *Rationale: Provides baseline to determine changes in soft tissue after treatment.*
2 Assess surrounding skin for integrity, adequacy of circulation, color, temperature, and sensitivity to touch. *Rationale: Provides baseline for determining change in condition of injured tissues.*
3 Determine time of injury. *Rationale: Cold reduces edema and soft tissue injury. Cold applications are most effective within the first 24 to 48 hours of injury (Airaksinen and others, 2003).*
4 Assess client's pain on scale of 0 to 10. *Rationale: Provides baseline to determine pain relief.*
5 Assess client's understanding of procedure.

PLANNING

Expected Outcomes focus on decreasing pain, edema, bleeding, and bruising while preventing ischemia.
1 Client reports decreased pain.
2 There is decreased edema and/or bleeding at site of injury.
3 Surrounding skin is slightly pale and cool to touch.

Delegation Considerations

Assessment of the client's condition may not be delegated; however, the skill of applying cold or dry heat applications may be delegated. The nurse directs personnel by:
- Explaining any mobility restrictions caused by the injury
- Reviewing what to observe (e.g., expected mobility, pain, wound status) and report back to nurse

Equipment
All Compresses, Bags, and Packs
- Soft cloth covering, stockinette, towel, or pillowcase
- Cloth tapes or ties
- Bath towel
- Bath blanket for warmth
- Waterproof pad

Cold Compress
- Towel or gauze
- Prescribed solution, ice
- Basin

Ice Bag or Gel Pack
- Ice bag
- Ice chips and water
- Reusable commercial gel pack (cold pack)
- Disposable commercial chemical cold pack

Electrically Controlled Cooling Device
- Gauze roll or elastic wrap
- Cool water flow pad or cooling pad and electrical pump

IMPLEMENTATION *for Cold Applications*

STEPS	RATIONALE
1 See Standard Protocol (inside front cover).	
2 Provide warm covering for client.	To prevent chilling.
3 Position client comfortably, keeping affected body part in proper alignment. Expose only the area to be treated and drape client with bath blanket.	Prevents further injury to area. Avoids unnecessary exposure of body parts, maintaining client's warmth, comfort, and privacy.

> **NURSE ALERT** In cases of strains, sprains, or fractures, extremity or body part should remain aligned to prevent further injury.

STEPS	RATIONALE

4 Place towel or absorbent pad under area to be treated.

5 **Apply cold compress.**

a. Place ice and water into basin.

b. Test temperature of solution, place gauze into basin, and wring out excess moisture.

Extreme temperature can cause tissue injury. Dripping gauze is uncomfortable to client.

c. Apply compress to affected area, molding it gently over site.

Ensures that cold is directed over the site of injury.

COMMUNICATION TIP Tell client that there is a normal progression of sensation changes during cold therapy: cold, then pain relief, followed by burning skin pain, and finally numbness.

---

6 **Apply ice pack or bag.**

a. Fill bag with water, then empty.

Prevents skin maceration by testing bag for leaks.

b. Fill bag two-thirds full with ice and water.

c. Express air from bag, secure closure, and wipe bag dry.

Allows ice bag to conform to area and promotes maximum contact.

d. Commercial ice packs are squeezed or kneaded.

Releases alcohol-based solution to create cold temperature.

e. Wrap pack or body part with towel, stockinette, or pillowcase (see illustration). Wrap prepared ice pack directly over area.

Prevents direct exposure of cold against client's skin. Cold is applied directly over the site of injury.

f. Secure with elastic wrap bandage, gauze roll, or ties.

Secures therapeutic cold to area of injury.

NURSE ALERT Sterile supplies must be used with open wounds.

---

7 **Apply commercial gel pack.**

a. Remove pack from freezer.

b. Wrap pack in towel, stockinette, or pillowcase or cover client's skin with towel.

Prevents direct exposure of cold application to the skin, reducing risk of tissue injury.

c. Place gel pack on affected area (see illustration).

d. Secure with gauze roll, cloth tape, or ties as needed.

Secures therapeutic cold to area of injury.

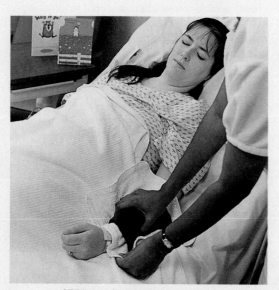

STEP 6e. Protecting client's skin.

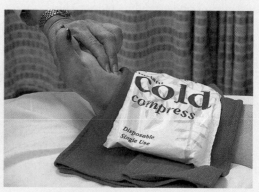

STEP 7c. Cold compress application.

STEPS	RATIONALE

8 Apply electrically controlled cooling device (see illustration).

a. Make sure all connections are intact and temperature (if adjustable) is set. (See agency policy and manufacturer's directions.)

Ensures safe temperature for application.

b. Wrap cool water flow pad around body part.

Ensures even temperature during cold application.

c. Set correct temperature.

d. Secure with elastic wrap bandage, gauze roll, or ties.

Secures therapeutic cold to area of injury.

9 Check condition of skin every 5 minutes for duration of application.

Determines presence of adverse reactions to cold, including mottling, redness, burning, blistering, and numbness (Stitik and Nadler, 1998).

a. If area is edematous, sensation may be reduced and extra caution must be used during cold therapy.

b. Numbness and tingling are common sensations with cold applications and indicate adverse reactions only when severe and coupled with other symptoms. Stop when client complains of burning sensation or skin feels numb.

Initially cold is sensed followed by pain relief. As treatment progresses, client may report burning sensation, pain in the skin, and finally numbness (Stitik and Nadler, 1998).

c. After 15 to 20 minutes (or as ordered by the physician), remove the compress or pad and gently dry off any moisture.

Drying prevents maceration of the skin. Prolonged application can result in tissue ischemia caused by diminished blood flow or compensatory vasodilation to provide warmth to the area being treated (Stitik and Nadler, 1998).

NURSE ALERT Areas with little body fat, such as knees and ankles, do not tolerate cold as well as fatty areas, such as thighs and buttocks. For bony areas reduce time of cold application.

---

10 See Completion Protocol (inside front cover).

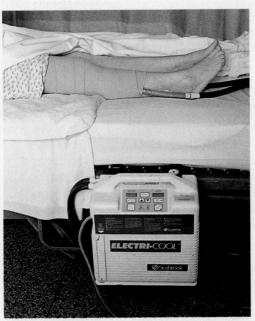

STEP 8 Electric cooling device.

EVALUATION

1 Inspect surrounding tissues for integrity, color, and temperature; ask client to describe sensitivity to touch. Re-evaluate after 30 minutes.

2 Palpate tissue or wound for edema, bruising, and bleeding.

3 Ask client to report pain level on scale of 0 to 10.

4 Ask client to apply cold application and discuss risks of treatment.

Unexpected Outcomes and Related Interventions

1 Skin appears mottled, reddened, or bluish purple appearance.

a. Stop treatment; symptoms indicate prolonged exposure.

b. Report to physician if symptoms are excessive or if they persist for more than 30 minutes.

2 Client complains of burning type pain and numbness.

a. Stop treatment; symptoms indicate possible ischemia.

b. Report to physician if symptoms are excessive or if they persist for more than 30 minutes.

Recording and Reporting

- Record pain level; presence of bleeding, bruising, and edema in area of injury; skin integrity, color, temperature, and sensitivity to touch; and temperature and duration of treatment.

- Report any sensations of burning, numbness, or unrelieved changes in skin color.

Sample Documentation

0930 Left ankle edematous and tender to touch after twisting injury. Ankle measures 32 cm at medial malleolus and 31 cm across metatarsal region of foot. Pain at 7 on 0 to 10 scale. Ecchymosis present, extending 8 cm on medial aspect with surrounding skin warm and pink. Dorsalis pedis and posterior tibialis pulses present and strong. Left extremity elevated with ice pack applied to ankle.

0950 Ice pack removed from ankle. Ankle measures 32 cm. Pain at 2 on 0 to 10 scale. Ecchymosis unchanged. Skin pink and cool; client reports numbness upon palpation.

Special Considerations
Pediatric Considerations

- A greater metabolic rate and larger trunk in relation to the rest of the body make children more prone to hypothermia (Nicoll, 2002). Exercise caution with young clients.

- Infants have an unstable temperature control mechanism, so mottling of extremities is common and may not indicate an adverse reaction if this symptom is seen alone.

- Further assessment in children with frequent soft tissue or musculoskeletal injuries may be necessary.

Geriatric Considerations

- Older clients are more at risk for tissue damage because of loss of temperature sensation (Nicoll, 2002). Check site frequently during all treatments.

- Anticipate shortening duration of treatment.

- Older clients may require more covering for warmth.

Home Care Considerations

- A bag of frozen vegetables conforms nicely to an affected area and is effective for brief periods of treatment. Place a thin towel between the bag and skin or place bag inside a pillowcase.

NCLEX® Style Questions

1 Which of the following clients would benefit most from the application of heat therapy?
1. One with joint inflammation and pain
2. One with a minor burn
3. One with suspected area of malignancy
4. One with an inflamed appendix

2 Why should the use of heat/cold therapy on confused clients be done with great caution?
1. Their skin may be very thin.
2. Therapy may increase their confusion.
3. Their perception of sensory stimuli may be reduced.
4. They are more sensitive to temperature variations.

3 Which of the following assessment findings is a contraindication for use of cold therapy?
1. A client with acute inflammation
2. A client with impaired circulation
3. A client with severe pain
4. A client suffering trauma within the past 24 hours

4 What is a major concern with the prolonged application of moist heat?
1. Maceration
2. Cramping
3. Erythema
4. Dermatitis

5 The nurse should intervene when observing another nurse applying moist heat in the following way:
1. Performing a neurovascular assessment prior to heat application.
2. Using a low setting on the microwave to heat the compress.
3. Checking affected joint range of motion after application.
4. Removing compress before 20 minutes have passed.

References for all chapters appear in Appendix D.

Special Mattresses and Beds

25

MEDIA RESOURCES

- **evolve** http://evolve.elsevier.com/Elkin

New federal legislation requires health care facilities to increase the assessment and documentation of client's risk for and presence of pressure ulcers. In addition, new interpretative guidelines of this legislation ask agencies to determine appropriate support surfaces to match the potential beneficial therapeutic benefit of a specific support surface and the client's risk for pressure ulcer formation (Merk, 2006).

The major cause of pressure ulcers is unrelieved pressure (see Chapter 22). The greater the pressure and the longer the pressure is applied, the greater the likelihood that a pressure ulcer will develop. Body tissues require adequate blood flow to supply oxygen and nutrients and remove carbon dioxide and other waste products (Brienza and Geyer, 2005; Mackey, 2005). When external pressure on the tissues exceeds 32 mm Hg (the capillary closing pressure), the network of capillaries collapses, and the supply of oxygen and nutrients to the cells, as well as removal of metabolic waste products, is interrupted. As a result, there is tissue ischemia and, if unrelieved, tissue death or necrosis.

Support surfaces reduce tissue capillary pressure and risk of pressure ulcers. These products reduce pressure over the bony prominences by redistributing pressure and shear and by controlling temperature and moisture (Brienza and Meyer, 2005). Although support surfaces reduce pressure, they must be used in conjunction with other pressure ulcer risk reduction strategies (see Chapter 22).

Support surfaces have differing purposes, including pressure reduction, pressure relief, repositioning, and support of the morbidly obese client. They are used in acute, rehabilitative, long-term, and home care settings. It is important to understand the difference between a pressure reducing and a pressure relieving support surface. Pressure reducing surfaces (e.g., fiber-filled and foam overlays, gel or water support systems, air-filled mattresses, low-air-loss and air-fluidized supports) increase the area of the body in contact with the surface, thereby spreading the load and reducing the effects of pressure. These devices maintain external skin pressures at a lower level than standard hospital mattresses (Merk, 2006).

Pressure relieving systems actually move under the client and thus reduce the amount of pressure applied to any one area at regular intervals. Pressure relieving devices consistently maintain external skin pressure at or below 32 mm Hg capillary closing pressure.

TABLE 25-1   Support Surfaces

CATEGORY AND MECHANISM OF ACTION	INDICATIONS FOR USE	ADVANTAGES	DISADVANTAGES
Support Surfaces and Overlays			
High-Specification Foam Overlays (available as an overlay or in a full mattress)			
Reduces pressure; the cover (top) can reduce friction and shear. Base height of 3-4 inches; see manufacturer's guidelines regarding the amount of body weight supported.	Use for moderate- to high-risk clients.	One-time charge. No setup fee. Cannot be punctured. Available in various sizes (e.g., bed, chair, operating room [OR] table). Little maintenance. Does not need electricity.	Increases body temperature. Traps moisture. Limited life span. Plastic protective sheet needed for incontinent clients or clients with draining wounds.
Water Overlays (available as an overlay or in a full mattress)			
Reduces pressure and pressure points because these surfaces provide flotation with pressure reduction by evenly redistributing client's weight over the entire support surface.	Use for high-risk clients.	Readily available. Some control over motion sensations. Easy to clean.	Easily punctured. Heavy. Fluid motion may make procedures (e.g., dressing changes, CPR) difficult. Maintenance needed to prevent microorganism growth. Client transfers out of bed are difficult. Difficult to raise and lower head of bed.
Gel Overlays			
Reduces pressure especially over pressure points because these surfaces provide flotation with pressure reduction by evenly redistributing client's weight over the entire support surface.	Use for moderate- to high-risk clients. Useful for clients who are wheelchair dependent.	Low maintenance. Easy to clean. Multiple-client use. Impermeable to needle punctures.	Heavy. Expensive. Lacks airflow for moisture control. Variable friction control.
Static Air-filled Overlays			
Overlays are pressure reducing and can lower the mean interface pressure between the client's tissue and the mattress.	Used for moderate- to high-risk clients. Used for clients who can reposition themselves.	Easy to clean. Multiple-client use. Low maintenance. Potential repair of some air-filled products. Durable.	Damaged by punctures from needles and sharps. Requires routine monitoring to determine adequate inflation pressure. Client transfers out of bed are difficult.
Low-air-loss Overlays (available in a full bed or overlay)			
Maintains a constant and slight air movement against the skin to prevent buildup of moisture and skin maceration.	Use for moderate- to high-risk clients.	Easy to clean. Maintains a constant inflation. Deflates to facilitate transfer and CPR. Controls moisture. Fabric covering the overlay is air permeable, bacteria impermeable, and waterproof. Reduces shear and friction. Setup provided by the manufacturer.	Damaged by needles and sharps. Noisy. Requires electricity.

Several support surfaces reduce friction, shear, and moisture (Table 25-1). Mattresses or beds with a slick surface help decrease friction and shear. Surfaces with porous covers allow airflow, which reduces moisture, resulting in decreased risk for skin maceration. Even though support surfaces are beneficial, frequent turning or repositioning of clients is the backbone of pressure ulcer preventive protocols. No bed or mattress eliminates diligent nursing care (Young and Clark, 2006). Although useful, turning devices can still injure soft tissues, requiring a nurse to be especially observant for signs of pressure formation.

TABLE 25-1 Support Surfaces—cont'd			
CATEGORY AND MECHANISM OF ACTION	**INDICATIONS FOR USE**	**ADVANTAGES**	**DISADVANTAGES**
Specialty Beds **_Air-Fluidized Beds_** Bed frame contains silicone-coated beads and incorporates both air and fluid support. The silicone-coated beads become fluidized when air is pumped through the beads.	Use for high-risk clients. Use for clients with stage III or IV pressure ulcers or burns.	Less frequent turning or repositioning. Improved client comfort. Quickly becomes firm for CPR or other treatments when the device is turned off. Reduces shear, friction, and edema to site. May facilitate management of copious wound drainage or incontinence. Setup provided by the manufacturer.	Continuous circulation of warm, dry air may increase client risk for dehydration, especially those with severe burns. Bed may increase room temperature. Client may experience disorientation. Transfer of clients is difficult. Heavy. Expensive. Width of bed may preclude use for obese clients or clients with contractures.
Low-Air-Loss Beds Bed frame with a series of connected air-filled pillows. The amount of pressure in each pillow is controlled and can be calibrated to client need.	Indicated in clients who need pressure relief, those who cannot be frequently repositioned, or those who have skin breakdown on more than one surface. Contraindicated in clients with unstable spinal column.	Head and foot of bed can be raised and lowered. Easy transfer in and out of bed. Less frequent turning schedule. Pillows can be transferred to stretcher with client. Setup provided by the manufacturer.	Requires a portable motor that is noisy. Bed surface material is slippery, and clients can easily slide down mattress or out of bed when being transferred.
Kinetic Therapy Provides continuous passive motion to promote mobilization of pulmonary secretions and provides low air loss, which provides pressure relief.	Primarily indicated for clients needing spinal stabilization. Should not be used when the client is hemodynamically unstable.	Reduces pulmonary complications associated with restricted mobility. Reduces the risk of urinary stasis and urinary tract infections (UTIs). Reduces venous stasis. Clients may have sensations of claustrophobia.	Does not reduce shear or moisture. Cannot be used with cervical or skeletal traction. Clients may have some motion sickness initially.

Data from Wound, Ostomy and Continence Nurses Society: _Guideline for prevention and management of pressure ulcers,_ Glenview, Ill, 2003, WOCN; Bryant RA: _Acute and chronic wounds: nursing management,_ ed 3, St Louis, 2007, Mosby; Morrison MJ: _The prevention and treatment of pressure ulcers,_ St Louis, 2001, Mosby; and Brienza D, Geyer MJ: Using support surfaces to manage tissue integrity, _Adv Skin Wound Care_ 18(3):152, 2005.

EVIDENCE IN PRACTICE

Cullum N and others: Support surfaces for pressure ulcer prevention, _Cochrane Database of Systematic Reviews,_ Hoboken, NJ, 2006, John Wiley & Sons.

Pressure ulcers occur in any setting and in all age-groups. When clients are at risk for pressure ulcer development, specialty beds and mattress overlays help reduce ulcer development or progression. There is sufficient evidence to support the effectiveness of high-specification foam over standard hospital foam. This foam evenly distributes the client's body weight over the surface and as a result reduces pressure. Clients with limited mobility have the lowest incidence of skin injury and pressure ulcers with alternating-pressure air mattresses, followed by low-pressure foam mattresses and water mattress overlays. There is also evidence to support the use of air-fluidized and low-air-loss devices as treatments to reduce pressure ulcer risk.

Although research offers no conclusive evidence of the effects of specialty beds, clinical data supports the use of specialty beds to reduce pressure ulcer formation in selected clients.

NURSING DIAGNOSES

Clients with actual or risk for **impaired skin integrity** or **impaired tissue integrity** may benefit from the use of pressure reduction/relief surfaces to counteract the combined effects of immobility, pressure, friction, shear, and moisture. Air-fluidized and air-suspension beds result in additional nursing diagnoses related to the pressure relief device rather than the pressure itself. For example, with air-fluidized beds, diaphoresis may go undetected and a **risk for deficient fluid volume** is possible. The client may experience **anxiety** and **fear,** especially with the use of kinetic beds. The constant turning and rigid structure may contribute to sympathetic stimulation, restlessness, increased tension, and apprehension.

SKILL 25.1 Using a Support Surface

There are numerous support surfaces designed to reduce pressure on tissues overlying bony prominences Most of the devices are easy to apply and keep clean. The extent to which the devices actually relieve pressure and prevent skin breakdown is highly variable. There are few systematic studies that consistently find one surface is better than others (Cullum and others, 2006).

Support surfaces are categorized as mattress (or wheelchair) overlays, mattress replacements, or specialty beds. An overlay rests on top of the hospital mattress and uses foam, air, water, gel, or combinations of these products to provide pressure relief. Mattress overlays and mattress replacements are considered to be either static (e.g., foam, gels) or dynamic (e.g., alternating-pressure surfaces).

A flotation pad is constructed of a silicone or polyvinyl chloride gel encased in a vinyl-covered square. The pad serves as an artificial layer of fat to protect bony surfaces such as the sacrum and greater trochanters.

One type of air mattress is fully integrated into the hospital bed. This bed surface is adjusted to the client's comfort level by adjusting pressures to the client's position and movement when in the automatic mode. A bedsheet always covers an air mattress to prevent skin from touching the plastic surface.

There are two types of foam mattresses. One is the foam mattress overlay, which may have either a flat smooth surface, foam rubber peaks ("egg-crate" variety, shown in Figure 25-1), or a cut surface. It is placed on top of the bed mattress, and usually the nurse places a sheet over the foam mattress pad overlay to prevent soiling and provide ease of cleaning. The second type is the foam specialty mattress, which completely replaces the hospital mattress and is covered by a loose-fitting cover intended to minimize friction and shear and protect the mattress. The foam mattresses are designed for comfort rather than pressure relief.

Air mattress overlays can be static or dynamic and consist of interconnected air cells or cushions inflated by the use of a motorized blower (Figure 25-2). These mattresses use a pressure-cycling device to intermittently inflate and deflate or to maintain a constant inflation and slight air movement in the mattress.

Replacement mattresses are denser, thicker, and more resilient to the client's weight; they evenly distribute pressure; minimize friction and shear forces; and provide comfortable, well-ventilated support (Collins, 2004; Merk, 2006). Replacement mattresses have foam, gel, air, or fluid sections that are customized to the needs of a specific client with moderate to high risk for skin breakdown. Another

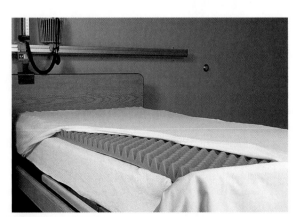

FIGURE 25-1 "Egg-crate" foam overlay is primarily for comfort.

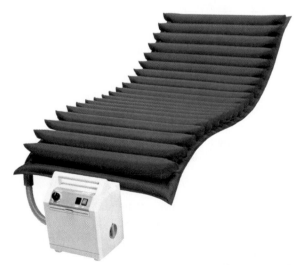

FIGURE 25-2 Dynamic air mattress overlay. (© 2006 Hill-Rom Services, Inc. Reprinted with permission. All rights reserved.)

available option is an air-integrated replacement mattress (Figure 25-3), which is used for clients with moderate to high risk for skin breakdown.

Other devices include a low-pressure seat cushion (Figure 25-4) overlaid on a wheelchair or a dry static floatation mattress system (Figure 25-5) overlaid on the bed or wheelchair. Through a system of controlled dynamics, low pressures are maintained by distributing pressure across the client's body surface. Thus friction and shear are minimized.

Support surfaces may reduce pressure on the client's skin. However, they do not replace regular repositioning, meticulous skin care, or range of joint motion. The decision to place a client on a support surface and the selection of this surface is a nursing responsibility. A support surface redistributes pressure and is comfortable. There are nine parameters to use when evaluating and selecting a support surface: life expectancy, skin moisture control, skin temperature control, redistribution of pressure, product service requirements, fall safety, infection control, flammability, and client-product friction (Maklebust, 2005).

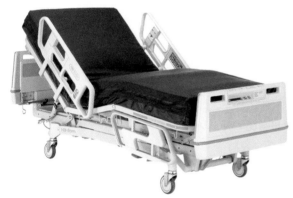

FIGURE 25-3 Air-integrated replacement mattress. (© 2006 Hill-Rom Services, Inc. Reprinted with permission. All rights reserved.)

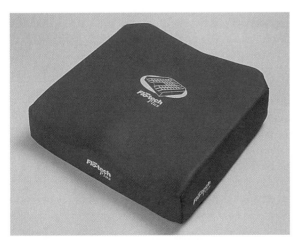

FIGURE 25-4 Low-pressure seat cushion. (Reproduced with permission from Invacare, Ltd.)

ASSESSMENT

1 Determine client's risk for pressure ulcer formation and the need for a pressure reduction surface, using a validated risk assessment tool such as the Braden scale (see Chapter 22). *Rationale: Risk assessment tools (e.g., Braden scale) provide an objective measure of risk consistent between evaluators over time (AHCPR, 1994). Assess risks by population: general population less than or equal to 16; intensive care unit (ICU) less than or equal to 15; older adult less than or equal to 18; and Black and Latino clients less than or equal to 18 (Bergstrom and others, 1998; Braden and Maklebust, 2005; Jiricka and others, 1995; Lyder and others, 1998).*

2 Perform routine skin assessment, especially over dependent sites and bony prominences. Look for changes in color (erythema or pallor), texture (edema or induration), temperature (warmth or coolness), blistering, or ulceration. Assess any areas of redness for normal reactive hyperthermia (area blanches and returns to pink color). *Rationale: Provides baseline data to determine change in skin integrity or change in existing pressure ulcer.*

3 Assess client's level of comfort using a 0 to 10 pain scale. *Rationale: Client may require pain medication to tolerate movement to another bed/mattress surface. Adequate pain control improves client's tolerance of position changes.*

4 Assess client's understanding of purposes of support surfaces. *Rationale: Facilitates client's cooperation in use of support surface.*

5 Verify physician's order for surface. *Rationale: A physician's order is usually required to obtain reimbursement.*

PLANNING

Expected Outcomes focus on maintenance of skin integrity and client comfort.

1 Client's skin remains intact without evidence of erythema, abnormal reactive hyperemia, or mottling.

2 Existing pressure ulcers show signs of healing.

3 Client rates comfort no greater than a 4 (on a scale of 0 to 10).

4 Client is removed from therapeutic surface when risk for pressure ulcer decreases.

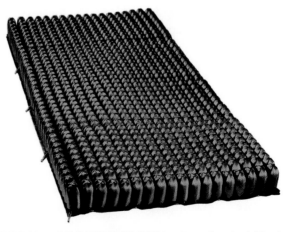

FIGURE 25-5 ROHO DRY FLOATATION mattress for a bed. (Courtesy The ROHO Group, Belleville, Ill.)

Delegation Considerations

Assessment of the client's need for a support surface may not be delegated. However, the skills of applying support surface mattresses or preparation of an alternative bed may be delegated. Some types of support surfaces require that the manufacturer's representative set up and maintain the support system. The nurse directs personnel by:

- Emphasizing the need to notify the nurse of any changes in the client's skin
- Monitoring regular turning and repositioning of the client and telling personnel to seek assistance for client position changes as necessary
- Explaining importance of reporting any changes in inflation or deflation cycles or leakage of air, water, or gel

Equipment

- Risk assessment tool (see Chapter 22)
- Foam overlay (see Figure 25-1)
- Air mattress overlay (see Figure 25-2)
- Replacement mattress (see Figure 25-3)
- Low-pressure seat cushion (see Figure 25-4)
- Flotation mattress for a bed (see Figure 25-5)
- Sheet(s)
- Clean gloves (if soiled linen is being handled)
- Standard bed frame (with mattress if overlay is to be used)

IMPLEMENTATION *for Using a Support Surface*

STEPS	RATIONALE
1 See Standard Protocol (inside front cover).	
2 Assist client to a chair when possible.	Eases application of device.
3 Obtain additional personnel as needed.	Assistance reduces the risk of friction and shear in transfer of client to new surface.
4 Apply support surface to bed or prepare alternative bed (bed may be occupied or unoccupied).	
a. Replacement mattress:	
(1) Apply mattress to bed frame after removing standard hospital mattress.	Hospital mattress needs to be stored, or mattress replacements may be used instead of hospital mattresses.
(2) Apply sheet over mattress. Keep layers between client and surface to a minimum.	Sheet reduces soiling. Multiple layers decrease surface effectiveness in reducing pressure (WOCN, 2003).
b. Air mattress/overlay:	
(1) Apply deflated mattress over surface of bed mattress. (There may be directions on pad indicating which side to place up.)	Provides smooth, even surface.

> **COMMUNICATION TIP** Tell client that the mattress may inflate and deflate periodically, may feel cool, and may require a period of adjustment.

STEPS	RATIONALE
(2) Bring plastic strips or flaps around corners of bed mattress.	Secures air mattress in place.
(3) Attach connector on air mattress to inflation device. Inflate mattress to proper air pressure determined by air pump or blower.	Mattresses vary as to requiring one-time or continuous inflation cycle. Manufacturer's directions indicate desired air pressure designed to distribute client's body weight evenly. Directions are included with each mattress.
(4) Place sheet over air mattress; eliminate all wrinkles. Do not tighten sheet.	Prevents soiling of mattress and reduces direct contact of skin against plastic surface. Tightened sheet reduces the effectiveness of the air mattress overlay.
(5) Check air pump to be sure pressure cycle alternates if alternating air is used.	Alternating airflow mattress produces intermittent cycling, inflating only parts of mattress at any one time. Intermittent cycle continually alternates pressure against skin and soft tissue (Whittemore, 1998).
(6) Assist client with transferring in and out of bed (see Chapter 6).	Mattress surface is less firm and may be slippery and is difficult for some clients to assist in transferring from bed to chair/stretcher.

STEPS	RATIONALE

c. Air-surface bed:

(1) Obtain and make bed.

Bed may be available in all client rooms; if not, see agency policy for ordering one.

(2) Place switch in the "Prevention" mode.

In the "Prevention" mode, surface pressures change automatically with client position to equalize pressure and eliminate points of pressure.

> **NURSE ALERT** This and other support beds are equipped with a cardiopulmonary resuscitation (CPR) switch to instantly lower head section from an elevated position and to deflate the mattress to provide a firm surface for chest compressions (see Figure 25-8, Skill 25.2).

d. Water mattress (supplemental and self-contained):

(1) Apply unfilled supplemental mattress flat over the surface of standard bed mattress. (Self-contained water mattress would replace bed mattress.)

Provides a smooth, even surface.

(2) Bring any plastic strips or flaps around corners of bed mattress.

Secures water mattress in place.

(3) Attach connector on water mattress to water source, and fill mattress to desired water level designed to distribute client's body weight evenly. Follow manufacturer's directions regarding level and temperature of water.

Proper water temperature prevents loss of body heat as client lies on mattress.

(4) Place sheet over water mattress, being sure to eliminate all wrinkles.

Reduces soiling of mattress and prevents direct contact of skin with plastic surface.

(5) Keep sharp objects away from mattress.

Tears and punctures result in loss of water, making mattress ineffective.

5 Position client comfortably as desired over support surface. Reposition routinely.

Location of existing pressure ulcer might influence type of client positioning required.

6 Instruct client to call for assistance to get in and out of bed.

Height of the bed may be increased with overlay, making getting in and out of bed difficult.

7 See Completion Protocol (inside front cover).

EVALUATION

1 Inspect condition of skin regularly (every 2 hours in high-risk client) to determine changes in skin and effectiveness of and need for support surface.

2 Observe and monitor existing pressure ulcers for evidence of healing.

3 Ask client to rate comfort on a 0 to 10 scale.

Unexpected Outcomes and Related Interventions

1 Client develops localized areas of abnormal reactive hyperemia for longer than 30 minutes (WOCN, 2003), mottling, swelling, and tenderness with evidence of breakdown. Existing pressure ulcers fail to demonstrate signs of healing.

a. Increase frequency of skin assessment.

b. Modify skin care regimen.

c. Increase types of pressure relief interventions.

d. Notify physician.

2 Client expresses discomfort.

a. Evaluate air level of surface.

b. Evaluate need for alternative surface.

c. Reposition client more frequently.

Recording and Reporting

- Record type of support surface applied, extent to which client tolerated procedure, and condition of client's skin in nurses' notes or skin assessment flow sheet.

- Report evidence of pressure ulcer formation to nurse in charge or to physician.

Sample Documentation

1000 Air mattress overlay applied to bed. Skin dry and intact without erythema. Comfort rated as 3 on a scale of 0 to 10.

Special Considerations

Pediatric Considerations

- Use pain assessment tools specifically developed for use in children.
- Parents are helpful in assisting the child in expressing pain and treatment preferences (Hockenberry and Wilson, 2007).

Geriatric Considerations

- Aging skin is drier, thinner, and less pressure sensitive, increasing the risk of skin breakdown (Meiner and Leuckenotte, 2006).

- Adding mattress overlays changes the bed height. Be careful when transferring and teaching family members to transfer from bed to chair.

Home Care Considerations

- Most of the devices in this procedure may be adapted for home use on a standard twin bed or hospital bed.
- Selection is based on client needs and environmental audit. For example, the client on total bed rest who smokes would not be an ideal candidate for a foam mattress because of the potential for fire; the client with pets that sleep in the bed may not be suited for a water- or air-filled mattress because of the risk of puncture.

SKILL 25.2   Using an Air-Suspension Bed

Air-suspension beds are indicated for clients who are immobile or otherwise confined to the bed. The air-suspension bed supports a client's weight on air-filled cushions. The bed minimizes pressure and reduces shear in a low-air-loss system (Figure 25-6). If a client has large stage III or stage IV pressure ulcers on multiple turning surfaces, a low-air-loss bed or air-fluidized bed may be indicated (AHCPR, 1994).

For clients requiring high air loss under a given body part, for example, under the buttocks, high-air-loss cushions may be substituted. High air loss provides for selective drying while not having the effect of substantially increasing insensible fluid losses.

It is possible to adapt the air-suspension bed to individual client needs with specialty cushions for positioning, foot support, and lateral arm supports. Clients usually require less analgesia while on the bed. Another adaptation of the air-suspension bed is the kinetic low-air-loss bed (Figure 25-7). This bed is marketed widely to intensive care areas and has the ability to provide a pressure relief surface while rotating continuously approximately 30 to 35 degrees. This surface is never used with a client who has an unstable spine or who is in traction.

These beds have CPR switches for immediate deflation to provide a hard surface for chest compressions (Figure 25-8). Scales may be built into the bed for ease in weighing. A battery system is necessary to maintain inflation during interruptions of power or during transport.

ASSESSMENT

1 Determine client's risk for pressure ulcer formation and the need for a pressure reduction surface, using a validated risk assessment tool such as the Braden scale (see Chapter 22). *Rationale: Risk assessment tools (e.g., Braden scale) provide an objective measure of risk consistent between evaluators over time (AHCPR, 1994). Assess risks by population: general population less than or equal to 16; ICU less than or equal to 15; older adult less than or equal to 18; and Black and Latino clients less than or equal to 18 (Bergstrom and others, 1998; Braden and Maklebust, 2005; Jiricka and others, 1995; Lyder and others, 1998).*

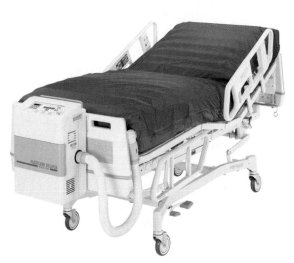

FIGURE 25-6 Low-air-loss bed. (© 2006 Hill-Rom Services, Inc. Reprinted with permission. All rights reserved.)

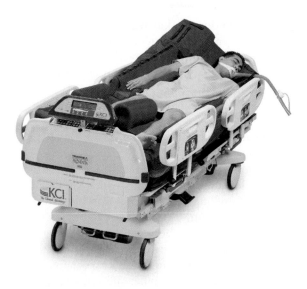

FIGURE 25-7 Lateral rotation bed. (TriaDyne® Proventa™ bed. Courtesy KCI, San Antonio, Tex.)

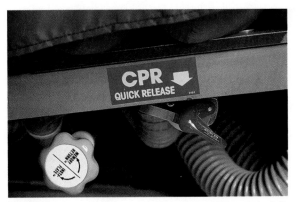

FIGURE 25-8 Cardiopulmonary resuscitation (CPR) switch deflates low-air-loss bed to provide hard surface.

2 Perform routine skin assessment, especially over dependent sites and bony prominences. Look for changes in color (erythema or pallor), texture (edema or induration), temperature (warmth or coolness), blistering, or ulceration. Assess any area of redness for normal reactive hyperthermia (area blanches and returns to normal pink color). *Rationale: Provides baseline data to determine change in skin integrity or change in existing pressure ulcer.*

3 Assess client's level of comfort and pain using a 0 to 10 scale. *Rationale: Client may require pain medication to tolerate movement to another bed/mattress surface. Adequate pain control improves client's tolerance of position changes.*

4 Assess client's understanding of purposes of support surfaces. *Rationale: Facilitates client's cooperation in use of support surface.*

5 Obtain client's baseline level of consciousness (LOC). *Rationale: Baseline is used to detect changes; clients may become confused or disoriented from the floating sensation of the bed.*

6 Review client's serum electrolyte and hematocrit levels, if available. *Rationale: The movement of air through the mattress increases the client's risk for dehydration (WOCN, 2003). Hemoconcentration results from dehydration.*

7 Verify client's medical orders. *Rationale: A physician's order is required to obtain reimbursement in the United States.*

PLANNING

Expected Outcomes focus on the maintenance of skin integrity and client comfort.

1 Client's skin remains warm, clean, and intact without evidence of abnormal reactive hyperemia or mottling.
2 Existing pressure ulcers show evidence of healing by formation of granulation tissue.
3 Client rates comfort no greater than a 4 (on a scale of 0 to 10).
4 Client remains alert and oriented.
5 Serum electrolyte and hematocrit values remain within normal limits or client's baseline.

Delegation Considerations

Assessment of the skin and underlying tissue may not be delegated. After the nurse completes the assessment, determines the need for a support surface, and selects the specific surface, the skill of placing the client on an air-suspension bed may be delegated. Some types of support surfaces require that the manufacturer's representative set up and maintain the support system. The nurse directs personnel by:

- Emphasizing the need to notify the nurse of any changes in the client's skin
- Reviewing regular turning and repositioning of the client and telling personnel to seek assistance for client position changes as necessary
- Reviewing what to report regarding any changes in inflation or deflation cycles or leakage of air, water, or gel
- Emphasizing the need to notify the nurse if the client becomes disoriented or restless, or complains of nausea

Equipment

- Air-suspension bed: low-air-loss (see Figure 25-6) or lateral rotation bed (see Figure 25-7)
- Gore-Tex sheet (supplied by distributor)
- Disposable bed pads, if indicated
- Clean gloves (if contacting body fluids)

IMPLEMENTATION *for Using an Air-Suspension Bed*

STEPS	RATIONALE
1 See Standard Protocol (inside front cover).	
2 Explain steps of transfer.	Reduces anxiety and helps client be a part of decision making during maneuvering.
3 Transfer client to bed using appropriate transfer techniques (see Chapter 6). Bed surface may be slippery; do not attempt to transfer client without assistance.	Appropriate transfer techniques maintain alignment and reduce risk of injury during procedure. Manufacturer's representative adjusts bed to client's height and weight.
4 After the client is transferred, release Instaflate or turn bed on by depressing switch; regulate temperature.	Pressure cushions will adjust automatically to preset optimal levels to minimize pressure, friction, and shear (Pieper, 2000).
5 Position client and perform range-of-motion (ROM) exercises as appropriate.	Promotes comfort and reduces contracture formation. The bed relieves pressure on skin, but clients must still be turned and exercised to avoid joint deformity or contractures (AHCPR, 1994).

STEPS	RATIONALE
6 To turn clients, position bedpans, or perform other therapies, set Instaflate. When procedure is complete, release Instaflate.	According to the manufacturer's instructions, Instaflate firms the bed surface to facilitate turning and handling client.

> **NURSE ALERT** Client will not receive pressure relief when bed is firm for procedures. Activate CPR switch to quickly deflate the bed in an emergency (see Figure 25-8).

STEPS	RATIONALE
7 Determine bed's special features, and use as needed.	
a. Scales.	Facilitates ease for obtaining routine weights.
b. Portable transport units to maintain inflation when primary power source is interrupted.	Provides continuous pressure relief.
c. Availability of specialty cushions for prone position, providing pressure relief, reducing moisture, preventing sliding down in bed, or relieving heavy weight from orthopedic devices.	Helps prevent friction and shearing forces.
d. Lateral rotation features that allow approximately 30 degrees of turning.	Helps prevent pulmonary and urinary complications of reduced mobility (Cullum and others, 2006; WOCN, 2003).
8 Provide adequate fluid intake.	Bed surface may be drying and contributes to dehydration.
9 See Completion Protocol (inside front cover).	

EVALUATION

1 Inspect condition of skin regularly (every 2 hours in high-risk client) to determine changes in skin and effectiveness of therapy.
2 Observe existing pressure ulcers for evidence of healing.
3 Ask client to rate comfort on a 0 to 10 scale.
4 Determine client's LOC and orientation.
5 Monitor client's serum and electrolyte values as available.

Unexpected Outcomes and Related Interventions
1 Client develops areas of new breakdown, or existing areas of breakdown worsen.
a. Modify skin care regimen.
b. Revise turning schedule as needed.
c. Notify physician.
2 Client experiences restlessness or nausea or becomes disoriented because of constant flotation.
a. Reposition client for comfort.
b. Notify physician. Symptomatic treatment, such as anti-anxiety medication, may be required while adjusting to the bed.
c. Evaluate the need for alternative support mattress.
3 Client becomes nauseated.
a. Provide short-term antiemetics.
b. Temporarily decrease frequency of lateral position.

Recording and Reporting
• Record transfer of client to low-air-loss bed or overlay, tolerance of procedure, and condition of skin in nurses' notes or skin assessment flow sheet.

• Report changes in condition of skin to physician: restlessness or change in orientation.

Sample Documentation
1000 Transferred onto air-suspension bed, low-air-loss bed without difficulty. Skin warm, dry, and intact without erythema or new areas of breakdown. Stage I pressure ulcer on left trochanter, no drainage present. Denies dizziness. Rates comfort as 3 on a scale of 0 to 10.

Special Considerations
Pediatric Considerations
• This bed is used commonly with older children. Instructions must be age appropriate and include any restrictions (e.g., raising the head of the bed, positioning).
• Younger children are usually easier to position, and thus the risk of pressure ulcers is easier to control.

Geriatric Considerations
• When hospitalized, some older adult clients may experience misperceptions of their environment that may be intensified by the constant flotation of the air-suspension bed. Proprioception abnormalities affecting older adults are the result of nervous system and muscle changes (Meiner and Lueckenotte, 2006).

Home Care Considerations
- A version of the bed is available for home use for rent or purchase; bed rental company is responsible for proper cleaning.

- Instruct family in importance of maintaining client hydration.
- Instruct family regarding the need to provide client's skin care.

SKILL 25.3 Using an Air-Fluidized Bed

An air-fluidized bed is a dynamic device designed to distribute a client's weight evenly over the support surface (Figure 25-9). The bed minimizes pressure and reduces shear force and friction through the principle of fluidization. Fluidization is created by forcing a gentle flow of temperature-controlled air upward through a mass of fine ceramic microspheres. The client lies directly on a polyester filter sheet that allows air to pass through but does not allow the microspheres to escape. Clients feel as though they are floating on a surface like a warm waterbed. The contact pressure of the client's body against the filter sheet stays at 11 to 16 mm Hg.

Air-fluidized beds are useful in the care of clients who require minimal movement to prevent skin damage by shearing force and for clients who experience significant pain when being turned or positioned, such as those with burns, skin grafts, pressure ulcers, or trauma. The surface of the filter sheet warms, causing clients to perspire. Moisture is then quickly absorbed into the circulating microspheres. Diaphoresis can go undetected, and thus insensible fluid loss may not be noticed until a client develops fluid and electrolyte imbalances. This surface is never used with a client who has an unstable spinal cord or severe pulmonary problems. Clients may also experience agitation, restlessness, or disorientation related to flotation.

Conventional fluidized beds do not allow for head-of-bed position changes. Foam wedges are used to elevate the head. There are combination air-fluidized/low-air-loss beds that allow head-of-bed elevation (Figure 25-10). These beds use air to lift the upper body, while the lower body stays in a fluidized bed surface. The weight of the bed structure makes transport extremely difficult.

ASSESSMENT

1 Determine client's risk for pressure ulcer formation and the need for a pressure reduction surface, using a validated risk assessment tool such as the Braden scale (see Chapter 22). *Rationale: Risk assessment tools (e.g., Braden scale) provide an objective measure of risk consistent between evaluators over time (AHCPR, 1994). Assess risks by population: general population less than or equal to 16; ICU less than or equal to 15; older adult less than or equal to 18; and Black and Latino clients less than or equal to 18 (Bergstrom and others, 1998; Braden and Maklebust, 2005; Jiricka and others, 1995; Lyder and others, 1998).*

2 Carefully inspect the skin for evidence of pressure and impending breakdown. Note condition of the skin over bony prominences, pressure sites, and existing pressure ulcers. Assess any areas of redness for reactive hyperemia (skin blanches and returns to pink color). *Rationale: This data provides a baseline to determine changes in client's skin.*

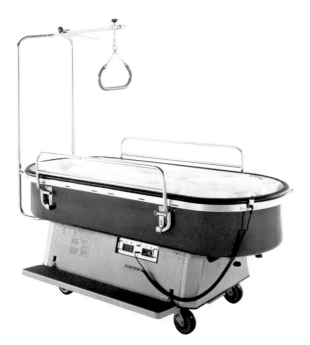

FIGURE 25-9 Air-fluidized bed. (© 2006 Hill-Rom Services, Inc. Reprinted with permission. All rights reserved.)

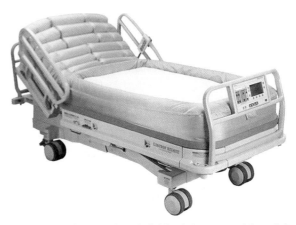

FIGURE 25-10 Combination air-fluidized therapy and low-air-loss bed. (© 2006 Hill-Rom Services, Inc. Reprinted with permission. All rights reserved.)

3 Determine client's level of comfort; ask client to rate pain on a scale of 0 to 10. *Rationale: Nerve endings related to pressure, touch, temperature, and limb position are located on the skin. Client comfort is one of the main purposes of support (Bryant, 2007; Maklebust, 2005).*

4 Review client's temperature and serum electrolyte and hematocrit levels. *Rationale: Body fluids may be lost through diaphoresis. Hemoconcentration results from dehydration.*

5 Assess client's emotional response and level of orientation. *Rationale: Flotation effect may cause altered sensory perceptions.*

6 Identify clients at risk for complications of air-fluidized therapy:

a. Older adult clients may become dehydrated from the airflow, increasing insensible fluid losses.

b. Clients receiving enteric tube feedings are at risk for aspiration from the inability to elevate head of bed other than with foam wedges under their back and shoulders.

c. Clients who have limited ability to change positions and who are susceptible to dehydration may have tenacious pulmonary secretions that are difficult to remove.

7 Determine client's and family member's understanding of the purpose of the bed. *Rationale: Family member's support and presence helps with implementing interventions. These beds generate noise, which may cause anxiety for the client and family.*

8 Review client's medical orders. *Rationale: A physician's order is required to obtain reimbursement.*

PLANNING

Expected Outcomes focus on maintenance of skin integrity, comfort, adequate fluid and electrolyte balance, and the client's comfort.

1 Client's skin remains warm, clean, and intact, and/or there is evidence of healing of pressure ulcers.

2 Client rates improved comfort and rates pain no greater than 4 (on a scale of 0 to 10).

3 Client's skin remains well hydrated, with good turgor; mucous membranes are moist.

4 Electrolyte levels are in the normal range.

5 Client remains alert and oriented or shows no change in LOC.

Delegation Considerations

Assessment of the need for an air-fluidized bed, choice of type to use, client education, and evaluation of effectiveness may not be delegated. Some types of specialty beds require that the manufacturer's representative set up and maintain the system. The nurse directs personnel by:

- Reviewing changes in skin and underlying tissue to be reported
- Monitoring regular turning and repositioning of the client
- Emphasizing the need to report changes in orientation, restless, or complaints of nausea

Equipment

- Air-fluidized bed (see Figures 25-9 and 25-10)
- Foam positioning wedges, if indicated
- Filter sheet (supplied by the rental company)
- Clean gloves (if contacting body fluids)

IMPLEMENTATION *for Using an Air-Fluidized Bed*

STEPS	RATIONALE
1 See Standard Protocol (inside front cover).	
2 Review manufacturer's instructions. Company representative may be in attendance. Premedicate client 30 minutes before transfer if needed. Obtain additional personnel as needed.	Ensures proper and safe use of bed. Promotes comfort during transfer for those clients in moderate to severe pain. Aids in ensuring client's safety. Company representatives ensure proper functioning of bed.
3 Transfer client onto air-fluidized bed using appropriate transfer techniques (see Chapter 6). A slide or lift may be used.	A slide or lift is needed to maneuver client over the rigid sides of the bed.

> **NURSE ALERT** Do not place a client in a prone position on an air-fluidized bed because of the risk of suffocation.

> **COMMUNICATION TIP** Tell client that there may be a sensation of floating or nausea when first placed on the bed.

4 Turn fluidization cycle on by depressing switch; regulate temperature.	Fluidization minimizes pressure against skin's surface and reduces friction and shear force when client moves.
5 Position client and perform ROM exercises routinely. Foam wedges may be needed to place client in Fowler's position.	Promotes comfort and reduces contracture formation. The bed reduces pressure on the skin, but clients must still be turned and exercised to avoid joint deformity or contracture (Pieper, 2000).

STEPS	RATIONALE

> **NURSE ALERT** Use foam wedges as needed (e.g. elevating the head, positioning). Areas supported by the foam wedges do not benefit from the pressure relief of the bed's surface.

6 Use fluidization switch to provide hard surface for turning, positioning bedpans, and other procedures. Remember to reactivate fluidization after procedure.

According to manufacturer's instructions, when fluidization is stopped, the bed becomes firm, allowing for ease in positioning. Reactivation of fluidization is necessary to minimize pressure.

> **NURSE ALERT** Activate CPR switch when resuscitation is necessary.

7 See Completion Protocol (inside front cover).

EVALUATION

1 Inspect condition of skin regularly (every 2 hours in high-risk client) to determine changes in skin and effectiveness of air-fluidized therapy.

2 Ask client to rate level of comfort on a scale of 0 to 10.

3 Observe moisture of client's skin and mucous membranes and skin turgor.

4 Monitor client's temperature and laboratory serum electrolyte and hematocrit levels.

5 Assess client's level of orientation.

Unexpected Outcomes and Related Interventions

1 Client develops areas of breakdown, or existing areas of breakdown worsen.
a. Evaluate and revise turning schedule as needed.
b. Keep skin clean and dry.
c. Reevaluate the client's risk factors affecting wound healing.
d. Notify physician. Advancement of existing pressure ulcer may be related to tissue necrosis, infection, nutritional deficiencies, or other systemic factors.

2 Client experiences agitation, restlessness, or disorientation related to flotation.
a. Provide reassurance and emotional support. Encourage client to verbalize concerns.
b. Notify physician. Symptomatic treatment may be necessary while adjusting to constant flotation.

3 Client's skin and mucous membranes are dehydrated and serum electrolyte levels are abnormal related to the temperature and evaporative effects of the bed.
a. Evaluate nutritional and fluid status, including intake and output (I&O).
b. Increase fluid intake unless contraindicated.
c. Collaborate with physician for other treatment modalities.

Recording and Reporting

- Record transfer of client to bed, tolerance to procedure, and condition of skin in nurses' notes or skin assessment flow sheet.
- Report changes in client's level of orientation, condition of skin, and electrolyte levels.

Sample Documentation

1600 Transferred onto air-fluidized bed without difficulty. Skin warm, dry, and intact. Mucous membranes moist. A 3-cm reddened area noted on sacrum with brisk capillary refill. Oriented to person, place, and time; no nausea. Rates comfort 4 on a scale of 0 to 10.

Special Considerations
Pediatric Considerations

- This bed is used commonly with children who are burn victims. Provide age-appropriate instructions and include any restrictions (e.g., raising the head of the bed, positioning).
- Tell parents that the child may initially have some dizziness or nausea when first placed on the bed. This is caused by the flotation sensation and will disappear as the child gets adjusted to the bed.

Geriatric Considerations

- Older adult clients are at increased risk for dehydration.
- When hospitalized, older adult clients may experience significant misperceptions of their environment that may be intensified by the flotation of the air-fluidized bed.

Home Care Considerations

- Beds weigh between 1700 and 2100 lb; therefore the company leasing the bed needs to inspect the home for accessibility and structural support.

SKILL 25.4 Using a Rotokinetic Bed

The rotokinetic bed maintains skeletal alignment while providing constant rotation (Figure 25-11). It is used in the care of spinal cord–injured and multiple-trauma clients. The support structure of the bed outlines the body parts and maintains proper alignment when secured properly. This bed improves skeletal alignment with constant side-to-side rotation up to 90 degrees (Tomaselli, Goldberg, and Wind, 2001). The bed rotates from side to side at a 60- to 90-degree angle every 7 minutes. Turning angles may be adjusted to meet the client's needs. Constant rotation reduces pressure ulcer development and stimulates body systems. It is recommended that the bed stay in the rotation mode for at least 20 hours a day. There is an emergency gatch that quickly interrupts rotation when needed. When CPR must be initiated, the bed is returned to the horizontal position and locked in place.

The constant motion may lead to sensory distress for the client. Older adults and confused clients may have difficulty adjusting to the constant kinetic stimulation, the limited visual field, and inner ear disequilibrium.

ASSESSMENT

1 Determine client's risk for pressure ulcer formation and the need for a pressure reduction surface, using a validated risk assessment tool such as the Braden scale (see Chapter 22). *Rationale: Risk assessment tools (e.g., Braden scale) provide an objective measure of risk consistent between evaluators over time (AHCPR, 1994). Assess risks by population: general population less than or equal to 16; ICU less than or equal to 15; older adult less than or equal to 18; and Black and Latino clients less than or equal to 18 (Bergstrom and others, 1998; Braden and Maklebust, 2005; Jiricka and others, 1995; Lyder and others, 1998).*

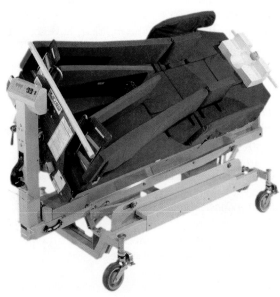

FIGURE 25-11 Rotokinetic bed. (RotoRest® Delta bed. Courtesy KCI, San Antonio, Tex.)

2 Carefully inspect the skin for evidence of pressure. Assess any areas of redness for normal reactive hyperemia (skin blanches and returns to pink color). *Rationale: Provides baseline of skin condition. Allows for proper positioning of pressure site.*

3 Assess the client's LOC, inner ear equilibrium, orientation, and anxiety. *Rationale: Establishes a baseline assessment to detect any change while client is on the bed. Constant motion may lead to sensory distress.*

4 Perform pulmonary assessment and obtain vital signs. *Rationale: Provides baseline data before using rotokinetic bed. Clients with severe injuries or spinal cord injuries are at risk for accumulation of pulmonary secretions. In addition, when these clients are first placed on the bed they are at risk of changes in vital signs caused by the motion of the bed.*

5 Assess the client's and family members' understanding of and response to the rotokinetic bed.

6 Determine client's level of comfort; ask client to rate pain on a scale of 0 to 10. *Rationale: Provides baseline data to determine client's comfort needs.*

7 Review client's medical orders. *Rationale: A physician's order is required to obtain reimbursement in the United States.*

PLANNING

Expected Outcomes focus on maintaining skin integrity and proper body alignment, promoting client comfort, decreasing client's anxiety, preventing pulmonary congestion, and maintaining skin integrity.

1 Client's skin remains intact, without abnormal reactive hyperemia or mottling.

2 Client's existing pressure ulcers show evidence of healing.

3 Client's musculoskeletal system is properly aligned and free of contractures.

4 Client's breath sounds improve or remain clear to auscultation.

5 Client remains alert, oriented, and cooperative.

6 Client denies nausea or dizziness.

7 Client's blood pressure remains consistent with baseline vital signs.

Delegation Considerations

The skill of placing a client on a rotokinetic bed may not be delegated to assistive personnel (AP). This type of bed is frequently used for clients with multiple trauma or spinal cord injuries, and the nurse must carefully determine what aspects of the client's care may be delegated to the appropriately skilled personnel. The nurse directs personnel by:

• Instructing to report any changes in the client's skin or tissue

• Instructing to maintain the exact rotation frequency of the bed and to stop the rotation only for selected aspects of care determined by the nurse (e.g., bathing, oral hygiene, enemas)

• Emphasizing to immediately notify the nurse for client confusion, nausea, and pain

Equipment

- Rotokinetic bed with support packs, bolsters, and safety straps (see Figure 25-11)
- Top sheet
- Pillowcases for bolsters
- Clean gloves (if contacting body fluids)

IMPLEMENTATION *for Using a Rotokinetic Bed*

STEPS	RATIONALE
1 See Standard Protocol (inside front cover) and review manufacturer's instructions.	
2 Place rotokinetic bed in horizontal position, and remove all bolsters, straps, and supports. Close posterior hatches.	
3 Unplug electrical cord. Lock gatch.	Prevents accidental rotation during transfer.
4 Maintaining proper alignment of the client and using appropriate transfer techniques (see Chapter 6), transfer client to rotokinetic bed.	Reduces risk of further tissue injury during transfer. May need physician available to assist in transfer.
5 Secure thoracic panels, bolsters, head and knee packs, and safety straps.	Maintains proper alignment and prevents sliding during rotation.
6 Cover client with top sheet.	Prevents unnecessary exposure.
7 Plug bed in.	
8 Have company representative set optional angle as ordered by physician. May gradually increase rotation.	Rotational angle is determined by physician based on the client's overall condition and tolerance to constant motion.
9 Increase degree of rotation gradually according to client's tolerance.	Gradually increasing rotation may reduce or prevent nausea, dizziness, and orthostatic hypotension (Tomaselli, Goldberg, and Wind, 2001).

> **NURSE ALERT** The bed must be stopped for CPR and bedside procedures (e.g., portable chest x-ray examination, dressing changes).

> **COMMUNICATION TIP** Tell the client that there may be a sensation of light-headedness or falling. Falls will not occur because of positioning of the pads, which are checked by two people to ensure proper placement.

STEPS	RATIONALE
10 It is difficult to maintain eye contact when talking with clients during rotation. Provide adequate space for caregivers and family to move around the bed to facilitate communication.	Allows opportunity to meet client's psychosocial needs.
11 The bed may be stopped for assessment and procedures. To stop the bed, permit bed to rotate to the desired position, turn the motor off, and push knob into a lock position. If necessary, the bed can be manually repositioned.	Allows nurse to assess client.
12 See Completion Protocol (inside front cover).	

EVALUATION

1 Inspect condition of skin (occipital, ears, axillae, elbows, sacrum, groin, and heels) and musculoskeletal alignment every 2 hours to determine changes in skin and effectiveness of rotokinetic therapy.

2 Inspect client's pressure ulcers for evidence of healing.

3 Observe alignment and ROM of all joints.

4 Auscultate lung sounds every shift, and compare with baseline.

5 Determine client's level of orientation at least once per shift.

6 Ask whether client is experiencing nausea or dizziness.

7 Monitor blood pressure.

Unexpected Outcomes and Related Interventions

1 Client develops areas of breakdown, or existing areas of breakdown worsen.

a. Revise rotation schedule; bed should stay in rotation for 20 hours a day to prevent breakdown.

b. Keep skin clean and dry. Change linen on bolsters as needed.

2 Client experiences hypotension.

a. If severe drop in blood pressure occurs, stop rotation. Notify physician. Monitor vital signs every 5 minutes.

b. For less severe blood pressure changes, decrease the rotational angle. Gradually increase the rotational angle as client adjusts to rotation.

3 Client becomes disoriented, confused, or uncooperative related to sensory/perceptual distortion.

a. Reorient client to person, place, and time.

b. Provide audio stimulation via radio or tape recorder.

c. Provide TV secured to bed frame (available from manufacturer).

d. Hang mirror on ceiling so that client may view surroundings.

e. Notify physician. Symptomatic treatment for motion sickness may be helpful.

4 Client develops crackles in lung fields.

a. Have client cough and deep breathe every 2 hours.

b. Notify physician. Incentive spirometry or other treatment measures may be warranted.

Recording and Reporting

• Describe the condition of skin before placement on the rotokinetic bed. A photograph may be taken to document skin condition and provide a baseline for later assessments for progress in healing.

• Record time of transfer to rotokinetic bed and the degree of rotation.

• Record and report subjective data indicating response to the constant rotation and presence/absence of dizziness, nausea, or blood pressure changes.

• A flow sheet may be used to document routine assessment and care, including the length of time the bed rotation is stopped. The bed needs to be rotating at least 20 hours out of every 24 hours and stopped for no more than 30 minutes at a time.

Sample Documentation

0930 Transferred to a rotokinetic bed; proper skeletal alignment maintained during transfer. Skin dry and intact. An area of redness noted on sacrum 4 inches in diameter, and both heels are reddened. Initial rotation begun at 30 degrees without C/O nausea or dizziness. BP stable at 130/74.

Special Considerations

Pediatric Considerations

• Provide age-appropriate education for the child. It is important that the child understand that he or she is secure in the bed and will not fall out as the bed turns.

• Distraction, such as talking books, videos, and music help the older child adjust to the bed and the restricted mobility.

Geriatric Considerations

• Older adults are at increased risk for sensation of lightheadedness or dizziness.

SKILL 25.5 Using a Bariatric Bed

A morbidly obese client may benefit from a bariatric bed, which is capable of allowing upright or sitting positioning, client transport, and provides in-bed scales (Figure 25-12). The bed is capable of supporting weights up to 850 pounds, providing a stable, balanced surface. The nurse changes the bed position to move the client to reduce risk of staff injury. The in-bed scale provides the nurse with a means of obtaining accurate weights, which is frequently a problem with the obese client. The bed is slightly wider than a standard hospital bed, yet it fits through the standard door width.

A full or double-wide bariatric bed accommodates a client weighing up to 1000 pounds. However, when this bed is selected it must be assembled in the client's room and cannot be used for transfers because this bed cannot move through a standard hospital doorway.

A limitation of this bed is the lack of pressure reduction or relief feature. Provide some type of pressure relief mattress placed on the bariatric bed for the at-risk obese client.

Choices for pressure relief include static air or gel type of mattresses. Several manufacturers have low-air-loss mattress replacement systems for the bariatric bed. These beds have CPR switches, which permit immediate deflation to provide a hard surface for chest compressions.

ASSESSMENT

1 Determine client's need for bed based on height and weight. This bed may not be used for clients with spinal cord injury. *Rationale: A bariatric bed provides a safe surface. Standard hospital bed frames are not designed to support obese clients safely.*

2 Determine client's risk for pressure ulcer formation and the need for a pressure reduction surface, using a validated risk assessment tool such as the Braden scale (see Chapter 22). *Rationale: Risk assessment tools (e.g., Braden scale) provide an objective measure of risk consistent between evaluators over time (AHCPR, 1994). Assess risks by population: general population less than or*

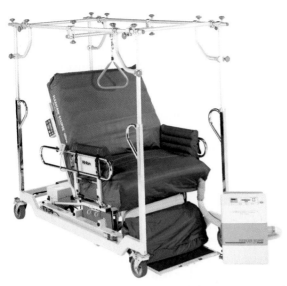

FIGURE 25-12 Bariatric bed with low-air-loss mattress replacement. (© 2006 Hill-Rom Services, Inc. Reprinted with permission. All rights reserved.)

equal to 16; ICU less than or equal to 15; older adult less than or equal to 18; and Black and Latino clients less than or equal to 18 (Bergstrom and others, 1998; Braden and Maklebust, 2005; Jiricka and others, 1995; Lyder and others, 1998).

3 Assess condition of skin. Note condition of skin between skinfolds. Note potential pressure sites. *Rationale: Determines need for client to have a low-air-loss or other pressure relieving surface on the bed.*

4 Assess client's and family members' understanding of purpose of bed.

5 Determine the frequency of routine weights. *Rationale: Scales are available in many bariatric beds or as underbed scales for beds without in-bed scales.*

6 Verify client's medical orders. *Rationale: A physician's order is required to obtain reimbursement in the United States.*

PLANNING

Expected Outcomes focus on safety, maximum independence, and maintaining skin integrity.
1 Client is able to reposition independently for comfort.
2 Client remains free of injury.
3 Client's skin remains intact without abnormal reactive hyperemia.

Delegation Considerations

After the nurse completes the assessment and determines the need for a specialty bed, the skill of placing the client on a bariatric bed may be delegated. Use of ceiling or heavy lifts is recommended. The number of people needed to assist in safe client transfer from traditional to bariatric bed must also be determined. Some types of specialty beds require that the manufacturer's representative set up and maintain the system. The nurse directs personnel by:

- Emphasing the need to notify the nurse of any changes in the client's skin or tissue
- Monitoring regular turning and repositioning of the client
- Reviewing specifics about applying, cleaning, and maintaining support surface
- Identifying number of staff needed to change client's position

Equipment

- Bariatric bed (see Figure 25-12)
- Pressure relief mattress overlay
- Sheets
- Overhead frame (optional)
- Heavy-duty lift (optional)
- Clean gloves (if contacting body fluids)

IMPLEMENTATION *for Using a Bariatric Bed*

STEPS	RATIONALE
1 See Standard Protocol (inside front cover).	
2 Explain steps of transfer.	Reduces anxiety and helps client be part of decision making during maneuvering.
3 Obtain assistance and use a heavy-duty lift.	Appropriate transfer techniques maintain alignment and reduce risk of injury to client and health care workers during procedure.
4 Place pullsheet, slide board, hydraulic lifts, or other assistive devices under the client, and transfer safely.	Reduces trauma from friction and shear to client's skin (Pieper, 2000).
5 Cover and position client, and place hand controls within reach. Be certain that the out-of-bed alarm is on, if needed. Attach overhead frame if needed.	Allows for maximal client independence. Alarm alerts caregiver that client has left the bed surface.
6 Encourage client to initiate frequent position changes and move in the bed as much as possible.	Morbidly obese clients quickly increase pressure over bony prominences. Frequent removal (e.g., every 30 to 60 minutes) of pressure from these points assists in reducing the risk for pressure ulcer formation.
7 See Completion Protocol (inside front cover).	

EVALUATION

1 Observe client's ability to move in bed.
2 Determine client's risk for injury.
3 Inspect condition of client's skin according to agency policy while client is on bed.

Unexpected Outcomes and Related Interventions

1 Client is unable to operate bed independently.
a. Assist client as needed.
b. Consult physician regarding physical therapy or occupational therapy evaluation to increase mobility or to provide facilitative devices.
2 Client develops areas of skin breakdown, or existing areas worsen.
a. Reevaluate need for support surface in use.
b. Evaluate turning schedule. May need to change or shift position more frequently than every 2 hours.

Recording and Reporting

- Record transfer of client to bed, subjective response, and condition of skin in nurses' notes or skin assessment flow sheet.
- Report changes in condition of skin.

Sample Documentation

1000 Transferred to bariatric bed. Demonstrated use of hand controls and trapeze bar. Skin dry, intact, and without erythema.

Special Considerations

Home Care Considerations

- Full-size bariatric beds (e.g., SIZEWise, Equitron) are available for rental or purchase.
- Persons of extreme obesity who are immobile need to alert their local emergency service personnel; ensures availability of adequate equipment and personnel.

NCLEX® Style Questions

1 An egg-crate mattress is appropriate for clients who:
   1. Have an existing pressure ulcer
   2. Are unable to move themselves
   3. Are immobilized with a spinal cord injury
   4. Have intact skin with risk for pressure ulcers
2 A client is at risk for dehydration and/or electrolyte imbalances when placed on which type of specialty bed?
   1. Air-suspension bed
   2. Air-fluidized bed
   3. Bariatric bed
   4. Rotokinetic bed
3 The nurse is caring for a client on a rotokinetic type bed. When the client complains of sudden dizziness; the nurse takes his blood pressure and notes that on lateral rotation the client develops orthostatic hypotension. What is the nurse's first action?
   1. Have the AP notify the doctor while you assess the client further.
   2. Stop the rotation of the bed and assess the client further.
   3. Assess for factors that make him hypotensive.
   4. Increase fluids and assess the client further.
4 A client is on an air-filled overlay on the mattress. The nurse notices skin breakdown over the coccyx and left hip in spite of meticulous skin care and routine repositioning. In addition, the client independently changes position when he feels pressure. What is the nurse's next action?
   1. Maintain the present mattress.
   2. Increase repositioning frequency.
   3. Check functioning and filling of mattress.
   4. Consider changing to a pressure relief device.
5 Which factor is not considered when determining the need to place a client on a bariatric bed?
   1. Client's ability to assist with transfer to the bed
   2. Availability of personnel to reposition client
   3. Ability of the environment to accommodate the bed
   4. Integrity of skin on pressure areas and in skinfold regions

References for all chapters appear in Appendix D.

Traction, Cast Care, and Immobilization Devices

26

MEDIA RESOURCES

- **evolve** http://evolve.elsevier.com/Elkin

Trauma or disease affecting the musculoskeletal system requires immobilization, stabilization, and support to the involved body part. Traction, casts, and immobilization devices are examples of methods used to accomplish these purposes to enhance the healing process.

Traction is prescribed for one or more of the following general uses: (1) correction of deformities, (2) gradual correction or improvement of a joint contracture, (3) treatment of a joint dislocation, (4) reduction, immobilization, and alignment of a fracture (Box 26-1), (5) prevention and management of muscle spasms, (6) prevention of further soft tissue damage, (7) preoperative and postoperative positioning and alignment, (8) maintenance of skeletal length and alignment, and (9) rest of a diseased joint (Schoen, 2000).

Traction involves a pulling force applied through weights to a part of the body while a second force, called countertraction, pulls in the opposite direction. Age, condition of the client, and purpose of the traction determine the amount of weight on the pulling force. A system of pulleys, ropes, and weights attached to the client provides this pulling force of traction. The client's body provides countertraction through the elevation of the foot or head of the bed. In straight or running traction, the traction force pulls against the long axis of the body while the client's body supplies the countertraction. In balanced traction, the amount of force in the traction is equal to the amount of force in the countertraction. A suspension is a mechanism that suspends a body part by using traction equipment, but it does not involve a pulling force. However, traction may be added to a suspension. In balanced-suspension traction, a sling or hammock and a system of weights attached to an over-bed frame support the affected part while weight is attached to the pin or wire traversing the bone.

Although there are many types of traction for different parts of the body, six general principles of traction care apply: (1) maintain the established line of pull, (2), maintain traction equipment, (3) maintain countertraction, (4) maintain continuous traction unless ordered otherwise, (5) maintain correct body alignment, and (6) prevent friction on the skin (Maher and others, 2002).

Two main types of traction are skin traction and skeletal traction. Skin traction noninvasively applies pull to an affected body structure by straps attached to the skin around the structure. Skel-

---

BOX 26-1 Types of Fractures

Closed fracture—skin intact over fracture
Open or compound fracture—skin punctured by bone ends
Comminuted—having three or more bone fragments
Compression—bone that is crushed (e.g., vertebra)
Depressed—bone fragments pushed inward
Displaced—two edges of fracture have moved out of alignment
Impacted—bone ends pushed into each other
Longitudinal—fracture runs parallel with bone
Oblique—fracture slants across bone
Pathologic—results from minor stress applied to pathologically weakened bone
Segmental—segment of bone fractured and detached
Spiral—around the bone
Transverse—across the bone

BOX 26-2 Assessment of Neurovascular Function (The Five P's)

Pain	Paresthesia
Pallor	Paralysis
Pulselessness	

---

etal traction is a type of traction applied by a physician under sterile conditions and used for treatment of fractures. It involves placement of a pin or wire through the bone. Weights are then attached to the device using ropes and pulleys. The entry through the skin provides a site for microorganisms to enter the soft tissues and bone. Meticulous skin care prevents the development of infection at these sites.

A second treatment method for immobilization involves the use of a cast. Applied externally, a cast immobilizes injured or deformed musculoskeletal tissues in proper position to promote healing. A cast prevents movement of injured tissues. Therefore correct application of the cast, with tissue structures in optimal position for healing, is imperative. An advantage of using a cast is that it permits early ambulation and in some cases partial-weight bearing.

A third treatment device used with musculoskeletal injury or disorder is the orthotic device. These devices immobilize a body part, prevent deformity, protect against injury, relieve pain and muscle spasm, maintain position until healing is complete, or assist with function. Immobilization devices are applied externally to the body. They are available in many variations ranging from arm slings to back braces and finger splints. They are made from a variety of materials such as rubber, leather, metal, and plastics.

Swelling from soft tissue trauma in the presence of a fracture creates pressure that affects circulation and neurological function. In addition, pressure exerted from tightly applied circumferential bandages, casts, or braces may result in neurovascular deficits. Cool skin temperature, pale skin color, diminished pulses, and increased capillary refill are evidence of decreased perfusion. Sensory complaints such as pain, numbness, tingling, and motor changes such as weakness or inability to move the extremity distal to the pressure may indicate a developing neurovascular problem (Box 26-2). Always promptly report development of compromised circulation to the physician.

EVIDENCE IN PRACTICE

Holmes SB, Brown SJ: Skeletal pin site care: National Association of Orthopaedic Nurses guidelines for orthopaedic nursing, *Orthop Nurs* 24(2):99-107, 2005.

Skeletal pin site care has been performed primarily based on tradition with very little research to support the practice. Holmes and Brown (2005) reviewed the research literature regarding skeletal pin site care and presented an analysis of the findings to a panel of five orthopedic experts for review. Four recommendations for skeletal pin site care were made. (1) Pins located in areas with considerable soft tissue are considered at greater risk for infection; (2) after the first 48 to 72 hours (when drainage may be heavy), pin site care should be done daily or weekly for sites with mechanically stable bone-pin interfaces; (3) chlorhexidine 2-mg/ml solution may be the most effective cleansing solution for pin site care; and (4) clients and/or their families should be taught pin site care before discharge from the hospital. Have clients demonstrate the care and provide them with written instructions that include signs and symptoms of infection.

NURSING DIAGNOSES

Nursing diagnoses for clients in immobilization devices focus on comfort and prevention of complications. **Acute pain** related to injury is appropriate when injury results in discomfort. **Anxiety** related to pain and/or immobility is appropriate when the immobilization results in muscle spasms or if it creates feelings of isolation, apprehension, and helplessness. **Bathing/hygiene self-care deficit, dressing/grooming self-care deficit,** and **toileting self-care deficit** are appropriate when the client is learning to adapt to limitations from impaired mobility; **risk for impaired skin integrity** and **impaired physical mobility** are appropriate if immobilization is maintained continuously for days to weeks. **Risk for peripheral neurovascular dysfunction** is appropriate when there is soft tissue swelling and/or the devices themselves put pressure on tissues. **Risk for infection** applies to clients with pin sites for the skeletal traction, external fixation, or halo traction or for clients with open wounds. **Impaired home maintenance** is necessary for the client going home with a cast or immobilization device. **Deficient knowledge** applies for clients who require information about care of a cast or immobilization device or cast removal.

SKILL 26.1 Care of the Client in Skin Traction

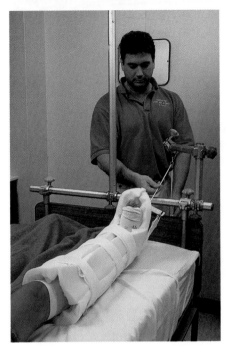

FIGURE 26-1 Buck's extension.

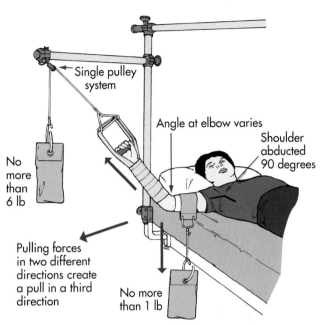

FIGURE 26-2 Dunlop's traction. (From Folcik MA, Carini-Garcia G, Birmingham JJ: *Traction: assessment and management,* St Louis, 1994, Mosby.)

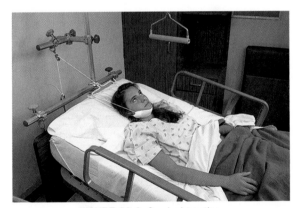

FIGURE 26-3 Cervical traction.

Skin traction is the application of a pulling force directly to the skin and soft tissue that indirectly pulls on the skeletal system. Skin traction immobilizes a fracture and relieves muscle spasms and pain; continuous application is required to achieve that goal. Skin traction usually provides temporary immobilization until the fracture can be surgically repaired by open reduction and internal fixation (ORIF) or skeletal traction can be implemented. Furthermore, skin traction maintains alignment and reduces contractures and dislocations. Clients need written physician orders for specific traction weights, bed position, and turning regimen.

There are several types of skin traction. The most common type of adult skin traction is Buck's extension. It is applied to one or both legs using straps or a commercially prepared foam boot with Velcro straps (Figure 26-1). Dunlop's traction is another form of skin traction. Dunlop's traction is applied to the forearm to treat fractures of the humerus (Figure 26-2).

Cervical traction using a head halter involves a halter with a cutout for the ears and face (Figure 26-3). The halter cradles the chin and has straps leading to a bar attached to ropes, pulleys, and weights. Cervical traction immobilizes arthritic conditions of the cervical vertebrae, not fractures. It can be removed periodically.

Bryant's traction is occasionally used to immobilize infants with congenital hip dislocation and fractures of the femur for children weighing less than 40 pounds (Figure 26-4). Traction to both legs maintains immobilization in a vertical position for 7 to 10 days followed by a spica cast.

Pelvic traction for low back pain is rarely used anymore. A pelvic sling for an open-book fracture of the symphysis pubis is occasionally used.

The more weight applied to the traction, the greater the chance of skin breakdown. No more than 7 pounds is used for Buck's extension traction. Cervical traction may use 7 to 10 pounds. Skin problems such as ulcers, dermatitis, burns, or abrasions prevent the use of skin traction because of the

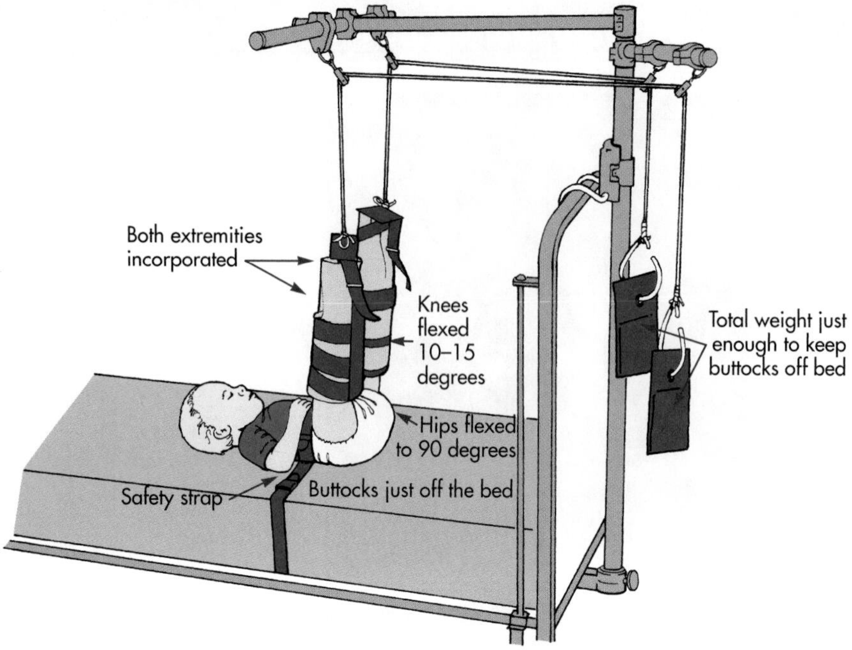

FIGURE 26-4 Bryant's traction. (From Folcik MA, Carini-Garcia G, Birmingham JJ: *Traction: assessment and management,* St Louis, 1994, Mosby.)

Both extremities incorporated

Knees flexed 10–15 degrees

Total weight just enough to keep buttocks off bed

Hips flexed to 90 degrees

Safety strap

Buttocks just off the bed

BOX 26-3 Traction Assessment (The Four *P's*)
Pounds: Is the correct weight in place and hanging freely? *Pull:* Is the direction of pull aligned with the long axis of the bone? *Pulleys:* Is the rope riding over the pulley and gliding smoothly? *Pressure:* Is each clamp and connection tight?

danger of exacerbation. Older clients and clients with diabetes are at increased risk of skin breakdown.

When caring for a client in traction, initially and regularly monitor clients for correct maintenance of the traction device. Hospital policy may specify a frequency of checks, which needs to be at least every 4 to 8 hours. Traction maintenance involves monitoring the weights, the direction of pull, the ropes and pulleys, and all connections (Box 26-3).

ASSESSMENT

1 Assess client's knowledge of the reason for traction. *Rationale: Determines concerns, fears, and need for further teaching.*
2 Assess integrity and condition of skin prior to traction application. *Rationale: Establishes baseline for skin integrity. Intact skin and local tissue have increased ability to tolerate traction's pulling forces.*
3 Assess client's overall health condition, including degree of mobility, ability to perform activities of daily living (ADLs), and current medical conditions. *Rationale: Determines client's ability to tolerate traction, self-care ability, and anticipated need for assistance.*
4 Assess client's position in bed: supine, perpendicular to the ends of the bed, with the affected limb in proper body alignment.

5 Assess client's level of pain using a scale of 0 to 10 and determine need for analgesics before procedure begins. *Rationale: Analgesics decrease client's discomfort while skin traction is being applied, and assessment also serves as the baseline for later comparison.*
6 Assess neurovascular status of extremity distal to the traction, including skin color, temperature, capillary refill, presence of distal pulses, sensation, and client's ability to move digits. *Rationale: Provides necessary baseline information for early detection of neurovascular deficit.*

PLANNING

Expected Outcomes focus on client's mental status, skin integrity, ADLs, comfort level, neurovascular status, and mobility.

1 Client will experience reduced anxiety levels as evidenced by a decrease in symptoms of apprehension, irritability, and/or helplessness.
2 Skin under traction boot or elastic wrap remains intact, without redness or breakdown.
3 Client will participate in ADLs as much as possible within limitations.
4 Client will verbalize an increased sense of comfort with a rating of 3 or lower on a scale of 0 to 10 after repositioning and administration of analgesics.
5 Client will be free of neurovascular deficit following application of circumferential dressing or boot.
6 Client will move all extremities independently by date of discharge.

Delegation Considerations

Neurovascular assessment of the client's condition cannot be delegated. The skill of assisting with application of skin traction may be delegated to assistive personnel (AP) who have had specific training. The nurse directs personnel by:

- Explaining how to adapt skill for specific client.
- Instructing personnel to inform the nurse if client demonstrates any change in skin condition or complains of discomfort.

Equipment for Buck's Extension

- Overhead frame for attachment of traction
- Traction bar
- Cross clamp and pulley
- Rope
- Buck's traction boot or moleskin and elastic bandages
- 1- to 5-pound weights
- Spreader bar

IMPLEMENTATION *for Care of the Client in Skin Traction*

STEPS	RATIONALE
1 See Standard Protocol (inside front cover).	
2 Administer analgesic for acute pain and muscle relaxant for spasms in advance of traction application.	Allows drugs to reach peak effect at time of traction application, thereby reducing pain and resultant muscle spasm. Analgesics do not effectively reduce muscle spasm pain.
3 Position client supine and nearly flat with no more than 30 degrees' elevation, with the affected leg halfway between the edge of the bed and middle of the bed.	

COMMUNICATION TIP Tell the client, "I will hold your extremity using slight tension." This will minimize any discomfort as traction is applied.

4 Wash affected leg (or legs) gently and pat dry. Do not shave legs.	Shaving may create micro nicks that could become inflamed under traction straps.

NURSE ALERT Do not place skin traction over irritated, damaged, or broken skin.

5 Apply foam boot, moleskin, or elastic bandages to affected leg, proceeding from distal to proximal.	Application distal to proximal prevents trapping of blood and promotes venous return (Maher and others, 2002).
a. Ensure that boot fits snugly.	Too tight leads to pressure to skin, peroneal nerve, and vasculature structures. Too loose leads to slipping and lack of traction force.
b. Seat heel properly in traction boot. Do not pad at heel.	Prevents pressure over heel.
c. Do not apply traction boot over sequential pneumatic compression devices. Instead use foot pumps.	Causes undue pressure on tissues and negates effects of compression device (Maher and others, 2002).

NURSE ALERT Skin traction that is too tight puts pressure on nerves and vascular structures that could result in an irreversible neurovascular deficit. Skin traction that is too loose will slip.

6 Attach weight to boot gradually and gently at the end of the bed. Physician determines exact amount of weight to be applied and position to be maintained.	Traction is slowly established to avoid involuntary muscle spasms or pain for client. Weight should create enough pull to overcome muscle spasms but does not cause marked increase in pain.

NURSE ALERT When applying Buck's extension, avoid pressure to the peroneal nerve at the neck of the fibula. Decreased sensation in the web space between the great toe and second toe, as well as inability to dorsiflex the foot and extend the toes, may indicate pressure to the nerve. Be alert to pressure over bony prominences about the ankle or the back of the heel.

STEPS	RATIONALE
7 Inspect traction setup: knots secure; ropes in pulleys and not frayed; weights hanging freely, not caught on bed or resting on floor; and bedclothes not interfering with traction apparatus. Check the four *P*'s of traction maintenance (see Box 26-3).	Routine observation of these checkpoints is necessary to maintain appropriate amount of tension and effective immobilization.
8 Before physician leaves, assess client's position and ask about additional permissible positions for client and bed. Client is primarily on back; may be allowed to turn to unaffected side for brief periods (10 to 15 minutes).	Positioning on side permits back care and relief of pressure to tissues.
9 Reassess neurovascular status of extremity distal to the traction, including skin color and temperature, capillary refill, presence of distal pulses, sensation, and client's ability to move digits.	Altered circulation, sensation, or motion indicate potential problems that can result in permanent neurovascular damage.

> **NURSE ALERT** If tissues distal to skin traction are cold or cool or if capillary refill is greater than 3 seconds, compare with unaffected extremity. If deficit is related to traction, wrap extremity, remove traction, and report neurovascular compromise.

10 Release and reapply traction boot every 4 to 8 hours and provide skin care according to physician's orders.

11 See Completion Protocol (inside front cover).

EVALUATION

1 Evaluate client's anxiety level for symptoms of apprehension, irritability, and/or helplessness.

2 Inspect skin tissues for signs of pressure, color changes, edema, or tenderness.

3 Evaluate client's ability to perform ADLs.

4 Ask client to rate discomfort on a scale of 0 to 10 and to report muscle spasms.

5 Evaluate neurovascular status every 30 minutes × 2, every 2 hrs for 24 hours, and then every 4 hrs thereafter (see agency policy).

6 Observe client's use of trapeze and unaffected limbs to reposition self correctly.

Unexpected Outcomes and Related Interventions

1 Client complains of increased pain after traction is applied.

a. Take the traction off (if allowed by physician), reposition client, and then reapply the traction. If not allowed, loosen traction slightly and reassess neurovascular status.

b. Administer analgesics as prescribed.

c. Realign body and/or limb.

d. If increased pain continues or pain occurs on passive motion, notify physician of possible neurovascular deficit.

2 Client has reddened areas on leg or heel under Buck's traction boot.

a. Obtain physician order to remove foam boot for 1 hour to relieve pressure.

b. Apply foam boot securely (you should be able to insert one finger between client's skin and Buck's traction boot). Recheck correct tightness frequently.

c. Increase frequency of skin checks to every hour.

d. Apply protective barrier agent (e.g., Aloe Vista or Sween cream) to affected limb for protection against skin breakdown.

e. Ensure that heels do not rest on bed or pillow.

Recording and Reporting

- Record assessment of skin integrity beneath traction, nursing interventions, and length of time client is in or out of specific traction in nurses notes.
- Record neurovascular assessments on flow sheet or nurses' notes.
- Report any neurovascular deficits to physician immediately.

Sample Documentation

0900 Buck's traction boot applied to client's left leg and attached to a 5-pound weight. No C/O pain, tingling, or numbness. Capillary refill 3 seconds in nail beds of toes bilaterally; able to wiggle toes; skin warm, dry, and pink to lower left leg. Side rails up, bed down, weights hanging freely. Knots tied, rope in pulley. In supine position with left leg in proper alignment.

1100 Assessed for comfort. States he is "hurting a lot"—reports an 8 on a 0 to 10 scale. Medicated with 5 mg morphine sulfate IV push. Buck's boot removed. Skin assessed, and no breakdown evident. Buck's reapplied. Client repositioned. No skin breakdown noted to heel, malleolus, coccyx, or back.

1200 Verbalized that pain medication helped and that pain is a 2 and reports feeling relaxed and comfortable.

Special Considerations

Pediatric Considerations

- Babies and young children are unable to remain still and in alignment.
- Bryant's traction is rarely used in children because of the risk for altered peripheral perfusion. Gravitational forces and circumferential wraps increase the risk for vasospasm and avascular necrosis (Hockenberry and Wilson, 2007).
- Do not remove Bryant's traction for sleep. Loosen the elastic wraps only when there is marked edema of feet.

Geriatric Considerations

- Older clients may have keratoses, rashes, or other lesions that could become irritated in skin traction.

- Older clients may have long-standing conditions of musculoskeletal tissues such as arthritis or gout that could lead to inflamed tissues and skin breakdown.
- Older and chronically ill clients may have increased need for position changes as a result of limitations from osteoporosis, osteomalacia, weakened muscles, or increased risk of skin breakdown.
- Older clients' skin heals more slowly and is more fragile, less elastic, and thinner than when they were younger (Stanley, Blair, and Beare, 2005). Use of alternating air pressure mattresses or foam overlays decreases the risk of impaired skin integrity (see Chapter 25).

Home Care Considerations

- If client is to be discharged to home, instruct relatives or caregivers in care needs (including home traction) and mode of ambulation.
- Teach family how to maintain integrity of traction by inspecting daily: weights hang freely, traction ropes rest in groove of pulley and hang freely, not caught on bed or resting on floor.

SKILL 26.2   Care of the Client in Skeletal Traction and Pin Site Care

Skeletal traction immobilizes fractures of the femur below the trochanter, fractures of the cervical spine, and some fractures of the bones of the arm or ankle. It also immobilizes the head of the femur in the case of acetabular fractures. Slow healing requires longer periods of traction (6 to 8 weeks) to promote bone repair. Skeletal traction is used less frequently as a result of new surgical repair procedures.

Skeletal traction involves puncturing the skin at the site where the pin enters and exits. In the case of external fixation or halo traction, the device attaches to the bone through the skin. Skeletal traction immobilizes clients for weeks or sometimes months until healing occurs. Prolonged immobilization influences nursing care, which focuses on supporting ADLs, maintaining traction, and preventing fat emboli and complications of immobility such as skin breakdown and pulmonary emboli.

A common form of skeletal traction is balanced-suspension skeletal traction (BSST), usually used for a fractured femur (Figure 26-5). BSST relieves muscle spasms, realigns the fracture fragments, and promotes callus formation. Callus formation is the development of new supportive bone around the injured site. BSST temporarily stabilizes the client's condition while waiting for surgical insertion of an internal fixation device such as a plate, screw, or nail. Balanced suspension involves a sling attached to splints around the leg and a Steinmann pin or Kirschner wire supplying the traction (Figure 26-6). Sufficient weight to overcome the quadriceps and hamstring muscle spasms may be 30 to 40 pounds.

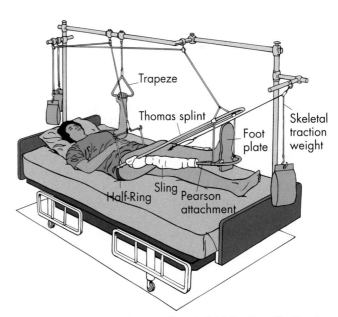

FIGURE 26-5 Balanced-suspension skeletal traction. Traction in long axis of right thigh is applied by means of Kirschner wire through proximal portion of tibia. Limb is supported by Thomas splint beneath thigh and Pearson attachment beneath leg. Footplate attachment prevents footdrop. Weights apply countertraction to upper end of Thomas splint and suspend its lower end. By using the left arm and leg as shown, client can shift position of the hips without change in amount of traction.

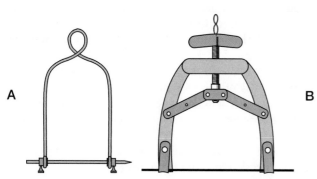

FIGURE 26-6 A, Kirschner wire and tractor. **B,** Steinmann pin and holder.

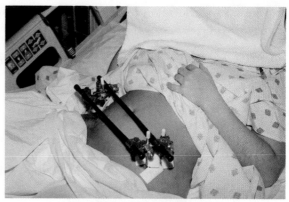

FIGURE 26-7 Pelvic AO fixator.

Other common forms of skeletal traction are sidearm traction (with a pin drilled through the lower humerus, external fixation (used for comminuted fractures with soft tissue injury, skull and facial fractures, and pelvic bones [Figure 26-7]). For cervical spine fractures, Crutchfield or Gardner-Wells tongs are inserted into the skull. Halo traction is frequently used for neurologically intact clients, stabilizing the spinal vertebra and preventing further injury to the spinal cord (Figure 26-8).

External fixation is a form of skeletal traction that consists of a frame or apparatus to hold pins placed into or through bones above and below a fracture site. External fixation devices promote early ambulation and use of other joints while maintaining immobilization of affected bones. A variety of external fixation frames are used for skull and facial fractures, ribs, bones of the extremities, and pelvic bones.

All skeletal traction involves placement of a device through the skin, called a *pin site*. Pin site care is believed to reduce the risk for pin tract infections. Procedures for pin site care must be kept current with evidence-based guidelines. Some institutions have policies outlining pin site care, such as cleanse site with Betadine swab every 4 hours. However, chlorhexidine 2-mg/ml solution has been identified as possibly being the most effective cleansing solution for pin site care (Holmes and Brown, 2005). Some agencies require specific physician's orders to specify frequency of pin site care and cleansing agent to use. Skeletal pin site care guidelines have been established by a panel of experts and published by the National Association of Orthopaedic Nurses (see Evidence in Practice, p. 572).

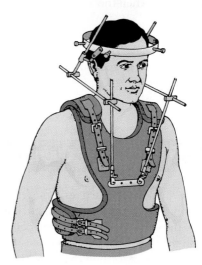

FIGURE 26-8 Halo vest. (Redrawn from Beare PG, Myers JL: *Principles and practice of adult health nursing,* ed 3, St Louis, 1998, Mosby.)

ASSESSMENT

1 Assess client's knowledge of the reason for traction, including nonverbal behavior and responses. *Rationale: Determines concerns, anxiety, and need for further teaching.*

2 Inspect integrity and condition of skin over bony prominences (e.g., use Braden scale to assess risk for pressure ulcers) and under devices in use. Consider need for spe-

cial bed or mattress (see Chapter 25). *Rationale: Provides baseline status of dependent tissues at risk for pressure ulcer formation.*

3 Assess client's degree of mobility, ability to perform ADLs, and current medical conditions. *Rationale: Determines client's health state and serves as baseline for further reference.*

4 Assess client's level of pain using a scale of 0 to 10 and determine the need for analgesics before procedure begins. *Rationale: Decreases client's discomfort while applying traction and serves as baseline for later comparison.*

5 Following application, assess traction setup: weights hanging freely, ordered amount of weight applied, ropes moving freely through pulleys, all knots tight in ropes and away from pulleys. *Rationale: Ensures accurate function of traction.*

6 Assess neurovascular status of extremity distal to the traction, including skin color, temperature, capillary refill, presence of distal pulses, sensation, and client's ability to move digits. *Rationale: Provides necessary baseline information and detects neurovascular deficits.*

7 Assess client's ability to reposition and participate in ADLs. *Rationale: Determines client's ability to change position and reduce risks for hazards of immoblity.*

8 Following application, assess pin sites for redness, edema, discharge, or odor. *Rationale: Identifies signs and symptoms associated with infection.*

9 Assess respiratory rate, rhythm, depth, and chest expansion. *Rationale: Pulmonary embolus can occur in the client who has associated spinal cord injury or who is on prolonged bed rest. Fat embolus syndrome (FES) can occur with long bone fracture. Halo vests are not recommended for clients with respiratory insufficiency because of the restricted chest expansion.*

PLANNING

Expected Outcomes focus on client's anxiety level, skin integrity, self-care abilities, comfort and mobility level, neurovascular status, infection risks, and pulmonary status.

1 Skeletal deformity is reduced, alignment is maintained, and injury is healed.

2 Client verbalizes decreased anxiety, irritability, and/or helplessness.

3 Skin over bony prominences or under halo vest remains intact, without redness or breakdown.

4 Client performs ADLs independently to all unaffected areas.

5 Client verbalizes a sense of comfort (3 or below on a scale of 0 to 10) after repositioning and administration of analgesics.

6 Client is free of neurovascular deficit following application of traction.

7 Skin around pin sites remains free of redness, swelling, or drainage.

Delegation Considerations

Skeletal traction is applied by the physician. The skill of assisting with insertion of skeletal pins and pin site care may be delegated to AP who are adequately trained in principles of surgical asepsis. Assessment for complications, including infection or inflammation at pin insertion site, may not be delegated.

Equipment
Balanced-suspension Skeletal Traction (see Figure 26-5)
- Ropes, pulleys, weights, weight holders
- Thomas splint
- Pearson attachment with sheepskin padding
- Footplate
- Trapeze

Halo Traction (see Figure 26-8)
- Halo ring with four pins
- Molded vest jacket
- Vertical metal bars connecting ring to jacket
- Tracheostomy tray (for emergency resuscitation)
- Allen wrench (allows removal of screws for resuscitation)

Pin Site Care Supplies
- Sterile cotton-tipped applicators
- Prescribed cleansing agent. Preferred agent is chlorhexidine 2 mg/ml solution. Sterile normal saline solution or Betadine solution may be used (check agency policy).
- Antiseptic ointment
- Split 2 × 2 dressings
- Clean gloves

IMPLEMENTATION *for Care of the Client in Skeletal Traction and Pin Site Care*

STEPS	RATIONALE
1 See Standard Protocol (inside front cover).	
2 Initial traction setup	Ensures proper alignment during and after traction application. Movement can cause severe pain or additional trauma.
a. Position client per physician direction. Support limb to be placed in traction. Do not move distal portion unnecessarily. Client will likely be placed in supine position with head of bed slightly elevated.	
b. Physician cleans skin over pin site and injects local anesthetic.	Anesthetic desensitizes area where pin site will be made. Client will feel pressure during drilling but should feel no pain.
c. Talk with client during the drilling procedure.	Distraction reduces client anxiety.
d. Attach weights and gently lower.	
3 Inspect traction setup: knots secure; ropes in pulleys; footplate in place; weights hanging freely, not caught on bed or resting on floor; and bedclothes not interfering with traction apparatus (see Box 26-3).	Routine observation of these checkpoints is necessary to maintain appropriate amount of tension and effective immobilization. Footplate prevents footdrop.

STEPS	RATIONALE

> **NURSE ALERT** Irreversible tissue death from ischemia occurs within 4 to 12 hours.

4 Reassess neurovascular status of distal aspects of involved extremities in comparison with corresponding body part.

  a. Inspect color and temperature.

Pink, warm tissues are adequately oxygenated. Whitish tissue indicates decreased arterial supply, and bluish color signifies venous stasis.

  b. Observe for edema.

May result from tissue trauma or venous stasis.

  c. Assess capillary refill by pressing on toe or fingernail, releasing, and noting "pinking" on nail within 3 seconds.

Normal refill indicates good perfusion.

5 Provide pin site care according to hospital policy or physician's orders.

  a. Remove gauze dressings from around pins and discard in receptacle. Remove and discard gloves.

  b. Inspect sites for drainage or inflammation.

Signs indicative of infection.

  c. Prepare supplies.

  d. Clean each pin site with prescribed solution by placing moistened sterile applicator close to the pin and cleaning away from the insertion site. Dispose of applicator.

> **NURSE ALERT** Touching one pin site with material used on another increases risk of transmission of microorganisms.

  e. Repeat the process for each pin site.

  f. Using a sterile applicator, apply a small amount of topical antibiotic ointment to pin site if this is the physician's orders or hospital policy.

Reduces development of infection.

  g. Cover with a sterile 2 × 2 split gauze dressing or leave site open to air as prescribed or according to hospital policy. Remove and discard gloves and perform hand hygiene.

6 Inspect skin (bony prominences, heels, elbows, sacrum, and areas under appliances) for signs of pressure, and lightly massage pressure areas every 2 hours unless evidence of beginning skin breakdown is evident (tenderness, reactive hyperemia).

Light massage increases circulation to area. Firm massage to compromised tissues increases tissue breakdown.

7 Provide nonpharmacological and pharmacological pain relief as indicated (see Chapter 10).

Pain may result from the traumatic injury and muscle spasms.

> **NURSE ALERT** Never ignore a client's complaint. Follow through and check it out.

8 Encourage the use of unaffected extremities for ADLs and active and passive exercises (see Chapter 6). Encourage use of trapeze bar for repositioning in bed.

Prevents muscle atrophy and maintains muscle tone for later ambulation.

9 For elimination provide a fracture pan (see Chapter 9).

Smaller bedpan is more comfortable for the client and easier to place under client.

10 See Completion Protocol (inside front cover).

EVALUATION

1 Inspect body part that is in traction for alignment.
2 Determine client's anxiety level in response to traction and immobilization.
3 Inspect skin overlying dependent areas and around the site for evidence of breakdown.
4 Ask client to rate participation in ADLs and use of unaffected extremities.
5 Have client rate level of pain and discomfort from muscle spasms.
6 Monitor neurovascular status and peripheral tissue perfusion every 2 hours for the first 24 hours and every 4 to 12 hours thereafter (see agency policy).
7 Monitor respiratory status for fat embolism syndrome, atelectasis, and pulmonary embolism every shift (see Chapter 12).
8 Observe for local and systemic indications of infection, including drainage and inflammation at pin sites, fever, elevated white blood cell count, continuous dull aching pain, redness, or warmth in extremity (possible osteomyelitis [i.e., bone infection]).

Unexpected Outcomes and Related Interventions

1 Client has severe edema, marked increase in pain, or inability to actively move joint or increased pain on passive movement, indicating compartment syndrome.
a. Prompt management is critical. Consult with physician.
b. Elevate extremity.
c. Reduce or eliminate compression caused by therapeutic devices.
2 Redness, increased swelling, and drainage develop at pin site(s) or fracture site (osteomyelitis).
a. Cultures of drainage may be indicated to identify infecting organism. (Physician's order is not usually required; see agency policy) (see Chapter 13).
b. Consult with physician for antibiotic orders.
3 Signs of osteomyelitis or systemic infection develop, including fever, elevated white blood cell count, general malaise. This is especially a concern with open fractures and extensive soft tissue injury.
a. Consult with physician. Orders may include irrigation of the site with antibiotic solution and/or intravenous (IV) antibiotics.
b. Encourage fluid intake and provide comfort measures for fever.
4 Evidence of nerve damage develops from pressure or trauma to nerves, depending on type of traction in place. For example, peroneal nerve: footdrop may develop with inability to evert and dorsiflex foot; radial or median nerve at wrist: inability to approximate thumb and fingers (radial) and numbness and tingling of thumb, index, middle fingers (medial) with wrist drop.
a. Eliminate pressure if possible according to type of traction in place.
b. Notify physician.

5 Client experiences FES (more common in fractures of pelvic and long bones) with symptoms of hypoxia, restlessness, mental changes, tachycardia, tachypnea, dyspnea, low blood pressure, and occasionally petechial rash over upper chest and neck.
a. This is a life-threatening emergency—50% of persons with fat emboli die.
b. Notify physician and initiate major resuscitation efforts.

Recording and Reporting

• Record in nurses' notes type of traction, site to which traction is applied, amount of weights, and client's response.
• Record on flow sheet specific routine assessments and frequency of assessment.

Sample Documentation

0700 BSST in place with 20-pound weight to left femur. Knots secure, ropes in pulleys, weights hanging freely. Neurovascular assessment to left foot—color pink, temperature warm, no numbness or tingling, wiggles toes on command, capillary refill 2 seconds. Reports pain at 2 on scale of 0 to 10. Lateral pin site dry, medial pin site draining small amount clear fluid (¼-inch diameter circle). No odor. No redness.

0900 Medial pin site drainage changed to yellow drainage (½-inch diameter circle). Pin site cultured. Reports pain of 6 on 0 to 10 scale. Dr. Breland notified of pin site drainage.

0915 Tylenol No. 3 tabs 2 administered PO. Medial and lateral pin sites cleansed with chlorhexidine 2-mg/ml solution, triple antibiotic applied, and split dressings applied. IV antibiotic started per order.

1000 Reports pain decreased to a 2. No drainage visible on medial or lateral pin site split dressing.

Special Considerations
Pediatric Considerations

• Blood loss from a fracture in a child poses a greater danger because the blood volume in a child is 70% to 85% of total body weight and only about 60% in the adult (Hockenberry and Wilson, 2007).
• Caregivers and parents work together to develop strategies to combat boredom of child in traction. Counseling regarding possibility of regressive type behaviors lessens the parents' anxiety. Interference with schoolwork is remedied by obtaining work from school as soon as the child is able to perform tasks.
• Assure children that someone will be there to assist them while they are in traction.

Geriatric Considerations

• Older clients are particularly prone to the development of altered skin integrity when they are immobilized and not repositioned frequently. This tendency results from a decreased amount of subcutaneous fat and skin that is less elastic, thinner, drier, and more fragile than that of a younger adult.

- Older clients may have long-standing conditions of musculoskeletal tissues such as arthritis or gout that could lead to inflamed tissues and skin breakdown.
- Older and chronically ill clients have increased need for position changes to prevent the complications of immobility and those resulting from limitations imposed by osteoporosis, osteomalacia, or weakened muscles. Severe varicose veins will prevent the use of skin traction in the older client because of the risk of skin breakdown.

Home Care Considerations

- Following removal of skeletal traction, teach client to ambulate slowly within medical guidelines, gradually increasing length of time out of bed and distance walked.

- Teach client to notify physician of undesirable signs such as marked increase in pain, muscle spasms, and increased numbness, indicating reinjury or insufficient healing.
- Teach family members to apply skin traction correctly if it is prescribed for home use following the removal of the skeletal traction.
- Teach client and family members the use of muscle relaxants and analgesics if prescribed for home use.

Long-Term Care Considerations

- Instruct clients in home safety methods to prevent further injuries.
- Instruct clients in dosage of vitamin D and the minimum amount of calcium needed in diet to promote strong bones.

SKILL 26.3 Care of the Client During Cast Application

A cast immobilizes an injured extremity to protect it from further injury, provides alignment of a fracture by holding the bone fragments in reduction and alignment during the healing process, and promotes comfort. In addition, it maintains a limb in alignment to prevent or correct structural abnormalities. Casts are used in many different ways (Figure 26-9). The use and type of application materials required depend on the anatomical area of injury.

Casts are made of one of two types of materials, plaster of Paris or synthetic material. The type of cast material selected depends on the number of cast changes anticipated and the type of musculoskeletal injury. Plaster of Paris is composed of open-weave cotton roll or strip covered with calcium sulfate crystals. When moistened with water, this material molds easily during application, but drying may require (1) 24 hours for a regular arm cast, (2) up to 48 hours before weight bearing or external pressure can be applied, and (3) 36 to 72 hours for large body casts (Schoen, 2000). During drying, the cast must be exposed to air to dry, be well supported on firm surfaces, handled with palms (not fingertips) to avoid indentations such as fingerprints, and turned regularly so that it will dry evenly. Lifting the cast by supporting the joints above and below the casted area prevents injury to underlying soft tissues. This type of cast is heavier than a synthetic cast.

Synthetic casting materials are composed of open-weave fiberglass tape covered with a polyurethane resin that is activated by water. This cast sets very quickly, in approximately 15 minutes, and can withstand pressure or weight bearing after 20 minutes (Table 26-1). It forms a lightweight, sturdy cast that is both radiolucent and waterproof. Different colors of this casting material are also available, ranging from fluorescent pink and green to navy blue and purple. Colors are often more appealing to children and aid

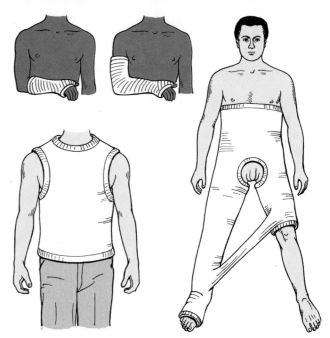

FIGURE 26-9 Types of casts. *Top left, short arm cast; top center,* long arm cast; *bottom left,* plaster body jacket cast; *far right,* one and one-half hip spica cast.

in maintaining the appearance of the cast (Figure 26-10). These casts are more expensive than plaster casts.

This skill includes assessment parameters before, during, and after cast application, including peripheral neurovascular status. Assisting with the application of the cast is also discussed. It is important to follow guidelines for care after application with respect to pressure against cast and weight bearing.

TABLE 26-1   Comparison of Casting Materials

	PLASTER OF PARIS	SYNTHETIC
Indications	Unstable or displaced fractures, edema, frequent cast changes	Stable fractures, long-term cast, clients who may abuse cast
Drying time	24-72 hours, depending on size of cast	7-15 minutes; can bear weight after 20 minutes
Drying method	Air dry	Air dry
Radiolucent	Minimal	Yes
Weight of cast	Heavy	Lightweight
Durability	May crumble and flake	Very sturdy
Bathing/immersibility	Must be kept dry	Can be immersed, as in swimming and bathing; must be thoroughly dried after exposure to water
Cleaning cast	Prevention of soiling is best approach. May use damp cloth and mild cleanser for slight soiling (do not wet cast)	May cleanse with warm water. Thoroughly dry after cleaning.
Choice of colors	No	Yes
Surface area	Smooth	Rough
Molding	Easy	Limited
Special equipment	None	May need special cast saw for cast removal
Padding	Cotton sheet wadding or Webril, stockinette	Nonabsorbent nylon stockinette and padding
Cost	Inexpensive	Expensive
Strength	Strong	Stronger than plaster of Paris

Data from Schoen DC: *Adult orthopaedic nursing*, Philadelphia, 2000, Lippincott.

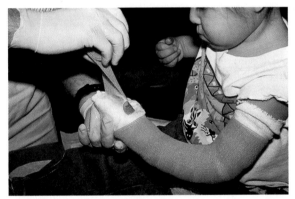

FIGURE 26-10 Synthetic casting materials are available in different colors that are appealing to children.

ASSESSMENT

1 Assess factors that may affect wound healing, such as diabetes, poor nutritional status, or steroid medication use. *Rationale: When there is a risk of slower healing, additional nutritional supplements may be required.*

2 Assess client's ability to cooperate and level of understanding concerning the casting procedure. *Rationale: Sudden movement during procedure could cause injury.*

3 Inspect condition of the skin that will be under the cast. Specifically note any areas of skin breakdown, rashes present, or incisional wound. *Rationale: Provides baseline for skin condition.*

4 Assess neurovascular status of the area to be casted (see Box 26-2). Specifically note presence or absence of motor and sensory function, skin color, temperature, and capillary refill. Compare with opposite extremity or surrounding tissues. Pay particular attention to tissues distal to cast. *Rationale: Changes in neurovascular status may occur after casting, possibly further compromising already injured tissues. It is important to note the baseline neurovascular status so that these changes, if they occur, can be accurately assessed.*

5 Assess client's pain status using a scale of 0 to 10.

6 Consult with physician to determine the extent to which client will be able to use the casted body part. *Rationale: Determines extent to which self-care will be impaired.*

PLANNING

Expected Outcomes focus on skin integrity, comfort, self-care, mobility, prevention of neurovascular complications, and maintenance of cast integrity.

1 Client's exposed skin distal to cast is warm and pink, with capillary refill less than 3 seconds.

2 Client exhibits no elevated temperature or other signs of infection.

3 Pulses distal to the cast are palpable, strong, and regular.

4 Cast remains clean, without indentations or fraying, until removal.

5 Client has edema of 1+ or less and demonstrates less than 25% decrease in active range of motion (ROM) of affected extremity after cast application.

6 Client verbalizes pain of 3 or less (scale of 0 to 10) after analgesic administration 20 to 30 minutes before the procedure.

7 Client requires minimal assistance with ADLs after an extremity is casted.

8 Client describes the steps of proper cast care.

Delegation Considerations

A complete assessment of the client before cast applications may not be delegated; however, the skill of assisting with cast application may be delegated. The nurse directs personnel by:

- Explaining the method to assist in positioning for specific client with mobility restrictions.

Equipment (may be on cast cart)
(Figure 26-11)

- Plaster cast
- Plaster rolls: 2, 3, 4, or 6 inch
- Padding material (felt, sheet wadding, Webril, stockinette, or gore lining)
- Clean gloves, apron, or protective cover
- Plastic-lined bucket or basin
- Water warmed at time of application
- Cart, chair, and fracture table scissors
- Paper or plastic sheets
- Synthetic cast

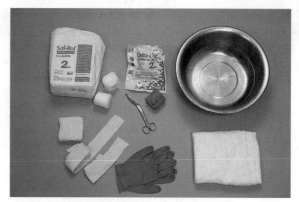

FIGURE 26-11 Casting materials.

- Synthetic rolls: 2, 3, or 4 inch
- Pail with water to dampen rolls
- Padding materials (nylon stockinette and synthetic padding)
- Cast cutter (to trim edge of cast, if needed)

IMPLEMENTATION *for Care of the Client During Cast Application*

STEPS	RATIONALE
1 See Standard Protocol (inside front cover).	
2 Administer analgesic before cast application: oral (PO), 30 to 40 minutes before; intramuscular (IM), 20 to 30 minutes before; IV, 2 to 5 minutes before.	Reduces pain during cast application. Provides optimal analgesic effect.
3 Use latex-free gloves if there is risk of an allergic reaction.	Synthetic cast can leave gluelike resin on hands. Prevents exposure to allergen (Yip and Roman, 2003).
4 Assist physician or certified technician in positioning client and injured extremity as desired, depending on type of cast to be used and area to be casted.	The parts to be casted must be supported and in optimal alignment.

> **COMMUNICATION TIP** Explain procedure to client, including how client is positioned, and how it will feel. "You may experience dampness and warmth under the cast during the cast application process and heat as it dries. This is normal and expected."

5 Prepare skin that will be enclosed in the cast. Change any dressing (if present), and cleanse the skin with mild soap and water.	Assists in maintaining skin integrity.

> **NURSE ALERT** Clients with skin damage or skin lesions may not be candidates for casting.

6 Assist with application of padding material around body part to be casted (see illustration). Avoid wrinkles or uneven thicknesses.	Decreases complications to the skin and prevents pressure points under the cast.
7 Hold body part or parts to be casted or assist with preparation of casting materials.	Support of body part may require application of slight manual traction.
a. *Plaster cast:* Mark the end of the roll by folding one corner of the material under itself. Hold plaster roll under water in a plastic-lined bucket or basin until bubbles stop; then squeeze slightly and hand roll to person applying the cast.	Once dampened, the end of the casting tape may be difficult to find. Dampened plaster rolls are unrolled and molded to fit the extremity or body part to be casted.

STEPS	RATIONALE

b. *Synthetic cast:* Submerge cast roll in lukewarm water for 10 to 15 seconds. Squeeze to remove excess water.

Submersion in water initiates the chemical reaction, which will eventually result in hardening of the cast (Maher and others, 2002).

8 Continue to hold the body parts as necessary as the cast is applied (see illustration), or supply additional rolls of casting tape as needed. When wrapping is done, gently compress with hands.

Positioning may require slight manual traction to maintain the necessary alignment. Thickness of the plaster cast determines strength of the cast. Compression promotes bonding of cast layers (Maher and others, 2002).

9 Provide walking heel, brace, bar, or other material to stabilize the cast as requested by the physician. An abduction bar or wooden post may be used to stabilize a spica cast.

Ambulation may be permitted with partial weight bearing on the affected extremity after cast has dried. Braces incorporated into a cast assist in joint motion and mobility.

NURSE ALERT Do not use abduction bar as a handle for positioning the client.

---

10 Assist with "finishing" the cast by folding the edge of the stockinette down over the cast to provide a smooth edge. Unroll a dampened plaster roll over the stockinette to hold it in place.

Smooth edges decrease the chance for skin irritation or tissue injury.

11 Using scissors, trim the cast around fingers, toes, or the thumb as necessary. Remove and discard gloves and perform hand hygiene.

The cast should not restrict joint movement or constrict circulation.

12 Depending on the tissue to be casted:

Pillows or other soft areas prevent indentation or other undesirable hardening of the cast.

Elevate to heart level the casted tissues on two to three cloth-covered pillows or in a sling. Avoid complete encasing of the cast. Air dry. If ice is ordered, place to side of cast to prevent indentation to top. When applying a sling, ensure that the sling supports but does not encase the cast.

Elevation enhances venous return and decreases edema. Covering of the cast delays drying. Plaster gives off heat from a chemical reaction when drying. Encasing cast restricts air movements and impedes drying.

13 Inform client to notify caregiver of any alteration in sensation, numbness, tingling, unusual pain, or inability to move fingers or toes in affected extremity.

Edema within a casted extremity causes pressure on nerves, blood vessels, and muscle tissues. This leads to neurovascular deficit, compartment syndrome, and necrosis of tissues.

14 Using palms of hands to support casted areas, assist client with transfer to stretcher or wheelchair for return to unit, or prepare for discharge. Use additional personnel to transfer client safely, especially with client in a spica or other large body cast.

Avoids indentations in cast that could cause pressure areas on underlying skin. Use pillows, restraints, and side rails to maintain principles of safe transport.

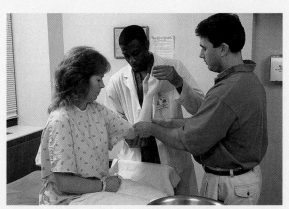

STEP 6 Padding under cast is smooth.

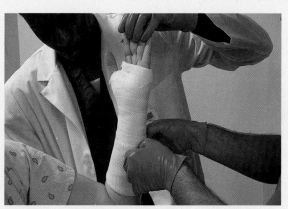

STEP 8 Support extremity during cast application.

STEPS	RATIONALE

> **NURSE ALERT** Client with wet large-limb or wet spica cast requires three people to assist in turning and transfer. Proper assistance prevents undue pressure on cast and prevents client injury.

15 Review all home care instructions with client and significant other (Box 26-4).

16 Explain to client the need to keep cast exposed until drying is complete; explain the use of elevation or ice.

Casts must dry from the inside out for thorough drying. Elevation and application of ice assist in decreasing edema formation.

17 Have client turn every 2 to 3 hours. Do not rest heel of cast on bed or pillow.

Avoids indentation and prevents continuous pressure to one area.

18 See Completion Protocol (inside front cover).

BOX 26-4　Cast Care Instructions

The First 24 Hours

- Follow the physician's instructions.
- Keep the cast and extremity above the level of the heart for at least 48 hours by propping your cast up on firm pillows.
- Put ice adjacent to the fractured area for 24 hours, but be sure to enclose the ice in a plastic bag to keep the cast dry. Do not place ice on the top of a damp cast.
- Move the parts of your body above and below the cast regularly to aid circulation and relieve stiffness. Massaging the joints and extremities gently around the cast will also improve circulation.
- Your cast needs at least 24 hours to dry if it is plaster. Avoid handling it as much as possible. When you do have to move the cast, such as when you change your body position, use only the palms of your hands and support the cast under your joints. You want to avoid putting indentations in the cast that will put pressure on the skin inside.
- Use a fan placed 18 to 24 inches from the cast to aid its drying in the first 24 hours. Be sure to expose the whole cast for drying, and do not cover it with linen for the first 24 hours.
- Never insert any object into your cast for any purpose; for example, do not try to scratch under cast when it itches.

How To Care for Your Cast

Plaster

- Do not get the cast wet because it will lose its strength. If cast does become wet, dry immediately. Use a towel to blot moisture off the cast and then dry it with a hair dryer set on low. When your cast does not feel cold and damp, it is dry.
- To keep the cast clean and dry, cover it with plastic when bathing, using the toilet (if it is a spica cast), or going out in rain or snow.
- Use a damp cloth and scouring powder to clean soiled spots on the cast. Be sure to brush away plaster crumbs or other objects from the edges of the cast, but do not remove or rearrange any padding. Do not break off or trim cast edges.

Synthetic

- If you have a fiberglass cast without wounds or incisions under it, you may be able to continue a more normal lifestyle (for example, bathing or swimming) if your doctor approves. A fiberglass cast can become wet.

- If you swim in a pool or a lake, be sure to rinse both the inside and outside of the cast to flush out any dirt and chemicals. You should use only a small amount of mild soap around your cast and rinse under your cast thoroughly.
- Washing or rinsing inside your fiberglass cast may reduce odor and irritation and improve the overall skin condition of the cast area. You may use a spray nozzle at a sink or a flexible shower head to rinse inside your cast with warm water.
- You must thoroughly dry the cast after wetting. Lightly towel off excess water and use a hair dryer on cool or low setting to dry inside cast. Do not cover the cast while it is drying.

Skin Care

- Skin care is very important during the time a cast is worn. Routinely inspect the skin condition around the cast.
- Do not insert objects under the cast because you could scrape the skin or add pressure and cause an infection or sore under the cast.
- You may use powders and lotions only outside the cast so that the skin stays clean and soft. Powder inside a cast can cake and cause sore areas.

Activity

- Do not walk on a leg cast for the first 48 hours. If you are allowed to walk on it, be sure to walk on the walking heel.
- If your arm is in a cast, be sure to use your sling for support and comfort.

Contact Your Doctor If

- You have pain, burning, or swelling
- You feel a blister or sore developing inside the cast
- You experience numbness or persistent tingling
- Your cast becomes badly soiled
- Your cast breaks, cracks, or develops soft spots
- Your cast becomes too loose
- You develop skin problems at the cast edges
- You develop a fever or foul odor under the cast
- You have any questions regarding your treatment

EVALUATION

1 Inspect exposed skin and check capillary refill by pressing on toe or finger if the cast is on an extremity (Figure 26-12).
2 Palpate the temperature of tissues around the casted area for warmth and assess for hot spots, which could indicate underlying localized infection.
3 Palpate any accessible pulses distal to the cast.
4 Inspect condition of the cast.
5 Observe for edema of tissues distal to the cast for signs of vascular compromise (whitish or bluish coloration).
6 Observe client for signs of pain or anxiety (hyperventilation, tachycardia, blood pressure elevation).
7 Observe client performing ADLs and ROM.
8 Observe client perform cast care.

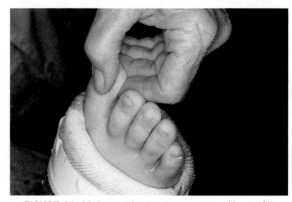

FIGURE 26-12 Inspecting toe to assess capillary refill.

Unexpected Outcomes and Related Interventions

1 Client experiences impaired physical mobility related to the cast.
a. Assist client with ROM exercises every 3 to 4 hours.
b. Teach isometric exercises.
2 Client reports increased severity in pain after application of the cast.
a. Reposition casted extremity or client. Adjust elevation of pillows as necessary.
b. Apply ice bags along sides of cast. Do not place heavy ice bags on top of damp cast because of risk of indentation.
c. Administer analgesics as ordered to maintain client's comfort level.
d. Perform neurovascular checks.
e. Assess tightness of the cast by checking with two fingers around the edges and checking with client. Cast should be snug but not tight.
f. If pain continues, notify physician.
3 Client develops compartment syndrome, with severe pain unrelieved by analgesics; change in neurovascular status, such as numbness, tingling, or decreased movement in distal skin and tissues; bluish color to distal parts; marked edema; diminished or absent pulse in area distal to casted extremity (pulselessness develops late in the syndrome); or capillary refill over 3 seconds.
a. Consult immediately with physician.
b. Prepare to bivalve cast using a cast cutter. Cut through underlying wadding and padding also.
4 Client reports a sensation of heat beneath the cast.
a. Assess for indications of localized and systemic infection.
b. Notify physician.

Recording and Reporting

- Record cast application, condition of skin, status of circulation (e.g., temperature, sensation), and motion of distal part.
- Record instructions given to client and family.

- Report abnormal or untoward findings from neurovascular checks; report signs and symptoms of compartment syndrome immediately.

Sample Documentation

0900 Left long arm synthetic cast applied and left arm placed in shoulder sling by Dr. Hill. Capillary refill of left index finger is 2 seconds. Skin warm, dry, and intact. Able to move all fingers of left hand, fingers warm to touch, nail beds pink, no swelling noted. Complains of pain at 5 (scale of 0 to 10).

0910 Tylox 1 tab administered PO. Left long arm cast and sling readjusted.

0945 Left long arm cast intact with sling. Capillary refill of left index finger unchanged. Moves all fingers of left hand, denies any numbness or tingling present, fingers warm to touch. No edema noted. Reports pain decreased to 1 (scale of 0 to 10).

Special Considerations

Pediatric Considerations

- Allow the child to choose the color of a synthetic cast.
- Teach caregivers to protect plaster cast from moisture and to ensure that synthetic casts are dried thoroughly if damp. Protect lower-extremity casts with plastic wrap during urination or defecation.
- Monitor children closely to ensure that objects are not placed beneath cast to scratch. Use medication, ice pack, and/or a hair dryer set to cool setting to control itching (Hockenberry and Wilson, 2007).
- Recognize that babies and young children demonstrate pain by restlessness and crying.
- Provide child with doll that has cast similar to child's cast to reduce anxiety and to use as a teaching tool.

Geriatric Considerations

- Lightweight, synthetic casts are better for older clients. Cast is less restrictive, and light weight helps clients maintain better balance.

- Plaster of Paris casts on older clients may have less plaster to aid in moving or lifting.
- Older clients may have reduced sensation and be less able to detect compression (Stanley, Blair, and Beare, 2005).
- Older clients may take longer for bone healing than younger clients.
- Older clients with age-related decreases in muscle strength may have difficulty in ambulating with a cast.

Home Care Considerations
- Reinforce cast care instruction (see Box 26-4).
- Instruct to elevate affected extremity when sitting to help reduce swelling.
- Remind to inspect cast daily for foul odor, which indicates skin excoriation or infection under cast.
- Remind to inspect skin daily for pressure or friction areas.
- Remind to inspect cast daily for cracks or changes in alignment.

SKILL 26.4 Care of the Client During Cast Removal

When caring for clients with casts, it is also important to understand the techniques for cast removal, which consist of removing the cast and padding, followed by skin care to the affected area. The cast is removed by use of a cast saw. The saw is noisy, but the procedure is painless because the saw vibrates and thus will not cut the skin. However, it is necessary, to prepare the client adequately for cast removal. A small child or confused adult may require gentle restraint during removal to avoid any injury. Careful removal of a synthetic cast (with gore lining) is important to prevent burns that may result from the heat generated by the vibrating saw. After cast removal, the client may experience tenderness, soreness, or muscle weakness.

ASSESSMENT

1 Assess client's understanding and ability to cooperate with cast removal. *Rationale: Cast removal may require a cast saw. Client needs to understand that the saw is noisy but does not cut skin.*
2 Assess client's readiness for cast removal (physician's orders, x-ray examination results, physical findings).
3 Ask if client feels itching or burning under the cast. *Rationale: Skin dryness or irritation normally may be present.*

PLANNING

Expected Outcomes focus on integrity of the underlying skin and client understanding of the cast removal procedure.

1 Client describes and demonstrates levels of activity and weight-bearing limitations.
2 There is no underlying tissue damage after cast removal.
3 Client can describe skin care measures and perform ADLs as appropriate.

Delegation Considerations
The skill of assisting with cast removal may be delegated to AP who have had specific training. The nurse directs personnel by:
- Reviewing with care provider proper positioning methods for specific clients.
- Reviewing skin care required following cast removal.

Equipment
- Cast saw
- Plastic sheets or paper
- Cold water enzyme wash
- Skin lotion
- Basin, water, washcloth, towels
- Scissors
- Eye protection (goggles, glasses) for client and health care professional

IMPLEMENTATION *for Care of the Client During Cast Removal*

STEPS	RATIONALE
1 See Standard Protocol (inside front cover).	
2 Assist with positioning of client.	Prevents accidental injury to skin during cast removal.
3 Describe the physical sensations to expect during cast removal (vibration of cast saw and generation of heat) (see illustration).	Knowledge of the procedure decreases level of anxiety.

> **COMMUNICATION TIP** Tell client, "You may feel warmth from the vibration of the saw, but the saw doesn't cut your skin. Here, let me demonstrate on my thumb."

STEPS	RATIONALE

4 Describe the expected appearance of the extremity. Skin under cast is often scaly with dead cells that slough off. Muscle atrophy occurs from disuse.

5 Describe and demonstrate the loud noise of the cast saw.

6 Apply eye goggles or protective glasses. Apply eye protection on client.

Prevents injury from saw.

7 Stay with client, and explain progress of procedure as cast and underlying padding are removed (see illustration).

8 Inspect tissues underlying the cast after removal.

9 If skin is intact, apply cold water enzyme wash (if available) to skin, and leave on for 15 to 20 minutes. Oil may be used to soften crust. Mild soap and water may also be used. Do not scrub the skin.

Areas of irritation or breakdown may require treatment. Enzyme wash assists in dissolving dead cells and fatty deposits. Vigorous scrubbing damages delicate tissues.

10 Gently wash off enzyme wash. Immerse tissues in basin or tub, if possible, to assist in dead cell removal.

11 Pat extremity dry, remove and discard gloves, perform hand hygiene, and apply generous coat of lotion to client's skin.

Rubbing may further traumatize the tissues. Lotion moistures dry skin.

12 After cast removal, explain and write out skin care procedures for client (Box 26-5).

Provides ongoing home care instruction for client and family.

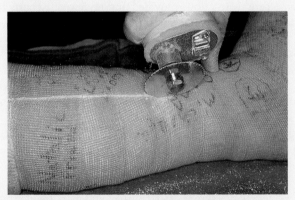

STEP 3 Vibration of cast cutter generates heat.

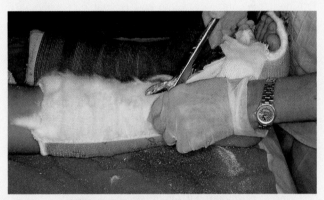

STEP 7 Removing padding beneath cast

BOX 26-5 Care After Cast Removal

Skin Care

Provide client written instructions concerning general care before discharge.

- Apply enzyme wash solution such as Woolite or Delicare and leave in place for at least 20 minutes. The enzymes in the solution loosen dead cells and help emulsify fatty or crusty lesions but cause no skin irritation.
- After 20 minutes, immerse the area in warm water and gently wash away the debris. Do not rub or scrub the skin areas, but gently swab the areas with a soft cloth.
- Rinse with clear warm water and pat dry.
- Apply a moisturizing skin lotion or apply a little oil, gently massaging it in to help maintain the integrity of the cells.
- Repeat the above steps in 24 to 48 hours, after which the area should need no special care.

Relieving Edema

- Apply cloth-covered ice bags if the edema is marked. Do not place ice directly on skin.
- Elevate the affected tissues for the next 24 hours or when swelling occurs.

Managing Tenderness, Weakness, Discomfort

- Take prescribed analgesic every 3 to 4 hours to build a therapeutic blood level, and continue the medication for 24 to 48 hours.
- Immerse the part or the entire body in warm water and gently exercise muscles under water.
- Wrap an elastic bandage from distal to proximal area if extra support is needed.
- Begin to reuse affected tissues and muscles slowly to avoid pain. Explain that usually it takes twice as long a time as the part was in a cast to regain full function.
- Perform prescribed muscle exercises with 5 to 10 repetitions every 4 hours to aid in regaining muscle strength. If muscle soreness persists, continue intake of prescribed nonnarcotic analgesic. Soak in warm water before exercise. Soreness should lessen as the muscle regains strength. Consult with therapist to prescribe appropriate exercises to increase mobility and strength.

STEPS	RATIONALE
13 Obtain physician's order to perform active and passive ROM and clarify level of activity allowed.	After immobilization, the involved joints and muscles will be weak, and ROM may be limited. Activity is resumed slowly to avoid reinjury.
14 Assist in transfer of client for return to unit or discharge.	
15 Instruct client to observe for swelling and to continue to elevate the extremity to control swelling.	
16 See Completion Protocol (inside cover).	

EVALUATION

1 Ask client to explain and demonstrate activity level and ROM exercises prescribed.

2 Inspect underlying skin for pressure areas, erythema (redness), or other signs of irritation or trauma.

3 Observe client perform skin care.

Unexpected Outcomes and Related Interventions

1 Client becomes very tense and is unable to cooperate during the cast removal.

a. Offer reassurance and support.

b. Reexplain the cast removal procedure and expected sensations during removal.

c. Demonstrate action of cast saw on personnel's hand.

2 Client experiences edema, pain, and difficulty moving affected tissues after removal of cast.

a. Assess neurovascular status of involved tissues.

b. Assess the type, length, site, amount, and severity of the pain, including onset.

c. Assess ability to perform active and passive ROM.

d. Contact physician with findings.

3 Client has scratch on underlying skin.

a. Inspect skin edges and severity of scratch.

b. Cleanse area and apply water-soluble lotion or ointment as ordered.

4 Client is unable to explain self-care measures or skin care.

a. Reassure client as necessary.

b. Reinstruct client in self-care after cast removal.

c. Instruct client in skin care measures, including gentle cleansing of the casted area (avoid scrubbing) and patting the area dry (avoid rubbing). Apply a water-soluble lotion or ointment to any scratches as ordered.

Recording and Reporting

- Record cast removal, condition of tissues formerly in cast, any skin care interventions, and name of person removing cast in nurses' notes.
- Record instructions given to client and family.

Sample Documentation

1000 Attempted to remove left long arm cast. Client began crying. Reexplained procedure and action of cast saw. Demonstrated vibration action.

1015 Left long arm cast removed without difficulty. Left arm soaking in basin of enzyme wash, rinsed. Skin intact. Lotion applied.

1045 Skin on left arm remains dry and soft. Written home care instructions provided and reviewed. Reports he understands and has no questions.

Special Considerations

Pediatric Considerations

- Demonstrate the cast saw on your own skin and on a doll before using on child. Allow the child to see that it does not cut to decrease anxiety.

Geriatric Considerations

- Older clients may experience marked stiffness or weakened muscles, depending on length of time in cast.
- Older client's skin is drier, thinner, and more fragile than that of a baby, child, or younger adult.

Home Care Considerations

- Elevate extremity with intermittent edema by using chair or bed with pillows.
- Suggest regular use of moisturizers for dry, scaly skin of casted extremity. Instruct client not to remove scaly skin by rubbing.
- Teach client to ambulate slowly and carefully until muscle strength is regained in affected extremity.
- Assess client's environment for potential safety risks.

SKILL 26.5 Care of the Client with an Immobilization Device—Brace, Splint

Immobilization devices increase stability, support a weak extremity, or reduce the load on weight-bearing structures such as hips, knees, or ankles. A splint immobilizes and protects a body part. Temporary splints reduce pain and prevent tissue damage from further motion immediately after an injury such as a fracture or sprain. Air splints, Thomas splints, and improvised splints from material on hand are examples of temporary splints applied in emergency situations. Upper extremity fractures are sometimes managed using splints such as hand and digital splints or sugar-tong splints. Slings support splints, casts, or injured upper extremities (Figure 26-13). They are commercially available or can be made for almost any body part (see Procedural Guideline 26-1). Velcro or buckle closures permit these devices to be adjusted to fit a body part of almost any size and shape. The abduction splint, used after hip replacement surgery, maintains the client's legs in an abducted position. This permits the client to be turned without changing the healing limb's position and prevents dislocation of the hip prosthesis. The device is easily removed for nursing care such as skin care, dressing changes, or neurovascular assessments. A posterior splint with elastic wraps is sometimes used to support an extremity.

Cloth and foam splints, known as immobilizers, provide long-term immobilization (Figure 26-14). Immobilizers treat sprains and dislocations that do not require complete and continuous immobilization in a cast or traction. Immobilizers are often used following orthopedic surgery. Other common types of immobilizers include cervical collars (soft or hard), belt type of shoulder immobilizers, and vinyl wrist forearm splints. Molded splints made of plastic provide support to clients with chronic injuries or diseases such as arthritis. They maintain the body part in a functional position to prevent contractures and muscle atrophy during the period of disuse. A splint goes into place and is removed quickly and easily when the skin or a wound is assessed.

Braces support weakened structures during weight bearing. For this reason, they are made of sturdy materials such as leather, metal, and molded plastic. Chest and abdominal braces such as the Milwaukee and Boston braces immobilize the thoracic and lumbar vertebral column to treat scoliosis (curvature of the spine). The brace does not correct the curve but instead prevents its progression. Lumbar braces support lumbar and sacral tissues after spinal surgery or fusion. Leg braces hold the thigh, leg, and foot in functional positions for weight bearing and ambulation. Both short leg and long leg braces support weak leg muscles, aid in control of involuntary muscle movement, or maintain surgical correction during the postoperative healing process. They are commonly used for clients with cerebral palsy, muscular dystrophy, multiple sclerosis, and after fractures and polio (Bakker and others, 2000).

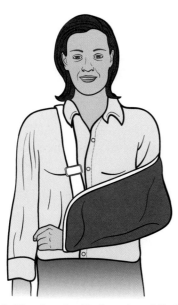

FIGURE 26-13 Sling for shoulder/arm immobilization. (Redrawn from Beare PG, Meyers JL: *Principles and practice of adult health nursing,* ed 3, 1998, Mosby.)

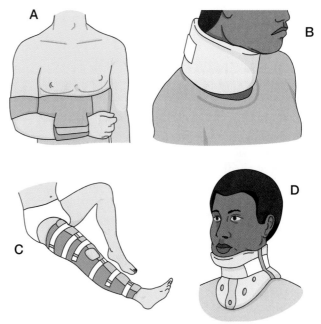

FIGURE 26-14 Examples of immobilizers. **A,** Shoulder immobilizer. **B,** Soft cervical collar. **C,** Knee immobilizer. **D,** Hard cervical collar. (Redrawn from Beare PG, Meyers JL: *Principles and practice of adult health nursing,* ed 3, 1998, Mosby.)

ASSESSMENT

1 Review client's medical history, previous and current activity level, and description of the condition requiring bracing or splinting. *Rationale: Reveals client's current and previous health status and purpose for brace/splint.*

2 Determine client's previous experience with braces or splints. *Rationale: Reveals client's baseline knowledge and need for instruction.*

3 Assess client's understanding of reason for brace/splint and its care, application, and schedule of wear. *Rationale: Determines need for further teaching.*

4 Inspect area of skin to be in contact with support device. *Rationale: Provides baseline to monitor client for skin breakdown. Immobile and older clients are particularly vulnerable.*

5 Obtain assessment of client's level of pain on a scale of 0 to 10. *Rationale: Provides baseline to determine if immobilization device affects comfort.*

6 Refer to occupational or physical therapy consultation to determine type of brace to be used, desired position, and amount of activity and movement permitted. *Rationale: Provides direction in proper use of brace.*

7 Assess client's additional need for an assistive device such as a cane, walker, or crutches (see Chapter 6). *Rationale: An assistive device may be needed to provide support and promote balance during ambulation.*

PLANNING

Expected Outcomes focus on maintaining skin integrity, improving client's knowledge, and preventing risk for injury.

1 Client's skin remains in good condition without circulatory impairment.

2 Client/significant other verbalizes purpose, correct application, and care of the device.

3 Client does not report an increase in pain on a 0-10 scale during device application.

4 Circulation and sensation distal to brace/splint are maintained.

5 Client uses the device correctly, including schedule of wear, activity limitations, and positioning.

Delegation Considerations

Assessment of the client's condition should not be delegated; however, the skill of caring for the client wearing a brace, splint, or sling may be delegated. The nurse directs personnel by:

- Reviewing correct application of the brace/splint and positioning of any ties or straps.
- Reviewing prescribed schedule of wear and activities permitted while in the brace.
- Instructing personnel to alert the nurse if client complains of pain, rubbing, or pressure from the brace or splint or if a change occurs in client's skin condition.

Equipment

- Brace/splint/commercially prepared sling or triangular bandage and safety pin
- Cotton shirt or gown

IMPLEMENTATION *for Care of the Client with an Immobilization Device—Brace, Splint*

STEPS	RATIONALE
1 See Standard Protocol (inside front cover).	
2 Explain reasons for brace or splint and demonstrate how device works.	Teaching and demonstration enhance learning, reduce anxiety, and encourage cooperation.
3 Assist client to a comfortable position: apply upper-extremity braces/splints with client sitting upright; apply lower extremity braces with client lying down.	Facilitates correct, aligned placement of brace.
4 Prepare skin that will be enclosed in brace/splint by cleaning skin with soap and water; rinse, pat dry, and change any dressings (if present). If applying a back brace, put a thin cotton shirt or gown on client. Ensure that there are no wrinkles causing pressure.	This protects skin, absorbs moisture, and keeps brace clean (Ball and Bindler, 2003).

> **COMMUNICATION TIP** Tell the client, "Be sure to let me know if you feel pressure, pain, numbness, or rubbing or if the skin becomes reddened."

STEPS	RATIONALE
5 Inspect device for wear, damage, or rough edges.	Potential for skin breakdown is decreased, and correct alignment is maintained.

STEPS	RATIONALE
6 Apply brace/splint as directed by physician, orthotist, physical therapist, or occupational therapist. If securing splint with elastic bandage:	Proper application of the brace/splint is important to avoid skin breakdown, pressure ulcers, neurovascular compromise, calluses, or worsening of the deformity.
a. Apply even tension as bandage is wrapped from distal to proximal.	Prevents trapping of blood distal to immobilization device.
b. Prevent padding from gathering or bunching.	Prevents irritation to underlying tissues.
7 Teach client prescribed schedule of wear and allowed activities while in brace/splint as directed by physician, physical therapist, or occupational therapist.	Proper use of brace/splint will facilitate healing and mobility and reduce pain and stress.
8 Reinforce signs of skin breakdown, pressure, or rubbing to report.	Brace/splint may need to be adjusted. Changes may also be required because of growth or atrophy, when muscles regain or lose strength, or after reconstructive surgery.
9 Teach client how to care for the brace/splint:	To maintain integrity of the brace/splint
a. When not in use, store metal braces upright in a safe but easily accessible location.	To prevent deformity or bending of the brace
b. Splints of molded materials should be stored away from heat.	To prevent melting and deformation of the splint
c. Leather materials should be treated with leather preservative.	To prevent drying or cracking
d. Keep brace clean, dry, and in good working order.	Plastic parts are cleaned with a damp cloth and thoroughly dried. Metal joints are cleaned with a pipe cleaner and oiled weekly. Remove rust with steel wool and clean metal parts with a solvent.
10 Assist client in ambulating with brace/splint in place.	Determines if client is able to ambulate safely.
11 Have client apply and remove the brace/splint.	Promotes client independence; demonstration confirms level of learning skill.

> **COMMUNICATION TIP** Let the client know that the brace/splint may seem awkward at first. Tell the client, "After you have had practice in using it, you will feel more comfortable and better able to move about." Also let the client know that assistance may be needed to apply and remove the brace/splint.

12 See Completion Protocol (inside front cover).

PROCEDURAL GUIDELINE 26-1

Sling Application

Equipment:
Commercially prepared sling or triangular bandage and safety pin.

Delegation Considerations
Assessment of the client's condition should not be delegated; however, the skill of applying a sling may be delegated. The nurse directs personnel or family members by:
- Reviewing the purpose of the sling.
- Reviewing correct application of the sling and positioning of any ties or straps.
- Reviewing prescribed schedule of wear and activities permitted while in the sling.
- Instructing personnel to alert the nurse if client complains of pain, rubbing, or pressure from the sling or if a change occurs in client's skin condition.

Procedural Steps
1   **See Standard Protocol (inside front cover).**
2   If commercial sling is used, follow directions on package for correct application.
3   If triangular bandage is used, position one end of the bandage over the shoulder of the unaffected arm.
4   Take the remaining bandage and place the material against the chest and then under and over the affected arm, cradling the arm.
5   Position the pointed end of the triangle toward the elbow.
6   Tie the two ends of the triangle at the side of the neck.
7   Fold the pointed end of the sling at the elbow in the front and secure with a safety pin, closing the end of the sling.
8   Adjust the length of the sling by adjusting the amount of material in the knot.
9   Ensure that the sling supports the limb comfortably without interfering with circulation.
10 Assess neurovascular status (see Box 26-2) after 20 to 30 minutes. Continue to monitor every 4 hours. Readjust sling as necessary.
11 Inspect areas of the skin underneath the sling for signs of pressure, including redness or breakdown.
12 Observe the client using the sling.
13 Ask the client to rate level of comfort on scale of 0 to 10 while the sling is in place.
14 Palpate pulse, skin temperature, observe skin color, and test sensation of extremity distal to position of sling.
15 Observe client perform ADLs while wearing the sling.
16 **See Completion Protocol (inside front cover).**

NCLEX® Style Questions

1 In the first 24 to 48 hours following the application of traction, when should the nurse perform a neurovascular assessment of a patient's foot?
1. Every 1 to 2 hours
2. Once a shift
3. Whenever the patient complains of pain
4. Whenever the weights are readjusted

2 The client develops severe pain and swelling in the tissues beneath his cast. The toes on the casted foot are cold, and capillary refill to the toes is 5-6 seconds. The nurse elevates the cast for 15 minutes with no change in pain level. The nurse's priority action will be to notify the physician and be prepared to do which of the following:
1. Cut in a window shape in the middle of the cast to allow visualization of the skin.
2. Bivalve the cast.
3. Apply warm compresses to the sides and top of cast.
4. Administer Tylenol No. 3 per written standing order.

3 A new plaster cast is applied to the client's ankle. Until it is fully dry, which is the best way to handle a newly applied cast?
1. Move carefully with the fingertips.
2. Move with the palms of the hands.
3. Move it in a sling.
4. Place it on a pillow.

4 During rounds, a nurse inspects the client's traction setup. Which of the following observations require a nursing intervention?
1. Traction is not exerting enough force.
2. Weights are not hanging freely at the end of the bed.
3. The pull of the ropes are at a 45-degree angle.
4. The Steinmann pin slipped slightly.

5 A resident in a skilled-nursing facility has just fractured her hip. The doctor orders Buck's skin traction until she can be admitted to the hospital for surgery the next day. Which assessment finding(s) indicates damage to the peroneal nerve, a complication of skin traction? Mark all that apply.
1. Cool temperature of the extremity
2. Inability to dorsiflex the foot
3. Inability to plantar flex the foot
4. Spasm of the calf muscle
5. Decreased sensation in the web space between the great toe and second toe

References for all chapters appear in Appendix D.

Intravenous Therapy

27

MEDIA RESOURCES

- **evolve** http://evolve.elsevier.com/Elkin

- **View Video!** Video Clips

- Nursing Skills Online

Delivery of infusion therapy is essential in the treatment of clients and requires your knowledge, professional accountability, and skill. You assess for and choose the most appropriate vascular access site and device, prepare the client, use the proper insertion technique, and closely monitor the infusion. You assume a primary role in safely and effectively delivering intravenous (IV) medications and fluids, as well as protecting clients from the potential complications associated with IV therapy. For all the skills in this chapter, follow the six rights of medication and IV fluid administration: **R**ight drug/solution, **R**ight dose/concentration, **R**ight client, **R**ight route, **R**ight date/time, and **R**ight documentation when providing IV therapy (Burke, 2005; Hodgson and Kizor, 2006).

The Infusion Nursing Standards of Practice includes evidence-based practice and are integrated throughout the skills in this chapter (INS, 2006). Additional guidelines published by the Joint Commission on Accreditation of Healthcare Organizations (JCAHO, 2005), Centers for Disease Control and Prevention (CDC, 2002), and the Occupational Safety and Health Administration (OSHA, 2001) are incorporated to support safe, efficient, and quality care when providing infusion therapy. Know and follow these standards, as well as agency standards and your state or government practice guidelines and standards when providing intravenous care.

Astute clinical management and specialized IV therapy skills are the norm for the delivery of infusion therapy. An IV device is invasive, thereby increasing the client's risk for infection. A client's previous experience with IV therapy affects how the nurse approaches his or her care. Infusion therapy requires critical thinking, including an assessment of a client's anatomy and physiology of the circulatory system, fluid and electrolyte balance, disease pathophysiology, type and duration of prescribed therapy, allergies, and the client's response to illness. Assessment also extends to the observation of the client's venous anatomy of the upper extremities, assessment of mobility or immobility, and previous attempts or procedures for IV therapy. The goal of all IV therapy is to maintain fluid and electrolyte balance or prevent fluid and electrolyte imbalance without complications associated with the delivery of IV medications or fluids (Burke, 2005).

EVIDENCE IN PRACTICE

O'Riordan GD and others: Optimal timing for intravenous administration set replacement. *The Cochrane Database of Systematic Reviews 2006*, Issue 4, www.cochrane.org/reviews/en/ab003588.html, accessed November 21, 2006.

Routine replacement of intravenous administration sets has been recommended to reduce intravenous infusion contamination and related bloodstream infection. A systematic review of 13 studies involving 4783 clients was conducted. Findings show that intravenous administration sets that do not contain lipids, blood, or blood products may be left in place for intervals of up to 96 hours without increasing the incidence of infection. There are no differences between clients with central versus peripheral catheters or between children and adults. In addition, the current recommendations that administration sets that contain lipids should be changed every 24 hours remains appropriate.

NURSING DIAGNOSES

A **risk for infection** is related to any invasive procedure. For the client receiving IV therapy for correction of fluid and electrolyte imbalance or with potential fluid alterations, actual **risk for imbalanced fluid volume** is appropriate. **Risk for injury** is created by the presence of an IV catheter acting as a foreign body and adverse events related to IV medications.

Psychological factors such as **fear** or **anxiety** related to the client's previous experience with infusion therapy may apply. **Acute pain** is applicable when painful IV-related complications develop. For clients receiving care in the home and needing to manage IV therapy, nursing diagnoses may include **impaired home maintenance** or **deficient knowledge.**

SKILL 27.1 Insertion of a Peripheral Intravenous Device

- **Nursing Skills Online:** IV Fluid Administration, Lessons 1 and 2

To maintain or correct fluid and electrolyte balance, isotonic, hypotonic, or hypertonic fluids are delivered through a variety of methods using continuous and/or intermittent infusion. Infusion therapy provides access to the venous system to deliver various medications in emergent and non-emergent situations and to infuse blood or blood products. Reliable venous access for infusion therapy administration is essential.

Successful IV therapy depends on client preparation, site selection, catheter selection, and catheter insertion. Several vascular access devices are available for use in peripheral veins (Table 27-1). Because potential for exposure to blood-borne pathogens is high during insertion and care of IV devices, adherence to asepsis and standard precautions is required (see Chapters 4 and 5).

Catheters are made of many materials such as silicone or a steel needle. Steel-winged infusion devices (butterfly needles) are used in limited, short-term situations. They are easier to insert but may easily infiltrate. Improved product design provides many choices: such as short, peripheral inside-the-needle and over-the-needle catheters (see Table 27-1). The Needlestick Safety and Prevention Act (OSHA, 2001), requires health care employers to identify and make use of effective and safer medical devices (see Chapter 17). Safer medical devices, such as sharps with engineered sharps-injury protections (e.g., sliding sheaths that cover needles after use, needles that retract into syringes) and needleless systems (e.g., IV medication systems with non-needle connections and ports), must be used when feasible (Deacon, 2004). In addition, the Infusion Nurses Society

TABLE 27-1 Intravenous Access Device Options

TYPE	USE
Winged infusion butterfly needle	One-time infusion, IV push administration
Short, over-the-needle catheter (less than 3 inches [75 cm])	Continuous infusion, intermittent infusion, short-term duration (less than 96 hours) (CDC, 2002)
Midline peripheral catheters (3- to 8-inch [7.5 to 20 cm])	Continuous infusion and intermittent infusion (7 to 14 days)

IV, Intravenous.

(INS) recommends that peripheral short catheters be equipped with a safety device with engineered sharps-injury protection (INS, 2006).

ASSESSMENT

1 Check accuracy and completeness of prescriber's original order. Check client's name; type and amount of intravenous solution and medication additives; and dose, ordered infusion rate, and length of time for therapy. *Rationale: Review ensures safe and correct administration of IV therapy by verifying order. Assists in selection of an appropriate access device and early placement of longer-term infusion devices and minimizes multiple venipunctures.*

2 Assess client's previous experience with IV therapy. *Rationale: Determines level of emotional support and instruction necessary.*

3 Determine if client is to undergo any planned surgeries or procedures. *Rationale: Allows nurse to place an adequate-size catheter and avoids placement in an area that will interfere with surgeries or procedures.*

4 Assess client's hand/arm dominance. *Rationale: Ensures that placement will not impair therapy or interfere with mobility and improves client's comfort and tolerance of IV therapy.*

5 Assess for clinical conditions such as dehydration, body weight, dry mucous membranes, altered vital signs, and lung sounds that will be affected by IV fluid administration. *Rationale: Provides baseline information to determine the effectiveness of IV therapy on the client's fluid and electrolyte balance.*

6 Assess laboratory data and client's history of allergies. *Rationale: May reveal information that affects insertion of devices, such as fluid volume deficit or anemia. Prepping agents, gloves, and plastic catheters may create a serious problem for clients with allergies to iodine, adhesive, or latex.*

7 Assess client's medical history for chronic illnesses and all prescribed and over-the counter medications. *Rationale: Chronic cardiac, respiratory, or renal diseases and subsequent medications (e.g., diuretics) indicate the need for electronic control of the infusion (see Skill 27.2, p. 606).*

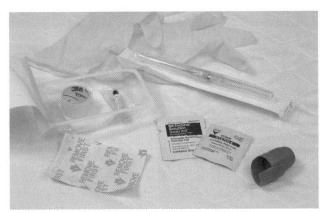

FIGURE 27-1 Intravenous start kit.

PLANNING

Expected Outcomes focus on minimal complications from IV therapy, minimal discomfort to the client, and restoration of normal fluid and electrolyte balance.

1 Fluid and electrolyte balance returns to normal.

2 Vital signs are stable and return to within normal limits for client.

3 Intake and output (I&O) are within normal limits for client's condition.

4 No swelling, pallor, pain, inflammation, or infiltration is present at venipuncture site.

5 IV line is patent, and infusion is delivered at prescribed rate and volume.

Delegation Considerations

The skill of IV insertion may not be delegated. The nurse directs personnel by:

- Reviewing what to observe, such as complaints of burning, bleeding or swelling at IV site and the report of this information back to the nurse.

- Reviewing when to inform the nurse when the volume of fluid is low in the IV bag or the electronic infusion device is sounding its alarm.

Equipment

- IV start kit (if available)—contains sterile tourniquet, sterile tape, sterile drape, antiseptic preps (Figure 27-1)
- Tourniquets (options: latex-free, single patient use, or blood pressure cuff)
- Clean gloves (latex-free for client with latex allergy)
- Antiseptic prepping agent(s) (2% chlorhexidine, povidone-iodine, 70% alcohol)
- IV fluids with time tape attached (if applicable)

For continuous infusion:

- Administration set with tubing
  - Injection cap or prn adapter with tubing
  - IV loop or short piece of extension tubing
  - 5-ml syringe for flush solution (e.g., sterile normal saline [NS] or heparin flush solution)

For intermittent infusion:

- Appropriate IV catheter (gauge appropriate to solution infusion type) (see Table 27-1)
- Sterile tape, 1 inch and ½ inch wide
- Transparent dressing or sterile 2 × 2 gauze
- Electronic infusion device (EID) and IV pole

IMPLEMENTATION *for Insertion of a Peripheral Intravenous Device*

STEPS	RATIONALE
1 See Standard Protocol (inside front cover).	
2 Verify client's identity by using at least two identifiers. Ask client to state name. Compare client's name on order sheet with one other identifier, such as hospital identification number on identification bracelet.	Ensures that correct client is receiving medication. At least two client identifiers, neither of which is the client's room number, are used when administering medications (JCAHO, 2006). Identification bracelets made at the time of admission are the most reliable source of identification.

STEPS	RATIONALE
3 Select appropriate-size catheter, prepare equipment for insertion and for continuous infusion, insert infusion set into fluid container, and prime IV tubing, maintaining sterility of closed system (see Skill 27.2). *Optional:* For intermittent infusion, prepare heparin or normal saline lock.	Smaller catheters (larger gauge) are less traumatizing. The catheter selected uses the smallest size and shortest length to accommodate prescribed therapy (INS, 2006).
4 Change client's gown to the more easily removed gown with snaps at the shoulder if available and position client in a comfortable supine position so you can extend the arm. Raise bed to your level and provide adequate lighting.	Provides proper body mechanics, reducing horizontal reach, and aids in successful vein location.
5 NOTE: Gloves can be left off to locate the vein but must be applied before prepping the site. Apply tourniquet around arm above antecubital fossa or 4 to 6 inches (10 to 15 cm) above the proposed insertion site (see illustration). Do not apply too tightly to cause injury or bruising to skin. Verify presence of a radial pulse. *Optional:* Apply blood pressure cuff instead of tourniquet. Inflate to a level just below client's normal diastolic pressure.	Tourniquet should be tight enough to impede venous return but not occlude arterial flow (see Chapter 13).

> **COMMUNICATION TIP** Encourage client to ask questions. Provide honest answers with a calm and reassuring manner. Tell client, "The stick will hurt some but will be less painful if you can hold still. It's OK to move the other arm." After site preparation and just before puncturing the skin, say, "There is going to be a stick now." Then proceed immediately with venipuncture.

STEPS	RATIONALE
6 Select the vein for device insertion.	
a. Use the most distal site in the client's nondominant arm, if possible (see illustration). Clip arm hair with scissors if necessary.	Venipuncture should be performed distal to proximal, which increases the availability of other sites for future IV therapy. Hair impedes venipuncture or adherence of dressing.

> **NURSE ALERT** Do not shave the IV site area. Shaving causes microabrasions and predisposes client to infections.

STEPS	RATIONALE
b. Avoid areas that are painful to palpation. Also avoid scars, rashes, or skin conditions.	May indicate inflamed vein. Difficult to discern IV site complication or previous skin condition.
c. Select a vein large enough for device placement.	Prevents interruption of venous flow while allowing adequate blood flow around the catheter.

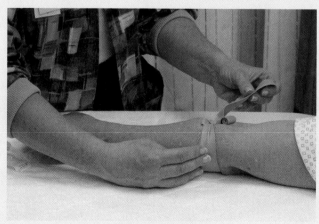

STEP 5 Apply tourniquet.

STEPS	RATIONALE
d. Choose a site that will not interfere with client's ADLs or planned surgery or procedures.	Maintains client's mobility as much as possible.
e. With the index finger palpate the vein by pressing downward and noting the resilient, soft, bouncy feeling as the pressure is released (see illustration).	Use of the same finger causes a development of sensitivity to better assess the vein condition. Fingers on nondominant hand tend to be more sensitive (Otto, 2005).
f. If possible, place client's arm in a dependent position and select the well-dilated vein.	Promotes venous distention.
g. Methods to faster venous distention include:	
(1) Stroking extremity from distal to proximal below the proposed venipuncture site.	Promotes venous filling.
(2) Applying warmth to extremity for several minutes (e.g., use a warm washcloth).	Heat increases blood supply through vasodilation.

> **NURSE ALERT** Vigorous friction and multiple tapping of the veins, especially in older adults, may cause hematoma and/or venous constriction.

STEPS	RATIONALE
h. Avoid sites distal to a previous venipuncture site, veins in the antecubital fossa or inner wrist, sclerosed or hardened cordlike veins, an infiltrated site or phlebotic vessels, bruised areas, and areas of venous valves or bifurcation.	Such sites increase risk of infiltration of newly placed IV line and excessive vessel damage. Veins in antecubital fossa are used for blood draws, and placement here limits mobility (Otto, 2005).

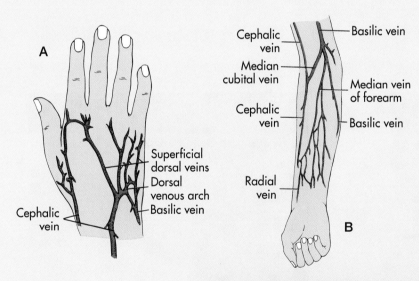

STEP 6a. Common IV sites. **A,** Dorsal surface of hand. **B,** Inner arm.

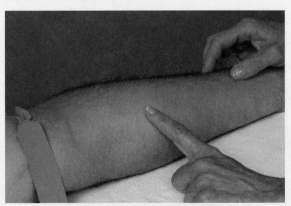

STEP 6e. Palpate vein for resilience.

STEPS	RATIONALE

i. Avoid fragile dorsal veins in older adult clients and vessels in an extremity with compromised circulation (e.g., in cases of mastectomy, dialysis graft, or paralysis).

Venous alterations can increase risk of complications (e.g., infiltration, decreased catheter dwell time).

7 Release tourniquet temporarily and carefully.

Restores blood flow while preparing for venipuncture.

8 Apply gloves if not done in step 5. Place adapter end of infusion tubing nearby on sterile gauze. Cleanse insertion site using friction in a horizontal plane, then a vertical plane, followed with a circular motion (moving from insertion site outward) (see illustration). Use antiseptic prep as a single agent or in combination. Allow to dry between agents if agents are used in combination. Reprep skin if touched after preparation (CDC, 2002).

Mechanical friction in this pattern allows penetration of antiseptic into epidermal layer of skin (Crosby and Mares, 2001). Drying prevents chemical reactions between agents and allows time for maximum microbicidal activity of agents (Rosenthal, 2004). 2% Chlorhexidine has recently been shown to be an effective agent (ONS, 2004; INS, 2006). Touching cleansed area would introduce organisms from nurse's hand to site.

9 Reapply tourniquet and verify presence of distal pulse. You may place tourniquet over client's gown sleeve.

10 Perform venipuncture. Anchor vein below proposed insertion site by placing thumb over vein and pulling skin against the direction of insertion 1½ to 2 inches distal to the site (see illustration). Instruct client to relax hand. Avoid placing fingers above site.

Stabilize vein for needle insertion. Provides ease for needle insertion for skin puncture and then into vein.

11 Warn the client of a sharp, quick stick. Puncture skin and vein, holding catheter at a 10- to 30-degree angle (see illustration).

Superficial veins require a smaller angle. Deeper veins require a greater angle.

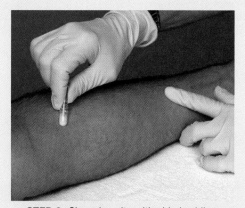

STEP 8   Cleansing site with chlorhexidine.

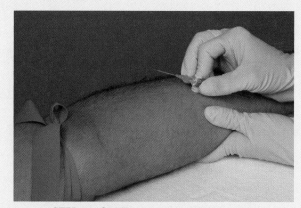

STEP 10   Stabilize vein below insertion site.

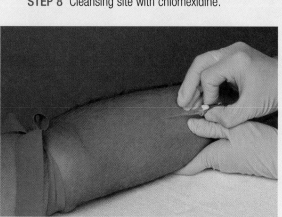

STEP 11 Puncture the vein with catheter at a 10- to 30-degree angle. Catheter enters vein.

STEPS	RATIONALE
12 Observe for a brisk, dark blood return in catheter's flashback chamber, lower catheter until almost flush with skin (see illustration), and slowly advance another ¼ inches into vein. Loosen stylet of over-the-needle catheter.	Allows for full penetration of vein wall, placement of catheter in inner lumen of vein, and easy advancement of catheter off stylet.
13 Advance catheter off stylet until catheter hub rests at venipuncture site (see illustration). Continue to hold skin taut. (If used, advance safety device on catheter by using push-tab to thread the catheter.)	Reduces risk of introduction of infectious microorganisms along catheter length.
14 Stabilize catheter with one hand and release tourniquet or blood pressure cuff with the other.	Restores blood flow to arm.
15 Apply gentle but firm pressure with index finger of nondominant hand 3 cm (1¼ inches) above insertion site (see illustration A). For the safety device, glide the catheter off the stylet while gliding the protective guard over the stylet. A click indicates device is locked over the stylet (see illustration B). (Techniques will vary with each IV device.) Remove the stylet.	Obstructs venous flow, minimizing blood loss.

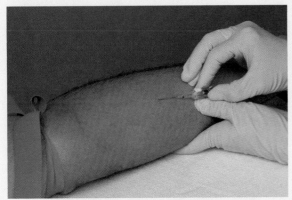

STEP 12 Blood return in flashback chamber.

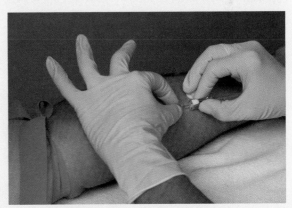

STEP 13 Advance catheter into vein.

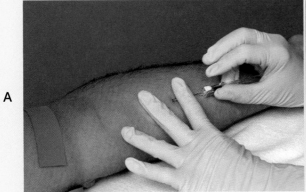

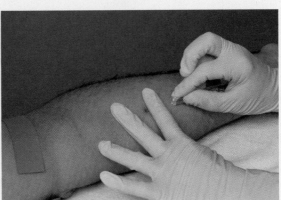

STEP 15 **A,** Apply pressure above insertion site with index finger of nondominant hand. **B,** Retract the stylet by pushing safety tab.

STEPS	RATIONALE

16 Intermittent infusion

Hold catheter firmly with dominant hand and attach sterile injection cap of prn adapter. Insert the prefilled 5-ml syringe containing flush solution into injection cap. Flush injection cap slowly with flush solution (see illustration). Withdraw syringe while still flushing or close slide clamp on extension tubing of injection cap while still flushing last 0.2 to 0.4 ml of flush.

"Positive-pressure flushing" allows fluid to displace removed needle, creates positive pressure in catheter, and prevents reflux of blood into catheter lumen. Stabilizing cannula prevents accidental withdrawal or dislodgment (INS, 2006).

17 Continuous infusion

Connect end of the IV tubing primed with fluid to catheter hub. Maintain sterile technique. Be sure connection is secure. Begin infusion by slowly opening the slide clamp or adjusting roller clamp of IV tubing.

Initiates flow of fluid through IV catheter, preventing clotting.

18 Secure catheter.

a. *Transparent dressing.* Secure catheter with nondominant hand while preparing to apply dressing.

Prevents accidental dislodgement of catheter.

b. *Gauze dressing.* Prepare a ½-inch-wide piece of sterile tape, about 4 inches long. Place sterile tape carefully under hub of catheter with adhesive side up (see illustration A). Criss-cross ends of tape over the hub (see illustration B) to make a chevron. Never apply over insertion site.

Securing the catheter and tubing prevents movement and tension on device, reducing mechanical irritation and possible phlebitis or infection. Regular adhesive tape is a potential source of pathogenic bacteria (INS, 2006). Allows easy visual inspection and recognition of complications. Taping around extremity could result in a "tourniquet effect" and impede venous return.

c. Avoid applying tape around the extremity.

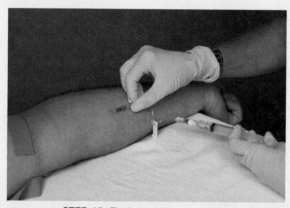

STEP 16 Flush injection cap slowly.

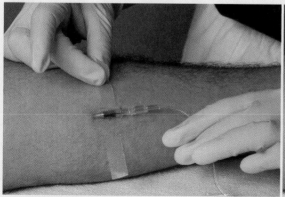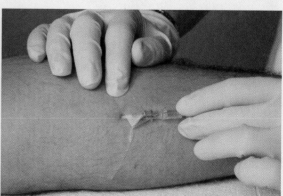

STEP 18b. **A,** Place tape under catheter hub. **B,** Criss-cross ends of tape over hub.

STEPS	RATIONALE

19 Apply sterile dressing over site.

a. *Transparent dressing:*

  (1) Carefully remove adherent backing. Apply one edge of dressing over IV site and then gently smooth remaining dressing. Leave connection between IV tubing and catheter hub uncovered (see illustration). Then remove outer covering and smooth dressing gently over site.

Transparent dressing allows continuous inspection of site, is more comfortable, and permits clients to bathe and shower without saturating dressing. Transparent dressings are occlusive to moisture and microorganisms (Hankins and others, 2004; INS, 2006).

  (2) Take a 1-inch piece of tape and place it from end of hub of catheter to insertion site, over transparent dressing (see illustration).

Gauze is less expensive than transparent dressing; may also be useful if there is bleeding from insertion site. All edges must be secured with tape to occlude air flow (Hankins and others, 2004).

> **NURSE ALERT** Insertion site should still remain visible.

  (3) Apply chevron and place only over tape, not transparent dressing (see illustration).

b. *Sterile gauze dressing:*

  (1) *Optional:* Fold 2 × 2 gauze in half and cover with a 1-inch-wide piece of tape extending about an inch from each side. Place under the tubing/catheter hub junction (see illustration).

Tape on top of tape makes it easier to access hub/tubing junction. Securing loop of tubing reduces risk of dislodging catheter from accidental pull.

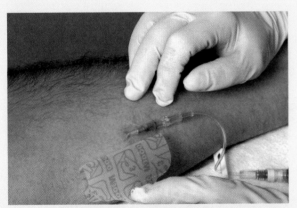

STEP 19a.(1) Apply transparent dressing.

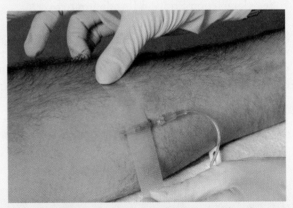

STEP 19a.(2) Place tape over transparent dressing.

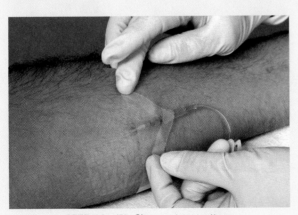

STEP 19a.(3) Chevron tape pattern.

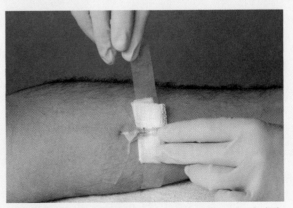

STEP 19b.(1) Place folded 2 × 2 gauze under cannula hub.

STEPS	RATIONALE

    (2) Place a 2 × 2 gauze pad over venipuncture site and catheter hub. Secure all edges with tape. Do not cover the connection between IV tubing and catheter bub (see illustration).

    (3) Curl a loop of tubing alongside the arm and place a second piece of tape directly over tubing and padded 2 × 2 (see illustration).

20 Remove and dispose of gloves.

21 Label the dressing, including the date, time, catheter gauge size and length, and nurse's initials (see illustration).

                                                   Allows for easy recognition of type of device and time interval for site rotation. INS standard for site rotation of peripheral IV access devices is every 72 to 96 hours (INS, 2006). CDC (2002) allows for replacement every 96 hours (observe agency policy).

22 Show client how to avoid placing pressure on venipuncture site and/or catheter dislodgment when attempting to reposition in bed or getting out of bed. Discuss signs and symptoms of possible infiltration or phlebitis to report (e.g., pain, swelling, burning, redness, or moisture on dressing).

23 Dispose of sheathed stylet and any uncapped sharps(s) in appropriate sharps container as soon as the device is secured.

24 See Completion Protocol (inside front cover).

NURSE ALERT If venipuncture is unsuccessful; always obtain a new catheter before a second attempt. Never reinsert the stylet (needle) into the catheter because this may damage catheter and cause catheter embolism. When the catheter is partially withdrawn through the stylet and/or reinserted, the damage can range from a small nick in the catheter to complete severing of the distal tip (INS, 2006). After a second unsuccessful attempt, ask another practitioner to perform venipuncture.

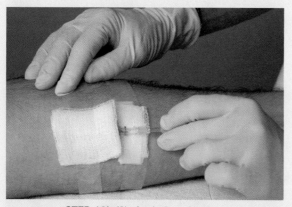

STEP 19b.(2) Apply 2 × 2 gauze.

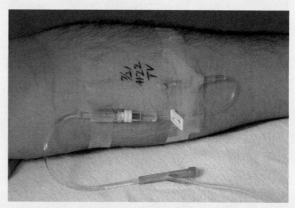

STEP 21 Label dressing.

EVALUATION

1 Observe client at least every 1 to 2 hours.

a. Check for patency of IV cannula.

b. Check that correct type/amount of IV solution has infused by comparing time tape or electronic infusion device (EID) record.

c. Count the infusion drip rate (if gravity drip) or check rate/volume on infusion pump.

2 Monitor client's (I&O), daily weights as indicated, skin turgor, mucous membranes, and vital signs for evidence of normal fluid volume.

3 Inspect client's IV site and extremity every 1 to 2 hours for the absence of pain, swelling, heat, or redness during the infusion.

TABLE 27-2	Phlebitis Scale
SCORE	**CLINICAL SIGNS**
0	No symptoms
1	Erythema at access site with or without pain
2	Pain at access site with erythema and/or edema
3	Pain at access site with erythema and/or edema
	Streak formation
	Palpable venous cord
4	Pain at access site with erythema and/or edema
	Streak formation
	Palpable venous cord >1 inch in length
	Purulent drainage

From Intravenous Nurses Society: 2006 Infusion nursing standards of practice, *J Infus Nurs* 29(1 Suppl):S1-92, 2006.

4 Ask client to describe one symptom of infiltration, phlebitis, and occluded infusion device complications (e.g., swelling, pain, tenderness, reduced flow) and to explain the action to take if such develops.

5 On completion of IV insertion and during IV infusion, ask if client is comfortable.

Unexpected Outcomes and Related Interventions

1 *Phlebitis:* Client complains of pain and tenderness at IV site with erythema at site or along path of vein. Insertion site is warm to touch, and rate of infusion may stop.

a. Stop the infusion and discontinue the IV. Restart IV if continued therapy.

b. Monitor previous site every 4 hours.

c. Document degree of phlebitis and nursing interventions per agency policy and procedure (Table 27-2).

2 *Infiltration:* Client's rate of infusion slows; insertion site is swollen, cool to touch, pale, and painful.

a. Discontinue existing IV line and restart in another site, preferably in opposite extremity.

b. Monitor previous insertion site every 4 hours until resolution of swelling.

c. Document degree of infiltration and nursing intervention (Table 27-3).

3 Infusion is completed before or after appropriate time frame.

a. Evaluate access device for position and patency; regulate remainder of infusion over prescribed time; assess need for EID (Macklin and Chernecky, 2004).

b. Monitor client with too-rapid infusion for fluid overload. Obtain vital signs, respiratory status, and I&O.

c. Notify health care provider.

5 *Positional IV infusion:* Client's flow rate is altered and changes with position of extremity.

a. Assess IV site for the need to restart the IV at another site.

b. Apply commercial protective device to protect the site (Figure 27-2).

TABLE 27-3	Infiltration Scale
GRADE	**CLINICAL CRITERIA**
0	No symptoms
1	Skin blanched
	Edema <1 inch in any direction
	Cool to touch
	With or without pain
2	Skin blanched
	Edema 1 to 6 inches on skin surface in any direction
	Cool to touch
	With or without pain
3	Skin blanched, translucent
	Gross edema >6 inches in any direction
	Cool to touch
	Mild-to-moderate pain
	Possible numbness
4	Skin blanched, translucent
	Skin tight, leaking
	Skin discolored, bruised, swollen
	Gross edema >6 inches in any direction
	Deep pitting tissue edema
	Circulatory impairment
	Moderate-to-severe pain
	Infiltration of any amount of blood product, irritant, or vesicant

From Intravenous Nurses Society: 2006 Infusion nursing standards of practice, *J Infus Nurs* 29(1 Suppl):S1-92, 2006.

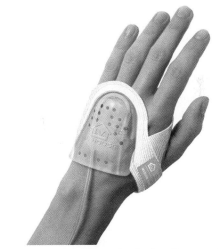

FIGURE 27-2 I.V. House Protective Device. (Courtesy I.V. House.)

c. Remove dressing, apply additional prepping agents, and resecure devices.

d. Continue hourly monitoring for proper rate of infusion.

Recording and Reporting

- Record number of attempts for insertion, type of fluid, insertion site by vessel, flow rate, size and type catheter or needle, and when infusion was begun. Use the agency's parenteral therapy flow sheet.

- Report any significant information such as infusion rate variance, positional IV site, or change in IV site due to phlebitis or infiltration.

Sample Documentation

1500 After procedure explained, site prepped with 2% chlorhexidine, left cephalic vein accessed with 20-gauge 1¼-inch Insyte catheter. Positive brisk blood return in flashback chamber after full advancement. Catheter flushed with 1 ml normal saline, and saline lock attached for IV antibiotics. Stated insertion was nonpainful and "felt fine" after insertion.

Special Considerations

Pediatric Considerations

- In addition to usual venipuncture sites, the four scalp veins and the dorsum of the foot are used in infants. Needle selection is based on age: 26 to 24 gauge for neonates; 24 to 22 gauge for children (McNally, 2005).
- Apply a Penrose drain or rubber band or use a blood pressure cuff inflated to just below the client's diastolic blood pressure. In accessing scalp veins, aim the catheter downward, toward the heart, so the flow of infusion can follow venous return (Hankins and others, 2004).

Geriatric Considerations

- Older adults arm muscles become less firm with aging. There is loss of dermal skin thickness, which leads to paper-thin skin. Anchor catheters carefully to avoid skin tear and IV infiltration. Loss of subcutaneous fat makes tendons and veins prominent. The catheter should be inserted without the use of a tourniquet if the skin is fragile and veins are visible and palpable (Otto, 2005). Place tourniquet, if used, over the client's sleeve to decrease shearing on fragile skin.

Home Care Considerations

- Ensure the client/caregiver's ability and willingness to administer and monitor IV therapy in the home. Determine if client or caregiver has the manual dexterity and cognitive ability to manage the infusion and/or seek assistance in an emergency.
- Ensure that all sharps and equipment contaminated by blood are disposed in leak-proof, puncture-resistant containers with lids.
- Ensure availability of 24-hour assistance with provider of home infusion therapy pharmaceuticals and equipment.

SKILL 27.2 Regulating Intravenous Infusion Flow Rates

- **Nursing Skills Online: IV Fluid Administration, Lesson 2**

Accurate infusion rates in IV therapy are essential to deliver infusion volumes and medications. Complications associated with IV therapy (e.g., infiltration, phlebitis, clotting of device, or circulatory overload) are reduced or eliminated with a properly regulated IV infusion. Various factors interfere with infusion rates (Table 27-4). Hourly observation of the flow rate and IV system assist in achieving the therapeutic outcome and reducing complications.

Numerous methods ensure an accurate hourly infusion rate for IV therapy. Fluids that run by gravity are adjusted through use of a flow control/regulator clamp. Fluids infused by an electronic infusion device or rate controller are regulated by a mechanical pump set at the prescribed rate. Health care providers usually order the volume of fluid a client is to receive within a specific time frame. For example, "1 L of D$_5$ NS over 8 hours." The nurse must be able to calculate hourly flow rates to ensure the prescribed amount of fluid to be infused over 8 hours. Regardless of whether gravity infusion or infusion via an electronic device is used, the nurse must assess infusion rates hourly. Infusion pumps are necessary when administering low hourly volumes (e.g., 5 ml/hr or less, 20 ml/hr) to neonatal or pediatric clients or other clients who are at increased risk for volume overload.

TABLE 27-4 Factors That Alter Intravenous Flow Rates

CLIENT FACTORS	MECHANICAL FACTORS
Change in client position	Height of parenteral container (should be higher than 36 inches [90 cm] above heart)
Flexion of involved extremity	Positional access device
Partial or complete occlusion of IV device	Viscosity or temperature of IV solution
	Occluded air vent
Venous spasm	Occluded in-line filter
Vein trauma (phlebitis)	Improperly placed restraints
Manipulated by client or visitor	Crimped administration set tubing
	Tubing dangling below bed
	Low battery of an electronic device

IV, Intravenous.

In addition, when infusing high volumes of IV fluids (more than 150 ml/hr) to clients with impaired renal clearance, older adults, or pediatric clients, or when infusing drugs or IV fluids that require specific hourly volumes, electronic infusion pumps permit accurate, on-time infusion. EIDs deliver the infusion via positive pressure. A rate controller used on gravity infusions regulates the infusion but, unlike the electronic pump, can be affected by many mechanical

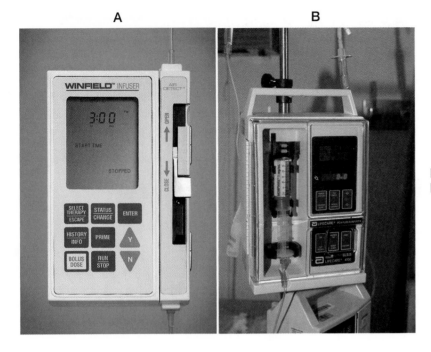

FIGURE 27-3 A, Electronic infusion device. **B,** Patient-controlled analgesia infusion pump.

and client factors. Recent advances in infusion technology have resulted in a variety of devices available for use to ensure accurate delivery (Macklin and Chernecky, 2004).

Many devices have operating and programming capabilities that allow for single- and multiple-solution infusions at different rates (Figure 27-3, A). A variety of detectors and alarms respond to air in IV lines, completion of infusion, high and low pressure, low battery power, occlusion, and the inability to deliver at a preset rate. An anti–free flow safeguard (preventing bolus infusion in the event of machine malfunction) is an important element of an electronic infusion pump. Know and follow the agency and manufacturer's recommendations for selecting infusion pump controls: infusion volume, rate, alarm settings, and or pump malfunction.

Clients in alternative care settings achieve infusion accuracy with ambulatory infusion pumps. Most pumps weigh less than 6 pounds and range from palm size to backpack size. They function on battery power, allowing the client freedom to return to normal life. Programming capabilities include automatic rate adjustments, remote site adjustments via a telephone modem, and therapy-specific settings such as patient-controlled analgesia (Figure 27-3, B). Follow the manufacturer's recommendations for specific device features.

ASSESSMENT

1 Verify provider's order in client's medical record for client's name and correct solution: type, volume, additives, rate, and duration of IV fluid order. Apply the six rights of medication administration. *Rationale: Ensures that correct IV fluid is administered (Ketchum, 2005).*

2 Assess client's knowledge of how positioning of IV site affects flow rate.

3 Inspect IV site, verify patency, and verify with client how the site feels (e.g., determine if there is pain, burning or tenderness at site. *Rationale: Pain or burning may be early indicators for phlebitis.*

4 Identify client's risk for fluid imbalance (e.g., child, older adult, history of heart, renal or respiratory disease; electrolyte imbalance). *Rationale: Strict infusion volume control will be required.*

PLANNING

Expected Outcomes focus on normal fluid and electrolyte balance and administration of IV fluids at the prescribed rate and correct dosage.

1 Client receives prescribed volume of fluid/medication over desired time interval.

2 Serum electrolytes remain within normal limits.

Delegation Considerations

The skill of regulating IV flow rates may not be delegated. The nurse directs personnel to report:

- Delayed or sudden emptying of IV bag.
- Sounding of the alarm on the infusion pump.
- Client complaints of burning, bleeding, or swelling at IV site.

Equipment

- Watch with a second hand
- Calculator, paper, and pencil
- Tape
- Label
- IV regulating device: EID (optional); volume control device (optional)

IMPLEMENTATION *for Regulating Intravenous Infusion Flow Rates*

STEPS	RATIONALE

1 See Standard Protocol (inside front cover).

2 Check the client's identification: ask name and client identification number on ID bracelet. Use two identifiers.

Ensures correct client is receiving correct IV fluids. At least two identifiers, neither of which is the client's room number, are used (JCAHO, 2006).

3 Obtain IV fluid and appropriate tubing and know calibration (drop factor) in drops per milliliter (gtts/ml) of infusion set used by agency:

Use of correct tubing ensures more accurate infusion delivery. Macrodrip tubing allows for higher infusion volumes.

a. *Macrodrip:* Used to deliver rate *greater than* 100 ml/hr. (Drip factor is 10 to 20 gtts/ml, depending on equipment used. Drop factor is printed on box.) For example:

> Travenol Laboratories: 10 gtts/ml
> Abbott Laboratories: 15 gtts/ml
> McGraw Laboratories: 15 gtts/ml

b. *Microdrip:* Used to deliver rates *less than* 100 ml/hr. Microdrip: 60 gtts/ml

Microdrip tubing is used for slow delivery and smaller volumes.

4 Calculate desired flow rate (hourly volume) of prescribed infusion:

$$\text{Flow rate (ml/hr)} = \frac{\text{Total infusion (ml)}}{\text{hours of infusion}}$$

Example: 1000 ml/8 hr = 125 ml/hr

5 Calculate the drop rate based on drops per minute.

$$\frac{\text{gtts factor}}{60} \times \frac{\text{flow rate}}{1} = \text{drop rate}$$

Example: infuse 120 ml/hr via 10 gtts/ml drop factor:

$$\frac{10}{60} \times \frac{120}{1} = 20 \text{ gtts/min}$$

Via 15 gtts/ml:

$$\frac{15}{60} \times \frac{120}{1} = 30 \text{ gtts/min}$$

Via 20 gtts/ml:

$$\frac{20}{60} \times \frac{120}{1} = 40 \text{ gtts/min}$$

Via 60 gtts/ml (microgtts):

$$\frac{60}{60} \times \frac{120}{1} = 120 \text{ gtts/min}$$

6 Time-tape the IV bottle or bag by securing marked adhesive tape or fluid indicator tape along side of fluid container (see illustration). Document each IV fluid bag sequentially and note type of fluid, client's name, infusion span, and beginning and expected end of infusion.

Gives a visual scale to assess progress of infusion hourly. Avoid use of felt-tip pens or permanent markers on plastic bag; these can contaminate IV solutions. In some agencies all fluids, including those on pumps, should be labeled and time-taped (follow agency policy).

7 Close rate-controlling clamp on IV tubing.

8 Insert infusion set into fluid bag: remove protective cover from IV bag port without touching opening, remove cap from spike and insert spike into port of IV bag, being careful not to puncture side of opening (see illustration). Hang bag from IV pole.

Maintains sterility of solution.

STEPS	RATIONALE
9 Fill drip chamber of tubing until half full by gently squeezing and releasing (see illustration).	Creates vacuum, allowing fluid to enter drip chamber.
10 Open rate-controlling clamp and slowly fill remainder of tubing (see illustration). Invert Y connector sites to displace air. Most tubings can be fully filled or primed without removing the cover on the end of the IV tubing. Tap on the Y-connector to displace the air.	Tubing must be fully filled with fluid before connecting to client to avoid air embolus. Too-rapid filling promotes development of tiny air bubbles within tubing.
11 Close rate-controlling clamp on tubing.	

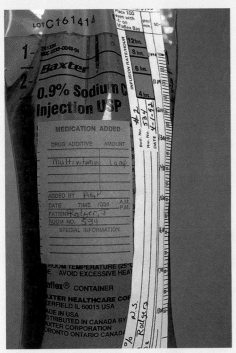

STEP 6 IV bag with time tape.

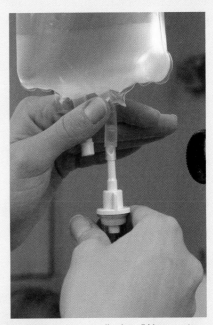

STEP 8 Insert spike into IV bag port.

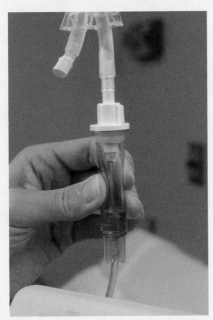

STEP 9 Squeeze drip chamber. Release as chamber fills.

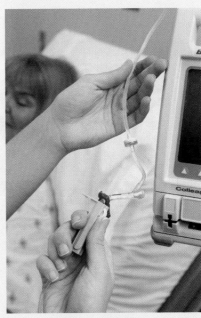

STEP 10 Open rate-controlling clamp to fill tubing.

STEPS	RATIONALE

12 Perform venipuncture (see Skill 27.1) and attach catheter to end of IV tubing or connect end of IV tubing to existing IV catheter (Skill 27.3), maintaining sterility.

13 With IV fluid bag a minimum of 36 inches (90 cm) above IV insertion site, adjust rate-controlling clamp to deliver drops per minute. *Optional:* A dial-a-flow device may be attached to IV tubing to regulate flow rate (see illustration).

Fluid container heights of 36 to 48 inches usually are sufficient to overcome venous pressure and other resistance from tubing and catheter (INS, 2006).

If an EID is used for infusion, do not use a dial-a-flow device, to prevent a disruption of EID flow mechanism.

14 *Optional:* Attach to EID or rate controller.

a. Place electronic eye on half-filled drip chamber below origin of drop and above fluid line if required (see illustration). NOTE: Some devices do not use an electronic eye.

Positioning necessary for accurate drip count.

b. Insert IV tubing into chamber of control mechanism (see illustration). (Consult manufacturer's instructions for use of pump.)

Pump chamber moves fluid through IV tubing.

c. Secure portion of IV tubing through "air in line" alarm system.

Allows for detection of air in tubing, which can enter vascular system, causing an embolus.

d. Close door to control chamber. Turn on pump and select rate per hour and total volume to be infused (see illustration).

Follow pump instructions. Ensures that correct volume will be administered.

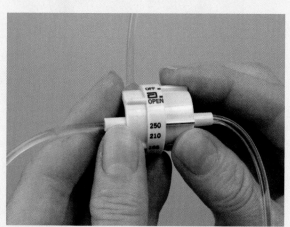

STEP 13 Dial-a-flow device.

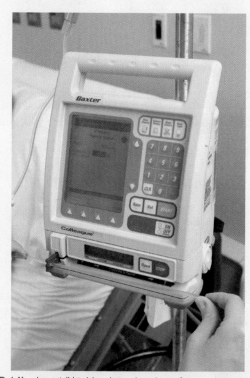

STEP 14b. Insert IV tubing into chamber of control mechanism.

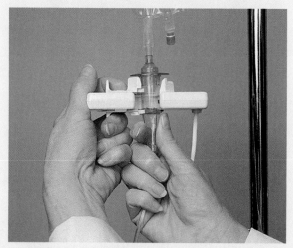

STEP 14a. Electronic eye placed over drip chamber.

STEPS	RATIONALE
e. Open rate-controlling clamp on tubing if closed, and press start button (see illustration).	Rate control clamp should be open completely while infusion controller or pump is in use to ensure accurate volume of infusion.
f. Monitor infusion on a scheduled frequency to assess patency of system when in alarm mode and monitor for proper infusion rate and infiltration.	
15 *Optional:* Attach IV tubing to volume control device.	
a. Place volume control device between IV bag and insertion spike of infusion set using sterile technique (see illustration).	Delivers small volume but must be refilled as it empties.

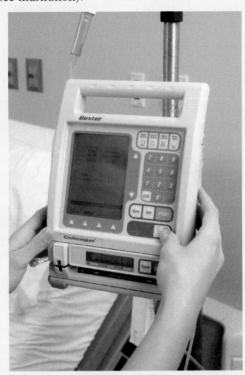

STEP 14d. Select rate and volume to be infused.

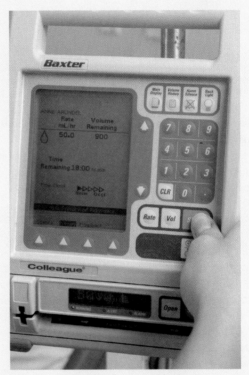

STEP 14e. Press start button.

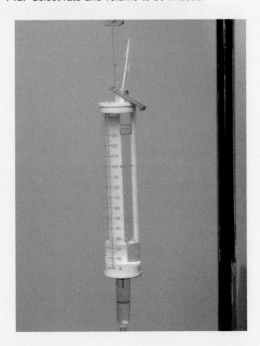

STEP 15a. Volume control device between IV bag and infusion tubing.

STEPS	RATIONALE
b. Fill IV tubing with fluid by opening regulator clamp.	
c. Place 2 hours of fluid allotment in chamber device.	This prevents infusion from running dry if 60 minutes elapse before nurse returns. Should infusion rate accidentally increase, will only allow 2 hours of fluids to infuse.
16 Instruct client about the following:	
a. To avoid raising hand or arm to a position that will affect flow rate.	Instruction informs client on how to protect IV site and importance of not altering rate control
b. To avoid manipulation of rate control clamp.	
c. Purpose and significance of alarms.	
17 See Completion Protocol (inside front cover).	

EVALUATION

1 Monitor IV infusion at least every 1 to 2 hours, noting volume of IV fluid infused and rate.
2 Observe client and monitor client's laboratory values for signs of fluid and electrolyte imbalance.
3 Observe for signs of infiltration, inflammation at site, clot in catheter, kink or knot in infusion tubing, and/or infusion pump malfunction.

Unexpected Outcomes and Related Interventions

1 Sudden infusion of large fluid volume of solution occurs with client having symptoms of dyspnea, crackles in lung, and increased urine output, indicating fluid overload.
a. Temporarily slow the infusion rate to 10 drops per minute and notify the health care provider.
b. Place client in high-Fowler's position; client may require diuretics.
c. New IV orders will be required.
2 The IV infusion is slower than prescribed.
a. Assess client for positional change that might affect rate, such as IV catheter or tubing obstruction.
b. If volume is deficient, consult with health care provider for new prescribed order to provide required volume.

Recording and Reporting

- Record rate of infusion, drops per minute, and ml/hr in client's medical record; any ordered change in fluid rates; and use of any EID or controlling device.
- At the change of shift or break time, report rate of infusion to nurse in charge or next nurse assigned to care for client.

Sample Documentation

1700 Complaining of SOB. HOB elevated. Lungs auscultated with inspiratory crackles bilaterally. Dr. Lee notified. Order noted to decrease IV to 25 ml/hr. Positive brisk, dark blood return noted via 20-gauge IV right cephalic vein. Changed to IMED Gemini infusion pump at 25 ml/hr. Purpose of fluid restriction and symptoms of pulmonary edema reviewed with client and wife, who verbalized understanding. O₂ at 4 L/min per nasal prongs applied.

Special Considerations
Pediatric Considerations

- Children are not small adults. Physiological differences must be remembered, particularly focusing on total body weight (85% to 90% water). Dehydration is a common cause of fluid and electrolyte imbalance; assessment of fluid needs includes meter-squared, weight, or caloric method (Otto, 2005).
- Containers exceeding 150 ml should not be connected to children younger than 2 years of age; no more than 250 ml for children younger than 5 years; and no more than 500 ml for children younger than 10 years. ALWAYS use tamper-resistant volume-controlled infusion pumps to ensure accurate fluid delivery.

Geriatric Considerations

- Common alterations in fluid and electrolytes affecting the cardiovascular client include hypovolemia, potassium and calcium imbalance, heart failure, and arrhythmias.
- Use an EID with microdrip tubing. Carefully monitor the client's clinical status, laboratory results, vital signs, weight gain or loss, and I&O (Otto, 2005).
- Dextrose infused too rapidly may cause cerebral edema more readily in older clients. normal saline given to an older client with impaired renal function can cause hypernatremia (Otto, 2005).

Home Care Considerations

- Ensure that client/caregiver is able and willing to operate the ambulatory infusion pump. Assess any physical or visual limitations with ability to connect/disconnect infusion therapy and problem solve pump malfunction (Cox and others, 2005).
- The nurse should be in the home during initiation of IV therapy to ensure correct pump settings regarding solution, rate, time, and alarms.
- Provide telephone numbers for 24-hour service and emergencies with written instructions regarding infusion procedure and pump use.

SKILL 27.3   Maintenance of Intravenous Site and Removal of IV Access

- Nursing Skills Online: IV Fluid Therapy Management, Lessons 3 and 4
- Nursing Skills Online: IV Fluid Administration, Lesson 3

Peripheral IV catheters and infusion therapy are frequently associated with complications such as local or systemic infections, phlebitis, and infiltration. Appropriate management of IV sites will prevent or minimize these complications (Nakazawa, 2005).

The skin insertion site is the most common source of colonization and infection for vascular catheters (Hadaway, 2005a). Therefore catheter dressings must be securely applied and changed when loose, wet, or soiled. A transparent membrane dressing or sterile gauze secured with tape is used to cover the site (Curchoe, 2002). A transparent dressing is changed with catheter site rotation and immediately if integrity of dressing is compromised (Masooli, 2005a). Gauze dressings are changed every 48 hours and immediately if integrity is compromised. When gauze is used in conjunction with transparent dressing, it is considered a gauze dressing and changed every 48 hours (INS, 2006; CDC, 2002).

Fluid containers include plastic bags, plastic bottles, and glass bottles. These containers are changed frequently, depending on the rate of infusion and the volume in the container (Gillies, 2004). The CDC (2002) does not make a recommendation for the hang time of IV fluids, but the INS recommends that each container be changed within 24 hours after the administration set is added (INS, 2006). Fluid containers on ambulatory infusion devices may remain longer than 24 hours if aseptic technique is used, the system remains closed without injection ports or add-on tubing, and the medication is stable for the anticipated infusion time (Hankins and others, 2004; INS, 2006). Always allow adequate time for this procedure, follow proper technique to prevent infection, and adhere to the specific agency policy (Rickard, 2004).

Changing infusion tubing is much simpler and more efficient if changed when hanging a new fluid container. The CDC (2002) recommends changing tubing no more frequently than every 96 hours. The INS (2006) recommends 72-96-hour intervals for continuous tubing changes, adding that 48-hour tubing changes may be considered if the rate of catheter-related infection and phlebitis in an institution exceeds 5%. The INS also recommends changing tubing used for intermittent infusion through an injection/access port every 24 hours because both ends of this tubing are manipulated more frequently than tubing used for continuous infusion. The CDC has no recommendation for changing of intermittent tubing.

An injection cap or prn adapter on a peripheral catheter is used to administer IV fluids or medications intermittently.

Change the injection cap when the catheter is changed. A short extension tubing or loop may be placed between the catheter hub and injection cap, which allows manipulation of the injection cap without movement of the catheter. This extension tubing remains attached to the peripheral catheter and is changed when the catheter is changed. For midline and central venous catheters, these caps should be changed at least every 7 days (INS, 2006). The fluid pathway and capped ends on all infusion tubing, stopcocks, extension tubing, and injection caps are sterile. The nurse must exercise caution to prevent contamination of these surfaces during changes (INS, 2005).

You may need to assist the client with many aspects of hygiene, such as gown changes, while the client is receiving IV therapy. Gowns with snaps across the shoulders are best, especially for multiple infusions. When using a regular gown or the client's clothing, thread the fluid container and tubing through the sleeve of the gown in the same manner as the client's arm. Infusion tubing is *never* disconnected to change a gown or any article of clothing. Coordinate care so that bathing or hygiene activities are done after removal of an old infusion site and before another venipuncture is made.

ASSESSMENT

1   Changing a peripheral IV dressing:
a. Determine when the dressing was last changed by checking the dressing label. *Rationale: This labeling provides instant identification for assessing and determining status of the site (Jones, 2004).*
b. Observe present dressing for moisture and occlusiveness. Determine if moisture is from leakage from the puncture site or from an external source. *Rationale: A soiled or wet dressing should be changed immediately.*
c. Observe IV system for proper functioning or complications (tubing or catheter kinks). Palpate the catheter site through the intact dressing for complaints of tenderness, pain, or burning. *Rationale: Unexplained decrease in flow rate may indicate problems with catheter placement or patency. Pain is associated with phlebitis and infiltration.*
d. Inspect exposed catheter site for swelling, redness, drainage, or blanching. *Rationale: Signs are indicative of phlebitis or infiltration.*
e. Monitor body temperature. *Rationale: Rise in body temperature could be sign of infection at IV site.*
f. Determine client understanding of the need for continued IV infusion.
2   Changing infusion tubing:
a. Determine when new infusion set is needed (e.g., according to agency policy or after contamination or puncture of infusion tubing). *Rationale: CDC (2002) and the INS (2006) recommend tubing changes every 72 to 96 hours.*

b. Observe for occlusions in tubing such as kinking, drug or mineral precipitate, and blood. *Rationale: Infusion of incompatible medications can lead to precipitate formation. Blood may flow retrograde from vein and adhere to tubing. Infusion of viscous blood components may cause adherence to walls of tubing and decrease size of lumen.*

c. Determine client's understanding of the need for continued IV infusions.

3 Changing infusion solution:

a. Verify prescriber's original order. Check client's name, intravenous solution name and any medication additives and dose, rate, route, and time of administration. *Rationale: The original order is the more reliable source of infusion and medication information. Review ensures safe and correct administration of IV therapy by verifying order.*

> **NURSE ALERT** If an order is written for KVO, contact the health care provider for clarification of solution and the rate of infusion (INS, 2006).

b. Determine the compatibility of all IV fluids and additives by consulting appropriate literature or the pharmacy. *Rationale: Patency of the inside of catheter depends on prevention of chemical interactions. Precipitation can occur because of concentration of drugs in solution. When pH changes by contact between solutions or medications, a precipitate can occur (Otto, 2005).*

c. Determine client's understanding of need for continuing IV therapy.

d. Verify patency of current IV access site. Carefully adjust roller clamp to see an increase in flow rate and then regulate back to ordered rate. Lowering IV container below level of IV site for blood return is an unreliable indicator. *Rationale: If patency is not verified, a new IV access site may be needed.*

e. Palpate site for swelling, coolness, or tenderness around IV site. *Rationale: These symptoms are consistent with infiltration.*

4 Discontinuing IV medications:

a. Observe fluid container for complete infusion of all medication.

b. Review care plan for any blood samples required after medication infusion. *Rationale: Monitoring of serum concentrations of some IV medications is required to avoid reaching toxic levels. Dosage adjustments or alterations of timing for next dose may be required (observe agency policy).*

5 Discontinuing peripheral IV access:

a. Observe existing IV site for signs and symptoms of infection, infiltration, or phlebitis (see Tables 27-2 and 27-3). *Rationale: Indications for discontinuing IV.*

b. Review physician's order for discontinuation of IV therapy. *Rationale: Health care provider order is required to discontinue IV therapy. The specific wording may not include removal of the catheter, but this is implied.*

PLANNING

Expected Outcomes focus on reducing the risk of infection and phlebitis, minimizing client discomfort, reducing risk of overhydration, and maintaining a patent IV catheter.

1 IV site will remain free of infection, redness, swelling, pain, or exudate.

2 Client's IV catheter and tubing will be patent.

3 IV solution is correct.

4 IV will be removed with minimal trauma to client.

5 Client's temperature remains normal.

Delegation Considerations

The skills of maintaining an IV site may not be delegated. The nurse directs personnel by:

- Explaining appropriate position for client to maintain to avoid injury at insertion site.
- Instructing staff to observe changes in client's temperature, pain, and tenderness at IV site and report back to the nurse.

Equipment

Changing a Peripheral IV Dressing

- Antiseptic swabs (2% chlorhexidine, 70% alcohol, povidone-iodine)
- Skin protectant solution
- Adhesive remover (optional)
- Clean gloves
- Strips of sterile, precut tape (or 36-inch roll of tape)
- Transparent dressing or sterile 2 × 2 gauze pads and tape
- Arm board or commercially available IV site protector (optional)

Changing Infusion Tubing

- Clean gloves
- Sterile 2 × 2 gauze pads (optional)
- If a new IV dressing must be applied, assemble additional equipment (see Skill 27.2).

Continuous infusion:

- Microdrip or macrodrip infusion tubing, as appropriate
- 0.22-μ filter and extension tubing if necessary
- Tubing label

Intermittent saline/heparin lock:

- 5-ml syringe filled with normal saline or heparin flush solution (observe agency policy)
- Loop or short extension tubing (if necessary), injection cap or prn adapter
- Antiseptic swab

Changing Infusion Container

- Bottle/bag of IV solution as ordered by physician or appropriate prescriber
- Time tape
- Pen

Discontinuing IV Medications

- Clean gloves
- Sterile 2 × 2 or 4 × 4 gauze sponge

- 5-ml syringe filled with normal saline or heparin flush solution (follow agency policy)
- 10-ml syringe filled with normal saline or heparin flush solution (follow agency policy)
- Antiseptic swabs
- Injection cap replacement (if needed)

Discontinuing Peripheral IV Access
- Clean gloves
- Sterile 2 × 2 or 4 × 4 gauze pad
- Tape
- Antiseptic swab

IMPLEMENTATION *for Maintenance of Intravenous Site and Removal of IV Access*

STEPS	RATIONALE
1 See Standard Protocol (inside front cover).	
2 Changing peripheral IV dressing	
a. Remove any overlying tape. Then remove transparent membrane dressing by picking up one corner and pulling the side laterally while holding catheter hub. Repeat for other side. *Or*	Technique minimizes discomfort during removal. Use alcohol swab on transparent dressing next to client's skin to loosen dressing.
b. Remove gauze dressing and tape from old dressing one layer at a time by pulling toward the insertion site. Leave chevron tape securing catheter to skin (follow agency policy).	Prevents accidental catheter displacement.
c. Observe insertion site for redness, swelling, tenderness, exudate, pallor, or pain. If present, discontinue infusion (Step 6).	Catheter moved during dressing change could accidentally dislodge and puncture blood vessel.
d. Have tape prepared for use. If IV is infusing properly, gently remove tape securing catheter. Stabilize cannula with one finger. Use adhesive remover to cleanse skin and remove adhesive residue, if necessary.	Exposes venipuncture site and prevents accidental displacement of cannula. Adhesive residue decreases ability of new tape to adhere securely to the skin.
e. Cleanse insertion site with antiseptic using friction in a horizontal plane, then in a vertical plane, followed with a circular motion, moving from insertion site outward (see illustration). Allow antiseptic solution to dry completely.	Friction in this pattern allows penetration of antiseptic into epidermal layer of skin (Crosby and Manes, 2001). Antimicrobial solutions should be allowed to air-dry completely to effectively reduce microbial counts (INS, 2006). If antiseptic agents are used in combination, allow each to air-dry separately.
f. *Optional:* Apply skin protectant solution such as Skin Prep or No Sting Barrier Film to the area where the tape or dressing will be applied. Allow to dry.	Coats the skin with protective solution to maintain skin integrity, prevents irritation from the adhesive, and promotes adhesion of the dressing.

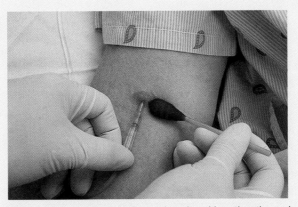

STEP 2e. Cleanse peripheral insertion site with antiseptic swab.

STEPS	RATIONALE
g. Tape or secure catheter	Prevents accidental catheter dislodgment.
(1) Transparent dressing: Secure catheter with non-dominant hand while preparing to apply dressing.	
(2) Gauze dressing: Place a narrow piece (½ inch) of tape under cannula hub with adhesive side up; cross tape over hub to make a chevron. Place tape on the cannula, never over the insertion site.	Chevron secures cannula.
h. Apply sterile dressing over site.	
(1) *Transparent dressing:*	Transparent dressing allows inspection of site.
(a) Carefully remove adherent backing and apply one edge of dressing and then gently smooth remaining dressing over IV site. Leave connection between IV tubing and catheter hub uncovered. Remove outer covering; smooth dressing over site.	Access to catheter hub is needed in times of emergency and when changing tubing.
(b) Take a 1-inch piece of tape and place it from end of catheter hub to insertion site, over transparent dressing. Apply chevron and place only over tape, not transparent dressing (see Skill 27.1, p. 603).	
(2) *Gauze dressing:*	
(a) *Optional:* Fold 2 × 2 gauze in half and cover with 1-inch-wide piece of tape extending about an inch from each side of gauze. Place under the tubing/catheter hub junction.	Gauze prevents pressure of cannula hub against skin. Securing loop of tubing reduces risk of dislodging catheter from accidental pull.
(b) Place another 2 × 2 gauze over venipuncture site and catheter hub. Secure all edges with tape. Do not cover the connection between IV tubing and catheter hub with the dressing.	Gauze dressings must be occlusive to prevent air flow (Hankins and others, 2004). Access to catheter hub is needed in times of emergency and when changing tubing.
(c) Curl a loop of tubing alongside the outside of the arm, and place a second piece of tape directly over tubing and padded 2 × 2 gauze.	
i. *Optional:* Apply short arm board or commercial protective device if venipuncture site or dressing is affected by the motion of the wrist.	Reduces the risk of phlebitis and infiltration from motion of the joint.
j. Anchor IV tubing with additional pieces of tape if needed. When using transparent dressing, avoid placing tape over dressing.	
k. Label the dressing with date and time of insertion, date and time of dressing change, gauge and length of catheter, and identification of nurse.	Allows easy recognition of type of device and time interval for site rotation.
3 Changing infusion tubing	
a. Open new infusion set and connect add-on pieces such as filters or extension tubing. Keep protective covering over spike and distal adapter. Secure all. Avoid the use of tape.	Separation of infusion tubing increases the risk of air emboli, hemorrhage, and infection. Protective covers reduce entrance of microorganisms.
b. If catheter hub is not visible, remove IV dressing. Do not remove tape securing catheter to skin (if gauze dressing was used).	Movement of catheter may cause it to dislodge.

NURSE ALERT If transparent dressing has to be removed, place small piece of sterile tape across hub to temporarily anchor catheter during disconnection.

STEPS	RATIONALE
c. For continuous IV infusion:	
(1) Move roller clamp to off position of new tubing.	
(2) Slow rate of infusion to existing IV rate by regulating roller clamp on old tubing.	
(3) Compress and fill drip chamber of old tubing.	Ensures fluid chamber remains full until new tubing is changed.
(4) Remove old tubing from IV container. *Optional:* Tape old drip chamber to IV pole without contaminating spike.	Fluid in drip chamber will run slowly to keep catheter patent.
(5) Place insertion spike of new tubing into old fluid container opening. Hang container on IV pole, compress and release drip chamber on new tubing, and fill drip chamber one-third to one-half full.	Permits drip chamber to fill and promotes rapid, smooth flow of solution through tubing.
(6) Slowly open roller clamp, remove protective cap from adapter (if necessary), and flush new tubing with solution. Stop infusion and replace cap. Place end of adapter near client's IV site.	Removes air from tubing and replaces it with fluid. Position equipment for quick, smooth connection of new tubing.
(7) Turn roller clamp on old tubing to "off" position.	Prevents spillage of fluid.
d. For saline/heparin lock	
(1) If a loop or short extension tubing is needed because of an awkward IV site placement, use sterile technique to connect the new injection cap to the loop or tubing.	
(2) Swab injection cap with antiseptic swab. Insert syringe with 1 to 3 ml of saline or heparin flush solution and inject through the injection cap into the loop of short extension tubing.	Maintains patency of lock.
e. *Optional:* Place 2 × 2 gauze under catheter hub.	Prevents tubing from accidentally contacting skin and collects blood that may leak from catheter hub.
f. Stabilize hub of catheter with nondominant hand and apply pressure over vein just above catheter tip (at least 1½ inches above insertion site). Gently disconnect old tubing from catheter hub and quickly insert adapter of new tubing or saline lock into catheter hub (see illustrations).	Minimizes loss of blood as tubing is changed.
g. For continuous infusion, open roller clamp on new tubing, allowing solution to run rapidly for 30 to 60 seconds, and then regulate IV drip rate (see illustration).	Clears catheter of any blood in lumen, preventing occlusion.
h. Attach a piece of tape or a preprinted label with date and time of tubing change onto tubing below the drip chamber.	Provides reference to determine next time for tubing change.
i. Form a loop of tubing and secure it to client's arm with a strip of tape.	
j. Remove and discard 2 × 2 gauze (if used) and old IV tubing. If necessary, apply new dressing (see Step 2).	Avoids accidental pulling against site and catheter movement.
4 Changing fluid container	
a. Prepare next solution at least 1 hour before needed. If prepared in pharmacy, be sure it has been delivered to the client's location. Review prescriber's order. Ensure that the solution is correct and properly labeled. Follow six rights of drug administration. Verify solution expiration date. Observe for precipitate and discoloration.	Ensures no disruption in fluid therapy to client.
b. Check client's identification using two identifiers.	Ensures correct client is receiving correct IV fluids.

STEPS	RATIONALE
c. Change solution when fluid remains only in neck of container or when new type of solution has been ordered.	Prevents waste of solution.
d. Move roller clamp to stop flow rate, and remove old IV fluid container from IV pole.	

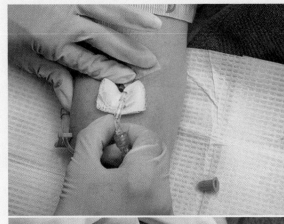

A

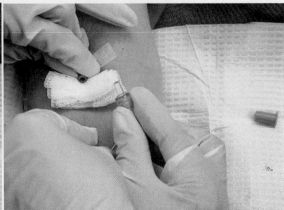

B

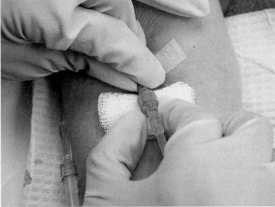

C

STEP 3f. A, Disconnect old tubing. **B,** While compressing vein, attach end of new tubing. **C,** Ensure that connection is connected and secure.

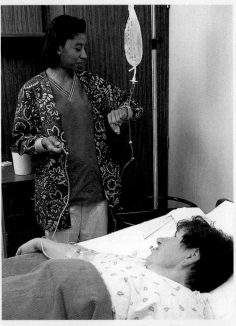

STEP 3g. Regulate flow of IV.

STEPS	RATIONALE

e. Quickly remove spike from old container, and without touching tip, insert spike into new container.

Maintains sterility of solution and reduces risk of solution in drip chamber running dry.

> **NURSE ALERT** If spike is contaminated, a new IV tubing set is required. Sterile IV tubing may be used for 72 hours unless compromised.

f. Hang new bag or bottle of solution on IV pole.

g. Check for air in tubing. If bubbles form, they can be removed by closing the roller clamp, stretching the tubing downward, and tapping the tubing with the finger (the bubbles rise in the tubing to the drip chamber) (see illustration). For larger amounts of air, swab port with antiseptic swab, allow to dry, connect a syringe to an injection port below the air, and aspirate the air into the syringe.

Infusion of air in tubing can result in air embolus, which can be fatal to client.

> **COMMUNICATION TIP** Tell client the "champagne type of bubbles" inside the tubing are not a problem.

h. Make sure drip chamber is one-third to one-half full. If drip chamber is too full, pinch off tubing below the drip chamber, invert the container, squeeze the drip chamber, hang container, and release the tubing (see illustration).

If chamber is completely filled, nurse cannot observe drip rate.

i. Regulate flow to prescribed rate.

j. Place time label on the side of container and label with the time hung, the time of completion, and appropriate interval. If using plastic bags, mark only on the label and not the container.

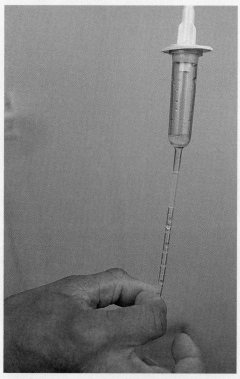

STEP 4g. Remove air bubbles from tubing.

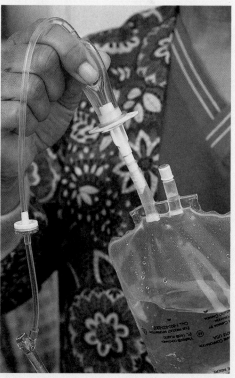

STEP 4h. Remove excess fluid from drip chamber.

STEPS	RATIONALE

5 Discontinuing IV medications

a. 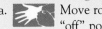 Move roller clamp on infusion tubing to the "off" position. — Prevents spillage of fluid.

b. Remove any clasping devices and disconnect medication delivery tubing from injection port.

> **NURSE ALERT** If the tubing spike, connector end, fluid pathway, or fluid container is contaminated, a new tubing set or fluid container is required.

c. Remove the needle or needleless adapter on the infusion tubing; discard appropriately in receptacle and replace with a sterile cap or cover, as required. — Infusion tubing can be reused with next ordered medication.

d. Swab injection port or prn adapter on main IV tubing with antiseptic swab (see illustration). — Ensures sterility of port.

e. For intermittent medication piggybacked into a continuous infusion, attach 5-ml saline-filled syringe to injection port and flush the line gently. Regulate fluid flow of the continuous infusion as ordered. — Saline flush prevents incompatible medications from coming into contact in the infusion tubing. There is no way to know how much pressure is exerted inside catheter lumen (Hadaway, 2005a). A 5-ml syringe generates less pressure than a 3-ml syringe. Do not force irrigation if resistance is felt.

f. For intermittent medications through a saline or heparin lock, attach saline-filled 5- to 10-ml syringe to injection port and flush catheter gently, or attach heparin flush solution-filled syringe to injection port and flush gently, if necessary (follow agency policy). Attach sterile injection port cover, if necessary. — Flushing with 3 to 10 ml of saline after each medication is crucial. Volume of flush depends on lumen size, catheter length, and medication infused (Hadaway, 2006).

> **NURSE ALERT** Flushing of any IV catheter must be approached carefully. If resistance is met, first assess mechanical causes (e.g., closed clamps, kinked tubing, and extremity position). Never forcefully attempt to flush. Fibrin formation, drug precipitates, and blood clots can occlude catheter lumen. Forceful flush against these occlusions can cause fracture of catheter and possible embolization. Size of syringe used for flushing should be in accordance with manufacturer's guidelines for pounds per square inch (INS, 2006).

g. Prepare client for obtaining blood samples after medication infusion, if necessary.

6 Discontinuing peripheral IV access

a. Explain procedure to client. Explain to client to hold the affected extremity still during cannula/needle removal. — Minimizes client's anxiety and discomfort.

b. Turn IV tubing roller clamp to "off" position. Remove tape securing tubing.

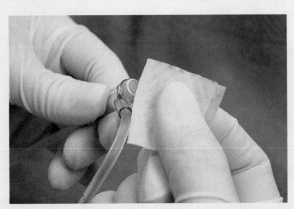

STEP 5d. Cleanse injection port.

STEPS	RATIONALE

c. Remove IV site dressing and tape while stabilizing catheter.

Movement of catheter will cause discomfort.

> **NURSE ALERT** Never use scissors to remove the tape or dressing because the catheter could accidentally be cut.

d. With dry gauze or alcohol swab held above site, apply light pressure and withdraw the catheter, using a slow, steady movement, keeping the hub parallel to the skin (see illustration).

Changing the angle of the catheter inside the vein could cause additional vein irritation, increasing the risk of post infusion phlebitis.

e. Apply pressure to the site for 2 to 3 minutes, using a dry, sterile gauze pad. Secure with tape. NOTE: More time is necessary if client is on anticoagulants.

Dry pad causes less irritation to the puncture site. Subcutaneous hematoma is a common complication. When needle is removed, vein wall contracts to stop bleeding. Contraction is enhanced by pressure to the site for at least 2 to 3 minutes (Otto, 2005). Anticoagulants increase clotting time.

f. Inspect the catheter for intactness, noting tip integrity and length.

Tips of catheter can break off, causing an embolus and emergency situation. Notify physician if tip is sheared or broken.

g. Instruct client to report any redness, pain, drainage, or swelling that may occur after catheter removal.

Post infusion phlebitis may occur within 48 to 96 hours after catheter removal.

7 See Completion Protocol (inside front cover).

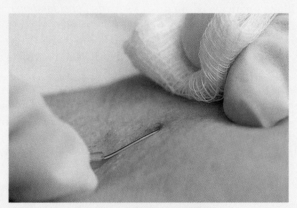

STEP 6d. Withdraw IV catheter.

EVALUATION

Changing Peripheral IV Dressing
1 Observe functioning, patency of IV system, and flow rate after changing dressing.
2 Inspect condition of IV site, noting color. Palpate for skin temperature, edema, and tenderness.
3 Monitor client's body temperature.

Changing Infusion Tubing
1 Observe flow rate of flush and observe connection site for leakage.

Changing Fluid Container
1 Observe client for signs of fluid volume excess or deficit to determine response to IV fluid therapy.
2 Monitor laboratory values and I&O.

Discontinuing IV Medications
1 Observe IV site for redness, pain, drainage, or swelling.
2 Observe continuous infusion for correct rate.
3 Observe tubing for leakage.

Discontinuing Peripheral IV Access
1 Observe IV site for evidence of bleeding.
2 Observe IV site for redness, pain, drainage, or swelling.

Unexpected Outcomes and Related Interventions
Changing Peripheral IV Dressing
1 IV catheter is infiltrated; phlebitis is present; or site is red, edematous, painful, and/or has presence of exudate.
a. Stop the infusion and discontinue IV.
b. Notify health care provider to evaluate client for source of infection; antibiotic therapy may be prescribed.

c. Culture of cannula may be ordered; confirm before IV removal.

d. Restart new IV in other extremity if continued therapy is required. Follow agency policy for complication management.

Changing Infusion Tubing

1 Decreased or absent flow of IV fluid indicated by a slowed or obstructed flow.

a. Open roller clamp, slide clamps, and recalibrate drip rate. Check for kinks in tubing.

b. Evaluate any pain or discomfort at the site for infiltration or temporary venous spasm.

Changing Fluid Container

1 Flow rate is incorrect; client receives too little or too much fluid.

a. Regulate to the correct rate.

b. Determine and correct the cause of the incorrect flow rate (e.g., change in client position, change in catheter position, kinked tubing).

c. Use electronic infusion device when accurate flow rate is critical.

d. Notify health care provider if client's anticipated infusion is less than or greater than 100 to 200 ml as expected (follow agency policy).

Discontinuing IV Medications

1 Solution in tubing below piggyback site turns cloudy because of precipitate formation, indicating medication incompatibility.

a. Stop all infusions.

b. Change tubing on continuous infusion.

Discontinuing Peripheral IV Access

1 Hematoma formation.

a. Apply a pressure dressing to the site; monitor site for additional bleeding.

b. Assess circulatory, motor, and neurological function of the extremity.

2 Catheter tip is missing

a. Apply tourniquet high on the extremity to restrict mobility or emboli.

b. Notify physician or licensed independent practitioner immediately.

Recording and Reporting

- Record time peripheral dressing was changed, reason for dressing change, type of dressing material used, patency of system, and observation of venipuncture site.
- Record tubing change, infusion solution type, volume, and rate of infusion on client's record. A special IV flow sheet may be used for parenteral fluids.
- Record time of discontinuing medication; tubing/catheter flush with type, volume, and concentration of flush solution; and the IV site condition.
- Record time peripheral IV was discontinued. Include site assessment information and gauge and length of catheter removed.
- Report to charge nurse or oncoming nurse dressing change, any significant information about the IV site or system, the time the medication or IV was discontinued, and the time and type of blood sample collections.

Sample Documentation

1300 IV dressing became wet during shower; new transparent dressing applied; insertion site without redness, edema, or drainage. Infusing at 125 ml/hr. No report of discomfort or tenderness in the hand or extremity.

1700 Gentamicin infusion complete; line flushed with 5 ml normal saline. D₅W with multivitamins infusing at 125 ml/hr. IV site without redness or edema; states there is no pain or discomfort at the site. Laboratory notified to obtain blood sample at 1745.

Special Considerations
Pediatric Considerations

- Use commercially available IV site protectors to cover and protect the IV site in young active children. Ensure that ID band is visible and nonrestricting.

Geriatric Considerations

- Infiltration in older adults may go unnoticed because of the skin's decreased integrity and loose skin folds. Because of decreased tactile sensation, a large amount of fluid may infiltrate before client experiences pain (Otto, 2005).
- In older adults, because of the decreased skin elasticity, skin turgor may not be a good indicatory of fluid balance; the best assessment sites are the forehead and sternum.
- Phlebitis may develop without pain but with significant inflammation resulting from the decreased sensitivity of the skin's nerve endings (Hankins and others, 2004).

Home Care Considerations

- Demonstrate with return demonstration hand hygiene and aseptic technique for changing IV site dressing. If the catheter comes out, apply gauze pressure dressing and notify home care agency nurse (Cox, 2005).
- Teach client to keep site dry during bath (preferred) or shower by wrapping in plastic bag and taping occlusively. Ensure EID or ambulatory infusion pump safety during hygiene activity.
- Discuss the signs and symptoms of possible infiltration or phlebitis such as swelling, pain, redness, or moisture at dressing site.

SKILL 27.4 Administering Intravenous Medications

- Nursing Skills Online: IV Medication Administration, Lessons 1-4

Because of technological advances and the efficacy, concentration, absorption, and rapid onset of medication, there is an increase in the use of IV medications. The IV route is often required if the client is unable to take oral medications. There are certain medications that can only be administered by the IV route. Because of the principles that make IV medication administration the preferred route (e.g., rapid onset, improved serum drug concentrations), the nurse is required to have greater knowledge and skills to prevent potentially dangerous complications. Parenteral administration of any drug is invasive and poses greater risk to the client.

When administering IV medications, the principles associated with delivery of any medication remain the same. Use the six rights of medication administration while applying the principles of IV therapy. Physical incompatibilities of IV medications, osmolarity of drug admixtures, and potential for IV therapy–related complications are considered before administering any medication intravenously (Hodgson, 2006).

A variety of methods are available for IV medication delivery. Dosages and admixtures vary and are usually calculated based on the client's weight, drug distribution and absorption, safety of administration, excretion, and solubility in solution. IV medications can be administered mixed in large admixture volumes (e.g., addition of 40 mEq KCl to 1000 ml IV fluid), by piggyback infusion (e.g., administration of an antibiotic concurrently with an IV infusion), or by bolus injection (delivery of an admixture or IV push medication through an existing IV access device). In all three methods of IV medication administration, the client is required to have an IV access device, either a continuous infusion or an access site such as a saline lock.

Because the liver and kidneys metabolize and excrete by-products of the IV medication, systemic diseases such as liver and renal impairment affect absorption. Older adults may have diminished renal and liver function and are more likely to experience toxicity related to IV drug administration. Clients with lower plasma proteins have more adverse effects when receiving IV medications because therapeutic response to the drug is related to the amount of drug not bound to a plasma protein or tissue. Drug binding influences both the effectiveness of the drug given and the duration of the effect.

Some drugs such as heparin are required to be given by continuous infusion to maintain a therapeutic action. The efficacy of therapeutic drugs given intermittently (e.g., antimicrobials) is determined by monitoring therapeutic drug serum levels. Serum drug levels such as peak and trough levels of aminoglycosides (e.g., gentamicin, tobramycin, amikacin, and vancomycin) are performed at specific intervals during IV medication therapy to monitor response and to protect the client from adverse effects if excretion of the metabolized drug is reduced. Serum drug levels reveal if drug doses are too high or low. Dosages are adjusted by increasing or decreasing the time between administrations or by increasing or decreasing the drug amount to provide therapeutic levels within a narrow range. Monitoring therapeutic drug levels is an additional responsibility of the nurse when administrating IV medications and is crucial in safe and effective delivery of care to the client (Ketchum and others, 2005).

When administering IV medications, the nurse assesses clients for hypersensitivity (allergic) reactions. Because of the rapid absorption of IV medications, an allergic response or delayed hypersensitivity occurs quickly and is exhibited by reactions ranging from a mild skin rash to anaphylaxis. The extent of the reaction is related to the hypersensitivity to the drug and the amount actually infused. If an allergic reaction occurs, stop the medication, keep the IV line open with an isotonic fluid infusion (such as 0.9% NS), stay with the client and monitor for respiratory distress and changes in vital signs, notify the health care provider, and be prepared to administer emergency medications and resuscitative measures if necessary (Scarlet, 2006).

The Needle Safety and Prevention Act of 2001 (OSHA, 2001; Deacon, 2004) resulted in more institutions using manufactured needleless systems or use of a system with catheter ports or Y connector sites designed to contain a needle housed in a protective covering. Needleless infusion lines allow a direct connection with the IV line via a recessed connection port or a blunt-ended cannula or shielded needle device (Figure 27-4).

ASSESSMENT

1. Check accuracy and completeness of MAR or computer printout with prescriber's original order. Check client's name; intravenous solution name and any medication additives; and dose, rate, route, and time of administration. *Rationale: The MAR or computer printout is the more reliable source of medication information. Review ensures safe and correct administration of IV therapy by verifying order.*

2. Review client's history for presence of diseases or conditions that might impair drug absorption, metabolism, or excretion.

3. Assess client's history of drug allergies. *Rationale: Ensures that a contraindicated medication is not administered.*

4. Review information about drug, including action, purpose, peak onset, normal dose, side effects, and nursing implications. Note appropriate time for infusion (e.g., mg/min). *Rationale: Nurse must be able to anticipate drug's effects and take appropriate action as client's condition changes.*

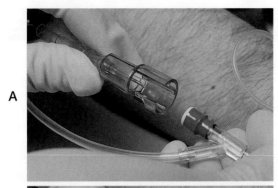

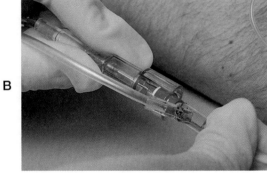

FIGURE 27-4 A, Needleless infusion system. **B,** Connection into an injection port.

5 When more than one medication is added to the IV solution, assess for compatibility. Observe institutional reference or pharmacy for drug compatibility list (Ketchum, 2005).
6 Assess appropriate laboratory values (e.g., creatinine, peak and trough levels). *Rationale: Determines drug efficacy and toxicity.*
7 Assess existing IV line for patency and note rate of infusion of main IV line. *Rationale: Patent line necessary for medication administration.*
8 Assess insertion site and for signs of infiltration or phlebitis (pain, tenderness, redness, swelling, heat on palpation). *Rationale: Administration of hyperosmolar drugs by IV route increases risk of phlebitis.*
9 Assess client's understanding of purpose for drug therapy.

PLANNING

Expected Outcomes focus on ensuring therapeutic response of drug with minimum adverse reactions.
1 Drug infuses within desired period.
2 IV site remains free of phlebitis or infiltration.
3 Client's laboratory values for therapeutic drug monitoring reveal desired response without renal toxicity.
4 Client does not show evidence of hypersensitivity, allergic reaction, or other side effects to IV medication.
5 Client/family is able to explain drug's purpose, action, side effects, and dosage.

Delegation Consideration
The skill of administering IV medications may not be delegated. The nurse directs personnel by:
- Reviewing what to observe (such as rapid heart rate, skin rash, dyspnea) and report back to the nurse.

Equipment
- IV medication
  Vial or ampule of prescribed medication
  Small-volume admixture (normal saline, dextrose and water, sterile water) in either syringe or 50- to 250-ml IV fluid bag
- *Optional:* Container for admixture diluent (Volutrol, Soluset, Burette)
- Sterile 21- to 23-gauge needle, 1 inch in length only if needleless system is not available. Use needleless system whenever possible.
- Label, if needed (Many small-volume admixtures are premixed and dispensed from pharmacy.)
- Syringe pump, if applicable
- Secondary administration set (needleless system preferred)
- Clean gloves
- 5-ml syringes
- NS or 0.9% solution in vial for injection
- One 3-ml syringe filled with heparin flush solution (10 units/ml) (follow agency protocol)
- Antiseptic swabs
- Tape (optional)
- IV pole
- Medication administration record or computer printout

IMPLEMENTATION *for Administering Intravenous Medications*

STEPS	RATIONALE
1 See Standard Protocol (inside front cover).	
2 Assemble medications in medication room using aseptic technique (see Chapter 15).	
3 Verify client's identity by checking identification bracelet and asking client's name. Compare with medication administration record.	Ensures that correct client is receiving medication. At least two client identifiers, neither of which is the client's room number, are used when administering medications (JCAHO, 2006). Identification bracelets made at the time of admission are the most reliable source of identification.

STEPS	RATIONALE

4 Explain procedure, and encourage client to report any symptoms of discomfort at IV site during infusion.

Keeps client informed.

5 IV push (bolus) (through existing continuous infusion line)

a. Prepare medication from ampule or vial (Chapter 17).

b. 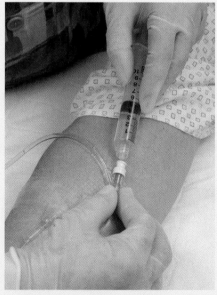 Select injection port closest to client. If add-on 0.22-μ filter is used, administer IV push medications below the filter next to client, preventing medication from being absorbed in filter.

Ensures that small-volume bolus enters vein quickly and directly.

c. Prepare injection site or cleanse connection port with antiseptic swab. Allow to dry.

Maintains aseptic technique.

d. Connect syringe of medication to IV line.
   (1) *Needleless system:* Remove cap of needleless injection port, if present. Connect tip of syringe directly.
   Or
   Insert blunt cannula through appropriate injection cap (see illustration).
   (2) *Needle system:* Insert short, small-gauge needle through center of injection port.

e. Occlude IV system by pinching tubing above injection port (see illustration).

Prevents reflux of medication up tubing and inadvertent bolus when infusion is resumed.

f. Aspirate gently on syringe plunger, observing for blood return.

In some cases, blood return may not be aspirated, even with patent IV. If IV is infusing well and has no signs of infiltration, proceed with medication administration. (McKnight, 2004).

NURSE ALERT Checking for a blood return is not a reliable method of determining catheter patency (Masoorli, 2005b). Absence of a positive blood return does not always indicate infiltration. There may be no blood return because fibrin is occluding catheter tip or tip is pressed against vein wall. Likewise, a positive blood return does not always ensure that the catheter is in correct position because blood return may be present even when there is infiltration. This may occur when catheter tip has eroded through vein, yet tip remains partially inside lumen of vessel (ONS, 2004). Absence of blood return requires further assessment before proceeding with therapy.

STEP 5d.(1) Insert syringe with blunt cannula tip into injection cap on existing infusion line.

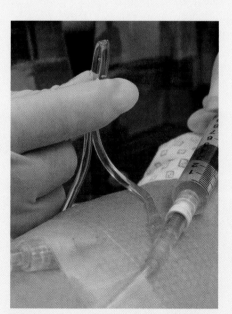

STEP 5e. Pinch IV tubing above injection port.

STEPS	RATIONALE
g. After observing for blood return, continue to occlude IV tubing and inject medication slowly over appropriate time (see illustration). Note if client reports any discomfort; if so, it may be necessary to stop administration. Use watch to time administration.	IV medications must be delivered at rate recommended by manufacturer. Infusion rate is available in drug pamphlet or handbook. Discomfort indicates chemical phlebitis.
h. Release tubing, withdraw syringe, and recheck fluid infusion rate.	Fluid infusion may need to be readjusted if injection changed drip rate.
i. If using a needleless system with injection caps, replace injection port cap with new sterile cap.	
6 IV push (through saline/heparin flush IV lock)	
a. Prepare medication from ampule or vial (see Chapter 17).	
b. Fill syringes with NS 0.9% (one containing 3 ml, the other containing 5 ml). Attach blunt cannula or remove needle from syringe as indicated by the type of needleless system.	One syringe flush will be used to clear lock before medication administration, the other to be used after medication is given.
c. Cleanse injection port of IV lock with antiseptic swab after removing cap if present.	Ensures aseptic technique.
d. Insert syringe of 3 ml NS 0.9% through injection port of IV lock (see illustration).	
e. Aspirate gently and observe for blood return.	In some cases blood return may not be aspirated. In this case assess carefully for infiltration.
f. If lock is intact and patent, flush gently with normal saline while assessing for resistance. If resistance is felt, never continue to apply force. Stop and evaluate cause.	Ensures catheter patency and prevents dislodging blood clot or drug precipitate into bloodstream. If resistance is felt and if more pressure is applied to overcome it, catheter fracture could result (ONS, 2004). Amount of flush should be equal to at least twice the volume capacity of the catheter and any add-on device (INS, 2006). For short peripheral catheters, 1 ml of flush is adequate (Hadaway, 2006).
g. Detach normal saline syringe, repeat cleansing of port with antiseptic swab, and attach syringe filled with medication.	
h. Inject medication slowly over appropriate time, using a watch to ensure proper time of delivery.	IV medication must be delivered at rate recommended by manufacturer.
i. Remove medication syringe.	

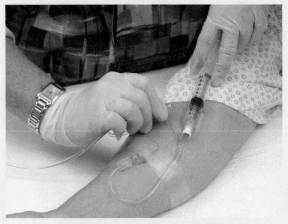

STEP 5g. Inject IV push medication.

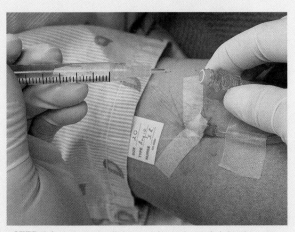

STEP 6d. Insert needleless syringe through injection port.

STEPS	RATIONALE
j. Recleanse cap or port with antiseptic swab and attach syringe with 5 ml 0.9% NS. Inject normal saline flush at same rate IV medication was delivered.	Irrigation with normal saline prevents occlusion of IV access device. Flushing at same rate as medication ensures that any medication remaining within IV is delivered at correct rate. Flushing with 3 to 10 ml of saline after each medication is crucial (Masoorli, 2005b).
k. *Optional* (if agency protocol): Inject syringe with heparin flush solution, maintaining positive pressure in IV access device. Using SASH method: Saline Administration Saline Heparin	Prevents incompatibility of heparin with drug administered because 0.9% NS is isotonic.

> **NURSE ALERT** Studies that have compared the use of saline versus heparin flush solutions in maintaining patency recommend saline for use with peripheral venous access devices (Hankins and others, 2004). The INS (2006) recommends flushing intermittently used peripheral catheters with 0.9% saline at established intervals. Use of heparin flush solution is more costly; requires an additional step with line manipulation; and carries potential for bioincompatibilities, alteration in clotting factors, and allergic reactions (follow agency policy).

7 IV piggyback (IVPB) or syringe pump through existing line

a. Attach tubing of administration set to prepared admixture container.

(1) *Piggyback infusion:* Small-volume admixture (50 to 250 ml) in a minibag that dilutes and administers drug. Insert spike of tubing into port of minibag (see illustration).

(2) *Syringe pump:* Small-volume admixture in a syringe (10 to 60 ml) to dilute and administer drug. Place prefilled syringe into miniinfusor pump (see illustration) (follow manufacturer's directions). Attach tubing to end of syringe.

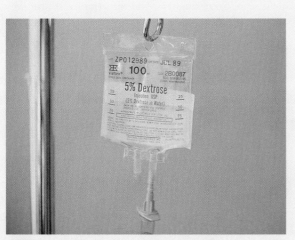

STEP 7a.(1) Small volume minibag for piggyback infusion.

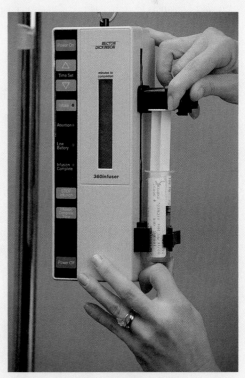

STEP 7a.(2) Syringe inserted into syringe pump.

STEPS	RATIONALE
b. Fill tubing with IV fluid.	Infusion tubing should be fluid filled and free of air bubbles to prevent air embolism.
(1) *Piggyback infusion:* Close roller clamp, squeeze drip chamber, and fill half full. Open roller clamp and prime remaining tubing.	
(2) *Syringe pump:* Gently push plunger of syringe to fill tubing completely.	
c. Administer IVPB.	
(1) Attach needle to end of IV minibag tubing and insert into injection port at upper end of main IV tubing after cleansing port with antiseptic swab; or, for needleless system, attach tubing to recessed connection port above backcheck valve (see illustration).	Use of injection port closest to drip chamber of primary IV line allows piggyback to infuse while stopping the flow of primary IV line through backcheck valve.
(2) Lower primary IV line. (Hook may be used to lower primary IV line.) NOTE: This step is not necessary if minibag is connected to EID.	Allows infusion of minibag and prevents infusion of primary line.
(3) Open regulator or clamp on minibag infusion. Regulate flow rate of infusion with roller clamp on primary tubing to deliver medication over 20 to 90 minutes (refer to agency policy or pharmacy instruction). If connected to EID, set rate and hit start button.	
(4) After medication has infused, check flow rate of primary infusion.	Backcheck valve prevents infusion of primary line while medication is infusing. Primary infusion will automatically begin to flow when tandem (piggyback) infusion is empty.

COMMUNICATION TIP If client complains of burning or stinging during infusion of hyperosmolar drugs (e.g., erythromycin, vancomycin) or highly alkaline drugs, assess IV site for symptoms of chemical phlebitis. IV infusion of drug greater than 650 mOsm/L is known to cause chemical phlebitis. If client has no signs of phlebitis, slow infusion and decrease rate to infuse over maximum time allowed. Consider option of further dilution of medication (confer with health care provider). Continue vigilance in assessing IV. Discuss with client importance of communicating further symptoms.

(5) Re-regulate primary infusion to desired IV rate.	Prevents infusion of excess fluid.
(6) Leave secondary bag and tubing in place for future drug administration or discard in appropriate container.	Establishment of secondary line produces route for microorganisms to enter main line. Repeated changes in tubing increase risk of infection. Follow agency policy and procedure for frequency of administration set tubing change (Gilles, 2004).

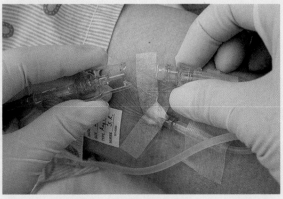

STEP 7c.(1) Attach tubing to recessed connection port.

STEPS	RATIONALE
d. Administer miniinfusion or syringe pump.	
(1) Attach blunt end of tubing to designated needleless port or insert sterile needle into injection port of existing IV line after cleansing injection port with antiseptic swab.	Maintains aseptic technique.
(2) Hang miniinfusor pump with syringe on IV pole with primary IV line. If required by type of syringe pump, set pump to deliver medication within time recommended by policy, pharmacist, or medication reference manual. Press button to "on" position. The infusion-complete alarm in "on" position should be used if available and if infusing via saline/heparin lock.	Prevents delay in flushing after completion of infusion, maintaining patency of access device.
(3) After medication infuses, turn off pump. Check flow rate of primary IV infusion and regulate to desired rate. (If stopcock is used, turn to "off" position after infusion is complete, and cap.)	Prevents infusion of excess fluid. Maintains sterility of system.
(4) Leave infuser tubing attached to primary line. Disconnect and cover end with sterile cap or disconnect and discard in appropriate container.	Tubing can be safely reused.

8 IVPB: saline/heparin lock

STEPS	RATIONALE
a. Take minidrip (60 gtt/ml) IV tubing and insert spike into minibag of medication.	Minidrip used to regulate small-volume infusion.
b. Close roller clamp and squeeze drip chamber to fill half full.	
c. Open roller clamp and fill remaining tubing.	Flushes air from tubing, preventing an embolus.
d. Attach sterile needle (e.g., 20-gauge, 1-inch) to tubing *or* attach sterile cap to end of primed tubing if using needleless system.	Needle should be changed with each administration. Keep end of tubing sterile.
e. Prepare injection port of needleless system or the saline/heparin stopper with antiseptic swab.	
f. Insert 5-ml syringe filled with 4 ml NS 0.9% and gently aspirate. Check for blood return, then flush normal saline slowly. Note any pain, swelling, or burning at IV site. Remove syringe.	In some cases blood return may not be aspirated. Assess lock carefully. Symptoms may suggest phlebitis or infiltration and the need to restart peripheral IV line.
g. Recleanse port or stopper with antiseptic swab. Attach end of tubing to port (needleless system) or insert sterile needle attached to tubing.	Ensures safe medication delivery.
h. Open flow clamp and regulate IV medication to infuse 20 to 90 minutes. (Follow agency policy or pharmacy instructions.)	Ensures safe infusion rate of medication.
i. Continue to observe infusion periodically until complete. When complete, disconnect, maintaining aseptic technique.	Ensures early identification of adverse effects.
j. Prep injection port with antiseptic swab, insert syringe with 5 ml normal saline and gently flush, maintaining positive pressure in IV access device.	Always flush port to prevent drug incompatibilities (see Step 6k). Flushing with 3 to 10 ml of saline after each medication is crucial. Volume of flush depends on lumen size and catheter length (Otto, 2005).
k. *Optional:* Recleanse port and inject heparin flush solution (follow agency policy), repeating procedure and using positive pressure.	Use of heparin may be recommended by agency.
l. Apply new sterile needle and cap to minibag tubing and retain for next administration.	Maintains sterility of IV tubing for future reuse.

STEPS	RATIONALE

9 Dispose of syringe, needles, and used tubing in appropriate container. Do not recap needles. Remove gloves.

10 See Completion Protocol (inside front cover).

> **NURSE ALERT** In instances of both phlebitis and infiltration, prompt removal of catheter is indicated. The duration and severity of phlebitis depends on how long catheter remains in place after first symptoms appear (ONS, 2004; INS, 2006). Treatment standard for phlebitis includes application of warm or cold compresses to affected site. Use of warm compresses to treat infiltration has become controversial. Cold may be better for some infusates, and warm may be more effective for others (INS, 2006). Follow agency policy for treatment options.

EVALUATION

1 Observe client's infusion for prescribed administration rate and note time of completion.

2 Inspect client's IV site and tubing for symptoms of IV complications (e.g., swelling, pain, tenderness, redness at site).

3 Monitor therapeutic drug levels (e.g., aminoglycosides, vancomycin, aminophylline, phenytoin).

4 Monitor client during infusion for allergic response or adverse reaction (e.g., urticaria, respiratory distress, tachycardia, hypotension).

5 Ask client to name IV medication, purpose, side effects, dosage, and frequency.

Unexpected Outcomes and Related Interventions

1 Client experiences burning, irritation, redness, or pain during infusion.
a. Reinspect site and check for blood return.
b. If phlebitis is present, discontinue infusion and reinsert another catheter, preferably in the opposite extremity, if IV therapy is still necessary.

2 Client experiences adverse reaction or allergic reaction during infusion of drug.
a. Stop the infusion.
b. Maintain existing IV line with NS 0.9% or prescribed solution.
c. Notify health care provider.
d. Stay with client and monitor vital signs and respiratory status.
e. Administer medications as prescribed.
f. Be prepared to perform cardiac or respiratory resuscitation.
g. After acute episode subsides, advise client of allergy and necessity for future reporting to health care personnel; advise client of significance of allergy; advise client as to the availability of medical alert identification tags. Document the incident in the medical record and report such information to pharmacy. Update allergy band and place on client.

Recording and Reporting

- Record drug, dose, route, amount/type of diluents (e.g., 1 g in 50 ml D_5W), with time/date of medication administration in the medical record or electronic documentation system.
- Record volume of fluid on client's I&O record.

Sample Documentation

0810 During initial 5 minutes of infusion of 100 ml NS and 1 g ampicillin, complained of sudden onset of "can't catch my breath," clutching at throat; high-pitched inspiratory stridor noted. Macular rash generalized over face and upper extremities noted. Ampicillin stopped immediately, IV fluids infused at 125 ml/hr. VS 98/60, 120, 26. Dr. Wills notified. Epinephrine 0.5 mg IV push given, with inspiratory distress subsiding within 30 seconds of administration. Allergy band applied.

0830 VS 120/84, 96, 18. States "breathing feels normal." Expressing some fear over "how fast it came on." Significance of allergy, implications for future administration, and notification of dentists, physicians, and other health care providers discussed. Aware that vital signs will continue to be monitored and to notify nurse immediately for any signs of respiratory distress.

Special Considerations
Pediatric Considerations

- Understand drug calculations with reference to age, height, weight or body surface area, dosage, and volume limitations (INS, 2006).
- Calculation of medication administration in children is most often based on body weight and body surface area, by use of a nomogram (Hankins and others, 2004).
- Use small-volume infusion tubing with pumps and controllers to infuse drugs and solutions. Ensure that these same pumps have alarms and tamper-proof or locking features.
- Adhere to the prescribed or recommended infusion rates.

Geriatric Considerations

- Therapeutic and toxic ranges of medications in older adults are very close, partially due to impaired renal function. Monitor serum drug levels carefully (Otto, 2005).
- Due to the concurrent use of multiple medications in the geriatric population, it is important to realize the potential for drug interactions (Ketchum, 2005; INS, 2006).
- The older adult may not be aware of his or her surroundings and may be slower to report symptoms of infiltration and phlebitis.
- Minimize excessive use of extension tubing and use Luer-Lok connections to avoid mishaps with an older client who might become confused or hyperactive.

Home Care Considerations

- Inform the client/caregiver that usually the initial dose of a new medication is given in the physician's office, clinic, or acute-care setting.

- Instruct the client/caregiver to know drug name, purpose for drug infusion, schedule, and drug side effects and the importance of reporting immediately to the physician/home care agency symptoms such as shortness of breath, rash, itching, hives, fever, abdominal cramps, or nausea/vomiting (Cox, 2005).
- Discuss issues regarding medication preparation, storage (drugs that require refrigeration), supply, and proper disposal of needles, syringes, and medication containers.

Long-Term Care Considerations

- An adverse outcome of inappropriate IV antimicrobial use in long-term care is the promotion of antimicrobial resistance and transmission of resistant microorganisms to other high-risk clients (Hankins and others, 2004).

SKILL 27.5   Transfusions of Blood Products

The transfusion of blood and blood components is a major factor in restoring and maintaining quality of life for the client with hematological disorders, cancer, injury, or surgical intervention. Caring for the client receiving blood or blood components is a nursing responsibility. However, the nurse should never view the transfusion of blood products as routine; overlooking a minor detail is dangerous and life threatening to the client (Scarlet, 2006).

Transfusions of blood and blood products is closely regulated and monitored. Standards of operations for all blood bank centers are set by the American Association of Blood Banks (AABB), OSHA, the U.S. Food and Drug Administration (FDA), and the American Red Cross. These standards include the collection of donor blood, distribution of the product, and standards for transfusion. Always verify specific agency policy regarding specific procedural requirements before any transfusion.

Blood and blood component therapies treat and restore hemodynamic homeostasis. A written health care provider's order to transfuse should always include which component to transfuse and the duration of the transfusion. A single unit of whole blood or blood components should be infused within a

4-hour period (INS, 2006). If more than one blood product is to be given, the sequence or order of transfusion should be specified. Any additional medications, such as an antihistamine (given when the history shows previous allergic response), antipyretics (given when the history shows previous febrile nonhemolytic response), or diuretics (given when the history shows potential for congestive heart failure) or other special treatment of the components should also be included in the written order for the transfusion (Otto, 2005).

Three blood typing systems, ABO, Rh, and most recently HLA typing (such as single donor), are used to ensure that transfusion products match the recipient's blood as closely as possible (Table 27-5). Before transfusion in nonemergent situations, the client's blood type and Rh factor must always be verified to be compatible with the donor transfusion.

There is increasing public awareness of the possible transmission of infectious diseases through transfusion of blood products. Because of improved testing of donor blood, the risk of the blood recipient developing an infectious disease is lower than ever before. However, viral, bacterial, and parasitic diseases can still be transmitted through blood. Screening of blood donors is one of the most important

TABLE 27-5 ABO System						
CLIENT'S BLOOD TYPE	RED BLOOD CELLS ANTIGEN	TRANSFUSION WITH TYPE A	TRANSFUSION WITH TYPE B	TRANSFUSION WITH TYPE AB	TRANSFUSION WITH TYPE O	TRANSFUSION OPTIONS
A	A	Yes	No	No	Yes	A, O
B	B	No	Yes	No	Yes	B, O
AB	AB	Yes	Yes	Yes	Yes	A, B, AB, O Universal recipient
O	None	No	No	No	Yes	O Universal donor

steps to identify persons with a medical history, behavior, or events that put them at risk of transmissible disease. All donor blood is tested for ABO grouping; Rh type antibody screening; rapid plasma reagin; syphilis; hepatitis B surface antigen; hepatitis C core antibody; and the presence of antibodies to hepatitis C, human immunodeficiency virus (HIV) 1 and 2, anti-HIV-1 and 2, anti-hepatitis C virus, anti-hepatitis B core, HIV-1 and HIV-2, HTLV-1 and HTLV-2, cytomegalovirus, and West Nile virus. Currently there are screening mechanisms to eliminate donors who might be at high risk for severe acute respiratory syndrome and mad cow disease (Otto, 2005).

Nurses must be prepared to inform the client thoroughly about the options, benefits, and risks of transfusion and reassure him or her that every effort is taken to ensure a safe blood supply and transfusion. Clients should know that there is never a completely risk-free transfusion.

One avenue for preventing the transmission of infectious diseases during blood transfusion is the use of autologous blood (i.e., the client's own blood). This can be done in several ways; however, the most frequent method is preoperative collection from the client. AABB standards establish the process for determining client eligibility, collecting, testing, and labeling the blood product unit. Before transfusion, ABO and Rh typings of the client are performed. Autologous units must be used before units from the general blood supply. Identification and verifying processes and methods of administration for autologous units are the same as those used for other units of blood.

The skill of transfusing blood or blood products requires you to know thoroughly and follow the policy and procedure of your agency or institution. To ensure the safe administration of the product, closely monitor your client before, during, and after the transfusion.

ASSESSMENT

1 Verify health care provider's order for specific blood or blood product with appropriate date, time of transfusion duration, and pretransfusion or posttransfusion medications to be given. *Rationale: Correct identification of ordered blood product is the first step to ensure safe administration.*

2 Obtain client's transfusion history, including previous transfusion reaction. Verify that type and crossmatch have been completed within 72 hours of transfusion and that consent for transfusion is provided. *Rationale: Identifies client's prior response to blood/blood product transfusion. If client has experienced a reaction in the past, anticipate a similar reaction and be prepared to rapidly intervene.*

3 Verify that IV catheter is patent and site is without complications such as infiltration or phlebitis. In emergency situations that require rapid transfusions, a 16- or 18-gauge cannula is preferred. However, transfusions for therapeutic indications may be infused with cannulas ranging from 20 to 24 gauge. *Rationale: Catheters used for blood transfusion must be patent and large enough to accommodate the appropri-*

ate flow rate but not large enough to damage the vein. The major concern is completing the transfusion within the recommended 4-hour time frame. If a smaller-gauge catheter is used, consider requesting split blood units to ensure timely administration.

4 Know the indications or reasons for a transfusion (e.g., low hematocrit secondary to postoperative bleeding). *Rationale: Allows nurse to anticipate client's response to therapy.*

5 Obtain and record pretransfusion baseline vital signs (blood pressure, pulse, respiration, temperature). If client is febrile (temperature greater than 100° F [37.8° C]), notify physician or licensed independent practitioner before initiating transfusion (follow agency policy). *Rationale: This provides comparison to detect change in client's condition during transfusion.*

6 Assess client's level of comfort and understanding of the procedure and rationale. *Rationale: Clarifying client's need for and associated benefits of therapy may alleviate some of the anxiety client may have.*

PLANNING

Expected Outcomes focus on safe, complication-free transfusion therapy, restoration of normal cell count, and improvement in oxygenation and tissue perfusion.

1 Client's systolic blood pressure improves, urine output is 0.5 to 1 ml/kg/hr, and cardiac output returns to baseline.

2 Client's laboratory values will reflect improvement in targeted areas (hematocrit and hemoglobin values).

3 Mucous membranes are pink, and client has brisk capillary refill.

4 Client will verbalize understanding of rational for therapy.

Delegation Considerations

Blood product administration may not be delegated. The nurse directs personnel by:

- Reviewing what to observe such as complaints of shortness of breath, hives, and/or chills and report this information back to the nurse.
- Reviewing to inform the nurse when volume of blood is low in the blood bag.

Equipment

- Blood administration set with standard 170-μ filter
- Prescribed blood product
- IV solution: NS 0.9%
- Clean gloves
- Tape
- Antiseptic wipes/swabs
- Vital sign equipment: thermometer, blood pressure cuff, stethoscope, and pulse oximeter
- Signed transfusion consent

Optional equipment
- Infusion pump (Verify that infusion pump can be used to deliver blood or blood products.)
- Use prescribed leukocyte-depleting filter (Institution may irradiate blood products within its blood bank facility.)
- Blood warmer (used mainly when large volume or rapid transfusion is needed)
- Pressure bag (used for rapid infusion in acute blood loss)

IMPLEMENTATION *for Transfusions of Blood Products*

STEPS	RATIONALE
1 **See Standard Protocol (inside front cover).**	
2 Obtain blood bag from laboratory following agency protocol. Blood transfusions must be initiated within 30 minutes after release from laboratory, blood bank, or controlled environment (INS, 2006).	Agencies differ as to personnel who can release a blood bag from a blood bank, but they always require two witnesses and some form of client identification. Usually only one unit is released at a time.
3 Open blood administration set and prime the tubing with NS 0.9% (see illustration), completely filling filter with saline. Maintain sterility of system and close lower clamp.	If filter is not completely primed with saline, transfusion will slow because of collection of debris in partially primed filter. Saline is used to wet the filter, dilute red blood cells to reduce their viscosity if necessary, and flush blood components from the tubing. If a reaction occurs, a separate bag of saline with a separate infusion tubing must be hung to decrease the amount of blood given to the client.

NURSE ALERT IV medications cannot be added to a blood bag or infused through a transfusion administration set. An additional IV site may be required if IV medications cannot be delayed or adjusted during blood transfusion(s). *Only NS 0.9%* can be used as a priming solution for blood and blood products.

COMMUNICATION TIP While preparing for blood administration, explain to client, "I will be staying with you for the first few minutes of the transfusion and will be checking you frequently while the blood is infusing. I'll take your blood pressure and temperature frequently. If you feel discomfort of any type while the blood is infusing, please let me know immediately."

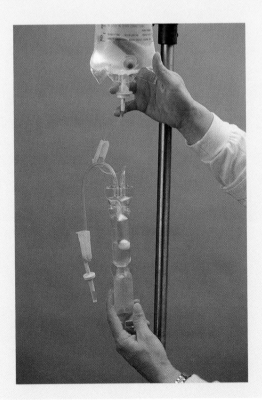

STEP 3 Blood administration set primed with normal saline.

STEPS	RATIONALE
4 Correctly verify blood product and identify client with a person considered qualified by your agency (e.g., RN, LPN, follow agency policy).	Strict adherence to verification procedures before administration of blood or blood components reduces the risk of administering the wrong blood to the client. Most hemolytic transfusion reactions are caused by clerical errors (AABB, 2005).
a. Check client's first and last names by having client state name, if able. Also check client's identification number and date of birth on armband and client record.	Verification process ensures right client receives correct blood product.

> **NURSE ALERT** When a discrepancy is noted during verification procedure, do not administer the product. Notify blood bank and appropriate personnel as indicated by agency policy. Most severe transfusion reactions occur from identification error, mislabeled blood samples, and mislabeled units (Hankins and others, 2004); verification of client, product, product type, and crossmatch may be the most important step of the entire procedure.

STEPS	RATIONALE
b. Verify that component received from blood bank is component ordered by physician.	Ensures client receives correct blood product.
c. Check that client's blood type and Rh type are compatible with donor blood type and Rh type. Be sure that transfusion is not discolored, clotted, or leaking and does not have bubbles present.	Verifies accurate donor blood and Rh type. Air bubbles, clots, or discoloration may indicate bacterial contamination or inadequate coagulation of the stored component. These are contraindications for transfusion of the product.
d. Check that unit number on unit of blood and form from blood bank match.	Further verification prevents accidental administration of wrong blood component.
e. Check expiration date and time on unit of blood.	Expired blood should never be used, because the cell components deteriorate and may contain excess citrate ions.
f. Record verification process as directed by agency policy.	Documentation of process on legal medical record.
5 Have client void or empty urinary drainage collection container.	If transfusion reaction occurs, urine specimen obtained must be recent and preferably taken after transfusion is initiated to assess for presence of red blood cells from a hemolytic reaction.
6 Review with client the purpose of the transfusion. Ask client to report immediately any signs and symptoms (during or after transfusion), including chills, low back pain, shortness of breath, nausea, excessive perspiration, rash, itching, or even a vague sense of uneasiness (Scarlett, 2006).	Once transfusion reaction occurs, staff must respond immediately with treatment.
7 Inspect blood product for signs of leakage or unusual appearance, including clots, bubbles, or purplish color. Gently invert bag 2 to 3 times.	Verifies quality of blood product. If signs of contamination are present, return blood product to laboratory. Inversion equally distributes cells throughout preservative solution.
8 Attach blood product to IV administration set by inserting spike of Y tubing located next to NS 0.9% tubing (see illustration). Close normal saline clamp above filter and open clamp above filter to blood product.	Prevents blood product from entering normal saline bag.
9 Turn off existing IV. Disconnect and cap tubing. Then quickly connect normal saline-primed blood administration tubing directly to client's IV site.	Ensures aseptic technique.
10 Open lower clamp and regulate blood infusion to allow only 2 ml/min to infuse in the initial 15 minutes. Remain with client for the first 5 to 15 minutes of the transfusion. Remove and discard gloves. Perform hand hygiene.	Most transfusion reactions occur within the first 5 to 15 minutes. Infusing a small amount of blood component initially minimizes the amount of incompatible blood to which the client is exposed, thereby minimizing the severity of a reaction.

STEPS	RATIONALE

11 Obtain vital signs (temperature, pulse, respiration, blood pressure) 5 minutes after initiation of transfusion and per agency policy after that.

Change from baseline vital signs may indicate transfusion reaction.

12 If there is no transfusion reaction, regulate rate according to physician's orders and infuse the remaining volume of blood as ordered. PRBCs are usually infused over 2 hours, and whole blood over 3 to 4 hours. Drop factor for blood tubing is 10 gtts/ml; check blood tubing package.

Careful regulation prevents adverse response. Client's condition and health care provider's orders dictate rate of blood infusion.

> **NURSE ALERT** Blood must be transfused within 4 hours of spiking the blood bag. Even if infusion is not complete, blood must be discontinued. This reduces the potential for exposure to bacterial infection from blood. Blood bank can split blood units if client is at risk for fluid overload.

13 After blood has infused, close roller clamp above filter to blood and open normal saline and infuse until blood administration is completely clear. Restart primary IV fluids as ordered only after assessing IV site for patency and signs and symptoms of phlebitis.

Normal saline infusion clears IV catheter of blood product.

> **NURSE ALERT** If transfusing more than one unit of blood or blood product, maintain NS 0.9% via blood administration set at prescribed infusion rate until second unit is started. Because of the risk of bacterial growth, blood administration sets and add-on filters should be changed after each unit or at the end of 4 hours, whichever comes first (INS, 2006).

14 Discontinue infusion and appropriately dispose of all supplies.

15 **See Completion Protocol (inside front cover).**

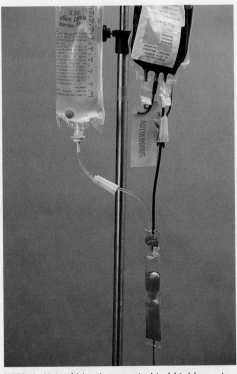

STEP 8 Unit of blood connected to Y tubing setup.

EVALUATION

1 Observe for any changes in vital signs and for chills, flushing, itching, hives, dyspnea, or tachycardia or any sign of transfusion reaction.
2 Monitor I&O and laboratory values (hemoglobin, hematocrit, prothrombin time, partial thromboplastin time, and platelet count) after transfusion. (In the hematologically stable adult, one unit of PRBCs should increase the hemoglobin by 1 g/100 ml and the hematocrit by 3%. A unit of platelet concentrate prepared from a single unit of whole blood should increase the client's platelet count by 5000 to 10,000 per milliliter) (Otto, 2005).
3 Monitor IV site and status of infusion each time vital signs are taken.

Unexpected Outcomes and Related Interventions

1 Client displays signs and symptoms of transfusion reaction.
a. Stop the transfusion. Stay with client and **notify** the physician.
b. A new normal saline infusion solution should be connected to the IV access site to prevent any subsequent blood from infusing from original blood tubing. Keep vein open with slow infusion at 10 to 12 drops/min to ensure patency and maintain venous access for medication and/or to resume transfusion.
c. Monitor vital signs.
d. Send entire blood setup back to blood bank (per agency policy).
2 Rate of infusion slows in the absence of infiltration.
a. Verify patency of IV catheter and that all clamps and stopcocks are open.
b. Ensure that blood bag is elevated to proper height and that filter is completely primed.
c. Gently flush IV line with normal saline or use a pressure bag or EID that permits blood transfusion.
3 Client experiences pain, swelling, or discoloration at IV site.
a. Stop the transfusion and discontinue the IV infusion and catheter.
b. Reinsert a new IV catheter in another site.
4 Fluid overload occurs, and/or client exhibits difficulty breathing or has crackles on auscultation.
a. Slow or stop the transfusion, elevate the head of the bed, and notify physician.
b. Administer prescribed diuretics, analgesics, and/or oxygen as prescribed.
c. Continue frequent assessments and closely monitor vital signs and I&O.

Recording and Reporting

- Record pretransfusion medications, vital signs, and location and condition of the IV system.
- Record the type/volume of blood component, blood unit/donor/recipient identification, compatibility, and expiration date according to agency policy.
- Record volume of normal saline and blood component infused.
- Record vital signs obtained before, during, and after transfusion.
- Report signs and symptoms of a transfusion reaction immediately.

Sample Documentation

1000 Early AM CBC noted. Physician aware of Hct 22. Type and crossmatch drawn with two witnesses per phlebotomy.

1230 Voided 320 ml clear, amber urine. 18 angiocath inserted left cephalic vein. NS 0.9% initiated at KVO. 1 unit PRBCs started at 40 ml/hr, after witnessed by J. Doe, RN.

Special Considerations
Pediatric Considerations
- Blood and blood products may be administered via 27-, 26-, or 24- gauge peripheral IV access in the neonate and via 24- or 22- gauge peripheral access in older children.
- Pediatric blood units are prepared in special units (Pedipacks) and usually equal half the volume of a conventional adult unit.
- Initiate the transfusion slowly (5 ml/min for initial 15 min). Remain with the child during this period of time and monitor vital signs and the infusion process.

Geriatric Considerations
- Older adults may have compromised cardiac, renal, and respiratory systems. Adjust the flow rate if the client cannot tolerate the prescribed flow rate. Flow rate should be 1 ml/kg/hr in the client at risk for circulatory overload.
- Vigilance in monitoring an access site during transfusion is vital in an older adult who may be less sensitive to the symptoms of infiltration, as well as the generalized symptoms of a transfusion reaction.

Home Care Considerations
- Clients who have had prior transfusion reactions, acute angina, or congestive heart failure are not considered good candidates for home transfusion.
- Nursing personnel must be present for the entire transfusion process and for 30 to 60 minutes after transfusion.
- Whole blood must not be administered in the home.
- Blood and blood products must be transported in a container with appropriate coolant. Verify and record the temperature at the time of delivery.
- Posttransfusion instructions must be given in writing, and the client/caregiver must be provided with names/phone numbers of individuals available to be called in the event of a delayed problem (unexplained fever, malaise, jaundice). Complications may occur days to weeks after transfusion.
- The container, empty bags, and tubing should be returned to the home care agency on completion of the transfusion.

NCLEX® Style Questions

1 Phlebitis is identified as the presence of two or more of which of the following sets of clinical features:
1. Tenderness, pitting edema, dyspnea, cough
2. Chest pain, cyanosis, hypotension, weak pulse
3. Headache, nausea, diarrhea, chills
4. Pain, erythema, induration, swelling

2 A client is receiving a blood transfusion following a total hip replacement. The client's blood type is type B+. Which of the following blood types for RBCs can this client safely receive (choose more than one answer)?
1. A+
2. O+
3. B−
4. AB+
5. B+

3 Considerations for IV catheter selection include which of the following?
1. Selecting the longest catheter with a larger gauge
2. Selecting the longest catheter with the smallest gauge
3. Selecting the shortest catheter with a larger gauge
4. Selecting the shortest catheter with the smallest gauge

4 A client that develops fluid volume excess will have which of the following clinical changes?
1. Tachycardia, flat jugular vein, infrequent edema
2. Tachycardia, distended jugular vein, toneless tense skin
3. Tachycardia, distended jugular vein, good skin turgor
4. Tachycardia, distended jugular vein, output greater than intake

5 The intravenous solution most compatible with blood or blood products is:
1. 0.33% saline
2. 0.45% saline
3. 0.9% normal saline
4. Ringer's lactate

6 A client returning from surgery has an order for 1000 ml D_5NS to infuse at 100 ml/hr. The drop factor on the client's infusion tubing is 10 gtts/ml. The correct infusion rate would be:
1. 34 gtts/min
2. 10 gtts/min
3. 60 gtts/min
4. 17 gtts/min

References for all chapters appear in Appendix D.

28

Fluid, Electrolyte, and Acid-Base Balance

MEDIA RESOURCES

- **evolve** http://evolve.elsevier.com/Elkin

Fluid, electrolyte, and acid-base imbalances occur to some degree in most clients with a major illness or injury. A variety of factors increase the risk for these imbalances, and several imbalances in the same client are common (Box 28-1). Many fluid, electrolyte, and acid-base imbalances are directly related to illness or disease such as diabetes, burns, renal failure, or congestive heart failure (CHF) (Box 28-2). Therapeutic measures such as major surgery, intravenous (IV) fluid therapy, dietary restrictions, medications (e.g., diuretics), or mechanical ventilation indirectly influence fluid, electrolyte, and acid-base balance (Lewis and others, 2004). To effectively monitor and respond to fluid and electrolyte imbalances, nurses need knowledge of the distribution, composition and regulation of body fluids, as well as of fluid and electrolyte balance.

DISTRIBUTION AND COMPOSITION OF BODY FLUIDS

Body fluids contain water, electrolytes, and nonelectrolytes (e.g., glucose, bilirubin, minerals, and urea). They are distributed in two distinct compartments: intracellular fluids and extracellular fluids. The fluid environment inside the cells (intracellular fluid [ICF]) must remain stable to maintain healthy cellular function. The fluid environment outside the cells (extracellular fluid [ECF]) includes both intravascular fluid (within the blood vessels) and interstitial fluid (between the cells and the blood vessels). Fluids in these compartments interact with the outside environment, providing the cells with a steady delivery of nutrients and removal of metabolic wastes.

Movement of Body Fluids

Fluids and electrolytes constantly shift to and from intracellular and extracellular compartments to meet the body's metabolic needs. Movement across these compartments depends on cell membrane permeability. Fluids and electrolytes move across these membranes by means of four processes: osmosis, diffusion, filtration, and active transport.

Osmosis involves the movement of water across a semipermeable membrane from an area of lesser concentration to an area of greater concentration (Figure 28-1). Osmolality (number of solutes in solution) of serum refers to its osmotic pressure, which is normally 280 to 295 mOsm/kg. For example, increases in ECF osmolality cause fluid to shift from ICF to ECF.

Diffusion is the process in which a solute (gas or substance) in a solution moves from an area of higher concentration to an area of lower concentration (Figure 28-2). An example of diffusion is the

---

BOX 28-1 Risk Factors for Fluid Imbalances

Deficient Fluid Volume
- Gastrointestinal losses such as from diarrhea, vomiting, or drainage from fistulas or tubes
- Loss of plasma or whole blood such as with burns or hemorrhage
- Excessive perspiration
- Fever
- Decreased oral intake of fluids
- Use of diuretics

Excess Fluid Volume
- Renal failure
- Congestive heart failure
- Cirrhosis
- Cushing's syndrome: increased serum aldosterone and steroid levels
- Excessive sodium (dietary intake or medications)

Third-Space Syndrome
- Portal hypertension
- Sepsis
- Small bowel obstruction
- Peritonitis
- Traumatic injuries
- Ascites
- Burns
- Nephrosis (nephrotic syndrome)

BOX 28-2 Clinical Applications of Alterations in Fluid Balance

Surgery

The stress of surgery causes fluid imbalances. In 24 to 48 hours after surgery, aldosterone and glucocorticoid hormones are increased, resulting in sodium, chloride, and fluid retention and potassium excretion. Increased antidiuretic hormone (ADH) secretion results in decreased urinary output, which helps maintain blood volume and blood pressure. After the second postoperative day, a diuretic phase begins as ADH levels return to normal and excess sodium and water are excreted.

Burns

In clients with severe burns, the body loses fluids in several ways. The greater the body surface burned, the greater the fluid loss. Plasma leaves the intravascular space and enters the interstitial fluid as trapped edema. This phenomenon is also called *third-spacing*. Plasma and fluids are lost as burn exudate (weeping tissues). Sodium and water shift into the cells, depleting extracellular fluid volume.

Congestive Heart Failure

In congestive heart failure decreased cardiac output results in decreased kidney perfusion and decreased urine output. The client retains sodium and water, resulting in circulatory overload, leading to pulmonary and peripheral edema.

Chronic Obstructive Pulmonary Disease

Alterations in respiratory function interfere with the elimination of carbon dioxide. Thus the body's buffers are unable to manage the carbon dioxide, resulting in a chronic acidosis. In chronic conditions the kidneys conserve bicarbonate to compensate. When assessing levels of arterial blood gases with chronic obstructive pulmonary disease, it is important to compare present values with a client's baseline.

Kidney Failure

Kidney failure results in abnormal retention of sodium, chloride, potassium, and water in the extracellular fluid and increased plasma levels of waste products such as blood urea nitrogen and creatinine. Hydrogen ions are retained, resulting in metabolic acidosis. Because of the disease process, compensation by bicarbonate reabsorption in the kidneys is not possible.

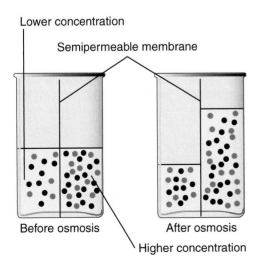

FIGURE 28-1 Osmosis through a semipermeable membrane. (Modified from Lewis SM and others: *Medical-surgical nursing: assessment and management of clinical problems,* ed 6, St Louis, 2004, Mosby.)

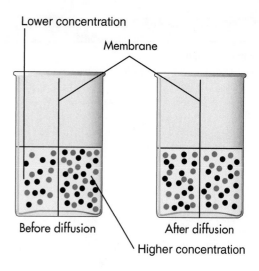

FIGURE 28-2 Diffusion. (Modified from Lewis SM and others: *Medical-surgical nursing: assessment and management of clinical problems,* ed 6, St Louis, 2004, Mosby.)

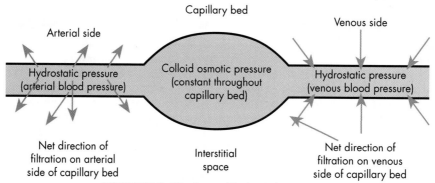

FIGURE 28-3 Filtration and hydrostatic pressure.

movement of oxygen and carbon dioxide between the alveoli and the blood vessels in the lungs.

Filtration is the process in which water and diffusible substances move together from an area of higher pressure to an area of lower pressure. The force behind filtration is hydrostatic pressure from the pumping action of the heart (Metheny, 2000). This process is active in capillary beds, where hydrostatic pressure differences determine the movement of water (Figure 28-3). An example of filtration is the movement of water and electrolytes from the arterial side of the capillary bed to the interstitial fluid. However, in CHF there is increased hydrostatic pressure on the venous side of the capillary bed, and the normal movement of water is reversed. This causes an accumulation of excess fluid (edema) in the interstitial space.

Active transport is the movement of molecules or ions "uphill" against an osmotic pressure to areas of higher concentration. It requires energy in the form of adenosine triphosphate (ATP). An example is the sodium-potassium-ATPase pump, which moves sodium to the outside of the cell and then returns potassium to the inside of the cell (Figure 28-4). The sodium-potassium pump keeps a higher concentration of potassium in the ICF and a higher concentration of sodium in the ECF.

When illness or injury disrupts fluid and electrolyte imbalances, medical treatment may involve administration of IV

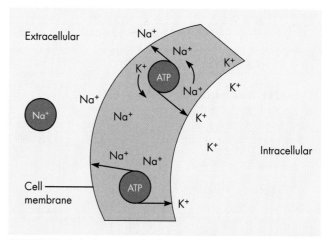

FIGURE 28-4 Sodium-potassium pump. (From Lewis SM and others: *Medical-surgical nursing: assessment and management of clinical problems,* ed 6, St Louis, 2004, Mosby.)

fluids (see Chapter 27). Nurses administer IV fluids and monitor the client's response to fluid therapy. Nurses must be aware of the contents of IV fluids, the intended purposes, and related contraindications and complications. An *isotonic* IV solution such as 0.9% normal saline (NS) has the same osmolality as blood plasma and will increase intravascular fluid volume without causing fluid to move to other compartments. A *hypotonic* IV solution such as 0.45% saline has a lesser concentration of solutes than plasma and moves water into the cells. *Hypertonic* solutions such as those containing 3% saline have a greater concentration of solutes than plasma and move water out of the cells and into the blood vessels.

Regulation of Body Fluids

Because fluid imbalances affect multiple systems, such as the heart and kidneys, there are often systemic results. These imbalances relate to excess loss of fluids or dehydration, excess fluid volume or retention of fluids, or third-space syndrome, when fluids are held within the body but are not accessible for normal body function (see Boxes 28-1 and 28-2).

Fluid intake is regulated primarily through the thirst mechanism, controlled by the hypothalamus. The thirst mechanism is affected by increased plasma osmolality, excess fluid loss, dry mucous membranes, and other factors. Clients who are unable to perceive or respond to the thirst mechanism are at risk for dehydration. This includes infants, frail elderly, clients with neurological impairment or those who are unconscious for any reason, and clients who are immobilized or restrained. The average daily fluid gains and losses in adults are 2200 to 2700 ml (Table 28-1).

In adults the kidneys produce about 60 ml/hr (1.5 L) of urine per day. Insensible water losses are not perceptible to the person and total about 400 ml/day. For example, water loss from the skin occurs in the form of sweat, which is increased with exercise, exposure to a warm environment, and fever. Excessive perspiration or diaphoresis may result in losses of 1000 ml or more in 24 hours. Insensible fluid losses are also increased substantially with an increased respiratory rate and depth. Normal fluid loss via the gastrointestinal tract is 100 ml/day. Vomiting or diarrhea increases gastrointestinal fluid loss substantially.

Third-space fluid losses occur when there is a shift from the vascular space into interstitial spaces of the body such as the pleural and peritoneal spaces. Although the fluid remains in the body, it does not participate in normal function of the ECF and is therefore considered a fluid "loss." It is difficult to observe or measure third-space fluid losses.

Fluid output is primarily regulated by retention and excretion of sodium and water by the kidneys. The kidneys regulate the glomerular filtration rate. Output is also regulated by hormonal factors, including the antidiuretic hormone (ADH), the renin-angiotensin-aldosterone (RAA) system, and the atrial natriuretic peptide (ANP) hormone.

Hormone Regulation

ADH is secreted by the hypothalamus and stored in the posterior pituitary. The hormone is released in response to a decrease in blood volume or increased sodium concentration. ADH decreases the production of urine by causing reabsorption of water by the kidney tubules. ADH helps the body retain water and is sometimes referred to as the "water conserving" hormone (Metheny, 2000). In the presence of defi-

Table 28-1 Adult Average Daily Fluid Gains and Losses

FLUID GAINS		FLUID LOSSES	
Oral fluids	1100-1400 ml	Kidneys	1200-1500 ml
Solid foods	800-1000 ml	Skin	500-600 ml
Metabolism	300 ml	Lungs	400 ml
		Gastrointestinal	100-200 ml
TOTAL GAINS	2200-2700 ml	TOTAL LOSSES	2200-2700 ml

cient fluid volume, as with vomiting and diarrhea or extreme sweating, ADH levels increase, resulting in conservation of water.

Aldosterone, a hormone produced by the adrenal cortex, regulates sodium and thus potassium and water balance. The RAA system stimulates secretion of aldosterone when there is decreased blood flow to the kidneys as in CHF. In response to the presence of aldosterone, the kidneys excrete potassium and reabsorb sodium; as a result, water is retained. Fluid deficits such as those produced by hemorrhage or gastrointestinal losses cause increases in aldosterone levels. The result of excessive aldosterone secretion is fluid volume overload due to excessive sodium retention. In the event of acute fluid losses, it often takes 2 or 3 days for both ADH and aldosterone to make corrective changes.

Another hormone, ANP, is released in the right atrium in the presence of atrial distention of the heart. It acts on the kidneys to initiate diuresis of sodium and water. The result is a decrease in intravascular volume. The diuretic effect of ANP may be beneficial to the client in acute heart failure and fluid volume overload (see Box 28-2).

NURSING DIAGNOSES

Nursing diagnoses relating to fluid and electrolyte imbalance include two major categories: **deficient fluid volume** and **excess fluid volume**. **Deficient fluid volume** occurs when there is prolonged or high decreased intake or prolonged or excessive fluid loss with high fever, sweating, diarrhea, vomiting, or third-space fluid losses. **Excess fluid volume** may be related to excessive intake of fluids, especially rapid IV infusion and excess sodium intake and fluid retention. **Hyperthermia** (associated with systemic infection, septicemia, or draining wounds) and **impaired skin integrity** (associated with burns) also contribute to fluid loss and electrolyte imbalance.

EVIDENCE IN PRACTICE

Stotts NA and Hopf HW: The link between tissue oxygenation and hydration in nursing home residents with pressure ulcers: preliminary data, *J WOCN* 30:84-190, 2003.

In a study of eight nursing home residents with stage II and IV pressure ulcers, low tissue oxygen saturation was measured in 6 of the 8 residents. Following supplemental IV fluid administration, a rise in tissue oxygenation was measured in a majority of the study group. Low tissue oxygen delivery may be an important factor in healing of pressure ulcers and other wounds. Tissue oxygen delivery is dependent on adequate fluid status. Therefore fluid balance and appropriate hydration status appears to be important to enhance wound healing in frail elderly clients.

SKILL 28.1   Monitoring and Maintaining Fluid Balance

Many factors change the distribution of body fluids. Thus nurses monitor clients for actual and potential fluid and electrolyte imbalances. During assessment the nurse considers factors influencing the fluid status and whether the change is normal and adaptive or the result of a pathological process.

ASSESSMENT

1 Consult the medical record or complete a nursing history with the client and family to identify risk factors for fluid volume imbalances (see Box 28-1). *Rationale: Current illness or disease processes, medications, treatments, and dietary restrictions can disrupt fluid and electrolyte balance.*

2 Monitor cardiovascular status for the following changes at least every 4 hours.

a. Hypovolemia (decreased circulating volume):

   (1) Falling blood pressure, especially orthostatic hypotension. Compare blood pressure lying, sitting, and standing (see Chapter 11). *Rationale: In the presence of decreased circulating blood volume, there is a drop in blood pressure and a compensatory rise in pulse rate when changing from a recumbent to a sitting or standing position.*

   (2) Increased pulse rate, weak pulse, and capillary filling time longer than 3 seconds.

   (3) Flat neck veins when supine.

   (4) Slow venous filling of dependent hands (longer than 3 to 4 seconds).

b. Hypervolemia (increased circulating volume)

   (1) Palpate for bounding pulse and inspect for increased venous pressure and jugular venous distention (JVD) when client is sitting upright (see Chapter 12). *Rationale: Indicates compromised ability of the right atrium to receive blood and pump it throughout the circulatory system.*

   (2) Monitor for increased respiratory rate, orthopnea, shortness of breath, or cough. Auscultate lungs for crackles (rales) and rhonchi (see Chapter 12). *Rationale: Indicates fluid buildup in the lung interstitial tissue (pulmonary edema), which requires immediate medical intervention.*

3 Check daily weights for changes, using same scale each time (see Procedural Guideline 8-1). *Rationale: Daily weight is the most effective way to evaluate fluid balance. Rapid weight loss or gain of 5% to 10% of body weight suggests moderate imbalance; greater than 10% alteration suggests severe fluid imbalance. Each kilogram of weight loss equals 1 L of fluid loss.*

a. Compare fluid intake and output (I&O) over 24 to 48 hours (see Skill 9.1). Monitor for intake significantly greater or less than output. *Rationale: In the presence of fluid excess and normal kidney function, urine is pale and dilute, and output increases. In the presence of kidney failure, oliguria intensifies the accumulation of fluids in the body, and urine is dark and concentrated.*

b. Intake includes *all* liquids taken by mouth, including ice chips, liquid medications, IV fluids, IV piggyback medications, tube feedings, and blood or blood components. *Rationale: Intake includes all sources of fluid; when intake exceeds output over time, it may result in fluid excess.*

c. Output includes urine, diarrhea, vomitus, diaphoresis (excessive sweating), gastric suction, and drainage from surgical tubes. Observe urine for oliguria, dark, concentrated (tea-colored) appearance. *Rationale: Output greater than intake over time results in fluid deficit in which the body conserves water. Concentrated urine is apparent.*

4 Inspect oral mucous membranes. *Rationale: Sticky, dry membranes; dry, cracked lips; and decreased saliva production suggest dehydration.*

5 Inspect skin for temperature and moisture. *Rationale: Dryness and flushed appearance suggest dehydration. Cool, clammy skin suggests hypovolemia.*

a. Palpate skin for inelastic turgor (tenting) over the sternum or forearm in adults or the abdomen in infants. *Rationale: Tenting indicates significant fluid deficit related to dehydration. The back of the hand is not a reliable place to test skin turgor because of loose, thin skin, especially in older adults.*

b. Assess for peripheral or central edema, periorbital edema, and blurred vision. Palpate dependent body parts such as feet/ankles for pitting edema (+1 to +4) (see Chapter 12). Measure abdominal girth every 12 to 24 hours for distention and possible fluid buildup. *Rationale: Presence of edema indicates fluid excess. Pitting edema indicates fluid excess of 10 pounds (20 L) or more. Clients on bed rest develop edema in sacral area when supine. Edema may shift from side to side as the client is turned.*

6 Assess mental status and level of consciousness (LOC). *Rationale: Dizziness, restlessness, confusion, lethargy, and coma may be related to dehydration or decreased cardiac output with hypovolemia.*

7 Monitor laboratory values for increased hematocrit (Hct), blood urea nitrogen (BUN), and urine specific gravity. *Rationale: Increased Hct suggests hemoconcentration caused by plasma or intravascular fluid loss. Increased BUN suggests hemoconcentration in the presence of normal kidney function. Increased urine specific gravity indicates concentrated urine. Decreased Hct suggests hemodilution caused by fluid retention. Decreased urine specific gravity indicates dilute urine.*

8 Assess client's and family's understanding of fluid imbalances and the importance of accurate assessment data.

PLANNING

Expected Outcomes focus on early identification of fluid imbalances. Treatment often needs to begin quickly to avoid potentially life-threatening complications.

1 Client will achieve or maintain normal fluid balance.
2 Causes of imbalance are identified and corrected.
3 Complications are prevented or managed promptly.

Delegation Considerations

The skill of monitoring fluid balance may not be delegated. The nurse directs personnel by:

- Explaining when to measure and record oral intake and urinary output for specific clients.
- Reviewing to observe and report back changes in urinary output volume, vomiting, and diarrhea.

Equipment

- Stethoscope
- Sphygmomanometer

IMPLEMENTATION *for Monitoring and Maintaining Fluid Balance*

STEPS	RATIONALE
1 See Standard Protocol (inside front cover).	
2 Provide oral hygiene every 2 to 4 hours and keep lips moist with water-soluble gel (see Chapter 7).	Fluid and electrolyte imbalances, especially fluid volume deficit, result in dry, cracked oral mucosa. Frequent oral hygiene increases client comfort and helps to maintain integrity of oral membranes.
3 Provide thorough skin care for comfort, turn and reposition frequently.	Dry or edematous skin is easily injured, which can lead to other impaired skin integrity problems (e.g., pressure ulcers).
4 Provide for client safety during transfer and position changes.	Clients with fluid deficit are at risk of orthostatic hypotension and subsequent falls.
5 Implement specific interventions to improve fluid status.	
a. Deficient fluid volume	
(1) If oral intake is not restricted, encourage fluids. Offer client's preferred fluids. If client is allowed nothing by mouth or is unable to tolerate oral fluids, administer parenteral fluids as indicated (see Chapter 27).	Fluid administration will restore fluid volume.

> **NURSE ALERT**   Surgical procedures trigger neuroendocrine, metabolic, and immunological responses, which may affect normal fluid distribution. Perioperatively anticipate shifts in the distribution of fluids from the vasculature space to the tissues, which may result in a vascular volume deficit or hypovolemia 48 to 72 hours later. The sequestered fluid commonly returns to the venous system (vanWisen and Breton, 2004).

(2) During IV therapy, monitor carefully for fluid overload, including daily weights, I&O, vital signs, orthopnea, shortness of breath or cough associated with crackles (rales) and rhonchi, JVD, and hyponatremia (decreased serum sodium).	Too rapid of an infusion can result in overhydration and sodium imbalance manifested by increased respiratory distress and cardiovascular changes.
(3) Initiate measures to control diaphoresis, emesis, or diarrhea.	Prevents further fluid loss.

> **NURSE ALERT**   When administering rapid rates of infusion, assess client frequently for fluid volume excess, especially in the presence of cardiac, renal, or neurological problems.

b. Excess fluid volume	
(1) Monitor IV infusion hourly for appropriate rate of administration and effectiveness.	Clients are at risk for cardiac and pulmonary complications if fluid overload develops.
(2) In the presence of circulatory or respiratory changes elevate the head of the bed. Oxygen therapy may be indicated (see Chapter 29).	

STEPS	RATIONALE
(3) Administer medications such as diuretics as prescribed.	Diuretics act on the renal tubules to assist in excretion of excess fluid and electrolytes.
(4) Restrict fluids to 1200 to 1500 ml/day as prescribed.	Clients with renal and cardiovascular diseases may have impaired renal clearance and therefore retain fluid. Restricting fluid intake is necessary to optimize physiological functioning.

6 See Completion Protocol (inside front cover).

EVALUATION

1 Monitor I&O each shift. Assess client's fluid status and appropriate electrolytes.

2 Measure client's weight daily.

3 Observe for physical signs of fluid imbalance (e.g., orthopnea, shortness of breath); auscultate lungs.

4 Monitor appropriate laboratory values (e.g., electrolytes, hematocrit, BUN, urine specific gravity).

Unexpected Outcomes and Related Interventions

1 After IV therapy for fluid deficit, client remains either hypovolemic or dehydrated.

a. Notify physician.

b. Adjust fluid therapy as ordered (e.g., increase volume or rate of ordered fluids either orally or intravenously) or seek orders for appropriate medications such as antiemetics to decrease losses.

2 After IV therapy, client shows signs of hypervolemia.

a. Notify physician.

b. Adjust fluid therapy as ordered (e.g., decrease the infusion rate of parenteral fluids) and administer diuretics as ordered.

Recording and Reporting

- Record assessment findings and interventions implemented, including oral or IV fluids, medications, and comfort measures.
- Report significant alterations in vital signs, oliguria, laboratory results, and mental status to the physician promptly.

Sample Documentation

1000 States nausea, vomiting ×3 days at home. Vital signs: temperature 98.4° F, HR 100 and regular, R 12, supine BP 118/80 mm Hg, standing BP 90/60 mm Hg. Alert; oriented to person, place, time. Complains of dizziness, thirst, nausea. Oral mucous membranes dry, jugular veins flat with head of bed flat, inelastic skin turgor, capillary refill longer than 5 seconds. Urine output 240 ml in 8 hr. IV of D_5LR infusing at 125 ml/hr via infusion pump left forearm. Antiemetic given as ordered.

Special Considerations
Pediatric Considerations

- Infants and small children have a greater need for water and are at greater risk for fluid and electrolyte imbalances because of their relatively greater surface area, their high rate of metabolism, and their immature kidney function. As much as 80% of an infant's body weight is water (Hockenberry and Wilson, 2007).
- When measuring output in infants, diapers may be weighed in grams. One gram of wet diaper weight equals 1 ml of urine.
- Children frequently respond to illness with fevers of higher temperature or longer duration than adults, resulting in increased insensible water losses (Hockenberry and Wilson, 2007).
- Tachycardia, dry skin and mucous membranes, sunken fontanels, and signs of circulatory failure are clinical indicators of dehydration in a child (Hockenberry and Wilson, 2007).
- In the presence of fluid deficit in infants, inspection will reveal depressed or sunken fontanels, and in fluid excess bulging fontanels are apparent.

Geriatric Considerations

- The amount of fluid in the body decreases with age. A person over 70 years of age may have as little as 45% to 50% of body fluid.
- Older adults tend to have decreased thirst sensation or may have altered ability to request or obtain needed fluids.

- Inability to obtain adequate fluids, difficulty swallowing, and an inability to evaluate medications that affect I&O may contribute to fluid imbalance (Ebersole and others, 2005).
- After age 65 years the kidneys begin to lose nephrons. Therefore the ability to concentrate urine declines.
- Atrophy of adrenal glands results in altered regulation of sodium and potassium and predisposes the client to fluid and electrolyte imbalance.

Home Care Considerations

- Household measures may be used, and totals calculated accordingly.
- Emphasize the importance of daily weights. Report changes to a health care professional. When instructing clients on daily weights, it is important to emphasize to use the same scale, wear the same clothing articles, and weigh themselves at the same time each day to maintain consistency with results.

SKILL 28.2 Monitoring Electrolyte Balance

Disturbances in electrolyte balance seldom occur alone and often are related to fluid imbalances. Various risk factors are associated with electrolyte imbalances (Table 28-2). Basic types of electrolyte imbalances include sodium, potassium, calcium, and magnesium imbalances. Electrolytes are substances that separate in solution into negatively charged ions (anions) and positively charged ions (cations). The numbers of positive and negative charges must be equal in body fluids. Electrolytes are vital to many body functions, including neuromuscular function, cardiac rhythm and contractility, mental processes, and gastrointestinal function. Most serum electrolytes are measured in milliequivalents (mEq) per liter.

Sodium is the most abundant cation in the ECF. Water follows sodium so that when the kidneys excrete sodium, water is excreted. This is the therapeutic action for some diuretics. Hyponatremia is a low serum sodium level, associated with many conditions, including kidney disease, gastrointestinal losses, increased sweating, and certain diuretics to name a few. Severe hyponatremia can result in seizures, vascular collapse, and shock. Dilutional hyponatremia occurs in the presence of water excess. Hypernatremia is caused by extreme water loss or overall sodium excess (Metheny, 2000).

Potassium, the predominant intracellular cation, regulates neuromuscular excitability and muscle contraction and is primarily regulated by the kidneys. Because the normal range for serum potassium is a narrow one (3.5 to 5 mEq/L), relatively small deviations from normal can be very serious. Hypokalemia is a low serum potassium level and is commonly caused by excessive fluid losses related to potassium-depleting diuretics, gastrointestinal losses, or diabetic ketoacidosis. Severe hypokalemia can affect cardiac conduction and function. Hyperkalemia is an elevated serum potassium level, which may be caused by altered kidney function because any condition that decreases urine output also decreases potassium excretion. Hyperkalemia may also be related to massive cell damage such as from burns, myocardial infarction, crushing injuries, and cell destruction after chemotherapy and radiation therapy. Severe hyperkalemia can cause cardiac conduction abnormalities.

Calcium contributes to the transmission of nerve impulses, cardiac contractions, muscle contractions, blood clotting, and formation of teeth and bone (Lewis and others, 2004). Hypocalcemia, a decrease in serum calcium levels, is associated with surgical removal of the parathyroid glands, acute pancreatitis, renal failure, decreased dietary intake, and excess loss with laxative abuse. Hypocalcemia results in altered blood clotting, anxiety, muscle cramps, and a tendency toward tetany. Hypercalcemia, an increase in the total serum calcium level, is frequently a symptom of an underlying disease, resulting in excess bone resorption with release of calcium. The most common cause of hypercalcemia is malignancy. Prolonged immobilization also promotes calcium loss from the bone and may cause a serum rise in calcium levels. Hypercalcemia can cause flabby muscles, depression, skeletal fractures, renal stones, and cardiac arrest.

Magnesium imbalances directly influence neuromuscular function and cardiovascular tone. Hypomagnesemia, a decrease in magnesium levels, results in increased neuromuscular and central nervous system activity. Magnesium deficit may be caused by excess losses via vomiting and diarrhea; large urine output; nasogastric suction; and decreased dietary intake because of chronic alcoholism, malnutrition, or inadequate absorption. Hypermagnesemia, an increase in magnesium levels, causes a diminished excitability of muscle cells and contributes to hypertension, cardiac dysrhythmias, ischemic heart disease, and sudden cardiac death. Elevated magnesium levels are associated with renal failure, adrenal insufficiency, and overdose associated with IV administration for the prevention of seizures in toxemia of pregnancy.

ASSESSMENT

1 Consult the medical record or complete a nursing history with the client and family to identify disease processes/conditions that affect or are influenced by electrolyte imbalances (see Table 28-2). *Rationale: Electrolyte imbalances frequently occur with underlying diseases and require anticipatory nursing interventions. For example, the client with CHF is at risk for sodium retention. An anticipatory intervention is a reduction in dietary sodium.*

TABLE 28-2 Common Risk Factors for Electrolyte Imbalances

ELECTROLYTE DEFICIT	ELECTROLYTE EXCESS
Hyponatremia Renal disease Adrenal insufficiency Gastrointestinal losses Excessive sweating Use of thiazide diuretics, especially along with low-sodium diets Metabolic acidosis Syndrome of inappropriate antidiuretic hormone	**Hypernatremia** Water deprivation Increased insensible water los,(e.g., burns, hyperventilation, fluidized beds) Administration of hypertonic intravenous saline solution Excessive sodium intake Excess aldosterone secretion Diabetes insipidus
Hypokalemia Use of potassium-depleting diuretics Diarrhea, vomiting, or other gastrointestinal losses Alkalosis Cushing's syndrome or adrenal hormone-producing tumors Excessive sweating Polyuria Excessive use of potassium-free IVs	**Hyperkalemia** Renal failure and oliguria Hypertonic dehydration Massive cellular injury (e.g., burns, trauma) Excessive administration of intravenous potassium Adrenal insufficiency Acidosis Rapid infusion of stored blood Use of potassium-retaining diuretics
Hypocalcemia Rapid administration of blood containing citrate Hypoalbuminemia Hypoparathyroidism Vitamin D deficiency Pancreatitis Alkalosis	**Hypercalcemia** Hyperparathyroidism Malignancies Paget's disease Osteoporosis Prolonged immobilization Acidosis
Hypomagnesemia Malnutrition/alcoholism Excessive dietary calcium (competes with magnesium) Inadequate gastrointestinal absorption of magnesium Excessive gastrointestinal losses Aldosterone excess Polyuria	**Hypermagnesemia** Renal failure Excessive oral or IV administration of magnesium

IV, Intravenous.

2 Assess current illness, health practices, medications, treatments, and dietary restrictions that can disrupt electrolyte balance.

3 Check electrolyte laboratory results for abnormalities. *Rationale: Provides current and/or baseline laboratory data from which to measure the success of interventions aimed at restoring electrolyte balance.*

4 Assess client's and family's understanding of the risk for electrolyte imbalances. *Rationale: Helps to determine prior client experience and adherence to interventions to maintain electrolyte balance.*

PLANNING

Expected Outcomes focus on early identification of a high risk for an actual electrolyte imbalance. Treatment is initiated quickly because complications can be life threatening.

1 Client will achieve or maintain a normal serum electrolyte level.

2 Complications of electrolyte imbalance are prevented or managed promptly.

Delegation Considerations

The skill of monitoring electrolyte balance may not be delegated. The nurse directs personnel by:

- Explaining when to obtain daily weights, I&O, vital signs.
- Reviewing what to observe and report back to nurse any changes in client's status, such as changes in vital signs, LOC, and orientation.

Equipment

- Stethoscope
- Sphygmomanometer

IMPLEMENTATION *for Monitoring Electrolyte Balance*

STEPS	RATIONALE

1 See Standard Protocol (inside front cover).

2 *Sodium balance:*

a. *Hyponatremia:* Assess for evidence of hyponatremia (serum sodium level less than 135 mEq/L):

  (1) Assess for abdominal cramps, nausea, and vomiting.

  (2) Observe mental status for personality change, irritability, apprehension, anxiety, convulsions, or coma.

  (3) Monitor vital signs for weak, rapid pulse and hypotension and orthostatic hypotension.

Hyponatremia causes hypoosmolality with a shift of water into cells (Lewis and others, 2004).

Early manifestations of hyponatremia.

Neurological symptoms are caused by fluid shift into brain cells (Lewis and others, 2004). Severe hyponatremia (less than 120 mEq/L) can result in neurological changes.

Severity of symptoms with hyponatremia depends on the magnitude, rapid onset, and cause (Metheny, 2000).

b. *Hypernatremia:* Assess for evidence of hypernatremia (serum sodium level greater than 145 mEq/L).

  (1) Assess for thirst, lethargy, weakness, agitation, and irritability.

  (2) Inspect mouth for dry tongue and mucous membranes.

  (3) Palpate for dry, flushed skin.

  (4) Monitor urine output for oliguria or anuria.

Hypernatremia causes hyperosmolality with a shift of water out of the cells into the hypertonic ECF, cellular dehydration in brain cells, and potential changes, including tissue trauma or hemorrhage to cerebral vessels.

Early signs of hypernatremia. Severe hypernatremia (concentrations greater than 160 mEq/L) may lead to seizures or coma (Metheny, 2000).

c. Provide comfort and safety measures, such as mouth care, including preparation for potential convulsions in severe cases (see Chapter 3).

d. Refer to a dietician when a low-sodium diet is prescribed. Instruct client about consuming less salt and sodium.

  (1) Read the nutrition labels and minimize the use of processed foods.

  (2) Request no added salt when eating out or traveling.

  (3) Use spices and herbs rather than salt.

  (4) Choose fresh fruits and vegetables as snacks rather than salted chips, nuts, or popcorn.

  (5) Avoid over-the-counter medications that contain sodium.

Processed foods contain high levels of sodium.

Enhances flavor of food.

3 *Potassium balance:*

a. *Hypokalemia:* Assess for evidence of hypokalemia (serum potassium level less than 3.5 mEq/L).

  (1) Monitor vital signs for a weak, irregular pulse; shallow respirations; and hypotension.

  (2) Observe for electrocardiogram (ECG) changes (depressed ST, T wave inversion or flattening, and U waves), and ventricular arrhythmias.

The most common cause of hypokalemia is the use of potassium-depleting diuretics such as thiazides and loop diuretics. Alkalosis may cause a temporary hypokalemia by a shift of serum potassium into the cells (Metheny, 2000).

> **NURSE ALERT** Severe hypokalemia (less than 2.5 mEq/L) can result in death from cardiac or respiratory arrest (Metheny, 2000).

  (3) Assess for generalized fatigue, weakness, decreased muscle tone, or decreased reflexes.

STEPS	RATIONALE

(4) Auscultate abdomen for decreased bowel sounds and palpate for abdominal distention.

(5) Assess extremities for muscle cramps and paresthesias.

b. Maintain adequate dietary intake of potassium (e.g., potatoes, spinach, broccoli, winter squash, dates, bananas, dried apricots, orange and grapefruit juice, dry beans, and yogurt).

c. Administer IV fluids with KCl as ordered. Urine output must be present, and, if there is no urine output, potassium replacement is not used.

Extreme caution is used with potassium replacement therapy due to risk of cardiac irritability.

NURSE ALERT
- The rate of administration of IV fluids containing KCl should not exceed 20 mEq of potassium per hour.
- KCL is always administered via an IV pump. Some facilities may require continuous ECG monitoring when K^+ replacement is infusing.
- When an IV fluid bolus is ordered, IV solutions containing K^+ must not be administered to avoid too rapid infusion of K^+.

---

d. *Hyperkalemia:* Assess for evidence of hyperkalemia (serum potassium level greater than 5.5 mEq/L)

The primary cause of hyperkalemia is renal failure, resulting in decreased excretion of potassium, massive tissue damage, or acidemia, which causes a shift of potassium out of the cells into the plasma. It can also be caused by rapid IV administration or massive oral ingestion of potassium.

(1) Observe for ECG changes, including peaked T waves, prolonged PR interval, widening of QRS, complete heart block, ectopic beats, and ventricular fibrillation leading to cardiac arrest.

(2) Assess for nausea, vomiting, diarrhea, and cramping pain.

(3) Assess for muscle twitching, paresthesias or paralysis, or seizures.

e. In the presence of hyperkalemia, collaborate with the physician to prescribe Kayexalate, an administration of IV dextrose along with IV Regular Insulin, or consider the possibility of renal dialysis.

Kayexalate exchanges sodium for potassium, and potassium is excreted in stool. In the emergent treatment of hyperkalemia, an IV infusion of dextrose along with IV Regular Insulin may be ordered to force potassium into the cells and lower the serum potassium level. The excretion of potassium is achieved rapidly with dialysis.

4 *Calcium balance.*

a. *Hypocalcemia:* Assess laboratory reports for hypocalcemia (total serum calcium level less than 8.5 mg/dl).

Hypocalcemia results from thyroid alterations as well as renal insufficiency. Kidneys are unable to excrete phosphorous, causing phosphorus levels to rise and calcium levels to fall.

(1) Assess for muscle cramps, numbness, and tingling circumorally and in fingers and toes.

(2) Observe for ECG changes, including prolonged QT interval, bradycardia, ventricular tachycardia, or asystole.

(3) Observe for laryngeal spasm and prepare for possible respiratory arrest.

NURSE ALERT Severe hypocalcemia is a medical emergency, particularly if laryngeal spasms and respiratory arrest are imminent. It is treated with IV calcium gluconate.

---

(4) Assess for colicky discomfort or diarrhea.

STEPS	RATIONALE

(5) Assess for Chvostek's sign, a contraction of facial muscles in response to a light tap over the facial nerve in front of the ear (see illustration).

(6) Assess for Trousseau's sign, carpal spasm induced by inflating a BP cuff above the systolic pressure for as long as 3 minutes (see illustration).

(7) Prepare for possible seizures and tetany (see Chapter 3).

b. *Hypercalcemia:* Assess laboratory reports for hypercalcemia (total serum calcium level greater than 11 mg/dl).

(1) Assess for decreased gastrointestinal motility, including nausea, vomiting, constipation.

(2) Assess for lethargy, fatigue, malaise, and muscle weakness.

(3) Observe for confusion, impaired memory, sudden psychosis, or coma.

(4) Monitor for weight loss, dehydration, increased thirst, and polyuria.

(5) Determine presence of hypertension or ECG changes.

(6) Assess for decreased muscle strength, hypoventilation, and depressed deep tendon reflexes.

(7) Auscultate abdomen for hypoactive bowel sounds or paralytic ileus.

c. Increase fluid intake to 3000 to 4000 ml of fluid daily (if allowed) or administer a loop diuretic as ordered.

5 *Magnesium balance:*

a. *Hypomagnesemia:* Assess for evidence of magnesium level less than 1.5 mEq/L or 1.8 mg/dl.

(1) Assess for hyperexcitability with muscular weakness or tremors, tetany, seizures, positive Chvostek's or Trousseau's sign (see illustrations for Steps 4a(5) and 4a(6)).

Rationale column:

Hypercalcemia frequently results from underlying diseases that cause excess bone resorption with release of calcium.

Promotes the excretion of calcium in urine.

Hypomagnesemia may occur with and contribute to the persistence of hypokalemia and hypophosphatemia (Metheny, 2000).

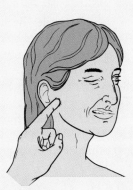

STEP 4a.(5) Chvostek's sign. (From Lewis SM and others: *Medical-surgical nursing: assessment and management of clinical problems,* ed 6, St Louis, 2004, Mosby.)

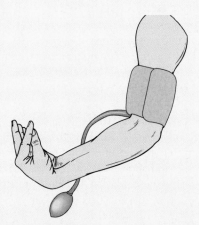

STEP 4a.(6) Trousseau's sign. (From Lewis SM and others: *Medical-surgical nursing: assessment and management of clinical problems,* ed 6, St Louis, 2004, Mosby.)

STEPS	RATIONALE

(2) Observe mental status for sudden changes, including confusion, ataxia, vertigo, depression, and psychosis.
(3) Monitor for cardiac dysrhythmias, which can be life threatening.
b. *Hypermagnesemia:* Assess for evidence of magnesium level greater than 2.5 mEq/L.
   (1) Observe for hypotension, lethargy, and drowsiness.
   (2) Assess for hyporeflexia.
   (3) Assess for nausea and vomiting.
   (4) Observe for ECG changes such as shortening QT interval, prolonged QRS and PR interval, and T wave changes.
6 See Completion Protocol (inside front cover).
	Hypermagnesemia is common in renal failure.

EVALUATION

1 Check laboratory values and physical signs to identify trends in response to medical treatment.

2 Monitor for evidence of complications related to treatment resulting in the opposite imbalance (e.g., treatment for hypokalemia may result in hyperkalemia).

Unexpected Outcomes and Related Interventions

1 After treatment, client has a persistent electrolyte imbalance.

a. Analyze the available data supporting the imbalance.

b. In collaboration with other health care team members, administer appropriate therapies to restore electrolyte balance.

Recording and Reporting

• Record time electrolytes were drawn and results, assessment findings, interventions, and outcomes. Note when physician was notified of significantly abnormal results.

• Immediately report abnormal electrolyte laboratory results and action taken.

Sample Documentation

1100 Serum Na 135, K 3.0. HR 110, weak and irregular, R 28. Client reports weakness, fatigue, nausea, and anorexia. Dozing and arouses easily. States, "My legs have been aching since yesterday." Client instructed to stay in bed. Dr. Johnson notified. Orders received.

Special Considerations

Pediatric Considerations

• Sodium is an important nutrient for premature infants. It is associated with protein synthesis, bone mineralization, and maintenance of ECF volume.

• Infants of mothers with diabetes are at risk of hypomagnesemia.

• If the mother was treated with magnesium sulfate for preterm labor, the infant is at risk for hypermagnesemia.

• Hyperkalemia may occur in premature infants because of a shift of potassium from the cells to the extracellular space.

Geriatric Considerations

• Atrophy of adrenal glands results in altered regulation of sodium and potassium and predisposes the older adult to fluid and electrolyte imbalance.

• Older adults have different laboratory "normals" than younger adults, as well as complex health histories that can affect the overall responses of their bodies to fluid and electrolyte alterations. Laboratory tests and their results need to be considered within context and not in isolation from the overall clinical picture (Meiner and Lueckenotte, 2006).

• Dehydration is the most common form of electrolyte imbalance in older adults. This is usually attributed to excess loss of water or impaired water ingestion (Meiner and Lueckenotte, 2006).

SKILL 28.3 Monitoring Acid-Base Balance

Regardless of the client's age, injury, or illness, optimal cellular function depends on adequate oxygenation and a balanced acid-base ratio.

Simply stated, acidosis results from either accumulation of acid or loss of base, and alkalosis results from either accumulation of base or loss of acid. Measurement of arterial blood gases (ABGs) assists in detecting disturbances in acid-base balance (Table 28-3).

The body's metabolic processes constantly produce acids, which are neutralized and excreted to maintain acid-base balance. Normally the body maintains an arterial pH between 7.35 and 7.45. The pH represents the concentration of hydrogen (H^+) in solution and indicates whether the imbalance is more acidic or more alkaline. It does not reflect the nature of the imbalance. Normally the ratio is 1 part acid to 20 parts base (Figure 28-5). The three regulatory mechanisms that protect the body against fluctuations in pH are the buffer mechanism, the respiratory system, and the renal system. The buffer mechanism reacts immediately to absorb or release hydrogen ions to maintain acid-base balance. The respiratory system responds within minutes, and the renal system takes 2 to 3 days to respond.

The respiratory system functions to excrete carbon dioxide (CO_2) and water. The amount of CO_2 in the blood is directly related to the carbonic acid concentration. With increased respirations, more CO_2 is eliminated at the alveolar level, which results in less carbonic acid. With decreased respirations, more CO_2 remains in the blood, which results in more carbonic acid.

The alkaline portion of the balance is maintained under normal conditions because the kidneys reabsorb and conserve bicarbonate. The kidneys can generate additional bicarbonate and eliminate excess hydrogen ions as compensation for acidosis. The body normally excretes acidic urine to help maintain acid-base balance. An acid-base imbalance is produced when the ratio between acid and base content of the blood is altered.

The primary types of acid-base imbalance are (1) respiratory acidosis related to carbon dioxide excess, (2) respiratory alkalosis related to carbon dioxide deficit, (3) metabolic acidosis related to bicarbonate deficit, and (4) metabolic alkalosis related to bicarbonate excess. To assess acid-base balance, a specimen of arterial blood is analyzed to determine the pH, the amount of carbon dioxide, and the amount of bicarbonate. This test, called an ABG, gives some information about the cause of acid-base imbalances (respiratory or metabolic) and whether the imbalance is being compensated for by the respiratory or renal system. ABG values also include the oxygenation status of the arterial blood. Normal ABG values are listed in Table 28-4.

ASSESSMENT

1 Assess client's risk factors for acid-base imbalances (see Table 28-3).

2 Assess factors that influence ABG measurements.

a. Suctioning. *Rationale: During suctioning a short-term oxygen desaturation may occur; wait until client's pulse oximetry reading returns to baseline status.*

b. Oxygen therapy. *Rationale: Enter the percentage of inspired oxygen concentration on the client's laboratory requisition information. This value is taken into account when evaluating ABG results.*

c. Ventilator setting change. *Rationale: Ventilator changes are done to improve the client's oxygenation status. However, ABG levels obtained immediately after a ventilator change may be false. Allow the client's physiology to compensate for these changes and wait 20 to 30 minutes following ventilator changes before obtaining a new series of ABGs.*

d. Body temperature. *Rationale: Body temperature affects the affinity of oxygen for hemoglobin and subsequently affects tissue oxygenation.*

3 Identify medications that may affect acid-base balance, such as diuretics, aspirin. *Rationale: Certain medications increase client's risk for acid-base imbalances, especially in the presence of other acute or chronic illnesses.*

4 Assess client for use of anticoagulant medications. *Rationale: Drugs increase bleeding following arterial puncture.*

PLANNING

Expected Outcomes focus on identifying risks for or an actual acid-base imbalance.

1 Client's extremity distal to puncture site remains warm and pink, has adequate capillary refill, and is free of pain.

2 Client will maintain or achieve normal acid-base balance.

3 Complications will be prevented or minimized.

Delegation Considerations

The skills of drawing arterial blood samples and monitoring acid-base balance may not be delegated. The nurse directs personnel by:

• Reviewing to observe and report back any changes in vital signs, LOC, restlessness.

Equipment

• 3-ml heparinized syringe
• 23- to 25-gauge needle
• Syringe cap
• Alcohol swabs (2)
• 2 × 2 gauze pad
• Tape
• Cup or plastic bag with crushed ice
• Label with client information
• Laboratory requisition
• Clean gloves
• Protective eyewear

NOTE: Commercial blood gas kits may be available.

TABLE 28-3 Acid-Base Imbalances

CAUSES	SIGNS AND SYMPTOMS
Respiratory Acidosis	
Hypoventilation Resulting from Primary Respiratory Problems	
Atelectasis (obstruction of small airways often caused by retained mucus)	*Physical examinations:* confusion, dizziness, lethargy, headache, ventricular dysrhythmias, warm and flushed skin, muscular twitching, convulsions, and coma
Pneumonia	
Cystic fibrosis	*Laboratory findings:* arterial blood gas alterations: pH <7.35, partial pressure of carbon dioxide in arterial blood ($Paco_2$) >45 mm Hg, arterial partial pressure of oxygen (Pao_2) <80 mm Hg, and bicarbonate level normal (if uncompensated) or >26 mEq/L (if compensated)
Respiratory failure	
Airway obstruction	
Chest wall injury	
Hypoventilation Resulting from Factors Outside of the Respiratory System	
Drug overdose with a respiratory depressant	
Paralysis of respiratory muscles caused by various neurological alterations	
Head injury	
Obesity	
Respiratory alkalosis	
Hyperventilation Resulting from Primary Respiratory Problems	
Asthma	*Physical examinations:* dizziness, confusion, dysrhythmias, tachypnea, numbness and tingling of extremities, convulsions, and coma
Pneumonia	
Inappropriate mechanical ventilator settings	*Laboratory findings:* arterial blood gas alterations: pH >7.45, $Paco_2$ <35 mm Hg, Pao_2 normal, and bicarbonate level normal (if short lived or uncompensated) or <22 mEq/L (if compensated)
Hyperventilation Resulting from Factors Outside of the Respiratory System	
Anxiety	
Hypermetabolic states	
Disorders of the central nervous system (head injuries, infections)	
Salicylate overdose	
Metabolic Acidosis	
High Anion Gap	
Starvation	*Physical examination:* headache, lethargy, confusion, dysrhythmias, tachypnea with deep respirations, abdominal cramps, and flushed skin
Diabetic ketoacidosis	
Renal failure	*Laboratory findings:* arterial blood gas alterations: pH <7.35, $Paco_2$ normal (if uncompensated) or <35 mm Hg (if compensated), Pao_2 normal or increased (with rapid, deep respirations), bicarbonate level <22 mEq/L, and oxygen saturation normal
Lactic acidosis from heavy exercise	
Use of drugs (methanol, ethanol, formic acid, paraldehyde, aspirin)	
Normal Anion Gap	
Renal tubular acidosis	
Diarrhea	
Metabolic Alkalosis	
Excessive vomiting	*Physical examination:* dizziness; dysrhythmias; numbness and tingling of fingers, toes, and circumoral region; muscle cramps; tetany
Prolonged gastric suctioning	
Hypokalemia or hypercalcemia	*Laboratory findings:* arterial blood gas alterations: pH >7.45, $Paco_2$ normal (if uncompensated) or >45 mm Hg (if compensated), Pao_2 normal, and bicarbonate level >26 mEq/L
Excess aldosterone	
Use of drugs (steroids, sodium bicarbonate, diuretics)	

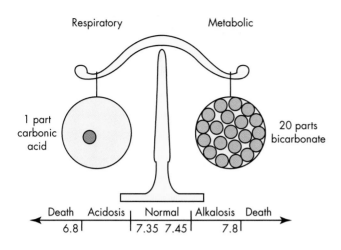

Respiratory   Metabolic

1 part carbonic acid

20 parts bicarbonate

Death | Acidosis | Normal | Alkalosis | Death
6.8 | | 7.35 7.45 | | 7.8

FIGURE 28-5 Carbonic acid/bicarbonate ratio and pH.

TABLE 28-4 Normal Arterial Blood Gas Values		
COMPONENT	**NORMAL VALUE**	**SIGNIFICANCE**
pH	7.35-7.45	Indicates acid-base status of the body
$Paco_2$	35-45 mm Hg	Pressure exerted by dissolved CO_2 in the blood
		Under control of the lungs
		Respiratory component
HCO_3	22-26 mEq/L	Buffers' effect of acid in the blood
		Under control of kidneys
		Metabolic component
Base excess (BE)	+/−2	Reflects status of all bases in blood
Pao_2	90-100 mm Hg	Pressure exerted by dissolved O_2 in blood
		Indicates effectiveness of oxygenation by lungs

IMPLEMENTATION *for Monitoring Acid-Base Balance*

STEPS	RATIONALE

1 See Standard Protocol (inside front cover).

2 Collect ABG sample by arterial puncture.

Arterial blood reflects accurate measurement of oxygen saturation and content of acid-base status.

a. Have heparinized syringe with attached needle, alcohol swab, syringe cap, and cup of ice ready at bedside. Select an appropriate site. The radial, femoral, or brachial arteries are commonly used.

Factors that contraindicate use of arterial site include amputation, contractures, localized infection, dressings or cast, mastectomy, or arteriovenous shunts.

b. Assess collateral blood flow to the hand using Allen's test:

Ensures circulation to extremity will not be compromised by an arterial puncture.

  (1) Have client make a tight fist.

  (2) Use fingers to apply direct pressure to both radial and ulnar arteries.

  (3) Have client open and close hand into a tight fist.

  (4) Release pressure over ulnar artery; observe color of fingers, thumbs, and palm of hand.

Flushing can be seen immediately when flow through ulnar artery is good, which confirms that the radial artery can be used for access.

NURSE ALERT If there is no flushing within 15 seconds; circulation is inadequate, and the radial artery should not be punctured or canulated. This test must be repeated on the other arm (Pullen, 2005). If both arms give a negative result, the femoral or brachial artery is usually chosen.

STEPS	RATIONALE

c. Palpate selected site with fingertips.

d. Stabilize artery by hyperextending wrist slightly.

e. Clean area of maximal impulse with alcohol swab, wiping in circular motion.

Determines area of maximal impulse for puncture site.

Facilitates insertion of the needle.

> **COMMUNICATION TIP** Tell client when you will insert the needle and that it will be painful for a short time.

f. Hold needle bevel up and insert at 45-degree angle, observing for blood return.

g. Stop advancing needle when blood is observed and allow arterial pulsations to pump 2 to 3 ml of blood into the heparinized syringe.

h. When sampling is complete, hold 2 × 2 gauze pad over puncture site and quickly withdraw needle, applying pressure over and just proximal to puncture site.

i. While applying pressure with one hand, expel air bubbles from syringe with other hand.

j. Maintain continuous pressure on and proximal to site for 3 to 5 minutes or longer.

k. Inspect site for signs of bleeding or hematoma formation.

l. Palpate artery distal to puncture site.

m. Place identification label on syringe, place syringe in ice, and attach appropriate laboratory requisition. If the client is receiving supplemental oxygen, note this on the requisition. Indicate client's body temperature.

n. Transport specimen to the laboratory immediately.

3 Interpret ABG report using a systematic approach: Check the Pao_2 (normal is 80 to 100 mm Hg) and the Sao_2 (normal is 95% to 100%).

Needle position facilitates flow of blood into syringe.

Maintains accurate results.

Avoids hematoma formation.

If client is receiving anticoagulant therapy or has bleeding disorder, pressure may be needed for up to 15 minutes.

Verifies that arterial circulation to the hand has not been compromised.

Supplemental oxygen influences results of testing. Elevated body temperature decreases the oxygen saturation results.

Laboratory report includes whether supplementary oxygen was being administered when blood sample was drawn. Hypoxemia refers to low levels of oxygen in the arterial blood, whereas hypoxia refers to low tissue oxygenation. Hypoxia can exist with normal ABG levels when the oxygen-carrying capacity of the blood is compromised (low hemoglobin) or there is low cardiac output and inadequate perfusion.

4 Check the pH to determine the presence of alkalosis (greater than 7.45) or acidosis (less than 7.35).

5 Determine the primary cause of the change in the pH. Check the $Paco_2$ to determine if it is high, within normal limits (WNL), or low (normal is 35 to 45 mm Hg).

a. If the $Paco_2$ is high, the client is hypoventilating and retaining carbonic acid, resulting in respiratory acidosis (see illustration). In collaboration with other health care team members, determine ways to improve the client's ventilation to eliminate excess CO_2 (e.g., deep breathing, pursed-lip breathing, bronchodilators).

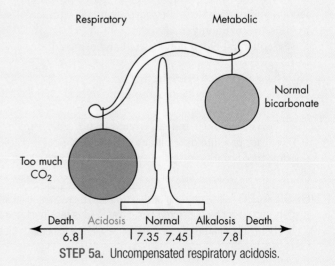

STEP 5a. Uncompensated respiratory acidosis.

| STEPS | RATIONALE |

b. If the $Paco_2$ is low, the client is hyperventilating and too much CO_2 is eliminated, resulting in respiratory alkalosis (see illustration). In collaboration with other health care team members, determine ways to promote retention of CO_2 (e.g., minimize anxiety, slow rate of breathing and breathe less deeply, breathe into a paper bag).

c. If the $Paco_2$ is WNL, the client is ventilating adequately.

6 Check the HCO_3 to determine if it is high, WNL, or low (normal is 22 to 26 mEq/L).

a. If the HCO_3 is high, there is a bicarbonate excess, which can result from retention of bicarbonate or a metabolic loss of acids (see illustration). For example, prolonged vomiting or gastric suction can result in metabolic alkalosis. In collaboration with other health care team members, determine ways to minimize the metabolic loss of acids.

b. If the HCO_3 is low and the CO_2 is normal, there is most likely a bicarbonate deficit from an accumulation of acids caused by a metabolic process (see illustration). Examples include such conditions as diabetic ketoacidosis and shock (with accumulation of lactic acid). With physician's orders, sodium bicarbonate may be given intravenously as an emergency measure. It is important to correct the condition that is causing abnormal production of acids, thereby decreasing acid production. NOTE: Acidosis can be caused by carbon dioxide excess or by a bicarbonate deficit, and alkalosis can be caused by a carbon dioxide deficit or bicarbonate excess.

7 Determine if there is evidence of the body attempting to compensate for the pH change.

a. If the primary problem is respiratory acidosis (pH less than 7.4 with an elevated $Paco_2$), the kidneys may compensate by retaining bicarbonate, which will cause the pH to trend toward the normal range (7.35 to 7.39). This process may take hours or days (see illustration).

b. If the primary problem is metabolic acidosis (pH less than 7.4 with a bicarbonate deficit), the body may compensate by hyperventilating immediately and eliminating carbon dioxide, causing the pH to trend toward the normal range (7.35 to 7.39) (see illustration).

c. If the primary problem is respiratory alkalosis (pH greater than 7.45 with low CO_2), the body may compensate by decreasing renal absorption of bicarbonate. The pH trends toward the normal range (less than 7.45). This begins in 8 hours and is maximal in 3 to 5 days (see illustration).

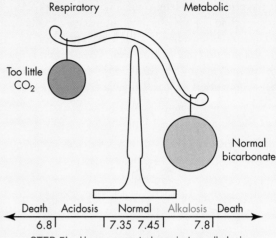

STEP 5b. Uncompensated respiratory alkalosis.

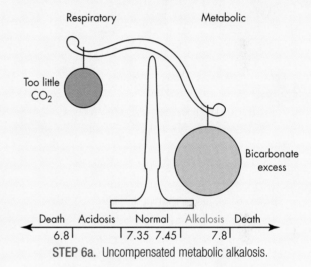

STEP 6a. Uncompensated metabolic alkalosis.

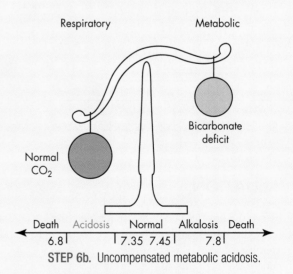

STEP 6b. Uncompensated metabolic acidosis.

STEPS	RATIONALE

d. If the primary problem is metabolic alkalosis (pH greater than 7.4 with bicarbonate excess), the body may compensate immediately with hypoventilation to promote retention of carbonic acid. The pH trends toward the normal range (less than 7.45) (see illustration).

8 See Completion Protocol (inside front cover).

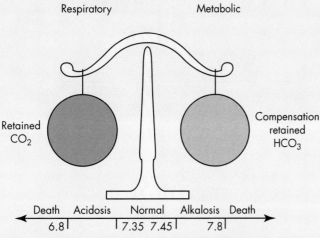

STEP 7a. Compensated respiratory alkalosis.

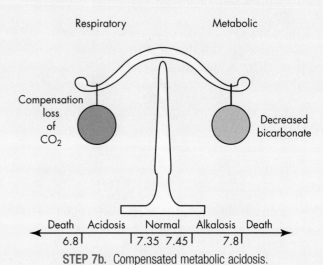

STEP 7b. Compensated metabolic acidosis.

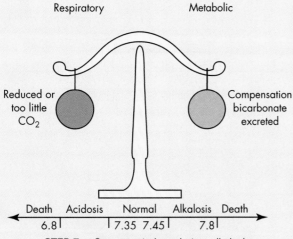

STEP 7c. Compensated respiratory alkalosis.

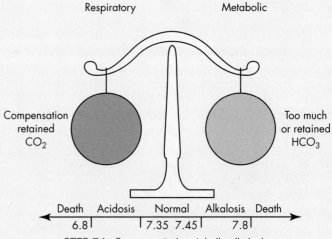

STEP 7d. Compensated metabolic alkalosis.

EVALUATION

1 Observe the arterial puncture site for bleeding.
2 Palpate distal pulse and verify intact circulation to distal extremity.
3 Evaluate ABG results to determine if acid-base imbalance exists.
4 Observe for complications.

Unexpected Outcomes and Related Interventions

1 Client continues to have persistent acid-base imbalance.
a. Notify physician.
b. Identify ways to correct imbalance, such as consulting a nutritionist for diet modification.

Recording and Reporting

- Record ABG values, condition of puncture site, interventions, and client response. Record specimens sent to the laboratory stat.
- ABG results must be reported to the physician as soon as available.

Sample Documentation

2300 Admitted in acute respiratory distress. Vital signs: HR 112, R 36. BP 148/84 mm Hg. Reports dyspnea at rest and speech interrupted to breathe. Alert and oriented ×3. Lung sounds reveal coarse crackles and wheezing throughout all lobes. Oxygen at 2 L per nasal cannula. Head of bed elevated. ABGs: Pao_2 68, pH 7.32, $Paco_2$ 50, and HCO_3 24. Dr. Lindsay notified. Orders received.

Special Considerations

Geriatric Considerations

The complex health histories presented by older adults and underlying conditions, especially pulmonary diseases, affect the overall responses to acid-base imbalance. Laboratory tests and results need to be considered within context of underlying diseases and not in isolation from the overall clinical picture (Meiner and Lueckenotte, 2006).

Long-Term Care Considerations

Treatment for alterations in acid-base balance, similar in long-term care as in the gerontologic population, may require transport of client to acute care setting.

NCLEX® Style Questions

1 A client is admitted to a medical unit with renal failure and congestive heart failure. During an assessment, the nurse notices that the client's ECG pattern differs from what it was 2 hours ago. Suspecting the client has an electrolyte imbalance, which of the following conditions are possible? (Choose more than one.)
1. Hyponatremia
2. Hypocalcemia
3. Hypernatremia
4. Hyperkalemia

2 A 40-year-old man presents to the emergency department with food poisoning and frequent vomiting. He complains of muscle weakness, abdominal pain, and cramping. ECG results show irregularities. The nurse would expect to administer medications to correct which electrolyte imbalance?
1. Hypernatremia
2. Hyponatremia
3. Hypokalemia
4. Hyperkalemia

3 A nurse receives a physician order to administer Kayexalate to reduce the serum potassium level of a client with hyperkalemia. This drug works by:
1. Forcing potassium into the cells
2. Depleting gastrointestinal absorption of potassium
3. Promoting renal excretion of potassium
4. Pulling potassium into the bowel for excretion

4 As part of a client's treatment for asymptomatic hypokalemia, an IV potassium supplement is prescribed. Which action is essential for correct administration of postassium? What is the correct administration rate?
1. Set the infusion rate at 20 mEq of potassium or lower per hour.
2. Set infusion rate at 40 mEq per hour.
3. Give the client extra oral fluids containing potassium.
4. Set infusion rate based on the client's urine output.

5 A client with kidney disease is at risk for hyponatremia. Which serum sodium level indicates hyponatremia?
1. 125 mEq/L
2. 135 mEq/L
3. 140 mEq/L
4. 145 mEq/L

References for all chapters appear in Appendix D.

29

Promoting Oxygenation

MEDIA RESOURCES

- **evolve** http://evolve.elsevier.com/Elkin

- **View Video!** Video Clips

- Nursing Skills Online

P hysiological needs such as food, water, and air are the primary stimuli for behavior according to Maslow's hierarchy of human needs. Ineffective respirations are a cause of distress that will not allow humans to focus on any other event. Respirations are effective when sufficient oxygenation is obtained at the cellular level and when cellular waste and carbon dioxide are adequately removed via the bloodstream and lungs. When this system is interrupted, such as by lung tissue damage, obstruction of airways by inflammation and excess mucus, or impairment of the mechanics of ventilation, intervention is required to support the client or death may occur.

NURSING DIAGNOSES

Nursing diagnoses directly related to problems affecting optimum oxygenation include **ineffective airway clearance** resulting from an ineffective cough or excessive secretions and **ineffective breathing pattern** exhibited by clients with respiratory muscle weakness and fatigue or abnormal breathing pattern. In addition, **impaired gas exchange** resulting from altered oxygen supply or alveolar hypoventilation and **impaired spontaneous ventilation** may be present for clients who exhibit an imbalance between ventilatory capacity and increased ventilatory demand. **Risk for infection** and **risk for aspiration** are present in these clients due to the damaged defense systems of the lungs. Any problem with oxygenation may also predispose the client to **fatigue,** as well as **imbalanced nutrition: less than body requirements** due to their inability to cope with an increased metabolic rate brought on by the increased demand for oxygenation.

Clients with breathing problems may also be at risk for **disturbed thought processes** from inadequate oxygenation and carbon dioxide retention. **Activity intolerance** related to imbalance between oxygen supply and demand may lead to a **self-care deficit.** Psychosocial nursing diagnoses such as **anxiety, fear,** and **hopelessness** may be related to dyspnea and feelings of suffocation, as well as the fear of dying. **Impaired verbal communication** applies when a client is severely dyspneic or has an artificial airway such as a tracheostomy.

SKILL 29.1 Oxygen Administration

- Nursing Skills Online: Airway Management, Lesson 1

Hypoxia is a condition in which insufficient oxygen is available to meet the metabolic needs of tissues and cells. Oxygen therapy refers to the administration of oxygen to a client to prevent or relieve hypoxia. Hypoxia results from hypoxemia, which is a deficiency of oxygen in the arterial blood. Supplemental oxygen for the relief of hypoxemia may be temporary, until the cause of the problem is corrected, or long term, when it is required for a chronic condition.

Room air has an oxygen concentration, or fraction of inspired oxygen (FiO_2), of 21%. Supplemental oxygen delivery is based on the FiO_2 required to maintain adequate oxygenation (Table 29-1), whether hospital or home use, and the portability desired.

ASSESSMENT

1 Perform a complete assessment of the respiratory system (see Chapter 12). Assess for impaired gas exchange (hypoxia or hypercapnia), during both rest and activity, including:

a. Behavioral changes, apprehension, anxiety, decreased ability to concentrate, decreased level of consciousness, fatigue, and dizziness. *Rationale: Decreased levels of oxygen (hypoxia) or increased levels of carbon dioxide (hypercapnia) affect a person's cognitive abilities, interpersonal interactions, and mood. These slight changes may be early indicators of problems with oxygenation.*

b. Assess vital signs, including rate, rhythm, and depth of respirations. *Rationale: Provides baseline of oxygenation status and enables early detection of hypoxia.*

c. Assess SpO_2 via pulse oximetry (see Chapter 11). *Rationale: In the presence of hypoxemia, the percent of hemoglobin saturated with oxygen declines, and the client's pulse oximetry level declines.*

d. Assess skin and mucosa for changes in color: pallor, cyanosis, or flushing. *Rationale: Pallor may occur when client's oxygen levels decline. Cyanosis is a late sign of hypoxia. Flushing may be noted when hypercapnia is present.*

2 Check arterial blood gas (ABG) results. *Rationale: Objectively quantifies changes in oxygen and carbon dioxide that affect acid-base balance (see Chapter 28).*

TABLE 29-1 Oxygen Delivery Systems			
DELIVERY SYSTEM	**FiO_2* DELIVERED**	**ADVANTAGES**	**DISADVANTAGES**
Nasal cannula	1-6 L/min: 24%-45%	Safe and simple Easily tolerated Effective for low concentrations Does not impede eating or talking Inexpensive, disposable	Unable to use with nasal obstruction Drying to mucous membranes Can dislodge easily May cause skin irritation or breakdown around ears or nares Client's breathing pattern will affect exact FiO_2
OXYMIZER	1-15 L/min: 24%-100% (see Skill 29-1, Step 5d, p. 661)	Higher concentrations without mask Releases O_2 only on inhalation Conserves O_2, increased portability Does not require humidification; however, may be used at flow rates of 6 L and up Two types available with nasal reservoir and pendant reservoir	Nasal reservoir type may interfere with drinking from cup Potential reservoir membrane failure
Simple mask	5-10 L/min: 30%-60%	Usually well tolerated.	Contraindicated for clients who retain CO_2
Venturi mask	4-12 L/min: 60%-80%	Delivers exact preset FiO_2 despite client's breathing pattern Does not dry mucous membranes Can be used to deliver humidity	Hot and confining, mask may irritate skin FiO_2 may be lowered if mask does not fit snugly Interferes with eating and talking
Partial rebreathing mask	8-12 L/min: 40%-70%	Delivers increased FiO_2 Easily humidifies O_2 Does not dry mucous membranes	Hot and confining, may irritate skin, tight seal necessary Interferes with eating and talking Bag may twist or kink; should not totally deflate
Nonrebreathing mask	10-15 L/min: 60%-80%	Delivers highest possible FiO_2 without intubation Does not dry mucous membranes	Requires tight seal, difficult to maintain and uncomfortable May irritate skin Bag should not totally deflate

*FiO_2, Fraction of inspired oxygen concentration.

PLANNING

Expected Outcomes focus on optimum oxygenation, safe application of oxygen therapy, and an understanding of and compliance with the oxygen prescription.

1 Client's oxygen saturation (SpO_2) and ABGs return to or remain within normal limits or baseline levels.
2 Client verbalizes improved comfort; and subjective experiences of anxiety, fatigue, and breathlessness return to normal.
3 Client's pulse, respirations, and color return to normal.
4 Client is able to state the indications for supplemental oxygen by discharge.
5 Client follows safety guidelines for supplemental oxygen therapy by discharge.
6 Client uses supplemental oxygen as prescribed by discharge.

Delegation Considerations

Assessment of the client's condition and setup of oxygen therapy liter flow cannot be delegated; however, the skill of nasal cannula or mask placement may be delegated. The nurse directs personnel by:

- Explaining how to adapt a skill for a specific client and reviewing what to observe and report back to the nurse.
- Instructing assistive personnel (AP) to immediately report any vital sign changes or other unexpected outcomes associated with the oxygen delivery device.

Equipment

- Delivery device ordered by physician
- Oxygen tubing (consider extension tubing)
- Humidifier, if indicated
- Sterile water for humidifier
- Oxygen source
- Oxygen flowmeter
- "Oxygen in use" sign

IMPLEMENTATION *for Oxygen Administration*

STEPS	RATIONALE

1 See Standard Protocol (inside front cover).

> **COMMUNICATION TIP** Explain to client the purpose of oxygen administration and safety precautions (Table 29-2). Also explain to the client the possibility of continued dyspnea because of the etiology of the breathing problem (e.g., narrowed airways, fever).

STEPS	RATIONALE
2 Attach delivery device (e.g., cannula, mask) to oxygen tubing. Consider extension tubing for clients who are not confined to bed.	Extension tubing increases client's ability to move about and assists in avoiding complications of bed rest.
3 Attach appropriate flowmeter to oxygen source, then attach oxygen tubing (see illustration).	Flowmeters with smaller calibrations may be safer for clients requiring low-dose oxygen when larger doses may be harmful, as in clients with chronic obstructive pulmonary disease (COPD).
4 Adjust oxygen flow rate to prescribed dosage. Verify that water is bubbling when using a humidifier.	Oxygen is a medication; correct dose is required and must be prescribed by physician.
5 Observe for proper fit, function, and FiO_2 of delivery device.	
a. *Nasal cannula:* Place tips of cannula into client's nares and adjust headband or plastic slide until cannula fits snugly and comfortably (see illustration).	Effective mechanism of oxygen delivery up to 6 L/min. Useful for low oxygen concentration for clients with chronic lung disease.

TABLE 29-2 Oxygen Safety Guidelines	
GUIDELINE	**EXPLANATION**
"Oxygen in use" sign is on client's door.	Notifies all personnel of oxygen in client's room.
Make sure oxygen is set at prescribed rate.	Oxygen is a medication and should not be adjusted without a physician's order.
Smoking is not permitted. Avoid electrical equipment that may result in sparks.	Oxygen supports combustion. Delivery systems must be kept 10 feet from open flames and at least 5 feet from electrical equipment.
Store oxygen cylinders upright. Secure with chain or holder.	Prevents tipping and falling while stationary or when client is being transported.
Check oxygen available in portable cylinders before transporting or ambulating clients.	Gauge on cylinder should register in green range, indicating that oxygen is available. Have backup supply available if level is low.

STEPS	RATIONALE

b. *Venturi Mask:* Oxygen delivered by turning barrel to preset intervals (see illustrations). Setting should correlate with prescribed dosage.

Delivers exact preset Fio_2 despite client's breathing pattern.

c. Partial rebreathing mask: 40% to 70% oxygen delivered using flow rates of 8 to 12 L/min (Pruitt and Jacobs, 2003). Mask seals tightly around mouth. Reservoir fills on exhalation and almost collapses on inhalation (see illustration). At 8- to 12-liter flow, should deliver 40% to 70% Fio_2.

Easily humidifies oxygen and does not dry mucous membranes. Delivers higher concentrations and is useful for short-term therapy of 24 hours or less. Client may not be able to tolerate the fit of the mask (Pruitt and Jacobs, 2003).

d. *Reservoir nasal cannula (OXYMIZER):* Fit as for nasal cannula. Reservoir is located under nose or as a pendant (see illustration).

Delivers higher flow of oxygen than cannula without changing to a mask, which is claustrophobic for some clients. Delivers a 2:1 ratio (e.g., 6-L nasal cannula is approximately equivalent to 3.5-L reservoir device or OXYMIZER).

NURSE ALERT Observe the reservoir bag to ensure that client's inspiratory demands are being met. It should not collapse completely on inspiration.

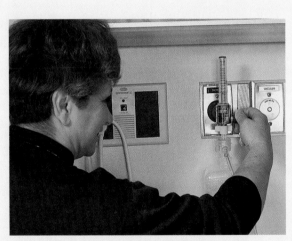

STEP 3 Flowmeter attached to oxygen source.

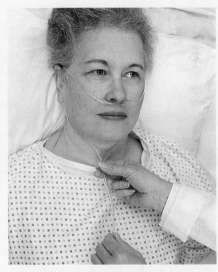

STEP 5a. Nasal cannula adjusted for proper fit.

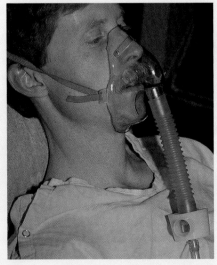

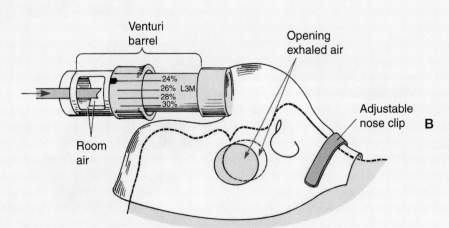

STEP 5b. **A,** Venturi mask. **B,** Oxygen is delivered by turning barrel to preset intervals.

STEPS	RATIONALE

e. *Nonrebreathing mask:*
   Contains one-way valves with a reservoir. Can be combined with a nasal cannula to provide higher FiO_2. A tight seal around the mouth is necessary to prevent room air from entering and decreasing the FiO_2.

Device of choice for short-term high FiO_2 delivery.
Valve prevents exhaled air from entering the reservoir. Client may not be able to tolerate mask (Pruitt and Jacobs, 2003). A leak-free nonrebreathing mask with competent valves and enough flow (10 to 15 L/min) should deliver FiO_2 of 60% to 80% (Pruitt and Jacobs, 2003).

f. *Simple face mask:*
   Place securely over client's nose and mouth (see illustration).

A simple face mask can deliver concentrations of 30% to 60% using flow rates of 5 to 10 L/min. It is a little easier to tolerate than other masks (Pruitt and Jacobs, 2003).

6 Post an "Oxygen in use" sign on wall behind bed and at entrance to room.

Alerts visitors and care providers that oxygen is in use.

7 Obtain an order for ABGs or pulse oximetry 10 to 15 minutes after initiation of therapy or change in oxygen concentration.

ABGs provide objective data regarding blood oxygenation and acid-base status (see Chapter 28).

8 Consult with physician regarding the need for continuous pulse oximetry if client's oxygen level is not stable.

Oximetry provides objective data regarding blood oxygenation and is used for trending (see Chapter 11).

9 **See Completion Protocol (inside front cover).**

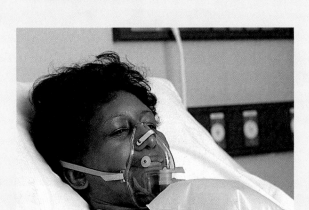

STEP 5c. Partial rebreathing mask.

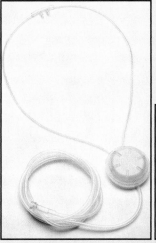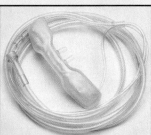

STEP 5d. Two types of OXYMIZER tubings, nasal reservoir (left) and pendant device (right). (CHAD, OXYMIZER, OXYPneumatic and TOTAL 02 are registered trademarks of CHAD Therameutics, Inc., www.chadtherapeutics.com)

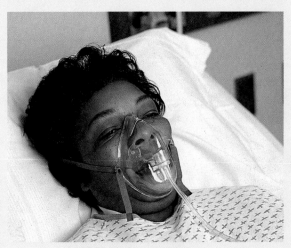

STEP 5f. Simple face mask.

EVALUATION

1 Observe repeat ABGs and/or pulse oximetry for objective measurement of improvement after initiation or change in therapy. Evaluate response both at rest and with activity (if possible).

2 Observe client for decreased anxiety, improved level of consciousness and cognitive abilities, decreased fatigue, and absence of dizziness.

3 Assess pulse and respirations; expect a decreased pulse with regular rhythm, decreased respiratory rate, and improved color.

4 Ask client to verbalize indications for supplemental oxygen.

5 Observe if client follows safety guidelines in present setting and ask client to verbalize safety guidelines for home use.

6 Observe client or caregiver demonstrate use of supplemental oxygen.

Unexpected Outcomes and Related Interventions

1 Client experiences nasal irritation, drying of nasal mucosa, sinus pain, or epistaxis.

a. Apply a water-soluble lubricant to areas of irritation around nares.

b. Recommend use of an isotonic saline nasal spray.

c. Determine if a reservoir cannula is appropriate (decreased liter flow without reducing FiO_2, oxygen delivery on inspiration only); if so, obtain order.

d. Consider humidification.

2 Client develops irritation of the face or posterior surfaces of the ear.

a. Apply ear protectors, or reposition nasal cannula so that it does not contact irritated areas.

3 Client has continued hypoxia: increased and/or irregular heart rate, SpO_2 declines.

a. Monitor ABGs and/or pulse oximetry.

b. Perform a complete respiratory assessment.

c. Notify physician.

d. Identify methods to decrease oxygen demand (e.g., total bed rest, positioning).

4 Client develops carbon dioxide retention with confusion, headache, decreased level of consciousness, flushing, somnolence, carbon dioxide narcosis, or respiratory arrest.

a. Monitor ABGs.

b. Notify physician of symptoms.

c. Attempt to maintain oxygen pressure (PaO_2) at 55 mm Hg. Hypoxia must be treated, but PaO_2 levels that exceed 60 to 70 mm Hg may worsen hypoventilation.

Recording and Reporting

- Record the respiratory assessment findings.
- Record method of oxygen delivery and flow rate.
- Record and report client's response and any adverse reactions.

Sample Documentation

0800 Alert and oriented. Respirations 20, even and non-labored. Lungs clear to auscultation. Mucous membranes pink. O_2 4-L/min nasal cannula. SpO_2 90%. Cough productive of yellow sputum. Fluids encouraged as tolerated.

10:00 Reddened area noted behind right ear. Foam ear protector added to nasal cannula tubing.

12:00 Denies discomfort from cannula. No further redness noted behind ears.

Special Considerations

Pediatric Considerations

- Oxygen hoods are transparent enclosures that surround the head of the neonate or small infant and deliver continuous humidified oxygen. Larger "tents" are available for larger children (Myers, 2002).

Geriatric Considerations

- Decrease in the partial pressure of oxygen (PaO_2) that occurs with aging is about 0.3% per year. After age 75, healthy nonsmokers do not show a noticeable decline. The decrease in oxygen is related to the loss of elasticity in the lungs and the increase in physiological dead space (Beers and others, 2005).
- The drive to breathe in clients who have chronically increased CO_2 levels is based on their oxygen levels. Providing oxygen flow rates greater than 2 L/min may increase oxygen levels to a degree that would decrease spontaneous respirations.

Home Care Considerations

- Teach the client and family how to correctly administer oxygen based on which system is used and the safety measures to be followed (see Chapter 38).
- Stress the dangers of changing the oxygen flow rate from the prescribed flow.
- Emphasize that the client may be short of breath because of reasons other than hypoxemia and to contact the physician if increased shortness of breath occurs.
- Teach the client and family signs and symptoms of hypoxia.

Long-Term Care Considerations

- Oximetry may be used to monitor clients during rehabilitation services, requiring different flow rates and/or delivery systems for activity versus rest.

SKILL 29.2 Airway Management: Noninvasive Interventions

The airways must remain open and free of obstruction to decrease resistance of airflow to and from the lung. Airway clearance techniques to maintain airway patency such as increasing fluids to assist in the removal of thick secretions depend on the pathophysiology responsible for the obstruction. Noninvasive interventions include positioning, deep breathing, coughing, medications, and hydration. Postoperative noninvasive procedures are addressed in Chapter 20.

Positioning enhances airway patency in all clients. A Fowler's or semi-Fowler's position promotes a client's chest expansion with the least amount of effort. A client with COPD who is short of breath may gain relief by sitting with his or her back against a chair and rolling the head and shoulders forward or leaning over a bedside table while in bed.

Deep breathing and coughing techniques help clients to effectively clear their airway while maintaining their oxygen levels. Teach a client "controlled coughing" by having him or her take a deep breath in and cough deeply with the mouth slightly open. If a client has difficulty coughing, teach the huffing technique. This involves taking a medium breath and then making a sound like "ha" to push the air out fast with the mouth slightly open. This is done three or four times, and then the client is instructed to cough.

Many devices assist with secretion clearance, such as vests that inflate with large volumes of air and vibrate the chest wall and hand held devices that assist in providing positive expiratory pressure to prevent airway collapse in exhalation (Garvey, 2005). Usefulness of these therapies is decided based on the individual client situation and preference of both the client and care provider.

Pharmacological management is essential for clients with respiratory disease. Medications such as bronchodilators effectively relax smooth muscles and open airways in certain disease processes such as COPD. Glucocorticoids relieve inflammation and also assist in opening air passages. Mucolytics and adequate hydration decrease the thickness of pulmonary secretions so that they can be expectorated more easily (Cigna and Turner-Cigna, 2005).

Clients with obstructive sleep apnea (OSA) may be unable to maintain a patent airway. In OSA, nasopharyngeal abnormalities that cause narrowing of the upper airway produce repetitive airway obstruction during sleep, with the potential for periods of apnea and hypoxemia. Pressure can be delivered during the inspiratory and expiratory phases of the respiratory cycle by mask to maintain airway patency during sleep. The process requires consideration of each individual's needs to obtain compliance (Beers and others, 2005).

For clients who have measurable changes in the flow of their airways, such as clients with asthma or reactive airways disease, peak expiratory flow rate (PEFR) measurements are useful. The PEFR is the maximum flow that a client forces out during one quick forced expiration and is measured in liters. Use these measurements as an objective indicator of the client's current status or the effectiveness of treatment. Decreased PEFR may indicate the need for further interventions such as increased doses of bronchodilators or antiinflammatory medications (Zoidis, 2005). Normal values vary according to a person's age, sex, and size. The National Institutes of Health (NIH) has a peak flow zone system organized in a "traffic light" pattern to help the client know what to do when the peak flow number changes. For helpful information, the client can be referred to the NIH government website (see http://www.nhlbi.nih.gov).

ASSESSMENT

1 Assess work of breathing, sense of breathlessness, and ability to clear copious or tenacious secretions by coughing. *Rationale: Indicates risk for impaired airway clearance. Secretions can plug the airway, decreasing the amount of oxygen available for gas exchange in the lung.*

2 Assess lung sounds for adventitious sounds such as wheezing. Assess for shortness of breath, use of accessory muscles of respiration, pallor, or cyanosis. *Rationale: Indicators of distress from airway obstruction, ranging from mild to life threatening. A decrease in adventitious sounds may indicate plugging of the airway from mucus rather than an improvement in condition.*

3 Assess client's SpO_2 with oximetry or collect ABGs. *Rationale: Establishes baseline for determining response to therapy.*

4 Assess for interrupted sleep, snoring respirations. Ask client about history of sleep apnea. *Rationale: Indications for use of continuous positive airway pressure (CPAP) or bilevel positive airway pressure (BiPAP). Refer client for evaluation.*

5 Monitor PEFR initially and with changes in therapy. Assess client's baseline knowledge of when and how to use PEFR and correct response to results. *Rationale: Client may monitor PEFR for early detection of problems after discharge; teach client the "red yellow green" method of evaluation.*

PLANNING

Expected Outcomes focus on client's airway patency, comfort, and ability for self-care.

- Client maintains a position that promotes maximum lung expansion and comfort.
- Client's airways are clear of retained secretions.
- Client's periods of sleep apnea are reduced to fewer than two episodes in 6 hours.
- Client's ABGs and pulse oximetry readings improve or remain normal.

- Client and family demonstrate correct use of CPAP/BiPAP and express comfort using equipment by discharge.
- Client and family demonstrate correct technique and verbalize an appropriate action plan based on PEFR values obtained by discharge.
- Client verbalizes the benefits of positioning, CPAP, and/or PEFR by discharge.

Delegation Considerations

Assessment of the client's condition cannot be delegated. The skills of positioning, therapeutic coughing, CPAP/BiPAP mask application, and follow-up PEFR measurements can be delegated. The nurse is responsible for the initial PEFR measurement. The nurse directs personnel by:

- Reviewing assessment findings to report back to the nurse, such as difficulty breathing and signs of distress and hypoxia.

Equipment
CPAP/BiPAP

- CPAP or BiPAP mask (Figure 29-1)
- Mask straps (face or nasal)
- Valve (CPAP or BiPAP)
- Oxygen source
- Generator (CPAP or BiPAP)
- Appropriate signs

PEFR

- Peak flowmeter
- Client diary/action plan, if appropriate

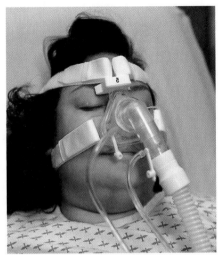

FIGURE 29-1 CPAP mask/BIPAP mask.

IMPLEMENTATION *for Airway Management: Noninvasive Interventions*

STEPS	RATIONALE

1 See Standard Protocol (inside front cover).

> **COMMUNICATION TIP** Explain to client that you are aware of the discomfort he or she is experiencing (i.e., breathlessness, pain) and that correct positioning will assist them.

2 Positioning

a. *Sitting:* Assist to semi-Fowler's or high Fowler's, sitting on side of bed or in chair with elbows resting on knees. Clients with COPD may benefit from leaning over table with arms propped up (see illustration).

Promotes optimum lung expansion and maximizes use of accessory muscles. Decreases client's work of breathing.

b. *Leaning:* Have client lean forward over the back of a chair or against the wall.

Leaning forward allows the lungs to expand with less transdiaphragmatic pressure (Jantarakupt and Porock, 2005).

c. *Supine:* Most clients are more comfortable supported by two pillows or with the head of the bed up at least 30 degrees.

Decreases orthopnea. Obese clients may experience decreased abdominal interference of full lung expansion when lying flat.

d. *Turning:* Turn at least every 2 hours. Use turning maneuvers to drain areas of lungs with retained secretions by gravity if tolerated by client. If unilateral reexpansion is needed (e.g., after general surgery), have client lie with side requiring expansion up: "good side down, affected lung up."

Encouragers drainage of secretions and promotes lung expansion on the affected side.

> **NURSE ALERT** Following some types of thoracic surgery (e.g., lobectomy), specific side-lying positions may be ordered to facilitate hemostasis and intrathoracic wound healing, whereas other positions may be contraindicated.

STEPS	RATIONALE

3 Controlled coughing

> **COMMUNICATION TIP** Explain to client that controlled coughing clears secretions that may obstruct the airway by allowing air behind the mucus to move during the cough.

a. Place client in upright position. High-Fowler's, leaning forward, or with knees bent and a small pillow or hand to support the abdomen may augment expiratory pressure.	Facilitates inhalation and lung expansion during coughing maneuver.
b. Instruct client to take two slow, deep breaths, inhaling through the nose and exhaling through the mouth.	Control of respiratory rate facilitates coughing and minimizes risk of paroxysms of coughing.
c. Instruct client to inhale deeply a third time, hold this breath, and count to three; then to cough deeply for two or three consecutive coughs without inhaling between coughs. Instruct the client to push air forcefully out of the lungs.	Ensures full, effective cough.
d. Have clients with difficulty coughing use a "huff" cough by taking a medium breath and then making a sound like "ha" to push the air out fast with their mouths slightly open. Repeat three or four times and then instruct client to cough.	Assists clients to generate more pressure to force secretions through airways.

4 CPAP/BiPAP administration

a. Position client comfortably with head elevated.	Allows for maximum lung expansion.

> **COMMUNICATION TIP** Before placing CPAP or BiPAP mask on the client, explain that a tight seal around the face is needed.

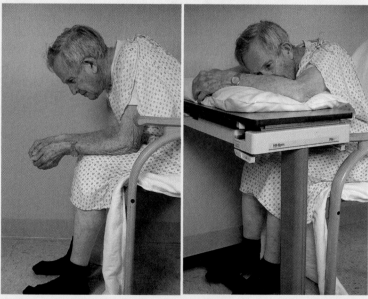

STEP 2a. Positioning optimizes chest expansion and reduces the work of breathing. Leaning position allows lungs to expand.

STEPS	RATIONALE
b. Position face mask or nasal mask tightly and adjust head strap until seal is maintained and client is able to tolerate (see Figure 29-1). *Several types of masks are available because of the difficulties in achieving a comfortable fit.*	Client may experience claustrophobic sensations and feelings of discomfort from continuous pressure. Support and education help client develop tolerance.
c. Instruct client to breathe normally.	Reduces hyperventilation and fatigue. Promotes optimum lung expansion.
d. Apply at ordered setting for prescribed length of time.	Like oxygen, administer CPAP/BiPAP at prescribed level.
5 PEFR measurements	
a. Instruct client about purpose and rationale.	
b. Assist client to high-Fowler's position.	Promotes optimum lung expansion.
c. Slide mouthpiece into base of the numbered scale.	Enables client to objectively monitor airway improvements during expiration.
d. Instruct client to take a deep breath.	
e. Have client place meter mouthpiece in the mouth and close lips, making a firm seal (see illustration).	Tight seal ensures all expired breath will be measured for accurate reading.
f. Have client blow out as hard and fast as possible through the mouth only.	Maximum effort is required for an accurate reading. Air expelled through nares will not be measured and will decrease PEFR readings.
g. Repeat maneuver two additional times, with the highest number recorded on chart.	
h. If client is to record PEFR at home, have client demonstrate PEFR technique independently and assess ability to record PEFR accurately on chart using "traffic light" pattern.	Return demonstration is an effective method to evaluate learning. Green zone (80% to 100% of the personal best number) indicates that no asthma symptoms are present. Yellow zone is 50% to 80% of personal best number and signals caution. The client may need treatment and may be having an attack. The red zone or less than 50% of personal best number signals a medical alert, and the client should take medication and call physician immediately (Zoidis, 2005).

> **COMMUNICATION TIP** Help client implement an appropriate action plan as prescribed by physician. Explain that PEFR is just one objective measure that can be used to judge symptom severity.

i. **See Completion Protocol (inside front cover).**

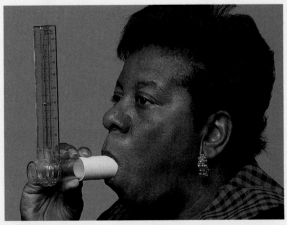

STEP 5e. Positive end-expiratory pressure measurement.

EVALUATION

1 Observe client's body alignment and position whenever in visual contact with client.
2 Auscultate lung fields for adventitious lung sounds.
3 Assess client's respiratory status during sleep to determine response to CPAP.
4 Review repeat ABGs and/or pulse oximetry.
5 Observe client and caregiver's use of CPAP/BiPAP mask and compliance with therapy.
6 Observe a return demonstration by client or family to determine if correct technique is being used with PEFR.
7 Determine client's PEFR and compare with the client's personal best.
8 Ask client to explain purpose and benefits of positioning and CPAP/BiPAP or PEFR.

Unexpected Outcomes and Related Interventions

1 Client is unable to maintain a patent airway.
a. Evaluate positioning. Consider suctioning and use of artificial airway (see Skill 29.3).
b. Monitor ABGs/pulse oximetry.
2 Client experiences worsening dyspnea with bronchospasm and hypoxemia.
a. Notify physician.
b. Monitor ABGs/pulse oximetry.
c. Medicate as ordered.
d. Evaluate for methods to decrease oxygen demand (bed rest, positioning).
3 Client is unable to tolerate CPAP/BiPAP.
a. Mask fit: Check fit of delivery device. Consider alternative (alternate type of mask, nasal pillows) if difficulties continue. If skin breakdown occurs across bridge of nose, apply a Band-Aid until skin becomes adjusted to the pressure. If generalized breakdown occurs, consider a reaction to the mask material (i.e., latex).
b. Pressure: Feelings of suffocation, shortness of breath, and discomfort related to pressure from CPAP/ BiPAP. Determine if another pressure setting will give similar results with more comfort or if BiPAP is required. If client is able to continue trying, he or she usually can adapt to these feelings over time.

c. Dryness: If a saline nasal spray is not effective, consider obtaining an order for a humidifier.
4 Client is unable or unwilling to give maximum effort for PEFR.
a. Encourage and reeducate client.
b. If unable to achieve adequate readings, contact physician immediately, medicate as ordered, and give support.

Recording and Reporting

- Record activity level, including assistance needed with positioning.
- Record cough effectiveness and respiratory assessment.
- For CPAP/BiPAP, record client compliance and tolerance, mask fit and skin assessment beneath mask, effectiveness of therapy, witnessed periods of apnea, and status of daytime hypersomnolence.
- For PEFR, record measurement before and after therapy and client's ability and effort to perform PEFR.

Sample Documentation

2400 Observed sleeping. Respirations 18, even and easy without snoring. Lungs clear to auscultation. No jerking movements noted. CPAP continues per face mask with good seal at 7.5 cm H_2O.

Special Considerations

Pediatric Considerations

- PEFR is an effective assessment for assisting the school-age child and adolescent in management of their asthma. Instruct parents and child to notify school nurse of use of PEFR and any related action plans (U.S. Environmental Protection Agency, 2004).

Home Care Considerations

- Frequent follow-up may be necessary to enhance CPAP/ BiPAP compliance and address unexpected outcomes promptly.
- PEFR may be incorporated into an "action plan" for the client at home as an objective measure of when a change in therapy is required.

SKILL 29.3 Airway Management: Suctioning

- **Nursing Skills Online: Airway Management, Lessons 3-5**

For some clients noninvasive techniques and medications are insufficient to maintain a patent airway. In these cases, suctioning is appropriate. Choose a method of suctioning, depending on the level of the secretions to be removed, the presence of an artificial airway, and the client's condition.

Suction the oral cavity by oropharyngeal suctioning, using a rigid plastic catheter (called a "Yankauer") with one large and several small eyelets to remove mucus (Figure 29-2). The catheter supplies continuous suction once you connect it to a suction source. Teach clients how to use this catheter to clear secretions from their oral cavity.

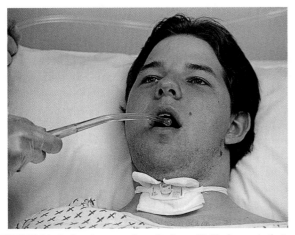

FIGURE 29-2 Oropharyngeal suctioning with Yankauer catheter.

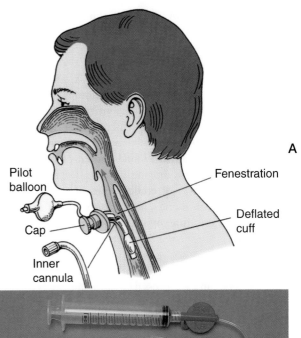

A

Pilot
balloon

Fenestration

Deflated
cuff

Cap

Inner
cannula

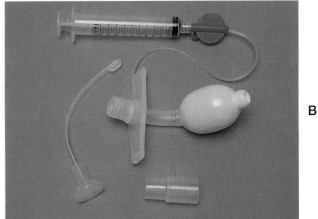

B

FIGURE 29-4 **A,** Tracheostomy tube in lower trachea. **B,** Tube with obturator for insertion. Syringe inflates balloon.

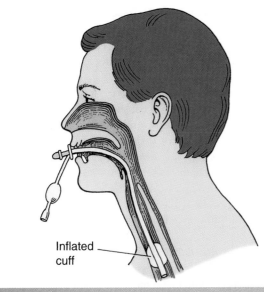

A

Inflated
cuff

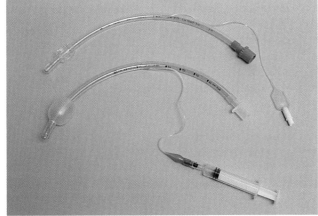

B

FIGURE 29-3 **A,** Endotracheal tube with inflated cuff. **B,** ET tubes with uninflated and inflated cuffs with syringe for inflation.

Suctioning of the lower airway using sterile technique may be necessary if clients cannot cough forcefully enough to clear secretions. Endotracheal (ET) (Figure 29-3) and tracheostomy (Figure 29-4) tubes allow direct access to the lower airways for suctioning. Physicians or certified personnel insert these artificial airways to create a route for mechanical ventilation, relieve mechanical airway obstruction, or protect the airway from aspiration because of impaired cough or gag reflexes.

EVIDENCE IN PRACTICE

Joanna Briggs Institute, 2000.

Proper methods of airway management and secretion removal are the topic of countless research studies. Unfortunately many studies lack good research design, involve small numbers of subjects, and inadequately or incompletely report findings. Proven clinical indicators for suctioning include adventitious breath sounds, noisy breathing, changes in pulse rate, changes in respiratory rate, changes in blood pressure, and prolonged expiratory breath sounds. There are interventions commonly used in years past and proven to be ineffective, such as instilling sodium chloride into the airway and entering the airway more than two times. Be familiar with advances in interventions to maintain a patient airway.

ASSESSMENT

1 Assess for clinical indicators for suctioning: coarse breath sounds, noisy breathing or adventitious breath sounds, increased or decreased pulse, increased or decreased respirations, increased or decreased blood pressure, prolonged expiratory breath sounds, and decreased lung expansion. Secretions in the airway, decreased oxygen saturations or level of consciousness, anxiety, lethargy, unilateral breath sounds, and cyanosis may also indicate a need for suctioning. *Rationale: Physical signs and symptoms result from airway obstruction and decreased oxygen to tissues. Individual client assessment is necessary before suctioning. Suctioning should never be performed as a "routine" without assessment (Joanna Briggs Institute, 2000).*

2 Assess upper airway: assess nasal and oral cavity: gurgling on inspiration or expiration, obvious nasal or oral secretions, drooling, gastric secretions or vomitus in mouth. *Rationale: Removal of oral secretions prevents aspiration pneumonia, especially in mechanically ventilated clients (Finder, 2005).*

3 Assess carefully clients with an increased risk for ineffective airway clearance (e.g., clients with a decreased level of consciousness or other neuromuscular or neurological impairment, those with decreased swallowing ability or dysphagia, and those with ineffective cough). *Rationale: Changes in neurological status and neuromuscular impairment increase the likelihood that the client may need to be suctioned.*

4 Identify contraindications to nasotracheal suctioning: facial trauma or surgery, bleeding disorder, nasal bleeding, epiglottitis or croup, laryngospasms, and irritable airway (AARC, 2004). *Rationale: Passage of catheter can cause additional trauma, increased bleeding, or servere bronchospasm.*

5 Assess client's understanding of procedure. *Rationale: Procedure can be distressing.*

PLANNING

Expected Outcomes focus on airway patency, avoidance of infection, and client's comfort and understanding.

1 Client's airways are cleared of secretions.

2 Adventitious breath sounds are decreased or cleared.

3 Client reports easier breathing.

4 Lung expansion improves.

5 Client performs correct oropharyngeal suctioning technique.

6 Absence of indication of aspiration.

Delegation Considerations

The skill of deep tracheal suctioning in acutely ill clients cannot be delegated. Oropharyngeal suctioning with a Yankauer or suction catheter can be delegated. The skill of performing tracheostomy tube suctioning in stable chronically ill clients with permanent tracheostomy tubes may also be delegated. The nurse directs personnel by:

- Instructing personnel to avoid mouth sutures and applying suction to sensitive tissues.
- Explaining how to vary the procedure for clients on home ventilators.
- Reviewing signs and symptoms of respiratory distress that might be exhibited during the procedure.
- Reviewing signs and symptoms that must be reported to the RN.

Equipment
Oropharyngeal (Nonsterile) and Nasotracheal (Sterile) Suctioning

- Sterile suction catheter 12 to 16 Fr (smallest diameter that will effectively remove secretions) for nasotracheal suctioning
- Clean, nonsterile suction catheter or Yankauer suction tip catheter for oropharyngeal suctioning
- Sterile gloves or one sterile and one clean
- Sterile basin (e.g., sterile disposable cup)
- Sterile water or normal saline (about 100 ml)
- Clean towel or paper drape
- Portable or wall suction
- Connecting tubing (6 feet)
- Face shield, if indicated

Endotracheal or Tracheostomy Suctioning

- 12 to 16 Fr catheter (approximate, adult: size of the suction catheter should be no more than half of the internal diameter of the artificial airway to minimize decrease in Pao_2 (AARC, 2004).
- Bedside table
- Two sterile gloves or one sterile and one clean glove
- Sterile basin
- Sterile normal saline (about 100 ml)
- Clean towel or sterile drape
- Portable or wall suction machine
- Connecting tubing (6 feet)
- Face shield, if indicated

Closed-system or In-line Suctioning

- Closed-system or in-line suction catheter
- 5 to 10 ml NS in syringe or vials
- Portable or wall suction apparatus
- Connecting tubing (6 feet)
- Two clean gloves

IMPLEMENTATION *for Airway Management: Suctioning*

STEPS	RATIONALE

1 See Standard Protocol (inside front cover).

2 Position client in semi-Fowler's or Fowler's position.

Aligns the airway and aids in maximal lung expansion.

3 Preparation for all types of suctioning

a. Open suction kit or catheter using aseptic technique. If sterile drape is available, place it across client's chest. Do not allow suction catheter to touch any nonsterile surfaces.

Prepares catheter and prevents transmission of microorganisms.

b. Fill basin or cup with approximately 100 ml of sterile water or normal saline (see illustration).

Sterile water or saline is used to both lubricate the suction catheter and check the patency of the tube.

c. 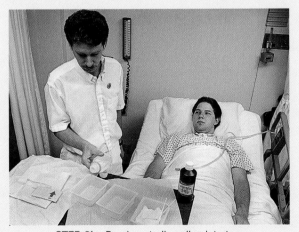 Connect one end of connecting tubing to suction machine or port. Check that suction is functioning properly by suctioning a small amount of water or saline from basin.

Always check for proper functioning of equipment before starting procedure.

d. Set regulator to appropriate negative-pressure: wall suction, 100 to 150 mm Hg (for adults), 80 to 100 mm Hg for infants, and 100 to 120 mm Hg for children is suggested (AARC, 2004).

Elevated pressure settings increase risk of trauma to mucosa. None of these recommendations for specific suction pressures are, as yet, evidence based. Follow facility guidelines and clinical judgment (Carroll, 2003).

4 Oropharyngeal suctioning

a. Apply mask or face shield if applicable. Attach suction catheter to connecting tubing. Remove oxygen mask if present, but keep near client's face.

Suction may cause splashing of body fluids. CDC guidelines suggest that masks or shields should be used whenever there is the risk of airborne bodily fluids.

Reduces chance of hypoxia.

b. Insert catheter into client's mouth, along gum line to pharynx. With suction applied, move catheter around mouth until secretions are cleared.

If catheter does not have a suction control to apply intermittent suction, take care not to allow suction tip to damage oral mucosal surfaces with continuous suction.

c. Encourage client to cough and repeat suctioning if needed. Replace oxygen mask if used.

Coughing moves secretions from lower and upper airways into mouth.

d. Suction water or saline from basin through catheter until catheter is cleared of secretions.

Clearing secretions before they dry reduces probability of transmission of microorganisms and clears catheter.

e. Place catheter in a clean, dry area for reuse with suction turned off or within client's reach or with suction on if client is capable of suctioning self.

Facilitates prompt removal of airway secretions when suctioning is needed in the future.

STEP 3b. Pouring sterile saline into tray.

STEPS	RATIONALE
5 Nasotracheal suctioning	
a. Apply mask or face shield as appropriate. **Apply sterile gloves** or clean glove to nondominant hand and sterile glove to dominant hand. Attach nonsterile suction tubing to sterile catheter, keeping hand holding catheter sterile.	Suction may cause splashing of body fluids. CDC guidelines suggest that masks or shields should be used whenever there is the risk of airborne bodily fluids. Reduces transmission of microorganisms and allows you to maintain sterility of suction catheter.
b. Secure catheter to suction tubing aseptically. Coat distal 6 to 8 cm (2 to 3 inches) of catheter with water-soluble lubricant from suction kit.	Eases passage of catheter.
c. If indicated, increase supplemental oxygen therapy as ordered by physician. Have client deep breathe with oxygen delivery device in place. If client is unable to take deep breaths, hyperoxygenate client with ventilation bag with mask attached.	Hyperoxygenation before suctioning can minimize post-suctioning hypoxemia (Moore, 2003).
d. Remove oxygen delivery device, if present, with nondominant hand. Insert catheter into nares during inspiration without applying suction. Do not force catheter through nares. Have client extend neck slightly (if not contraindicated).	Forcing the catheter causes trauma to the airway tissues. Extending client's neck may facilitate passage of the catheter.

NURSE ALERT Keep oxygen delivery device readily available in case client exhibits symptoms of hypoxemia.

e. Advance catheter to just above entrance into trachea. Allow client to take a breath. Quickly insert catheter approximately 16 to 20 cm (6 to 8 inches in adults) into trachea. Client will begin to cough. One method of approximating the correct length of catheter to insert is to use the distance from the client's nose to the base of the earlobe as a guide.	Ensures proper placement of catheter in airway to remove secretions.
f. Advance catheter until resistance is felt as client coughs. Apply intermittent suction no longer than 15 seconds (AARC, 2004). Withdraw catheter by placing and releasing nondominant thumb over vent of catheter. Slowly withdraw catheter while rotating it back and forth between dominant thumb and forefinger. Encourage client to cough. Replace oxygen device, if applicable. Do not perform more than two passes with the catheter during *any suctioning session*.	Intermittent suction and rotation of catheter prevent injury to tracheal mucosa. Suctioning longer than 15 seconds can worsen existing hypoxemia (AARC, 2004). Observe client for any signs of distress during suctioning. Stop suctioning and apply oxygen. Close observation is necessary after the procedure to assess for cardiovascular, respiratory, and neurological adverse effects (AARC, 2004; Joanna Briggs, 2000).

NURSE ALERT If catheter "grabs" mucosa, remove thumb to release suction.

f. Rinse catheter and connecting tubing by suctioning water or normal saline from the basin until tubing is clear.	
g. Assess need to repeat suction procedure. Observe for alterations in cardiopulmonary status. Allow adequate time (1 to 2 minutes) between suction passes.	
6 ET or tracheostomy tube suctioning	
a. Apply mask or face shield as appropriate. **Apply sterile gloves** or clean glove to nondominant hand and sterile glove to dominant hand. Attach nonsterile suction tubing to sterile catheter, keeping hand holding catheter sterile (see illustration).	Suction may cause splashing of body fluids. CDC recommends wearing mask or shield when there is risk of airborne bodily fluids. Reduces transmission of microorganisms and allows you to maintain sterility of suction catheter.
b. Check that equipment is functioning properly by suctioning small amounts of saline from basin.	Lubricates catheter and tubing.

STEPS	RATIONALE

c. Hyperoxygenate client before suctioning, using manual resuscitation bag and increasing Fio_2 for several minutes; or, if mechanically ventilated, use the ventilator to provide additional breaths without increasing tidal volume. Up to 2 minutes may be necessary to provide for time for the increased oxygen to reach the mechanically ventilated client.

Hyperoxygenation before suctioning decreases suctioning-induced hypoxemia. Most sources recommend hyperoxygenating with 100% Fio_2, yet no clear guidelines are established for clients with COPD, who may not tolerate increased levels of oxygenation. Use hyperinflation with caution in the client who has or is at risk for increased intracranial pressure or who is hemodynamically unstable. Instillation of normal saline before suctioning has been shown to possibly increase infections and is not effective in removing secretions (Joanna Briggs, 2000).

NURSE ALERT If mucus is visible at tracheostomoy or ET tube opening, suction to remove secretions *prior* to hyperoxygenation. This prevents secretions from being pushed back into the trachea.

---

d. Open swivel adapter or tracheostomy or ET tube or, if necessary, remove oxygen or humidity delivery device with nondominant hand.

Exposes artificial airway.

e. Without applying suction and using dominant thumb and forefinger, gently but quickly insert catheter into artificial airway (time catheter insertion with client's inspiration) until resistance is met or client coughs; then pull back 1 cm (½ inch).

Application of suction pressure while introducing catheter into trachea increases risk of damage to tracheal mucosa.

f. Apply intermittent suction by placing and releasing nondominant thumb over vent of catheter (see illustration). Slowly withdraw catheter while rotating it back and forth between dominant thumb and forefinger. If catheter "grabs" mucosa, remove thumb to release suction. The maximum time catheter may remain in airway is 15 seconds (AARC, 2004). Encourage client to cough.

Intermittent suction and rotation of catheter prevent injury to tracheal mucosal lining. Hypoxia related to removal of oxygen in airway and secretions will occur during suctioning procedure. No more than two passes with the suction catheter is recommended during any one suctioning session. Repeated suctioning can result in significant changes in cardiac output, heart rate, and intracranial pressure (Joanna Briggs, 2000).

g. Close swivel adapter or replace oxygen delivery device. Encourage client to deep breathe. Some clients respond well to several manual breaths from the mechanical ventilator or resuscitation bag.

Reoxygenates and reexpands alveoli. Suctioning can cause hypoxemia and atelectasis. Monitor client for signs of postsuctioning distress.

h. Rinse catheter and connecting tube with sterile water or normal saline until clear. Use continuous suction.

Removes catheter secretions. Secretions left in tubing decrease suction and provide environment for growth of microorganisms.

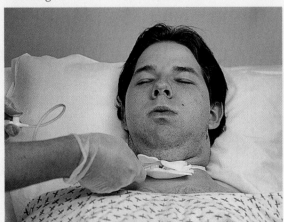

STEP 6a. Attaching catheter to suction.

STEP 6f. Suctioning tracheostomy.

STEPS	RATIONALE
i. Assess client's cardiopulmonary, neurological, and hemodynamic status for secretion clearance and complications. Repeat Steps d through h one time if you determine that secretion clearance was inadequate. Allow adequate time (up to 2 minutes) between suction passes to reestablish baseline oxygenation.	The effects of hypoxia from suctioning can cause dysrhythmias, hemodynamic instability, and increased intracranial pressure, among other complications. A maximum of two suction passes is recommended to minimize effects of hypoxemia (Joanna Briggs, 2000).
j. Perform nasopharyngeal and oropharyngeal suctioning to clear upper airway of secretions. After suctioning upper airway, the catheter is contaminated and should not be reinserted into the lower airway.	Removes upper airway secretions. Upper airway is considered "clean," whereas lower airway is considered "sterile." Therefore same catheter can be used to suction from sterile to clean areas, but not from clean to sterile areas.
k. Disconnect catheter from connecting tubing. Roll catheter around fingers of dominant hand. Pull glove off inside out so that catheter remains in glove. Pull off other glove in same way. Discard into appropriate receptacle. Perform hand hygiene. Turn off suction device.	Reduces transmission of microorganisms. Clean equipment should not be touched with contaminated gloves.
l. Place new, unopened suction kit at bedside.	
7 ET or tracheostomy tube suctioning with a closed-system (in-line) catheter (see illustration)	
a. Attach suction.	
(1) 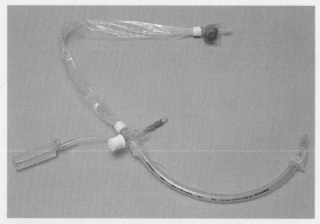 In many institutions, catheter is attached to mechanical ventilator circuit by personnel from respiratory therapy. If not already in place, open suction catheter package using aseptic technique. Attach closed-suction catheter to ventilator circuit by removing swivel adapter and placing closed-suction catheter apparatus on ET or tracheostomy tube. Connect Y on mechanical ventilator circuit to closed-suction catheter with flex tubing.	Catheter becomes part of the circuit and is often changed by respiratory therapist with each circuit change, when contaminated, or per agency policy.
(2) Connect one end of connecting tube to suction machine. Connect other end to end of closed-system or in-line suction catheter if not already done. Turn suction device on and set vacuum regulator to appropriate negative pressure (100 to 150 mm Hg for adults) (AARC, 2004).	Prepares suction apparatus. Excessive negative pressure damages tracheal mucosa and can induce greater hypoxia.

STEP 7 Closed-system suction catheter attached to an ET tube.

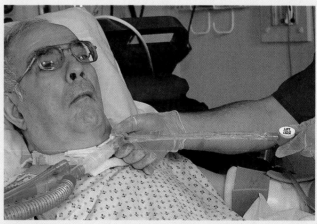

STEP 7e. Suctioning tracheostomy with closed-system suction.

STEPS	RATIONALE
b. Hyperinflate (1 to 2 lung inflations with an increased volume) and/or hyperoxygenate (increase Fio_2) client using resuscitation bag or manual breathing mechanism on mechanical ventilator according to institution protocol and clinical status (100% oxygen usually recommended).	Decreases atelectasis caused by negative pressure and increases oxygen available to tissues during suctioning. Using the ventilator for hyperinflation and hyperoxygenation may result in more hemodynamic stability (Joanna Briggs, 2000). Both hyperinflation and hyperoxygenation are recommended before and after suctioning (AARC, 2004).
c. Unlock suction control mechanism if required by manufacturer. Open saline port and attach saline syringe or vial.	
d. Pick up suction catheter enclosed in plastic sleeve with dominant hand.	Catheter sterility and secretion containment are provided by plastic sheath.
e. Wait until client inhales to insert catheter, using a repeating maneuver of pushing catheter and sliding (or pulling) plastic back between thumb and forefinger until resistance is felt or client coughs (see illustration). (NOTE: Some catheters contain depth markings that are useful in positioning catheter.)	Mechanical ventilator breaths, oxygen, and positive end-expiratory pressure are not interrupted during suctioning. Catheter slides within plastic sheath. Coughing occurs or resistance is felt when catheter touches carina.
f. Encourage client to cough and apply suction while withdrawing.	Removes secretions from airway.

> **NURSE ALERT**   Be sure to withdraw catheter completely into plastic sheath so it does not obstruct airflow!

STEPS	RATIONALE
g. Reassess cardiopulmonary status, including pulse oximetry, to determine need for subsequent suctioning or complications. If cardiac monitoring is available, observe rhythm during suctioning. Repeat Steps b through f, 1 or 2 more times to clear secretions. Allow adequate time (at least 1 full minute) between suction passes for ventilation and reoxygenation.	Repeated passes clear airway of secretions to promote ventilation and oxygenation. Suctioning can cause complications such as irregular heartbeats, hypoxia, and bronchospasm.
h. When airway is clear, withdraw catheter completely into sheath. Be sure black line on catheter is visible in sheath. Squeeze vial or push syringe while applying suction to rinse inner lumen of catheter. Use at least 5 to 10 ml of normal saline to clear catheter of retained secretions. Lock suction mechanism, if applicable, and turn off suction.	Black line is reference point to determine correct position of catheter when not in use. Inability to see black line suggests catheter is in airway and may be impeding airflow. Interior of catheter must be rinsed to prevent bacterial growth (Fretag and others, 2003).

> **NURSE ALERT**   Failure to lock mechanism can result in inadvertent continuous suction and serious complications.

STEPS	RATIONALE
i. Client may require suctioning of oral cavity (see step 4).	Separate suction catheter is necessary for oral cavity.
j. Place new, unopened suction kit on suction machine or at head of bed.	Provides immediate access to suction catheter when needed.
8 See Completion Protocol (inside front cover).	

EVALUATION

1 Auscultate lung fields and compare client's respiratory assessments before and after suctioning.

2 Ask client if breathing is easier and if congestion is decreased.

3 Observe client's respirations, color, and measure pulse oximetry (Spo_2).

4 Observe client's oropharyngeal suctioning technique.

Unexpected Outcomes and Related Interventions

1 Client becomes cyanotic or restless or develops tachycardia, bradycardia, or other abnormal heart rhythm.

a. Discontinue attempt at suctioning until stabilized, unless client's condition is deteriorating because of secretions in airway. Provide supplemental oxygen.

b. Monitor vital signs and pulse oximetry.

c. Hyperoxygenate before and after suctioning.

2 Bloody secretions are returned, which may indicate trauma.

a. Evaluate technique and frequency of suctioning.

b. If bleeding continues, notify physician of potential hemorrhage and monitor vital signs.

3 Client has episodes of coughing.

a. Reassure client.

b. Instruct client about relaxation techniques.

c. Medicate as needed.

4 No secretions are obtained.

a. Reassess respiratory system for presence of secretions.

b. Stimulate client's cough.

c. Check that suction system is functioning.

d. Reassess lung sounds.

5 Thick secretions are present and difficult to suction.

a. Monitor client's hydration status. Dehydration contributes to thick secretions.

b. Increase fluids if not contraindicated.

c. Notify physician if signs and symptoms of infection are present.

Recording and Reporting

• Record respiratory assessments before and after suctioning; size of catheter used; route; amount, consistency, and color of secretions obtained; frequency of suctioning.

• Report client's intolerance to procedure or worsening of oxygenation.

Sample Documentation

1200 Occasional productive cough. Requires hourly suctioning per ET tube. Moderate amount (5 ml or less) of thick yellow sputum. Able to use Yankauer catheter to suction mouth with good technique. Lungs clear after cough and suctioning. Spo₂ 92% to 94%. Respirations nonlabored after suctioning, 14 per minute.

Special Considerations
Pediatric Considerations

• Diameter of suction catheter should be no more than one-half the internal diameter of the child's tracheostomy or other artificial airway (Hockenberry and Wilson, 2007).

• Vacuum pressure should range from 40 to 60 mm Hg for preterm infants and from 60 to 100 mm Hg for infants and children. Unless secretions are thick, lower range of negative pressure is recommended (Hockenberry and Wilson, 2007).

• Closed suction systems are used only on older children. Care must be used so that the weight of the closed system does not displace the child's ET tube.

Geriatric Considerations

• Older adults with ischemic cardiac or obstructive pulmonary disease may benefit from maintenance of oxygen supply during suctioning to reduce the risk of irregular heartbeats.

• Due to increased fragility of tissues, older adults may have bloody secretions on suctioning. Monitor the suction return for clearing and avoid unnecessary suctioning.

Home Care Considerations

• In the home adhere to best practices for infection control while weighing the necessity of cost-effectiveness in a chronic situation. For example, clean suctioning techniques may be acceptable, and the secretion collection container may be cleaned and disinfected every 24 hours.

• Assess the knowledge level of the client and caregivers to determine the amount of instruction and frequency of visits required for safe, effective practices.

• Portable suction machines are more common in the home or long-term care settings; as the secretion jar fills, efficiency of the suction decreases.

SKILL 29.4 Airway Management: Endotracheal Tube and Tracheostomy Care

• **Nursing Skills Online:** Airway Management, Lessons 7 and 8

An artificial airway places the client at high risk for infection. However, correct care of the artificial airway helps to prevent infection. Artificial airways also make clients susceptible to airway injury. Harm may occur to the client if an artificial airway is not maintained in the correct position.

ET tubes are short-term artificial airways used to administer mechanical ventilation, relieve upper airway obstruction, protect against aspiration, or clear secretions (see Figure 29-3). ET tubes are generally removed within 14 days. If the client requires continued assistance from an artificial airway, a tracheostomy is considered for long-term use. A surgical incision is made into the trachea, and a tracheostomy tube is inserted (see Figure 29-4, A).

ASSESSMENT

1 Observe condition of tube and inspect around mouth/skin. ET tube: soiled or loose tape; pressure sores on naris, lip, or corner of mouth; unstable tube; excessive secretions. Tracheostomy tube: soiled or loose ties or dressing; unstable tube; excessive secretions. *Rationale: A client with an artificial airway is at risk for impaired skin integrity and infection due to difficulty controlling secretions and due to pressure points of the artificial airway.*

2 Identify factors that increase risk of complications from ET tubes: type and size of tube, movement of tube up and down trachea, amount of inflation of tube cuff, and duration of placement. *Rationale: Tube moving up and down trachea predisposes client to tracheal trauma or dislodgement. Cuff underinflation may allow aspiration, whereas overinflation may cause ischemia or necrosis of tracheal tissue. Use of tubes for longer periods of time increases the risk of lower airway complications such as pneumonia.*

3 Auscultate lungs bilaterally. *Rationale: Provides baseline confirming bilateral lung inflation.*

4 Determine proper ET tube depth as noted in centimeters to lip of gum line. Record in client's chart at time of intubation. *Rationale: Ensures tube is at proper depth to adequately ventilate lungs.*

5 Assess client's knowledge and comfort with procedure. *Rationale: Facilitates client's learning, and participation in care and may help to decrease anxiety.*

6 If applicable, assess client's understanding of and ability to perform own tracheostomy care. *Rationale: Increases client's feeling of autonomy and decreases feelings of lack of control over condition/secretions.*

PLANNING

Expected Outcomes focus on the prevention of infection and breakdown of skin and mucosa around the artificial airway.

1 Client's artificial airway/tube is in correct position and properly secured.

2 Client remains afebrile without signs and symptoms of infection.

3 Client's oral mucous membrane/stoma remains free of breakdown or accumulation of secretions.

4 Client's artificial airway is intact without persistent dried secretions.

5 Client cooperates with care.

6 Client is able to demonstrate correct technique of tracheostomy care when appropriate.

Delegation Considerations

The skill of ET tube care cannot be delegated. The skill of tracheostomy care can be delegated to AP when a permanent or long-term tracheostomy is in place in chronically ill clients. The nurse directs personnel by:

- Explaining how to adapt the skill for a specific client.
- Reviewing what to observe and report back to the nurse.
- Teaching emergency procedures for acutely ill clients in case the tracheostomy tube inadvertently becomes dislodged when ties are being changed by the RN.

Equipment
Endotracheal Tube Care

- Towel
- ET and oropharyngeal suction equipment
- 1 to 1½-inch adhesive or waterproof tape (not paper tape) or commercial ET stabilizer (follow manufacturer's instructions for securing)
- Two pairs of clean gloves
- Adhesive remover swab or acetone on a cotton ball
- Mouth care supplies (e.g., pediatric-size toothbrush, sponge toothette for edentulous clients, toothpaste, and nonalcohol based mouthwash)
- Face cleanser (e.g., wet washcloth, towel, soap, shaving supplies)
- Clean 2 × 2 gauze
- Tincture of benzoin or liquid adhesive
- Face shield (if indicated)

Tracheostomy Care

- Bedside table
- Towel
- Tracheostomy suction supplies
- Sterile tracheostomy care kit, if available, or:
  - Three sterile 4 × 4 gauze pads
  - Sterile cotton-tipped applicators
  - Sterile tracheostomy dressing
  - Sterile basin
  - Small sterile brush (or disposable cannula)
  - Tracheostomy ties (e.g., twill tape, manufactured tracheostomy ties, Velcro tracheostomy ties)
- Hydrogen peroxide
- Normal saline
- Scissors
- Pair of sterile and clean gloves
- Face shield

IMPLEMENTATION *for Airway Management*

STEPS	RATIONALE
1 See Standard Protocol (inside front cover).	
2 ET tube care	
a. Initiate ET suction (see Skill 29.3).	Removes secretions. Diminishes client's need to cough during procedure.

> **NURSE ALERT** Keep an oral airway immediately accessible in the event that the client bites down and obstructs the ET tube.

> **COMMUNICATION TIP** Instruct client not to bite or move ET tube with tongue or pull on tubing; removal of tape can be uncomfortable.

STEPS	RATIONALE
b. Connect oral Yankauer suction catheter to suction source.	Prepares for oropharyngeal suctioning.
c. Prepare method to secure ET tube.	
(1) Tape method: Cut piece of tape long enough to go completely around client's head from naris to naris plus 15 cm (6 inches): adult, about 30 to 60 cm (1 to 2 feet). Lay the tape adhesive side up on bedside table. Cut and lay 8 to 15 cm (3 to 6 inches) of tape, adhesive sides together, in center of long strip.	Adhesive tape must be placed around head from cheek to cheek below ears. Placing adhesive sides together in center of strip prevents the tape from adhering to hair.
(2) Commercially available ET tube holder: Open package and set device aside with the head guard in place and Velcro strips open.	
d. Have an assistant apply a pair of gloves and hold ET tube firmly so that tube does not move. Note the number marking once again on the ET tube at the gum line.	Reduces transmission of microorganisms. Maintains proper tube position and prevents accidental extubation.
e. Remove old tape or commercial tube holder.	Provides access to skin under tape for assessment and hygiene. Reduces transmission of microorganisms.
(1) Tape: Carefully remove tape from ET tube and client's face. If tape is difficult to remove, moisten with water or adhesive tape remover. Discard tape in appropriate receptacle or place tape on bedside table or on distant end of towel.	
(2) Commercial tube holder: Remove Velcro strips from ET tube and remove tube holder.	Devices are latex free, fast, and convenient.
f. Use adhesive remover swab to remove excess adhesive left on face after tape removal; then wash adhesive remover from face.	Adhesive can cause damage to skin and prevent adhesion of new tape.
g. Remove oral airway or bite block if present and place in towel.	Provides access to and complete observation of client's oral cavity.

> **NURSE ALERT** Do not remove oral airway if client is actively biting ET tube. This may result in occlusion of the airway!

STEPS	RATIONALE
h. Clean mouth, gums, and teeth opposite ET tube with nonalcohol based mouthwash solution (e.g., chlorhexidine) and 4 × 4 gauze, sponge-tipped applicators, or soft toothbrush. Suction fluid from oral cavity with Yankauer catheter or use toothbrush made to be connected to suction.	Take care to not allow aspiration to occur. Keeping the cuff inflated on the ET tube assists in preventing aspiration. Alcohol-based mouthwashes dry oral mucosa (Lewis and others, 2004). Orally intubated clients are at risk for ventilator-associated pneumonia because of pathogens found in plaque. Toothbrushes remove plaque and tartar (Garp and others, 2005).

STEPS	RATIONALE
i. *Oral ET tube only:* Note "cm" ET tube marking at lips or gums. With help of assistant, move ET tube to opposite side or center of mouth. Do not change tube depth.	Prevents pressure sore formation at sides of client's mouth. Ensures correct position of tube.
j. Repeat oral cleaning as in Step h on opposite side of mouth.	Removes secretions from oropharynx; removes plaque from teeth.
k. Clean face and neck with soapy washcloth; rinse and dry. Shave male client as necessary.	Moisture and beard growth prevent adhesive tape adherence.
l. Secure ET tube (assistant continues holding tube).	
(1) Tape method:	Positions tape to secure ET tube in proper position.
(a) Pour small amount of tincture of benzoin on clean 2 × 2 gauze and dot on skin above upper lip (oral ET tube) or across nose (nasal ET tube) and cheeks to ear. Allow to dry completely.	Protects and makes skin more receptive to tape.
(b) Slip tape under client's head and neck, adhesive side up. Take care not to twist tape or catch hair. Do not allow tape to stick to itself. It helps to stick tape gently to tongue blade, which serves as a guide while sliding under neck. Center tape so that double-faced tape extends around back of neck from ear to ear.	
(c) On one side of face, secure tape from ear to nares (nasal ET tube) or edge of mouth (oral ET tube). Tear remaining tape in half lengthwise, forming two pieces that are ½- to ¾-inch wide. Secure bottom half of tape across upper lip (oral ET tube) or across top of nose (nasal ET tube) (see illustration A). Wrap top half of tape around tube and up from bottom. Tape should encircle tube at least two times for security (see illustration B).	Secures tape to face. Using top tape to wrap prevents downward drag on ET tube.
(d) On other side of face, gently pull tape firmly to pick up slack and secure to remaining side of face (see illustration). Assistant can release hold when tube is secure. You may want assistant to help reinsert oral airway.	Secures tape to face and tube. ET tube should be at same depth at the lips. Check earlier assessment for verification of tube depth in centimeters.

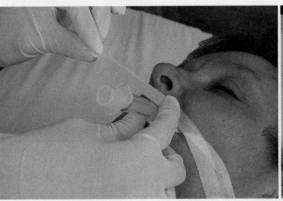 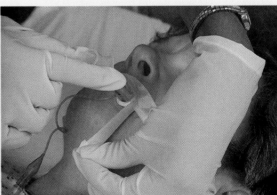

STEP 2I.(1)(c) A, Securing bottom half of tape across client's upper lip. **B,** Securing top half of tape around tube.

STEPS	RATIONALE
(2) Commercially available device	
(a) Thread ET tube through opening designed to secure ET tube. Be sure that the pilot balloon is accessible. Place strips of ET holder under the client's head at the occiput.	Commercial holders have a slit in the front of the holder designed to secure the ET tube.
(b) Verify that ET tube is at the established depth, using the lip or gum line marker as a guide. Attach Velcro strips at the base of the client's head. Leave 1 cm (½ inch) slack in strips. Verify that tube is secure.	Ensures that ET tube remains at correct depth as determined during assessment.
m. Clean oral airway in warm water and rinse well. Shake excess water from oral airway.	Promotes hygiene. Reduces transmission of microorganisms.
n. Reinsert oral airway without pushing tongue into oropharynx by initially inserting upside down until the tip is beyond the end of the tongue and then rotating 180 degrees into place.	Prevents client from biting ET tube and allows access for oropharyngeal suctioning by sliding catheter along outer edge.
3 Tracheostomy care	
a. Suction tracheostomy (see Skill 29.3). Remove soiled tracheostomy dressing, discard in glove with coiled catheter, remove gloves, and perform hand hygiene.	Removes secretions so as not to occlude outer cannula while inner cannula is removed.
b. Have client deep breathe or use AMBU bag to deliver supplemental oxygen. Prepare equipment on bedside table.	
(1) Open sterile tracheostomy kit. Open three 4 × 4 gauze packages using aseptic technique and pour normal saline on one package and hydrogen peroxide on another. Leave third package dry.	Replenishes oxygen lost in suctioning of tracheostomy.

> **COMMUNICATION TIP** Explain the importance of routine tracheostomy care to prevent infection, occlusion, and crusting of secretions around stoma. Explain that the procedure is not painful but that movement of the tracheostomy may promote coughing.

STEPS	RATIONALE
(2) Open two packages of cotton-tipped swabs and pour normal saline on one package and hydrogen peroxide on the other. Do not recap bottles.	Preparation and organization of equipment allows you to complete procedure efficiently and then reconnect client to oxygen source in a timely manner.
(3) Open sterile tracheostomy dressing package.	
(4) Unwrap sterile basin and pour about 2 cm (¾ inch) hydrogen peroxide into it with equal parts normal saline. Open small sterile brush package and place aseptically into sterile basin.	Half strength peroxide removes dried secretions in the inner cannula.

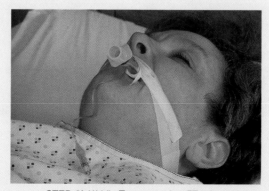

STEP 2l.(1)(d) Tape securing ET tube.

STEPS	RATIONALE

(5) Prepare length of twill tape long enough to circle around client's neck twice (about 60-75 cm or 24-30 inches for an adult). Cut ends on diagonal.

(6) If using commercial tracheostomy tube holder, open package.

c. **Apply sterile gloves.** Keep dominant hand sterile throughout procedure.

Reduces transmission of microorganisms.

d. Remove oxygen source.

> **NURSE ALERT** It is important to stabilize the tracheostomy tube at all times during tracheostomy care to prevent injury, discomfort, and accidental extubation. Use assistant if available.

e. If a nondisposable inner cannula is used:

(1) While touching only the outer aspect of the tube, remove the inner cannula with nondominant hand. Drop inner cannula into ½ strength hydrogen peroxide in basin.

Half strength hydrogen peroxide loosens crusted secretions from inner cannula.

(2) Place tracheostomy collar or T tube and ventilator oxygen source over or near outer cannula. NOTE: T tube and ventilator oxygen devices cannot be attached to most outer cannulas when inner cannula is removed. A new inner cannula may be quickly inserted so that the oxygen source may be maintained. The old inner cannula can then be cleaned in the half-strength peroxide, rinsed in the normal saline, and then stored in a sterile container for use the next time the tracheostomy is cleaned (two cannulas would be on hand at all times).

Maintains supply of oxygen to client to prevent desaturation.

This allows quick reconnection to oxygen source.

(3) To prevent oxygen desaturation in affected clients, quickly pick up inner cannula and use small brush to remove secretions inside and outside cannula (see illustration).

Brush removes thick or dried secretions.

(4) Hold inner cannula over basin and rinse with normal saline, using nondominant hand to pour.

Removes secretions and hydrogen peroxide from inner cannula.

(5) Replace inner cannula and secure "locking" mechanism (see illustration). Reapply ventilator or oxygen sources once inner cannula is in place.

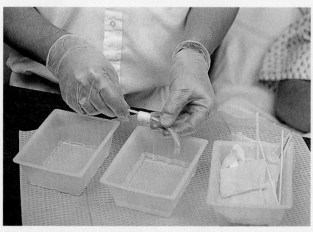

STEP 3e.(3) Cleansing the tracheostomy inner cannula.

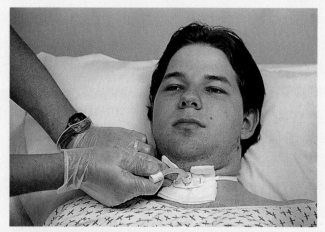

STEP 3e.(5) Reinserting the inner cannula.

STEPS	RATIONALE

f. If a disposable inner cannula is used:

(1) Remove new cannula from manufacturer's packaging.

(2) While touching only the outer aspect of the tracheostomy tube, withdraw old inner cannula and replace with new cannula. Lock into position.

(3) Dispose of contaminated cannula in appropriate receptacle.

g. Using hydrogen peroxide–saturated cotton-tipped swabs and 4 × 4 gauze, clean exposed outer cannula surfaces and stoma under faceplate, extending 5 to 10 cm (2 to 4 inches) in all directions from stoma (see illustration). Clean in circular motion from stoma site outward, using dominant hand to handle sterile supplies.

h. Using normal saline–prepared cotton-tipped swabs and 4 × 4 gauze, rinse hydrogen peroxide from tracheostomy tube and skin surfaces.

i. Using dry 4 × 4 gauze, pat skin and exposed outer cannula surfaces lightly.

j. Secure tracheostomy.

(1) Instruct assistant, if available, to apply clean gloves and to hold tracheostomy tube securely in place.

Rationale column:

Maintains sterility of the inner aspect of the new cannula.

Aseptically removes secretions from stoma site. Half-strength hydrogen peroxide may decrease skin irritation.

Prevents possible irritation from hydrogen peroxide.

Dry surfaces decrease growth of microorganisms and skin excoriation.

Promotes hygiene, reduces transmission of microorganisms, and secures tracheostomy tube.

> **NURSE ALERT** Assistant must not release hold on tracheostomy tube until new ties are firmly attached to reduce risk of accidental extubation. If no assistant is present, do not remove old ties until new ties are in place and secured. (Follow manufacturer's guidelines for Velcro ties.) Secure tracheostomy ties with one-finger slack.

(2) Insert one end of prepared tie through faceplate eyelet (see illustration) and pull ends even.

(3) Slide both ends of tie behind head and around neck to other eyelet and insert one tie through second eyelet. Cut old ties and remove.

(4) Pull new ties snugly.

(5) Tie ends securely in double square knot, allowing space for only one finger in tie.

(6) Insert fresh tracheostomy dressing under clean ties and faceplate (see illustration).

Rationale column:

Prevents tube displacement.

One-finger slack prevents ties from being too tight. Knot should be to the side of the neck. Foam and Velcro tracheostomy holders are also commonly used.

Absorbs drainage. Dressing prevents pressure on clavicle heads.

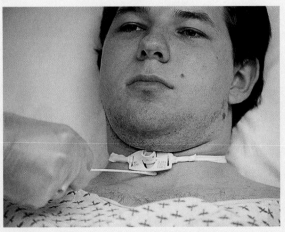

STEP 3g. Cleansing around stoma.

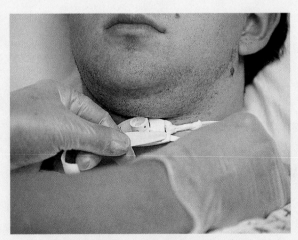

STEP 3j.(2) Replacing tracheostomy ties.

STEPS	RATIONALE
k. Position client comfortably and assess respiratory status.	Promotes relaxation. Some clients may require post-tracheostomy care suctioning.

NURSE ALERT For accidental extubation, call for assistance and manually ventilate client with resuscitation bag, if necessary. Tracheostomy obturator should be kept at bedside with a fresh tracheostomy to facilitate reinsertion of the outer cannula, if dislodged. An additional tracheostomy tube of the same size and shape should be kept on hand for emergency replacement.

4 See Completion Protocol (inside front cover).

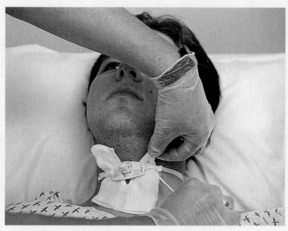

STEP 3j.(6) Applying tracheostomy dressing.

EVALUATION

1 Auscultate lungs and observe that airway is in proper position with tape/ties secure and comfortable for client. ET tube should be at the same depth as before care (as per physician order), with the same centimeter marking at lips and equal bilateral breath sounds.

2 Measure client's temperature; observe stoma for signs of infection.

3 Compare oral mucosa and airway assessments before and after artificial airway care. Observe for signs of tissue breakdown or persistent dried secretions.

4 Observe client's actions to determine compliance with the procedure.

5 Have client indicate when tracheostomy care is required and independently demonstrate the technique for tracheostomy tube care.

Unexpected Outcomes and Related Interventions

1 Tube is not secure, and artificial airway moves in or out or is coughed out by client.

a. Adjust or apply new ties.

2 Breath sounds not equal bilaterally with an ET tube in place.

a. Evaluate ET tube for proper depth. If incorrect, arrange for ET tube to be repositioned as allowed by institution.

b. Obtain order for chest x-ray study to verify placement if applicable.

c. Assess client's respiratory status and observe for the presence of mucus plugs.

3 Breakdown, pressure areas, or stomatitis (tracheostomy tube) develop.

a. Increase frequency of tube care.

b. Make sure skin areas are clean and dry.

4 Hard, reddened areas with or without excessive or foul-smelling secretions develop, indicating infection.

a. Notify physician.

b. Increase frequency of tube care.

c. Remove inner cannula, if applicable, for cleaning and suctioning.

5 Accidental extubation

a. Call for assistance and keep head of bed elevated.

b. Maintain patent airway by replacing old tracheostomy tube with new tube.

c. Observe vital signs and signs of respiratory distress.

Recording and Reporting

• Record respiratory assessments before and after care, and ET tube care: depth of ET tube, frequency and extent of care, client tolerance, and any complications related to presence of the tube.

- Record tracheostomy care: type and size of tracheostomy tube, frequency and extent of care, client tolerance, and any complications related to presence of the tube.
- Report signs of infection or displacement of ET or tracheostomy tube immediately.

Sample Documentation

0800 Routine ET tube care done. Size 7.5-cm tube remains with 22-cm marking at lips. No irritation or skin breakdown noted. Mouth care given. Respirations even and easy at a rate of 16 breaths per minute. Clear breath sounds bilaterally.

Special Considerations
Pediatric Considerations
- Monitor children with new tracheostomy for complications such as hemorrhage, edema, accidental decannulation, and airway obstruction (Hockenberry and Wilson, 2007).

Geriatric Considerations
- Older adult skin may be more fragile and prone to breakdown from secretions or pressure or to tearing when tape is removed.

Home Care Considerations
- Caregivers in the home must know signs and symptoms of respiratory and stomal infections.

SKILL 29.5 Managing Closed Chest Drainage Systems

- **Nursing Skills Online: Chest Tubes, Lessons 1-4**

Trauma, disease, or surgery can interrupt the closed negative-pressure system of the lungs, causing lung collapse. Air (pneumothorax) or fluid (hemothorax) may leak into the pleural cavity. A chest tube is inserted, and a closed chest drainage system is attached to promote drainage of air and fluid from the pleural space so the lungs can reexpand (see Figure 29-8). This type of tube is also called a thoracostomy tube or thoracic catheter. Suction may be added to assist gravity in draining fluid.

The placement of the chest tube depends on the type of drainage that is needed. Because air rises, apical and anterior chest tube placement (Figure 29-5, A) promotes removal of air. Chest tubes are placed low and posterior or lateral (Figure 29-5, B) to drain fluid. Mediastinal chest tubes are placed just below the sternum (Figure 29-6) and drain blood or fluid, preventing its accumulation around the heart (e.g., after open heart surgery).

Although single-bottle systems are available, single-unit water-seal or waterless systems are most often used. The water-seal system contains two or three compartments or chambers (Figure 29-7). Fluid drains into the first chamber. The second chamber contains the water seal, which allows air to escape because of the force of expiration but not to reenter on inspiration. If suction is needed, a third chamber is used. The amount of suction depends on the amount of sterile water in the suction chamber.

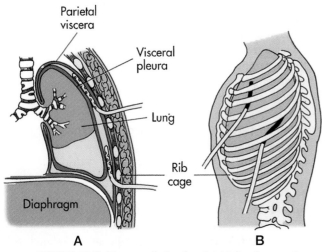

FIGURE 29-5 Diagram of sites for chest tube placement.

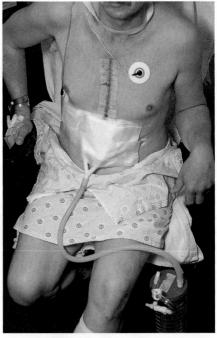

FIGURE 29-6 Mediastinal chest tube following open heart surgery.

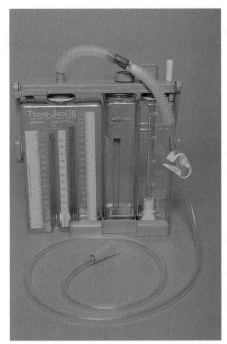

FIGURE 29-7 Disposable chest drainage system.

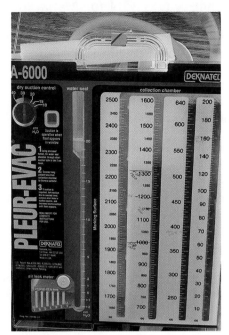

FIGURE 29-8 Waterless drainage system.

The waterless system (Figure 29-8) follows the same principles, except that sterile water is not required for suction. The suction control chamber is replaced by a one-way valve located near the top of the system. The drainage chamber takes up most of the space in the drainage unit. The suction control chamber contains a suction control float ball that is set by a suction control dial after the suction is connected and turned on.

ASSESSMENT

1 Perform a complete respiratory assessment (see Chapter 12) and baseline vital signs and oximetry (see Chapter 11). *Rationale: Baseline vitals signs are essential for any invasive procedure. Chest tube insertion often causes respiratory distress.*
2 Assess client's comfort level on a scale of 0 to 10.
3 Assess if client is able to breathe deeply and comfortably. *Rationale: Detects early signs and symptoms of complications. Promotes reexpansion of the lung.*
4 Review client's hemoglobin and hematocrit levels. *Rationale: Parameters reflect if blood loss is occurring, which may affect oxygenation.*
5 Measure client's oxygen saturation level using oximetry: *Rationale: Provides baseline to determine response to tube insertion.*

PLANNING

Expected Outcomes focus on removal of air and fluid from the pleural space and reexpansion of the lung with maximum client comfort.

1 Client's respirations are nonlabored.
2 Client's breath sounds are present in all lobes.
3 Client's lung expansion is symmetrical.
4 Client's vital signs, hemoglobin level, and hematocrit are within normal ranges by discharge.
5 Client performs breathing exercises correctly.
6 Client reports improved comfort on a scale of 0 to 10.
7 Chest tube remains in place, and chest drainage system remains airtight and functioning properly.
8 Client's oxygen saturation is within client's normal range.

Delegation Considerations
The skill of chest tube management cannot be delegated.

Equipment
- Local anesthetic, if not an emergent procedure
- Prescribed drainage system
- Water-seal system versus waterless system: sterile water or normal saline per manufacturer's directions
- Suction, if used
- Chest tube tray (all items are sterile), typically: knife handle, chest tube clamp, small sponge forceps, needle holder, knife blade, suture, sterile drape, two clamps, 4 × 4 sponges, suture scissors
- Dressings: petroleum gauze, large dressing of choice, additional 4 × 4 dressings, tape
- Two rubber-tipped hemostats for each chest tube
- 1-inch adhesive tape for taping connections
- Face mask/face shield
- Sterile gloves

IMPLEMENTATION *for Managing Closed Chest Drainage Systems*

STEPS	RATIONALE
1 See Standard Protocol (inside front cover).	
2 Set up water-seal system.	
a. Obtain a chest drainage system. Remove wrappers and prepare to set up as a two- or three-chamber system.	Maintains sterility of system for use under sterile operating room conditions.
b. While maintaining sterility of the drainage tubing, stand system upright and add sterile water or normal saline to appropriate compartments.	Reduces possibility of contamination.
(1) For a two-chamber system (without suction), add sterile solution to water-seal chamber (second chamber), bringing fluid to the required level as indicated.	Water-seal chamber acts as a one-way valve so that air cannot enter pleural space.
(2) For a three-chamber system (with suction), add sterile solution to the water-seal chamber (second chamber). Add amount of sterile solution prescribed by physician to the suction control (third chamber), usually 20 cm H_2O pressure. Connect tubing from suction control chamber to suction source. Tailor length of drainage tube to client. Suction control chamber vent must be without occlusion when suction is used.	Depth of rod below fluid level dictates highest amount of negative pressure that can be present within system. For example, 20 cm of water is approximately 20 cm of water pressure. Any additional negative pressure applied to system is vented into the atmosphere through suction control vent. This safety device prevents damage to pleural tissues from an unexpected surge of negative pressure from suction source.
	Excessively long drainage tube may result in occlusions.
	Provides safety factor of releasing excess negative pressure into the air through suction control vent.
3 Set up waterless system.	
a. Remove sterile wrappers and prepare to set up.	Maintains sterility of system for use under sterile operating room conditions.
b. For a two-chamber system (without suction), nothing is added or needs to be done to system.	Waterless two-chamber system is ready for connecting to client's chest tube after opening wrappers.
c. For a three-chamber system with suction, connect tubing from suction control chamber to suction source.	Suction source provides additional negative pressure to system.
d. Instill 15 ml sterile water or normal saline into diagnostic indicator injection port located on top of system.	Allows for observation of a rise and fall in water in diagnostic air leak window. This is not necessary for mediastinal drainage because there will be no tidaling. In an emergency, system **does not** require water for setup.
4 Tape all connections between the client and the chest tube collection unit in a double spiral fashion using 1-inch adhesive tape. Then check systems for patency by:	Prevents atmospheric air from leaking into system and client's intrapleural space. Provides chance to ensure airtight system before connecting it to client. Allows correction or replacement of system if it is defective before connecting it to the client.
a. Clamping the drainage tubing that will connect the client to the system.	
b. Connecting tubing from float ball chamber to suction source.	

> **NURSE ALERT** Bubbling will be seen at first because there is air in tubing and system. This should stop after a few minutes unless other sources of air are entering system. If bubbling continues, check connections and locate source of air leak as described in Table 29-3.

STEPS	RATIONALE
c. Turning on suction to prescribed level.	
5 Turn off suction source and unclamp drainage tubing before connecting client to system. Make a second check to be sure drainage tubing is not excessively long.	Having client connected to suction when it is initiated could damage pleural tissues from sudden increase in negative pressure. Suction source is turned on again after client is connected. Tubing that is coiled or looped becomes clotted, impeding drainage, and may potentially cause a tension pneumothorax (Allibone, 2003).
6 Position the client for tube insertion so the side in which the tube will be placed is accessible to physician.	

STEPS	RATIONALE

7   Assist physician with chest tube insertion by providing needed equipment and analgesic and offering client support and instruction. Physician will clamp tube, suture it in place, and apply occlusive dressing.

8   Help physician attach drainage tube to chest tube; remove clamp.

Connects drainage system and suction (if ordered) to chest tube.

9   Tape tube connection between chest and drainage tubes. One method: One long strip of tape on each side with an overlapping tape wrapped spirally enables connections to be observed and remain secure.

Secures chest tube to drainage system and reduces risk of air leaks that cause breaks in airtight system.

10   After tube placement, position client:

a. Using semi-Fowler's to high-Fowler's position to evacuate air (pneumothorax) (see illustration).

Permits optimum drainage of fluid and/or air. Air rises to highest point in the chest.

b. Using high-Fowler's position to drain fluid (hemothorax)

Permits optimum drainage of fluid.

11   Check patency of air vents in system.

a. Water-seal vent must have no occlusion.

Permits displaced air to pass into atmosphere.

b. Suction control chamber vent must not be occluded when using suction.

Provides safety factor of releasing excess negative pressure into atmosphere.

c. Waterless systems have relief valves without caps.

12   Position tubing on mattress next to client. Secure with clamp provided so that tubing is not obstructed.

Excess tubing hanging over the edge of mattress may form a dependent loop where drainage could pool, causing a blockage.

13   Adjust tubing to hang in a straight line from top of mattress to drainage chamber.

Promotes drainage.

TABLE 29-3 Problem Solving With Chest Tubes

ASSESSMENT	INTERVENTION
1 Air leak can occur at insertion site, connection between tube and drainage device, or within drainage device itself. Continuous bubbling is noted in water-seal chamber.	Locate leak by clamping tube at different intervals. Leaks are corrected when constant bubbling stops.
2 Assess for location of leak by clamping chest tube with two rubber-shod or toothless clamps close to the chest wall. If bubbling stops, air leak is inside client's thorax or at chest insertion site.	**NURSE ALERT** Unclamp tube, reinforce chest dressing, and notify physician immediately. *Rationale: Leaving chest tube clamped can cause collapse of lung, mediastinal shift, and eventual collapse of other lung from buildup of air pressure within the pleural cavity.*
3 If bubbling continues with the clamps near the chest wall, gradually move one clamp at a time down drainage tubing away from client and toward suction control chamber. When bubbling stops, leak is in section of tubing or connection between the clamps.	Replace tubing, or secure connection and release clamps.
4 If bubbling still continues, this indicates the leak is in the drainage system.	Change the drainage system.
5 Assess for tension pneumothorax: • Severe respiratory distress • Low oxygen saturation • Chest pain • Absence of breath sounds on affected side • Tracheal shift to unaffected side • Hypotension and signs of shock • Tachycardia	Make sure chest tubes are patent: remove clamps, eliminate kinks, or eliminate occlusion. Notify physician immediately and prepare for another chest tube insertion. A flutter (Heimlich) valve or large-gauge needle may be used for short-term emergency release of pressure in the intrapleural space. Have emergency equipment, oxygen, and code cart available because condition is life threatening.
6 Water-seal tube is no longer submerged in sterile fluid because of evaporation.	Add sterile water to water-seal chamber until distal tip is 2 cm under surface level.

STEPS	RATIONALE
14 Place two rubber-tipped hemostats (for each chest tube) in an easily accessible position, such as taped to the top of client's headboard. These should remain with client if ambulating.	Chest tubes are double-clamped under specific circumstances: (1) to assess for an air leak (see Tables 29-2 and 29-3) to empty or change collection bottle or chamber or disposable systems. Have new system ready to be connected before clamping tube so that transfer can be rapid and drainage reestablished.
15 Care for client with chest tubes	
a. Assess vital signs; oxygen saturation; skin color; breath sounds; and rate, depth, and ease of respirations.	Provides data to compare with baseline and information about procedure-related complications.
b. Monitor color, consistency, and amount of drainage every 15 minutes for the first 2 hours. Indicate level of drainage fluid, date, and time on chamber's write-on surface.	Provides baseline for continuous assessment of type and quantity of drainage. Ensures early detection of complications.
(1) From a mediastinal tube less than 100 ml/hr is expected and a total of approximately 500 ml in first 24 hours.	Sudden gush of drainage may result from coughing or changing client's position; releasing blood rather than indicating active bleeding.
(2) From a posterior chest tube between 100 and 300 ml is expected during first 2 hours after insertion, with a total of 500 to 1000 ml expected in the first 24 hours.	
(3) From an anterior chest tube that is inserted for a pneumothorax, little or no output is expected.	

> **COMMUNICATION TIP** Discuss client's continued participation in care, as appropriate. Medicate as needed.

c. Observe chest dressing for drainage.	Drainage around tube may indicate blockage.
d. Palpate around the tube for swelling and crepitus (subcutaneous emphysema) as evidenced by crackling.	Indicates presence of air trapping in subcutaneous tissues. Small amounts are commonly absorbed. Large amounts are potentially dangerous.

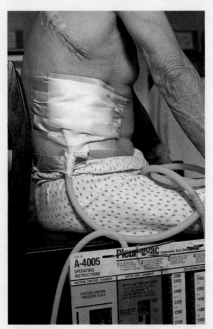

STEP 10a. Pleural chest tube in place.

STEPS	RATIONALE
e. Check tubing to ensure that it is free of kinks and dependent loops.	Promotes drainage.
f. Observe for fluctuation of drainage in the tubing and water-seal chamber during inspiration and expiration. Observe for clots or debris in tubing.	If fluctuation or tidaling stops, it means that either the lung is fully expanded or the system is obstructed.
g. Keep drainage system upright and below level of the client's chest.	Promotes gravity drainage and prevents backflow of fluid and air into the pleural space.
h. Check for air leaks by monitoring the bubbling in the water-seal chamber: Intermittent bubbling is normal during expiration when air is being evacuated from the pleural cavity, but continuous bubbling during both inspiration and expiration indicates a leak in the system.	Absence of bubbling may indicate that the lung has fully expanded if client had pneumothorax.

> **NURSE ALERT** Stripping the chest tube is controversial and is generally not recommended as it greatly increases negative pressure within the tube, causing lung injury. Gentle milking of a chest tube by squeezing and releasing one hand at a time is sometimes performed on tubes with high volumes of bloody drainage. Research is inconclusive in this area, and the nurse should refer to hospital policy (Lazzara, 2002).

16 Assist in chest tube removal.	
a. Administer prescribed medication for pain relief about 30 minutes before procedure.	Reduces discomfort and relaxes client by allowing time for medication to take effect.
b. Assist client with sitting on edge of bed or lying on side without chest tubes.	Physician prescribes client's position to facilitate tube removal.
c. Physician prepares an occlusive dressing of petroleum gauze on a pressure dressing and sets it aside on a sterile field.	Essential to prepare in advance for quick application to wound during tube withdrawal.
d. Physician asks client to take a deep breath and hold it or exhale completely and hold it.	Prevents air from being sucked into chest as tube is removed.

> **COMMUNICATION TIP** Support client physically and emotionally while physician removes dressing and clips sutures.

e. Physician holds prepared dressing at point of tube insertion and quickly pulls out chest tube.	Prevents entry of air through chest wound.
f. Physician quickly and firmly secures it in position with elastic bandage (Elastoplast) or wide tape. Physician sometimes uses skin clips or draws purse-string sutures together before applying dressing.	Keeps wound aseptic. Prevents entry of air into chest. Wound closure occurs spontaneously. Clips or sutures aid in skin closure.
17 See Completion Protocol (inside front cover).	

EVALUATION

1 Assess client for decreased respiratory distress and chest pain.
2 Auscultate client's lungs and observe chest expansion.
3 Monitor vital signs, hematocrit, and hemoglobin level.
4 Evaluate client's ability to use deep-breathing exercises while maintaining comfort.
5 Reassess client level of comfort (on a scale of 0-10) comparing level with comfort before chest tube insertion.
6 Monitor continued functioning of system as indicated by reduction in the amount of drainage, resolution of the air leak, and complete reexpansion of the lung.
7 Monitor client's oxygen saturation.

Unexpected Outcomes and Related Interventions

1 Air leak is unrelated to client's respiration.
a. See Table 30-3 for determining the source of an air leak and problem solving.
2 Chest tubes become obstructed by a clot or kinked tube.
a. Observe client for mediastinal shift or respiratory distress, which may constitute a medical emergency.
b. Determine source of obstruction, as noted by lack of flow through tube or clot detected in system. If kinked, straighten tubing and adjust to prevent continued problems.
c. If clot is identified, notify physician.

3 Chest tube becomes dislodged.

a. Immediately apply pressure over chest tube site with anything that is within immediate reach (e.g., several layers of client's hospital gown, bed sheet, towel, gauze dressings).

b. Have assistant obtain a sterile petroleum dressing. Apply as client exhales. Secure dressing with a tight seal.

c. Notify physician.

4 Substantial increase in bright-red drainage is observed.

a. Observe for tachycardia and hypotension.

b. Report to physician because this may indicate that client is actively bleeding.

5 Drainage system is knocked on side or damaged.

a. Observe for signs of increasing pneumothorax, which would indicate that water-seal is not being maintained. Notify physician.

b. Obtain a second unit and change system after following setup guidelines.

Recording and Reporting

- Record respiratory assessment; amount of suction, if used; amount of drainage since the previous assessment; type of drainage in chest tubing; and presence or absence of an air leak, including amount if present.
- Record integrity of dressing and presence of drainage on dressing.
- Record client comfort and tolerance.

Sample Documentation

0800 Resting comfortably, denies complaint. Respirations even and easy. Lungs clear with breath sounds heard over all lung fields. Left posterior chest tube and dressing intact with tidaling present in water-seal chamber. No air leak noted. 50 ml serous drainage collected in past 8 hours. Taking deep breaths as instructed without complaints of discomfort.

NCLEX® Style Questions

1 The nurse is beginning a respiratory assessment on a client who is short of breath. Which action is the first step for this assessment?

1. Ask the client about his respiratory history by asking short-answer questions.
2. Auscultate posterior lung sounds while he is flat on his side.
3. Obtain pulse oximeter to assess oxygenation.
4. Listen to client's anterior lung sounds.

2 The RN is observing the LPN suctioning the client through an ET tube. Which of the following indicates acceptable technique? The LPN:

1. Hyperventilates client with 21% oxygen before suctioning
2. Uses a clean catheter for suctioning
3. Inserts catheter with nurse's thumb covering the suction control port
4. Dips catheter in saline before suctioning

3 The nurse realizes that suctioning the client may cause: (Select all that apply.)

1. Hypoxia
2. Dysrhythmias
3. Irregular pulse rate
4. Thick secretions

4 Which of the following activities could a nurse delegate to assistive personnel?

1. Suctioning of an ET tube
2. Tracheostomy care for a chronically ill client on humidified oxygen
3. Sputum collection via suctioning
4. Tracheostomy care on a mechanically ventilated client

5 The nurse is caring for a client requiring supplemental oxygen therapy. It is determined that the client needs an Fio₂ of 60%. Which of the following oxygen delivery devices does the nurse anticipate will be provided?

1. Nasal cannula at 6 liters per minute
2. Venturi mask at 10 liters per minute
3. Nonrebreathing mask at 6 liters per minute
4. Partial rebreathing mask at 6 liters per minute

6 The nurse is assessing a client with an artificial airway. Which of the following would indicate that the client might need to be suctioned? (Select all that apply.)

1. Crackles auscultated on inspiration
2. Decreased breath sounds in the bases
3. Weak cough
4. Thick secretions

References for all chapters appear in Appendix D.

Gastric Intubation

MEDIA RESOURCES

- **evolve** http://evolve.elsevier.com/Elkin
- **Video Clips**
- **Nursing Skills Online**

A nasogastric (NG) tube is a flexible tube passed through the client's nares, nasopharynx, and esophagus and into the stomach (Figure 30-1). An NG tube is inserted for selected surgical procedures, when vomiting and gastric distention occur, and for irrigation of the stomach. There are also times following major surgery or trauma when normal peristalsis temporarily slows or is absent and eating or drinking fluids causes abdominal distention. Temporary insertion of an NG tube serves to decompress the stomach, keeping it empty until peristalsis returns.

When used for decompression, the NG tube is usually attached to low intermittent suction to facilitate the removal of secretions. Decompression of the stomach with removal of fluids and gas promotes abdominal comfort, decreases the risk of aspiration, and allows surgical anastomoses to heal without distention. For clients who are unable to swallow, the NG tube is used for the administration of medications and may be used as a temporary feeding tube. The tube is also used to irrigate the stomach and to remove toxic substances, such as in poisoning.

NG tubes are typically a larger diameter (12 to 18 Fr) than feeding tubes (see Chapter 31) to enhance the removal of thick secretions or to instill fluids rapidly. Their stiffer composition and larger diameter make these tubes more uncomfortable for the client and cause more irritation of the sensitive nasopharyngeal mucosa. Types of NG tubes include a single lumen tube (Levin) or a tube with a central lumen and a separate air vent lumen (Salem sump).

Nursing interventions for clients with an NG tube include measures to maintain patency of the tube such as irrigation; and measures to promote comfort such as positioning the tube to prevent pressure on the nares, cleansing around the nares, and lubrication of the oral and nasal membranes.

EVIDENCE IN PRACTICE

Ellett M L.C and others: Gastric tube placement in young children, *Clin Nurs Res* 14(3):238-252, 2005.

There are specific measures to verify placement of NG tubes. These measures include gastrointestinal aspirate of pH ≤5.0 and abdominal radiograph. These measures are also reliable indicators for tube placement in children. In 72 children pH verification documented correct placement of NG

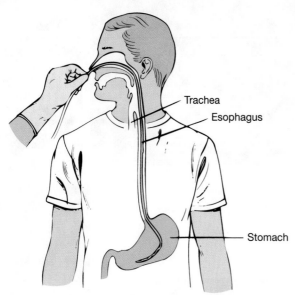

FIGURE 30-1 Placement of nasogastric tube.

Trachea

Esophagus

Stomach

tubes in 85% of the children. The remaining children's tube placement was verified with an abdominal radiograph. When caring for any client with an NG tube, it is necessary to accurately verify the location of the tube immediately after insertion and when assessing tube functioning or administering irrigations, medication, and tube feedings.

NURSING DIAGNOSES

Nursing diagnoses for clients with NG tubes may include **impaired oral mucous membrane,** which occurs from the irritation of the tube and the drying of the mucous membranes caused by mouth breathing, and **impaired tissue integrity,** which occurs from the pressure of the tube on the nasal mucosa. Removal of gastric secretions can create the risk for **deficient fluid volume** associated with altered electrolyte imbalance.

SKILL 30-1 Inserting Nasogastric Tube—Includes Checking Placement of Nasal Tube

---

• Nursing Skills Online: Enteral Nutrition, Lesson 2

Placement of an NG tube requires a physician's order. Clean technique is recommended for NG tube insertion. The procedure is uncomfortable. Clients complain of a burning sensation as the tube passes through the nasal mucosa.

Clients may also have dry, irritated nasal mucosa, and the nares may become excoriated. Provide frequent oral hygiene because clients with NG tubes frequently breathe through their mouths. The tube can accidentally migrate into the pulmonary system, in the distal esophagus or gastric antrum, or kink on itself in the stomach. Other complications include sinusitis, earache, esophagitis, gastric or esophageal ulceration and bleeding, and pulmonary aspiration. NG tubes are contraindicated when the client has severe facial or head trauma or certain types of head and neck surgery because of the risk of inserting the tube into brain tissue.

ASSESSMENT

1 Ask client about past history of nasal surgery or trauma or the presence of a cold or allergy. Inspect client's nares and oral cavity for deviated nasal septum, nasal surgery, inability to breathe well when either nasal opening is occluded, and nasal or oral irritation or bleeding. *Rationale: Determines proper naris for tube insertion, provides baseline data about the condition of nasal and oral cavity, and determines the need for special measures for oral hygiene or comfort after the tube is inserted.*

2 Auscultate for bowel sounds, then palpate client's abdomen for distention or pain. *Rationale: Provides baseline information about presence of abdominal sounds and the client's level of comfort and level of abdominal distention.*

3 Determine if client has had an NG tube insertion in the past. *Rationale: Procedure is uncomfortable; client's previous experience will complement any explanation.*

4 Assess client's level of consciousness and ability to cooperate or assist with the procedure and the need for special positioning during insertion.

5 Check medical record for physician's order, type of NG tube to be placed, and whether tube is to attach to suction or drainage bag. *Rationale: Physician's order is required. Adequate stomach decompression depends on NG suction.*

PLANNING

Expected Outcomes focus on decompression of the stomach, comfort, adequacy of fluid volume, adequacy of nutrition, and prevention of complications related to NG intubation.

1 Client's abdomen remains soft without distention.
2 Client's level of comfort improves or remains the same.
3 Client's NG tube remains patent.
4 Client's nasal mucosa remains moist and intact.

Delegation Considerations

The skill of inserting and maintaining an NG tube may not be delegated. The nurse directs personnel by:

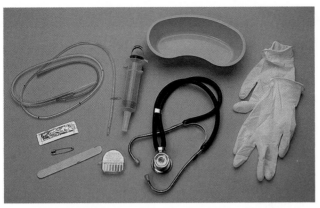

FIGURE 30-2 Nasogastric tube insertion equipment.

- Explaining when to measure and record the drainage from an NG tube.
- Emphasizing the need for frequent oral and nasal hygiene measures and comfort measures such as positioning and offering ice chips if allowed.
- Reviewing the need to observe for and report increases, decreases, or changes in NG drainage or client discomfort.

Equipment (Figure 30-2)

- 14- to 16-Fr NG tube (smaller-lumen catheters are not used for decompression in adults because they are not able to remove thick secretions)
- Water-soluble lubricating jelly
- pH test strips (measure gastric aspirate acidity)
- Tongue blade
- Flashlight
- Emesis basin
- Asepto bulb or catheter tip syringe
- 2.5-cm (1-inch) wide hypoallergenic tape or commercial fixation device

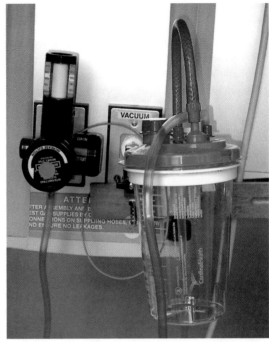

FIGURE 30-3 Suction equipment. (Photo courtesy Constance Maxey, Barnes-Jewish Hospital, St Louis, Mo.)

- Safety pin and rubber band
- Clamp, drainage bag, or suction machine or pressure gauge if wall suction is to be used
- Towel
- Glass of water with straw
- Facial tissues
- Normal saline for irrigation
- Tincture of benzoin (optional)
- Suction equipment (Figure 30-3)
- Clean gloves

IMPLEMENTATION *for Inserting Nasogastric Tube—Includes Checking Placement of Nasal Tube*

STEPS	RATIONALE

1 See Standard Protocol (inside front cover).

> NURSE ALERT Have suction equipment and emesis basin within reach in case of vomiting.

2 Prepare equipment at bedside. Cut a piece of tape about 10 cm (4 inches) long and split one half of it into two pieces to form a Y, or have NG tube fixator device available.	Tape or fixator device holds the NG tube in place after insertion.
3 Position client in high-Fowler's position with pillows behind head and shoulders. Raise bed to a horizontal level comfortable for the nurse.	Promotes client's ability to swallow during procedure. Positioning of bed prevents horizontal reach by nurse, which can cause injury.
4 Place bath towel over client's chest; give facial tissues to client. Have client blow nose.	Prevents soiling of client's gown. Tube insertion through nasal passages may cause tearing and coughing with increased salivation. Removes existing nasal secretions.
5 Stand on client's right side if right-handed, left side if left-handed.	Allows easiest manipulation of tubing.

STEPS	RATIONALE

6 Instruct client to relax and breathe normally while occluding one naris. Then repeat with other naris. Select nostril with greater airflow.

Tube passes more easily through naris that is more patent.

7 Measure distance to insert tube:

a. *Traditional method:* Measure distance from tip of nose to earlobe to xiphoid process (see illustration).

Tube extends from naris to stomach; distance varies with each client.

b. *Hanson method:* Mark a 50-cm point on the tube and then measure traditionally. Tube insertion is midway between 50 cm (20 inches) and previous method.

8 Mark this distance on tube with a piece of tape or an indelible marker.

Marks amount of tube to be inserted from naris to stomach.

9 Curve 10 to 15 cm (4 to 6 inches) of end of tube tightly around index finger and then release.

Curving tube tip aids insertion and decreases tube stiffness.

10 Lubricate about 7.5 to 10 cm (3 to 4 inches of the distal end of the tube with a water-soluble lubricant.

Minimizes friction against nasal mucosa and aids in tube insertion. Water-soluble lubricant is less toxic than oil-soluble if aspirated.

COMMUNICATION TIP Tell the client to raise his hand if he needs you to stop. Then stop and allow him to rest before proceeding again. Explain to client that sensation of tube will decrease over time.

---

11 Tell client that insertion is about to begin and instruct client to extend neck back against pillow.

Promotes comfort and reduces friction during insertion. Position facilitates initial passage of tube through naris and maintains clear airway for open naris.

12 Insert tube slowly through naris, aiming end of tube downward (see illustration). Continue to insert tube along floor of nasal passage aiming down toward ear. If resistance is felt, apply gentle downward pressure to advance tube. (Do not force past resistance.)

Minimizes discomfort of tube rubbing against upper nasal turbinates. Resistance is caused by posterior nasopharynx. Downward pressure helps tube curl around corner of nasopharynx.

13 If resistance is met, try to rotate the tube and see if it advances. If still resistant, withdraw tube, allow client to rest, relubricate tube, and insert into other naris.

Forcing against resistances can cause trauma to mucosa. Helps relieve client's anxiety.

NURSE ALERT If unable to insert tube in either naris, stop procedure and notify physician.

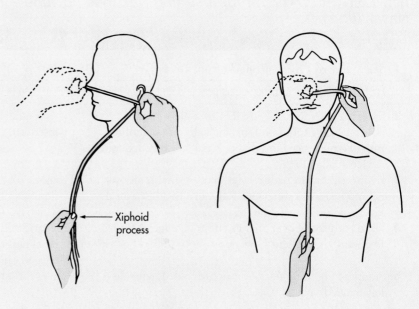

STEP 7a. Technique for measuring distance to insert nasogastric tube.

Xiphoid process

STEPS	RATIONALE
14 Continue insertion of tube until just past nasopharynx by gently rotating it toward the opposite nostril and then pass the tube just above oropharynx.	Helps prevent coiling of tube in oropharynx.
a. Stop tube advancement, allow client to relax, and provide tissues.	Relieves anxiety; tearing is a natural response to mucosal irritation, and excessive salivation may occur because of oral stimulation.
b. Explain to client that next step requires that client swallow. Give client glass of water with straw unless contraindicated.	Sipping of water aids passage of NG tube into esophagus.
15 With tube just above oropharynx, instruct client to flex head forward and swallow small sips of water. Advance tube 2.5 to 5 cm (1 to 2 inches) with each swallow. If client is not allowed fluids, instruct to dry swallow or suck air through straw. Advance tube with each swallow.	Flexed neck position closes off upper airway to trachea and opens esophagus. Swallowing closes epiglottis over trachea and helps move the tube into the esophagus. Swallowing water reduces gagging or choking. Water is removed later from stomach by suction.
16 If client begins to cough, gag, or choke, withdraw slightly and stop tube advancement. Instruct client to breathe easily and take sips of water.	Tube may accidentally enter larynx and produce coughing, and withdrawal of the tube reduces risk of laryngeal entry. Gagging is eased by swallowing water, which must be given cautiously to reduce the risk of aspiration.

> **NURSE ALERT** If vomiting occurs, assist client in clearing airway; oral suctioning may be needed. Do not proceed until airway is cleared.

STEPS	RATIONALE
17 If client continues to gag and cough or complains that tube feels as though it is coiling in back of throat, check back of oropharynx using flashlight and tongue blade (to compress client's tongue). If tube has coiled, withdraw it until the tip is back in the oropharynx. Then reinsert with client swallowing.	Tube may coil around itself in the back of throat and stimulate gag reflex.
18 After client relaxes, continue to advance tube with swallowing until tape or mark is reached. Temporarily anchor tube to cheek with a piece of tape until placement is checked.	Tip of tube must be well within stomach to decompress properly. Anchoring of tube prevents accidental displacement while the tube placement is verified.
19 Verify tube placement: Check agency policy for preferred methods for checking NG tube placement.	
a. Ask client to speak.	Client is unable to talk if NG has passed through vocal cords.
b. Inspect posterior pharynx for presence of coiled tube.	Tube is pliable and can coil up in back of pharynx instead of advancing into esophagus.

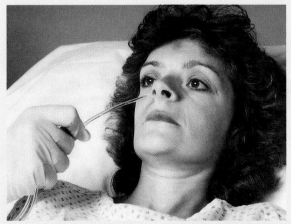

STEP 12 Insert nasogastric tube with curved end pointing downward.

STEPS	RATIONALE
c. Attach the catheter-tipped syringe to end of tube and aspirate gently back on syringe to obtain gastric contents, observing color, usually cloudy and green, off-white, tan, bloody, or brown.	Aspiration of contents provides a means to measure fluid pH and determine tube tip placement in gastrointestinal tract (Cottrell and Asturi, 2004).
d. Measure pH of aspirate with color-coded pH paper with range of whole numbers at least 1 to 11 (see illustration).	Gastric secretions are usually highly acidic, preferably 4 or less, compared with intestinal aspirates, which are usually greater than 4, or respiratory secretions, which are usually greater than 5.5 (Metheny and Titler, 2001).

> **NURSE ALERT**   Be sure to use gastric (Gastrocult) pH and not Hemoccult test.

e. Have ordered x-ray examination performed of chest/abdomen.	X-ray film verifies initial placement of the tube (Metheny and Titler, 2001).
f. If tube is not in stomach, advance tube by about 2.5 to 5 cm (1 to 2 inches) and repeat steps a through d to verify tube placement.	Tube must be in stomach to provide decompression.

> **NURSE ALERT**   Insufflating air into tube and listening with a stethoscope is not a reliable method to determine tube placement. In studies with feeding tubes, tubes inadvertently placed in lungs, esophagus, or even the brain can transmit sounds similar to that of air entering the stomach (Metheny and others, 1998a; Metheny and others, 1998b).

STEPS	RATIONALE
20 Anchor tube.	
a. After tube is properly inserted and position verified, either clamp distal end or connect tube to drainage bag or suction source.	Drainage bag is used if gravity drainage is ordered. Intermittent suction is most effective for gastric decompression. If the client is going to the operating room, the tube may be clamped.
b. Tape tube to nose; avoid putting pressure on nares. (Option: wipe nose off with alcohol swab.)	Prevents tissue necrosis. Tape anchors tube securely. Swab cleanses skin so tape will adhere better.
(1) Apply small amount of tincture of benzoin to lower end of nose and allow it to become "tacky" (optional).	Benzoin secures tape by preventing loosening of tape if client perspires.
(2) Apply tape to nose, leaving the split end free. Be sure end of tape over nose is secure.	.
(3) Carefully wrap two split ends of tape around tube (see illustration).	
(4) *Alternative:* Apply tube fixation device using shaped adhesive patch (see illustration).	
(5) Fasten rubber band to end of NG tube in a slip knot and pin rubber band to client's gown, allowing slack for movement of head.	Stabilizes the tube and decreases friction and pressure, which can irritate nasal mucosa.
21 Keep head of bed elevated at least 30 degrees unless physician orders otherwise.	Helps prevent esophageal reflux and minimizes irritation of tube against posterior pharynx.

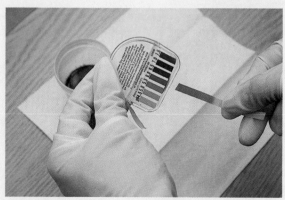

STEP 19d. Checking pH of gastric aspirate.

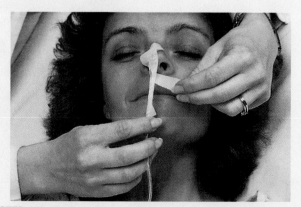

STEP 20b.(3) Tape is crossed over and around nasogastric tube.

STEPS	RATIONALE

22 Once placement of tube is confirmed, place a mark on the tube to indicate where the tube exits the nares or measure tube length from nares to connector. Document findings, measurement.

23 Provide regular oral hygiene (see Chapter 7) every 2 to 3 hours.

24 **See Completion Protocol (inside front cover).**

Mark provides a visual guide to indicate whether tube displacement may have occurred.

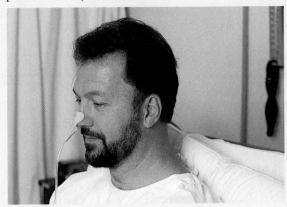

STEP 20b.(4) Client with tube fixation device.

EVALUATION

1 Turn off suction and auscultate for bowel sounds. Palpate client's abdomen for distention and pain.

2 Ask client to describe any discomfort and rate comfort (using a scale of 0-10).

3 Observe color and amount of gastric secretions and check patency of NG tube.

4 Observe client's oral and nasal mucosa.

Unexpected Outcomes and Related Interventions

1 Client develops abdominal distention, vomiting, or absence of drainage from tube.

a. Assess patency of tube and irrigate tube as needed. Caution: never irrigate an NG tube in a client who has had stomach surgery unless there is a physician's order.

b. Verify that suction is on as ordered.

c. Determine if suction ordered will drain secretions. If drainage not seen, irrigate tube (see Skill 30.2) and reevaluate.

2 Client develops chronic inflammation and erosion of nasal mucosa.

a. Provide frequent skin care to area.

b. Retape tube to avoid pressure on naris.

c. Consider removal of tube and reinsertion into opposite naris (physician's order necessary).

3 Client develops signs and symptoms of pulmonary aspiration: fever, shortness of breath, pulmonary congestion.

a. Perform complete respiratory assessment.

b. Contact physician to report symptoms.

c. Prepare for chest x-ray examination.

Recording and Reporting

• Record length, size, and type of gastric tube inserted in chosen nares, and verification methods; include client's response and level of comfort, description of NG drainage (e.g., color, amount, insertion distance), whether tube is connected to drainage or to suction, and amount of suction applied.

• Report insertion procedure and any complications.

Sample Documentation

1000 Inserted 16-Fr NG tube into left nares, advanced to 50-cm mark. Client assisted with insertion by swallowing and states he is comfortable. NPO status acknowledged. 50 ml of light-green secretions aspirated with a pH of 3.0. Tube secured with tape and attached to low intermittent suction. Bowel sounds absent.

Special Considerations
Pediatric Considerations

• For children, the use of sedation and analgesia should be considered prior to tube insertion (Hockenberry and Wilson, 2007).

• The amount of preprocedure preparation is dependent on the child's developmental level, as well as the health care needs. Never surprise the child with this procedure (Hockenberry and Wilson, 2007).

Geriatric Considerations

• Geriatric clients may have sensory deficits that affect their ability to assist with NG tube insertion. If the client has hearing impairment, make sure that the client's hearing aid is in place and adjusted appropriately so that the client will be able to hear instructions.

• Check for ill-fitting dentures and remove them for the client's safety and comfort during the insertion.

• Oral and nasal mucosal drying may be present. Be sure that the tube is adequately lubricated for insertion.

Home Care Considerations
- If long-term decompression of the stomach is required, such as when the bowel is obstructed, a permanent decompression tube such as a gastrostomy tube is surgically

inserted. Teach clients and caregivers how to take care of the gastrostomy tube and suction device. A portable, intermittent suction device is usually used in the home.

SKILL 30.2 Irrigating Nasogastric Tube

Irrigating an NG tube maintains the tube's patency. The most common causes of NG tube occlusion is failure to flush at regular intervals (Colagiovanni, 2000). An NG tube is generally used for decompression so medications and tube feedings are not administered. However, if a medication is given, irrigation is necessary. Indications of occlusion include decreased volume of gastric secretions or abdominal distention, pain, or nausea. The NG tube is irrigated before and after the administration of medications. Before irrigating the NG tube, always verify tube placement.

ASSESSMENT

1 Assess the volume, color, and character of gastric secretions. *Rationale: Thick secretions and a reduced volume of secretions may indicate the need to irrigate the NG tube. Color can also be an indicator of tube placement (Figure 30-4).*
2 Assess client's abdomen for distention or pain. *Rationale: Abdominal distention indicates that NG tube may not be patent.*
3 Turn off gastric suction and auscultate for bowel sounds and note any passage of flatus. *Rationale: Determines presence of peristalsis. Gastric suction noise will obliterate bowel sounds.*

PLANNING

Expected Outcomes focus on maintenance of nasogastric drainage to ensure adequate decompression of the stomach.
1 Client's NG tube remains patent.
2 Tube remains in proper position.
3 Client denies abdominal discomfort or nausea.
4 Abdomen remains nondistended.

Delegation Considerations
The skill of irrigating an NG tube may not be delegated. The nurse directs personnel by:
- Reviewing the need to observe for and report increases, decreases, or changes in NG drainage or client discomfort.

Equipment (Figure 30-5)
- 60-ml catheter tip syringe
- Normal saline for irrigation
- Towel
- Clean gloves
- Stethoscope

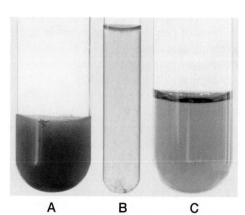

FIGURE 30-4 Gastric contents. **A,** Stomach. **B,** Stomach. **C,** Intestinal. (Courtesy Dr. Norma Metheny, St Louis University School of Nursing.)

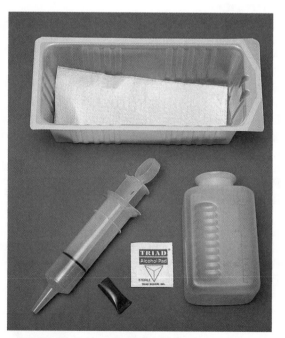

FIGURE 30-5 Nasogastric tube irrigation equipment.

IMPLEMENTATION *for Irrigating Nasogastric Tube*

STEPS	RATIONALE

1 See Standard Protocol (inside front cover).

2 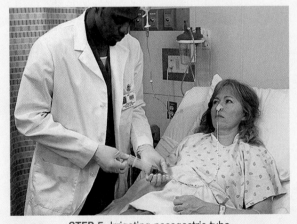 Verify that NG tube is properly placed (see Skill 30.1, Steps 19 a-d). Once tube position is verified, proceed with irrigation.

Prevents accidental entrance of irrigating solution into lungs.

3 Draw up 30 ml of normal saline into Asepto or catheter-tip syringe.

Saline minimizes potential loss of electrolytes from stomach fluids.

4 Pinch or clamp NG tube and disconnect from connection tubing. Lay end of connection tubing on towel.

Reduces soiling of client's gown and bed by drainage of gastric secretions.

5 Insert tip of irrigation syringe into end of NG tube and unclamp tubing. Hold syringe with top pointed at floor and inject water slowly and evenly (see illustration). Do not force solution.

Position of syringe prevents introduction of air into vent tubing, which could cause gastric distention. Solution introduced under pressure can cause gastric irritation or gastric trauma.

> **NURSE ALERT** Do not inject water through blue "pigtail" air vent on Salem sump tube.

6 If resistance occurs, check for kinks in tubing. Reposition client on left side and try again. Repeated resistance is reported to physician.

Tip of tube may be against stomach wall. Repositioning may dislodge tube away from stomach lining.

7 After instilling irrigant, immediately aspirate fluid by pulling back gently on syringe to withdraw fluid. Calculate the difference in amount between that instilled and withdrawn.

Irrigation clears tubing, so stomach remains empty. Fluid remaining in stomach is measured as intake.

8 Reconnect NG tube to suction. (If solution does not return, repeat irrigation.) If tube fails to drain secretions, it may become necessary to increase amount of suction pressure. This requires a physician's order.

Reestablishes gastric drainage system; may repeat irrigation or repositioning of tube until NG tube drains properly.

9 Option: take syringe, draw up 10 ml air, insert tip into end of blue pigtail and inject air.

Maintains patency of air vent for promoting drainage.

10 See Completion Protocol (inside front cover).

STEP 5 Irrigating nasogastric tube.

EVALUATION

1 Auscultate bowel sounds.
2 Inspect client's abdomen for distention; palpate for distention, pain, and rigidity.
3 Inspect amount and color of returned irrigant.
4 Verify correct position of tube.
5 Determine client's level of comfort.

Unexpected Outcomes and Related Interventions

1 Client's NG tube cannot be irrigated and is no longer patent.
a. Contact physician. The buildup of secretions poses a risk for aspiration.

2 Client's NG tube can be irrigated, but irrigation fluid cannot be withdrawn, and the tube continues to drain poorly.
a. Contact physician.
b. Position of tube may need to be confirmed.

Recording and Reporting

* Record verification of tube placement, volume, and color of drainage before irrigation of the tube; any symptoms of discomfort that the client is having; ease of irrigation and the amount and type of irrigant. Include the difference in volume instilled and volume withdrawn as intake or output. Record the client's response to irrigation, including any discomfort or relief of symptoms.
* Report any difficulty with irrigation.

Sample Documentation

0800 NG tube draining scant amounts of green liquid. Position of tube verified, pH 3.0. Irrigated with 30 ml NS. Initially NG tube irrigated sluggishly but became easier to irrigate. Withdrew 20 ml light green fluid at end of irrigation. Client stated he had been feeling mild nausea.

1000 Increased volume of light-green gastric secretions draining from NG tube at low suction. Client states he no longer feels nauseated. Abdomen remains soft and nontender.

SKILL 30-3 | Removing Nasogastric Tube

An NG tube is removed when it is no longer needed for decompression of the stomach and gastric secretions empty normally into the duodenum through the pyloric sphincter and when intestinal motility returns. A physician's order is required for this procedure.

The client's ability to handle gastric secretions is sometimes evaluated by removing the NG tube from suction and putting it to gravity drainage or by clamping the NG tube for a specified number of hours per day. If the client does not have a return of gastric or intestinal motility, the symptoms of abdominal distention, discomfort, or nausea may return.

ASSESSMENT

1 Turn off gastric suction and auscultate abdomen for bowel sounds. Also note if client has had bowel movements or is passing flatus. *Rationale: Return of flatus, bowel sounds, and bowel movements confirms the presence of peristalsis and bowel functioning. Gastric suction noise will obliterate bowel sounds.*

2 Palpate for pain and abdominal distention. *Rationale: Abdominal distention and pain may contraindicate tube removal; contact physician before proceeding.*

3 Ask client about nausea and to describe abdominal pain.

PLANNING

Expected Outcomes focus on minimizing the discomfort caused by removal of the tube.

1 Client remains comfortable after removal of the tube.

2 Client's abdomen remains soft and nontender, and bowel sounds are normal.

Delegation Considerations

The skill of removing an NG tube may not be delegated. The nurse directs personnel by:

* Emphasizing the need for frequent oral and nasal hygiene measures after the removal.
* Reviewing the need to observe for and report any nausea, vomiting, or changes in client discomfort.

Equipment

* Tissues
* Towel
* Clean gloves
* 60-ml catheter tip syringe
* Measurement container

IMPLEMENTATION *for Removing Nasogastric Tube*

STEPS	RATIONALE
1 See Standard Protocol (inside front cover).	Physician's order is required.
2 Verify physician's order.	

COMMUNICATION TIP Tell client that removal of tube is less distressing than the insertion.

| **3** Place towel over client's chest to protect gown and cover tube. | Towel will protect client's gown and bed linens. |
| **4** ✋ Turn off suction and disconnect NG tube from drainage bag or suction. Remove tape or NG tube fixation device from bridge of client's nose and unpin tube from client's gown. | Tube is free of connections before removal. |

STEPS	RATIONALE
5 Stand on client's right side if right-handed, left side if left-handed.	Allows for easy manipulation of tube.
6 Draw up 30 ml of air into catheter-tip syringe, attach syringe to end of NG tube, flush tube with air.	Clears gastric fluids from tube that could irritate esophagus and mouth during the removal.
7 Hand the client facial tissue and ask client to take a deep breath and hold it as tube is removed.	Client may wish to blow nose after tube is removed. Airway is partially occluded during removal of tube.
8 Clamp or kink tube securely and pull tube out steadily and smoothly onto towel while client holds breath.	Kinked tube is less likely to expel gastric contents (if present) into throat or trachea. Breath holding minimizes risk of aspirating gastric contents if spilled from tube during removal.
9 Measure volume of drainage, and note character of content. Record on Intake and Output Summary (see Chapter 9). Dispose of NG tube, remove and discard gloves, and perform hand hygiene.	Maintains accurate intake and output.
10 Clean nares and provide mouth care.	Promotes comfort.
11 See Completion Protocol (inside front cover).	

EVALUATION

1 Ask client about level of comfort after removal of the tube and provision of mouth care.
2 Palpate client's abdomen and auscultate for bowel sounds.

Unexpected Outcomes and Related Interventions

1 Client complains of nares or throat pain after removal of the NG tube.
a. Consult with physician about the use of topical anesthetics to reduce pain from irritated nasal mucosa.
b. Encourage client to ingest warm, soothing liquids if able. Be alert for any swallowing problems that may indicate erosion of the esophagus.
2 Abdominal distention and pain occur.
a. Notify physician.
b. Prepare to reinsert NG tube and/or obtain abdominal x-ray examination.

Recording and Reporting

- Record abdominal assessment findings (e.g., absence of distention or presence of bowel sounds before tube removal); include if there was any difficulty removing the NG tube; include client's level of comfort and any symptoms after removal of the tube.
- Report any return of nausea, vomiting, abdominal distention, or decrease in client's level of comfort.

Sample Documentation

1300 Removed NG tube without difficulty. Mouth care provided after the removal. Bowel sounds auscultated in all four quadrants. Abdomen remains soft, nontender. Skin at left naris red and intact.

NCLEX® Style Questions

A client was admitted to the medical nursing unit with severe vomiting and abdominal pain. The physician has ordered a nasogastric tube inserted.

1 The client tells you he broke his nose in a fight 20 years ago. Based on this information, which of the following steps should be followed to insert an NG tube?
1. Tell Mr. Smithers that will prevent the tube insertion.
2. Call Dr. Lang for an order for local anesthetic.
3. Assess patency of each nostril.
4. Add extra lubricant to the tube during insertion.

2 When measuring length of insertion for a nasogastric tube, which is the correct measure?
1. Corner of mouth to earlobe to xyphoid process
2. Tip of nose to earlobe to xyphoid process
3. 50 cm from tip of tube
4. Tip of nose to umbilicus

3 Once the tube is passed, which of the following indicates that the tube is properly placed in the stomach?
1. Tan aspirate with pH 3.2
2. Yellow aspirate with pH 5.5
3. Clear aspirate with pH 6.7
4. Light brown aspirate with pH 4.3

4 The client calls you to his room and complains of abdominal pain and severe nausea. You are aware that the NG output has decreased over the past 3 hours and determine the tube may not be draining properly. You should implement which of the folllowing?
1. Notify the physician.
2. Turn the client to his left side to promote drainage.
3. Withdraw the tube 2 to 3 inches.
4. Irrigate the tube with saline and withdraw the fluid instilled.

5 After removal of the nasogastric tube, which of the following may indicate that the tube needs to be replaced?
1. Abdominal pain
2. Abdominal distention
3. Lack of appetite
4. No bowel movement for 24 hours

References for all chapters appear in Appendix D.

Enteral Nutrition

31

MEDIA RESOURCES

- **evolve** http://evolve.elsevier.com/Elkin
- **View Video!** Video Clips
- Nursing Skills Online

Enteral nutrition is the administration of nutrients directly into the gastrointestinal (GI) tract. The most desirable and appropriate method of providing nutrition is the oral route; unfortunately this is not always possible. When oral feedings are not possible, yet the stomach or intestine is able to digest nutrients, enteral tube feeding is an option. Enteral feeding is preferred over parenteral nutrition because it improves use of nutrients, is generally safer for clients, maintains structure and function of the gut, and is less expensive (ASPEN, 2002). A variety of enteral feeding formulas are available in whole protein or partially digested form. Special enteral formulas for renal disease, hepatic disease, pulmonary disease, or diabetes, as well as adult and pediatric formulas, are also available. The skills presented in this chapter focus on the administration of nutritional feedings directly into the GI tract with the goal of restoring the client's nutritional status. Nurses will administer enteral feedings most commonly via small-bore (diameter) tubes (8 Fr to 12 Fr) inserted through the nose and advanced to either the stomach or proximal small intestine (Metheny and Titler, 2001) (Figure 31-1).

A rare yet potentially fatal complication associated with the insertion of a feeding tube is inadvertent placement into another part of the body. Placement into the respiratory tract reportedly occurs in approximately 5% of the cases in intensive care settings. To avoid this problem, initial placement of a feeding tube should be verified with an abdominal x-ray before the instillation of any substance into the tube (American Association of Critical Care Nurses [AACN], 2005).

A nurse administers tube feedings in several ways: as a bolus amount via gravity given several times a day through a large-bore syringe, as an intermittent gravity drip given over 30 minutes to 1 hour several times per day using a pouch to hang the feeding, or as a continuous drip given per infusion pump given over a 24-hour period.

Verifying placement of a feeding tube before administering medication or tube feeding is critical to safe client care. A feeding tube is improperly positioned when it is accidentally placed in the lung, esophagus, or even the stomach when it should be in the small bowel (Metheny and Titler, 2001). Tubes are easily misplaced as a result of normal movements, excessive coughing, or move-

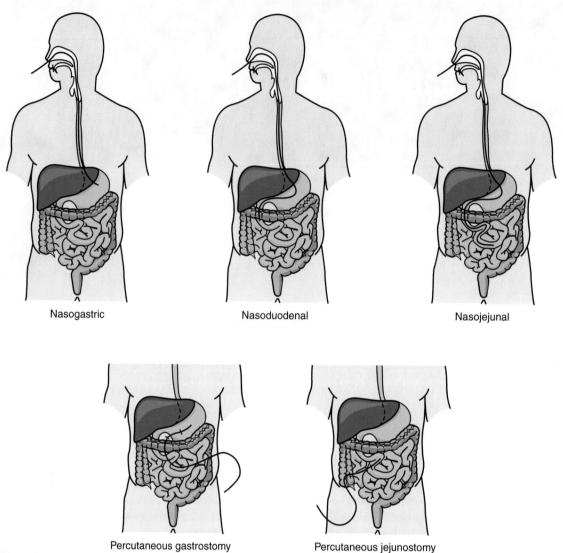

Nasogastric

Nasoduodenal

Nasojejunal

Percutaneous gastrostomy

Percutaneous jejunostomy

FIGURE 31-1 Tube feeding routes. (From Beare PG, Myers JL: *Principles and practice of adult health nursing,* ed 3, St Louis, 1998, Mosby.)

ments of a confused or agitated client. In addition, the distal tip can migrate upward or downward from its original correct position, even when the external portion of the tube is taped in place (Metheny, 2002; Metheny and Titler, 2001). When a tube migrates to the lung, complications such as aspiration, pneumonia, pneumothorax, and peritonitis can develop if feedings are administered.

Placement of a nasogastric (NG) or nasointestinal (NI) feeding tube should be verified by x-ray examination to determine that the tube is in the stomach or intestine rather than in the airways (AACN, 2005; Metheny and others, 1998a). Abdominal x-ray films are the standard of care. Unfortunately, not all institutions have policies mandating this method. X-ray examinations are also not usually performed for large-diameter NG tubes because clinicians usually believe the tubes are less likely to enter the lung undetected (Metheny and others, 1998a). A pH measurement is the next best method for confirming feeding tube placement. By

testing the pH of fluid aspirated from a newly inserted feeding tube, it is possible to make reliable judgments about the tube's location (Metheny and others, 1998b).

Traditionally the location of the tip of a feeding tube was determined by using a syringe to instill air through the tube. Using a stethoscope, you would listen for a gurgling sound over the epigastric region to indicate proper tube placement. The reliability of this method is highly questionable and is not to be used to rule out inadvertent respiratory positioning of feeding tubes (AACN, 2005; Metheny and others, 1998a).

Many potential complications arise from prolonged intubation, including nasal erosion, sinusitis, esophagitis, gastric ulceration, and pulmonary aspiration (Baskin, 2006). The cost of managing the ensuing complications and infections is expensive. Complications are related to the tube itself, such as placement in the lung, frequent tube clogging, or the tube being inadvertently pulled out. Complications also occur when the administered feeding causes delayed gastric emptying, bloating, or diarrhea (Metheny and others, 2005; Lebak and others, 2003).

EVIDENCE IN PRACTICE

Metheny NA, Schallom ML, Edwards SJ: Effect of gastrointestinal motility and feeding tube site on aspiration risk in critically ill patients: a review, *Heart Lung* 33:131, 2004.

Aspiration is a risk in critically ill tube-fed clients. Many of these clients have a decreased level of consciousness, which leads to depressed cough and gag reflexes. Researchers reviewed the literature to determine if the location of the feeding tube (i.e., gastric versus intestinal feeding tube or tube placement through the nose or percutaneously) increased the risk of aspiration. Although multiple factors affect the risk of aspiration, one cannot conclude that the type of or placement of the feeding tube is the cause. How-

ever, these researchers noted that the clinical assessment of greatest interest was the evaluation of gastric emptying, usually measured through residual volumes. Clients with higher gastric volumes had a greater aspiration risk.

NURSING DIAGNOSES

Imbalanced nutrition: less than body requirements related to inability to ingest or digest food or absorb nutrients is appropriate when clients have weight loss, a reduction in food intake, and physical signs of malnutrition. **Impaired swallowing** related to neuromuscular impairment makes a client a candidate for tube feedings. **Risk for aspiration** is another indication for use of tube feedings, but it is also a condition that a client receiving tube feedings is predisposed to. Clients may experience **diarrhea** or be at **risk for constipation** related to altered intake associated with tube feedings.

SKILL 31.1 Intubating the Client with a Small-Bore Nasogastric or Nasointestinal Feeding Tube

- **Nursing Skills Online: Enteral Nutrition, Lesson 2**

Small-bore NG and NI feedings are used for short-term management of nutritional problems during acute illness and recovery. Clients often require tube feedings because of ineffective swallowing or a weakened gag reflex causing a risk for aspiration. Some clients have an increased metabolism as a result of sepsis or burns and are unable to ingest enough calories to meet their metabolic needs. After a feeding tube is inserted, clients remain at risk for aspiration and need careful nursing assessment and intervention to avoid this complication. Avoid using large-bore NG tubes for tube feedings because they carry increased risk of aspiration and are more irritating to the nasopharyngeal and esophageal mucosa (ASPEN, 2002).

Small-bore feeding tubes are available in weighted (tungsten) or unweighted designs (Figure 31-2). Weighted tubes were thought to pass more easily into the duodenum or jejunum via peristalsis; however, research does not show an advantage of the weight in promoting intestinal passage. Nonetheless, clinicians use weighted tubes more frequently than nonweighted tubes for nasoduodenal and nasojejunal feedings because they are believed to remain in correct position longer than nonweighted tubes. Aside from the weighted tip, small-bore tubes are made of a softer material. Thus small-bore tubes can be left in place for an extended period with less irritation to the nasopharyngeal, esophageal, and gastric mucosa. Because the tubes are flexible, a guide wire or stylet provides rigidity to facilitate insertion and positioning and then is removed once correct place-

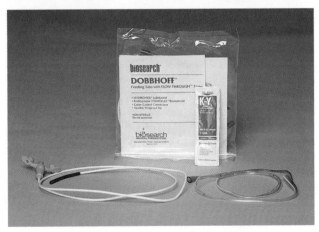

FIGURE 31-2 Small-bore feeding tubes.

ment is verified. Placing a NG or NI feeding tube requires a physician's order.

Assessment

1 Verify client's need for enteral tube feedings and intubation: impaired swallowing, head or neck surgery, decreased level of consciousness, surgeries involving upper GI tract, or facial trauma. Obtain order after consultation with physician. *Rationale: Recent head or neck surgery, esophageal surgery, or facial trauma may necessitate tube placement by a physician. It is important to identify clients before they become nutritionally depleted; approximately 40% of hospitalized patients are malnourished (Pearce and Duncan, 2002).*

2 Assess client's weight, height, hydration status, input and output (I&O), electrolyte balance, and metabolic needs. *Rationale: Provides baseline information to measure nutritional improvement once enteral feedings are initiated.*

3 Determine patency of nares. Have client close each nostril alternately and breathe. Examine each naris for patency and skin breakdown. *Rationale: Nares may be obstructed or irritated. Assessment determines most patent naris for tube insertion.*

4 Review client's medical history: nosebleeds, nasal surgery, deviated septum, anticoagulant therapy, and coagulopathy. *Rationale: Requires nurse to seek a physician's order to change route of nutritional support.*

5 Assess client for gag reflex. Place tongue blade in client's mouth, touching uvula. *Rationale: Identifies client's ability to swallow and determines if risk for aspiration exists.*

6 Assess client's mental status. *Rationale: An alert client is better able to cooperate with procedure. If vomiting occurs, an alert client can usually expectorate vomitus, which can help reduce the risk of aspiration.*

7 Auscultate bowel sounds (notify physician if sounds are absent). *Rationale: Absence of bowel sounds may indicate decreased or absent peristalsis and increased risk of aspiration or abdominal distention.*

8 Determine if the physician wants a prokinetic agent administered before placement of an NI tube. *Rationale: Prokinetic agents such a metoclopramide given **before** NI tube placement help advance the tube into the intestine (Silva, Saconarto, and Atallah, 2006; Kittinger, Sandler, and Heizer, 1987).*

PLANNING

Expected Outcomes focus on safe insertion of feeding tube with placement in stomach, duodenum, or jejunum.

1 Placement of tube in stomach or intestine is verified.

2 Feeding tube remains patent.

3 Client does not develop respiratory distress (e.g., increased respiratory rate, coughing, gagging, poor color) or signs of discomfort or nasal trauma.

Delegation Considerations

The skill of intubating the client with a small-bore NG or NI feeding tube cannot be delegated. The nurse directs personnel by:

- Explaining how to assist with positioning client during intubation.
- Reviewing what to observe (e.g., gagging, choking) following tube insertion and ordering to report this information back to the nurse.

Equipment

- NG or NI tube (8 to 12 Fr) with guide wire or stylet
- 60-ml Luer-Lok or catheter-tipped syringe
- Stethoscope
- Hypoallergenic tape and tincture of benzoin with cotton-tipped applicator or tube fixation device
- pH indicator strip (scale 0.0 to 14.0)
- Glass of water and straw
- Emesis basin
- Safety pin
- Rubber band
- Towel
- Facial tissues
- Clean gloves
- Suction equipment in case of aspiration
- Penlight
- Tongue blade

IMPLEMENTATION *for Intubating the Client with a Small-Bore Nasogastric or Nasointestinal Feeding Tube*

STEPS	RATIONALE
1 See Standard Protocol (inside front cover).	
2 Explain procedure to client and how to communicate during intubation (e.g., raise a finger to indicate gagging or discomfort).	It is important for client to have a method for communication during the procedure to alleviate stress. Nurse may need to pause during insertion to decrease gagging.

> **COMMUNICATION TIP** To help the client have a chance to participate and feel a sense of control, explain how to try to relax and communicate during tube insertion. "Now I will explain each step as we go along. The tube will cause a slight burning pain as it passes through your nose. I want you to raise one finger to tell me if it's too uncomfortable so that I can be gentle and at the same time get this done as quickly as possible."

3 Place towel over client's chest and position client in sitting or high-Fowler's position. If client is comatose, place in semi-Fowler's position with head propped forward using a pillow. It may be necessary to have an assistant help with positioning of confused or comatose clients.	Position reduces risk of pulmonary aspiration in event client vomits. Assists with closure of airway and passage of the tube into the esophagus. When inserting the tube into the nose, avoid tipping the client's head back because it opens the airway and increases risk for aspiration.

> **NURSE ALERT** Place tissues and emesis basin within client's reach.

STEPS	RATIONALE
4 Check feeding tube for flaws: rough or sharp edges on distal end and closed or clogged outlet holes.	Flaws in feeding tube hamper tube intubation and can injure client.
5 Determine length of tube to be inserted and mark with tape or indelible ink (see illustration).	Determines approximate depth of insertion.

> **NURSE ALERT** Tip of tube must reach stomach. Measure distance from tip of nose to earlobe to xiphoid process of sternum (see illustration). Add an additional 20 to 30 cm (8 to 12 inches for NI tube (Hanson, 1979; Lord and others, 1993; Welch, 1996).

6 Prepare NG or NI tube for intubation:	
a. Perform hand hygiene.	Reduces spread of microorganisms.
b. Inject 10 ml of water from 60-ml Luer-Lok or catheter-tipped syringe into the tube.	Aids in guidewire or stylet insertion.
c. Make certain to securely position guidewire against weighted tip and to snugly fit both Luer-Lok connections.	Promotes smooth passage of tube into GI tract. Improperly positioned stylet can induce serious trauma.
7 Cut adhesive tape 10 cm (4 inches) long or prepare tube fixation device.	
8 Dip tube with surface lubricant into a glass of room temperature water or apply water-soluble lubricant. Do not place tubes in cold or ice water.	Activates lubricant to facilitate passage of tube into naris to GI tract. Ice or cold water causes tubes to become inflexible, causing trauma to mucous membranes.

> **COMMUNICATION TIP** Explain that you are now about to insert the feeding tube. Let client know how he or she can assist. "I will insert the tube through your nose toward the back of your throat. Swallowing will help advance the tube. Once the tip is in the back of your throat, I will ask you to begin to swallow. The water (ice chips) may help if you find it hard to swallow. I will tell you when to stop swallowing."

9 Hand the alert client a glass of water with straw or glass with crushed ice (if able to swallow).	Client is asked to swallow to facilitate tube passage.
10 Gently insert tube through nostril to back of throat (posterior nasopharynx). This may cause client to gag. Aim back and down toward ear (see illustration).	Natural contour facilitates passage of tube into GI tract.
11 Have client flex head toward chest after tube has passed through nasopharynx.	Closes off glottis and reduces risk of tube entering trachea.
12 Emphasize need to mouth breathe and swallow.	Helps facilitate passage of tube.

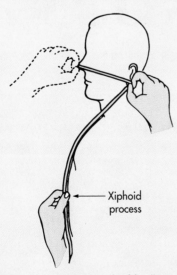

STEP 5 Determining length of feeding tube.

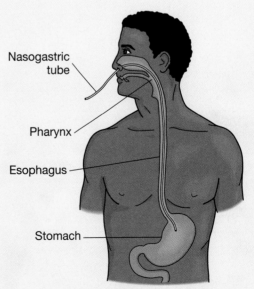

Nasogastric tube

Pharynx

Esophagus

Stomach

STEP 10 NG tube inserted through nose and esophagus into stomach.

STEPS	RATIONALE

13 When you insert tube to tip of the carina (approximately 25 cm [10 inches] in the adult), stop and listen for air exchange from distal portion of the tube.

If air can be heard, tube could be in respiratory tract; remove tube and begin again (Metheny and Titler, 2001).

> **NURSE ALERT** Do not force tube. If resistance is met or client starts to cough, choke, or become cyanotic, stop advancing tube and pull tube back.

14 Advance tube each time client swallows until desired length has been passed.

Reduces discomfort and trauma to client.

15 Check for position of tube in back of throat with penlight and tongue blade.

Tube may be coiled, kinked, or entering trachea.

16 Temporarily anchor tube to nose with small piece of tape and verify placement of tube (see Skill 31.2).

Movement of tube stimulates gagging. Assesses general position before anchoring tube more securely.

17 After verifying tube placement by gastric aspirates, anchor tube to nose and avoid pressure on nares. Mark exit site on tube with indelible ink. Use one of the following options for anchoring:

Properly secured tube allows client more mobility and prevents trauma to nasal mucosa.

a. Apply tape
   (1) Apply tincture of benzoin sparingly to nose and allow it to become "tacky."
   (2) Remove gloves and split one end of the adhesive tape strip lengthwise 5 cm (2 inches).
   (3) Wrap each of the 5-cm strips around tube as it exits nose (see illustration).
b. Apply tube fixation device
   (1) Apply wide end of shaped adhesive patch to bridge of nose (see illustration).
   (2) Slip connector around feeding tube as it exits nose (see illustration).

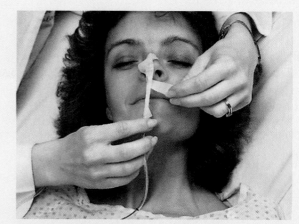

STEP 17a.(3) Wrapping tape to anchor nasoenteral tube.

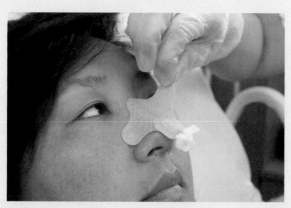

STEP 17b.(1) Applying fixation device patch to bridge of nose.

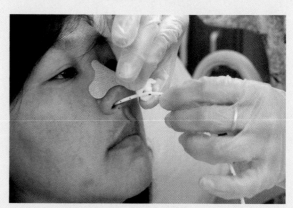

STEP 17b.(2) Slip connector around feeding tube.

STEPS	RATIONALE
18 Fasten end of NG tube to client's gown using piece of tape (see illustration). Do not use safety pins to pin tube to client's gown.	Reduces traction on naris when tube is moved. Safety pins can become unfastened and cause injury to client.
19 Assist client to comfortable position. NOTE: Positioning client on right side does not facilitate intestinal placement.	Researchers indicate that placing patient on right side does not promote passage of tube into the small intestine (Kittinger and others, 1987).

> **NURSE ALERT** Leave guidewire or stylet in place until x-ray confirmation of correct position is obtained. Never attempt to reinsert partially or fully removed guidewire or stylet while feeding tube is in place. Guidewire or stylet may perforate GI tract, especially the esophagus or nearby tissue, and seriously injure client.

20 Obtain x-ray film of abdomen.	X-ray verifies placement of tube (AACN, 2005).
21 Apply gloves and administer frequent oral hygiene. Cleanse tubing at nostril.	Promotes client comfort and integrity of oral and nasal mucous membranes.
22 See Completion Protocol (inside front cover).	

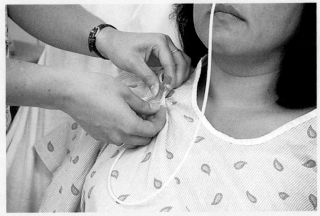

STEP 18 Fasten feeding tube to client's gown.

EVALUATION

1 Have client speak; observe for persistent gagging or paroxysms of coughing.

2 Confirm x-ray film results and auscultate lung sounds. Remove the guidewire or stylet after x-ray film verification of correct placement.

3 Routinely assess location of external exit site marking on the tube, as well as color and pH of fluid withdrawn from NG or NI tube.

4 Inspect nasal mucosa at least every 8 hours.

Unexpected Outcomes and Related Interventions

1 Client has severe and persistent coughing, shortness of breath.
a. Place client in high Fowler's position.
b. Auscultate lung sounds.
c. Verify placement of feeding tube.

2 Persistent gagging leads to vomiting with aspiration of GI contents.
a. Position client on side, remove feeding tube if gagging continues, and suction airway as needed (see Skill 31.3).
b. Contact physician and consider need for immediate chest x-ray film.

3 Nasal mucosa becomes inflamed, tender, and/or eroded.
a. Retape tube to relieve pressure on mucosa.
b. Consider removal of tube, and reinsert in opposite naris (physician order required).

Recording and Reporting

- Record in nurses' notes type and size of tube placed, length of tube insertion, client's baseline respiratory rate and depth, presence of lung sounds, and tolerance of procedure, confirmation of tube position by x-ray film, and pH and appearance of aspirate.
- Report to physician any incidence of aspiration or suspected change in tube position.

Sample Documentation

1000 10 Fr small-bore feeding tube inserted into right naris, advanced approximately 60 cm. No gagging or vomiting. Abdominal x-ray film confirmed duodenal placement. Intestinal aspirate tested at pH 7.0, bile colored in appearance.

Special Considerations

Pediatric Considerations

- Premature infant and neonate: measure from nose or mouth to earlobe and then to the xiphoid process (Hockenberry and Wilson, 2007).
- Older child: Measure from (a) nose to bottom of the earlobe and then to the lower end of the xiphoid process, or (b) nose to earlobe and then to a point midway between the xiphoid process and the umbilicus (Hockenberry and Wilson, 2007).
- In infant, observe for vagal stimulation during insertion, evidenced by decreased heart rate.

Geriatric Considerations

- Ensure adequate lubrication of tube to decrease discomfort for the older adult who may have decreased oral or nasopharyngeal secretions.

Home Care Considerations

- Assess client or primary caregiver's ability to maintain tube and feeding program.
- Assess environmental safety and sanitation of client's home to determine potential for infection or injury if tube is to be inserted for ongoing nutritional support.
- See Home Care Considerations for Skill 31.2.

Long-Term Care Considerations

- Clients who require prolonged enteral feedings in the long-term care setting frequently have gastrostomy or jejunostomy tubes in place (see Skill 31.3).

SKILL 31.2 Verifying Tube Placement for a Large-Bore or Small-Bore Feeding Tube

- **Nursing Skills Online: Enteral Nutrition, Lesson 3**

Nasally or orally placed small-bore feeding tubes are inserted into the stomach for either intermittent or continuous feedings. The tubes are also inserted into the small intestine (duodenum or proximal jejunum). Large-bore tubes are not suitable for small bowel feedings. Intermittent feedings are boluses administered over a short time period; therefore they are only given into the stomach because it is a natural reservoir for fluid (ASPEN 2002).

It is possible for an NG or NI enteral feeding tube to move into a different location (from the stomach to the intestine or from the intestine into the stomach) without any external evidence that the tube has moved (Chen and others, 2000). The risk for aspiration of regurgitated gastric contents into the respiratory tract is increased when the tip of an NI tube accidentally dislocates upward into the stomach or when the tip of either an NG or NI tube dislocates upward into the esophagus.

Following initial x-ray film verification that a tube is positioned in the desired site (either the stomach or small intestine), the nurse is responsible for ensuring that the tube has remained in the intended position before administering formula or medications through the tube. Therefore the nurse verifies tube position every 4 to 12 hours and as needed according to agency policy. Because it is not feasible to have frequent x-ray films, other methods of determining tube placement are under review. Certain characteristics of fluid aspirated from feeding tubes are helpful in assessing placement of the tube. Color may differentiate gastric from intestinal placement. Because most intestinal aspirates are stained by bile to a distinct yellow color and most gastric aspirates are not, the difference can often distinguish the sites (Metheny and others, 1998a). The pH of an aspirate also offers valuable data in assessing placement of a feeding tube (Gharpure, Meert, and Sarnaik, 2000; Metheny and others, 1999). Bedside testing of pH using pH paper covering a range from 0 to ≥11 is sufficient for this purpose and aids in the assessment of feeding tube placement (Metheny and others, 1994).

ASSESSMENT

1. Review agency policy and procedure for frequency and method of verifying feeding tube placement.
2. Identify signs and symptoms of accidental respiratory migration of feeding tube: coughing, choking, or cyanosis. *Rationale: Signs and symptoms indicate accidental insertion of tube into airway. However, absence of signs and symptoms does not ensure nonrespiratory placement, especially in clients with decreased level of consciousness and/or altered cough and gag reflexes.*
3. Identify conditions that increase risk of spontaneous tube dislocation from intended position: retching/vomiting, nasotracheal suctioning, severe bouts of coughing. *Rationale: Feeding tubes may become dislocated by increases in intraabdominal pressure.*
4. Observe for external portion of the tube marked in ink to indicate tube placement. Observe if the mark has moved away from the naris. *Rationale: Increased external length of tube may indicate distal tip is no longer in correct position.*
5. Auscultate client's bowel sounds. *Rationale: Determines if normal peristalsis is present.*

6 Review client's medication record for gastric acid inhibitors and proton pump inhibitors. *Rationale: H₂ receptor antagonists reduce volume of gastric acid secretion and concentration (acid content) of secretions, thus causing pH value to be higher; thus the secretions are more alkaline (basic) (Metheny and Stewart, 2002).*

7 Review client's history for previous tube displacement. *Rationale: History places client at increased risk.*

PLANNING

Expected Outcomes focus on correct placement of feeding tube tip.

1 Gastric fluid aspirated from point of tip insertion tests at a pH of 1.0 to 4.0.

2 Intestinal fluid aspirated from point of tip insertion tests at a pH greater than 6.0.

Delegation Considerations

The skill of verification of feeding tube placement may not be delegated. The nurse directs personnel by:

- Explaining proper tube position and distance from client's nose and ordering to report back to the nurse if the feeding tube appears dislodged.
- Reviewing what to observe (e.g., gagging, vomiting, coughing, change in respiratory rate, complaints of shortness of breath) and ordering to report this information back to the nurse.
- Reviewing what to observe (e.g., irritation, bleeding or redness at nares, or dried oral mucous membranes) and ordering to report this information back to the nurse.

Equipment

- 60-ml or Luer-Lok or catheter-tip syringe (check feeding tube for syringe compatability)
- Stethoscope
- Clean gloves
- pH indicator strip (scale of 0.0 to ≥11.0 preferred)
- Irrigation solution (normal saline or tap water; check agency policy)

IMPLEMENTATION *for Verifying Tube Placement for Large-Bore or Small-Bore Feeding Tube*

STEPS	RATIONALE
1 See Standard Protocol (inside front cover).	
2 Perform measures to verify tube placement at the following times:	Establishes placement with initiation of treatment.
a. When tube is initially inserted.	
b. For intermittently fed clients, test placement immediately before feeding and before medications.	More frequent checking has been associated with increased clogging of small-bore tubes. To avoid this problem, flush tube with water after checking residual volume (Edwards and Metheny, 2000).
c. For continuously tube-fed clients, test at least once every 4 to 12 hours and before medication administration.	
d. Wait at least 1 hour after medication administration by tube or mouth.	Premature aspiration of gastric fluid will remove medication, reducing dose delivered to client. Medication may also interfere with pH testing and appearance of aspirate (Metheny and others, 1994).
3 Draw up 30 ml of air into a 60-ml syringe and then attach to end of feeding tube. Flush tube with 30 ml of air before attempting to aspirate fluid. Repositioning client from side to side may be helpful. More than one bolus of air may be needed in some cases.	Burst of air aids in aspirating fluid more easily (Metheny and others, 1993). Smaller syringes generate unnecessarily high pressures inside the tube.
4 Draw back on syringe slowly and obtain 5 to 10 ml of gastric aspirate for pH testing (see illustration). Observe appearance of aspirate to help assess position of tube. (NOTE: If you need to check for gastric residual, see Skill 31.3, Step 7.)	Drawing back quickly increases intratubular pressure and may cause the tube to collapse. Four to 5 ml is sufficient quantity for pH testing. Aspirates of NG and NI continuously tube-fed clients often have appearance of curdled formula. Aspirates for NI tubes are often stained yellow from bile. Gastric aspirates from intermittently tube-fed clients are not typically bile stained (unless intestinal fluid has refluxed into the stomach).

STEPS	RATIONALE

5 Gently mix aspirate in syringe. Measure pH of aspirated GI contents by dipping pH strip into cup of the fluid or by applying a few drops directly to test strip. Compare color of strip with color on chart provided by manufacturer (see illustration) (Metheny and others, 1998a).

Mixing ensures equal distribution of contents for testing. pH paper covering a wide range provides most accurate readings of gastric pH levels (Metheny and others, 1994).

a. Gastric fluid from client who has fasted for at least 4 hours usually has pH range of 1.0 to 4.0.

Range of 1 to 4 is reliable indicator of stomach placement, especially when gastric acid inhibitor is not being used (Baskin, 2006).

b. Fluid from NI tube of fasting client usually has pH greater than 6.0.

Intestinal contents are more basic (alkaline) than stomach contents (Metheny and others, 1999).

c. Client with continuous tube feeding may have pH of 5.0 or higher.

Formulas contain solutions that are basic (alkaline).

d. pH of pleural fluid from tracheobronchial tree is generally greater than 6.0.

The pH of pleural fluid makes it difficult to differentiate between respiratory and intestinal placement (Metheny and others, 1999).

NURSE ALERT Auscultation of insufflated air is no longer considered a reliable method for verification of tube placement because a tube inadvertently placed in lungs, pharynx, or esophagus can transmit a sound similar to that of air entering the stomach (Metheny and others, 1998b, 1998c).

---

6 If after repeated attempts it is not possible to aspirate fluid from a tube that was originally established by x-ray examination to be in desired position, and (a) there are no risk factors for tube dislocation, (b) tube has remained in original taped position, and (c) client is not experiencing difficulty, assume tube is correctly placed (Metheny and others, 1993).

When abdominal x-ray films are obtained for clinical reasons, the nurse can take advantage of reports to monitor tube location.

7 Irrigate tube. Irrigate before medications, between different medications, and after the final medication before feedings are restarted.

Irrigation prevents mixing of medications in tube, which may predispose tube to clogging. Flushes medication completely through tube so medications do not mix with enteral nutrition inside tube and clog.

a. Verify tube placement (see Steps 3–6).
b. Draw 30 ml of irrigating solution into syringe.

Provides sufficient amount to flush the length of the tube.

c. Kink feeding tube while disconnecting it from feeding bag tubing or while removing plug at end of tube.

Prevents leakage of gastric secretions.

d. Insert tip of catheter into end of feeding tube. Release kink and slowly instill irrigating solution.

Irrigation of solution clears tubing.

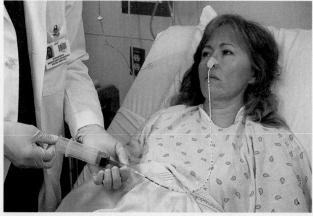

STEP 4 Aspirate gastric contents.

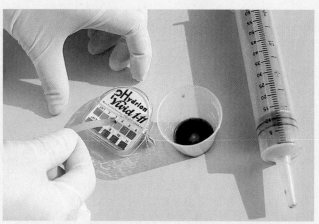

STEP 5 Compare color on test strip with color on pH chart.

STEPS	RATIONALE

> **NURSE ALERT** If unable to instill fluid, reposition client on left side and try again because tubing may be against abdominal wall.

e. When solution is instilled, remove syringe. Reinstitute tube feeding or administer medication as ordered.	Maintains tube patency.

8 See Completion Protocol (inside front cover).

EVALUATION

1 Verify that color, pH, and appearance of aspirate are consistent with the initial tube placement according to x-ray film results..

2 Observe flow rate of enteral formula.

3 Observe client for respiratory distress: persistent gagging, paroxysms of coughing, respiratory patterns (e.g., rate) inconsistent with baseline.

Unexpected Outcomes and Related Interventions

1 Client develops respiratory distress evidenced by dyspnea and changes in arterial blood gas or oxygen saturation values.

a. Contact physician immediately.

b. Be prepared to obtain chest x-ray examination and initiate oxygen therapy.

c. Turn off feeding pump or withhold intermittent feedings.

2 Unable to aspirate fluid or pH is greater than or equal to 6.0.

a. Determine client's risk of dislodgement (retching, vomiting, severe coughing, or frequent nasotracheal suctioning). If risk is low and tube has remained taped in original position, start next feeding. If risk is high and tube has moved, consider need to verify placement with an x-ray film (Metheny and Titler, 2001).

Recording and Reporting

• Record type of tube, pH, appearance of aspirate, condition of naris, and client's tolerance to tube feeding.

Sample Documentation

1430 Feeding tube placement confirmed, aspirant pH 3.0 of dark green bile colored fluid. Skin of naris clear and intact. Active bowel sounds auscultated over 4 quadrants.

Special Considerations
Pediatric Considerations

• In infant, inject 0.5 to 1 ml of air before aspiration of gastric secretions for pH measurement.

Geriatric Considerations

• Older adults frequently take medications that may affect pH, including H_2 receptor antagonists, proton pump inhibitors, or antacids.

Home Care Considerations

• Instruct client or family caregiver to check that tube is in correct position before administering feedings or medications, why this is important, and to withhold administration of any fluid if placement is in doubt.

SKILL 31.3 Administering Tube Feedings for Nasogastric, Gastrostomy, and Jejunostomy Tubes

• Nursing Skills Online: Enteral Nutrition, Lesson 4

Enteral tube feeding is preferred over parenteral nutrition (see Chapter 36) because it improves use of nutrients, is generally safer for clients, maintains structure and function of the gut, and is less expensive. Enteral feedings are most commonly given via small-bore tubes inserted through the nose and advanced to either the stomach or small intestine. NG feedings are the most common, allowing tube-feeding formulas to enter the stomach and then pass more gradually through the intestinal tract to ensure absorption.

NI tubes allow for successful postpyloric feeding, in which formula is placed directly into the small intestine beyond the pyloric sphincter of the stomach. The advantage of NI feedings is decreased gastric reflux, which reduces the risk of aspiration.

When clients cannot tolerate nasoenteral feeding tubes or require permanent enteral feeding or when nasoenteral feeding tubes interfere with rehabilitation, there are other options. One such option is gastric feeding. Gastric feedings permit the delivery of partially digested nutrients to the stomach or intestine at a normal physiological rate. Gastric

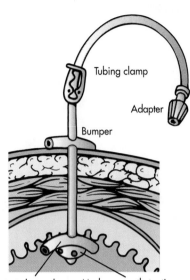

FIGURE 31-3 Placement of PEG tube into stomach.

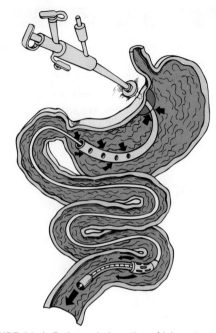

FIGURE 31-4 Endoscopic insertion of jejunostomy tube.

feedings via a gastrostomy feeding tube are relatively safe to administer, provided the client has normal gastric emptying and there is not excessive residual volume. A gastrostomy tube is surgically placed in the stomach and exits through an incision in the upper left quadrant of the abdomen, where it is sutured in place. A more current practice is a percutaneous endoscopic gastrostomy (PEG) tube, which is inserted during endoscopic viewing of the stomach. This tube exits through a puncture wound in the upper left quadrant of the abdomen, but it is held securely in place by virtue of its design (Figure 31-3).

When clients have a gastric ileus (decreased or absent peristalsis that affects the stomach but not the intestines), delayed gastric emptying, gastric resections, or neurological impairments that place them at greater risk of aspiration, enteral nutrition may be delivered via a percutaneous endoscopic jejunostomy (PEJ) tube (Baskin, 2006). Jejunostomy tubes, like gastrostomy tubes, are inserted during surgery or endoscopy. Endoscopic insertion is done through a PEG tube. After insertion of the large-bore PEG tube, the PEJ tube is passed through the PEG and advanced into the jejunum (Figure 31-4). A Y-connector attached to the jejunostomy tube caps the PEG tube and closes the system. This Y-connector labels the gastrostomy tube and designates the jejunostomy tube for feeding. Tne nurse must know which tube is gastric and which tube is jejunal.

This skill includes the administration of tube feeding via bolus, intermittent and continuous drip by both gravity and infusion pump. It is very important to check placement of NG and NI tubes before initiating feedings (see Skill 31.2). Using good hand hygiene and clean equipment and hanging formula only for the recommended time (8 hours in open system, 24 hours in closed system) prevents spoiling and avoids contamination of the system and subsequent infection in the client.

ASSESSMENT

1 Assess client's need for enteral tube feedings: unable to eat, unwilling to eat, or has increased energy requirements.
2 Identify signs and symptoms of malnutrition, including baseline weight, height, and laboratory values (e.g., albumin, protein, lymphocyte). *Rationale: Provides baseline to measure effectiveness of enteral feedings.*
3 Assess for food allergies.
4 Assess abdomen for distention or tenderness. Auscultate for bowel sounds before each feeding. *Rationale: Abdominal distention may indicate increased gastric residual. Absent bowel sounds indicate inability of GI tract to digest or absorb nutrients.*
5 Verify physician orders for tube feeding formula, rate, and frequency. Laboratory data and bedside assessments such as finger-stick blood glucose measurements are also ordered by the physician.

PLANNING

Expected Outcomes focus on safe administration of tube-feeding formula, client tolerance of formula, and avoidance of complications related to tube feeding administration.

1 Client's nutritional status improves (e.g., laboratory values return to normal, increased weight, improved I&O) by discharge.
2 Client experiences no aspiration or signs of respiratory distress.

3 Skin surrounding stoma site is dry, intact, and without signs of infections (gastrostomy or jejunostomy feeding tube only).

Delegation Considerations

The skill of administration of enteral tube feeding may be delegated. The assessment for the presence of peristalsis and verification of tube placement is performed by the nurse before initiating the tube feeding. The nurse directs personnel by:

- Explaining to position client upright in bed or chair.
- Reviewing what to observe, such as any difficulty in infusing feeding or any distress experienced by client, such as gagging, paroxysms of coughing, vomiting, or choking, and ordering to report this information back to nurse.
- Explaining when to irrigate tube after tube feedings.

Equipment

- Disposable feeding equipment:
  Bolus syringe: 60-ml bulb or plunger syringe
  Gavage/intermittent infusion: plastic feeding bag with drip chamber and tubing, *or*
  Continuous infusion: infusion pump with plastic feeding bag and appropriate drip chamber and tubing for pumps; use pump designed for tube feedings
- 60-ml Luer-Lok or catheter-tip syringe (check feeding tube for syringe compatibility)
- Stethoscope
- pH test strip (range 0.0 to ≥11.0)
- Prescribed enteral feeding
- Clean gloves
- Equipment to obtain blood glucose by finger-stick
- Towel

IMPLEMENTATION *for Administering Tube Feedings for Nasogastric, Gastrostomy, and Jejunostomy Tubes*

STEPS	RATIONALE
1 See Standard Protocol (inside front cover).	
2 Prepare enteral feeding solution. Check expiration date on formula and have formula at room temperature.	Ensures GI tolerance of formula. Cold formula causes cramping and discomfort because the solution is not warmed by mouth and esophagus.
	Prevents leakage of tube feeding.
3 For continuous and intermittent feeding by feeding bag: Prepare administration set and check integrity of feeding bag container.	
a. Connect tubing to feeding bag container, using aseptic technique	The feeding system, including the bag, connections, and tubing, must be free of contamination to prevent bacterial growth (Padula and others, 2004).
b. Shake formula container well and fill feeding bag with formula (see illustration). Open regulator clamp on tubing and fill tubing with formula to remove air (prime tubing). Hang bag on intravenous (IV) pole.	Filling tube with formula prevents excess air from entering GI tract once infusion begins.
4 For intermittent or bolus feeding, have syringe ready for administration.	
5 Elevate head of bed to high-Fowler's or to at least 30 degrees. For client forced to remain supine, place in reverse Tredelenburg position.	Reduces risk of aspiration during feeding with head higher than stomach.
6 [image] For NG and NI tube feedings verify placement of feeding tube (see Skill 31.2). Consider together the results from pH testing and appearance of aspirate (see illustration).	Feedings instilled into a misplaced tube may cause serious injury or death. On occasion, color alone may differentiate gastric from intestinal placement because most intestinal aspirates are stained by bile to a distinct yellow color and most gastric aspirates are not (Metheny and others, 1999).

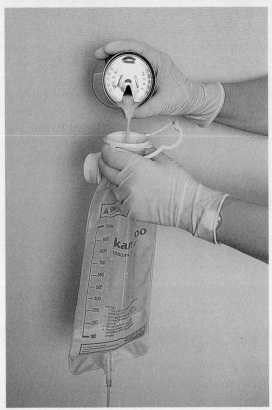

STEP 3b. Fill feeding bag with formula.

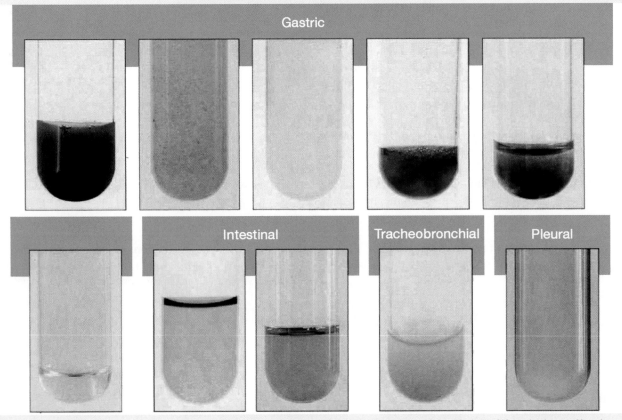

STEP 6 Typical color of aspirates from stomach, intestine, and airway. (Used with permission from Metheny NA and others: pH, color, and feeding tubes, *RN* 61:25, 1998.)

STEPS	RATIONALE

7 Check for gastric residual. Assess residual volume before each feeding. Residual volume is also assessed every 4 to 12 hours for continuous feedings (check agency policy).

a. NG/NI tubes: Connect catheter-tip syringe to end of feeding tube; pull back evenly to aspirate total amount of gastric contents (see illustration). Return aspirated contents to stomach unless volume exceeds 100 ml or as defined by agency policy.

For adults, a residual volume in excess of 200 ml may indicate intolerance to the feeding or delayed emptying (ASPEN, 2002). Return of aspirate prevents fluid and electrolyte imbalance.

b. Gastrostomy tube: Attach syringe, and aspirate gastric secretions as above. Return aspirated contents to stomach unless volume exceeds 100 ml. If volume is greater than 100 ml on several occasions, hold feedings and notify physician (McClave and others, 1992).

For adults, a volume in excess of 100 ml for gastrostomy/jejunostomy tubes raises concern about intolerance to the feeding. However, feedings may continue while further examinations are conducted (ASPEN, 2002). Fluids aspirated from the GI tract contains electrolytes, and if withheld, may cause electrolyte imbalances.

c. Jejunostomy tube: Aspirate intestinal secretions, observe volume, and return contents as above.

8 Irrigate feeding tube with 30 ml of water (see Skill 31.2, Step 7).

Irrigation clears tubing. Tip of tube may lie against stomach wall. Changing client's position may move tip away from stomach wall. Notify physician if unable to irrigate.

9 Initiate feeding:

a. Bolus or syringe feeding

(1) Pinch proximal end of feeding tube.

(2) Remove plunger from syringe and attach barrel of syringe to end of tube.

Prevents air from entering client's stomach.
Barrel receives formula for feeding.

(3) Fill syringe with measured amount of formula (see illustration). Release tube; elevate syringe to no more than 18 inches (45 cm) above insertion site and allow it to empty gradually by gravity. Repeat steps 1 to 3 until prescribed amount is delivered.

Height of syringe allows for safe, slow, gravity drainage of formula. Total delivery of feeding may take several minutes, depending on the amount of the bolus. Administering the feeding too quickly may cause abdominal discomfort to client or increase risk for aspiration.

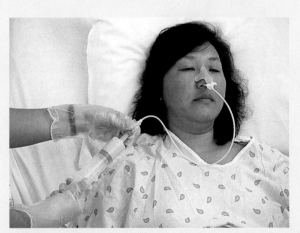

STEP 7a. Check for gastric residual (small-bore tube).

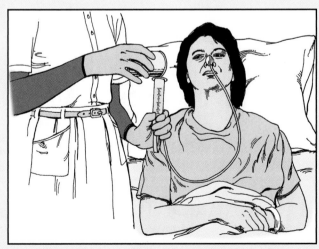

STEP 9a.(3) Fill syringe with formula for bolus feeding.

STEPS	RATIONALE

b. Intermittent feeding using a feeding bag (see illustration).

  (1) Attach tubing of administration set to proximal end of feeding tube.

  (2) Set rate by adjusting roller clamp on tubing. Allow bag to empty gradually over 30 to 60 minutes.
         Gradual emptying of tube feeding by gravity from feeding bag reduces risk of abdominal discomfort, vomiting, or diarrhea induced by bolus or too-rapid infusion of tube feedings.

  (3) Label bag with tube feeding type, strength, and amount. Include date, time, and initials. Change bag every 24 hours.
         Helps decrease bacterial colonization.

c. Continuous drip method

  (1) Connect tubing of administration set to proximal end of feeding tube.

  (2) Connect tubing through infusion pump and set rate (see illustration).
         Continuous feeding delivers prescribed hourly rate of feeding, thus reducing abdominal discomfort.

> **NURSE ALERT** Maximum hang time for formula is 8 hours in an open system and 24 hours in closed, ready-to-hang system, which was supplied from pharmacy.

10 Advance rate of concentration of tube feeding gradually (Box 31-1).
         Helps to prevent diarrhea and gastric intolerance to formula.

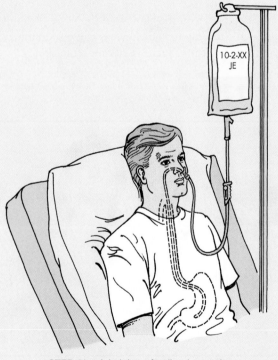

STEP 9b. Administer feeding by gravity.

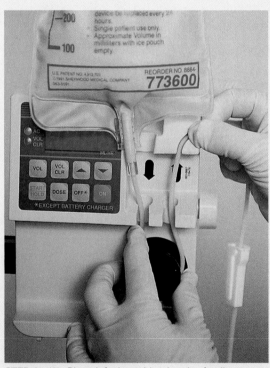

STEP 9c.(2) Place infusion tubing in tube-feeding pump.

STEPS	RATIONALE
11 Administer any free water via feeding tube as ordered or between feedings.	Maintains tube patency.
12 Irrigate feeding tube as ordered (see Skill 31.2).	Provide client with source of free water to help to maintain fluid and electrolyte balance. Assists with tube patency.
13 When tube feedings are not being administered, cap or reclamp proximal end of feeding tube.	Prevents air from entering stomach between feedings.
14 Rinse syringe or bag and tubing with warm water whenever feedings are completed.	Rinsing removes formula left in equipment, reduces potential for bacterial growth, and allows for reuse of equipment. Most institutions require replacement with new equipment every 24 hours.
15 The gastrostomy/jejunostomy exit site of the tube is usually left open to air. However, if a dressing is needed because of drainage, change as needed.	Leaking or gastric drainage may cause irritation and excoriation to skin. Skin around feeding tube is cleansed daily with warm water and mild soap. The area must be dried completely before apply a dressing.
16 See Completion Protocol (inside front cover).	

BOX 31-1 Advancing the Rate of Tube Feeding

Intermittent

1 Start formula at full strength for isotonic formulas (300 to 400 mOsm) or at ordered concentration.

2 Infuse formula over at least 20 to 30 minutes via syringe or feeding container.

3 Begin feedings with no more than 150 to 250 ml at one time. Increase by 50 ml per feeding per day to achieve needed volume and calories in six to eight feedings. (NOTE: Concentrated formulas at full strength may be infused at slower rate until tolerance is achieved.)

Continuous

1 Start formula at full strength for isotonic formulas (300 to 400 mOsm) or at ordered concentration. Usually hypertonic formulas are also started at full strength but at a slower rate.

2 Begin infusion rate at designated rate.

3 Advance rate slowly (e.g., 10 to 20 ml/hr) per day to target rate if tolerated (tolerance indicated by low gastric residuals and absence of nausea and diarrhea).

EVALUATION

1 Measure residual volume per agency policy.
2 Monitor finger-stick blood glucose level every 6 hours until maximum administration rate is reached and maintained for 24 hours (check agency policy).
3 Monitor I&O every 8 hours.
4 Weigh client daily until maximum administration rate is reached and maintained for 24 hours and then weigh client three times per week.
5 Monitor laboratory values such as electrolytes, albumin.
6 Observe client's level of comfort.
7 Auscultate client's lungs and observe respiratory rate and character.
8 Auscultate bowel sounds.

Unexpected Outcomes and Related Interventions

1 Excessive gastric residual volume.
a. Hold feeding and notify physician.
b. Maintain client in semi-Fowler's or at least have head of bed elevated 30 degrees.
c. Recheck residual in 1 hour.

2 Client aspirates formula. Respirations are rapid and shallow; color is ashen. Breath sounds full of rhonchi. Client coughs up secretions that are similar to tube feeding.
    Notify physician.
    Turn off tube feeding immediately.
    Position client in Fowler's position, suction, and notify physician immediately.
    Prepare for chest x-ray examination.
3 Client's feeding tube becomes clogged.
a. For a newly inserted tube, notify physician and obtain x-ray film confirmation of placement (Metheny and others, 1998a).
b. Attempt to flush tubing with large-bore syringe and warm water. (Avoid using a small-bore syringe because this exerts large amount of pressure and may rupture tube.)
c. Notify physician if unable to clear feeding tube.
d. If tube cleared, keep patent by flushing every 4 hours, before clamping off each time, and before and after each feeding and medication infusion.

Recording and Reporting

- Record residual volume, amount and type of feeding, client's response to tube feeding, patency of tube, and any adverse effects.
- Record volume of formula and any additional water on I&O form.
- Report type of feeding, status of infusion and feeding tube, client's tolerance, and any adverse effects.

Sample Documentation

0900 NG feeding tube placement confirmed, aspirant pH 3.0. 50 ml of residual volume aspirated and returned to the stomach. Active bowel sounds in all four quadrants. Abdomen soft and nondistended. Full-strength Osmolyte hung per infusion pump at 60 ml/hr. Head of bed elevated 45 degrees. Lungs clear to auscultation. Denies abdominal discomfort.

Special Considerations

Pediatric Considerations

- When giving intermittent feeding to small child, administration may take approximately 20 to 30 minutes or as long as it would take to bottle-feed the child.
- Hold infant and offer pacifier during feeding to stimulate more natural feeding experience (Hockenberry and Wilson, 2007).

Geriatric Considerations

- Assess client regularly for hyperglycemia because older adults may be more susceptible to high glucose concentration in enteral formulas.
- Assess routinely for gastric residual because older adults may have decreased transit time so that formula remains in stomach longer.
- Use of intestinal feeding tubes may reduce the risk of aspiration of feedings for the older adult.

Home Care Considerations

- Teach client or primary caregiver to check placement of tube and method of measurement before administering any formula.
- Instruct client or primary caregiver not to administer a feeding if there is any doubt concerning tube placement.
- Reinforce importance of giving feeding at room temperature.

Home Care Considerations

- May be used as nighttime feedings to supplement resident's nutritional status; this is especially true in rehabilitation settings.

NCLEX® Style Questions

1 What is the most important fact that is documented on any nasally or orally placed feeding tube prior to the instillation of any solution?
   1. Radiographic confirmation of feeding tube location
   2. Confirmation that the tube is in the stomach
   3. Confirmation that the tube is in the intestine
   4. The type and location of the feeding tube placement

2 A new order for nasointestinal enteral nutrition has been written. The client has not yet received any feeding. The nurse checks placement of the small-bore nasally placed feeding tube. The following results were obtained: 10 ml of yellow-stained fluid, pH of 7.0. What is the next action of the nurse?
   1. Administer the feeding at ½ the prescribed rate.
   2. Assess the client's lungs for abnormal lung sounds associated with aspiration.
   3. Administer the food at the prescribed rate.
   4. Hold feedings and notify physician.

3 A new order for enteral nutrition has been written. The client has not yet received any feeding. The nurse checks placement of the small-bore nasally placed feeding tube. The following results were obtained: 20 ml of clear fluid, pH of 4.0. Based on these findings, where is the tip of the tube most likely positioned?
   1. Respiratory tract
   2. Stomach
   3. Intestine
   4. Esophagus

4 As a result of a motor vehicle accident, the client has had multiple facial fractures and suffered a stroke. Based on these facts, what type of tube feeding should the nurse administer?
   1. Nasogastric
   2. Nasointestinal
   3. Gastrostomy
   4. Jejunostomy

5 Which intervention is best to prevent nosocomial infections associated with enteral nutrition?
   1. Insert NG tubes sterilely.
   2. Perform hand hygiene.
   3. Wear sterile gloves when handling the feeding system.
   4. Boil the tube feedings and allow them to cool before administration.

References for all chapters appear in Appendix D.

Altered Bowel Elimination

32

MEDIA RESOURCES

- **evolve** http://evolve.elsevier.com/Elkin
- **Video Clips**
- **Nursing Skills Online**

An understanding of normal bowel elimination and factors that promote, impede, or cause alterations in elimination is necessary to provide individualized client care. Supportive nursing care respects the client's privacy. In addition, interventions designed to promote normal bowel elimination are performed in a way to minimize physical and emotional discomfort.

Disorders of the bowel requiring direct nursing intervention include diarrhea, constipation, and impaction and conditions resulting from surgical removal of portions of the bowel. Left unrecognized, constipation progresses to fecal impaction, in which stool blocks the intestinal lumen. Stasis of bowel contents produces abdominal distention and pain. In some cases liquid stool passes around the obstruction, which can be misinterpreted as diarrhea. Enemas (see Skill 9.5) and suppositories (see Skill 16.7) may facilitate passage of stool. If these are unsuccessful, the impaction may need to be removed manually (see Skill 32-1).

Certain diseases prevent the normal passage of intestinal contents throughout the small and large bowel. The treatment for these disorders results in the need for a temporary or permanent artificial opening, a stoma, in the abdominal wall. An enterostomy is any surgical procedure that produces an artificial stoma in a portion of intestine through the abdominal wall (see Skill 32-2). The fecal drainage from the stoma is often called *effluent*. The forms of enterostomy are ileostomy, which involves the ileum of the small intestine, and colostomy, which involves various segments of the colon (Figure 32-1). Depending on the reason for the surgery, an enterostomy is either permanent or temporary. Ostomies of the genitourinary (GU) tract are discussed in Chapter 33.

EVIDENCE IN PRACTICE

Bliss DZ, Fischer LR, Savik K: Managing fecal incontinence: self care practices of older adults, *J Gerontol Nurs* 31(7):35, 2005.

There is increasing evidence that low fat intake and increased dietary fiber and bulk-forming foods reduce the client's risk of colorectal cancers, fecal incontinence, digestive diseases, and other cancers. Constipation and fecal incontinence are especially troublesome in older adults. Assisting clients and their families in selecting different foods helps to reduce the incidence of these problems. Encourage the client to drink 2000 to 3000 ml of fluids daily, if not contraindicated by other

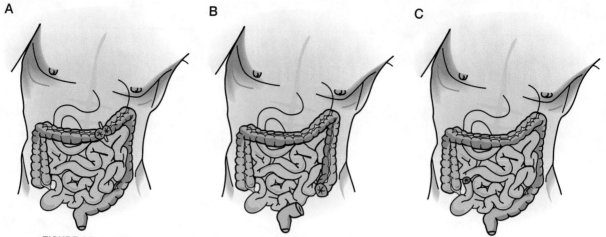

FIGURE 32-1 Types of colostomies. **A,** Transverse (double-barrel) colostomy. **B,** Sigmoid colostomy. **C,** Ileostomy.

medical conditions. A high-fiber diet (25 to 30 g/day) reduces constipation; as fiber passes through the colon, it acts as a sponge. As a result, bulkier and softer stools develop. In addition, the waste moves through the body easier and results in more regular bowel movements, thus reducing constipation and incontinence.

NURSING DIAGNOSES

A nursing diagnosis associated with clients who have constipation or an impaction includes **constipation** related to factors such as dehydration, decreased activity, postsurgical ileus, opioid use, or inadequate dietary fiber. **Acute pain** and/or **chronic pain** may be related to bowel distention. Common diagnoses associated with clients who have ostomies include **deficient knowledge** related to ostomy management, **disturbed body image** related to presence of the ostomy, and **risk for impaired skin integrity** related to irritation of peristomal skin. **Anxiety** may be related to altered bowel function and the associated foul-smelling odors or spillage or leakage of liquid stools.

SKILL 32.1 Removing Fecal Impactions

This skill is performed when the administration of enemas (e.g., oil retention) or suppositories are unsuccessful at removing impacted stools. Fecal impaction occurs in all age-groups. Physically and mentally incapacitated persons and institutionalized older adult clients are at greatest risk (Prather, 2004). Digital removal of an impaction is embarrassing and uncomfortable for the client. Excessive rectal manipulation may cause irritation to the mucosa and subsequent bleeding or vagus nerve stimulation, which can produce a reflex slowing of the heart rate.

Fecal impaction occurs when there is a history of constipation. Constipation is defined as infrequent stools. However, a consensus definition of functional constipation includes two or more of the following factors noted for at least 3 months: (1) straining with defecation at least one fourth of the time, (2) lumpy or hard stools (or both) at least one fourth of the time, (3) sensation of incomplete evacuation at least one fourth of the time, or (4) two or fewer bowel movements in a week (Coggrave and others, 2005; Dosh, 2002; Lembo and Camilleri, 2003). A variety of interventions (e.g., diet and exercise) successfully relieves constipation and reduce the risk for impaction.

ASSESSMENT

1 Ask client about normal and current bowel elimination pattern including frequency and characteristics of stool, use of laxatives, enemas, and other medications; level of regular exercise; urge to defecate but inability to do so; presence of hemorrhoids; abdominal discomfort, especially when attempting to defecate; feelings of incomplete emptying; and sensations of bloating, cramping, or excessive gas (Eberhardie, 2003). *Rationale: This information is valuable in determining contributing factors and preventing recurrence of this problem.*

2 Inspect client's abdomen for distention before palpation. *Rationale: Observation initially identifies any distended or asymmetrical areas, which are further investigated on palpation or auscultation.*

3 Auscultate all four quadrants for presence of bowel sounds. *Rationale: Hypoactive bowel sounds may result from partial ob-*

struction of the gastrointestinal (GI) tract as with constipation or masses. Hyperactive bowel sounds may be present due to intestinal irritation, as with diarrhea, or partial obstruction of GI tract or before defecation.

4 Palpate client's abdomen for distention, discomfort, or masses. *Rationale: Symptoms are related to accumulation of feces in intestinal tract. When severe constipation occurs, a palpable mass may be felt.*

5 Observe consistency of stool, seepage of liquid stool, or continual passage of small amounts of hard stool. *Rationale: Seepage of stool is symptomatic of an impaction high in colon. Client may be able to pass small pieces of hard stool or have episodes of passing small amounts of liquid stool (Prather, 2004).*

6 Observe the anal area for signs of irritation from passing stool or hemorrhoids. *Rationale: Indicates possible straining on defecation.*

7 Measure client's current vital signs and level of pain on pain scale. *Rationale: Establishes a baseline for detecting slowing in heart rate from vagus nerve stimulation during digital stimulation.*

> **NURSE ALERT** Because of the risk of vagus nerve stimulation, clients with a history of dysrhythmias or heart disease have a greater risk of changes in heart rhythm. Be sure to monitor client's pulse before and during procedure. If in doubt whether to perform this procedure on a cardiac client, consult with client's physician.

8 Determine if client is receiving anticoagulant therapy. *Rationale: Procedure may be contraindicated because irritation and manipulation of the rectum may cause bleeding of rectal mucosa.*

9 Check client's record for physician's order for digital removal of impaction. *Rationale: A physician's order is necessary because of possible vagus nerve stimulation.*

PLANNING

Expected Outcomes focus on removal of the impaction and prevention of further occurrences.
1 Client's rectum is free of stool.
2 Client's vital signs remain normal during and after procedure.
3 Bowel sounds return to normal.
4 Client is free of abdominal discomfort.
5 Anal area is free of tissue damage.
6 Client experiences minimal discomfort.
7 Client/family verbalizes ways to prevent constipation.

Delegation Considerations

The skill of removing an impaction may not be delegated. The nurse directs personnel by:
- Explaining how to assist in positioning the client for the procedure.
- Reviewing what to observe for (e.g., color and consistency of any evacuated stool, rectal bleeding or bloody mucus) and to report back to nurse.

Equipment
- Clean gloves
- Water-soluble local anesthetic lubricant (NOTE: Some institutions require use of water-soluble lubricant without anesthetic when nurse performs procedure.)
- Waterproof, absorbent pads
- Bedpan
- Bedpan cover (optional if available)
- Bath blanket
- Washbasin, washcloths, towels, and soap

IMPLEMENTATION *for Removing Fecal Impactions*

STEPS	RATIONALE
1 See Standard Protocol (inside front cover).	
2 Keeping far side rail raised, assist client to left side-lying position with knees flexed and back toward nurse.	Promotes client safety. Provides access to rectum.
3 With near side rail lowered, drape client's trunk and lower extremities with bath blanket and place waterproof pad under client's buttocks.	Maintains client's sense of privacy and prevents unnecessary exposure of body parts.

> **COMMUNICATION TIP** At this time, instruct client to take slow, deep breaths during procedure.

STEPS	RATIONALE
4 Lubricate gloved index finger of dominant hand with lubricant.	Reduces discomfort and permits smooth insertion of finger into anus and rectum.
5 Instruct client to continue to take slow deep breaths, gradually and gently insert gloved index finger, and feel anus relax around the finger. Then, if necessary, insert middle finger.	Slow deep breaths may help to relax the client. Gradual insertion of index finger helps to dilate anal sphincter.
6 Explain your action and then gradually advance fingers slowly along rectal wall toward umbilicus.	Allows nurse to reach impacted stool high in rectum.

STEPS	RATIONALE
7 Gently loosen fecal mass by moving fingers in a scissors motion to fragment fecal mass. Work fingers into hardened mass.	Loosening and penetrating mass allows nurse to remove it in small pieces, resulting in less discomfort to client.
8 Work stool downward toward end of rectum. Remove small sections of feces and discard into the bedpan.	Prevents need to force finger up into rectum and minimizes trauma to mucosa.
9 Periodically assess heart rate and look for signs of fatigue.	Vagal stimulation slows heart rate and may cause dysrhythmia. Procedure may exhaust client.

> **NURSE ALERT** Stop procedure if heart rate drops or rhythm changes or if rectal bleeding occurs.

10 Continue to clear rectum of feces and allow client to rest at intervals. If needed, use tissue.	Rest improves client's tolerance of procedure.
11 After removal of impaction, provide perineal hygiene.	
12 Remove bedpan and dispose of feces. Remove gloves and perform hand hygiene.	Reduces transmission of microorganisms.
13 If needed, assist client to toilet or clean bedpan. (Procedure may be followed by enema or cathartic.)	Disimpaction may stimulate defecation reflex.
14 See Completion Protocol (inside front cover).	

EVALUATION

1 Perform rectal examination for stool.
2 Measure vital signs and compare to baseline values. Continue to monitor the client for bradycardia for 1 hour.
3 Auscultate bowel sounds.
4 Palpate abdomen to determine if it is soft and nontender.
5 Observe anal and perianal area for irritation or skin breakdown
6 Ask client to describe comfort level on pain scale.
7 Ask client/family to identify ways to prevent constipation.

Unexpected Outcomes and Related Interventions

1 Client experiences bradycardia, decrease in blood pressure, and decrease in level of consciousness as a result of vagus nerve stimulation.
a. Stop procedure and retake the vital signs.
b. Notify physician immediately.
c. Remain with client and monitor vital signs and level of consciousness.
d. Be prepared for potential emergency intervention.
2 Client has seepage of liquid fecal material after removal of impaction.
a. Assess client for continuing impaction.
b. Contact physician. A suppository or an enema may be needed to remove hardened feces higher in the rectum.
c. Increase fluids (if allowed), fiber in diet, and activity level to increase peristaltic activity.
3 Client has trauma to the rectal mucosa, as evidenced by blood on the gloved finger.
a. Stop procedure if bleeding is excessive.
b. If bleeding continues, notify physician for further treatment measures.

Recording and Reporting
- Record client's tolerance to procedure, amount, and consistency of stool removed, as well as adverse effects.
- Report any adverse effects to nurse in charge or physician.

Sample Documentation
1600 Ten pieces, ranging from 1-2 cm, of hard, dark brown, lumpy stool removed from rectum without rectal bleeding, pain, or fatigue. Pulse 80-88 strong and regular. Normal bowel sounds present in all four quadrants. No abdominal distention or complaints of pain.

Special Considerations
Pediatric Considerations
- Digital removal of stool is not recommended in pediatrics due to risk of anal fissures and pain that may trigger stool withholding (Hockenberry and others, 2003).

Geriatric Considerations
- Many older adult clients are especially prone to dysrhythmia and other problems related to vagal stimulation; monitor heart rate and rhythm closely.
- At least 28% of older adult clients are constipated as a result of insufficient dietary bulk, inadequate fluid intake, laxative abuse, diminished muscle tone and motor function, decreased defecation reflex, mental or physical illness, and presence of tumors (Ebersole and others, 2004).
- For older adults, instituting a diet adequate in dietary fiber (6 to 10 g/day) adds bulk, weight, and form to stool and improves defecation (Ebersole and others, 2004).

- Consider development of regular toileting routine that includes responding to the urge to defecate (Meiner and Lueckenotte, 2006).

Home Care Considerations

- Consider having client or family member keep a week's diary of meals and fluid intake. Determine if dietary pattern contributes to constipation. Recommend a diet adequate in fiber that includes client's food choices.
- Have client or family member maintain a weekly bowel diary.

Long-Term Care Considerations

- In long-term care, maintenance of activity and adequate hydration are very important in maintaining peristalsis.
- Individualized bowel programs developed following a stroke, brain, or spinal cord injury help reduce the occurrence of constipation and subsequent impaction.

SKILL 32.2 Pouching an Enterostomy

- Nursing Skills Online: Ostomy, Lesson 4

Immediately after bowel diversion surgery, a pouch is placed over the newly created stoma because incontinent ostomies may drain effluent (fecal drainage) immediately. The pouch collects all effluent and protects the skin from irritation. A pouch with its skin barrier must fit comfortably, cover the skin surface around the stoma, and create a good seal. The postoperative pouch is clear to allow for visibility of the stoma.

Pouching a newly formed stoma differs from techniques used to pouch a stoma several days or weeks old. The new stoma is edematous during the postoperative healing process. An incision line from a bowel resection may lie close to the stoma. The stoma itself often has a series of small stitches around its perimeter. A pouch and its skin barrier are applied so as not to constrict the stoma or traumatize healing tissues (Thompson, 2000). Initially the pouch over a postoperative colostomy does need to be emptied frequently because drainage is diminished or lacking. Several days may pass before a client's normal elimination pattern returns. In the case of an ileostomy, the client will have frequent loose or watery stools when peristalsis returns (Black, 2000).

Many types of pouches and skin barriers are available (Schiff, 2000). Some pouches have skin barriers directly preattached and are called one-piece pouching systems. The manufacturer precuts some of these one-piece pouches to size, whereas others must be custom cut to the client's specific stoma size. Other systems are two separate pieces. The pouch is applied to the skin barrier by attaching it to the flange (a plastic ring) on the barrier. Often the skin barrier needs to be custom cut. For two-piece systems the skin barrier with flange must be used with the corresponding size pouch that fits that flange from the same manufacturer; otherwise leakage occurs. The nurse caring for a client with an ostomy needs to understand how to use each of these different pouching systems. Modifications for preventing complications related to leakage of feces or urine are essential (Erwin-Toth, 2001; Thompson, 2000).

ASSESSMENT

1 Observe existing skin barrier and pouch for leakage. Check length of time in place. *Rationale: Helps to determine pouch and barrier selection.*

2 Auscultate for bowel sounds. *Rationale: Documents presence of peristalsis.*

3 If you cannot observe stoma through pouch, apply gloves and remove existing pouch by gently pushing skin from adhesive barrier. Properly dispose of soiled pouch (save clamp if attached to pouch). Observe stoma for the following characteristics:

a. *Size:* Use measuring card to determine correct size of client's stoma (Figure 32-2). *Rationale: Accurate stoma size is critical for planning and selecting stoma pouch size. Stoma opening needs to be 1/8 to 1/16 inch larger than the client's stoma. During the 6- to 8-week postoperative phase the client's ostomy will change size and shape. Thus the new stoma needs to be remeasured with each pouch change. If there is no change in measurement for 2 to 3 weeks, stoma edema is probably resolved, and stoma size will remain constant (Colwell, Goldberg, and Carmel, 2004).*

b. *Shape:* If the stoma is round, use precut, presized pouches as an option. *Rationale: Irregularly shaped stomas (Figure 32-3) require a custom-cut shape made on skin barrier to match the shape of the stoma.*

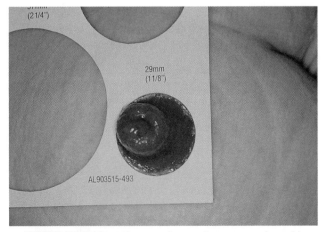

FIGURE 32-2 Measuring an ostomy using a measuring grid.

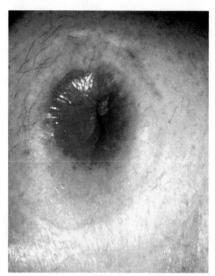

FIGURE 32-3 Irregular stoma (flush on right side, raised on left with skin irritation).

c. *Type:* Determine whether stoma is flush to skin, protruding, or indented. *Rationale: Type of stoma is important when selecting skin barrier, pouch, and accessories such as paste, strips, or binders.*

d. *Color:* Stoma should be pink-red in color. *Rationale: Dark-colored stoma can indicate stoma necrosis, which is most common in the first 3 to 5 postoperative days.*

e. *Effluent:* Determine amount and consistency of fecal drainage from stoma. *Rationale: Consider differences in drainage from different types of ostomies when selecting the ostomy pouch. Pouches are available in different sizes and closed or open ended. Only a pouch designed for stool is used.*

Rationale: Determines if problems with stoma exist. Stoma characteristics are one of the factors to consider when selecting an appropriate pouching system (WOCN, 2005). Determines need for barrier paste to increase adherence of pouch to skin or to fill in irregularities. Many enterostomal pouch systems have a flexible adhesive, a pectin, karaya, or synthetic wafer flange to prevent leakage.

> **NURSE ALERT** When a new ostomy is present, it is important to measure the stoma with each pouching system change to determine correct size of equipment needed (see step 7). The system may need modifications as the stoma size changes (WOCN, 2005). Follow each ostomy pouch manufacturer's directions and measuring guide to determine which size ostomy pouch to use based on client's actual stoma measurement size (Erwin-Toth, 2000).

4 Observe peristomal skin for blistering, redness, irritation, cuts, rash, presence of stones, or skin breakdown (Table 32-1). *Rationale: Improper ostomy fit may cause pressure on skin, ostomy adhesives may cause skin irritation, and moisture can further increase risk of skin breakdown.*

> **NURSE ALERT** Intact skin barriers with no evidence of leakage do not need to be changed daily and can remain in place for 3 to 5 days (Erwin-Toth, 2001).

5 Observe abdominal contour, pressure areas, and abdominal incision (if present). *Rationale: Relationship of abdominal contour to stoma determines proper placement of pouch. The presence of pressure areas from the pouching system may necessitate the use of a new pouching system (WOCN, 2005).*

6 Assess abdomen for best type of pouching system to use. Consider: abdominal contour and peristomal plane, presence of scars, incisions, and location and type of stoma. *Rationale: Determines pouching system selection and need for other equipment. A firm/flat and round/hard abdomen usually needs a flexible or soft pouching system, whereas a flabby or soft abdomen usually needs a firmer system. Stomas that are retracted or in skin folds need convexity (curving outward), and different pouching systems are necessary to prevent leaking.*

7 Assess client's self-care ability to determine the best type of pouching system to use. Assess client's vision, dexterity or mobility, and cognitive function. *Rationale: Clients with poor vision will benefit by using yellow-tinted sunglasses to reduce glare and improve contrast and by using magnification mirrors (Jeffries and MacKay, 1997). Clients who also have mobility problems or spinal cord injuries will benefit by using equipment that has a longer pouch, which is easier to empty independently when sitting (Erwin-Toth, 2003; Thompson, 2000). Clients who have difficulty using their hands or who have limited vision will find a one-piece system or a precut pouch and skin barrier more desirable to use.*

PLANNING

Expected Outcomes focus on preventing peristomal and stoma skin breakdown, containing effluent, and helping client adjust to life with an ostomy, emotionally and physically, when performing ostomy self-care.

1 Stoma is moist and reddish pink. Skin is intact and free of irritation; sutures are intact (in the presence of a postoperative stoma).

2 Client denies burning around stoma.

3 Stoma is functioning with moderate amount of liquid or soft stool and flatus in pouch. Bowel sounds are present. (Flatus is noted by bulging of pouch in absence of drainage; flatus initially indicates return of peristalsis after surgery.)

4 Skin barrier and pouching system is intact without evidence of leakage.

5 Client observes stoma and steps of procedure carefully.

6 Client indicates readiness to learn and begin self-care.

Delegation Considerations

The skill of pouching a stoma may not be delegated. In some agencies the pouching of an established enterostomy (6 weeks after surgery) may be delegated. The nurse directs personnel by:

- Explaining about the expected appearance of the stoma, amount, color, and consistency of drainage from the ostomy.
- Reviewing what to observe for, such as changes in effluent and stoma (e.g., color, presence of blood) and ordering to report back to the nurse.

Equipment

- Pouch, clear drainable colostomy/ileostomy in correct size for two-piece system or custom cut-to-fit one-piece type with attached skin barrier (Figure 32-4)
- Pouch closure device, such as a clamp
- Ostomy measuring guide
- Adhesive remover (optional)
- Clean gloves
- Ostomy deodorant
- Gauze pads or washcloth
- Towel or disposable waterproof barrier
- Basin with warm tap water
- Scissors
- Skin barrier such as sealant wipes or wafer
- Stoma paste or Stomahesive (optional)
- Stethoscope
- Tape or ostomy belt

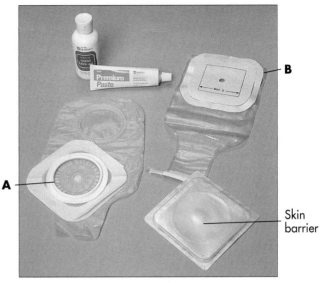

FIGURE 32-4 Ostomy pouches and skin barriers. **A,** Two-piece detachable system. (NOTE: Skin barrier would need to be custom cut according to stoma size.) The pouch opening is already precut by the manufacturer to fit the size of the flange on the skin barrier. **B,** One-piece pouch with skin barrier attached.

TABLE 32-1 Peristomal Skin Damage		
TYPE OR CAUSE OF DAMAGE	**APPEARANCE**	**TREATMENT PRINCIPLES**
Chemical Damage Effluent in contact with skin Incorrect use of adhesives or solvents	Erythematous and denuded areas corresponding to leakage of effluent *or* areas of product use (adhesives, solvents)	Eliminate effluent contact with skin; allow adhesives to dry and remove solvents from skin. *Topical:* Skin barrier powder; sealants if needed
Mechanical Damage (Figure 32-5, *A*) Inappropriate skin care (scrubbing or "picking") Incorrect tape removal or fragile skin, resulting in "stripping" of epidermis	Patchy areas of erythema or denudation corresponding with areas subjected to trauma or "taped" areas	Eliminate cause; teach atraumatic skin care, appropriate tape removal, and use of sealants when indicated. *Topical:* Skin barrier powder; sealant as indicated
Fungal Rash *(Candida)* (Figure 32-5, *B*) Antibiotics resulting in fungal overgrowth Persistent skin moisture	Maculopapular rash with satellite lesions	Keep skin dry; eliminate pooled urine; restore normal flora. *Topical:* Antifungal powder and sealant as indicated
Allergic Reaction Can be caused by any product	Areas of erythema or pruritus corresponding to area of skin exposed to allergen	Use patch test if needed to determine allergen; eliminate contact with allergen. *Topical:* Corticosteroid agent if needed for control of pruritus (cream or spray, not ointment, which would interfere with pouch adherence)

Modified from Hampton BG, Bryant RA: *Ostomies and continent diversions: nursing management,* St Louis, 1992, Mosby.

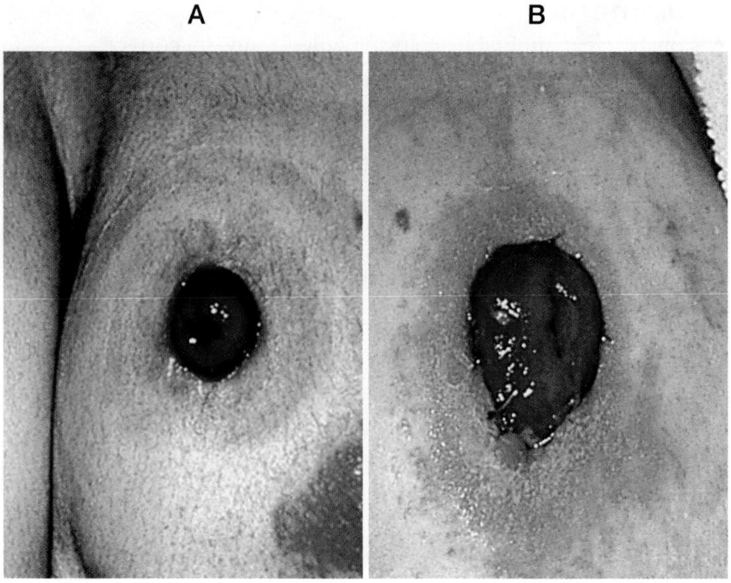

A   B

FIGURE 32-5 **A,** Mechanical injury. **B,** Candidiasis. (Permission to use and/or reproduce this copyrighted photo has been granted by the owner, Hollister Incorporated.)

IMPLEMENTATION *for Pouching an Enterostomy*

STEPS	RATIONALE
1 See Standard Protocol (inside front cover).	
2 Position client either standing or supine and drape. If seated, position client either on or in front of toilet.	When client is supine, there are fewer skin wrinkles, which allows for ease of application of pouching system; maintains client's dignity.
3 Place towel or disposable waterproof barrier under client.	Protects bed linen.

> **NURSE ALERT** If portions of skin barrier remain after pouch removal, use an adhesive remover to gently remove them. Improper removal of barrier will irritate client's skin, cause skin tears, and result in poor adherence of the new pouch.

STEPS	RATIONALE
4 Cleanse peristomal skin gently with warm tap water using gauze pads or clean washcloth; do not scrub skin; dry completely by patting skin with gauze or towel.	Avoid use of soap because it leaves a residue on skin that interferes with pouch adhesion to skin. Skin needs to be dry. Skin barrier and pouch do not adhere to wet skin and moisture increases client's risk for fungal infections. If blood appears on gauze pad, do not be alarmed. If rubbed, stomas ooze some blood as a result of cleaning process. Stoma's surface is highly vascular mucous membrane. Bleeding into pouch is abnormal (WOCN, 2004a).

> **NURSE ALERT** Do not use adhesive removers routinely. However, adhesive removers may be necessary when client's skin tears easily or there is buildup of sticky residue over peristomal skin. When using an adhesive remover, follow up with washing skin with water and mild soap to remove oily coating on skin from adhesive remover (WOCN, 2004b).

> **COMMUNICATION TIP** While caring for the stoma, talk in a pleasant tone and use normal facial gestures to convey acceptance. Provide information about the stoma and wound healing.

STEPS	RATIONALE
5 Measure stoma as needed for correct size of pouching system needed (see Figure 32-2). Remove gloves.	Ensures accuracy in determining correct size pouch. A new stoma shrinks and does not reach usual size for 6 to 8 weeks (Thompson, 2000).

STEPS	RATIONALE

6 Select appropriate pouch for client based on client assessment. With a custom cut-to-fit pouch, use an ostomy guide to cut opening on pouch ¹⁄₁₆ to ¹⁄₈ inch larger than stoma before removing backing. Prepare pouch by removing backing from barrier and adhesive. With an ileostomy, apply thin circle of barrier paste around opening in pouch; allow to dry (see illustrations).

Appropriate size of pouch opening keeps drainage off skin and lessens risk of damage to stoma during peristalsis or activity. Pouch and skin barrier are changed whenever leaking. Change pouch when client is comfortable; before a meal is better because this avoids increased peristalsis and chance of evacuation during pouch change. Paste facilitates seal and protects skin.

7 Apply skin barrier and pouch. If creases next to stoma occur, use barrier paste to fill in; let dry 1 to 2 minutes.

a. For one-piece pouching system:

(1) Use skin sealant wipes on skin that will be directly under adhesive skin barrier or pouch; allow to dry. Press adhesive backing of pouch and/or skin barrier smoothly against skin, starting from the bottom and working up and around sides.

Ensures smooth, wrinkle-free seal. Be aware of any irritated or open areas because the skin sealant wipes often contain alcohol (WOCN, 2004b).

(2) Hold pouch by barrier, center over stoma, and press down gently on barrier; bottom of pouch points toward client's knees when sitting (see illustration).

A different positioning of the pouch may be necessary to allow better gravity flow. For example, a client confined to bed may need to have pouch positioned horizontally over the side of the abdomen (Thomason, 2000).

(3) Maintain gentle finger pressure around barrier for 1 to 2 minutes.

Gentle pressure and body heat assist in adhesion.

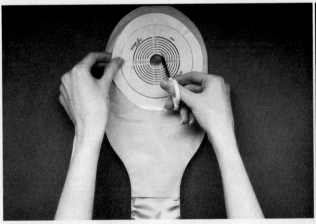

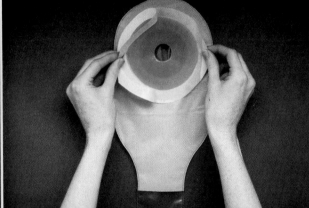

STEP 6 **A,** Cut-to-fit, one-piece drainable ostomy pouch. **B,** Removing the backing paper for the barrier on a one-piece pouch. **C,** Applying barrier paste to a one-piece ostomy pouch. (Courtesy ConvaTec, Princeton, NJ.)

STEPS	RATIONALE

b. If using two-piece pouching system:

(1) Apply barrier-paste flange (barrier with adhesive) as in steps above for one-piece system (see illustration). Then snap on pouch, and maintain finger pressure.

Creates wrinkle-free, secure seal; decreases irritation from adhesive on skin. Some two-piece pouching systems may have a snapping or clicking sound that occurs when attaching pouch to skin barrier.

c. For both pouching systems gently tug on pouch in a downward direction.

Determines that pouch is securely attached.

8 Gently press on pectin or karaya flange to facilitate adhesion.

A pectin, karaya, or synthetic skin barrier keeps pouch system attached securely (Erwin-Toth, 2001). Some clients may prefer a belt attached to the pouch for extra security.

9 Although many ostomy pouches are odor-proof, some nurses and clients like to add a small amount of ostomy deodorant into pouch. Do not use "home remedies," which can harm stoma, to control ostomy odor. Do not make hole in pouch to release flatus.

Causes damage to pouch and defeats purpose of odor-proof pouch. A hole for flatus may also allow effluent to leak.

NURSE ALERT Aspirin is never added to ostomy pouch. It can cause stomal bleeding.

---

10 Fold bottom of drainable open-ended pouch up once and close using a closure device such as a clamp (or follow manufacturer's instructions for closure).

Maintains secure seal to prevent leaking.

11 Properly dispose of old pouch and soiled equipment. Client may also request spraying of room air freshener in room if needed.

Lessens odors in room.

12 Change one- or two-piece pouch every 3 to 5 days or longer unless leaking; pouch can remain in place for tub bath or shower; after bath, pat the pouch and underlying skin dry.

Avoids unnecessary trauma to skin from too-frequent changes. If pouch is removed for bathing or shower, have client use a mild soap without oils or deodorants. Make sure all soap residue is rinsed off. Drying ensures adhesion of pouch and prevention of skin irritation under pouch (Erwin-Toth, 2001).

13 See Completion Protocol (inside front cover).

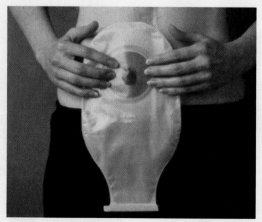

STEP 7a.(2) Client applying a one-piece pouch. (Courtesy ConvaTec, Princeton, NJ.)

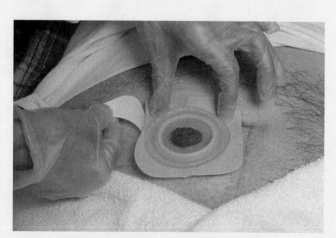

STEP 7b.(1) Application of barrier-paste flange.

EVALUATION

1 Observe appearance of skin around stoma and existing incision (if present) for color, swelling, trauma, and healing. Ask if client feels burning around stoma.

2 Auscultate bowel sounds and observe amount, color, consistency, and frequency of fecal elimination (effluent) from stoma.

3 Observe integrity of skin barrier and pouching system. Inspect edges of pouch for "tracking" of effluent under edges, which may indicate a potential leak due to skinfold or wrinkle.

4 Observe client's behavior when looking at stoma and handling equipment. Note whether client talks about stoma.

5 Ask client to discuss steps to use in pouching ostomy.

Unexpected Outcomes and Related Interventions

1 Client's peristomal skin is irritated, and/or client complains of a burning sensation.

a. Assess stoma as mucosal layer of stoma separates from skin.

b. Leaking may be caused by undermining of pouch seal by effluent. Remeasure stoma size.

c. If burning and irritation occur directly under pouch or skin barrier, consider possible allergic response.

d. Obtain referral for enterostomal therapy.

2 Necrotic stoma is manifested by purple or black color, dry instead of moist texture, failure to bleed when washed gently, or presence of tissue sloughing.

a. Observe stoma for color, moisture, bleeding.

b. Determine presence of excessive edema or excessive tension on bowel suture line.

3 Client's skin barrier and pouch leak.

a. Assess if client is waiting too long (e.g., if pouch more than half full of stool) to empty pouch.

b. Remeasure stoma and reevaluate pouch and skin barrier size (Thompson, 2000).

c. Determine if client is cutting out the correct size on the skin barrier.

d. Evaluate if stoma is in a skinfold or whether other irregularities exist.

e. Determine whether a convex disk, skin barrier paste, or other measures are needed to prevent leakage.

4 Client cannot perform ostomy-pouching change.

a. Determine if client lacks the physical or mental ability to do ostomy self-care.

b. Eliminate distractions and other factors (e.g., pain) that might interfere with client's performance of ostomy self-care (Ball, 2000).

c. Reevaluate client's understanding of ostomy self-care (Ball, 2000).

d. Reevaluate client's problems with self-image, coping skills, and support systems (Ball, 2000).

Recording and Reporting

- Record condition of peristomal skin, stoma, and sutures. Record size of stoma, type of pouch and skin barrier applied, amount and appearance of stool or drainage in pouch, and color and texture of stool.
- Document any abdominal distention and tenderness and nature and location of bowel sounds.
- Record client's level of participation and need for teaching.
- Report any of the following to nurse in charge and/or physician: abnormal appearance of stoma, suture line, or peristomal skin or character of output and absence of bowel sounds. No flatus in 24 to 36 hours and no stool by third day.

Sample Documentation

1600 Colostomy stoma is ½ in diameter, round, slightly swollen, and red in color. Peristomal skin intact. Stoma draining 1300 ml dark-brownish liquid stool. Active bowel sounds in all quadrants. Two-piece ostomy pouching system with hydrocolloid skin barrier in place without odor or other signs of leaks. Client has not yet looked at stoma. ET nurse began instruction of client's ostomy self-care technique.

Special Considerations
Pediatric Considerations

- Because most ostomy surgery done on neonates is for emergency situations, often no time is available for preoperative selection of stoma site. However, most stomas are temporary, with stoma being "taken down" (removed or closed) when baby is about 1 year old. Colostomies are the most frequent type of stomas in neonates. They are usually done because baby has necrotizing enterocolitis (NEC), Hirschsprung's disease, or imperforate anus (Colwell and others, 2001; Rogers, 2003).

- Although normal stoma color is red, a temporary change in stoma color to white or purple may occur when baby is crying (Colwell and others, 2001).

- If caring for a preterm infant, be aware that peristomal skin is not fully developed; thus never use skin sealants and adhesive removers because they damage the epithelium (Rogers, 2003).

- Usually a baby triples its birth weight in the first year. A stoma does not delay baby's growth. As baby grows in size, so does the stoma. Therefore stoma is measured frequently, and appropriate adjustments in pouching and skin barrier size are made accordingly.

- Whenever possible, adolescents requiring an ostomy benefit from presurgical contact with other adolescents who have an ostomy (Erwin-Toth, 1999).

Geriatric Considerations

- Evaluate older adult's cognitive status for understanding ostomy self-care instructions.
- Evaluate older adult's motor and visual ability to prepare ostomy equipment. For clients who are unable to custom cut the size of their skin barriers, consider having barriers precut by ostomy equipment supplier or using a precut two-piece system (Erwin-Toth, 2001).
- Older clients need teaching about change in number of eliminations (from an incontinent ostomy) that would be normal on a daily basis. Older clients may have some physical limitations, but most are able to learn self-care if given enough time (O'Shea, 2001).
- Financial concerns about cost of ostomy supplies and reimbursement may be an important issue for some clients on fixed income.

Home Care Considerations

- Client should understand that, although the nurse may have used sterile gauze to clean stoma, it is not necessary to use sterile gauze. In fact, gauze is not needed at all; a washcloth or any soft material can be used.
- Evaluate client's home toileting facilities. This includes:
  - Presence of adequate toileting facilities in client's home
  - Privacy
  - Flushing toilet facilities
  - Number and location of toileting facilities
  - Number of other people living with client who must share toileting facilities

NCLEX® Style Questions

1 A client comes to the clinic complaining of abdominal discomfort. Which of the following signs might suggest functional constipation?
1. Diarrhea and abdominal distention
2. Lumpy, hard stools and absent bowel sounds
3. Straining with defecation and sensation of incomplete evacuation
4. Hard stools and reduced fluid intake

2 One risk associated with digital removal of impacted stool is stimulation of the vagus nerve. When this nerve is stimulated what can occur?
1. Reflex vomiting
2. Reflex tachycardia
3. Reflex bradycardia
4. Reflex urination

3 Your postoperative client has a 4-day old ostomy. When changing the pouch for the first time, what is the reason for measuring the stoma?
1. Peristomal edema is present.
2. During the first 6 to 8 weeks post op, the stoma site changes.
3. The skin barrier is soiled with fecal matter.
4. The client wants to know the size of the stoma.

4 A client with an enterostomy pouch is complaining of an intense itching and burning around the stoma area. What is your first action?
1. Observe the stoma, peristomal skin, and pouching system.
2. Obtain a new skin barrier and paste system.
3. Obtain a physician's order for an antifungal powder.
4. Determine if stoma is in a skinfold.

References for all chapters appear in Appendix D.

Altered Urinary Elimination

33

MEDIA RESOURCES

- **evolve** http://evolve.elsevier.com/Elkin

- **View Video!** Video Clips

- Nursing Skills Online

Urinary elimination is a natural and private process that persons take for granted until a physical alteration occurs. Clients with alterations in urinary elimination require both physiological and psychological support. Physiological support includes use of an invasive procedure: the insertion of a catheter into the bladder or irrigation of a catheter. Psychological support involves assisting clients with body image changes or apprehension associated with caring for urinary diversions or ongoing elimination needs. As a nurse you must be competent in performing technical skills and in being sensitive to clients' psychological needs.

Urinary catheterization is the placement of a tube into the bladder to remove urine. The invasive procedure requires a medical order and strict sterile technique. Many conditions require the use of urinary catheters. For example, clients with fluid imbalance often need a temporary indwelling catheter to measure accurate intake and output (I&O). Clients with urinary retention accumulate urine in the bladder as a result of obstruction, trauma, paralysis, or inadequate bladder contraction. Because excessive accumulation of urine in the bladder increases risk for urinary tract infection and can cause backward flow of urine up the ureters to the kidneys causing kidney damage, indwelling or intermittent catheterization becomes necessary. Urinary incontinence, an involuntary leakage of urine, may require indwelling catheterization if the leaking urine interferes with skin integrity or wound healing. Regardless of the indication for catheterization, strict aseptic technique is required to prevent transmission of infection into the urinary system.

Clients may develop alterations that require the creation of alternate routes for urine elimination. When a client requires long-term urinary catheterization, a suprapubic catheter is a treatment option. The catheter is inserted through the abdominal wall directly into the bladder to provide a continuous route for urine drainage. In clients who develop bladder cancer requiring the removal of the bladder, urinary diversions are created. Urinary diversions involve the surgical implantation of the ureters into a portion of the bowel or directly onto the abdominal wall to maintain a route for urinary elimination. In all cases, when a client has an alternate route for urine elimination, it is important that you consider the effects this has on the individual's body image and ability to maintain a normal lifestyle.

EVIDENCE IN PRACTICE

Ryder, MA: Catheter-related infections: It's all about biofilm, *Topics Adv Pract Nurs eJournal* 5(3), 2005 Medscape http://www.medscape.com/viewarticle/508109, accessed October 23, 2005.

Urinary catheterization is associated with an increased incidence of nosocomial (health care associated) infections. The risk of infection is associated with the method and duration of catheterization, the quality of catheter care, and client susceptibility (Guidelines for Preventing Infections, 2004). Recently it has been found that these infections are directly linked to the formation of a biofilm on the catheter by microorganisms. The biofilm creates a positive growth environment for the microbes, helps them survive longer, and thus contributes to antimicrobial resistance and increased risk for serious, difficult-to-treat catheter-related bloodstream infections. Current research is focusing on prevention or disruption of this biofilm. In addition, research is also focusing on catheter materials, type and amount of catheter irrigations, and use of cranberry juice and routine care techniques and their relationship to infection (Gray, 2004; Brosnahan, 2004; Wilde, 2004).

NURSING DIAGNOSES

Urinary retention may be an appropriate nursing diagnosis for conditions such as urinary tract obstructions or inadequate bladder contraction. Unstable clients with **deficient** or **excess fluid volume** may need a temporary indwelling catheter to accurately measure I&O. **Risk for infection** is increased whenever a catheter is introduced into the normally sterile bladder. **Disturbed body image** applies to clients with urinary diversions or those requiring catheterization and who have a confused sense of their physical self.

SKILL 33.1 | **Urinary Catheterization with Straight or Indwelling (Retention) Catheter: Female and Male**

- Nursing Skills Online: Urinary Catheterization, Lessons 1 and 2

The steps for inserting an indwelling and a single-use straight catheter are the same. The difference lies in the inflation of a balloon to keep the indwelling catheter in place and the presence of a closed drainage system. Urinary catheters are made with one to three lumens (Figure 33-1). Single-lumen catheters (Figure 33-1, A) are used for intermittent catheterization (i.e., the insertion of a catheter for one-time bladder emptying). Double-lumen catheters, designed for indwelling catheters, provides one lumen for urinary drainage while a second lumen is used to inflate a balloon that keeps the catheter in place (Figure 33-1, B). Triple-lumen catheters (Figure 33-1, C) are used for continuous bladder irrigation or when it becomes necessary to instill medications into the bladder. One lumen drains the bladder, a second lumen is used to inflate the balloon, and a third lumen delivers fluid from an irrigation bag into the bladder.

A prescriber chooses a catheter on the basis of factors such as latex allergy, history of catheter encrustation, and susceptibility for infection. As a nurse, you must always assess clients carefully for latex allergies before inserting a catheter. Indwelling catheters are made of latex or silicone.

Some have special coatings that reduce urethral irritation and encrustation (Smith, 2003a). For example, antimicrobial catheters are coated with silver or an antibiotic to reduce the incidence of urinary tract infection (Newman, 2004). Straight or intermittent catheters are made of rubber (softer and more flexible) or polyvinyl chloride (PVC). Some PVC catheters are designed for client self-catheterization and are made with a hydrophilic coating that, when moistened, becomes slippery and thus does not require the application of a lubricant (Newman, 2004).

The size of a urinary catheter is based on the French (FR) scale, which reflects the internal diameter of the catheter. Most adults with an indwelling catheter should have a size 14-16 Fr to minimize trauma and risk for infection (Toughill, 2005; Smith, 2003a). Larger catheter diameters have higher risks for urinary tract infections (Gray and others, 2006). However, larger sizes are often needed in special circumstances such as after urological surgery. Smaller sizes are needed for children such as a 5-6 Fr for infants and an 8-10 Fr for children.

Indwelling catheters come in a variety of balloon sizes from 3 ml (for a child) to 30 ml for continuous bladder irrigation (CBI). The size of the balloon is usually printed on the catheter port (Figure 33-2). The recommended balloon size for an adult is a 5-ml balloon. Long-term use of larger

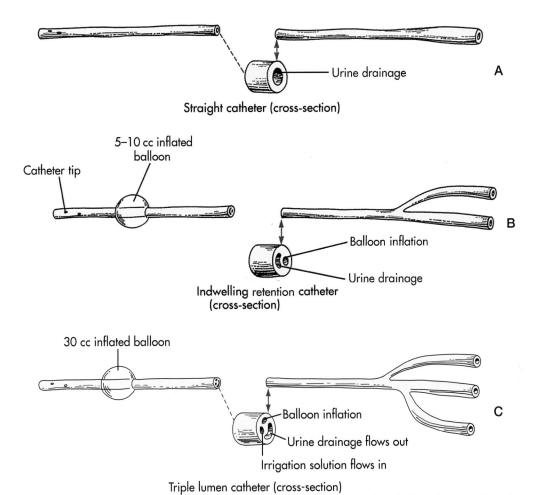

FIGURE 33-1 **A,** Straight catheter (cross-section). **B,** Indwelling retention catheter (cross-section). **C,** Triple-lumen catheter (cross-section).

balloons has been associated with ulceration of the bladder and urethra (Marklew, 2004). In addition a larger balloon (30 ml) increases the volume of urine that pools below the level of the catheter lumen and increases the risk of infection (Gray and others, 2006). For some clients (i.e., urinary retention or critical illness) long-term catheterization may be required, and it may be necessary to change the indwelling catheter periodically. Routine catheter changes are not recommended (Gray, 2004). Catheters should be changed for leaking, blockage, and before obtaining a sterile specimen for urine culture (Emr and Ryan, 2004; Gray, 2006). Long-term catheterization should be avoided due to its association with urinary tract infection (Trautner, Hull, and Daroviche, 2005). Make every attempt to remove catheters as soon as a client can void.

With an indwelling catheter a urinary drainage bag is attached to collect the continuous flow of urine. Always hang the bag below the level of the bladder on the bed frame or a chair so that urine will drain down, out of the bladder. The bag should never touch the floor. When a client ambulates, carry the bag below the level of the client's bladder. Urine in the bag and tubing is a medium for bacterial growth, and infection can develop if urine is allowed to reflux (return to the bladder). Most drainage bags

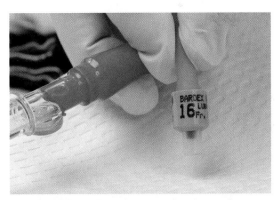

FIGURE 33-2 Size of balloon printed on catheter.

contain an antireflux valve to prevent urine from reentering the bladder.

ASSESSMENT

1 Review client's medical record, including presciber's order and nurses' notes. Note previous catheterization, including catheter size, response of client, and time of last catheterization. *Rationale: Identifies purpose of inserting catheter, previous catheter size, and potential difficulty with catheter insertion.*

2 Identify any condition that may impair passage of catheter (e.g., enlarged prostate gland in men, urethral strictures). *Rationale: Obstruction of the urethra may prevent passage of the catheter into the bladder.*

3 Ask client and check chart for allergies. *Rationale: Identifies allergy to antiseptic, tape, latex, and lubricant. Povidone-iodine allergies are common; if client is unaware of allergy, ask instead if allergic to shellfish.*

4 Assess client's knowledge and prior experience with catheterization. *Rationale: Reveals need for client instruction and likelihood of client cooperation.*

5 Assess client's weight, level of consciousness, ability to cooperate, and mobility of lower extremities. *Rationale: Are indicators of how much assistance is needed to properly position the client.*

6 Assess client's gender and age. *Rationale: Determines catheter size.*

7 Ask client the time of last voiding. Check I&O flow sheet. *Rationale: Determines time of last void and indicates if urinary retention is likely.*

8 Palpate bladder over symphysis pubis. *Rationale: Palpation of a full bladder will cause pain and/or urge to void, indicating a full or overfull bladder.*

9 Inspect perineal region, observing for perineal landmarks, erythema, drainage, or discharge. *Rationale: Determines the visibility of the urethra and need for cleansing the perineum.*

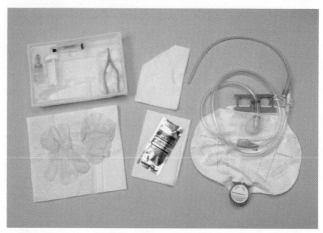

FIGURE 33-3 Catheter kit for indwelling catheterization (includes drainage bag with catheter attached, specimen cup, prefilled syringe for balloon inflation, cotton balls, forceps, cleansing solution, sterile gloves, lubricant, and sterile drapes). (Courtesy C R Bard, Covington, Georgia).

PLANNING

Expected Outcomes focus on emptying the bladder and on promoting client comfort.
1 Client's bladder is not palpable.
2 Client verbalizes absence of discomfort or bladder fullness.
3 Client has a urine output of at least 30 ml/hr of clear light yellow urine in urinary drainage bag.

Delegation Considerations
The insertion of an indwelling or straight urinary catheter may be delegated in some settings (see agency policy). Otherwise the nurse directs personnel to:
• Assist the nurse with positioning the client and directing the light source.

• Report any changes in the color, amount, and odor of the urine and if the indwelling catheter leaks or causes pain.

Equipment
• Catheter kit (Figure 33-3) and the appropriate-size catheter (Catheter kits vary. Check list of contents on the package. Basic equipment includes drapes [one fenestrated], lubricant, sterile cleansing solution incorporated in an applicator or to be added to cotton balls, and specimen container. Some kits contain a catheter with attached drainage bag; others contain only a catheter.)
• Nonallergenic tape or catheter strap (to secure catheter)
• Extra sterile gloves and catheter (optional)
• Clean gloves
• Washcloth, towel, soap, and basin for water
• Flashlight or other additional light source
• Flat sheet or bath blanket
• Measuring container for urine

IMPLEMENTATION *for Urinary Catheterization with Straight or Indwelling (Retention) Catheter: Female and Male*

STEPS	RATIONALE
1 See Standard Protocol (inside front cover).	

COMMUNICATION TIP Tell client that you will explain the procedure step by step as you proceed.

2 Arrange for extra nursing personnel to assist with positioning as needed.	Some female clients may have difficulty maintaining dorsal recumbent position.
a. *Position female* client dorsal recumbent (on back with knees flexed) and have client relax thighs. Drape with bath blanket so that only perineum is exposed.	Exposes perineum and allows hip joints to be externally rotated.

STEPS	RATIONALE

b. *Alternate female position:* position side-lying (Sims') position with upper leg flexed at knee and hip. Ensure that rectal area is covered with drape to reduce risk of contamination.

Alternate position is more comfortable if client cannot abduct leg at the hip joint (e.g., if client has arthritic joints or contractures). Support client with pillows if necessary to maintain position.

b. *Position male* client supine with legs extended and thighs slightly abducted. Cover upper body with small sheet or towel. Cover legs with separate sheet so that only genitals are exposed.

Aids in visualization of penis.

3 Cleanse client's perineal area with soap and water, rinse, and dry. Place waterproof pad under client. Remove and discard gloves.

COMMUNICATION TIP Encourage client to lie still to avoid accidental contamination of the sterile equipment. Explain each step as you proceed and especially before inserting the catheter.

---

4 Position light to illuminate perineum or have assistant available to hold flashlight to visualize urinary meatus.

5 Perform hand hygiene.

6 While standing on left side of bed (if right-handed) or right side of bed (if left-handed), place catheter kit tray on clean surface and open outer wrap using sterile technique (see Chapter 5) (see illustration).

Outer wrap serves as sterile work field.

a. Indwelling catheterization open system: Open the drainage system bag, close clamp, and place drainage bag over edge of bottom bed frame and drainage tube up between mattress and side rail. Open outer package of catheter, maintaining sterility of inner wrapper.

Closed systems have catheter preattached to drainage tubing and bag, which helps maintain a sterile system.

b. Indwelling catheterization closed system: Open the drainage bag with preattached catheter. Place bag near end of bed. Keep sterile catheter on sterile field.

c. Straight catheterization: Open outer package of catheter, maintaining sterility of inner wrapper.

7 Put on sterile gloves.

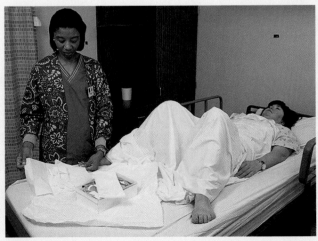

STEP 6 Client in dorsal recumbent position with nurse preparing catheter kit.

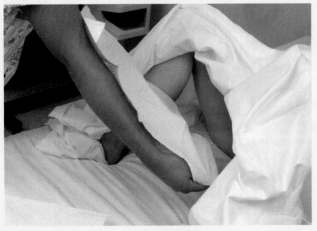

STEP 8a. Place sterile drape under buttocks as client lifts hips slightly off the bed.

STEPS	RATIONALE

8 Drape perineum keeping gloves sterile.

a. *Drape female:* Allow top edge of drape to form cuff over both hands. Place drape down on bed between client's thighs. Slip cuffed edge just under buttocks, taking care not to touch contaminated surfaces with sterile gloves (see illustration).

Outer surface of drape covering hands remains sterile. Sterile drape against sterile gloves maintains sterility of gloves and workspace.

b. Pick up fenestrated sterile drape. Allow drape to unfold without touching unsterile surfaces. Drape over perineum, exposing the labia (see illustration).

c. *Drape male:* Apply drape over thighs, just below penis. Place fenestrated drape with opening centered over penis (see illustration).

9 Arrange supplies on sterile field, maintaining sterility of gloves. Place sterile tray with cleaning medium (premoistened cotton-tipped applicator or cotton balls, forceps, and solution) lubricant, catheter, and prefilled balloon inflation syringe (indwelling catheterization only) on the sterile drape close to the perineum. Open sterile specimen container if specimen to be obtained (see Skill 33.2). Open inner sterile wrapper of catheter.

Provides easy access to supplies during catheter insertion and helps to maintain aseptic technique. Appropriate placement is determined by size of client and position during catheterization.

10 Indwelling catheterization

a. Test integrity of catheter balloon according to manufacturer's recommendations. This may include injecting solution into balloon port (see illustration). Withdraw if no leakage.

If leakage is present, a different catheter will be needed. NOTE: Some manufacturers do not recommend this step because balloon may stretch, increasing trauma on insertion.

b. Lubricate catheter with water-soluble gel 2.5 cm to 5 cm (1 to 2 inches) for women and 12.5 to 17.5 cm (5 to 7 inches) for men (see illustration).

Facilitates insertion of catheter with minimal tissue irritation. Female urethra is shorter.

c. Pour antiseptic solution over all but one cotton ball or open package of premoistened antiseptic applicators.

Dry cotton ball is used to remove excess antiseptic solution from meatus.

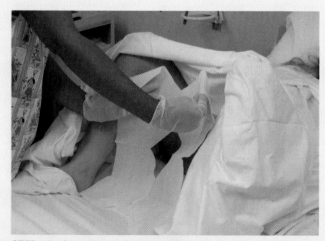

STEP 8b. Place sterile fenestrated drape (with opening in center) over perineum with labia exposed.

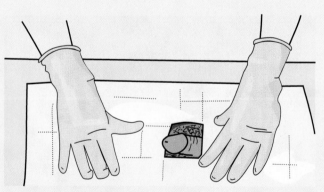

STEP 8c. Draping male.

STEPS	RATIONALE

d. Cleanse urinary meatus with antiseptic solution.
  (1) *Cleansing female:* (a) Separate labia with fingers of nondominant hand (now contaminated) to fully expose urinary meatus. (b) Maintain position of nondominant hand until catheter has been inserted. (c) Use the forceps to hold one cotton ball or one applicator at a time. Clean labia and urinary meatus from clitoris toward anus. (i) Use first cotton ball or applicator to clean along side farthest from nurse along meatus in a single stroke. (ii) Use second cotton ball or applicator to clean labia and meatus nearest nurse. (iii) Use third cotton ball or applicator to clean midline, directly over the meatus (see illustration).

Reduces risk of introducing microorganisms into sterile bladder. Front to back cleansing is cleaning from area of least contamination toward highly contaminated area. Dominant hand remains sterile.

  (2) *Cleansing male:* (a) With nondominant hand (now contaminated) retract foreskin (if uncircumcised) and grasp penis at shaft just below glans. Hold shaft of penis at right angle to body. This hand remains in this position for remainder of procedure. (b) Using uncontaminated dominant hand and forceps to hold cotton balls (or applicator), cleanse meatus with circular strokes, beginning at the meatus and working outward in a spiral motion. (c) Repeat with three cotton balls (or applicators) (see illustration).

When grasping shaft of penis, avoid pressure on dorsal surface to prevent compression of urethra.

> **COMMUNICATION TIP** As you prepare to cleanse the area, tell the client, "This will feel cold and wet." Explain that catheter insertion will not hurt but pressure is usually felt and may be uncomfortable.

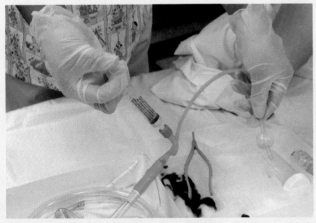

STEP 10a. Inflating balloon on double-lumen catheter to test balloon integrity.

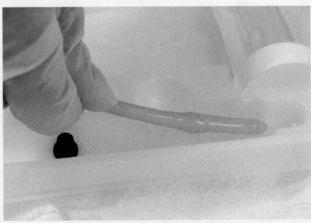

STEP 10b. Lubricating catheter.

STEPS	RATIONALE

e. Hold catheter 7.5 cm to 10 cm (3 to 4 inches) from tip. Hold end of catheter loosely coiled in palm of dominant hand. If catheter is not attached to a drainage bag, make sure to position urine tray so that end of catheter can be placed there once insertion begins.

(1) *Inserting catheter (female):* (a) Ask client to bear down gently and insert catheter (see illustration). (b) Advance catheter slowly a total of 5 to 7.5 cm (2 to 3 inches) or until urine flows out catheter's end. (c) As soon as urine appears, advance catheter another 2.5 to 5 cm (1 to 2 inches) Do not force catheter if resistance is met. (d) Release labia but maintain secure hold of catheter with nondominant hand.

Bearing down may help visualize urinary meatus and promotes relaxation of external urinary sphincter, aiding in catheter insertion.

Indicates that catheter tip is in bladder or lower urethra. Advancement ensures correct bladder placement. Prevents expulsion of catheter.

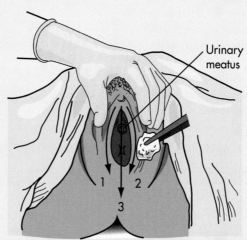

STEP 10d.(1)(c)(iii) Cleansing female perineum.

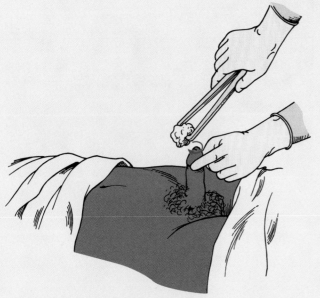

STEP 10d.(2)(c) Cleansing male urinary meatus.

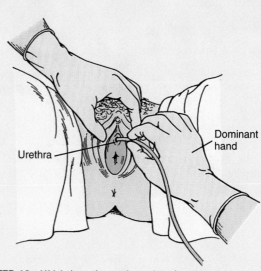

STEP 10e.(1)(a) Inserting catheter into female urinary meatus.

STEPS	RATIONALE

(2) *Inserting catheter (male):* (a) Gently apply upward traction to penis. (b) Ask client to bear down as if to void and then slowly insert catheter through the meatus (see illustration). (c) Advance catheter 17 to 22.5 cm (7 to 9 inches) or until urine flows out end of catheter. (d) When urine appears, advance catheter to bifurcation of drainage and balloon inflation port (see illustration). **Do not force catheter insertion.** (e) Lower penis and hold catheter securely in nondominant hand.

It is normal to meet resistance at the prostate. When resistance is met, hold catheter firmly against sphincter without forcing. After a few seconds, sphincter may relax and catheter can be advanced.

Further advancement of catheter to bifurcation of drainage and balloon inflation port ensures proper placement (Daneshgari and others, 2002).

NURSE ALERT   Stop catheter insertion if resistance is felt. Do not use force to insert catheter.

---

f. Allow bladder to empty fully unless institution policy restricts maximum volume of urine drained (see agency policy). Collect urine specimen as needed. Fill specimen container to desired level (20 to 30 ml) by holding end of catheter in dominant hand over cup.

Retained urine may serve as reservoir for growth of microorganisms.

g. While holding catheter in place with nondominant hand, inflate catheter balloon with amount of fluid designated by manufacturer (see illustration).
   (1) Continue to hold catheter with nondominant hand.
   (2) With free dominant hand, attach prefilled syringe in injection port at end of catheter.
   (3) Slowly inject total amount of fluid (see illustration). If client complains of sudden pain, stop injection, withdraw fluid from balloon, advance catheter further, reinflate balloon.
   (4) After inflating catheter balloon, release catheter from nondominant hand. Gently pull catheter until resistance is felt. Then advance catheter slightly. If not previously connected, attach catheter to drainage bag.

Indwelling catheter balloons should not be underinflated because underinflation causes balloon distortion and potential bladder damage (Fallis, 2005; Toughill, 2005).
By moving catheter slightly back into bladder, pressure on bladder neck is avoided.

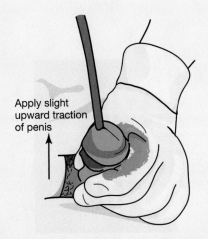

Apply slight upward traction of penis

STEP 10e.(2)(b) Inserting catheter into male urinary meatus.

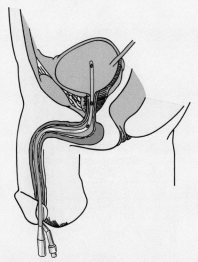

STEP 10e.(2)(d) Male anatomy with correct catheter insertion to the bifurcation of the drainage and balloon inflation port.

STEPS	RATIONALE
h. Secure indwelling catheter with hypoallergenic tape or catheter strap.	Minimal tension on catheter reduces accidental dislodgement, prevents trauma to the bladder and urethra, and reduces bladder neck irritation (Gray and others, 2006; Toughill, 2005).
(1) *Female:* Secure catheter to inner thigh with tape or catheter strap, allowing enough slack to prevent tension (see illustration).	
(2) *Male:* Secure to lower abdomen with tape or catheter strap (see illustration). If retracted, replace foreskin over the glans penis.	Anchoring catheter to lower abdomen maintains the urethra in a straight position and reduces pressure on urethra at junction of penis (Gray and others, 2006). Tension or pulling on indwelling catheters can damage and erode through urethra (Toughill, 2005).
i. Position drainage bag lower than bladder by attaching to bed frame. Do not attach to side rails of bed (see illustration).	Maintains closed system urine drainage, minimizing risk for infection (Marklew, 2004). Placement on side rails could result in bag being raised above bladder.
11 Straight catheterization	
a. Follow steps 10b through 10e. Allow urine to flow out catheter end. Do not advance catheter further.	Allows complete drainage of bladder. Catheter will not remain in bladder and thus does not require advancement.
b. Collect urine specimen as needed. Fill specimen container to desired level (20 to 30 ml) by holding end of catheter in dominant hand over cup.	Sterile urine measured for culture and sensitivity to determine microorganism growth and type of antibiotics that will be effective in treatment.

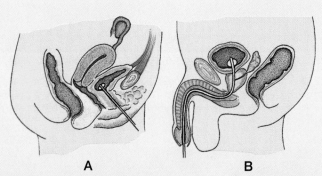

STEP 10g. Placement of inflated balloon in bladder. **A,** Female. **B,** Male.

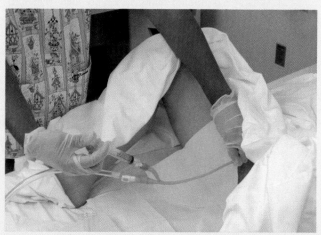

STEP 10g.(3) Hold catheter in place with nondominant hand while inflating balloon.

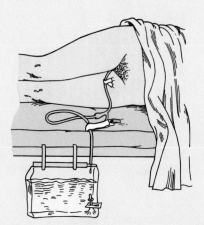

STEP 10h.(1) Securing the female indwelling catheter.

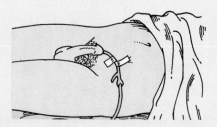

STEP 10h.(2) Securing the male indwelling catheter.

STEPS	RATIONALE

c. When urine stops flowing, withdraw catheter slowly and smoothly until removed.

12 Wash and dry perineal area as needed.   Cleansing solutions can be irritating to skin.

13 Remove and dispose of equipment, drapes, and urine in proper receptacles.   Reduces transmission of microorganisms.

14 Label specimen according to agency policy and send to laboratory immediately.   Fresh urine specimen ensures more accurate findings.

15 Measure urine and record.   Monitors output as baseline assessment.

> **NURSE ALERT** Drainage bag should be emptied at least every 3 to 4 hours or when bag is one half to two thirds full to avoid over-production of biocontaminants (Gray and others, 2006).

16 See Completion Protocol (inside front cover).

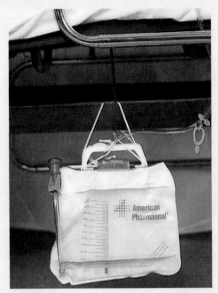

STEP 10i. Drainage bag below level of bladder and secured to the bed frame.

EVALUATION

1 Palpate bladder and observe amount, color, and clarity of urine.

2 Evaluate client's level of comfort.

3 Observe character and amount of urine in drainage tubing and bag or collection container.

Unexpected Outcomes and Related Interventions

1 Client complains of discomfort during inflation of balloon.
a. Stop inflation immediately; allow inflation fluid to return to syringe.
b. Advance another 1 inch (2.5 cm) and retry inflation.
c. If client still complains of pain, remove catheter and report to prescriber.

2 Catheter cannot be advanced into urethra.
a. Have client take deep breaths to relax and attempt reinsertion.
b. If catheter cannot be advanced, do not use force. Remove catheter and report to prescriber.

3 Catheter goes into vagina.
a. Leave catheter in vagina.
b. Recleanse urinary meatus. Using another catheter kit or another sterile catheter, insert catheter into meatus (check agency policy).
c. Remove catheter in vagina after successful insertion of second catheter in bladder.

4 Sterility is broken during catheterization by nurse or client.
a. Replace gloves if contaminated and start over.
b. If client touches sterile field but equipment remains sterile, avoid touching that part of sterile field.
c. If equipment is contaminated, replace it with sterile items or start over again with new kit.

Recording and Reporting

- Record the following in nurses' notes: reason for catheterization; type and size of catheter inserted; amount of fluid used to inflate balloon; specimen collection (if applicable); color, consistency, and amount of urine obtained with initial catheterization; client's response to procedure.
- Empty drainage bag and record in I&O flow sheet amount of urine every 8 hours or as ordered.
- Report any difficulties with insertion or abnormal appearance of urine to physician or other prescriber.

Sample Documentation

0800 Bladder distended. C/O full sensation but unable to void. 16 Fr catheter inserted without difficulty, 700 ml of clear yellow urine returned. Balloon inflated with 10 ml sterile solution. Catheter to bedside drainage. Denies discomfort or pain.

Special Considerations

Pediatric Considerations

- When caring for an infant or young child, explain procedures to parents. Describe procedure to child at level the child is able to understand (Hockenberry and Wilson, 2007).
- Children and adolescents will experience some discomfort during catheterization. Assistance and gentle holding may be necessary, especially with younger children. Most children prefer to have the parents remain with them during the procedure. Ask adolescents if they would like a parent to remain with them.
- Catheterization in infants and children may be made easier by use of a generous amount of lubricant containing 2% lidocaine (xylocaine) (Hockenberry and Wilson, 2007).
- Teaching young children to blow into a straw or pinwheel can aid in relaxing pelvic muscles (Hockenberry and Wilson, 2007).

Geriatric Considerations

- The older adult client who is physically compromised is at high risk of developing septicemia, a life-threatening infection that has spread to the blood. Avoid catheterization unless required for diagnostic testing or accurate I&O or when using a bedpan or toilet would cause excessive pain or retention of urine that endangers the upper urinary tract (Wilde, 2004).
- Symptoms of a urinary tract infection in the older adult may be difficult to recognize and limited to a change in mental status (Wilde, 2004).
- The use of urinary catheters in older adults has been shown to increase the incidence of pressure ulcer development (Horn and others, 2004).
- The presence of a urinary catheter can interfere with already compromised mobility of the older adult (Trautner, Hull, and Daroviche, 2005).

Home Care Considerations

- Clients who are at home may use a leg bag during the day and switch to a larger-volume bag at night.
- Male clients may prefer to secure their catheter on the upper thigh as a way to more easily disguise the catheter under clothing (Hanchett, 2002).
- Educate clients with indwelling catheters on the care of the catheter, signs of urinary tract infection, and troubleshooting techniques for a leaking catheter (Emr and Ryan, 2004).

Long-Term Care Considerations

- Urinary catheters contribute to functional disability by interfering with transfers and ambulation.
- Long-term care regulations dictate that long-term (>30 days) urinary catheters should only be used (1) to avoid urine contamination of stage 3 or 4 pressure ulcers, (2) treat documented urinary retention, (3) when coma or terminal illness is present, and (4) if exact measurement of urine output is needed (CMS, 2003; Gray, 2006).

SKILL 33.2 Removal of an Indwelling Catheter

- Nursing Skills Online: Urinary Catheterization, Lesson 5

Removal of an indwelling catheter is a skill requiring clean technique. When removing the catheter, you must avoid trauma to the urethra. Be sure that the catheter balloon is fully deflated to prevent trauma and subsequent swelling of the urethra, which could interfere with the ability to independently void. Clamping a catheter prior to removal is not recommended because there is no clear evidence that this practice will improve bladder function after removal (Fernandez and Griffiths, 2005). Clinicians have clamped catheters to

cause a buildup of urine in the bladder with the aim of promoting better bladder muscle tone after catheter removal. This practice has not been shown to be effective.

All clients need to have their voiding monitored after catheter removal. Clients whose catheters have been placed for an overdistended bladder, urinary retention due to an enlarged prostate or a urethral stricture, or other urinary retention should have their voiding monitored for at least 24 to 48 hours by using a voiding record or bladder diary. The bladder diary should record the time and amount of each voiding, including any incontinence. Abdominal pain and distention, a sensation of incomplete emptying, incontinence, constant dribbling of urine, and voiding in very small amounts can indicate inadequate bladder emptying.

Indwelling catheters increase the risk of urinary tract infection that can develop 2 to 3 or more days after catheter removal. All clients need to be informed of the risk for infection, prevention measures, and signs and symptoms that need to be reported to the primary care provider.

ASSESSMENT

1 Check physician's order.
2 Note length of time catheter was in place. *Rationale: Catheters in place for more than a few days are more likely to cause urethral irritation and buildup of encrustation.*
3 Assess urine color, clarity, odor, and amount. Note any urethral discharge or the presence of encrustation. *Rationale: May be an indicator of inflammation or urinary tract infection and a source of pain during catheter removal.*
4 Assess client's knowledge of removal procedure. *Rationale: Reveals need for client instruction.*
5 Determine size of catheter inflation balloon. *Rationale: Determines size of syringe required to deflate balloon.*

PLANNING

Expected Outcomes focus on client comfort, adequate bladder emptying, and client's learning about early detection of urinary tract infection.

1 Client will void at least 150 ml with each voiding no more than 6 to 8 hours after catheter removal.
2 Client will verbalize feeling of comfort after catheter removed.
3 Client will identify signs and symptoms of urinary tract infection.

Delegation Considerations

Assessment of the client's condition should not be delegated; however, the skill of removing a urinary catheter may be delegated. The nurse instructs personnel to:

- Report to the nurse how the client tolerated the procedure, the exact time the catheter was removed, and the time and amount of subsequent voiding.

Equipment

- 10-ml syringe or larger without a needle or (size depends on volume of solution used to inflate the balloon)
- Waterproof pad
- Clean gloves
- Toilet, bedside commode, urine "hat," urinal, or bedpan

IMPLEMENTATION *for Removal of an Indwelling Catheter*

STEPS	RATIONALE
1 See Standard Protocol (inside front cover).	
2 Position client supine and place waterproof pad under buttocks. Females will need to abduct legs with a second waterproof pad between thighs. Pad can lie on male's thighs.	Position provides access to catheter.
3 Move syringe plunger up and down to loosen and then withdraw plunger 0.5 ml from end of syringe. Insert hub of syringe into inflation valve (balloon port). Allow balloon fluid to drain into syringe by gravity. Make sure that entire amount of fluid is removed by comparing removed amount to volume needed for inflation.	Many manufacturers recommend that fluid return to syringe by gravity to avoid development of creases or ridges in balloon (Smith, 2003a). A partially inflated balloon causes trauma to urethral wall as catheter is removed.

NURSE ALERT Do not cut balloon inflation valve to drain water.

| 4 Pull catheter out smoothly and slowly. Examine catheter to ensure that catheter is whole. | Non-whole catheter means pieces of catheter may still be in bladder. Notify prescriber immediately. |

NURSE ALERT Catheter should slide out very easily. Do not use force. If any resistance is noted, repeat step 3 to remove remaining water. Notify prescriber.

5 Wrap catheter in waterproof pad. Unhook collection bag and drainage tubing from bed.
6 Measure urine and empty drainage bag. Record output.
7 Cleanse perineum with soap and water and dry area thoroughly.

STEPS	RATIONALE
8 Encourage client to maintain or increase fluid intake (unless contraindicated).	Maintains normal urinary output

> **COMMUNICATION TIP** Instruct client to tell you when the need to empty the bladder occurs and that all urine needs to be measured. Make sure client understands how to use the collection container.

STEPS	RATIONALE
9 Explain that many clients experience mild burning, discomfort, or small-volume voiding with first voiding, which soon subsides.	Burning is result of urethral irritation from catheter.
10 Inform client to report any signs of urinary tract infection, which are most likely to develop in 2 to 3 days.	Will increase likelihood of timely treatment.
11 Ensure easy access to toilet, commode, bedpan, or urinal. Place urine "hat" on toilet seat if client is using toilet. Place call bell within easy reach.	
12 Initiate voiding record or bladder diary if indicated.	Evaluates bladder function.
13 See Completion Protocol (inside front cover).	

EVALUATION

1 Observe time (less than 6 to 8 hours) and amount of first voiding (at least 150 ml).
2 Ask client to describe comfort level.
3 Ask client to list signs and symptoms of urinary tract infection.

Unexpected Outcomes and Related Interventions
1 Water from inflation balloon does not return into syringe.
a. Reposition client, ensure that catheter is not pinched or kinked.
b. Remove syringe. Attach new syringe and allow enough time for passive emptying.
c. Attempt to empty balloon by gently pulling back on the syringe plunger.
2 Client is unable to void after catheter removal, having had adequate fluid intake. Bladder is distended.
a. Assist to normal position for voiding.
b. Provide privacy.
c. Notify prescriber. Client may need to be catheterized.
3 Client voids small amounts frequently and states that bladder does not feel empty.
a. Consider possible urinary retention with overflow.

b. Obtain prescriber's order for catheterization for residual urine.
c. Perform bladder ultrasound or catheterize within 5 to 10 minutes of voiding. Depending on the volume obtained, the prescriber may order an intermittent catheterization schedule or replacement of indwelling catheter.

Recording and Reporting
- Record in nurses' notes: time catheter was removed; teaching related to increasing fluid intake and signs and symptoms of urinary tract infection; and time, amount, and characteristics of first voiding.
- Record intake times and amounts and voiding times and amounts on voiding record or bladder diary as indicated.

Sample Documentation
1600 Urinary catheter removed without difficulty. Client encouraged to increase fluids and that first voiding will be measured. Informed that first void may be uncomfortable and voiding within 6 to 8 hours is to be expected. Instructed to report signs and symptoms of UTI.

1930 Voided 350 ml of clear yellow urine. Complained of mild burning with voiding.

SKILL 33.3 Inserting Straight Catheter for Specimen Collection or Post-Void Residual (PVR) Urine

- Nursing Skills Online: Urinary Catheterization, Lessons 2 and 4

Straight catheterization empties a distended bladder when a client cannot void, to collect a urine specimen, or to measure post-void residual (PVR), which is the amount of urine left in the bladder after voiding. PVR can also be measured using a portable bladder ultrasound, which provides accurate measurement of urine in the bladder and reduces the risk for infection related to catheterization (Sparks and others, 2004; Teng and others, 2005; Stevens, 2005). Urinary retention is the inability of the bladder to fully empty such as with obstruction of the urethra by an enlarged prostate, bladder neuropathy caused by diabetes mellitus, or nerve damage related to spinal cord injury. Clean intermittent catheterization (CIC) using a straight catheter is a program of regularly scheduled catheterizations. Clients usually perform CIC under clean technique to promote regular emptying of the bladder.

A client's ability to void depends on the ability to perceive the urge to void, to relax the urethral sphincter, and on the bladder contracting enough to completely empty. If a client is unable to void, every effort is made to promote urinary elimination before performing catheterization. This involves assisting the client to assume the normal voiding position. Females need to assume a sitting position, and males may find it helpful to stand. Other measures to promote voiding include having the client listen to running water, putting a client's hand in warm water, or stroking a female client's inner thigh. Give clients privacy and do not rush them. Comfort and adequate fluid intake are also important factors in facilitating voiding.

ASSESSMENT

1 Review I&O flow sheet for frequency and amount of each voiding. *Rationale: Will identify the usual volume of voided urine.*

2 Ask client to describe any difficulty or discomfort experienced while voiding. *Rationale: Pain is associated with a urinary tract infection, and difficulty passing urine such as the need to strain may indicate a urethral obstruction.*

3 Identify time client voids. *Rationale: PVR urine determinations need to be performed no more than 5 to 10 minutes after voiding to obtain accurate data.*

4 Assess client's knowledge and experience with urinary retention and catheterization. *Rationale: Reveals need for client education and support.*

PLANNING

Expected Outcomes focus on monitoring quantity of residual urine, promoting comfort, and preventing urinary tract infection.

1 Successive catheterizations result in decreasing amount of residual urine.

2 Urine remains clear, dilute, and without foul odor.

3 Client reports voiding without difficulty or discomfort.

4 Client explains the purpose of the procedure and what is expected.

Delegation Considerations

Assessment of the client's condition should not be delegated; however, the skill of obtaining catheterized specimens or measuring residual urine may be delegated in some settings (see agency policy). The nurse directs personnel to:

• Report to the nurse the time of catheterization and volume of voided and catheterized urine.

Equipment

• Catheterization kit for straight catheterization: contains collection chamber, single-lumen catheter, disinfectant applicators (cotton balls, antiseptic solution, forceps), drapes (one is fenestrated with center hole), sterile gloves, lubricant, and specimen container. (NOTE: Contents vary. Read contents on outer package and add necessary items.)

• Wash cloth, towel, soap, and basin for water

• Clean gloves

IMPLEMENTATION *for Inserting Straight Catheter for Specimen Collection or Post-Void Residual (PVR) Urine*

STEPS	RATIONALE
1 See Standard Protocol (inside front cover).	

> COMMUNICATION TIP Explain to clients requiring a PVR that their bladder may not empty completely and that the amount of urine left in the bladder needs to be measured.

STEPS	RATIONALE
2 Ask client to void completely and measure volume of urine.	Helps determine how effectively client is emptying bladder.
3 Immediately after client voids, position and drape client as in Skill 33.1.	Urine is being produced and collected in the bladder continuously. A delay in the procedure would give inaccurate information about client's ability to empty the bladder.
4 Insert straight catheter following steps in Skill 33.1.	
5 Allow bladder to empty fully into collection container unless institution policy restricts maximum volume of urine drained (see agency policy). Collect urine specimen in sterile container (if indicated).	Retained urine may serve as reservoir for growth of microorganisms.
6 Steadily and smoothly remove straight catheter.	
7 Assist client to a comfortable position. Wash and dry perineal area.	Promotes comfort.
8 See Completion Protocol (inside front cover).	

EVALUATION

1 Measure amount of residual urine and each subsequent void.
2 Note if urine appears clear, dilute, and without foul odor.
3 Ask client to describe any difficulty or discomfort when voiding.
4 Ask client to explain the purpose of the procedure and what is expected.

Unexpected Outcomes and Related Interventions

1 Residual volume is greater than 100 ml of urine, indicating inadequate bladder emptying.
a. Continue ordered catheterization schedule and notify prescriber.
2 Client has signs and symptoms associated with a bladder infection (fever; chills; dysuria; frequent voiding in small amounts; incontinence; dull or aching pain localized in flank, back, lower abdomen, or groin; and cloudy, bloody, or foul-smelling urine).
a. Monitor vital signs and notify the prescriber.
b. Prepare to obtain a urine specimen for urinalysis and culture and sensitivity (if ordered).
c. Encourage increased fluid intake (if appropriate).

Recording and Reporting

• Record in the nurses' notes: amount of urine voided, time of catheterization, amount and characteristics of urine obtained from catheterization, and client's response to procedure.

Sample Documentation

1300 Voided 200 ml clear urine without discomfort. Catheterized 5 minutes after voiding for a residual of 125 ml of clear yellow urine. Reported minimal discomfort during the procedure; however, expresses concern about how many more times this procedure needs to be done.

Special Considerations
Pediatric Considerations

• Neonates and small children need shorter lengths of catheters to prevent catheter knotting as the bladder compresses (Smith, 2003b).
• See Pediatric Considerations for Skill 33.1.

Geriatric Considerations

• Urinary incontinence and retention are not considered a normal part of aging.
• Older adults are at higher risk for the development of serious infection, including septicemia from urinary retention. Avoid frequent catheterizations.
• Intermittent catheterization (IC) can be taught to older adults as long as they are motivated and have the cognitive and motor abilities to perform the skill (Newman, 2004).

Home Care Considerations

• IC is the recommended method for managing urinary retention. It is associated with lower risk of urinary tract infection.
• Some clients who are prone to infection choose to use sterile technique.

Long-Term Care Considerations

• IC performed by a nurse in the long-term care setting should be done using aseptic technique (Newman, 2004).

SKILL 33.4 Closed and Open Intermittent Urinary Catheter Irrigation

Urinary catheter irrigations are performed on an intermittent or continuous basis to maintain catheter patency. There are two types of irrigation: closed catheter irrigation and open irrigation. Closed catheter irrigation provides intermittent or continuous irrigation of the urinary catheter without disrupting the sterile connection between the catheter and the drainage system (Figure 33-4). Continuous bladder irrigation (CBI) is an example of a continuous infusion of a sterile solution into the bladder, usually using a three-way irrigation closed system with a triple-lumen catheter. CBI is often used following genitourinary surgery to keep the bladder clear and free of blood clots or sediment.

Open catheter irrigation is used when intermittent irrigation of the catheter and bladder is required. The skill in-

volves breaking or opening the closed drainage system at the connection between the catheter and the drainage system. Strict asepsis is required throughout the procedure to minimize contamination and subsequent development of a urinary tract infection. Both open and closed irrigation can be used to irrigate the bladder with medication.

ASSESSMENT

1 Verify in the medical record the order for type (continuous or intermittent) and amount of irrigant. *Rationale: An order is required to initiate therapy. Frequency and volume of solution used for irrigation may be in the order or standardized as part of agency policy. Each type of irrigation requires different equipment.*

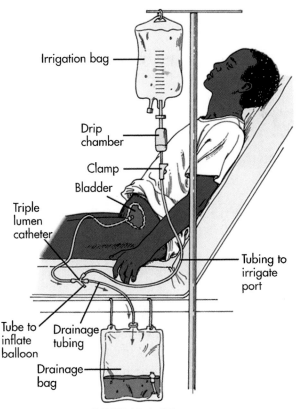

Irrigation bag

Drip chamber

Clamp

Bladder

Triple lumen catheter

Tubing to irrigate port

Tube to inflate balloon

Drainage tubing

Drainage bag

FIGURE 33-4 CBI setup.

2 Type of catheter in place. *Rationale: Single- and double-lumen catheters used with open irrigation. Triple-lumen catheters used for both intermittent and continuous closed irrigation.*

3 Palpate bladder for distention and tenderness. *Rationale: Bladder distention indicates that flow of urine may be blocked from draining.*

4 Ask client to describe bladder pain or spasms. *Rationale: Accumulation of blood clots or catheter blockage can increase bladder spasms. Offers baseline to determine if therapy is successful.*

5 Observe urine for color, amount, clarity, and presence of mucus, clots, or sediment. *Rationale: Indicates if client is bleeding or sloughing tissue, which would require increased irrigation rate or frequency of catheter irrigation.*

6 Measure client's body temperature. *Rationale: Establishes baseline to detect fever from infection.*

7 Assess client's knowledge regarding purpose of performing catheter irrigation. *Rationale: Reveals need for client instruction.*

PLANNING

Expected Outcomes focus on continuous urine flow and client comfort.

1 Urine output is greater than volume of irrigating solution instilled.

2 Client's urine output has decreased blood clots and sediment. (NOTE: Urine will be bloody following bladder/urethral surgery, gradually becoming lighter and blood tinged in 2 to 3 days.)

3 Client reports relief of bladder pain or spasms.

4 Client remains afebrile.

Delegation Considerations

The skill of catheter irrigation may not be delegated. The nurse directs personnel to:

- Report to nurse if the urinary catheter stops draining or if client reports pain and any symptoms of urinary tract infection.

Equipment

- Clean gloves
- Bag of irrigation solution at room temperature as prescribed
- Irrigation tubing with clamp to regulate irrigation flow rate (closed continuous or intermittent)
- Y connector (optional) to connect irrigation tubing to double-lumen catheter (closed continuous or intermittent)
- Intravenous (IV) pole (closed continuous or intermittent)
- Sterile 30- to 50-ml irrigation or catheter-tipped syringe (open intermittent)
- Screw clamp (closed and open intermittent)
- Disposable sterile irrigation kit that contains solution container, collection basin, and sterile drape (open intermittent)
- Sterile catheter plug
- Antiseptic swabs
- Tape

IMPLEMENTATION *for Closed and Open Intermittent Catheter Irrigation*

STEPS	RATIONALE
1 See Standard Protocol (inside front cover).	
2 Closed catheter irrigation	
a. Place label on irrigation solution bag with client's name, room number, date and time, type of solution, and any additives. Clearly mark bag for GU IRRIGATION ONLY. If replacing a bag, discard any sterile solution not used within 24 hours (see agency policy).	Bag may be prelabeled by pharmacy. Follows principles of medication safety. Clear labeling indicates fluid is not to be infused intravenously. Discarding minimizes possibility of fluid contamination.
b. Identify client by checking identification bracelet and asking client's name. Use two identifiers.	Ensures correct client receives ordered medication. At least two identifiers (neither to be the client's room number) are to be used when administering medications (JCAHO, 2004).

STEPS	RATIONALE

c. Hang bag on IV pole.

d. Using aseptic technique, insert (spike) tip of sterile irrigation tubing into bag containing irrigation solution (see illustration).

e. Close clamp on tubing and fill drip chamber one-half full by squeezing the chamber. Open clamp to completely fill tubing and remove air. Close clamp.

Air in tubing may cause bladder fullness and spasms.

f. Using aseptic technique, wipe off irrigation port of triple-lumen catheter with antiseptic swab and connect the irrigation tubing.

Prevents transmission of infection.

> **NURSE ALERT** Be sure the drainage tubing from indwelling catheter is patent (not clamped or obstructed). If irrigation solution continues to infuse rapidly and drainage from the bladder is blocked by a blood clot, overdistention can result in extreme discomfort and bladder damage or rupture.

g. For continuous irrigation: Calculate drip rate and adjust rate at roller clamp. If urine is bright red or has clots, increase irrigation rate until drainage appears pink (according to ordered rate or agency protocol).

Continuous drainage is expected. It assists with prevention of clotting in presence of active bleeding in bladder and flushes clots out of bladder.

h. For intermittent irrigation: Clamp tubing on drainage system, open clamp on irrigation tubing, allow prescribed amount of fluid to enter bladder, close irrigation tubing clamp, and then open drainage tubing clamp.

Fluid is instilled through catheter in a bolus, flushing the system. Fluid drains out after irrigation is complete.

i. Replace bag of irrigation solution as needed.

j. Empty catheter drainage bag as needed.

Bag will fill rapidly and may need to be emptied every 1 to 2 hours.

k. Compare urine output with infusion of irrigation solution every hour.

Determines urinary output and ensures that irrigant is draining freely.

3 Open intermittent catheter irrigation

a. Open sterile irrigation tray: Establish sterile field (see Chapter 4) and pour ordered amount of sterile solution into sterile solution container. Replace cap on large container of solution. Add sterile syringe to field.

Adheres to principles of surgical asepsis.

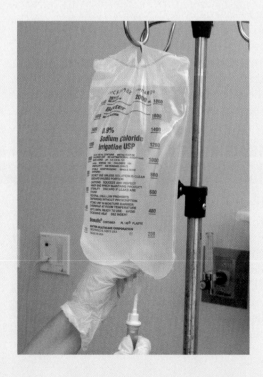

STEP 2d. Spiking bag of sterile irrigation solution for CBI.

STEPS	RATIONALE
b. Position drape under catheter.	Prevents soiling of bed linen.
c. Aspirate 30 ml of solution back and forth into irrigating syringe. Dispel solution back into container. Then place syringe in sterile solution container until ready to use.	Clears syringe, making it easy to move plunger back and forth. Maintains sterility of irrigating syringe.
d. Move sterile collection basin close to client's thigh.	
e. Wipe connection point between catheter and tubing with antiseptic wipe before disconnecting.	Reduces transmission of microorganisms.
f. Disconnect catheter from drainage tubing, allowing any urine to flow into sterile collection basin; cover open end of drainage tubing with sterile protective cap and position tubing so it stays coiled on top of bed.	Maintains sterility of inner aspects of catheter lumen and drainage tubing. Reduces potential of infection by way of microorganism contamination.
g. Take syringe and aspirate 30 to 50 ml of solution. Insert tip of syringe into lumen of catheter and gently push plunger to instill solution (see illustration).	Many manufacturers of irrigation solutions recommend gentle fluid instillation to minimize trauma to bladder (Getliffe, 2003).

NURSE ALERT Do not force the irrigation. Catheter may be completely occluded and needs to be changed.

STEPS	RATIONALE
h. Remove syringe, lower catheter, and allow solution to drain into basin. Drainage solution amount should be equal to or greater than amount instilled. If ordered, repeat instilling solution and drain until drainage is clear of clots and sediment.	If clot has been removed, solution will drain freely into basin.
i. Irrigation with clamping: After irrigating, clamp catheter with screw clamp for prescribed time, remove syringe from catheter and apply a sterile plug. Remove clamp and allow solution to drain into basin.	Some irrigation solutions require time in the catheter and bladder to exert therapeutic effect. Clamped drainage tubing and bag should not be left unattended.
k. After irrigation is complete, remove protector cap from urinary drainage tubing adapter, cleanse adapter with antiseptic wipe, reinsert adapter into lumen of catheter.	

4 Anchor catheter (see Skill 33.1).

5 See Completion Protocol (inside front cover).

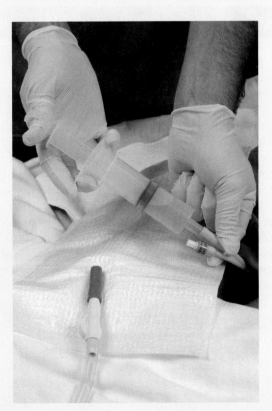

STEP 3g. Gentle instillation of fluid irrigates catheter.

EVALUATION

1 Measure actual urine output by subtracting total amount of irrigation fluid infused from total volume drained.
2 Observe that catheter is draining and inspect urine for blood clots and sediment.
3 Review I&O flow sheet to verify that hourly output into drainage bag is in appropriate proportion to irrigating solution entering bladder. Expect more output than fluid instilled because of urine production.
4 Ask if client is experiencing pain.
5 Monitor body temperature for fever.
6 Inspect drainage tubing for kinks, incorrect clamping, or looping.

Unexpected Outcomes and Related Interventions

1 Irrigation solution will not infuse or is slower than previously set.
a. Examine drainage tubing for clots, sediment, or kinks.
b. Notify prescriber if irrigant is retained, client complains of severe pain, or bladder is distended.
2 Drainage output is less than amount of irrigation solution infused.
a. Examine drainage tubing for clots, sediment, or kinks.
b. Inspect urine for presence of or increase in blood clots and sediment.
c. Evaluate client for pain and distended bladder.
d. Notify prescriber.

3 Bright-red bleeding with irrigation drip wide open.
a. Assess for hypovolemic shock (vital signs, skin color and moisture, anxiety level).
b. Leave irrigation drip wide open and notify prescriber.
4 Client experiences pain with irrigation.
a. Examine drainage tubing for clots, sediment, or kinks.
b. Evaluate urine for presence of or increase in blood clots and sediment.
c. Evaluate for distended bladder.
d. Notify prescriber.

Recording and Reporting

• Record amount and type of solution used as irrigant, amount infused, amount returned as drainage, and characteristics of output.
• Report catheter occlusion, sudden bleeding, infection, or increased pain to prescriber.
• Record I&O.

Sample Documentation

0800 Lower abdomen soft and flat. Catheter drainage of 225 ml of bright-red urine with moderate-size dark bloody clots. 3000 ml of NS infusing at 60 gtt per minute. Client rates bladder spasms at 5 on a 0 to 10 scale. Lying on left side, knees flexed.

SKILL 33.5 Suprapubic Catheter Care

A suprapubic catheter is a urinary drainage tube inserted surgically into the bladder through the abdominal wall above the symphysis pubis (Figure 33-5). The catheter may be sutured to the skin, secured with an adhesive material, or retained in the bladder with a fluid filled-balloon similar to an indwelling catheter.

Suprapubic catheters are placed when urethral catheterization is difficult such as when there is blockage of the urethra (e.g., enlarged prostate, urethral stricture) or in clients with spinal cord injury. They may be used as a temporary measure to manage urinary retention until normal bladder function returns. Long-term nursing care of suprapubic catheters includes client or caregiver education about maintaining catheter patency and how to empty the drainage bag, clean the site, and observe for infection.

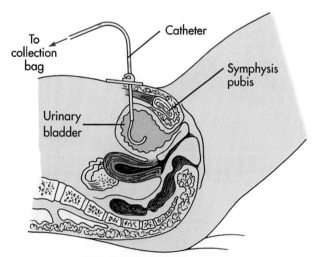

FIGURE 33-5 Suprapubic catheter in female client.

ASSESSMENT

1 Assess catheter insertion site for inflammation: pain, erythema, edema, and drainage. *Rationale: If insertion site is new, slight inflammation may be expected as part of normal wound healing but can also indicate infection.*

2 Assess urine in catheter or bag for amount, color, clarity, and sediment. *Rationale: Abnormal findings may indicate potential complications such as blockage or urinary tract infection.*

3 Assess for fever and chills. *Rationale: Indicates urinary tract infection or site infection.*

4 Assess tape site for signs of irritation. *Rationale: Repeated taping can cause skin irritation and breakdown.*

5 Check for allergies. *Rationale: Client may be sensitive to tape, latex, or antiseptic solution.*

6 Assess client's and/or caregiver's knowledge of purpose of catheter and its care. *Rationale: Determines level of instruction required.*

PLANNING

Expected Outcomes focus on maintaining flow of urine, client comfort, and prevention of infection.

1 Client's catheter is patent, and output is 30 ml or greater per hour.

2 Client's catheter site is free of signs of infection: erythema, edema, discharge, or tenderness.

3 Client remains afebrile; and urine is clear, free from odor, sediment, and bacteria.

4 Client verbalizes no pain or discomfort at insertion site.

5 Client and/or caregiver can explain purpose and demonstrate care for catheter.

6 Client and/or caregiver identify indications of infections of the urinary tract and site.

Delegation Considerations

Assessment of client's condition should not be delegated; however, the skill of caring for an established suprapubic catheter may be delegated (see agency policy). The nurse instructs personnel to:

- Report any change in the client's comfort from the tube, any drainage around insertion site, change in the amount and character of the urine, or any foul odors or fever.

Equipment

- Gloves: sterile and clean
- Sterile gauze for cleaning site
- Cleansing agent
- Drain (split) gauze
- Tape
- Velcro tape holder (optional)
- Dressing bag

IMPLEMENTATION *for Suprapubic Catheter Care*

STEPS	RATIONALE
1 See Standard Protocol (inside front cover).	
2 Remove dressing; discard gloves.	
3 Prepare supplies and cleansing agent for applying a dry, sterile dressing. Established catheters are often cleansed with mild soap and water (see agency policy).	The catheter insertion site is considered a surgical incision and should be treated similarly to other incisions.
4 Apply sterile gloves.	
5 Inspect insertion site and patency of catheter.	Reveals how catheter is held in place. Sutures should be clearly seen wrapped around catheter and secured to skin. Urine should be seen draining in tubing.
6 Without creating tension, hold catheter erect with nondominant hand while cleaning. Cleanse in circular motion, starting near catheter insertion site and continuing in outward widening circles for approximately 5 cm (2 inches) (see illustration).	Moves from area of least contamination to area of most contamination. Tension on catheter may cause discomfort or damage to wall of bladder or cause the catheter to slip out of place.

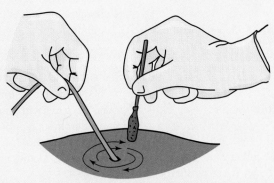

STEP 6 Cleansing around suprapubic catheter, avoiding tension on catheter.

STEPS	RATIONALE
7 With fresh, moistened gauze, gently cleanse base of catheter, moving up and away from site of insertion (proximal to distal).	Removes microorganisms and any drainage that adheres to tubing.
8 With sterile gloved hand, apply drain dressing (split gauze) around catheter and tape in place (see illustration).	Serves to collect secretions.
9 Secure catheter to abdomen with tape or Velcro multipurpose tube holder to reduce tension on insertion site.	Secures catheter and reduces risk of excessive tension on suture and/or body seal.
10 Coil excess tubing on bed and secure it to dressing. Keep drainage bag below level of bladder at all times.	Prevents kinking and backflow of urine from the tubing into the bladder.
11 See Completion Protocol (inside front cover).	

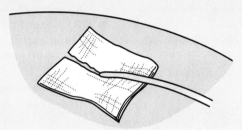

STEP 8 Split drain dressing for suprapubic catheter.

EVALUATION

1 Monitor suprapubic catheter output.
2 Observe catheter insertion site for erythema, edema, discharge, or tenderness.
3 Monitor for signs of infection (e.g., fever, elevated white blood cell count) and observe client's urine for clarity, sediment, or unusual odor.
4 Ask client whether there is any pain or discomfort from suprapubic catheter.
5 Ask client or caregiver to explain purpose and demonstrate care of insertion site and drainage bag.
6 Ask client or caregiver to state signs and symptoms of urinary tract infection and insertion site infection.

Unexpected Outcomes and Related Interventions

1 Catheter becomes obstructed (blood clots or sediment form, tip of catheter in bladder is positioned against bladder wall).
a. Increase fluids (if not contraindicated) to at least 1500 ml/day.
b. If ordered, irrigate catheter. Do not use force (see Skill 33.4).
c. Notify prescriber.
2 Client has urinary tract infection or catheter site infection.
a. Increase fluids to at least 1500 ml/day (if not contraindicated).
b. Administer antiinfectives as prescribed.

c. Monitor vital signs; observe amount, color, consistency of urine; assess site.
3 Urine leaks around catheter.
a. Monitor vital signs; assess urine for signs of infection.
b. Change dressing frequently; protect skin from moisture.
c. Notify prescriber.
4 Catheter becomes dislodged.
a. Apply sterile gauze to site.
b. Apply pressure if bleeding.
c. Reassure client.
d. Notify physician.

Recording and Reporting

• Record in nurses' notes character of urine and dressing changes, including assessments of wound and client's comfort level.
• Record urine output on I&O flow sheet.

Sample Documentation

0800 Catheter draining 100 ml of clear yellow urine in 2 hours. Dressing with small amount of dark brown drainage removed from suprapubic catheter site. No redness, edema, or drainage at the site. Insertion site cleansed and dressed with drain dressing. Denies any pain at insertion site.

Special Considerations
Home Care Considerations
- Before discharge from the hospital, the client must be able to clean and dress the suprapubic site and empty the drainage bag, observing characteristics of the urine.
- Teach clients signs of catheter obstruction, urinary tract infection, and wound infection.

SKILL 33.6 Pouching an Incontinent Urinary Diversion

A urinary diversion involves a surgical procedure in which the bladder is bypassed or removed (Figure 33-6). The most common indications for permanent urinary diversions are malignancy, trauma, and bladder conditions involving neurological dysfunction or pain (Dixon, Wasson, and Johnson, 2001). Continent cutaneous diversions involve the creation of an internal pouch or reservoir for urine from a segment of bowel (Figure 33-6, A). The stoma has a muscular closure or valve similar to the sphincter at the urinary meatus to prevent urine leakage. Clients perform self-catheterization of the diversion every 4 to 6 hours and do not need to wear an external collection pouch. Periodic irrigation of the reservoir may be necessary because of mucus secretion from the bowel mucosa. A small gauze pad may be used to cover the stoma to protect clothing from mucus drainage. A second type of continent urinary diversion is the orthotopic bladder replacement or "neobladder." This surgical procedure involves creating a reservoir for urine from a portion of the ileum or colon. The urethra is then fastened to the reservoir. Clients learn to relax the urinary sphincter to allow emptying of the reservoir. A sigmoidostomy involves attachment of the ureters to a portion of the large intestine or ileum (Figure 33-6, B). Urine is excreted into the intestine, allowing for continence but predisposing the client to bowel incontinence.

Incontinent urinary diversions include the ileal conduit (Figure 33-6, C) and the ureterostomy. The ileal conduit is surgically created by transplanting the ureters into a closed-off portion of the ileum and creating an opening through the abdomen through which urine drains continuously. A ureterostomy drains urine continuously as an opening through the skin and abdominal wall from one or both ureters that have been rerouted from the bladder to this abdominal opening (Figure 33-6, D). The stoma of either of these incontinent diversions is normally red or pink and protrudes slightly above the skin (Colwell, Goldberg, and Carmel, 2004). Pouches are attached to the skin surrounding the stoma to collect the urine and prevent skin damage. Ureteral stents (Figure 33-7) maintain patency of ureters. Stents usually remain in place 5 to 7 days (Colwell, Goldberg, and Carmel, 2004).

ASSESSMENT

1. Inspect pouch for amount and color of urine, leakage, and length of time in place. *Rationale: Expect output of at least 30 ml/hr. Empty when one-third to one-half full. Weight of urine in pouch weakens the seal, resulting in leakage.*

2. Inspect stoma and all external suture lines for healing progress. *Rationale: Stoma should be moist and reddish pink; in postoperative period stoma may be edematous and have ureteral stents in place (see Figure 33-7).*

3. Observe skin around stoma for erythema and skin breakdown. *Rationale: Determines presence of urine leakage and need to replace skin barrier.*

4. Assess level of comfort on a scale of 0 to 10. *Rationale: In postoperative period increased pain could indicate that urine is entering the peritoneum.*

5. Observe abdomen for abdominal contours, folds, and suture line. *Rationale: Helps to determine proper pouch type and size.*

6. Assess client's emotional response, knowledge, and understanding of ostomy. *Rationale: Helps to determine client readiness to learn self-management of urinary diversion.*

7. Assess client's visual acuity and manual dexterity. *Rationale: Determines client's ability to change pouch and type of pouch system to use.*

PLANNING

Expected Outcomes focus on maintaining urine output, a healthy stoma, skin integrity, and promoting self-care.

1. Urine drains freely from stents or stoma at least 30 ml/hr. No leaking is seen around pouch.

2. Stoma remains red, shiny, and moist.

3. Skin around stoma is free of irritation and breakdown. If in postoperative stage, sutures are intact, and incision is well approximated; stents in place.

4. Client rates discomfort at less than baseline assessment (scale of 0 to 10).

5. Client and/or primary caregiver are able to care for stoma, skin, and pouch.

A **Ileal reservoirs** divert urine into a surgically created pouch, or pocket, that functions as a bladder. The stoma is continent, and the client removes urine by regular self-catheterization.

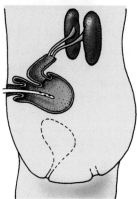

Continent internal ileal resevoir (Kock's pouch)

B **Sigmoidostomies** divert urine to the large intestine, so no stoma is required. The client excretes urine with bowel movements, and bowel incontinence may result.

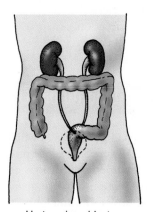

Ureterosigmoidostomy

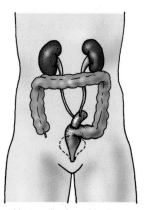

Ureteroiliosigmoidostomy

C **Conduits** collect urine in a portion of the intestine, which is then opened onto the skin surface as a stoma. After the creation of a conduit, the client must wear a pouch.

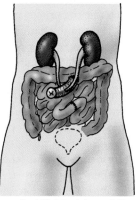

Ileal (Bricker's) conduit

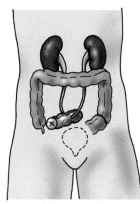

Colon conduit

D **Ureterostomies** divert urine directly to the skin surface through a ureteral skin opening (stoma). After ureterostomy, the client must wear a pouch.

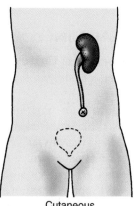

Cutaneous ureterostomy

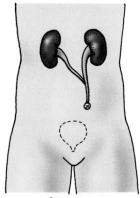

Cutaneous ureteroureterostomy

FIGURE 33-6 Urinary diversion procedures used in the treatment of bladder cancer. (From Ignatavicius DD, Workman ML: *Medical-surgical nursing: critical thinking for collaborative care,* ed 4, Philadelphia, 2002, Saunders.)

Delegation Considerations

Assessment of client's condition should not be delegated; however, the skill of pouching a stable urinary diversion may be delegated in some settings (see agency policy). In some agencies a stoma nurse specialist is available to guide care, assist with product selection, and assist with problems. The nurse directs personnel to:

- Report any leakage of urine and/or breakdown of skin or stoma integrity.

Equipment

- Clean gloves
- Underpad, washcloth, towel, and warm water
- Scissors with pointed end
- Measuring guide
- Gauze pad
- New pouch, skin barrier, and adhesive if required
- Urinary drainage bag (many products are available)
- Mirror (optional for client self-care)

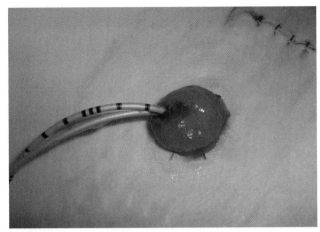

FIGURE 33-7 Viable ileal conduit stoma with stents present and normal peristomal skin and pouch. (Permission to use this copyrighted photo has been granted by the owner, Hollister Incorporated.)

IMPLEMENTATION *for Pouching an Incontinent Urinary Diversion*

STEPS	RATIONALE
1 See Standard Protocol (inside front cover).	
2 Position client to allow for easy access to stoma so that abdomen is as smooth or flat as possible. Place a towel or disposable waterproof pad under client. Provide a mirror when client is ready to observe pouching process.	Skin wrinkles on the abdomen complicate pouch application and increase tendency for leaking.
3 Prepare pouch by removing backing from barrier and adhesive; if using a cut to fit; cut opening $\frac{1}{16}$ inch (1.6 mm) to $\frac{1}{8}$ inch (3 mm) larger than stoma before removing backing (see illustration). Some pouches have a standard opening that attaches to plastic ring. Some urinary pouches have special skin barrier that melts and forms secure seal around base of stoma.	Barrier facilitates seal and protects skin. Correct size of opening keeps urine off skin and reduces risk of maceration and skin irritation. New stoma will shrink and does not reach optimal size for 6 to 8 weeks. The stoma nurse may leave a template of the stoma to use when cutting the opening.
4 Tightly roll several gauze pads separately to form "wicks."	Used to absorb urine during pouch change. Urine drains almost continuously.
5 Remove used pouch gently by pushing skin away from barrier, avoiding any tension on stents (if present). Immediately place a wick or gauze pad over stoma (see illustration). If stents are present, place gauze pad underneath tips.	Gauze keeps urine from leaking onto skin.

> **NURSE ALERT** Ureteral stents in place after surgery allow healing for ureteroenteric anastomoses. Use care to avoid tension or accidental dislodgement.

STEPS	RATIONALE
6 Cleanse skin around stoma gently with warm tap water using gauze pads. Do not scrub skin. Hold a gauze wick over stoma opening continuously	Avoid soap, lotions, or creams, which interfere with pouch adhesion. Wick prevents skin surrounding stoma from becoming wet with urine. Pouch does not adhere to wet skin.
7 If creases form near stoma, gently lift skin to smooth surface or use barrier strips or seal to fill in.	Creates smooth surface for pouch placement and prevents leaking.

STEPS	RATIONALE
8 *Apply one-piece pouch.* Hold pouch by barrier, center over stoma, and press down gently (see illustration). If stents are present, feed stents through opening in skin barrier and into pouch and then press down gently. If bedside urinary drainage bag is used, angle pouch to facilitate urine drainage.	Angling pouch avoids uneven twisting, which can disrupt seal and irritate the skin.
a. Press adhesive tape backing smoothly against skin, starting from bottom and working up and around sides.	Ensures closure completely around stoma.
b. Maintain gentle finger pressure around barrier for 1 to 2 minutes.	Ensures molding and adherence of skin barrier.

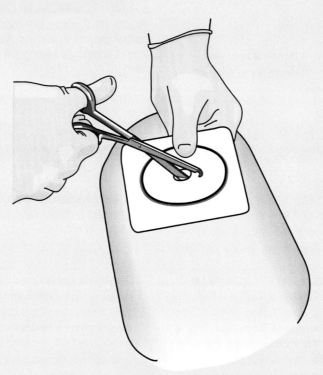

STEP 3 Cutting opening of pouch to fit stoma.

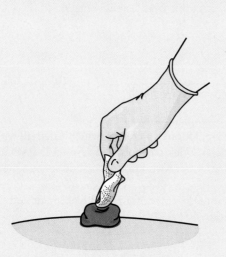

STEP 5 Holding wick in place to prevent leaking.

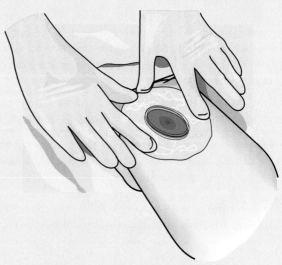

STEP 8 Press pouch firmly to secure in place.

STEPS	RATIONALE
9 *Apply two-piece pouch.* Apply flange (barrier with adhesive) as above and then snap on pouch. If client is mostly ambulatory and upright, apply pouch vertically.	Weight of urine in bag is pulled down by gravity. Pulling at an angle can disrupt the seal and create leakage.
11 Dispose of used pouch and soiled equipment in a plastic bag and place it in appropriate trash receptacle (see agency policy).	Avoids odor in the room.
12 Empty pouch when one-half to two-thirds full of urine. Measure and record urine output and characteristics. Secure valve or plug used to close pouch (see illustration).	Prevents tension on bag that can irritate skin and disrupt the seal. Pouches can be attached at night to a large drainage bag.
13 See Completion Protocol (inside front cover).	

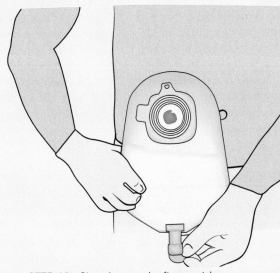

STEP 12. Clamping pouch after emptying.

EVALUATION

1 Observe urine output through stoma. Urine should be clear yellow with whitish mucus. Inspect for leakage around pouch.

2 Inspect and palpate stoma for color, shine, moistness, edema, or tenderness.

3 Observe skin for erythema or breakdown. If suture line is present, inspect for approximation and signs of inflammation.

4 Ask client to rate discomfort using pain scale.

5 Observe client performing pouch care.

Unexpected Outcomes and Related Interventions

1 Output from pouch is less than 30 ml/hr or 240 ml per 8 hours.

a. Assess for pressure or fullness in stoma region.

b. Observe for pouch leakage.

c. Stents or stoma could be blocked by blood clot or debris. Irrigation may be indicated. Notify wound care/enterostoma nurse and/or prescriber.

2 Pouch leaking urine or skin around stoma is irritated, itching, or burning.

a. Change pouch.

b. Consult wound care/enterostoma nurse.

3 Client will not participate in care of stoma.

a. Listen to client's feelings with empathy.

b. Guard against displaying disapproval or disgust while caring for client.

c. Consider if client is willing to have family member assist.

Recording and Reporting

• Record in nurses' notes type of pouch, time of change; condition and appearance of stoma and peristomal skin; character of urine; time of irrigation; and client response, including verbal and nonverbal reaction to stoma and level of participation in care.

• Record actual urinary output and characteristics of urine.

• Report abnormalities in stoma or peristomal structures and absence or decrease in urinary output to enterostoma nurse and/or prescriber.

Sample Documentation

0800 Ileal conduit stoma shiny, moist, and beefy red. 250 ml clear yellow urine with whitish mucus present in pouch. Peristomal skin intact. Suture line dry and approximated. Pouch changed with client assisting. Client correctly reapplied pouch with verbal cues. Client verbalized understanding of procedure for emptying pouch.

Special Considerations

Pediatric Considerations

- Stomas created in infancy that are placed above the umbilicus will grow with the body and will stay in the same relative anatomic position (Colwell, Goldberg, and Carmel, 2004).
- When applying a pouch on a preterm infant, use care in removing skin barrier adhesives because the skin has decreased ability to stretch (Colwell, Goldberg, and Carmel, 2004).
- Carefully assess stoma location in infants and toddlers still in diapers. Lower abdomen pouches may require rolling down the diaper so that the pouch can be placed outside the diaper (Colwell, Goldberg, and Carmel, 2004).

- Parents can help a child adjust to an ostomy through developmental stages by making stoma care a normal part of life (Colwell, Goldberg, and Carmel, 2004).

Geriatric Considerations

- Limitations in physical and visual ability may require adaptation and assistance in self-ostomy routine.

Home Care Considerations

- Referral to ostomy specialist is essential.
- Stress importance of reporting fever, chills, or back or flank pain or cloudy, foul-smelling urine to nurse or physician as soon as possible.
- At home, pouch spout should be opened and connected to larger drainage bag at night.
- All disposable pouches are odor proof. Inform clients of pouching systems available that best fit their needs.
- Pouch covers are available or can be made easily. Special underwear and sleep garments are also available.
- Advise clients when they travel to always keep spare ostomy supplies with them in case luggage gets lost.

NCLEX® Style Questions

1 What nursing action is the most important to ensure an accurate measurement of post-void residual urine?
1. Have the client void before and after catheterization.
2. Catheterize the client 30 minutes after voiding.
3. Ask the client to void and catheterize within 5 minutes.
4. Add the volumes of voided and catheterized urine.

2 Correct nursing intervention to prevent injury before removal of an indwelling catheter is demonstrated by which of the following?
1. Applying sterile gloves
2. Positioning the client in the prone position
3. Emptying urine collection bag
4. Deflating the catheter balloon

3 When should the balloon be inflated during insertion of an indwelling catheter in a male?
1. When urine appears in the tubing
2. When urine flow stops
3. After insertion of the catheter to the bifurcation point
4. After advancing the catheter a total of 3 to 4 inches

4 What should be the initial nursing action when administering an open intermittent catheter irrigation?
1. Irrigate the catheter to dislodge any encrustation.
2. Ensure that the catheter is not kinked or clamped off.

3. Wipe the connection site between the catheter and tubing with antiseptic.
4. Use catheter-tipped syringe and withdraw urine from catheter.

5 When cleansing a suprapubic catheter insertion site, what is the first nursing action?
1. Cleanse the skin close to the catheter using a circular motion.
2. Wipe the catheter nearest the skin and then up the catheter.
3. Cleanse the skin farthest away from the catheter, using a circular motion.
4. Wipe the catheter starting away from the skin down the catheter to the skin.

6 The nurse is changing the pouch on an ileal conduit. Place the following steps in correct order:
1. Smooth any creases near stoma by lifting skin or using barrier strips.
2. Dispose of used pouch and soiled equipment.
3. Hold pouch by barrier, center over stoma, and press down gently.
4. Maintain gentle finger pressure around barrier for 1 to 2 minutes.
5. Cleanse skin around stoma with warm tap water and gauze pad.
6. Press adhesive tape backing smoothly against skin, starting from the bottom and working up.

References for all chapters appear in Appendix D.

Altered Sensory Perception

34

MEDIA RESOURCES

- **evolve**   http://evolve.elsevier.com/Elkin

Meaningful sensory stimuli allow a person to learn about the environment and are necessary for healthy functioning and normal development. Many clients seeking health care have preexisting sensory alterations, whereas others might develop alterations after medical treatment. As the nurse, you play an important role in educating clients to care for sensory aids such as eye prosthetics and hearing aids. In addition, you provide care, such as eye or ear irrigations, that promotes the integrity of sensory organs.

Whenever you care for clients with sensory alterations, safety is a priority. You must be able to anticipate how the client's sensory alteration places the client at risk for injury. Orientation to any new environment, arranging an existing living environment to minimize safety hazards, and educating family and friends about ways to help clients adapt to sensory loss are just some of the interventions you may use.

In an acute care environment you may need to provide clients with more direct supervision and communicate the client's sensory loss to other health care professionals. When assisting with ambulation for a visually impaired client, stand on the client's nondominant side approximately one step ahead and have the client lightly hold your arm. Place items such as the call light, over-bed table, and telephone within the client's reach and describe their locations to the client. Do not move items without telling client.

If a client has a hearing deficit, be sure that he or she understands the communication. Always face the client before beginning to speak and make sure there is enough light for the client to see your lips. Eliminating external noises; speaking in a slow, clear, normal tone of voice; and accentuating facial gestures help the client to hear correctly. Ask clients what communication styles they prefer. Sign language, lipreading, writing with pad and pencil, or use of communication boards may be necessary for hearing-impaired clients. Teach family or friends these same techniques so that they can become a source of support.

Clients may be very sensitive about lens or prosthetic care. Accidental breakage or malfunction of the client's sensory aids may seriously impair sensory function and threaten self-esteem if the client becomes dependent on others for assistance. Most clients have established routines for cleaning contact lenses or eye prostheses. Adapt to these routines as much as possible when administering care to clients. Likewise, encourage clients to participate in care of sensory aids as much as possible. Careful handling of these devices is vital to avoid damage or injury.

A visual or hearing impairment may be caused by the presence of foreign bodies, irritants, or secretions. In the older adult or in clients who wear hearing aids, cerumen impaction can cause discomfort and further hearing loss. Inflammation or infection of the eyes may produce drainage or secretions that reduce vision. Irrigation of the eye or ear may help restore or maintain existing function. The presence of a foreign body or irritant in the eye or ear requires immediate intervention to restore function and prevent permanent sensory loss.

EVIDENCE IN PRACTICE

Boyd-Monk H: Bringing common eye emergencies into focus, *Nursing 2005* 35(12):46-51, 2005.

Chemical exposures to the eye require immediate flushing of the eye. The primary intervention is to initially irrigate the eye with tap water or milk for at least 15 minutes and bring the individual and the chemical container to the nearest emergency department (ED). Within the ED use normal saline to continue the eye irrigation. Use Litmus paper to assess the pH of the conjunctiva. The pH of the eye should be between 7.3 and 7.6 before irrigation is stopped. While acids can cause superficial corneal damage, alkalis such as ammonia can permanently impair vision by damaging the cornea and other parts of the eye.

NURSING DIAGNOSES

An appropriate nursing diagnosis associated with a visual or hearing impairment is **disturbed sensory perception** (visual/auditory), how they perceive and respond to environmental stimuli. Clients with a hearing loss may also have **impaired verbal communication,** depending on their ability to use and understand language. Clients requiring irrigations of the eye or assistance with eye prostheses may be at **risk for infection** if the client does not use the proper technique. A client with a sensory impairment in an unfamiliar environment such as a hospital room is especially at **risk for injury. Pain (acute** or **chronic)** may apply when injury or infection involves the eye or ear. Clients who are unable to demonstrate proper care techniques may have **deficient knowledge.** Visual or hearing impairments also affect psychosocial status, resulting in **impaired social interaction, social isolation, fear,** or **anxiety.**

SKILL 34.1 | Caring for an Eye Prosthesis

As a result of tumor, infection, congenital blindness, or severe trauma to the eye, clients need an enucleation, a procedure involving the complete removal of the eyeball. All that remain are the socket and eyelids. For obvious cosmetic purposes, clients who had an enucleation are often fitted with an artificial eye, or prosthesis.

Artificial eyes are made of glass and plastic and fit just behind the client's eyelids. Each prosthesis is designed to take on the appearance of the client's natural iris, pupil, and sclera. Prostheses are relatively easy to remove and insert and can be worn day and night. The prosthesis can be cleaned with soap and water daily or any time up to several months based on client preference.

ASSESSMENT

1 Assess client's routines for prosthetic care: frequency, method of cleaning, and type of cleaning solution. *Rationale: Determines compliance with and knowledge of self-care.*
2 Inspect eyes to determine which eye is artificial (no movement or pupillary reaction to light).
3 Assess client's ability to remove, clean, and reinsert prosthesis. *Rationale: Identifies if further education is needed.*
4 Inspect surrounding tissues of eyelid and eye socket for inflammation, tenderness, swelling, or drainage after prosthesis removal. Wear gloves during this evaluation. *Rationale: Infections can spread easily to neighboring eye, underlying sinuses, or brain tissue.*

PLANNING

Expected Outcomes focus on client's comfort, prevention of infection, and understanding of prosthetic care.
1 Client verbalizes feelings regarding prosthesis removal.
2 Client's eyelid margins and eye socket are clean and of normal pink color, with lashes turned away from prosthesis.
3 Client demonstrates no signs of infection such as redness, tenderness, swelling, or discharge of socket or eyelid margins.
4 Client verbalizes that prosthetic eye fits comfortably.
5 Client demonstrates proper technique for removing, cleaning, and reinserting prosthesis.

Delegation Considerations
The skills of removal, cleansing, and insertion of an eye prosthesis may be delegated. The nurse directs personnel by:
• Stressing the importance of careful handling of the device.
• Informing care provider of types of findings to report (e.g., inflammation, drainage).

Equipment

- Soft washcloth or cotton gauze square
- Washbasin with warm water or saline
- 4 × 4 gauze pads
- Mild soap
- Bath towel
- Suction device (e.g., rubber bulb syringe, medicine dropper bulb) (*Optional:* bulb syringe removes prosthesis by suction if manual removal is not successful.)
- Clean gloves
- Covered plastic storage case

IMPLEMENTATION *for Caring for an Eye Prosthesis*

STEPS	RATIONALE
1 See Standard Protocol (inside front cover).	
2 Place towel just below client's face.	Catches prosthesis if accidentally dropped and avoids breakage or scratching. Absorbs excess irrigation fluid.
3 Have client look up. With thumb, gently retract lower eyelid against lower orbital ridge (see illustration).	Exposes lower edge of eye prosthesis.
4 Exert slight pressure below eyelid (see illustration). If prosthesis does not slide out, use bulb syringe or medicine dropper bulb to apply direct suction to prosthesis.	Maneuver breaks suction, causing prosthesis to rise and slide out of socket (Kolberg Ocular Prosthetics, 2005).
5 Place facecloth in bottom of basin or sink. Place prosthesis in palm of hand and clean with mild soap and water or plain saline by rubbing between thumb and index finger.	Provides cushion to prevent breakage of prosthesis. Tears and secretions containing microorganisms may collect on surface of prosthesis. Soap is less irritating than detergents.

> **COMMUNICATION TIP** During this time make client feel at ease by using a calm, gentle approach. Now is a good time to ask, "Tell me how often you find it necessary to clean your artificial eye. Have you ever had difficulty with that?"

STEPS	RATIONALE
6 Rinse well under running tap water or rinse with normal saline and dry with soft washcloth (see illustration).	Soft cloth maintains shiny appearance of prosthesis. Paper towel may dull finish. Removes stubborn deposits.
7 If client is not to have prosthesis reinserted, store in sterile saline or water in plastic storage case. Label with client's name and room number.	Proper storage prevents damage, infection, and loss (Kolberg Ocular Prosthetics, 2004).
8 Clean eyelid margins and socket.	
a. Retract upper and lower eyelids with thumb and index finger. (Inspection can be done at this time.)	Exposes eye socket.
b. Wash socket with washcloth or gauze square moistened in warm water or saline.	Removes secretions that may contain microorganisms.

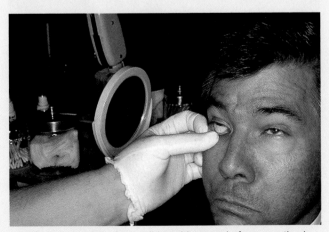

STEP 3 Retraction of lower lid to aid removal of eye prosthesis.

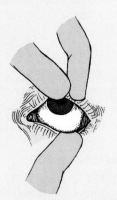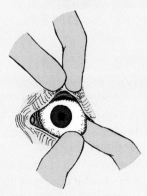

STEP 4 Exertion of pressure below eyelid and removal of prosthesis.

STEPS	RATIONALE

c. Thoroughly pat dry, removing excess moisture with gauze pads.

Removes moisture that can harbor microorganisms.

d. Wash eyelid margins with mild soap and water. Wipe from inner to outer canthus, using a clean part of cloth with each wipe. Dry eyelids by patting.

Prevents secretions from entering tear duct in inner canthus. Prevents trauma to mucous membranes.

> **NURSE ALERT**   If crusts are difficult to remove, place moistened cloth over eyelids for several minutes during cleaning. This will help to remove crusts.

9 Moisten prosthesis with water or saline.

Makes insertion easier because dry plastic rubs against tissue surfaces.

10 Retract client's upper eyelid with index finger or thumb of nondominant hand (see illustration).

Eases prosthesis insertion.

11 With dominant hand, hold prosthesis so that notched or pointed edge is positioned toward nose. Iris faces outward. Note presence and orientation of colored dot at margin of prosthesis.

Correct positioning of prosthesis ensures proper fit (Kolberg Ocular Prosthetics, 2004).

A colored dot usually indicates "up" on an artificial eye.

12 Slide prosthesis up under upper eyelid as far as possible. Then push down lower lid to allow prosthesis to slip into place.

Prosthesis will fit evenly into socket.

> **NURSE ALERT**   Do not force prosthesis into socket.

13 Gently wipe away excess fluid if necessary.

Wipe toward nose to prevent dislodgement. Reduces transmission of microorganisms.

14 See Completion Protocol (inside front cover).

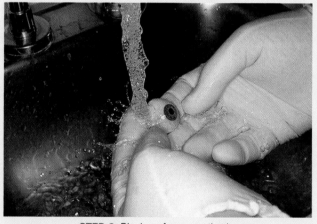

STEP 6 Rinsing of eye prosthesis.

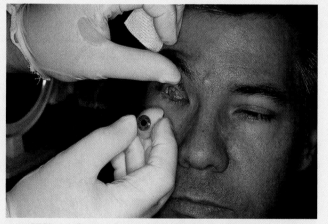

STEP 10 Replacement of eye prosthesis into eye socket.

EVALUATION

1 Ask client about feelings regarding prosthesis removal.
2 Inspect eyelids and eye socket for cleanliness, color, and position of eyelashes.
3 Inspect eyelids and socket for signs of infection.
4 Ask client if prosthesis fits comfortably.
5 Observe client demonstrating technique for prosthesis care.

Unexpected Outcomes and Related Interventions

1 Client states prosthesis feels uncomfortable.
a. Reposition prosthesis.
b. Remove prosthesis. Inspect for any rough areas.
c. Notify physician or advanced practice nurse of assessment findings.

2 Inflammation develops in tissues of socket or lid margins.

a. Remove prosthesis for a few days if necessary. Clean eyelid and socket.

b. Provide client with comfortable eye patch until inflammation subsides.

3 Client develops excessive, purulent, or foul-smelling drainage.

a. Wearing clean gloves, remove prosthesis and clean area. Inspect socket and surrounding tissue.

b. Place prosthesis in appropriate cleaning and storage solution.

c. Provide eye patch if desired.

d. Instruct client on proper handwashing and procedures to use to help reduce infection.

e. Notify physician or advanced practice nurse of assessment findings.

4 Client is unable to perform prosthesis care correctly.

a. Teach and demonstrate prosthetic care to client and significant other.

b. Provide literature or media regarding prosthetic eye care.

c. Observe return demonstration until correctly performed.

Recording and Reporting

- Document prosthetic eye on admission assessment note.
- Record appearance and condition of eye socket.
- Record and report any signs and symptoms of infection involving eye socket.
- Record removal of prosthesis and storage location if not reinserted after cleaning.

Sample Documentation

1400 Client reports tenderness around left artificial eye. Prosthesis removed. No scratches or rough edges noted on prosthesis. Slight redness and edema noted at outer canthus. Socket and eyelids cleaned with normal saline. Client agrees not to wear prosthesis until symptoms improve. Prosthesis cleaned, stored, and labeled. Eye patch provided.

Special Considerations
Pediatric Considerations

- Prostheses are easily removed; the child may accidentally dislodge this during play. Encourage to explain to child that this "special eye" may fall out but can be easily put back in place after it has been properly cleaned (Hockenberry and Wilson, 2007).

Geriatric Considerations

- Older adults normally experience a reduction in visual function. With only one eye, the older adult may require greater assistance with respect to safety precautions.
- If an older adult has underlying thyroid disease and has some exophthalmos, recommend that an oculist determine if the prosthesis fits appropriately (Ebersole, Hess, and Luggen, 2004).

Home Care Considerations

- If a client becomes disabled and suffers an inability to perform self-care measures on a regular basis, be sure the prosthesis is cleaned regularly to prevent possible infection.
- Assess client's home environment for resources needed to perform cleaning.
- Determine if client is able to use equipment available in the home to care for prosthesis.

SKILL 34.2 Eye Irrigations

Eye irrigations effectively flush out exudates, irritating solutions, or foreign bodies from the eye. The procedure is typically used in emergency situations when a foreign object or some other substance has entered the eye. When a chemical or irritating substance contaminates the eyes, irrigate immediately with copious amounts of water or milk (Phipps and others, 2003). In addition, contact lens wearers may need eye irrigation to wash out particles of dust or fibers causing eye irritation.

ASSESSMENT

1 Assess reason for eye irrigation by obtaining a history of the injury from the client. *Rationale: Determines amount, type of solution, and immediacy of treatment.*

2 Assess eye for redness, excessive tearing, and discharge. Assess eyelids and lacrimal glands for edema. Assess visual acuity before and after treatment. Ask client about itching, burning, pain, blurred vision, or photophobia (Phipps and others, 2003). *Rationale: Provides baseline for condition of eye. Topical anesthetic drops may need to be administered to provide comfort.*

3 Assess client's ability to cooperate. *Rationale: Extra assistance may be needed.*

PLANNING

Expected Outcomes focus on client's physical and psychological comfort and improving vision.

1 Client verbalizes reduced pain/burning/itching after eye irrigation.

2 Client demonstrates minimal anxiety during and after irrigation.

3 Client verbalizes improved visual acuity after eye irrigation.

4 Client maintains normal pupillary reaction and eye movement after irrigation.

Delegation Considerations

The skill of eye irrigation cannot be delegated. The nurse directs personnel by:

- Instructing to report any client complaint of discomfort or excess tearing.

Equipment

- Prescribed irrigating solution: volume usually varies from 30 to 180 ml at 90° to 100° F (about 32° to 38° C). (For chemical flushing, use tap water or prescribed intravenous [IV] fluid in volume to provide continuous irrigation over 15 minutes.)

- Sterile basin for solution
- Curved emesis basin
- Waterproof pad or towel
- 4 × 4 inch gauze pads
- Soft bulb syringe, eye dropper, or IV tubing
- Clean gloves
- Penlight

IMPLEMENTATION *for Eye Irrigations*

STEPS	RATIONALE
1 See Standard Protocol (inside front cover).	
2 Remove contact lenses (if possible) before beginning irrigation (Box 34-1).	Prompt removal of lenses is needed to safely and completely irrigate foreign substances from client's eyes.
3 Assist client to side-lying position on the same side as the affected eye. Turn head toward affected eye.	Irrigation solution will flow from inner to outer canthus, preventing contamination of unaffected eye and nasolacrimal duct.

> **COMMUNICATION TIP** Reassure client that eye can be closed periodically and that no object will touch eye.

4 Place waterproof pad under client's face.	
5 With 4 × 4 gauze moistened in prescribed solution (or normal saline), gently clean eyelid margins and eyelashes from inner to outer canthus.	Minimizes transfer of debris from lids or lashes into eye during irrigation.
6 Place curved emesis basin just below client's cheek on side of affected eye.	Catches irrigation fluid.
7 Explain next steps to client and encourage relaxation. With gloved finger, gently retract upper and lower eyelids to expose conjunctival sacs. To hold lids open, apply gentle pressure to lower bony orbit and bony prominence beneath eyebrow. Do not apply pressure over eye.	Retraction minimizes blinking and allows irrigation of conjunctiva.

BOX 34-1 Removal of Contact Lenses

Soft Lenses (Wear Gloves)

- If possible, have client look straight ahead. Retract lower eyelid and expose lower edge of lens.
- Using pad of index finger, slide lens off cornea to white of eye.
- Pull upper eyelid down gently with thumb of other hand and compress lens slightly between thumb and index finger.
- Gently pinch lens and lift out without allowing edges to stick together.
- If lens edges stick together, place lens in palm and soak thoroughly with sterile saline.
- Place lens in storage case.
- Follow procedure for cleansing and disinfecting.

Rigid Lenses (Wear Gloves if Drainage Is Suspected or Present)

- Be sure lens is positioned directly over cornea. If it is not, have client close eyelids. Place index and middle fingers of one hand beside the lens and gently but firmly massage lens back over cornea.
- Place index finger on outer corner of client's eye and draw skin gently back toward ear.
- Ask client to blink. Do not release pressure on lids until blink is completed.
- If lens fails to pop out, gently retract eyelid beyond edges of lens. Press lower eyelid gently against lower edge of lens.
- If client is unable to assist, use a specially designed suction cup. Place cup on center of lens and, while applying suction, gently remove lens off client's cornea.
- Place lens in storage case.
- Follow procedure for cleansing and disinfecting.

STEPS	RATIONALE

8 Hold irrigating syringe, dropper, or IV tubing approximately 1 inch (2.5 cm) from the inner canthus.

If irrigator touches eye, there is risk of injury.

> **COMMUNICATION TIP** Use a calm, confident, soft voice when talking with client and reinforcing importance of the procedure. For example, "You are doing great; just relax; that's it. We need to flush this out of your eye as completely as possible to lessen the chance of an eye injury."

9 Ask client to look up. Gently irrigate with a steady stream toward lower conjunctival sac, moving from inner to outer canthus (see illustration).

Allows irrigation solution to flow freely, washing out irritant from eye.

10 Allow client to close the eye periodically.

Lid closure moves secretions from upper to lower conjunctival sac. This also gives client a break while reducing anxiety.

11 Continue irrigation until you use all solution or secretions have been cleared. (NOTE: An irrigation of 15 minutes or more is needed to flush chemicals.)

Assessment of eye secretion pH may be necessary if eye was exposed to an acidic or basic solution during injury (Boyd-Monk, 2005).

12 Dry eyelids and facial area with sterile cotton ball.

13 See Completion Protocol (inside front cover).

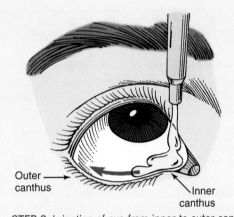

STEP 9 Irrigation of eye from inner to outer canthus.

EVALUATION

1 Assess client's comfort level after eye irrigation.

2 Observe for verbal and nonverbal signs of anxiety during irrigation.

3 Ask client if vision is blurred after irrigation.

4 Complete post-irrigation visual acuity.

5 Observe pupillary reaction (to light and accommodation) and extraocular eye movement.

Unexpected Outcomes and Related Interventions

1 Client demonstrates extreme anxiety during irrigation.

a. Reinforce rationale for irrigation.

b. Allow client to close eye periodically during irrigation.

c. Instruct client to take slow, deep breaths.

d. Seek extra assistance if needed to prevent injury.

2 Client complains of pain and foreign body sensation in eye after irrigation. Excessive tearing and photophobia noted.

a. Advise client to close the eye and avoid eye movement.

b. Notify physician or advanced practice nurse of findings.

Recording and Reporting

- Record in nurses' notes condition of eye, type and amount of solution used for irrigation, length of time for irrigation, and client's report of pain and visual status.

- Report continued symptoms of pain and visual blurring to physician or advanced practice nurse.

Sample Documentation

0800 Client states having blurred vision and tenderness in left eye. Yellow, crusty drainage noted on eyelids with slight edema and redness of conjunctiva. Eyelids cleaned and eye irrigated with 30 ml warm, sterile, normal saline for 10 minutes. Neosporin ophthalmic ointment applied.

0900 Client states that eye "feels better." Vision clearer. Pupils equal, round, reactive to light, accommodation. Normal eye movements noted. Conjunctiva remains red with slight edema.

Special Considerations
Pediatric Considerations

- Children with foreign bodies or chemicals in the eye become panicked. You may need to use a mummy restraint (see Chapter 3) so that the eye can be irrigated safely and quickly and thus reduce the risk of injury (Hockenberry and Wilson, 2007).
- Parents need education and demonstration when having to continue eye irrigations at home (Hockenberry and Wilson, 2007).

Geriatric Considerations

- Due to changes in fine motor coordination or mobility, an older adult who needs eye irrigations in the home setting may need the assistance of a family member or friend. Therefore the significant other must be present for client teaching (Ebersole and others, 2004).

Home Care Considerations

- If client suffered injury in the home, instruct in ways to minimize chemical injuries in the future. Have client wear eye goggles when working with chemicals or in a dusty environment (Occupational Safety & Health Administration, 2005).
- Instruct client and family about how to perform emergency irrigation of the eye.

SKILL 34.3   Caring for Clients with Hearing Aids

Hearing is vital for normal communication and orientation to sounds in the environment. Sensorineural hearing loss is a major disabling condition in the United States, affecting 34 million people (Sommer and Sommer, 2002). For people with hearing loss, a proper hearing aid improves the ability to hear and understand spoken words. Hearing aids amplify sound so that it is heard at a more effective level. All aids have four basic components:

1. A microphone, which receives and converts sound into electrical signals
2. An amplifier, which increases the strength of the electrical signal
3. A receiver, which converts the strengthened signal back into sound
4. A power source (batteries)

In addition, programmable hearing aids are now available. The programmable hearing aids are in analog and digital formats. Clients seeking these aids need to be evaluated by a licensed audiologist to determine the type of aid and which frequencies are needed for the individual client (National Institute on Deafness and Other Communication Disorders [NIDCD], 2004). These aids input signals rather than just amplifying the sounds. An audiologist programs the aid with the use of a computer specific to a client's hearing impairment. These aids are adjusted to accommodate the range of the client's residual hearing. Programmable aids independently amplify high-frequency (soft-spoken consonants) from low-frequency (loudly spoken vowels) sounds; this process occurs rapidly and continuously (Ebersole and others, 2004). Several styles of hearing aids are available to clients today.

1. *In-the-ear* (ITE) hearing aids fit completely in the outer ear and are used for mild-to-severe hearing loss (Figure 34-1). The plastic case is large enough to hold internal circuitry and external controls. ITE aids can hold added technical mechanisms such as a telecoil, a small magnetic coil contained in the hearing aid that improves sound transmission during telephone calls. ITE aids can be damaged by earwax and ear drainage, and their small size can cause adjustment problems and feedback. They are not usually worn by children because the casings need to be replaced as the ear grows.
2. *Behind-the-ear* (BTE) hearing aids are worn behind the ear and are connected to a plastic earmold that fits inside the outer ear. The components are held in a case behind the ear. Sound travels through the earmold into the ear. People of all ages wear BTE aids for mild-to-profound hearing loss (Figure 34-2). Poorly fitting BTE earmolds can cause feedback, a whistling sound caused by the fit of the hearing aid. BTE aids are better protected from earwax.
3. *Canal aids* fit into the ear canal and are available in two sizes. The *in-the-canal* hearing aid is customized to fit the size and shape of the ear canal and is used for mild-to-moderately severe hearing loss. A *completely-in-canal* hearing aid is largely concealed in the ear canal and is used for mild-to-moderately severe hearing loss (Figure 34-3). Because of their small size, canal aids may be difficult for the user to adjust and remove and may not be able to hold additional devices, such as a telecoil. Canal aids can also be damaged by earwax and ear drainage. They are not typically recommended for children.

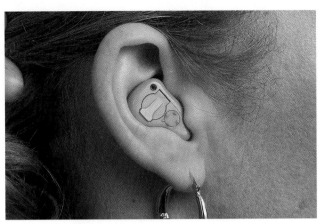

FIGURE 34-1 In-the-ear hearing aid.

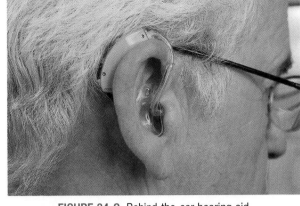

FIGURE 34-2 Behind-the-ear hearing aid.

4 *Body aids* are used by people with mild-to-profound hearing loss. The aid is attached to a belt or a pocket and connected to the ear by a wire. Because of its large size, it incorporates many signal processing options, but it is usually used only when other types of aids cannot be used (National Institute on Deafness and Other Communication Disorders [NIDCD], 2004).

ASSESSMENT

1 Observe whether client can hear clearly with use of aid by talking slowly and clearly in normal tone of voice. *Rationale: Inability to hear may indicate faulty function of hearing aid or may indicate that aid is no longer effective for client's auditory loss.*

2 Assess client's knowledge of and routines for cleansing and caring for hearing aid. *Rationale: Determines compliance with and knowledge of self-care.*

3 Assess if hearing aid is working by removing from client's ear. Close battery case and turn volume slowly to high. Cup hand over hearing aid. If squealing sound (feedback) is heard, it is working. If no sound is heard, replace batteries and test again. *Rationale: May indicate malfunctioning of hearing aid.*

4 Assess client for any unusual physical or auditory signs/symptoms (pain, itching, redness, discharge, odor, tinnitus, decreased acuity). *Rationale: May indicate injury, infection, or cerumen accumulation.*

5 Inspect earmold for cracked or rough edges. *Rationale: Poorly fitting hearing aids cause irritation and/or discomfort to external ear canal.*

6 Inspect for accumulation of cerumen around aid and plugging of opening in aid. *Rationale: Cerumen can block sound reception.*

PLANNING

Expected Outcomes focus on facilitating communication and promoting comfort and appropriate self-care.

1 Client hears conversation spoken in normal tone of voice and responds appropriately.

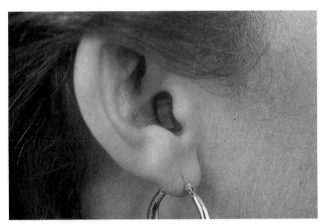

FIGURE 34-3 Completely-in-canal hearing aid.

2 Client responds appropriately to environmental sounds.

3 Client demonstrates proper care of the hearing aid.

4 Client verbalizes that the aid fits comfortably.

Delegation Considerations

The skill of caring for a hearing aid may be delegated. The nurse directs personnel by:

- Confirming that care provider knows proper way to care for prosthetic device.
- Clarifying communication tips to use for individual client while aid is being cleaned.
- Having care provider report presence of any drainage.

Equipment

- Soft towel and washcloth
- Warm soap and water
- Brush or wax loop
- Storage case
- Clean gloves (if drainage is present)

IMPLEMENTATION *for Caring For Clients with Hearing Aids*

STEPS	RATIONALE
1 See Standard Protocol (inside front cover).	
2 Have equipment at bedside for client to see.	Makes client a partner in care.
3 Remove hearing aid. Apply gloves if drainage is present.	Reduces transmission of microorganisms.
a. Have client turn hearing aid volume off. Grasp aid securely and gently remove device following natural ear contour.	Prevents feedback (whistling) during removal. Prevents dropping hearing aid. Prevents injury to ear.
4 Cleaning hearing aid	
a. Place towel over work surface. Wipe aid with soft washcloth while holding over towel. Use wax loop or brush (supplied with aid) to clean holes in hearing aid.	Prevents breakage if dropped. Impaction of wax blocks normal sound transmission.

> **NURSE ALERT** Caring for a hearing aid should protect the device from moisture, heat, breakage, and loss.

> **COMMUNICATION TIP** Ask client to share at this time any tips for care of the aid. Use the time to discuss whether the client is having any difficulty hearing or using the aid at home, at work, or in social situations. When clients are children, involve parents.

STEPS	RATIONALE
b. Open battery door and allow it to air dry.	Increases battery life and allows moisture to evaporate.
c. Wash ear canal with washcloth moistened in soap and water. Rinse and dry.	Removes cerumen from ear canal. Removes soap residue and water that may harbor microbes or damage hearing aid.
d. If hearing aid is to be stored, place in dry storage case with desiccant material. Label case with client's name and room number. If more than one aid, note right or left.	Protects hearing aid against damage, moisture, and breakage.
5 Inserting hearing aid	
a. Check batteries (see Assessment).	
b. Identify hearing aid as either right (marked "R" or red color coded) or left (marked "L" or blue color coded).	Proper orientation prevents damage and injury.
c. Hold aid so that canal—long portion with hole(s)—is at the bottom. Guide aid along client's cheek and bring it to the ear.	Proper orientation is important for hearing aid insertion.
d. Insert canal portion of aid into ear first. Use other hand to pull up and back on outer ear. Gently push aid into ear canal until it is in place and fits snugly in midline.	Ensures correct positioning of aid within ear canal.
e. Adjust or have client adjust volume gradually to comfortable level for talking to client in regular voice 3 to 4 feet away. Rotate volume control toward nose to increase volume and away from nose to decrease volume.	

> **NURSE ALERT** Programmable aids have the volume control located on the remote. For most clients, hearing aids work best at lower volume settings.

6 See Completion Protocol (inside front cover).

EVALUATION

1 Talk with client in a normal tone of voice and observe response.
2 Observe client's response to environmental sounds.
3 Observe client perform hearing aid care (removal, cleaning, and reinsertion).
4 Ask client about comfort after hearing aid insertion.

Unexpected Outcomes and Related Interventions

1 Client is unable to hear conversations or environmental sounds clearly. Client's verbal responses are inappropriate.
a. Remove hearing aid and check battery for power and correct placement.

b. Inspect earmold and ear canal for cerumen blockage.

c. Change volume setting as needed.

d. If problems persist, contact audiologist or hearing aid specialist.

2 Client is unable to perform care of hearing aid.

a. Demonstrate correct aid care and offer return demonstration.

b. Consider instructing family member or friend who will be available to client.

c. Have significant other present for client teaching.

3 Client complains of ear discomfort and may complain of whistling sound.

a. Remove aid and reinsert.

b. Assess external ear for signs of inflammation.

c. If problems persist, contact audiologist or hearing aid specialist.

Recording and Reporting

- Record that hearing aid is removed and stored if client is going for surgery or special procedure. Be sure to document where or with whom aid is stored.
- Report to nursing staff and document on plan of care tips that promote communication with client.
- Record client's preferred communication techniques.
- Record and report any signs or symptoms of infection or injury or sudden decrease in hearing acuity to physician or advanced practice nurse.

Sample Documentation

1000 Client responds inappropriately to questions. Unable to hear normal conversation tone. States he hears "an echo." Volume turned down on ITE aid in right ear. Daughter states that client frequently turns the volume up so he can "hear better." Reviewed proper volume settings and improved listening techniques with client and daughter.

Special Considerations

Pediatric Considerations

- As children grow older, they can become self conscious of a hearing aid. Changes in hair style may assist some children in overcoming self-consciousness (Hockenberry and Wilson, 2007).
- Changes in style and size occur as child gets bigger.

Geriatric Considerations

- The small size of some hearing aids may make it difficult for older adults to handle and manipulate the devices. Clients should contact their hearing aid specialist for assistance. Family members may be able to assist with care of device.
- High-pitched signals associated with consonants *f, p, t, k, ch, sh,* and *st* are more difficult to hear clearly as people age (Ebersole and others, 2004).
- Inappropriate responses to questions or situations, inattentiveness, difficulty following instructions, monopolization of conversation should alert you or family members that the client may have some hearing loss that needs to be evaluated. People incorrectly may assume the client is confused (Ebersole and others, 2004).
- Be alert for client assessment findings that may indicate some depression. Hearing loss and depression are common, and correction of hearing loss may actually resolve depression in some clients (Slaven, 2003).
- Age-related hearing loss, presbycusis, is common. Clients and their families can overcome this auditory change by speaking slowly and clearly. Not all clients with this type of hearing loss require a hearing aid (Ebersole and others, 2004).

Home Care Considerations

- Initial use of hearing aid should be restricted to quiet situations in the home. Clients need to adjust gradually to voices and household sounds (Ebersole and others, 2004).
- Avoid exposure of aid to extreme heat or cold. Do not leave in case near stove, heater, or sunny window. Do not use with hair dryer on hot settings or with sunlamp.
- Remove aid for bathing and when at hair stylist. Hair spray tends to clog hearing aid.

Long-Term Care Considerations

- Because of potential high number of hearing aids in long-term care facilities, clients and their families need to clearly label hearing aid to prevent loss.
- Always store hearing aid in the client's bedside table.
- When possible, request that family buy an extra battery to keep in client's bedside table.
- Instruct clients not to remove their aids in common rooms (e.g., sunroom, recreation areas).

SKILL 34.4 Ear Irrigations

The common indications for irrigation of the external ear are presence of certain foreign bodies and buildup of cerumen. The procedure is not without potential hazards. Damage to the external auditory meatus may occur by scratching the lining of the canal if the client suddenly moves or if there is inadequate control of the irrigating syringe (Phipps and others, 2003). Improperly drying the ear may lead to acute otitis externa (infection of the outer ear). If the client moves suddenly during irrigation, the tympanic membrane can be perforated. Water pressure can also cause perforation. The ear should never be irrigated if vegetable matter or an insect is present in the canal; the tympanic membrane is ruptured; or the client has otitis externa, myringotomy tubes, or a mastoid cavity (Phipps and others, 2003). Irrigations should be performed with liquid warmed to body temperature to avoid vertigo or nausea in clients (McKenry and others, 2006).

In addition to irrigation, cerumen can be removed by use of a curette, which is performed by a physician or advanced practice nurse. Instillation of ceruminolytic agents that soften and loosen the matter for cleaning is another alternative.

ASSESSMENT

1 Review prescriber's order, including solution to be instilled and affected ear(s) to receive irrigation. *Rationale: Ensures safe and correct administration of irrigation solution.*

2 Review medical history for ruptured tympanic membrane, myringotomy tubes, mastoid cavity, or surgery of auditory canal. *Rationale: These factors contraindicate ear irrigation.*

3 Inspect pinna and external auditory meatus for redness, swelling, drainage, abrasions, and presence of cerumen or foreign objects. *Rationale: Provides baseline information to monitor effects of irrigation.*

a. Attempt to remove foreign object in ear by straightening ear canal. *Rationale: Straightening of canal may cause object to fall out and negate need for irrigation.*

b. If vegetable matter (e.g., dried bean or pea) is occluding canal, do not perform irrigation. *Rationale: Irrigant may cause object to absorb solution and swell, causing further damage.*

4 Use an otoscope to inspect deeper portions of the auditory canal and tympanic membrane (Figure 34-4). *Rationale: If client's tympanic membrane (eardrum) is not intact, irrigation is contraindicated.*

5 Assess client's comfort level using a scale of 0 to 10. *Rationale: Provides baseline to evaluate changes in client's condition. Presence of pain is symptomatic of ear infection or inflammation.*

6 Assess client's hearing ability in the affected ear. *Rationale: Occlusion of canal by cerumen or foreign object can impair hearing.*

7 Assess client's knowledge of proper ear care. *Rationale: May indicate need for instruction regarding hygiene.*

PLANNING

Expected Outcomes focus on client comfort and improved auditory perception.

1 Client denies increased pain, using a scale of 0 to 10, during instillation.

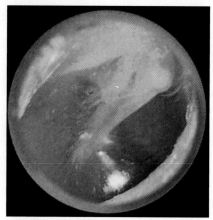

FIGURE 34-4 Normal tympanic membrane.

2 Client verbalizes increased comfort, using a scale of 0 to 10, after irrigation.

3 Client's ear canal is clear of discharge, cerumen, or foreign material after irrigation.

4 Client demonstrates improved hearing acuity in affected ear after irrigation.

5 Client describes proper ear care techniques.

Delegation Considerations

The skill of irrigating the external ear cannot be delegated. The nurse directs personnel by:

• Instructing to report any ear drainage or client's report of discomfort.

Equipment

• Clean gloves
• Otoscope (optional)
• Irrigation syringe
• Emesis basin
• Towel
• Cotton balls or 4 × 4 gauze
• Prescribed sterile irrigating solution warmed to body temperature or mineral oil, over-the-counter softener
• Medication administration record (MAR) or computer printout

IMPLEMENTATION *for Ear Irrigations*

STEPS	RATIONALE
1 See Standard Protocol (inside front cover).	
2 ✋ Assist client to a sitting or lying position with head tilted forward and toward the affected ear. Place towel or waterproof pad under client's head and shoulder. Have client help hold basin under affected ear (see illustration).	Position minimizes leakage of fluids around neck and facial area. Solution will flow from ear canal to basin.
3 Pour prescribed irrigating solution into sterile basin. Check the temperature of the solution (98.6° F [37° C]) by pouring a small drop on your inner forearm.	Solution that is too hot or too cold can cause nausea, vertigo, and vomiting (Phipps and others, 2003).

> **NURSE ALERT** Advise client to not make any sudden moves to prevent trauma to the ear.

STEPS	RATIONALE
4 Gently clean auricle and outer ear canal with moistened cotton applicator. Do not force drainage or cerumen into ear canal.	
5 Fill irrigating syringe with solution, and expel air.	Prevents sudden expulsion of fluid.
6 For adults and children over age 3 years, gently pull pinna up and back. In children 3 years or younger, pinna should be pulled down and back (Phipps and others, 2003; Hockenberry and Wilson, 2007). Place the tip of the irrigating device just inside the external meatus. Leave a space around the irrigating tip and canal.	Pulling of pinna straightens external ear canal. Prevents obstruction of canal with device, which can lead to increased pressure on tympanic membrane.
7 Direct the fluid slowly and gently toward the superior aspect of the ear canal. Brace hand holding syringe against other hand holding ear. Do not occlude canal with syringe.	Fluid is directed back behind impacted cerumen. Technique prevents syringe tip from going deep in canal should client move.

COMMUNICATION TIP Talk in a confident, calm voice to help the client relax. As you begin the irrigation, say, "Now you are going to feel the warm water. I am going to be sure to do this gently. If you feel any discomfort at all, let me know."

STEPS	RATIONALE
8 Maintain the flow of irrigation in a steady stream until you see pieces of cerumen flow from the canal.	Constant flow of fluid loosens cerumen.
9 Periodically ask if client is experiencing pain, nausea, or vertigo.	Symptoms indicate irrigating solution is too hot or too cold or instilled with too much pressure.
10 Drain excessive fluid from ear by having client tilt head toward affected side.	Excess fluid may promote microorganism growth.
11 Dry canal gently with a cotton-ball.	Drying prevents buildup of moisture that can lead to otitis externa.
12 See Completion Protocol (inside front cover).	

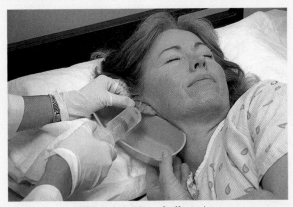

STEP 2 Irrigation of affected ear.

EVALUATION

1 Evaluate severity of pain using pain scale during and after irrigation.
2 Inspect condition of external meatus and ear canal.
3 Evaluate hearing acuity in affected ear after irrigation.
4 Ask client to describe proper ear care techniques.

Unexpected Outcomes and Related Interventions

1 Client complains of increased ear pain during irrigation.
  a. Discontinue irrigation and notify physician or advanced practice nurse.

2 Client's ear canal remains occluded. Client's hearing acuity has not improved in the affected ear.
a. Repeat irrigation if prescribed.
b. If condition persists, notify physician or advanced practice nurse.

Recording and Reporting

- Record procedure, amount of solution instilled, time of administration, and ear receiving irrigation. Do not chart medicated irrigation until *after* it is given to client.
- Record appearance of external ear and client's hearing acuity.
- Report adverse effects/client response to physician or advanced practice nurse.

Sample Documentation

1000 Client reports difficulty hearing in right ear. Cerumen plug noted in canal. Irrigated right ear with 50 ml warm normal saline. Return fluid clear with brown particles. No complaints of pain or discomfort. States that hearing "is fine." Responding appropriately to normal conversation tone. Right ear canal clear.

Special Considerations
Pediatric Considerations

- Be certain that child's head is immobilized to prevent puncturing eardrum.
- Ask parent to help calm child during procedure.

Geriatric Considerations

- Older adults often require ongoing ear care for cerumen removal. Use of a softening agent such as slightly warmed mineral oil (0.5 to 1 ml) twice daily for several days before irrigation is helpful (National Institute on Deafness and Other Communication Disorders [NIDCD], 2005).
- Older adults with higher risk of cerumen impaction include those with large amounts of ear canal hair, those with benign growths that narrow the ear canal, and those who habitually wear hearing aids (Ebersole and others, 2004).

Home Care Considerations

- Instruct client to clean ears with a damp washcloth wrapped around a finger. Do not use a cotton-tipped applicator.
- If client uses a ceruminolytic agent, instruct that these are softening products and that they will not remove the impaction (McKenry and others, 2006).

NCLEX® Style Questions

1 The nurse should question an order for an ear irrigation if the client has a history of:
1. Myringotomy tubes
2. Migraine headaches
3. Cerumen accumulation
4. Hearing impairment

2 How should the nurse position a 26-month-old child's ear during irrigation?
1. Without pulling on the earlobes
2. While pulling the pinna down and back
3. While pulling the tragus down and back
4. While pulling the auricle up and back

3 Which statement best explains nursing actions during an irrigation of the left ear?
1. Lean the client's head toward right side.
2. Hold the irrigation syringe approximately 1 inch from the inner canthus.
3. Delegate the procedure to assistive personnel.
4. Place the client in supine position with head elevated.

4 A client with bilateral in-the-ear hearing aids complains of diminished hearing in the left ear. The nurse decides to check the function of the hearing aid. Place the following steps in appropriate order for cleaning a hearing aid:
1. Wash ear canal.
2. Place hearing aid in storage case.
3. Apply gloves.
4. Grasp aid securely and remove from the ear.
5. Use brush to clean the holes in the aid.
6. Have client turn hearing aid volume off.
Which answer is the correct sequence for the above steps?
1. 6, 4, 3, 1, 2, 5
2. 3, 6, 4, 5, 1, 2
3. 3, 4, 1, 6, 5, 2
4. 6, 4, 3, 5, 1, 2

5 After caring for an eye prosthesis, the nurse's priority documentation includes which of the following?
1. Where the client stores the eye prosthesis at home
2. The client's feelings about wearing the eye prosthesis
3. Any signs and symptoms of inflammation or infection noted in the eye socket
4. Which family member was present during the procedure

References for all chapters appear in Appendix D.

Emergency Measures for Life Support in the Hospital Setting

35

MEDIA RESOURCES

- **evolve** http://evolve.elsevier.com/Elkin

The oxygen transport system consists of the respiratory (lungs) and cardiovascular (heart) systems. Adequacy of oxygen delivery depends on the amount of oxygen entering the blood and carbon dioxide leaving the lungs (ventilation), movement of oxygen to the red blood cells at the alveolar level (diffusion), and the blood flow to the lungs and tissues (perfusion). An emergency situation requiring life support occurs when one or more of the above mechanisms fail.

Respiratory and cardiac arrests are emergency situations that you must be prepared to handle. Respiratory arrest, or cessation of ventilation, results in the absence of oxygen delivery to the alveoli. Causes of a respiratory arrest may include airway obstruction, traumatic brain injury or other neurological causes, cardiopulmonary illnesses, or ingestion of toxic substances. Early intervention of a respiratory arrest may prevent a cardiac arrest.

Cardiac arrest is the cessation of circulating blood flow that eliminates oxygen transport and perfusion. An irregular heart rhythm or arrhythmia causes many cardiac arrests. Ventricular fibrillation or ventricular tachycardia without a pulse requires defibrillation, which is an externally applied electrical shock to attempt to restore a perfusing rhythm. Early defibrillation may return the heart quickly to a normal rhythm, and the client may not progress to a respiratory arrest. The majority of arrests involve the collapse of both the respiratory and cardiovascular systems. This is defined as a cardiopulmonary arrest. All clients receive cardiopulmonary resuscitation (CPR) in the event of an arrest unless otherwise indicated, such as a client having an advance directive for final health care or a "do not resuscitate" status.

Advance directives offer valuable information concerning resuscitation status and individual client decisions regarding resuscitation efforts. Although advance directives may be addressed before or during the client's hospital admission, you play an important role in encouraging clients to complete the document. Because of their unique relationship with clients and the associated high level of trust, nurses are the ideal facilitators for the initiation of advance directives. The American Nurses Association *Position Statement on Nursing and the Patient Self-Determination Acts* states that it is the nurse's responsibility to facilitate informed decision making for clients making choices about end-of-life care. Clients want to discuss end-of-life care, and they expect providers to initiate these conversations. Although further research is required on the degree of improvement of end-of-life care, there is some evidence that advance directives give a client a means of controlling treatment decisions about the end of his or her life (Ditto and others, 2001). An advance directive can minimize disagreements among family members regarding resuscitation status determination when the client is physically or mentally unable to make decisions. Many hospitals have a mechanism to assist the client and family regarding this issue. Social services and an ethics committee may be of assistance to the client and family.

TABLE 35-1 Adult, Child, and Infant CPR Techniques (Health Care Provider [HCP])

TECHNIQUE	ADULT	CHILD (1-8 YEARS OLD)	INFANT (UNDER 1 YEAR) DOES NOT INCLUDE NEWBORNS
Airway	Head tilt-chin lift (HCP: suspected trauma, use jaw thrust)	Head tilt-chin lift (HCP: suspected trauma, use jaw thrust)	Head tilt-chin lift (HCP: suspected trauma, use jaw thrust)
Initial breathing	2 breaths @ 1 second/breath	2 breaths @ 1 second/breath	2 breaths @ 1 second/breath
HCP: rescue breathing without chest compressions	10-12 breaths/min (approximate)	12-20 breaths/min (approximate)	12-20 breaths/min (approximate)
HCP: rescue breaths for CPR with advanced airway (endotrachael tube/tracheotomy)	8-10 breaths/min (approximately)	8-10 breaths/min (approximately)	8-10 breaths/min (approximately)
Foreign body airway obstruction	Abdominal thrusts	Abdominal thrusts	Back slaps and chest thrusts
Chest compressions: push hard and fast to allow complete recoil	Lower half of sternum, between nipples Heel of one hand, other hand on top 1½-2 inches One or two rescuers 30 compressions, 2 breaths (30:2)	Lower half of sternum, between nipples Heel of one hand or as for adults Approximately ⅓ to ½ depth of chest One rescuer: 30 compressions, 2 breaths (30:2) Two rescuers: 15 compressions, 2 breaths (15:2)	Just below nipple line (lower ½ of the sternum) Two fingers, two thumb (encircling hands) Approximately ⅓ to ½ depth of chest One rescuer: 30 compressions, 2 breaths (30:2) Two rescuers: 15 compressions, 2 breaths (15:2)

From American Heart Association: Part 3. Overview of CPR, *Circulation, 112*:IV-12: 2005b.

EVIDENCE IN PRACTICE

American Heart Association: Part 3: Overview of CPR, *Circulation 112*:IV-12, 2005b.

The American Heart Association continues to research cardiac arrest treatment and outcomes. The 2005 Consensus Conference reviewed current information and developed the *2005 AHA Guidelines for Cardiopulmonary Resuscitation (CPR) and Emergency Cardiac Care (ECC)*, thus simplifying the basic life support (BLS) steps (Table 35-1) (AHA, 2005a and 2005b). Sudden cardiac arrest (SCA) is the leading cause of death in the United Stated and Canada. Most victims of SCA also have ventricular fibrillation at some point during the arrest. When providing emergent care, it is important to initiate CPR and to convert ventricular fibrillation if present to normal sinus or perfusing rhythm by the use of an electrical shock delivered through a manual or an automatic external defibrillator (AED). CPR is important both before and after shock delivery. Client outcomes demonstrate that CPR can double or triple a victim's survival chance, and CPR should be continued until defibrillation is available.

NURSING DIAGNOSES

Nursing diagnoses that apply to clients who receive CPR include **ineffective breathing pattern,** which may be related to injury; paralysis affecting the diaphragm or phrenic nerve; a collapsed lung (pneumothorax); chest trauma with blood accumulation in the chest (hemothorax); or drug overdose. **Impaired gas exchange** is associated with cardiac and pulmonary disorders that interfere with the body's ability to exchange carbon dioxide and oxygen. **Impaired spontaneous ventilation** occurs when there is no respiratory activity initiated by the client, which occurs during a respiratory or cardiopulmonary arrest. **Decreased cardiac output** occurs when there is a cardiac arrest. Finally, **ineffective tissue perfusion** of vital organs (e.g., brain, kidney, heart) occurs if cardiopulmonary function is not maintained or restored.

SKILL 35.1 Code Management

This skill includes the initial response and management of cardiopulmonary arrest. All who respond to cardiopulmonary arrests should arrive well trained in a simple, easy-to-remember approach. The ACLS Provider Course teaches the primary and secondary survey approach to arrest situations. This memory aid describes two sets of four steps: A-B-C-D. With each step the responder performs an assessment and then, if the assessment so indicates, a management intervention. Initially, a code is managed by the first responder performing the basic skills of CPR, which includes the primary survey of A (airway), B (breathing), C (circulation), D (early defibrilation). This survey continues until the code team arrives. The initial process also includes the notification of the hospital's resuscitation team or code team. Most of the code team members have been trained in the ACLS guidelines and the performance of the secondary survey: A (airway intubation), B (confirmation of airway and ventilation), C (rhythm analysis of cardiac rhythm), D (differential diagnosis of the cause). Both surveys must be continually reassessed and managed as appropriate throughout the code situation.

The hospital response team usually includes a physician, intensive care nurse, respiratory therapy personnel, radiology and laboratory technologists, and other personnel. A representative from pastoral care may be available to be with the family. During an arrest the client's family may ask to wait in a nearby area. If the client is in a two-bed room and the roommate can be assisted to leave, this is appropriate. If the roommate cannot leave, it is appropriate for assistive personnel (AP) to remain with the person. Move excess furniture out of the way and bring resuscitation equipment into the room.

CPR is initiated and maintained by the discovering staff until the code team arrives. As soon as possible, the client's cardiac rhythm is determined, and, if appropriate, the client is defibrillated with a manual defibrillator or an AED. AEDs are now readily available in a majority of public places such as airports, shopping malls, and all health care settings. The advantage of the AED is that all people with basic cardiac life support training can defibrillate. AEDs eliminate the training in rhythm interpretation and make early defibrillation practical and achievable. The AED is an external defibrillator that incorporates a rhythm analysis system. The device attaches to a client by two adhesive pads and connecting cables. The pads relay the rhythm for interpretation and deliver the electric shock. A fully automatic defibrillator requires only that the operator attach the pads and turn on the device.

CPR certification is required of most nursing students or for entry into the nursing program. As a result, CPR will not be covered in detail in this chapter. A few summary points about CPR are presented in Table 35-1. This skill will focus on code management of the client with cardiac arrest.

ASSESSMENT

1 Determine if client is unconscious by shaking client and shouting, "Are you OK?" Assess client's unresponsiveness. *Rationale: Confirms that client is unconscious rather than asleep, intoxicated, or hearing impaired. Unconsciousness can also be caused by substance abuse, hypoglycemia, ketoacidosis, and shock.*

> **NURSE ALERT** If an unconscious client has adequate respirations and pulse, remain with him or her until further assistance is present. Place victim in a modified lateral recovery position (see illustration). Continue to determine presence of respirations and pulse because respiratory or cardiopulmonary arrest is still possible.

2 Activate emergency medical service in accordance with hospital policy and procedure (e.g., call a code blue or 99). *Rationale: The majority of adult victims are in ventricular fibrillation and need*

defibrillation and antidysrhythmic drugs as soon as possible. Early access to emergency cardiac care systems improves client outcomes (AHA, 2005a).

PLANNING

Expected Outcomes focus on the goals of care, which are restoration of cardiac and pulmonary function before irreversible organ damage occurs.
1 Client regains pulse and respirations or is assisted with a ventilator as long as a pulse exists.
2 No complications occur from the resuscitation.
3 Physician may terminate CPR and pronounce death.

Delegation Considerations
The skill of code management may not be delegated. However, AP who are certified in BLS techniques can perform the basic skills of CPR. Most APs are certified in BCLS and may use an AED. However, manual defibrillation is reserved for licensed personnel who have advanced cardiac life support (ACLS) certification. All other skills in the code situation are directed by the code team leader and performed by nurses, respiratory therapists, and other health care professionals.

Equipment
- Crash cart (Figure 35-1): Most adult crash carts have the following equipment:
  - Clean and sterile gloves, gown, protective eyewear
  - Oxygen source
  - Bag-valve-mask (BVM)
  - Laryngoscope, handle, straight and curved blades

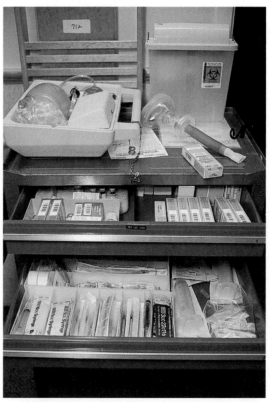

FIGURE 35-1 Emergency resuscitation cart.

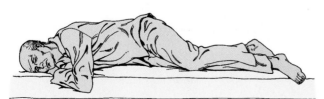

STEP 1 Recovery position.

- Endotracheal (ET) tube, various sizes (6 to 8 Fr)
- Carbon dioxide monitor (optional, see agency policy)
- Tape
- Backboard
- AED and/or manual defibrillator
- Intravascular needles (14- to 22-gauge)
- Central vascular access kit
- IV tubing, fluids (9% normal saline [NS], D₅W)

- Syringes
- Lab specimen tubes
- Arterial blood gas kit
- Code medications
- ACLS guidelines or algorithms
- Suction machine and suction equipment if not with crash cart

IMPLEMENTATION *for Primary Survey ABC*

STEPS	RATIONALE

Primary Survey: A (Airway)

> **NURSE ALERT** It may not always be possible to apply all personal protective equipment at the beginning of a code.

1 Open airway using:	Determines if client has spontaneous respirations. Tongue is most common cause of blocked airway in an unresponsive client.
a. Head tilt-chin lift (no trauma) (see illustration) *Or*	
b. Jaw thrust (spinal cord trauma suspected) (see illustration).	Suspect a spinal cord injury with any kind of trauma. Jaw thrust maneuver prevents head extension and neck movement and further paralysis or spinal cord injury.

> **NURSE ALERT** A cervical brace should be applied as soon as possible to maintain cervical-spine stability.

Primary Survey: B (Breathing)

2 Attempt to ventilate client using one of these methods.	
a. Mouth-to-mouth using barrier device	Forms airtight seal and prevents air from escaping through nose.
b. Mouth-to mouth using a pocket mask (see illustration)	Provides secure seal and permits use of supplemental oxygen.
c. BVM (see illustration)	

> **NURSE ALERT** Give breaths with enough force to make chest rise. Slow breaths deliver air at a low pressure to reduce the risk of gastric distention.

3 If readily available, insert oral airway (see Skill 35.2).	Maintains tone on anterior floor of mouth and prevents obstruction of posterior airway by tongue.
4 Suction secretions if necessary or turn victim's head to one side unless trauma is suspected.	Suctioning prevents airway obstruction. Turning client's head to one side allows gravity to drain any secretions, decreasing risk of aspiration.

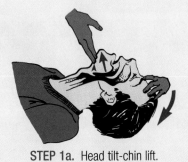

STEP 1a. Head tilt-chin lift.

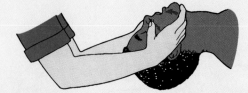

STEP 1b. Jaw-thrust without head tilt.

STEPS	RATIONALE

Primary Survey: C (Circulation)

5 Check carotid pulse on adult or child; use brachial pulse on an infant. Check for 3 to 5 seconds.

Carotid pulse is present when other peripheral pulses are not palpable. Because the neck of an infant is short, the carotid pulse is difficult to locate. Compressions are contraindicated when a pulse is present.

6 Place victim on hard surface such as floor, ground, or backboard. Victim must be flat. If necessary, logroll victim to flat, supine position using spine precautions.

Facilitates external compression of the heart. Heart is compressed between sternum and spinal vertebrae, which must be on hard, flat surface.

Primary Survey: D (Defibrillation)

7 If pulse is absent and an AED is available, apply AED immediately as appropriate.

Most successful defibrillation rates occur when AED is applied and used within 5 minutes following collapse. Survival rates decline when defibrillation is delayed (AHA, 2005b).

a. After one shock, resume CPR for 5 cycles and then begin rhythm analysis and shock sequence again.

One shock followed by chest compressions for 5 cycles provides sufficient blood movement and improved perfusion before another set of shocks is delivered (AHA, 2005b).

8 If pulse is absent and an AED is unavailable, immediately initiate chest compressions:

a. Assume correct hand position and compression ratio for client (see Table 35-1 and illustration).

Specific hand position, compression depth, and ratio are different for adult, child, and infant to avoid injury to heart, lung, or liver.

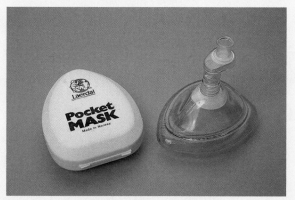

STEP 2b. Pocket mask.

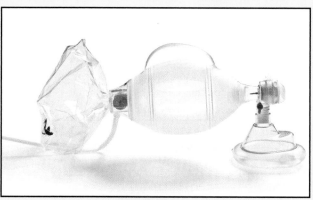

STEP 2c. Bag-valve-mask. (Courtesy AMBU USA.)

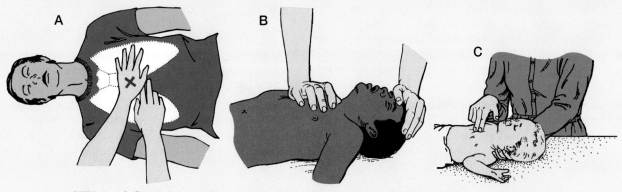

STEP 8a. **A,** Proper hand position: adult. **B,** Proper hand position: child. **C,** Proper hand position: infant.

STEPS	RATIONALE

> **NURSE ALERT** Ensure that fingers are off ribs and lowermost part of the xiphoid process. This reduces change of rib fractures that could result in punctured lung or liver lacerations, which can further compromise cardiopulmonary status. Continue chest compressions, ventilation, and AED use.

IMPLEMENTATION *for Secondary Survey ABCD*

STEPS	RATIONALE

1 Give code leader brief verbal report on events just before code, vital signs, medical diagnosis, and code interventions performed before code team's arrival.

This information is critical in the selection of appropriate treatment for the client.

2 On arrival of sufficient personnel, delegate tasks as appropriate.

Delegation of duties is essential to meet all needs of client and his or her family in a timely manner.

a. Assist victim's roommate or visitors away from code scene. Assign pastoral care or other nurses to communicate with family.

b. Delegate someone to remove excess furniture or equipment from room.

c. Have someone bring client's chart to bedside or be able to access client's electronic medical record.

Clarifies client's present medical condition, code status, and presence of any allergies.

d. Assign a nurse as recorder to record/document events of code.

Documents events of code and medications and treatments administered.

e. Assign another nurse as crash cart nurse to get medications and supplies from cart and to hand them off to code team members. The bedside nurse will be involved with medication administration, vital signs, assisting with procedures, etc.

Provides code personnel with appropriate medication and equipment in a timely manner.

Secondary Survey: A (Intubate, Airway)

3 If respirations are absent, assist code team with ET intubation.

Intubation provides patent airway and improves pulmonary ventilation.

a. Have available laryngoscope, handle, curved and straight blades, and ET tubes. Ensure that light source on laryngoscope is functional.

Functional laryngeal light facilitates visualization of the vocal cords and placement of the ET tube into the trachea.

> **NURSE ALERT** The use of a laryngeal mask airway or esophageal-tracheal combitube can also be used to provide advanced airway support (AHA, 2005b).

Secondary Survey: B (Confirmation of Airway and Ventilation)

4 Assist in confirmation of ET tube placement or advanced airway support by auscultating lungs for bilateral breath sounds and epigastric area for lack of breath sounds. Carbon dioxide (CO_2) detector or esophageal detector devices are used as secondary methods to confirm correct airway placement.

Auscultation of lungs and exhaled CO_2 monitoring or esophageal detector device further verifies correct airway placement and adequacy of ventilation and gas exchange.

5 Ventilate using a BVM on intubation.

BVM provides more oxygen delivery air for improved ventilation when administered through an ET tube or other advanced airway support system.

Secondary Survey: C (Analysis of Cardiac Rhythm)

6 Attach manual defibrillator/monitor to client using electrocardiogram electrodes, quick-look paddles, or "hands-off" defibrillation electrodes to visualize cardiac rhythm.

Cardiac rhythm monitor devices provide immediate rhythm display for analysis without disruption of rescue breathing and chest compression (AHA, 2005c).

STEPS	RATIONALE
7 If cardiac rhythm is "shockable," continue CPR and assist code team with manual defibrillation.	Manual defibrillation is performed by ACLS-certified personnel.
a. Turn defibrillator on and select proper energy level following agency policy and equipment directions.	Energy is delivered in prescribed dosages. Manual biphasic devices deliver shocks at a lower level (200 joules); monophasic waveforms use 360 joules (AHA, 2005c).
b. Apply conductive gel or gel pads to client's chest where defibrillator paddles will be placed. Some defibrillators use "hands-off pads" that are applied to client's chest and directly connected to the manual defibrillator.	Decreases thoracic impedance and helps minimize burns to client's skin (Craig, Hopkins-Pepe, 2006).
c. Paddles are placed on client's chest wall.	Placement ensures appropriate discharge of current.
d. Verify that no one is in physical contact with client, bed, or any item contacting the client during defibrillation. A warning must be called out before initiating the charge.	Prevents accidental delivery of shock or injury to personnel.
8 Establish IV access with large-bore needle (14- to 22-gauge) and begin infusion of 0.9% NS.	Provides a route for rapid drug administration, access for blood samples, and fluid administration. Physiological saline is isotonic.
9 Assist with procedures as needed.	Much of the equipment needed for special procedures during a code is on the crash cart. Knowledge of crash cart contents and their location is essential to provide personnel with appropriate equipment without delay.
10 Continue CPR until relieved, until victim regains spontaneous pulse and respirations, until rescuer is exhausted and unable to perform CPR effectively, or until physician discontinues CPR.	Artificial cardiopulmonary function is maintained. Interruption of CPR is planned and organized. Interruptions occur seamlessly during changing CPR personnel, defibrillation, and intubation. Interruptions must be kept to a minimum and not exceed 30 seconds.
Secondary Survey: D (Differential Diagnosis)	
11 Assist physician in obtaining laboratory and diagnostic studies.	Helps in determining cause of the arrest.
12 See Completion Protocol (inside front cover).	

EVALUATION

1 Reassess primary and secondary survey ABCDs throughout code event.
2 Palpate carotid pulse at least every 5 minutes after first minute of CPR.
3 Observe for spontaneous return of pulse or respirations.
4 Observe that CPR is not interrupted for more than 5 seconds unless an interruption is for AED application, manual defibrillator use, or intubation.

Unexpected Outcomes and Related Interventions

1 Client experiences skeletal injury such as fractured ribs or sternum or internal organ injury such as lacerated lung or liver.
a. Obtain appropriate diagnostic tests to document fractures.
b. Assess client's post-arrest breathing or symmetry and pain.
c. Observe for hemoptysis or gastrointestinal bleeding.
d. Observe for distended abdomen.

2 Client's CPR is unsuccessful.
a. Contact chaplain services, social worker, or other family support systems.
b. Provide for privacy for client's family to begin grieving process (see Chapter 37).
c. Complete postmortem care on client (see Chapter 37).

Recording and Reporting

- Immediately report arrest, indicating exact location of victim. In hospital setting, follow agency policy for alerting the code team. In community setting, activate emergency response system.
- Most hospitals use a form designed specifically for in-hospital arrests.
- Record in nurses' notes or on designated CPR worksheet: onset of arrest, time, and number of AED shocks (you will need to know the device specific energy level delivered by the AED), time and energy level of manual defibrillations, medications given, procedures performed, cardiac rhythm, use of CPR, and the client's response.

Sample Documentation
(Without Code Sheet)

0734 Client found pulseless and unresponsive in bed. Code team activated. Backboard under client. CPR begun. Pocket mask used for ventilation. AED indicates shock is needed; one shock at 200 J delivered. CPR continues.

0740 Code team arrives, quick-look paddles applied, ventricular fibrillation present, manually defibrillated at 360 J with monitor showing continued ventricular fibrillation. CPR continued.

0741 Intubated with No. 8 ET tube, left side of mouth at 26 cm. Securely taped. Bilateral breath sounds ausculated with BVM-assisted ventilations. CPR continues.

0745 20-gauge IV inserted in right and left antecubital sites. Blood sent to lab for electrolytes and complete blood count. NS wide open via right antecubital site.

0746 Ventricular fibrillation still present; repeat manual defibrillation at 360 J. Monitor shows sinus tachycardia. Carotid pulse palpated. Blood pressure 96/46 mm Hg.

0810 Transported to cardiac care unit with physician, RN, and respiratory therapist. Client remains intubated with monitor showing sinus tachycardia. Client is nonresponsive.

Special Considerations
Pediatric Considerations

- Infants and children experience respiratory arrest more frequently than full cardiopulmonary arrest.

Geriatric Considerations

- Older adults, especially those with osteoporosis, are at greater risk for rib fractures.
- Whenever possible, loose-fitting dentures would be removed to avoid airway obstruction during CPR and airway insertions. Properly fitting dentures should be left in place as they assist in ensuring a tight seal during artificial ventilation.

Long-Term Considerations

- It is important that a resident's code status be determined and documented when admitted to a long-term care facility.

SKILL 35-2 Inserting an Oropharyngeal Airway

An oropharyngeal airway is a semicircular-shaped, minimally flexible, curved piece of hard plastic (Figure 35-2). When inserted, it extends from just outside the lips, over the tongue, and to the pharynx (Figure 35-3). **Oral airways** allow you to suction through a central core or along the side of the airway, facilitate resuscitation, and maintain airway patency in the unconscious client.

The oral airway is sized for adults and children, varying in length and width. Pediatric sizes are 000, 00, 0, 1, 2, and 3. School-age children are usually size 3 or 4. Adult sizes are 4 through 10 or small, medium, and large. Choose the size of an oral airway on the basis of the client's age and the width and length of the client's mouth. Size is correct if, when the flange is held parallel to the front teeth with the airway against the client's cheek, the end of the curve reaches the angle of the jaw. General size guidelines for choosing an oral airway for children are provided in Table 35-2.

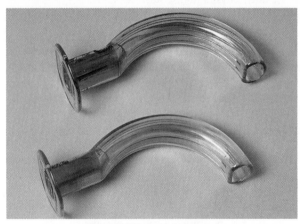

FIGURE 35-2 Oral airways.

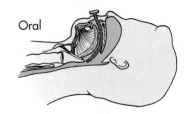

FIGURE 35-3 Placement of oral airway.

Oral

ASSESSMENT

1 Identify need to insert oral airway. Signs and symptoms include upper airway "gurgling" with respiratory cycle, absent cough or gag reflex, increased oral secretions or excretions, excessive drooling, grinding teeth, clenched teeth, biting of oral tracheal or gastric tubes, labored respirations, and increased respiratory rate. *Rationale: These conditions place clients at risk for obstruction of upper airway. This airway is*

TABLE 35-2 Oral Airway Guidelines for Size by Age	
SIZE	**AGE**
000	Premature neonates
00	Newborn
0	Newborn to 1 yr
1	1 to 2 yr
2	2 to 6 yr
3	6 to 18 yr
4 and larger	≥18 yr

only used with unconscious client because in a conscious client, the gag reflex causes vomiting or retching when something is placed in pharynx. Oral airways may stimulate vomiting or laryngospasm if inserted in semiconscious client.

2 Determine factors that normally influence upper airway functioning such as age (children have a proportionally larger tongue), presence of nasal and oral airway, and drainage tubes (swallowing is more difficult with tubes in place). *Rationale: Allows you to accurately assess need for oral airway. Clients at greater risk for upper airway obstruction are infants; children; and adults with cold and flu, loss of consciousness, seizure disorders, neuromuscular diseases, increased oral secretions or excretions, or facial trauma.*

3 In postoperative client assess for presence of cough or gag reflex; gently place tongue blade on back of client's tongue. *Rationale: Provides guide as to when oral airway can be safely removed following general anesthesia.*

> **NURSE ALERT** Never insert an oropharyngeal airway in a conscious client or a client with recent oral trauma, oral surgery, or loose teeth.

PLANNING

Expected Outcomes focus on the goals of care, which include improvement in airway patency and status.

1 Client's respiratory status improves, as evidenced by easier respirations with normal rate, easier removal of secretions, and lack of gurgling noise in throat with respirations.

2 Client is not able to grind teeth or bite tubes.

3 Client's tongue does not relax back into pharynx and obstruct airway.

Delegation Considerations

The skill of inserting an oropharyngeal airway may not be delegated. The nurse directs personnel by:

- Reviewing to observe for any signs of airway distress, vomiting, or change in level of consciousness and to report back to the nurse.

Equipment

- Appropriate-size oral airway
- Clean gloves
- Tissues or washcloths
- Suction equipment, if indicated
- Tape
- Face shield, if indicated
- Tongue blade

IMPLEMENTATION *for Inserting an Oropharyngeal Airway*

STEPS	RATIONALE
1 See Standard Protocol (inside front cover).	
2 Position unconscious client; semi-Fowler's position is preferred.	Provides easy access to oral cavity.

> **NURSE ALERT** Never insert an oral airway in a conscious client.

STEPS	RATIONALE
3 Apply clean gloves and face shield (when possible).	Reduces transmission of microorganisms.
4 Whenever possible use padded tongue blade to open client's mouth.	Provides access to oral cavity.
5 Insert oral airway.	When inserting airway, take care not to push client's tongue into pharynx.
a. Hold oral airway with curved end up, insert distal end until airway reaches back of throat; then turn airway over 180 degrees and follow natural curve of tongue. Nurse may also hold airway sideways, insert halfway, and then rotate airway 90 degrees while gliding it over natural curvature of tongue. Outer flange is just outside client's lips.	Provides patent airway and prevents displacement of client's tongue into posterior oropharynx.

STEPS	RATIONALE

> **NURSE ALERT** Secure airway temporarily with tape on the upper and lower flange. May need to insert an ET airway as soon as possible.

6 Suction secretions as needed.	Removes secretions; maintains patent airway.
7 Reassess client's respiratory status.	Directs nurse to initiate intervention.
8 Clean client's face with soft tissue or washcloth.	Promotes hygiene.
9 Administer frequent oral hygiene.	Increases client comfort and removes debris. It also provides moisture to oral mucosal tissues.

10 See Completion Protocol (inside front cover).

> **NURSE ALERT** Do not use lemon glycerin swabs for oral care because they are drying to mucosal tissues and promote bacterial growth. Oral airway may also need to be removed, cleaned, and reinserted in clients with a copious amount of oral mucous secretions. If secretions are left in place, they could occlude oral airway.

EVALUATION

1 Observe client's respiratory status and compare respiratory assessments before and after insertion of oral airway.

2 Assess that airway is patent, that client does not occlude airway by biting tube, and that client's tongue does not obstruct airway.

Unexpected Outcomes and Related Interventions

1 Client continually coughs and gags when airway is inserted.

a. Do not continue inserting airway if client begins to gag. Stimulation of gag reflex can cause vomiting and risk of aspiration.

b. Remove oral airway and position client on side. Replace with smaller-size airway.

c. Evaluate need for a different airway (e.g., nasopharyngeal airway).

2 Airway obstruction not relieved.

a. Obtain immediate assistance.

b. Reinsert airway.

3 Client pushes airway out of place or out of mouth.

a. If client is conscious and gagging, place in lateral recumbent (rescue) position and suction.

b. Determine client's need for oral airway.

Recording and Reporting

• Record and report assessment findings while inserting oral airway, size of oral airway, placement, any other procedures performed at same time, especially positioning, secretions obtained, client's tolerance of procedure.

Sample Documentation

1000: Nonresponsive, airway secretions increasing, upper airway gurgling auscultated. Gag reflex absent. Size 4 oropharyngeal airway inserted without trauma. Airway suctioned for yellow airway secretions. Bilateral lungs sounds, no adventitious sounds.

Special Considerations
Pediatric Considerations

• Oral airways are seldom used in treatment of airway obstruction in children and infants. Due to narrowness of child's airway, oral airways are often more occlusive than beneficial (Hockenberry and Wilson, 2007).

• For infants and small children sliding oral airway along side of mouth rather than with tip up is recommended because the soft palate is easily injured.

NCLEX® Style Questions

1 Place the following interventions in correct sequence for the major steps of CPR and AED.
   1. Call for help.
   2. Open the airway.
   3. Get the AED.
   4. Provide 2 breaths.
   5. If no pulse present attach the AED.
   6. Check for pulse.

2 Following one shock of AED, the nurse should do which of the following actions next:
   1. Palpate the carotid pulse.
   2. Perform CPR for 5 cycles.
   3. Perform a rhythm analysis.
   4. Place client in the recovery position.

3 Name the preferred technique to open the airway when there is no suspected trauma.
   1. Head tilt-chin lift
   2. Jaw thrust
   3. Lateral-lying position
   4. All of the above

4 _____ minutes is the ideal time goal from victim collapse to first defibrillation?
   1. Three
   2. Five
   3. Seven
   4. Ten

5 Which of the following is true about an oral airway?
   1. It eliminates the need to position the head of the unconscious client.
   2. It eliminates the possibility of an upper airway obstruction.
   3. It is of no value once an endotracheal tube is inserted.
   4. It may stimulate vomiting or laryngospasm in the semi-conscious client.

References for all chapters appear in Appendix D.

36

Care of the Client with Special Needs

MEDIA RESOURCES

- **evolve** http://evolve.elsevier.com/Elkin
- **View Video!** Video Clips
- Nursing Skills Online

Clients with special needs include those with complex medical and nursing diagnoses and those who require a variety of interventions involving the use of high technology. Such clients are often in acute care or intensive care settings. These interventions require a higher level of problem solving and coordination. Many of the interventions are performed in cooperation with physicians or allied health professionals. It is common for facilities to have certification programs that are required before implementation of these skills such as a peripherally inserted central catheter (PICC) program (Robinson and others, 2005). Nurses must be familiar with their facility's policies and standards of care.

Your role in assessment takes on special importance in these skills. Because you have more frequent and prolonged contact with clients requiring these skills, you have a unique perspective on their progress toward goals and outcomes. This includes positive factors such as family support and adequate resources, as well as factors that might have a negative impact on the outcome such as the development of complications or the presence of family stressors.

EVIDENCE IN PRACTICE

CDC: Guidelines for preventing health-care associated pneumonia, MMWR 2003/53RR03:1, May, 2004.

The nurse's role in reducing the client's risk for developing complications for clients receiving mechanical ventilation is key. Examples of nursing interventions to prevent ventilator-associated pneumonia (VAP) for patients receiving mechanical ventilation include frequent positioning and oral care. Elevating the client's head of bed to an angle >30 degrees reduces the risk of aspiration of oral or gastric secretions. In addition, nurses can provide oral care to reduce plaque. Better teeth cleansing can reduce aspiration of colonized oral secretions and reduce the risk of VAP.

NURSING DIAGNOSES

The following nursing diagnoses apply to clients requiring multiple skills in this chapter. Clients may exhibit **anxiety** related to the complexity of care. These skills are highly technical and specialized; therefore clients often demonstrate **deficient knowledge** related to inexperience with procedures. Clients are at **risk for injury, risk for impaired skin integrity,** and/or **risk for infection** related to the asso-

ciated disease processes, invasiveness of procedures, and altered fluid/nutritional balance. Clients requiring any of the skills may present with **deficient fluid volume, excess fluid volume,** and/or **risk for imbalanced fluid volume** related to disease process and/or side effects of medication or treatment. **Disturbed body image** is related to physical changes brought on by side effects of treatment. Apply critical thinking in selecting appropriate nursing diagnoses.

SKILL 36.1 Care of Clients with Central Venous Access Devices

• Nursing Skills Online: Vascular Access, Lessons 1 and 2

Long-term central venous access devices (CVADs) are indicated for some clients who will receive intravenous (IV) therapy or hemodialysis for longer than 7 days and up to several years. The devices are used to administer IV fluids, medications, blood products, and parenteral nutrition fluids. The access devices are also used for hemodialysis and temporary cardiac pacing procedures. The use of intravascular devices becomes complicated in instances of septic thrombophlebitis, endocarditis, and bloodstream infection. Catheter-related infections are associated with increased morbidity and mortality rates, prolonged hospitalization, and increased medical costs.

Physicians or credentialed advanced practice nurses insert central venous catheters through the subclavian or jugular veins (Figure 36-1) and in emergencies through the femoral veins. The chest and neck sites are preferred be-

cause they provide a flat, relatively immobile area and blood flows through the large veins at a high rate. However, the risk of infection is higher with internal jugular veins than with subclavian (Mermel and others, 2001). Double-, triple-, or quadruple-lumen catheters are used when the client requires several different infusions. Each port is labeled with the gauge size and position (e.g., 16-gauge distal). The largest gauge is used for blood therapy and colloid administration. If total parenteral nutrition (PN) is administered, the port remains designated for PN only throughout the life of the catheter. The middle port is used for central venous pressure (CVP) monitoring or IV infusions, and the proximal port is used for IV infusions. The proximal lumen should be used for obtaining blood specimens.

Specially trained nurses or physicians insert PICCs. The PICC extends from the insertion site at the antecubital fossa to the distal end of the catheter resting in the central circulation. These catheters may be inserted at the client's hospi-

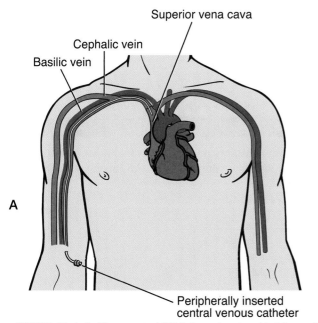

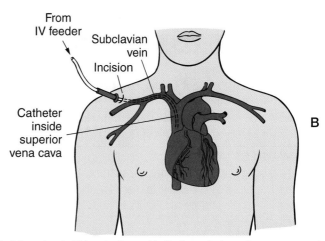

FIGURE 36-1 **A,** Placement of PICC through antecubital fossa. (Modified from Lewis SM and others: *Medical-surgical nursing: assessment and management of clinical problems,* ed 4, St Louis, 2000, Mosby.) **B,** Placement of central venous catheter inserted into subclavian vein.

tal bedside, in the outpatient department, or in the client's home. Other long-term devices include surgically tunneled catheters that are designed to have a portion lie within a subcutaneous (SQ) passage before exiting the body (e.g., Broviac, Hickman, or Groshong). Another long-term access device is a surgically implanted infusion port. These ports are placed in a vessel, body cavity, or organ and are attached to a reservoir placed under the skin (e.g., Port-a-Cath).

ASSESSMENT

1 Assess client for indications for long-term device:
a. IV therapy anticipated for longer than 7 days, including transfusions, PN administration, long-term antibiotics, or continuous infusions such as narcotics
b. Infusion of vesicants or irritants such as in chemotherapy
c. Altered peripheral venous circulation
d. Frequent long-term phlebotomy
2 Assess vital signs and intake and output (I&O). *Rationale: Provides baseline to determine client's response to fluid therapy.*
3 Assess catheter patency by testing for blood return in catheter and free infusion of IV fluid or manual flush. *Rationale: A patent line is necessary for the safe infusion of fluids, blood products, and PN.*
4 Assess insertion site for integrity of catheter and skin. *Rationale: Determine the presence of early signs of phlebitis or infiltration. Development of phlebitis or infiltration requires prompt removal of catheter.*

PLANNING

Expected Outcomes focus on maintaining a patent channel of venous access, maintaining fluid and electrolyte balance, and preventing complications related to maintenance of access devices.
1 I&O remains in balance with electrolytes within normal limits.
2 IV infusion setup is intact and functioning properly with infusion flowing freely.

3 Client has no evidence of complications: clotting, local inflammation or phlebitis, systemic infection, venous thrombosis, air embolus, extravasation (leaking of medication into tissues around the site), or migration of catheter.

Delegation Considerations
The skill of maintenance of CVADs may not be delegated. The nurse directs personnel to:
• Assist with positioning and handing off supplies.

Equipment
Site Care and Dressing Change
• Gloves (sterile and clean)
• Mask
• Combination antiseptic swabs (e.g., alcohol, chlorhexidine, and/or povidone-iodine)
• Transparent or gauze dressing
• Label
• Catheter stabilization device if catheter not sutured

Blood Drawing Through Central Venous Catheter
• Nonsterile gloves
• Chlorhexidine swabs
• 5-ml Luer-Lok syringes
• 10-ml Luer-Lok syringes
• Vacutainer system
• Preservative-free saline flush
• Heparin flush (10 to 100 μ/ml)
• Blood tubes, including waste tube
• Needleless injection cap

Removal of Central Venous Catheter
• Clean gloves
• Chlorhexidine swabs
• Suture removal set
• 4 × 4 gauze
• Tape

IMPLEMENTATION *for Care of Clients with Central Venous Access Devices*

STEPS	RATIONALE
1 Insertion site care: a. **See Standard Protocol (inside front cover).** Provide insertion site care every 48 hours and prn for gauze dressings, every 7 days and prn for transparent dressings (Infusion Nursing Standards of Practice, 2006).	Allows visual inspection of site for rapid detection of infection or other complications. An intact transparent dressing can remain in place longer without development of infection at site.

> **COMMUNICATION TIP** Explain to client the need for catheter site care on a regular basis and the nursing plan for maintaining the catheter, "I will be checking the catheter dressing every day to make sure it's in place and to check for infection. I will also be checking to make sure it remains in the right position and that it's still working correctly."

STEPS	RATIONALE
b. Don mask.	Minimizes exposure of microorganisms over IV site.

STEPS	RATIONALE

c. 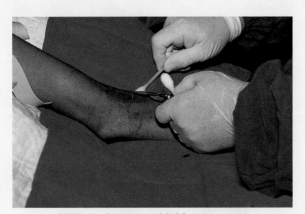 Remove old dressing and tape in direction catheter was inserted. Discard in receptacle.

d. Remove stabilization device if in use.

Allows for better inspection of skin surrounding catheter insertion (Infusion Nursing Standards of Practice, 2006). Provides baseline for condition of catheter site.

e. Inspect catheter, insertion site, sutures (if present), and surrounding skin.

f. Remove and discard gloves; open dressing kit in sterile manner and **apply sterile gloves.**

Sterile technique required to apply new dressing.

g. Using combination antiseptic swab, cleanse catheter and site, working outward in circular motion, or follow steps 2h and 2i if combination swab not available.

Removes resident microorganisms from skin.

h. Using combination swab, cleanse catheter and site, working outward in circular motion. Repeat × 2; allow to dry completely. Use chlorhexidine alone if client is allergic to alcohol, then use a back-and-forth scrub method.

Alcohol swabs defat the skin. Circular cleansing motions move bacteria on the skin away from the insertion site. Chlorhexidine reduces the skin surface bacteria.

i. Using combination swab, cleanse catheter and site, working in a horizontal plane with first swab, a vertical plane with second swab and a circular pattern moving outward with third swab (see illustration). Allow antiseptic to dry completely.

Allowing site to dry completely promotes maximum bactericidal effectiveness.

j. Apply new stabilization device if not sutured (see illustration).

Provides stabilization of catheter to minimize risk of accidental removal.

k. Apply sterile, clear occlusive dressing or gauze dressing (see illustration).

l. Write the date, time, and your initials on label.

Provides means to determine when next dressing change is due.

m. Clamp lumens to catheter one at a time and remove injection caps.

n. Cleanse ports with chlorhexidine or alcohol and allow to dry completely.

o. Put new caps in place and open clamps for infusion.

Routine cap changes decrease the risk of catheter-related infection.

p. **See Completion Protocol (inside front cover).**

STEP 1i. Cleansing of PICC catheter site.

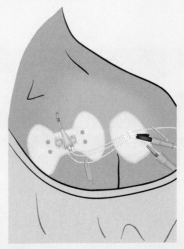

STEP 1j. Subclavian central venous access device secured with stabilization device and covered with transparent dressing. (Courtesy of C.R. Bard, Covington, Georgia.)

STEPS	RATIONALE

2 Blood drawing through central venous access device

a. **See Standard Protocol (inside front cover).**

b. Explain procedure to client.

c. Cleanse injection cap with alcohol or chlorhexidine and allow to dry completely.

If solution is not allowed to dry, new cap may be difficult to remove with next change.

d. Stop IV infusion. NOTE: If infusion is critical for client's well-being (such as vasopressor medications), draw blood through a different peripheral vein.

Prevents interruption of critical fluid therapy.

e. Flush catheter port with 5 ml normal saline (check agency policy).

Clears IV catheter.

f. Attach 5 ml syringe and aspirate 3 to 5 ml blood and discard or attach Vacutainer device and draw a red-top blood tube for discard.

Initial specimen is diluted with saline solution. Amount of discard will vary with catheter size and length; check manufacturer's guidelines. Vacutainer system reduces risk of blood exposure.

g. Attach appropriate-size syringe, aspirate proper amount of blood required for ordered specimen, and place in appropriate laboratory tube(s) or obtain specimens with Vacutainer system. If using syringes, a blood transfer device (see illustration) should be used to reduce the risk of needle stick exposure when transferring blood from syringe to laboratory tube.

Multiple specimens can be removed at one time and placed in various different tubes.

h. Flush catheter with 10 ml normal saline solution.

Reduces risk of clotting in catheter after procedure.

i. Flush catheter port with prescribed amount of heparin solution as heparin concentration varies (see agency policy).

Flush volumes will vary with type of catheter used. Heparin flush is believed to reduce incidence of clot formation at tip of catheter.

j. Clamp lumen, and remove cap.

k. Cleanse port with alcohol or chlorhexidine and allow to dry completely.

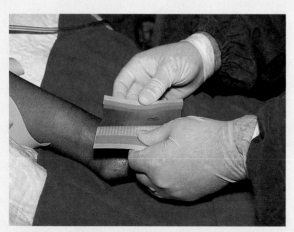

STEP 1k. Application of transparent dressing to PICC site.

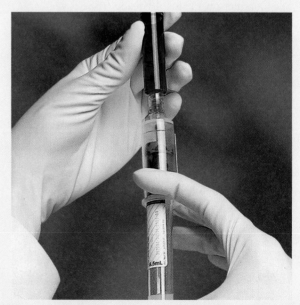

STEP 2g. Blood transfer device prevents needle sticks. (Courtesy Becton Dickenson.)

STEPS	RATIONALE

l. Put on new cap. Open clamps for infusion and resume IV infusion.

m. **See Completion Protocol (inside front cover).**

3 Removal of central venous catheter

a. **See Standard Protocol (inside front cover).**

b. Explain procedure to client.

c. Place client in Trendelenburg's or supine position.

    Trendelenburg's position reduces risk of air embolism entering cerebral circulation.

d. Place moisture-proof underpad beneath site.

e. Remove old dressing and tape. Discard in receptacle. Inspect catheter and insertion site.

    Provides baseline for condition of catheter site.

f. Cleanse site using combination antiseptic or chlorhexidine swabs (or according to institution policy). starting at site and working outward in circular motion or, with chlorhexidine, use a back-and-forth scrub method. Allow to air dry. Remove gloves.

    Removes microorganisms on surrounding skin.

NURSE ALERT Avoid pulling exposed part of suture through skin.

---

g. If sutures present, open suture removal set.

h. **Apply sterile gloves.** With nondominant hand, grasp suture with forceps. Using dominant hand, cut suture carefully with sterile scissors, making sure to avoid damage to skin or catheter. Lift suture out and discard.

    Damaged catheter may break off, leaving a portion of catheter in arm.

i. Using nondominant hand, apply sterile 4 × 4 gauze to site. Instruct client to take deep breath and hold it as catheter is withdrawn.

    Holding breath involves a Valsalva maneuver that reduces the risk of air embolus by decreasing negative pressure in respiratory system.

j. With dominant hand, remove catheter in a smooth, continuous motion. Apply pressure to site immediately and continue for 5 to 10 minutes. Observe for bleeding.

    Client is at risk for bleeding and needs direct pressure on site to prevent hematoma or hemorrhage.

k. Apply Betadine ointment and sterile gauze dressing to site. Write date, time, and initials on dressing.

    Antibiotic ointment reduces chance of bacterial growth at old insertion site.

l. Inspect catheter integrity and discard.

NURSE ALERT If catheter is removed because of suspected infection, send tip to laboratory for culturing per facility policy and procedure. In addition, draw two sets of blood samples for culture (Mermel and others, 2001). If catheter tip is broken or compromised in some way, place catheter in container and apply label with client's name and date. Risk management department of facility may need catheter for investigation.

---

m. **See Completion Protocol (inside front cover).**

EVALUATION

1 Monitor I&O every 8 hours for fluid balance and monitor laboratory values for electrolyte balance as ordered.

2 Inspect IV setup and catheter or port every 8 hours and prn for leaks or tears, secure connections, integrity of dressing, tubing free of obstruction or kinks, correct solution, tubing labeled, and electronic infusion pump functioning properly.

3 Evaluate for complications:

a. Evaluate for signs of clot formation in catheter: difficulty flushing, sluggish infusion, and absent or sluggish blood return.

b. Inspect insertion site every 4 hours for the first 48 hours and then every 8 hours for warmth, tenderness, swelling, drainage, or bruising or bleeding. Observe skin around the site for cellulitis. Check institution policies; more frequent inspection may be delineated.

c. Monitor for systemic infection every 12 hours, including fever, hypotension, tachycardia, increased white blood cell (WBC) count, confusion or change in level of consciousness, and decreased urinary output.

d. Observe for thrombosis every 8 hours, including pain, tenderness, or numbness in the neck, shoulder, or arm on affected side of the body.

e. Observe for air embolism every 8 hours, including dyspnea, respiratory distress, or cyanosis.

f. Observe for extravasation during infusions, including burning or swelling around insertion site or port (Port-A-Cath).

g. Observe for migration of catheter or port every 12 hours:
   (1) *All catheters:* irregular heart rate or dysrhythmia
   (2) *PICC:* frequent nausea and emesis; frequent, severe episodes of coughing
   (3) *Hickman/Groshong:* swelling, burning sensation

Unexpected Outcomes and Related Interventions

1 Client has broken or leaking catheter.

a. *Hickman/Broviac:*
   (1) Stop use of catheter.
   (2) Clamp with nonserrated instrument between broken area and exit site.
   (3) Cover the broken part with sterile gauze and tape securely.

b. *PICC:*
   (1) Stop use of catheter.
   (2) Cover the broken part with sterile gauze and tape securely.

2 Client has infiltration as evidenced by edema, blanched skin, skin cool to touch, pain, numbness, discoloration (Infusion Nurses Society [INS], 2006).

a. Stop infusion immediately.

b. Consult clinical pharmacist for antidote.

3 Client has air embolus as evidenced by new onset of shortness of breath or chest pain.

a. Close off open end of catheter.

b. Place client in Trendelenburg's position on left side.

c. Obtain immediate emergency assistance.

4 Client has bright-red blood filling syringe or tracheal compression with respiratory distress, indicating arterial laceration.

a. Notify physician.

b. Apply direct pressure to artery for 15 minutes.

Recording and Reporting

- Notify physician immediately of signs/symptoms of any physical complications; suspected catheter or port occlusion or migration; leaks, tears, or breaks in catheter.
- Notify physician or nurse who inserted PICC immediately for suspected phlebitis as evidenced by redness pain or edema of affected arm (INS, 2006); suspected catheter occlusion/migration; or leaks, tears, or breaks in catheter.
- Document catheter site care in nurses' notes: size of catheter, changing injection caps: appearance of site, catheter, and suture; date and time of dressing change.
- Document in nurses' notes catheter removal: client position (Trendelenburg's or supine), appearance of site, integrity of catheter on removal, client's tolerance of procedure, and presence/absence of bleeding every 15 minutes × 4.

- Document in nurses' notes: blood draw via injection cap: date, time, sample drawn.
- Document in nurses' notes unexpected outcomes, physician notification, and interventions.

Sample Documentation

1400 Central line dressing change to right subclavian triple-lumen catheter per protocol. No redness, drainage, or swelling to site. Stabilization device intact. All ports with good blood return and flush without difficulty. IV fluids infusing per distal port at 100 ml/hr without difficulty. Middle port attached to CVP monitoring. Injection cap to proximal port changed.

Special Considerations

Pediatric Considerations

- Flush volumes and discard volumes will be less due to smaller catheter length and circumference; check manufacturer's guidelines. Discard volumes are also less because pediatric clients have a smaller amount of total circulating blood volume.

Geriatric Considerations

- The older adult client is at greater risk for alterations in skin integrity, nutritional imbalance, and fluid and electrolyte imbalance.

Home Care Considerations

- Common indications for CVAD in the home setting include antibiotic/antiviral administration, pain control, parenteral nutrition, and hydration.
- Ensure that client or caregiver is able and willing to care for CVAD.
- Ongoing assessment by the home care provider is critical in the early detection of infection and the possible salvage of long term–use catheters.
- Instruct client or caregiver to notify the nurse/physician immediately for pain, swelling, burning, or numbness at site, affected arm, or side of body; bleeding or leaking; difficulty breathing; any perceived change in well-being; or pump alarming.
- Instruct client or caregiver in flushing technique, site care and dressing change, and emergency interventions.

Long-Term Care Considerations

- Long-term care facilities have varying levels of health care providers (e.g., licensed practical nurses, RNs, IV therapy provider, durable medical equipment provider); therefore coordination of CVAD responsibilities is essential.
- The acute care facility should discharge the client to the long-term care facility with instructions taught to the client and written instructions sent so that consistent care is provided.

SKILL 36.2 Administration of Parenteral Nutrition

- Nursing Skills Online: Vascular Access, Lesson 3

Parenteral nutrition (PN) is the administration through a central vein of a nutritionally complete formula, including amino acids, dextrose, fat emulsions, vitamins, electrolytes, minerals, and trace elements. Clients who receive PN have a nonfunctioning gastrointestinal tract from critical illnesses such as pancreatitis, sepsis, cardiac conditions, trauma, liver failure, GI conditions impairing absorption, or anorexia nervosa. A central vein is chosen for infusion, since the vein has a wide diameter and high blood flow, suitable for PN solutions with high osmolarities (e.g., 30% dextrose). This reduces the risk of a chemical phlebitis.

The common sites for PN infusions are the subclavian and internal jugular veins. The PN regimen is individually designed for a client; the prescription is ordered by the physician and reviewed daily, with special consideration given to the electrolyte, fluid, and nitrogen balance. Collaboration with the dietitian is also important.

ASSESSMENT

1 Assess indications of and risks for protein-calorie malnutrition: weight loss from baseline or ideal, muscle atrophy/wasting/weakness, edema, lethargy, failure to wean from ventilatory support, chronic illness, allergy to foods (especially eggs), and nothing by mouth more than 6 days. *Rationale: Clinical indications for parenteral nutrition.*

2 Assess levels of serum albumin, total protein, transferrin, prealbumin, triglycerides, glucose, and urine nitrogen balance as ordered by physician. *Rationale: Provides baseline measure of nutritional status and blood glucose level.*

3 Consult with physician and dietitian on calculation of calorie, protein, and fluid requirements for client. *Rationale: Provides multidisciplinary plan for client's nutritional support.*

4 Inspect condition of central vein access for presence of inflammation, edema, drainage, or tenderness at site. *Rationale: Identifies early signs of infection or infiltration.*

5 Assess baseline vital signs and weight. *Rationale: Provides measures to evaluate effectiveness of nutritional support.*

6 Verify physician's order for nutrients, vitamins, minerals, trace elements, electrolytes, and flow rate. *Rationale: Ensures safe and accurate PN administration.*

PLANNING

Expected Outcomes focus on adequacy of nutrition, adequacy of fluid volume, and prevention of complications related to PN therapy.

1 Client will achieve/maintain ideal body weight.
2 Client will achieve/maintain fluid and electrolyte balance.
3 Client will maintain serum glucose levels at less than 180 mg/dl.
4 Client will remain free of local and systemic infection.

Delegation Considerations

The skill of PN management may not be delegated. The nurse directs personnel to:

- Perform blood glucose monitoring and to report the results.
- Monitor client's urinary output and report the results.

Equipment

- Bedside glucose monitoring kit
- IV tubing
- IV solution of PN
- IV infusion pump
- IV filter (optional: 0.22 μ for dextrose/amino acids, 1.2 μ for three-in-one solutions)
- Alcohol swabs
- clean gloves

IMPLEMENTATION *for Administration of Parenteral Nutrition*

STEPS	RATIONALE
1 See Standard Protocol (inside front cover).	

> **COMMUNICATION TIP** Describe for client the nutrients contained in the solution. Also explain, "We will be checking your blood often to be sure your blood sugar level is just right and that other blood values are where we want them."

STEPS	RATIONALE
2 Initiate central line management protocol (see Skill 36.1).	
3 Inspect PN solution for particulate matter or separation of fat into a layer. Check label on PN solution bag with physician's order.	Presence of matter or lipid separation requires that solution be discarded. Notify pharmacy. Ensures client receives correct solution.
4 Check client's identification band; ask client to state name and compare to PN label.	Ensures that correct client receives correct PN solution. Use at least two client identifiers (neither to be client's room number) whenever administering medications (JCAHO, 2006).

STEPS	RATIONALE
5 Attach appropriate filter to IV tubing, prime tubing, connect it to dedicated port of multilumen central catheter, and label port.	Establishes patent, free-flowing line.
6 Use IV pump or volume controller (see illustration) to infuse solution at ordered rate.	Pump reliably delivers prescribed volume at ordered rate.
7 Assess appearance of central line site routinely (see agency policy) (see Skill 36-1).	
8 Change tubing and filter every 24 hours.	Client is at increased risk of infection because of impaired nutritional status. High concentration of glucose in infusion also increases risk of infection.

> **NURSE ALERT** If bag or tubing contamination is suspected or integrity of product may have been compromised, discard bag and tubing.

9 Do not add medications to PN solution.	In rare circumstances, medications may be administered via the Y-site below the PN filter if verified as compatible by pharmacy or nutrition support service and no other ports are available.

> **NURSE ALERT** Before the time PN solution is due to be totally infused, have backup fluids (D$_{10}$W) available if new PN solution cannot be obtained on time. This maintains blood glucose levels and ensures patency of line.

10 See Completion Protocol (inside front cover).

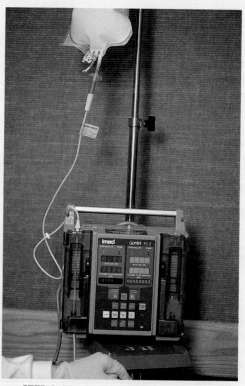

STEP 6 IV pump in use to infuse total PN.

EVALUATION

1 Monitor biweekly weights for fluid balance assessment and nutritional adequacy.

2 Monitor I&O and evaluate for fluid overload or dehydration (see Chapter 9).

3 Monitor blood glucose level every 6 hours or as ordered (see Chapter 13).

4 Monitor for signs and symptoms of infection at infusion site, including redness, swelling, tenderness or drainage; monitor for systemic signs of infection, including fever, elevated WBC count, and malaise.

Unexpected Outcomes and Related Interventions

1 Client develops hypoglycemia or hyperglycemia.

a. Client may need gradual adjustment of concentration of glucose in PN solution.

b. Insulin may be necessary to maintain proper blood glucose level.

2 Client has sharp chest pain, dyspnea, decreased breath sounds on one side, crepitus, cyanosis, or resonance to percussion. These indicate pneumothorax, hydrothorax, or hemothorax.

a. Stop infusion and notify physician immediately.

b. Obtain chest x-ray examination as ordered by physician.

c. Monitor vital signs.

d. Provide emotional support.

e. Assist with insertion of chest tube if necessary (see Chapter 29).

f. Assist with removal of catheter and insertion of replacement.

Recording and Reporting

• Report to physician deviation from baseline assessment or laboratory parameters and signs/symptoms of dehydration or fluid overload.

• Document assessment of physical condition, bedside blood glucose values, and IV solution on applicable flow sheet.

• Document I&O and weight on graphic sheet.

Sample Documentation

0700 Weight maintained at 58 kg for 1 week. Central line insertion site without redness, swelling, or drainage. Vital signs stable. Denies discomfort from catheter. Daily infusions continued with 2000 ml/day as ordered. 150 g dextrose, 42.5 ml amino acids, 200 ml fat emulsion, 50 mEq Na, 30 mEq K, 4.5 mEq Ca, 5 mEq Mg, 50 mEq Cl, 12 mEq PO_4, 10 ml multivitamins, 1 ml trace minerals, and 100 units heparin.

Special Considerations
Geriatric Considerations

• PN is appropriate treatment for older adults with the following conditions:

• Cachexia (chronic protein-calorie malnutrition), which is more common in older adults with cancer, hepatic disease, or chronic neurological disease. Manifestations of cachexia include emaciation, loss of SQ fat and lean body mass, brittle hair, and banded nails.

• Older adults may also have protein malnutrition. Malnutrition is primarily the result of protein losses (not reduced intake), as with burns, pemphigus, or albuminuria.

• Older adults are at higher risk for complications related to PN therapy.

Home Care Considerations

• Assess client's and caregiver's ability to manage parenteral feedings. Also assess environmental conditions: sanitation, equipment storage, power source. Make referral to home IV agency.

• Teach client and caregiver to report any of the following immediately: perceived change in physical condition, weight change, altered glucose values, or change in skin turgor or integrity; pain, redness, or swelling at infusion site; infusion pump alarm that cannot be corrected.

• Instruct client and caregiver in proper steps used to obtain capillary blood sample and measure glucose level.

SKILL 36.3 Care of Clients on Mechanical Ventilation

Mechanical ventilation controls or assists the client's respirations when the client is unable to maintain adequate gas exchange because of respiratory or ventilatory failure (Table 36-1). The ventilator takes over the physical work of moving air in and out of the lungs, but it does not replace or alter the physiological function of the lung. Mechanical ventilation maintains or improves ventilation, oxygenation, and breathing pattern. It corrects profoundly impaired ventilation that may be evidenced by hypercapnia and symptoms of breathing difficulty. Invasive mechanical ventilation typically requires the use of an endotracheal or tracheostomy tube (see Chapter 31) and delivers room air under positive pressure or oxygen-enriched air in concentrations of up to 100%. Noninvasive mechanical ventilation uses a special face or nasal mask (see Chapter 31).

Clients should remain on mechanical ventilation only as long as necessary. When it becomes time to discontinue or wean clients off mechanical ventilation, the goal is to avoid reintubation within 24 to 48 hours after discontinuation. Management of the client on mechanical ventilation and

TABLE 36-1 Overview of Mechanical Ventilation Types

TYPES	DESCRIPTION	NURSING CONSIDERATIONS
Positive-Pressure		
Continuous positive airway pressure (CPAP)	Applies positive pressure during entire respiratory cycle.	Used for clients who breathe spontaneously but have hypoxemic respiratory failure; also useful during weaning.
Positive end-expiratory pressure (PEEP)	Applies positive pressure during expiration.	Used for treating hypoxemic respiratory failure.
Volume-cycled	Delivers a preset volume to client; peak inspiratory pressure will vary.	Used in short-term ventilation and with ventilator weaning.
Pressure-cycled reached	Delivers volume to client until a preset pressure is reached; tidal volume will vary.	Useful when excessive inspiratory pressure could damage lungs, as in neonates; tidal volume varies with airway resistance and lung compliance.
High-Frequency		
High-frequency jet ventilation (HFJV)	Delivers gas rapidly under low pressure via special injector cannula. Delivers 100-200 breaths per minute with tidal volume of 50-400 ml.	Clients on any mode of high-frequency ventilation require continuous sedation and neuromuscular blocking agent administration.
High-frequency oscillatory ventilation (HFOV)	Delivers over 200 breaths per minute or 900-3000 vibrations, with tidal volume of 50-80 ml, airway pressures controlled.	Most common of high-frequency types; maintains alveolar ventilation with low airway pressure; useful for treating esophageal or bronchopleural fistulas or pneumothorax; may avert barotrauma in high-risk clients if used early in treatment.
High-frequency positive-pressure ventilation (HFPPV)	Delivers 60-100 breaths per minute, with tidal volume of 3-6 ml/kg.	Tidal volume is less than the normal 5-7 ml/kg.
Mode of Use		
Control	Fully regulates ventilation in client with paralysis or in arrest. Delivers set tidal volume at prescribed rate, using predetermined inspiratory/expiratory times.	Client may require sedation to reduce competition with ventilator.
Assist	Client initiates inspiration and receives preset tidal volume that augments ventilatory effort.	
Assist-control	Client initiates breathing, but backup control delivers a preset number of breaths at a set volume.	
Synchronized intermittent mandatory ventilation (SIMV)	Ventilator delivers set number of breaths at specified volume; client may breathe spontaneously between SIMV breaths at volumes differing from those set on machine; used for weaning.	Requires frequent monitoring during weaning process.

eventual discontinuation of treatment requires interdisciplinary collaboration among physicians, nurses, respiratory therapists, pharmacists, nutritionists, pastoral care personnel, and rehabilitation services. Nursing care for the client includes provision of emotional support, prevention of equipment failure, prevention of complications (e.g., pneumothorax, atelectasis, decreased cardiac output, pulmonary barotrauma, stress ulcer, or infection), and promotion of optimal gas exchange.

ASSESSMENT

1 Assess client's level of consciousness and ability to cooperate with the procedure and the need for special positioning and sedation during the intubation procedure.

Rationale: Combative behavior on part of client not only makes the procedure more difficult but also requires greater respiratory effort for client.

2 Assess the ability and willingness to communicate and establish an appropriate means to do so (e.g., use of notepad or alphabet board or hand signals). *Rationale: Decreasing apprehension and facilitating communication allows client to remain calmer and more cooperative during mechanical ventilation.*

3 Assess client's need for specialized nutritional support. *Rationale: Client will not be able to have any oral intake and will have increased nutritional needs from the stress related to the condition.*

4 Assess client's baseline vital signs and laboratory values (e.g., electrolytes, arterial blood gases [ABGs], hemoglobin [Hg]/hematocrit [Hct]) ordered by the physician. After initiation of mechanical ventilation, monitor and evaluate client's arterial Hg saturation (Spo_2) per pulse

oximetry and end-tidal carbon dioxide concentration (EtCO$_2$) continuously. *Rationale: Provides means to monitor client's response and tolerance to mechanical ventilation.*

PLANNING

Expected Outcomes focus on establishing and maintaining a patent airway, facilitating effective gas exchange, maintaining adequate fluid volume and nutrition, and preventing complications related to intubation and mechanical ventilation.

1 Client's airway remains clear of secretions.
2 Client's partial pressure of oxygen in arterial blood (Pao$_2$), respiratory pattern, Spo$_2$ and EtCO$_2$ remain within desired parameters.
3 Client's oral and nasal mucous membranes and lips remain moist and clear of abrasions, excoriations, or erosions.
4 Client maintains fluid and electrolyte balance.
5 Client maintains mental status and level of consciousness.
6 Client remains free of lung infection.

Delegation Considerations

The skill of caring for the client on mechanical ventilation may not be delegated.

Equipment

- In-line suction catheter
- Suction unit
- Clean gloves
- 10-ml syringe
- Stethoscope
- Manual resuscitation bag with oxygen tubing
- 1-inch adhesive tape
- Scissors
- Bite block
- Oral airway
- Pulse oximeter (Spo$_2$) sensor and monitor
- Capnography/end tidal CO$_2$ (EtCO$_2$) window and monitor
- Pediatric toothbrush, toothpaste, toothette with chlorhexidine mouthwash

IMPLEMENTATION *for Care of Clients on Mechanical Ventilation*

STEPS	RATIONALE
1 See Standard Protocol (inside front cover).	

> **COMMUNICATION TIP** Reduce anxiety by explaining the ventilator system to client, including anticipated experiences (e.g., suctioning, ventilator alarms) and benefits. Include family in discussion, especially when client is not responsive.

> **NURSE ALERT** Client cannot speak with endotracheal tube in place; be sure that communication device/system is always within reach and available to client.

STEPS	RATIONALE
2 If client does not have an endotracheal (ET) or tracheostomy tube, assist physician with insertion; verify placement with EtCO$_2$ and then order chest x-ray examination.	EtCO$_2$ verifies placement of tube in trachea and not esophagus (Ahrens and Sona, 2003). X-ray examination evaluates correct tube level placement in trachea.
3 Implement safety and infection-control measures:	
a. Check ventilator, EtCO$_2$, Spo$_2$, and cardiac alarms at beginning of each shift, after visits to bedside by others, and after examinations or treatments.	Monitors client's cardiopulmonary status during procedures. Movement during procedures could disrupt ET tube position.
b. Check for endotracheal tube position in centimeters every shift and secure stabilization of artificial airway with every client contact (see Skill 31.4).	Prevents accidental migration of tube into right or left bronchus or extubation of tube.
c. Keep airway, face mask, and manual resuscitation bag at bedside.	Necessary to ventilate client if endotracheal tube is inadvertently removed.
d. Ensure availability of emergency supplies on unit (e.g., extra endotracheal tubes, tracheostomy tube, chest tubes).	
e. Check endotracheal tube cuff, using minimal leak technique, every shift and after any change in tube position (see Chapter 29).	Ensures stable position of tube.
f. Physician verifies tube position after every chest x-ray examination.	Endotracheal tube must be placed through the vocal cords into the trachea. Ensures that the tube is not too close to carina or in the right mainstem bronchus (ACEP, 2001).

STEPS	RATIONALE
g. Using inline catheter, suction endotracheal or tracheostomy tube prn; suction oropharynx/nasopharynx after endotracheal suctioning and before any cuff manipulation (see Chapter 29).	Maintains patency of airway.
h. Use swivel adapter between endotracheal tube and ventilator.	Minimizes movement of endotracheal tube.
i. Move oral endotracheal tube from one side of mouth to the other every 24 hours; retape endotracheal tube every 24 hours when repositioned and prn, using skin prep pads (see Skill 29-4).	Helps to minimize oral mucosa irritation and erosion.
j. Perform oral hygiene every 2 hours with oral toothettes rinsed in chlorhexidine or antiseptic mouthwash. Have oral suction close at hand.	Keeps mucosa hydrated. Suction of secretions during oral care prevents risk of aspiration. Chlorhexidine is effective in reducing oral bacteria in oral cavity.
k. Brush teeth with soft pediatric-size toothbrush and toothpaste at least twice a day. Have suction at hand and remove excess secretions. Remove gloves.	Good oral hygiene through regular tooth brushing decreases plaque and therefore reduces oropharyngeal colonization. It can reduce the risk of VAP (Garp and others, 2003).
l. Monitor in-line temperature and humidity continuously.	Overheating can cause increase in client's body temperature.
m. Keep ventilator tubing clear of condensation and secretions. Always drain tubing away from client into fluid traps in ventilator tubing system before repositioning client.	Prevents accidental spillage into client's airway.
n. Place bite block if client is biting tube.	Prevents obstruction to air flow.
o. Administer sedatives or analgesics as ordered if client is fighting ventilator and ineffective ventilation occurs; observe carefully after administration.	Establishes more relaxed breathing pattern.
p. Troubleshoot high- and low-pressure alarms within 15 seconds. Intervene as necessary to correct cause.	Some causes for high-pressure alarms include tube obstruction from secretions, kinked tubing or airway, and increased airway resistance from bronchospasm or worsening lung disease (pneumothorax, decreased compliance). Possible causes for low-pressure alarms include accidental extubation, disconnection of tubing, or inadequate tracheal tube cuff inflation.
4 When possible, place client in semi-Fowler's position, minimum of 30 degrees' head of bed elevation.	Promotes lung expansion and prevents aspiration if client is on enteral feedings.
5 If client becomes confused or combative, consult physician on use of soft restraints. A time-limited physician's order is required.	Restraints are used to prevent the client from extubating self (see Chapter 3).

COMMUNICATION TIP Reassure client, "This is a way of helping you remember not to pull out the tube that you need to help you breathe."

6 Monitor EtCO$_2$ continuously and ABGs intermittently to detect possible overventilation or inadequate alveolar ventilation.	Overventilation causes respiratory alkalosis from decreased carbon dioxide. Inadequate ventilation may cause respiratory acidosis from increased carbon dioxide (Ahrens and Sona, 2003).
a. Monitor Spo$_2$ continuously (see Skill 11.2).	Provides ability to continuously assess pulmonary function.
b. Assess EtCO$_2$ and Spo$_2$ whenever ventilator settings are changed.	Confirms endotracheal tube placement and cardiopulmonary status and detects client's tolerance to ventilator changes.
c. Check ABGs when a sudden change in client's condition occurs.	Provides more accurate measure of O$_2$ saturation and partial pressure of oxygen.
7 Perform the following at least hourly:	
a. Make sure client can reach call light if able to use it.	Ensures mode of communication for client.
b. Check all connections between client and ventilator, making sure that alarms are turned on, including both high- and low-pressure alarms and volume alarms.	Maintains pressure within system.

STEPS	RATIONALE
c. Verify that ventilator settings are correct and that ventilator is operating at those settings. Compare client's respiratory rate with the setting. Make sure that spirometer reaches correct volume for volume-cycled mode; for pressure-cycled modes, assess exhaled tidal volume.	Maintains integrity of system and ensures that settings are consistent with current physician's orders.

NURSE ALERT Do not assume that ventilator settings are correct because they may be altered accidentally or intentionally by other personnel such as respiratory therapists or physicians. Do not assume that the machine is operating correctly because loose connections or obstructions in tubing can cause altered function despite ventilator settings.

STEPS	RATIONALE
d. Check humidifier and refill if necessary. Check corrugated tubing for condensation and then drain and discard any accumulation.	Do not return condensation to humidifier because of possible bacterial contamination. Responsibilities for ventilator management will vary by facility, check your facility's policy.
e. Check temperature gauges and make sure that gas is being delivered at correct temperature. The desired range of temperatures is between 89.6° F (32° C) and 98.6° F (37° C).	Maintain client's body temperature.
8 At least every 4 hours assess client for:	
a. Confusion, anxiety/restlessness, agitation/lethargy, headache.	Sign of inadequate ventilation/gas exchange.
b. Adventitious breath sounds, dyspnea, tachypnea, inability to move secretions.	Signs of inadequate gas exchange.
c. Decreased urine.	Sign of inadequate renal perfusion.
d. Nasal flaring, tracheal tug, intractable cough, use of accessory muscles.	Signs of ineffective breathing patterns, possibly related to problem with equipment.
e. Changes in respiratory depth, prolonged expiratory phase, or altered chest excursion during spontaneous breaths.	Signs of inadequate ventilation.
9 Auscultate for bilateral breath sounds. Note if they are decreased on left side. Arrange for chest x-ray films as ordered.	Determines whether tube has slipped into right main stem bronchus.
10 Auscultate over trachea for presence of air leaks.	
a. Using minimal occlusive pressure, inflate cuff with 10-ml syringe.	Excessive cuff pressure causes tissue necrosis.
b. Leave syringe attached to cuff of tubing or place on ventilator for easy access.	Cuff deflation destroys seal and results in inadequate ventilation.
11 Monitor fluid I&O and electrolyte balance. Weigh client as ordered.	Fluid retention can signal early pulmonary edema.
12 Using aseptic technique, change tubing only when needed, including humidifier, nebulizer, and ventilator. During tubing change ventilate client manually.	Changing ventilator circuit only with a mechanical failure or when visibly soiled is preferred over routine changing because it does not increase risk of VAP and minimizes circuit disruptions (AACN, 2004; CDC, 2004).
13 Change client's position frequently.	Avoids impaired circulation of both air and blood flow.
14 Perform chest physiotherapy (see Chapter 29) as necessary, including percussion and postural drainage as appropriate.	Promotes clearing of secretions from alveoli and tracheobronchial tree.
15 Monitor GI function to prevent complications:	Inactivity and stress can produce decreased bowel function.
a. Administer H₂ blockers and other medications as ordered.	Reduces gastric acid production to prevent stress ulcer.
b. Auscultate for decreased bowel sounds and check for abdominal distention, which may signal paralytic ileus.	Nasogastric tube may be needed to provide decompression.
c. Check nasogastric secretions for blood using Gastroccult or other agency-approved reagent.	Stress ulcer is a common complication of mechanical ventilation.

STEPS	RATIONALE
16 Provide emotional support to minimize stress.	Apprehension and anxiety can increase client's respiratory rate and effort.

> **COMMUNICATION TIP** Explain procedures even to clients who are unresponsive because they may still be able to hear and understand. "I am going to suction you now so that you can breathe better."

STEPS	RATIONALE
17 Develop activity plan: turning, up to chair, repositioning, or ambulation as tolerated.	
a. During night hours allow 2-hour intervals of uninterrupted sleep with activity during day and evening hours.	Prevents fatigue and helps client develop energy reserve.
b. Do passive/active range-of-motion (ROM) exercises.	Maintains joint mobility and venous return.
c. Change positions every 2 hours and prn.	Reduces incidence of skin breakdown.
d. Evaluate for rotational therapy.	Rotational therapy is a special form of positioning on a rotating bed that will turn in a constant cycle to reduce incidence of atelectasis and pneumonia.
e. Assist client to chair two to three times daily if tolerated.	
f. Assist client to stand and walk in place at bedside if tolerated.	Builds tolerance to exercise.
18 Assist with daily evaluation of client's readiness for a spontaneous breathing trial or ventilator weaning trial.	Daily evaluation of client's spontaneous breathing trial results in quicker liberation from mechanical ventilation (Ely and others, 2001).
19 Initiate interdisciplinary consults as indicated.	Client has potential need for nutritional and spiritual support, physical therapy, speech therapy, or other support.
20 See Completion Protocol (inside front cover).	

EVALUATION

1 Assess client for secretions and suction as needed to maintain airway patency.

2 Continuously evaluate SpO_2, $EtCO_2$, respiratory pattern and vital signs at least every 2 hours for acutely ill clients and at least every 4 hours in stable, chronically ill clients.

3 Monitor ABGs as ordered and prn with respiratory distress.

4 Inspect oral/nasal mucosa and lips for integrity and adequate moisture.

5 Monitor daily weights, I&O, and related laboratory values.

6 Use Glasgow Coma Scale to evaluate neurological status and measure level of consciousness.

7 Monitor for signs and symptoms of infection, including fever, elevated WBC count, and sputum characteristics.

Unexpected Outcomes and Related Interventions

1 Client develops signs/symptoms of inadequate ventilation/gas exchange/ineffective breathing pattern:

a. Remove from ventilator and ventilate with bag/mask device at 100% oxygen.

b. Search for reversible cause.

c. Have assistant call code blue or agency's cardiac/respiratory emergency system if indicated.

2 Client develops signs of inadvertent extubation/malposition of endotracheal tube or leak in cuff, characterized by vocalization/gurgling sounds, activated low-pressure alarm, decreased/absent breath sounds, gastric distention, asymmetrical chest expansion, increased/decreased peak inspiratory pressure (PIP), air leak around mouth/nose, loss of tidal volume, radiographic evidence of malposition.

a. Manually ventilate client with manual resuscitation bag at 100% fraction of inspired oxygen (FiO_2) until reintubation or repositioning of tube is achieved.

b. Have assistant notify physician.

c. Prepare for reintubation.

3 Client develops signs/symptoms of pneumothorax: absent/diminished breath sounds on affected side, acute chest pain, and possibly tracheal deviation or submucosal or mediastinal emphysema.

a. Remove from ventilator and ventilate with manual resuscitation bag/mask device at 100% FiO_2.

b. Prepare for chest tube insertion (see Chapter 29).

4 Client develops signs of atelectasis characterized by decreased or bronchial breath sounds, increased breathing

effort, tracheal deviation toward side of normal findings, increased PIP, decreased lung compliance, decreased Pao_2, Spo_2 in the presence of constant ventilator parameters, or localized consolidation on chest x-ray film.
a. Notify physician.
5 Client develops signs of VAP characterized by purulent secretions or change in consistency/color of secretions, decreased bronchial breath sounds, coarse crackles/wheezes, positive sputum per Gram stain, positive sputum and/or blood cultures, and progressive/persistent infiltrate on chest x-ray film.
a. Notify physician.
b. Administer antibiotics as prescribed.
c. Suction prn and obtain cultures as ordered.

Recording and Reporting

- Document the following on appropriate forms in client record:
  Date/time ventilatory support initiated, size of endotracheal tube, insertion depth in centimeters
  Ventilator settings and client mechanics, including Fio_2 delivered/exhaled tidal volume, minute ventilation, mode of ventilation, breaths per minute, positive end-expiratory pressure, inspiration/expiration ratio or inspiratory time, PIP, compliance, date/time of changes in ventilator parameters
  Physical assessment findings, weight, vital signs, lung sounds, and hemodynamic parameters and waveforms
  Spo_2 and $EtCO_2$ values and ABG values
  Interventions/comfort measures and client's response

Sample Documentation

0930 After discussion with client and physician, client elected to receive mechanical ventilation. Sedated with 2 mg midazolam IV push. Intubated with 7 Fr endotracheal tube by MD; insertion depth 24 cm. $EtCO_2$ level 39 with good waveform on intubation. Cuff inflated to minimum occlusive pressure as verified by auscultation for air leaks. 10-ml syringe at bedside. Tube placement verified with chest x-ray film; no epigastric gurgling noted; bilateral breath sounds auscultated. Fio_2 at 100%; will titrate down to maintain Spo_2 at or above 92%. Ventilator set on assist control, with respiratory rate at 12 and tidal volume at 700 ml. Sedation administered per sedation protocol if client is combative or fighting ventilator. Client tolerated procedure without adverse effects.

Special Considerations
Pediatric Considerations
- Endotracheal tubes used in neonates and small children are cuffless. Strict vigilance to placement is imperative.

Geriatric Considerations
- Older adults are at risk for complications with greater frequency and intensity than younger clients.
- Because of alterations in sensory capabilities, the older adult client has special considerations in communication techniques and emotional support.
- Alterations in electrolyte balance, nutritional status, or cardiovascular function can produce sudden changes in the client's cognitive and physical condition.
- Underlying medical conditions and the presence of multiple medications can have significant negative effects on client's progress.
- Older adults are at greater risk for infection because of diminished immune function.
- Use diligence in monitoring the older adult client's condition on an ongoing basis and perform interventions to limit or control complications quickly and aggressively.

Home Care Considerations
- If family caregiver is unable to accept responsibility for performing all procedures related to mechanical ventilation support, client will require management in long-term facility.
- Backup supplies must be present, including airways, oxygen supply, manual resuscitation bag, and tracheostomy tubes.
- The preparation for transition to the home must begin as soon as possible to allow maximum time to instruct family members and evaluate their return demonstrations.
- Outline emergency interventions clearly to prevent life-threatening complications of treatment.

Long-Term Care Considerations
- Long-term care facilities accepting clients on mechanical ventilation require placement of a tracheostomy for long-term airway management.

SKILL 36.4 Care of Clients Receiving Hemodialysis

The purpose of hemodialysis is to remove toxic wastes and other impurities from the blood in a client with renal failure. The blood is removed from the body through a surgically created access site, pumped though a dialyzing unit to filter out toxins, and returned to the body (Figure 36-2).

Hemodialysis is performed in an emergency in acute renal failure, or as an ongoing long-term therapy in end-stage renal disease. A client's condition determines the frequency and duration of dialysis. For example, a client in chronic renal failure may need treatments up to 3 to 4 hours in

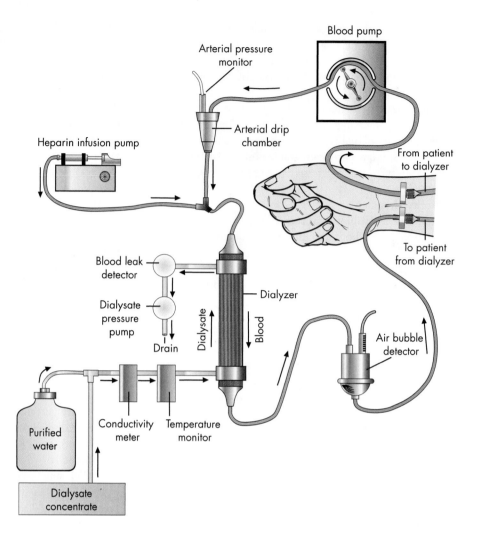

FIGURE 36-2 Components of a hemodialysis system. (Redrawn from Thelan LA, Davie JK, Urden LD: *Textbook of critical care nursing: diagnosis and management,* ed 3, St Louis, 1998, Mosby.)

length, 3 times a week. Hemodialysis helps to restore or maintain acid-base and electrolyte balance, prevent complications associated with uremia, and restore or maintain fluid balance. These goals are met by extracting by-products of protein metabolism (especially urea and uric acid), creatinine, excess water, and other unmeasured toxins from the blood.

A dialysis procedure involves having the client's blood flow between surfaces of semipermeable membranes. At the same time, the dialysis solution (called dialysate) is pumped around the other side of the apparatus using hydrostatic pressure. The dialysate is an aqueous fluid containing isotonic concentrations of sodium and chloride ions; low concentrations of potassium, calcium, and magnesium ions; and high concentrations of bicarbonate and glucose. The toxic wastes and excess water are removed as a result of the differing pressure and concentration gradients between the blood and the dialysate. Because the blood has greater concentrations of hydrogen ions and other electrolytes than the dialysate, the solutes diffuse across the semipermeable membrane into the solution. In the other direction, glucose and acetate are more highly concentrated in the dialysate;

thus they diffuse across the semipermeable membrane into the blood.

A vascular access route is needed for hemodialysis. Dialysis treatments require the easy availability of a large amount of blood flow—at least 250 to 300 ml/min (Ignatavicius and Workman, 2002). Normally the body cannot provide this type of circulation without surgical revision of blood vessels. For chronic, long-term dialysis a surgeon creates an arteriovenous (AV) fistula or graft. AV fistulas are formed by connecting an artery to a vein, usually the radial or brachial artery and the cephalic vein in the nondominant arm (Figure 36-3). To obtain access to a fistula, a dialysis nurse cannulates it or inserts two large-gauge needles, one toward the venous blood flow and one toward the arterial blood flow (Figure 36-4). In this way the hemodialysis machine draws blood out through the artery for filtering and returns it through the venous needle (Ignatavicius and Workman, 2002).

An AV fistula must develop or mature before it can be cannulated. As a fistula matures, the increased pressure of the arterial blood flow into the vein causes the vessel walls to thicken and thus strengthen. AV grafts are used when an AV fistula does not mature or if the fistula becomes clotted.

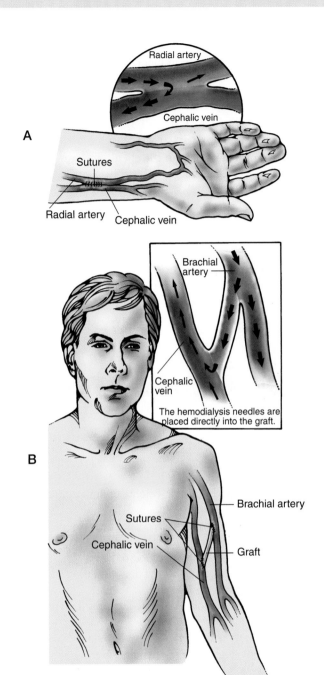

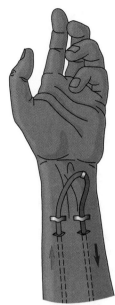

FIGURE 36-4 An arteriovenous shunt in the forearm. One part of the shunt cannula is in an artery; the other part in a vein. The ends of the shunt cannula are joined when dialysis is not in progress. (From Lewis SM and others: *Medical-surgical nursing: assessment and management of clinical problems,* ed 4, St Louis, 2006, Mosby.)

FIGURE 36-3 Options for long-term vascular access for hemodialysis. **A,** Surgically created venous fistula. **B,** Surgically placed straight vascular graft in the upper arm. The graft creates a shunt between arterial and venous blood. (From Lewis SM and others: *Medical-surgical nursing: assessment and management of clinical problems,* ed 4, St Louis, 2006, Mosby.)

A graft placed between the artery and vein is made of a synthetic material, gortex. Gortex can easily be cannulated with a needle.

Additional procedures using temporary dialysis catheters include hemofiltration and ultrafiltration. These therapies are termed continuous renal replacement therapies. Continuous arteriovenous hemofiltration (CAVH) and continuous venovenous hemofiltration (CVVH) are used to treat hemody-

namically unstable clients with fluid overload who do not need dialysis. CAVH and CVVH dialyze clients with unstable blood pressure and those who require both fluid removal and dialysis. These procedures mechanically filter toxic wastes and infuse a replacement fluid such as Ringer's lactate. Ultrafiltration is similar to CAVH but is slower.

Nurses who work in outpatient dialysis centers receive specialized training to administer dialysis. Clients visit these centers usually three times per week with treatment lasting 3 to 4 hours. When these clients become acutely ill and hospitalized, nursing staff must know how to monitor their status and provide appropriate supportive care.

ASSESSMENT

1 Assess client's weight and compare to most recent post-dialysis weight. *Rationale: Sudden weight gain can be caused by fluid retention.*

2 Assess client's vital signs with blood pressure taken in both supine and standing positions if able. *Rationale: Provides baseline to evaluate response to dialysis.*

3 Assess client for changes in mental status, speech, and thought processes. *Rationale: Change in cognition may be caused by fluid and electrolyte imbalances.*

4 Palpate client's distal pulses and auscultate or palpate over fistula or AV shunt for a bruit or thrill. *Rationale: Determines adequacy of circulation in fistula or shunt, as well as distal portion of extremity.*

5 Assess client's heart rate and rhythm. *Rationale: Determines adequacy of systemic circulation and establishes baseline for assessments after dialysis. Also assesses myocardial irritability secondary to possible hyperkalemia and increased blood toxins.*

6 Assess client's respiratory rate, rhythm, quality, and character of lung sounds. *Rationale: Determines baseline for assessing client's respiratory status after dialysis because of potential changes related to fluid overload.*

7 Inspect condition of skin around vascular access. If external device is present, inspect insertion site. *Rationale: Documents skin integrity and absence of infection at vascular access site.*

PLANNING

Expected Outcomes focus on improving client's quality of life, maintaining fluid and electrolyte balance, and preventing complications of the dialysis process.

1 Client relates a feeling of improved well-being.

2 Excess fluid and solute wastes are removed from blood with decreased weight, blood pressure within normal limits, and electrolyte balance.

3 Client is without nausea, vomiting, cardiovascular complications, or alteration in mental status.

4 Vascular access is patent and intact.

5 Client verbalizes understanding of dialysis purpose and procedure.

Delegation Considerations

The skill of providing care to the client receiving hemodialysis may not be delegated.

Equipment

- Stethoscope
- Antiseptic swabs
- 4 × 4 gauze squares or 2-inch gauze roll
- Nonallergenic tape (optional)
- Gloves (sterile and clean as needed)

IMPLEMENTATION *for Care of Clients Receiving Hemodialysis*

STEPS	RATIONALE
1 See Standard Protocol (inside front cover).	

> **COMMUNICATION TIP** Thoroughly review steps of procedure with client and family member. If client has received dialysis in the past, ask if there are any questions or if client wants to discuss the experience.

STEPS	RATIONALE
2 Restrict fluids to 1 to 1.5 L/day.	Reduced renal function limits volume of fluid that can be filtered by body.
3 Develop adequate diet plan in collaboration with dietitian and client. Encourage adherence on part of client.	Reduced renal function limits type and quantity of nutrients that can be metabolized/excreted by body.
4 Before dialysis, provide light meals.	Large meals cause shunting of blood to gut. Hemodynamics are altered during dialysis. Hypotension and vomiting may develop.
5 Alter or adapt routine administration of medications to avoid complications of dialysis.	Hemodialysis may remove some medications if given before dialysis.
a. Withhold antihypertensives per physician order until after treatment.	If client is normotensive before dialysis and medication is given, client might become hypotensive.
b. For IV fluids, do not use lactated Ringer's solution.	Solution has high potassium load. Hyperkalemia is serious risk for client in renal failure.
c. Give calcium used as a phosphate binder with meal, not just "around mealtime."	Calcium must be given with meal to act as phosphate binder rather than calcium supplement.
6 For care of fistula or shunt access.	
a. Inspect for bleeding, edema, warmth. For edema, elevate extremity. Instruct client on how to assess for bruit/thrill daily.	Bleeding may occur from previous needle insertion sites. A thrill on palpation or bruit on auscultation indicates patency of fistula or graft.

> **COMMUNICATION TIP** Be sure that client knows how to properly assess patency of access site by asking for return demonstration. "Please show me where you feel your shunt to be sure that it is not clotted."

STEPS	RATIONALE
b. If clotting is suspected or confirmed, declotting is usually performed in radiology department.	Risk of damage to access site; risk of clotting. Goal is to avoid stagnation of flow to decrease clotting and reduce risk of infection.

STEPS	RATIONALE
c. Use dual-lumen catheters for blood draws and IV fluids only with approval of nephrologist. Flush catheter with correct amount of heparin flush after blood draw.	Repeated access of catheters may result in clotting or catheter damage.

> **NURSE ALERT** If necessary to obtain blood specimen, apply clean gloves.

d. Post warning sign in prominent location and instruct client to refuse to allow others to perform venipuncture or blood pressure measurements on affected extremity.	

> **NURSE ALERT** No blood pressures, needle sticks, or any constricting procedure should be performed on access arm.

e. Clean AV graft limb with warm soap and water daily. Do not apply lotions over fistulas/grafts.	Use of lotion may promote bacterial growth over areas.
f. If access device is external and newly placed, clean around insertion site with antiseptic swab. Using sterile gloves, apply sterile gauze squares, gauze roll, or transparent dressing (see agency policy).	Reduces transmission of infection. Some agencies only allow dialysis staff to care for access sites.
7 See Completion Protocol (inside front cover).	

EVALUATION

1 Compare weight and blood pressure to preprocedure parameters. A weight change of 1 kg is equivalent to 1 L of fluid.
2 Ask client to describe general feeling of well-being.
3 Observe for nausea, vomiting, change in vital signs, or altered level of consciousness. NOTE: Temperature may rise because blood urea nitrogen is an antipyretic and is decreased with dialysis. Hypotension may indicate hypovolemia or a drop in Hct. Rapid respirations may indicate hypoxemia.
4 Inspect vascular access site.
5 Palpate AV shunt or fistula for thrill and auscultate for bruit.
6 Ask client to describe the purpose and process of hemodialysis.

Unexpected Outcomes and Related Interventions

1 Client develops internal bleeding manifested by apprehension; restlessness; pale, cold, clammy skin; excessive thirst; hypotension; rapid, weak, thready pulse; increased respirations; or decreased body temperature.
a. Report to physician immediately.
b. Prepare to transfuse if ordered.
2 Client develops excessive site bleeding.
a. Maintain pressure on site and notify physician.
3 Client develops fever.
a. Assess for sources and signs of infection.
b. Culture blood as ordered.
c. Administer antipyretics and antibiotics as ordered.
4 Client develops hypotension, which may be related to antihypertensive medications, inadequate sodium in diet, unstable cardiovascular disease, hypoalbuminemia, or hypovolemia from excessive fluid and sodium removal during dialysis.
a. Elevate client's feet.
b. Administer 100 to 500 ml normal saline boluses as ordered by physician.
c. Measure blood pressure frequently during episode.
d. Administer colloid osmotic agent as ordered.

Recording and Reporting

• After dialysis, record in the nurses' notes: client education given and client's ability to explain treatment and care responsibilities, assessment of vascular access before and after treatment.
• Record on appropriate flow sheet vital signs, laboratory data, client's weight before and after treatment, and all food and fluid intake before treatment.

Sample Documentation

1045 Client scheduled for hemodialysis. Discussed wife's concerns about patency of fistula. Demonstration with return demonstration by wife of fistula thrill palpation. AV fistula in left forearm has palpable thrill; able to auscultate bruit. Dry weight before treatment 91.2 kg. BP 170/102 mm Hg (sitting); 155/97 mm Hg (standing).

Special Considerations
Geriatric Considerations

• Older adults are at greater risk for complications, including systemic or peripheral circulatory problems such as hypotension and hypoxia that can be life threatening.

Home Care Considerations

- Teach client how to care for vascular access site, which includes keeping incision clean and dry to prevent infections and cleaning site with soap and water daily until healing is complete and sutures are removed; notifying health care team of pain, swelling, redness, or drainage in accessed arm; palpation technique to assess thrill daily; free use of arm after site has healed, with care not to exert excessive pressure on it; avoiding any treatments or procedures on the access arm; and use of exercises for access arm to promote vascular dilation and enhance blood flow.
- Client who will be performing hemodialysis at home must thoroughly understand all aspects of the procedure.

Specialized home care dialysis teams assist client with the transition to home. Client should be given phone number for contacting health care team for any questions or to report any problems. Client should be encouraged to have another person present during home dialysis sessions in case problems develop.

Long-Term Care Considerations

- Long-term care facilities providing hemodialysis often have specialized RNs similar to those in acute care settings to administer hemodialysis.
- Nocturnal hemodialysis is an alternative in long-term care setting.

SKILL 36.5 Care of Clients Receiving Peritoneal Dialysis

Peritoneal dialysis (PD) takes place within the peritoneal cavity. The peritoneum within the abdominal cavity acts like a dialysis machine membrane, filtering infused dialysate solution and blood from vessels in the abdominal cavity. The process is slower than hemodialysis. It removes toxins from the blood of a client with acute or chronic renal failure who does not respond to or tolerate hemodialysis. In addition, lifestyle and client choice may dictate the use of PD.

The surgical insertion of a silicon rubber (Silastic) catheter into the abdominal cavity is necessary to infuse PD solutions (Ignatavicius and Workman, 2002) (Figure 36-5). During PD a hypertonic dialysate solution is infused into the peritoneal cavity (Figure 36-6), and then diffusion moves the excessive concentrations of electrolytes and uremic toxins across the membrane into the dialysate. The solution is left for a specified period of time and then drained. The semipermeable peritoneal membrane filters excess water, electrolytes, and toxins from the blood. Excessive water is removed in the same way by osmosis. After an appropriate dwell time, the dialysate solution is removed, to be replaced by fresh solution. The procedure may be performed manually or by a cycler machine. Table 36-2 summarizes the types of peritoneal dialysis.

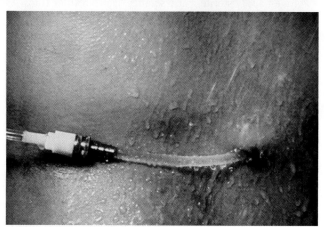

FIGURE 36-5 Tenckhoff catheter used in peritoneal dialysis. (From Lewis SM, Collier IC, Heitkemper MM: *Medical-surgical nursing: assessment and management of clinical problems,* ed 5, St Louis, 2000, Mosby.)

ASSESSMENT

1 Assess client's weight and vital signs before treatment. Blood pressure should be measured with client standing and supine. *Rationale: Provides predialysis baseline.*
2 Assess client's serum electrolyte levels, especially potassium. *Rationale: Determines amount of potassium to be added to dialysate, ordered by physician.*
3 Assess client's knowledge and compliance with diet plan. Review sources of high sodium, potassium, and phosphorous; these often require restriction. *Rationale: Foods high in sodium, potassium, and phosphorus increase client's risk for fluid and electrolyte imbalances.*

PLANNING

Expected Outcomes focus on successful filtering of toxic wastes from client's blood, maintaining fluid and nutritional balance, and prevention of complications related to the dialysis treatment.

1 Excess fluid and solute wastes are removed from blood and lymph as evidenced by decreased weight, blood pressure within normal limits, and electrolyte balance (especially potassium).
2 Client relates a feeling of improved well-being.
3 Client has no complications as evidenced by absence of nausea, vomiting, cardiovascular complications, respiratory distress, or alteration in sensorium.
4 Client's catheter remains patent and intact.
5 Client verbalizes understanding of PD purpose and procedure.

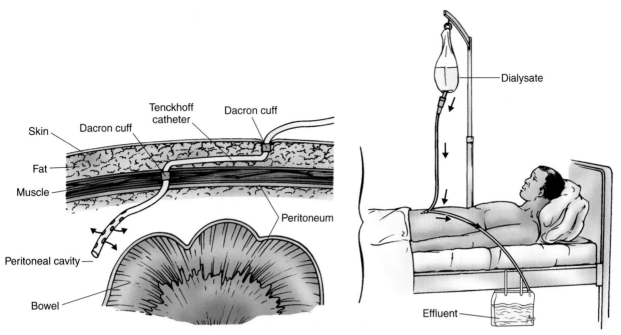

FIGURE 36-6 Manual peritoneal dialysis via an implanted abdominal catheter (Tenckhoff catheter). (From Lewis SM and others: *Medical-surgical nursing: assessment and management of clinical problems,* ed 4, St Louis, 2000, Mosby.)

TABLE 36-2 Methods of Peritoneal Dialysis	
TYPE	**DESCRIPTION**
Continuous ambulatory peritoneal dialysis (CAPD)	Manual; three to five exchanges daily; last bag of solution remains in abdomen overnight.
Continuous cycling peritoneal dialysis (CCPD)	Cycler machine changes solution 3-5 times or more overnight; last bag of solution remains in abdomen during daytime.
Intermittent peritoneal dialysis (IPD)	Manual or automated; connected for about 10 hours, with cycle changing every 30-60 minutes; abdomen left "dry" between sessions.

Equipment
Dialysis Infusion
- PD administration set (i.e., all-in-one combined drainage and infusion bag system)
  Medications to be added to PD infusion (may be added by pharmacy)
- Mask
- Graduated containers for measuring I&O or scale for weighing dialysate drained
- Stethoscope

Site Care
- Sterile gloves and masks
- Precut sterile 4 × 4 gauze
- Cotton swabs with povidone-iodine or other antiseptic solution

Delegation Considerations
The skill of performing peritoneal dialysis may not be delegated. The nurse instructs personnel to:
- Provide routine comfort measures throughout the procedure.

IMPLEMENTATION *for Care of Clients Receiving Peritoneal Dialysis*

STEPS	RATIONALE

1 See Standard Protocol (inside front cover).
2 Review client's understanding of treatment and provide emotional support.

COMMUNICATION TIP Client often is fatigued and may experience other symptoms because of blood toxins. Keep discussion simple and focused on client needs.

STEPS	RATIONALE
3 Warm dialysate solution to body temperature according to agency procedure.	Avoids hypothermia and shock during infusion.
4 Prepare any prescribed medications (e.g., heparin, potassium chloride, antibiotics) to be added to dialysate following the six rights of medication administration (see Chapter 15), then add medications to dialysate aseptically (see Chapter 27).	Ensures right client receives right medications. Some agencies require medications to be added in pharmacy.
5 Identify client by checking identification bracelet and asking client's name. Compare with medication administration record.	Ensures correct client receives medication. Use at least two client identifiers (neither to be client's room number) whenever administering medications (JCAHO, 2006).
6 Place client in supine position with head of bed elevated at client's comfort when equipment and solutions are ready.	Promotes comfort and relaxation. Abdominal distention from fluid instillation makes breathing difficult in Fowler's or semi-Fowler's position. If tube is new, supine position may help prevent hernias.
7 Apply mask and then prepare dialysis administration set. Have client and all persons in room wear mask during connection and disconnection of administration set.	Avoids introducing pathogens into peritoneal cavity.
a. Remove end cap or pull ring from PD system and remove cap from client's dialysis catheter. Immediately in sterile fashion, connect PD system to dialysis catheter (see Figure 36-6).	Nothing must touch end of catheter or dialysis system to prevent infection.
b. Hang drainage bag on bed frame below client.	Facilitates drainage by gravity.
c. Open any clamps on client drain line and let the peritoneal cavity drain. Client may need to change position; roll from side to side.	Position changes help to eliminate all of old dialysate.
d. When drainage complete (typically 15 to 30 minutes), close transfer set on dialysis catheter.	
8 Prime infusion side by allowing solution to fill drainage bag for approximately 5 seconds.	Maintains integrity of system and prevents air from entering line.

> **NURSE ALERT** Avoid introducing air into peritoneal cavity.

STEPS	RATIONALE
9 Clamp drain side.	
10 Open transfer set and infuse prescribed amount of dialysate solution into peritoneum. Remove gloves.	Allows for instillation of dialysate into peritoneal cavity.
11 Allow ordered solution to dwell for prescribed interval (10 minutes to 4 hours).	Fluid dwell time varies, dependent on concentration of electrolytes to be removed.
12 When dialysis treatment is completed, mask client, put on mask and gloves, and then clamp the catheter.	Sterile technique needed.
13 After carefully disconnecting inflow line from catheter, place a sterile (Betadine) cap over catheter end.	Avoid introducing pathogens into peritoneal cavity.
14 Measure volume of effluent/drainage using spring scale (1 g = 1 ml) or in graduated cylinder.	
15 **See Completion Protocol (inside front cover).**	
16 Repeat cycles of drainage-infusion-dwell (using a new dialysate system of solution for each cycle) until prescribed amount of dialysate and prescribed number of cycles have been achieved.	Prescribed cycling is necessary to achieve desired fluid and electrolyte balance.
17 Monitor vital signs every 15 minutes until stable and then every 2 to 4 hours as ordered.	Client is at risk for respiratory distress from fluid overload.
18 During treatment have client change positions frequently and perform ROM exercises and deep breathing.	Improves client comfort, reduces risk of impaired skin integrity, reduces risk of respiratory complications, and enhances dialysate drainage.

STEPS	RATIONALE
19 Maintain adequate nutrition, adhering to any prescribed diet.	Needed to replace protein lost during dialysis.
20 Maintain standard precautions when emptying collection bag and measuring solution.	Fluid is contaminated and may carry transferable diseases such as hepatitis.
21 Change dressing every day and prn.	Reduces development of infection at catheter insertion site.
a. See Standard Protocol (inside front cover).	
b. Mask yourself and client. Remove old dressing and contaminated gloves.	Prevents transmission of infection to peritoneum, which could lead to peritonitis.
c. Inspect site for signs of infection. Then prepare sterile field or open sterile kit: prepare dressing of two precut 4 × 4 gauze pads and three cotton swabs soaked in povidone-iodine or other antiseptic solution.	
d. Apply sterile gloves. Use cotton swabs to clean around catheter site. Use circular motion, starting from insertion site and moving away toward the abdomen.	Removes microorganisms on skin's surface.
e. Apply precut gauze pads over catheter site. Tape edges of gauze pads.	
22 See Completion Protocol (inside front cover).	

EVALUATION

1 Compare weight and blood pressure to preprocedure parameters. A weight change of 1 kg is equivalent to 1 L of fluid.

2 Monitor electrolytes (especially potassium).

3 Ask client to describe general feeling of comfort.

4 Observe for respiratory distress indicating fluid overload or leakage of dialysate into pleural cavity. Watch for abdominal pain, cloudiness of effluent, and fever, which can indicate peritonitis.

5 Observe catheter for kinks and observe outflow for cloudiness, blood, or blood clots. Clear fluid drainage should be present after a few fluid changes. Observe site for signs of infection.

6 Ask client to describe the purpose and process of peritoneal dialysis.

Unexpected Outcomes and Related Interventions

1 Client develops peritonitis manifested by abdominal pain and elevated temperature.
a. Notify physician.
b. Culture all sites to determine portal of entry: transluminal, periluminal, hematogenous, or through bowel wall.
c. Administer prescribed antibiotics.
d. Consult with physician for possible removal of catheter.

2 Client develops exit site infection manifested by redness, swelling, heat, and pain.
a. Notify physician.
b. Assess response to cleansing agents.
c. Continue thorough daily site care.
d. Administer antibiotics as ordered.

3 Client develops abdominal or shoulder pain.
a. Abdominal pain may be related to rapid inflow. Decrease rate of infusion during initial exchanges.
b. Pain may be related to abdominal distention and air in peritoneal cavity. Prime new tubing carefully and do not use vented systems.

4 Client develops increased body temperature or decreased body temperature due to inadequate management of temperature control of dialysate solution.
a. Drain solution.
b. Treat for hyperthermia or hypothermia.
c. Evaluate warming procedure.

5 Client develops fluid overload, manifested by dyspnea, altered mental status, and alteration in breath sounds.
a. Calculate fluid balance accurately.
b. Use a more hypertonic dialysate as ordered by physician.
c. Limit fluid intake.
d. Shorten dwell time.
e. Correct any catheter malfunction.
f. Monitor weight, vital signs, and cardiorespiratory status frequently.

6 Client develops fluid deficit manifested by alteration in fluid and electrolyte balances.
a. Calculate fluid balance accurately.
b. Discontinue use of hypertonic solution.
c. Replace fluid and sodium losses.
d. Monitor vital signs and weight closely.
e. Lengthen dwell time.

7 Client develops hypokalemia manifested by decreased levels of serum potassium.

a. Monitor serum potassium.

b. Add potassium to dialysate for clients with normal levels.

c. Instruct clients with chronic problems to increase dietary intake of potassium.

Recording and Reporting

- Document client's vital signs, weight, laboratory results, type of solution, number of cycles, and volume of infusion and return.
- Document any unexpected outcomes and interventions performed.
- Report any significant changes to physician.

Sample Documentation

1015 Weight after peritoneal dialysis is 70 kg. Electrolytes are WNL. Vital signs: BP 159/82 mm Hg, pulse 94 beats per minute, respirations 20 breaths per minute. Temperature 37° C. Inflow 2 L in 15 minutes, dwell time 4 hours, drained 2300 ml in 15 minutes. Effluent clear, pale yellow. Site nontender without redness or drainage. Client reports feeling much better. Denies questions or concerns about the procedure.

Special Considerations
Geriatric Considerations

- Older adults are at risk for complications related to metabolic and nutritional changes and difficulty in following through with instructions because of alterations in sensory perceptions and judgment.
- Monitor clients carefully to ensure that complications are prevented or minimized.

Home Care Considerations

- The client who will perform continuous ambulatory peritoneal dialysis (CAPD) or continuous cycling peritoneal dialysis at home will usually undergo a 2-week training program before performing the treatment independently.
- The client must be able to understand and perform all the necessary steps of the procedure, in addition to verbalizing when to report any untoward effects of treatment such as infection and fluid imbalance.
- A support group can be helpful in facilitating adjustment to client's new regimen.
- Home care nurses provide periodic supervision and assessment of client's performance of the treatment.
- Client should be able to verbalize the following items related to care of insertion site and catheter: avoid showers until exit site has healed; once site has healed, showering only; no bathing in tub or swimming in unchlorinated pools, lakes, or rivers; avoid running through fountains; no sports in which trauma to the abdomen is probable; and no heavy weight lifting.
- Client should carry emergency medical information and identification at all times, including phone number of dialysis center.
- Client should record vital signs, weight, and response to each treatment.
- Nurse stresses importance of follow-up visits with dialysis team to evaluate effectiveness of treatment and detect any problems that may arise.

Long-Term Care Considerations

- Staff of long-term care facilities may be trained in use of either the Y-bag or cycler system, with support from a continuous peritoneal dialysis unit (Carey and others, 2001).
- The transition from acute care to home care will be improved by consistent use of one system as selected by client and physician.

NCLEX® Style Questions

1 Place the following skills steps in proper sequential order for CAPD using an all-in-one combined system.
1. After drainage complete, close off PD catheter.
2. Remove cap from dialysis catheter and attach CAPD system to PD catheter.
3. Remove end cap from CAPD system.
4. Place drainage bag below client.
5. Clamp drainage bag.
6. Apply mask to self, client, and all persons in room.
7. Prime infusion side by allowing solution to fill drainage bag for approximately 5 seconds.
8. Open clamps on client's catheter and drain line.
9. Open PD catheter and infuse prescribed amount of dialysate solution.

2 Place the following skill steps in proper sequential order for removal of a central venous catheter.
1. Cleanse site with antiseptic and allow to air dry.
2. Using nondominant hand, apply sterile 4 × 4 gauze to site and instruct client to take deep breath and hold as catheter is withdrawn.
3. Open suture removal set.
4. Place client in Trendelenburg's or supine position.
5. With dominant hand, remove catheter in a smooth, continuous motion.
6. Wearing nonsterile gloves, remove old dressing and tape. Discard catheter in receptacle.
7. Apply sterile gloves and remove sutures.
8. Apply pressure to site immediately and hold pressure for 5 to 10 minutes.
9. Apply Betadine ointment and sterile gauze dressing to site; write date, time, and initials on dressing.

3 The client's central line transparent dressing has been in place for 4 days; however, the edges of the transparent dressing are loose. What is the appropriate action?
1. Assess site and tape down loose edges.
2. Assess site and apply another transparent dressing over the existing dressing.
3. Assess site, remove loose dressing, cleanse site per protocol, and apply new transparent dressing.
4. Assess site and apply gauze dressing over existing transparent dressing.

4 What is included when teaching clients with new hemodialysis AV fistulas?
1. How to check their blood pressure
2. How to check for fistula thrill
3. How to measure their heart rate
4. How to cleanse site with Betadine and cover with dressing

References for all chapters appear in Appendix D.

37

Palliative Care

MEDIA RESOURCES

- **evolve** http://evolve.elsevier.com/Elkin

A lthough much of health care is devoted to helping people who are seeking cure and recovery from acute diseases and injury, there is a dramatic increase in the number of people who are living with chronic, incurable illnesses. Furthermore, as good as technical medicine is, everybody dies and needs expert, sensitive nursing care throughout that process. Palliative care, a growing specialty in nursing, responds to this need for a shift in focus to the care of clients whose disease cannot be cured. The main goal of palliative care is to help clients and families achieve the best quality of life possible. It involves expert management of pain and the other symptoms clients experience physically, psychologically, and spiritually. Palliative care involves both the client and family and is used at any point during the course of an illness, acute or chronic, from diagnosis to death. It is important to know the differences between palliative and hospice care (Box 37-1).

Clients who have complex, serious illness may benefit from palliative care throughout the course of their illness, even while seeking treatment for their disease. As the goals of care change, the focus may shift to more palliative care strategies. Hospice care is a final phase of palliative care, designed for clients who can no longer benefit from treatment, who will likely not live more than 6 months, or who are actively dying (Figure 37-1). Making this distinction is important because some clients, family members, or health care professionals may refuse helpful palliative care interventions, believing that palliative care is only for the dying (Douglass, Maxwell, and Whitecar, 2004). Because end-of-life care provides an excellent example of palliative care, the remainder of this chapter will focus on nursing care of the dying client.

Shifting the focus of nursing care away from cure and toward improving quality of life is challenging. Symptoms or treatments considered appropriate when seeking cure for an illness may no longer be appropriate for a client approaching the end of life (Ferrell and Coyle, 2006). For example, consider nutritional therapies in curative versus end-of-life treatment. When clients try to recover from an illness, they may be encouraged to eat more foods to increase their strength and healing. However, when clients approach death, their body systems change. There is decreased blood flow to the gastrointestinal (GI) tract and decreased cardiovascular (CV) function. The effects of illness and treatment, fatigue, and decreased activity decrease a client's caloric needs and intake. Clients who are near death often lose their appetite or feel nauseated by food. Forcing food or fluid intake may stress the GI and CV systems, potentially creating increased discomfort (Ersek, 2003).

Providing relief of pain and suffering is a hallmark of palliative care nursing. Pain management at the end of life has some unique aspects (Paice and Fine, 2006). Offer accurate information and assurance to clients and family members unfamiliar with pain management drugs and their side ef-

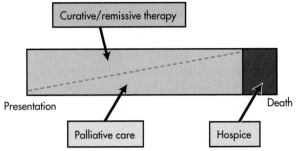

FIGURE 37-1 Palliative care and hospice. (From Emanuel L and others: *The EPEC Project,* Chicago, Il, Northwestern University.)

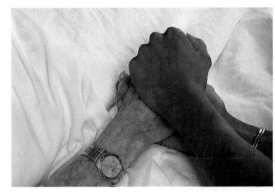

FIGURE 37-2 Touch can communicate caring and compassion.

fects. Because pain and other discomforts are what people say they are, you should make thorough, ongoing assessments without imposing judgments on the client's reports of pain (Wentz, 2003). The more you understand palliative care interventions, the better you are able to assist clients and families achieve a higher quality of life and symptom relief.

PSYCHOSOCIAL/SPIRITUAL CARE

In palliative care give priority to client and family emotional and spiritual experiences. In situations involving serious life-limiting illness, it is critical that you develop the ability to understand, acknowledge, and be present to people experiencing intense emotions. The experiences of death and dying have been extensively researched. In her classic study of emotional responses to death and loss, Kübler-Ross (1969) identified five stages: denial, anger, bargaining, depression, and acceptance. Even though Kübler-Ross describes the dying process in stages, the nurse must realize that each person does not necessarily pass through all of the stages in an orderly, sequential manner. Clients may not experience some stages, or they might move back and forth between them. Sometimes nurses or family members take the client's emotional expressions personally or try to protect the client from experiencing fear, anger, or depression. Remember that the client's emotions are not something you are expected to "fix." Instead, view emotional expression as a necessary part of the client's adjustment to significant life changes and development of effective coping skills. Clients may hesitate to express their

emotions for fear that others will abandon them. However, there is evidence that allowing clients to talk about their emotions and fears promotes hope and well-being (Buckley and Herth, 2004). Active listening and being available to others who are expressing intense emotions builds therapeutic, trusting relationships among the client, family members, and the nurse. Compassion and attentiveness may be conveyed in many ways, including the therapeutic use of touch (Figure 37-2), active listening, and sometimes simply sitting in silence with the client (Stanley, 2002).

The death of a loved one causes grief for the survivor(s). Grief is the emotional and behavioral response to loss. Survivors (and clients) experience grief in many different ways, including sadness, relief, denial, shock, guilt, or anger. People express grief differently, but most people gradually move through their grief and learn to adjust to life without their loved one. However, for some people the grief process becomes more prolonged and very difficult. For example, multiple losses or the loss of a child can be especially hard to understand or accept. Deaths by murder or suicide can leave survivors with questions that will never be answered. People without sufficient social supports may have a harder time functioning in daily life. These are examples of dysfunctional (or complicated) grief,

---

BOX 37-2 Spirituality Concepts

Meaning
- What gives your life meaning and purpose in your current situation?
- What are your goals, things you still want to achieve?
- What do you live for now?

Hope
- What do you hope for?
- How have your hopes changed?
- What gives you hope during difficult times?

Community
- Who are the people most important to you?
- Who gives you comfort in difficult times?
- Are you able to participate in community activities (i.e., church, family, friends, neighborhood)?

Sense of Holy Other or God
- What is your concept of that which is larger than yourself? What is God like for you?
- Is religion or God significant to you? If yes, can you describe how?
- Are there certain religious practices or rituals that are meaningful to you?

---

which often require ongoing bereavement support and/or referral for professional help.

Spiritual concerns often arise in situations of serious chronic illness and impending death. Clients and family members may face questions about the meaning of life, pain, suffering, life's limitations, and the loss of personal and environmental control. You need skills in spiritual assessment, planning, and intervention to offer palliative care in these situations. Begin by developing a working definition of spirituality. Although spirituality is defined many ways, four basic concepts may provide direction to spiritual assessment and interventions. Those concepts are: meaning, hope, community, and a sense of the Holy Other (Vandecreek and Lucas, 2001). A spiritual assessment helps you understand the client's spiritual strengths and needs and identify helpful interventions. Some questions that might help you better understand these spiritual concepts and complete a spiritual assessment are described in Box 37-2.

Since discussions about spiritual concerns may arouse feelings of discomfort or uncertainty, limit initial data collection to information most immediately helpful in assisting the client and family. Explain that these personal matters are being discussed to provide the most holistic care possible. Discuss spiritual questions at an appropriate time and approach the topic in a quiet and unrushed manner. Sometimes a spiritual assessment can be a spiritual intervention (i.e., the client or family may experience hope or connectedness while talking about spiritual strengths or needs with an attentive listener). Expand the assessment through quiet observation and explore spiritual concerns when they arise.

The spiritual concept of hope takes on great significance near the end of life. Clients with terminal illness may fear pain, loneliness, loss of control, being a burden to others, or the possibility of dying alone. Because hope and help are related, when clients believe no one is there to help them, they can become fearful and feel hopeless. Encouraging expression of fears supports the client's ability to feel hopeful and find meaning in his or her present circumstances. Dying clients and their families hope for different things over the course of their experience with illness and death. They may hope to attend a family wedding, sit at the table for meals, see an important person one last time, or have a peaceful death. Listen for shifts in what clients hope for and find ways to support those emerging sources of hope.

The terms spirituality and religion are often used interchangeably and for many people are closely related. However, there are important differences in these terms. Religion refers to a person's specific beliefs and behaviors associated with a religious tradition (Koenig, 2002). Spirituality is an awareness of one's inner self and a sense of connection to a higher being, nature, or a greater purpose (Mauk and Schmidt, 2004). All clients, including those who do not practice a particular religion, have spiritual strengths, needs, and practices. Clients and families who do not practice a religion may emphasize their values, relationships, and life accomplishments at the time of death or remember the deceased at a nonreligious service. If clients and their families have a religious tradition, honoring practices unique to their beliefs can be very important when providing individualized care. Involvement of a priest, rabbi, pastor, or hospital chaplain facilitates spiritual and religious care for people at the end of life.

Remember that often people within the same religion have varying beliefs or practices or adhere more or less strictly to their beliefs. However, there are some common understandings related to specific religious practices at the end of life that are helpful to consider (Box 37-3).

Cultural sensitivity is crucial in end-of-life care. Social and demographic trends in the United States show significant changes in ethnic, racial, and cultural characteristics of populations served by health care providers (Valente, 2004). The client's culturally influenced health care beliefs and practices, communication patterns, and family structures affect the dying process. The same is true for nurses and all caregivers. To provide appropriate care, look beyond your personal assumptions and preconceived ideas and focus on the needs and cultural practices of those in your care.

LEGAL/ETHICAL ISSUES

End-of-life care poses difficult ethical questions in health care. Ethical issues related to advance directives, aid-in-dying, use of artificial food and hydration, euthanasia, pain management, or the appropriate use of technology at the end of life demand careful attention and continued dialogue. Health care providers help families make difficult decisions at the end of life, making it imperative that you develop knowledge and insight on ethical and legal matters (Briggs and Colvin, 2002).

BOX 37-3 Some Religious Practices Related to Death and Dying

Judaism: The belief in an afterlife is held in some types of Judaism, as well as the belief that one's good deeds in life live on in the memory of loved ones. Because life is valued as a gift of God, efforts to continue life are supported, especially in Orthodox Judaism. After death there should be no preparation of the body until it is known whether members from the Jewish Burial Society are coming to the facility. A family member may stay with the body until burial. It is customary to be buried within 24 hours, but not on the Sabbath. Families participate in a mourning period during which grief is expressed openly and in keeping with ritual. In some, but not all types of Judaism, cremation, autopsy, and embalming are avoided.

Christianity: Christians believe in life after death and eternal life. Some may request rituals of confession, laying on of hands, anointing the sick, baptism, or holy communion. Prayer and reading from the Bible may be appropriate. There may be a period of viewing the body or a wake before burial. A funeral or memorial service is the norm. Cremation, autopsy, and embalming are usually allowed.

Islam: Muslims believe in eternal life and the will of God (Allah). Clients may wish to face Mecca (the East) as they are dying. Cleanliness and modesty are very important. Regular prayer five times a day should con-

tinue as long as possible. Honoring that schedule shows respect to the client, family, and the Muslim faith. Loved ones usually remain with the dying person 24 hours a day and may wish to prepare the body with ritual washing and wrapping in a white cloth at the time of death. Burial is usually in a Muslim cemetery within 24 hours.

Hinduism: Hindus believe in one supreme deity and in lesser gods with power and interest in specific areas of life. Beliefs include reincarnation and karma (how one has lived in this world affects how one might return in the next one). Clients may want the presence of a Brahmin priest who may chant prayers. Only the family should touch the body after death, and they are responsible for washing and preparing the body. Cremation is traditional.

Buddhism: There is no supreme deity. The "eightfold path" consists of maintaining right beliefs, intent, speech, conduct, endeavor, mindfulness, effort, and meditation. The goal of life and death is to reach the eternal state of nirvana, or inner peace and happiness. Death is a transition and part of life; there is a belief in rebirth. The client may want to remain conscious to be able to think right thoughts during the dying process. Cremation and autopsy are usually allowed.

Data from Kemp C, Bhungalia S: Culture and the end of life: a review of major world religions, *J Hospice Palliative Nurs* 4(4):235-242, 2002.

An important ethical-legal consideration in palliative and end-of-life care concerns the use of advance directives. Advance directives can take several written forms or can be negotiated by a client's representative, known as a durable power of attorney for health care. In an advance directive, a client communicates his or her values and wishes about future medical care to help guide decisions when the client can no longer participate (e.g., overwhelming illness, unconsciousness, or sedating drugs). Clients can express their wishes on the use of extraordinary medical procedures, artificial nutrition and fluids, comfort measures, life support interventions, or any other unique preference for care in their advance directive. Laws relating to advance directives vary from state to state; thus it is imperative to know those that apply. Institutions usually have written policies and sample forms for advance directives that can help clients and families in their deliberations. Copies of completed advance directives should be given to the physician, to responsible family members, and placed in the client's medical record. Even if a client's wishes regarding cardiopulmonary resuscitation (CPR) are outlined in an advance directive, a physician must also write a "do not resuscitate" order in the medical chart when a decision is made by the client or family to not initiate CPR. Because these discussions are very sensitive and emotional for clients and families, provide a quiet setting for dialogue and participate whenever your involvement is appropriate.

Some clients may desire to hasten their death and ask for aid-in-dying. This very controversial topic arouses intense feelings in clients, families, and caregivers. Although simple answers to this difficult question are impossible to give, you should talk to a client about fears of suffering, pain, and abandonment that may underlie the interest in aid-in-dying. Regardless of your own beliefs, you should listen nonjudgmentally to the client's concerns so that suitable interventions, such as more effective pain management or help with spiritual distress, can be offered. The involvement of the client, family, and all members of the interdisciplinary team is essential for discussing ethical concerns.

SELF-CARE

Nurses involved in palliative and/or hospice care are often affected, touched, and changed by their experiences with clients and families (Wakefield, 2000). Because of the deep personal connections experienced in palliative care, it is natural for nurses to share with clients and families feelings of sadness, helplessness, and loss. They may be reminded of their own personal losses or struggle with difficult ethical dilemmas. To nurture the insights necessary to remain present, helpful, and meaningfully engaged with clients experiencing suffering, death, or loss, you should consistently take care of yourself physically, spiritually, and emotionally and develop "personal power" (Sherman, 2004). Some self-care strategies include talking about feelings and experiences with trusted friends; humor; maintaining physical, emotional, mental, and spiritual health; getting adequate sleep; and using exercise, meditation, or prayer. You might also gain insight by reflecting on your own personal beliefs and feelings about death and loss (Box 37-4).

EVIDENCE IN PRACTICE

Harstäde C, Andershed B: Good palliative care: How and where? The patient's opinions, *J Hospice Palliative Nurs* 6(1):27-35, 2004.

This research describes clients' and families' perspectives on preferred end-of-life care, including relationships and tasks. Clients prefer care that helps them feel safe, encourages

---

BOX 37-4 Reflecting on Personal Feelings About Death

1 Do you believe it is part of your nursing role to talk with clients/families about death?
2 Are you able to be "present" with people when they express emotions?
3 What are your personal experiences with significant loss?
4 Are you experiencing grief in your life at this time? How might that affect your response to others' grief?
5 How do your personal spiritual beliefs affect caring for people who are dying?
6 How do you act when you are in situations that you feel powerless to change?

---

their participation, and gives them a sense of trust. They want to feel it is safe to express their thoughts and feelings, however difficult, with others. Clients' feelings of safety also increase when they believe their caregivers are clinically competent. Active client participation in treatment discussions and exploring options with trusted caregivers are also highly valued.

NURSING DIAGNOSES

Although appropriate nursing diagnoses will vary according to the disease process and individual client/family needs, the following are commonly associated with palliative care. The diagnosis of **acute pain** and/or **chronic pain** applies when pain is unrelieved and/or requires ongoing evaluation. **Risk for constipation** is related to use of opioid analgesia and immobility. **Risk for impaired skin integrity** is related to immobility, poor nutrition, and muscle wasting. **Anxiety** may apply when the client has difficulty sleeping or is agitated or restless. A client who is having difficulty finding or maintaining sources of strength, hope, community, or meaning may be at **risk for spiritual distress**. Because religious practices may be central to a client's spiritual well-being, being unable to engage in meaningful religious activities may place a client at **risk for impaired religiosity**. A client might also demonstrate a **readiness for enhanced religiosity** and experience a desire to strengthen religious beliefs for comfort and hope at the end of life. **Anticipatory grieving** occurs before the actual loss, sometimes leading to a greater ability to cope with the situation. **Dysfunctional grieving** applies when clients and families are unsuccessful in incorporating loss into their lives.

SKILL 37.1 Care of the Dying Client

Because suffering is so complex, palliative care at the end of life involves the care of the whole person—body, mind, and spirit. You can reduce client's and family members' fear and uncertainty throughout the active dying process by helping them understand and anticipate symptoms and events unfamiliar to them. Although a client can have impaired function of a body system and experience symptoms unique to the disease process, you can discuss with clients and family members some common, recognizable patterns in the dying process and involve them with care interventions (Table 37-1).

ASSESSMENT

1 Assess each symptom for onset, precipitating factors, quality, severity, and what has helped to relieve symptoms in the past (Wentz, 2003). If the client is nonverbal, look for cues such as facial grimacing and restlessness as indicators of distress. *Rationale: Determines level of distress for planning client-specific interventions.*
2 Listen for indications of spiritual distress such as, "I haven't accomplished what I wanted to in life," "I wasted so much of my life," or "Without him, my life doesn't mean anything." *Rationale: Spiritual matters are often expressed in "common" or nonreligious language and should be recognized for their deeper spiritual meanings.*
3 Determine barriers to expression of feelings. *Rationale: Lack of privacy, pain, stress, distrust, or fatigue may create barriers to self-expression.*

4 Gather information about the client's grief patterns and coping strengths. *Rationale: Clients' well established coping patterns will likely be of more use to them near the end of life than new strategies or those designed by others.*
5 Identify spiritual and or religious needs and strengths.

PLANNING

Expected Outcomes focus on promoting comfort, autonomy, family involvement, and dignity throughout the dying experience.
1 Client demonstrates relief from pain and other symptoms.
2 Client/family participate in decisions regarding end-of-life care, as desired.
3 Client/family are involved in care according to their abilities and preferences.
4 Client/family demonstrate satisfaction with all aspects of palliative care.

Delegation

Psychosocial/spiritual care cannot be delegated. The nurse instructs assistive personnel to:
- Position clients using approaches to minimize symptoms.
- Offer comfort measures (bathing, positioning, toileting, hygiene care) frequently.

TABLE 37-1 Physical Changes Commonly Associated with Impending Death

SIGNS AND SYMPTOMS	INTERVENTIONS
Coolness and color changes in extremities	Use slippers or socks; cover person with light blankets, not tucked tightly over toes.
Increased periods of sleeping/unresponsiveness	Sit with the client, perhaps holding a hand and talking quietly; encourage speaking to the client even though there may be a lack of response.
Bowel or bladder incontinence	Change bedding as appropriate, use bed pads, and frequent skin care. An indwelling urinary catheter may be indicated for client fatigue or skin breakdown.
Congestion/increased secretions	Elevate the head, gently turn the head to drain secretions. Use prescribed medication to help decrease secretions. Suctioning is rarely necessary.
Restlessness or disorientation	Speak calmly, reduce lights. Gently massage hands or feet. Play soothing music.
Decreased intake of food or fluids	Do not force client to eat or drink. Offer ice chips, popsicles, sips of fluid; apply lip balm; moisten mouth. Assure family about normal decline in intake.
Decreased urine output	Consider advocating for the removal of indwelling urinary catheters.
Altered breathing patterns (apnea, labored and irregular breathing)	Elevate the head, hold hand, use quiet voice tones. Administer prescribed anxiolytics and/or opioids for pain and apprehension.

Equipment

- Personal care items most preferred by client
- Comfort and hygiene products
- Clean gloves

IMPLEMENTATION *for Care of the Dying Client*

STEPS	RATIONALE
1 See Standard Protocol (inside front cover).	
2 Promote pain relief (see Chapter 10).	
a. Administer prescribed analgesics on an around-the-clock (ATC) schedule, including medications for breakthrough pain.	ATC dosing is most effective method for maintaining adequate pain control. Using breakthrough doses minimizes pain episodes without overmedicating (Whitecar, Maxwell, and Douglass, 2004).
b. Collaborate with physician to consider use of adjuvant pain medications (e.g., antidepressants and anticonvulsants for neuropathic pain and antiinflammatory drugs for bone pain (Whitecar, Maxwell, and Douglass, 2004).	Adjuvant medications can enhance opioid effectiveness or treat pain not relieved by opioids.
c. Advocate for the most effective, least invasive route for analgesic administration.	Best route is based on client's level of consciousness, GI and circulatory status, type of medication, and ease of delivery.
d. Monitor effectiveness of medication regimen and adverse side effects at regular intervals.	Clients may need larger opioid doses to get relief as disease progresses, drug tolerance builds, and symptoms increase. Treating symptom before it worsens enhances relief. Pain medication doses may have to be decreased as liver and kidney function decline in the actively dying client (Paice and Fine, 2006).
e. Monitor for constipation, sedation (usually transitory), nausea, vomiting, or dry mouth.	Side effects of opioids and sedatives. Excessive sedation may require decrease in dose.
f. Consider nonpharmacological methods of pain control such as relaxation, repositioning, heat/cold, massage, and diversion.	Nonpharmacological therapies enhance effectiveness of pain medication and/or allow clients to develop an ability to participate in their symptom management (Matzo and Sherman, 2006).
3 Promote skin integrity and implement actions to prevent pressure ulcers.	Skin integrity is compromised by immobility, poor nutrition, and weight loss.
a. Reposition q2h or more often for comfort.	Immobility and prolonged pressure on an area cause pain and joint stiffness.

STEPS	RATIONALE
b. Use pressure-reducing devices.	Dying clients have decreased movement or experience pain with movement.
c. Treat pressure ulcers promptly.	Pressure ulcers produce client discomfort.
d. Apply alcohol-free lotion as needed and desired.	Lotion massage of hands, feet, or back may increase client comfort (Kolcaba and others, 2004).

> **NURSE ALERT** Do not massage any reddened area on client's skin because massaging causes breaks in the skin's surface capillaries and increased risk of skin breakdown.

STEPS	RATIONALE
e. Cleanse perineal area frequently if incontinent.	Promotes skin integrity, dignity, well-being.
4 Encourage family involvement in providing care important to client such as nail and hair care (see illustration).	Individualized care according to client preferences facilitates a sense of autonomy, dignity, and well-being. Family feels valued and useful in client care.
5 Promote nutrition as tolerated.	
a. Offer food preferences	Anorexia and difficulty swallowing are common at end of life, so eating patterns will change. Clients are more likely to eat food they prefer.
b. Medicate as prescribed for nausea and vomiting on regular schedule.	Decreased blood flow and/or medications slow GI motility and can cause nausea.
c. 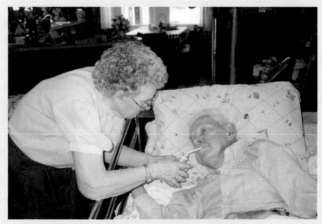 Provide oral care q2h or as requested.	Reduces oral bacteria, mouth odor, and bad taste.
d. Avoid foods with strong odors.	Strong smells can intensify nausea.
e. Offer small amounts of food and encourage client to identify food preferences. Do not push client to eat or drink.	Gradual dehydration may be a natural way for the body to decrease distressing symptoms such as congestion, excess secretions, shortness of breath, vomiting, and edema (Ersek, 2003).
f. Offer information to family about natural decrease in client appetite at end of life. Help family shift hope focus and find new ways to help.	Education can reduce family distress. Because offering food and fluid symbolizes life, love, and nurturing, no longer doing so can be difficult adjustment.
6 Maintain adequate elimination.	
a. Administer prescribed stool softeners and laxatives, especially when administering opioid analgesia.	Opioid analgesia, inactivity, and decreased fluid intake contribute to constipation.
b. Encourage use of bedside commode as long as possible.	Natural position for defecation promotes elimination and maintains client autonomy.
7 Promote oxygenation and comfortable ventilation.	
a. Elevate head of bed.	Diaphragm can move more easily in sitting position than when lying flat.
b. Increase air movement with fans or open windows.	Air flow stimulates trigeminal nerve in the cheek, which inhibits feelings of dyspnea. Use of oxygen is not routine at end of life unless for comfort (Pitorak, 2003).

STEP 4 Encourage family involvement in care.

STEPS	RATIONALE
c. Use actions that conserve energy and balance rest and activity.	Reducing activity decreases client oxygen use and minimizes shortness of breath.
d. Offer prescribed opioids for severe dyspnea and atropine to decrease secretions.	Air hunger is a very distressing, frightening symptom that may require medication use.
8 Promote emotional well-being.	A peaceful death is characterized by emotional comfort.
a. Talk with client about fears, stressors, anxieties, and care options.	Clients get a sense of purpose, safety, and hope when included in discussions (Harstäde and Andershed, 2004).
b. In nonverbal clients, observe for agitation and emotional distress.	Ensures more timely and appropriate therapies and helps distinguish pain from emotional distress (Panke, 2003).
c. Administer prescribed antianxiety medication in cases of significant depression or anxiety.	Sadness may be normal with significant loss, but severe anxiety and/or depression decrease quality of life. Professional psychological assessment and/or medication may be appropriate.
d. Consult interdisciplinary team for help with emotional, social, and psychological issues.	Creative and effective team care approaches can be identified. Client/family may benefit from professional counseling.
e. Facilitate communication between client and significant others. A social work referral may be helpful.	Intervention may be helpful if client and significant others are in conflicting stages of grieving or there is unresolved conflict (Kemp, 2002).
f. Involve family in providing care as desired and appropriate, such as assisting with bathing, feeding, and repositioning.	This is important to the client-family relationship before death and helps in the grieving process after death (Kemp, 2002).
g. Teach family what to expect as client's condition changes.	Family members cope better if they are prepared and involved.
9 Promote spiritual well-being.	
a. Facilitate spiritual activities (prayer, meditation, or reading client's spiritual texts).	Spiritually meaningful activities sustain client hope and help client experience peace and reconciliation.
b. Consult with spiritual care team when appropriate.	Complex spiritual issues are best evaluated by a spiritual care professional.
c. Involve others in client's care with activities such as reading, presence, comfort measures or help with meals. Encourage visits by clergy.	Promotes client's sense of meaningful community. Family participation in care promotes intimacy and meaning.
d. When client/family can express feelings and wishes, identify person(s) who will manage client's affairs and make funeral arrangements.	Preserves client/family autonomy in decision making.
10 See Completion Protocol (inside front cover).	

EVALUATION

1 Evaluate client's degree of relief from symptoms such as pain, constipation, nausea, fatigue, anxiety, depression, or spiritual distress.

2 Monitor progress in decision making regarding client's/family's important concerns.

3 Observe level of participation in care based on client/family preferences.

4 Evaluate client/family satisfaction with emotional/spiritual support.

Unexpected Outcomes and Related Interventions

1 Pain and/or other symptoms are not well managed with prescribed treatment plan.

a. Collaborate with interdisciplinary team for alternative medications or adjuvant therapies.

b. Talk with client/family about what actions they believe may be helpful.

c. Consider emotional or spiritual issues that may interfere with symptom management.

2 Client/family experience ethical conflicts or disagreements in decision making.

a. Clarify client wishes or consult client advance directives.

b. Use active listening to reflect feelings and clarify issues.

c. Offer self or other member of interdisciplinary team to intervene if desired.

3 Family members are not present or not participating in care.

a. Determine cause of nonparticipation; reinforce any teaching if appropriate.

b. Maintain a nonjudgmental attitude and support client/family coping styles and relationship patterns.

4 Client and/or family members appear to be in emotional/spiritual distress.

a. Use active listening and assessment skills to clarify issue.

b. Seek consultation with interdisciplinary team.

Recording and Reporting

- Record in nurses notes: interventions for pain and symptom management, including client response; changes in physical, mental, emotional, spiritual status; determinations of client/family preferences; family presence and involvement; and any unresolved issues and concerns.
- Report when a previously alert client becomes unresponsive.

Sample Documentation

1500 Client less responsive to verbal stimuli with occasional periods of restlessness. No oral intake this shift. Mouth care given every 2 hours. Unable to rate pain. Appears calmer when family present. Hospital chaplain and grandchildren visiting. Family members tearful and verbalizing awareness that client is nearing death. A family member plans to remain with client at all times.

Special Considerations

Pediatric Considerations

- Treat family and child as a unit. Encourage parents to stay with child and participate in care as much as desired or possible.

- Decisions to end treatment can be more difficult when children are involved.
- Consider child's age and developmental level of child in care planning, symptom management, and sibling support (Hellsten and Kane, 2006).

Geriatric Considerations

- Older clients may have more than one disease process (comorbidity).
- Many chronic illnesses have uncertain prognoses that complicate treatment decisions.
- Knowledge of multiple drug interactions and geriatric pharmacology is essential.
- Pain, respiratory distress, and confusion are most common symptoms in older adult who is dying (Derby and O'Mahony, 2006).
- Older adults have experienced multiple losses in their lives, which may impact their reactions to subsequent losses.

Home Care Considerations

- Family members assume primary care responsibility, necessitating ongoing teaching and support.
- Educate family members about symptom management approaches and when to seek help.
- Volunteers may be needed to give family respite time.

SKILL 37.2 Care of the Body After Death

After a client dies the designated health care provider, often a physician, certifies the death and records the time and actions taken at the time of death in the medical record. The physician may request permission from the family for an autopsy, or postmortem examination, although this is less likely with an anticipated death or when cause of death is known. An autopsy may be performed to confirm or determine the cause of death, gather data regarding the nature and progress of a disease, study the effects of therapies on body tissues, and provide statistical data for epidemiology and research purposes. An autopsy consent form must be signed by the appropriate family member and the physician or designated requestor. Autopsies normally do not delay burial.

The nurse is responsible for the dignified care of the body after death. Often family members wish to view the body before final preparations are made and/or they may wish to help with preparing the body. The nurse gives family members and significant others ample time to say good-bye before transferring the body to the morgue or funeral home.

ASSESSMENT

1 Assess for presence of family members or significant others and whether they have been informed of client's death by physician. Determine who is legally responsible for after-death procedures. *Rationale: Assists nurse in coordinating agency-based procedures for care at time of death.*

2 Assess family's grief response. *Rationale: Determines level of support and guidance needed.*

3 Determine if client is an organ or tissue donor. Call organ/tissue request and procurement team (consult agency policy). *Rationale: Trained requestors most often approach families for donation and manage organ retrieval. Successful recovery of tissues or organs depends on skillful and timely requesting.*

4 Assess client's religious preference and/or cultural heritage. *Rationale: Client's religious or cultural practices for body preparation may require changes in routine procedures.*

5 Determine if autopsy will be done. *Rationale: If autopsy is planned, some procedures such as removal of tubes and lines may be altered or prohibited.*

PLANNING

Expected Outcomes focus on preventing injury to the deceased's body and facilitating grieving of family and friends.

1 Survivors will have an opportunity to grieve consistent with their religious, cultural, and personal values.
2 Client's body is prepared in a dignified manner consistent with cultural and religious practices, with family involvement as desired.
3 Client's body will be free of new skin damage and optimally prepared for mortuary.

Delegation

Emotional and supportive care at time of death cannot be delegated. The nurse may delegate personnel to:
• Provide postmortem care of the body
• Prepare room and area for viewing of the body

Equipment

• Clean gloves, gown, and other protective clothing if needed
• Plastic bag for hazardous waste disposal
• Washbasin, washcloth, warm water, and bath towel
• Clean gown or disposable gown for body (consult agency policy)
• Absorbent pads
• Body bag or shroud kit (consult agency policy)
• Paper tape and gauze dressing
• Paper bag, plastic bag, or other suitable receptacle for client's clothing, belongings, and other items to be returned to family
• Valuables envelope
• Identification tags as specified by agency policy

IMPLEMENTATION for Care of the Body After Death

STEPS	RATIONALE
1 See Standard Protocol (inside front cover).	
2 Discuss routine postmortem care with family members and ask if they wish to include their own cultural or religious practices.	Seeking family input provides culturally sensitive care, honors the client's individuality, and communicates care.
3 Ask family members if they wish to be involved in final preparation of the body.	Facilitates grieving.
4 If tissue, body, or organ donation has been made, consult agency policy for specific guidelines.	Retrieval of tissues (e.g., corneas, skin) may require special body preparation. Federal law mandates that family members be given a chance to authorize tissue or organ donation (Ferrell and Coyle, 2006).
5 Prepare body in private room or move roommate to another area for this phase of end-of-life care.	Provides staff and family with privacy for rituals, body preparation, and expressions of grief.
6 Don't rush. Proceed at pace that honors family's cultural, spiritual, and personal preferences and expectations.	A rushed pace may seem disrespectful and increase family distress. A slow pace gives time for reflection and saying good-bye (Pitorak, 2003).
7 ▨ Apply gown or protective barriers as applicable.	Withdrawal of intravenous lines or tubes may cause minor bleeding or release of infectious body fluids.
8 Identify body and leave identification in place as directed in agency policy.	Ensures proper identification of body for delivery to morgue, autopsy room, and funeral home.
9 Remove all indwelling catheters, tubes, tape, and airways. With autopsy, policy may direct to leave devices in place.	Creates a normal, nonmedical appearance for family observation of body.
10 Remove soiled dressings and replace with clean gauze dressings using paper tape. Cover puncture wounds with a small dressing.	Changing dressings helps to control odors caused by microorganisms and creates more acceptable appearance. Paper tape minimizes skin trauma.
11 If person wore dentures, insert them. If mouth fails to close, place a rolled-up towel under chin.	It is difficult to insert dentures after rigor mortis occurs. Dentures maintain natural facial expression if body is to be viewed.
12 Position client as outlined in agency procedures. Avoid tightly tying hands together.	Client appears natural and comfortable. Tying hands together can cause skin discoloration.
13 Place small pillow or folded towel under head, or slightly elevate head of bed.	Prevents pooling of blood in face and subsequent discoloration.

STEPS	RATIONALE
14 Close eyes gently by grasping eyelashes and pulling lids over corneas of eyes.	Closed eyes present a more natural appearance. Pressure on lids can lead to discoloration.
15 Wash body parts soiled by blood, urine, feces, or other drainage. Place an absorbent pad under client's buttocks.	Prepares body for viewing and reduces odors. Relaxation of sphincter muscles may cause release of urine or feces.
16 Place clean gown on the client (agency policy may require removal after viewing).	Body in modest and dignified state for viewing.
17 Brush and comb client's hair. Remove any clips, hairpins, or rubber bands.	Client should appear well-groomed for family viewing. Hard objects can damage or discolor face and scalp.
18 Remove all jewelry and give to designated family member. Exception: If family requests that wedding band be left in place, place a small strip of tape around client's finger over the ring.	Prevents loss of client's valuables.
19 Place a sheet or light blanket over body with only head and upper shoulders exposed if the body will be viewed. Remove unneeded equipment from room. Provide soft lighting and offer chairs. Determine if those viewing body would like to be alone or have a staff person in room.	Maintains dignity and respect for client and limits exposure of body. People viewing body are provided with pleasant, comfortable environment for this important phase of grief process.
20 After body has been viewed, remove all linen and client's gown. Place body in body bag and cover with shroud in accordance with agency policy (see illustration).	
21 Place identification on outside of body bag as directed by agency policy.	Ensures proper identification of body.
22 Arrange transportation of body to morgue or mortuary.	Body should be cooled in morgue to delay tissue decomposition.
23 Respond to family questions or concerns before they leave.	
24 Remind family members to notify others of the death. Confirm name of funeral home.	Following a death, grieving people may have difficulty remembering details and may need guidance.
25 **See Completion Protocol (inside front cover).**	

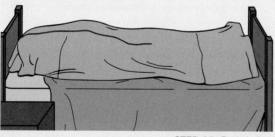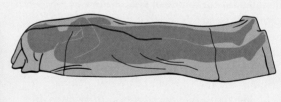

STEP 20 Body in body bag covered by shroud.

EVALUATION

1 Observe family/significant others' response to the loss.
2 Determine if family has received appropriate emotional/spiritual support after the death.
3 Note appearance and condition of client's skin during preparation of the body.

Unexpected Outcomes and Related Interventions

1 Grieving survivors become immobilized by grief and have difficulty functioning.
a. Maintain a nonrushed atmosphere. Allow time for questions and expressions of grief.
b. Offer spiritual or psychological consultation from interdisciplinary team.

2 Lacerations, bruises, or abrasions are noted on skin surfaces of deceased.

a. Cleanse areas thoroughly before family viewing.

b. Inform family of any notable bruises or lacerations that they may see.

c. Document any new skin tears or breakdown.

Recording and Reporting

- Record in nurses' notes date and time of death as determined by designated professional, or physician, time professional notified, name of professional pronouncing death, completion of postmortem care, identification of body, disposition of body, information provided to significant others, and whether autopsy consent was signed.
- Document any marks, bruises, or wounds on body before death or those observed during care of body.
- Document how valuables and personal belongings were handled and who received them. Secure signatures as required by agency policy.

Sample Documentation

0245 Pronounced dead by Dr. J. Anderson at 0213. Wife and other family members present at time of death and assisted with preparation of the body. Spiritual care provider was present, offering support. Two bruises on left forearm, both approximately 1 cm in diameter. Allen and Sons Funeral Home notified of death. Glasses and clothes sent with body to morgue with security personnel. White colored metal ring left in place at wife's request, taped to left hand ring finger.

Special Considerations
Home Care Considerations

- More people are choosing to die at home.
- Instruct family members on who to call if symptom control is needed, what to do and who to call at the time of death, and how body is to be transported.
- Nursing knowledge of home care reimbursement is essential, including Medicare and Medicaid hospice benefits.

Long-Term Care Considerations

- Less on-site physician involvement in long-term care facilities means that nurses have a primary responsibility in assessing and managing pain and other symptoms.
- Challenges include providing privacy and autonomy for client and family, involving family as much as possible or desired, individualizing care, keeping family members informed of changes, and keeping environment as home-like as possible.

NCLEX® Style Questions

1 A family member asks the nurse to explain what palliative care means. Which statement should be included in his or her discussion of palliative care?

1. It is designed only for persons at the end of life.
2. It has as its focus the seeking of cures and remission from disease.
3. It involves care of physical, psychosocial, and spiritual symptoms.
4. It is not appropriate for acute illness.

2 The nurse is caring for a dying client who feels fearful, isolated from his church community, and hopeless and forgotten. Which of the following nursing diagnoses may be most appropriate for this client? Select all that apply:

1. Dysfunctional grieving
2. Chronic pain
3. Impaired religiosity
4. Anxiety
5. Readiness for enhanced religiosity
6. Risk for spiritual distress

3 A nurse is providing family education regarding pain management. Which of the following statements would be appropriate to include in the discussion?

1. "Drugs are the only way to manage pain."
2. "We will be careful that she does not become addicted to the pain medications by using small doses."

3. "It's best to only give pain medication when she asks for it."
4. "The amount of medication she gets may change, depending on her responses to the medication."

4 The nurse begins to prepare for the body of a deceased client. Place all of the following actions in proper sequence, beginning with what the nurse should do first.

1. Wash body parts soiled by blood, urine, feces or other drainage.
2. Place a clean gown on the client.
3. Apply gloves, gown, or protective barriers as applicable.
4. Remove all indwelling catheters, tubes, tape, and airways.
5. Ask family members if they want to be involved in final preparation of the body.

5 Which of the following statements best describes the nurse's role in the ethical dilemmas that can occur in end-of-life care?

1. The nurse can facilitate important ethical conversations by listening and advocating for client and family values and wishes.
2. The nurse should leave ethical decisions to the physicians.
3. The nurse should express personal opinions and beliefs to give the client and family members alternative considerations.
4. The nurse should tell the client and family members what most people do in a similar situation.

References for all chapters appear in Appendix D.

38

Discharge Teaching and Home Health Management

MEDIA RESOURCES

- **evolve** http://evolve.elsevier.com/Elkin

The goals of discharge teaching and home health management are to promote healthy behaviors, to encourage the client's involvement in health care decisions, and to improve client outcomes (Joint Commission on Accreditation of Healthcare Organizations [JCAHO], 2004). Teaching begins at the time of admission to the health care facility and often includes multiple topics (Box 38-1). It is integrated throughout the client's stay in the health care facility and continues in the home and outpatient settings. To provide successful client teaching, begin by developing a trusting relationship with the client. Then assess the client's knowledge level and learning needs; psychosocial, spiritual, and cultural values; and physical and emotional readiness to learn (Redman, 2001). The client's literacy level, social support system (e.g., family or significant others), physical and cognitive limitations, language barriers and financial situation should also be assessed (JCAHO, 2004). To help clients learn, assess available client education programs and individualized client health education goals; and determine, individualize, and prioritize client's educational needs. In addition, encourage clients to provide feedback to ensure that the information provided is understood, appropriate, and useful. Document evidence of client education and achievement of outcomes as a result of education in the client's medical record.

Client teaching is an essential part of practice in state practice acts, in various federal and state regulations, and in accreditation criteria. Practice guidelines, which define the standard of practice and are research based, incorporate client education and are now widely used in health care settings to improve the quality of care (Redman, 2001).

You have an ethical responsibility to teach your clients. The *Patient Care Partnership* states that clients have the right to make informed decisions about their care (American Hospital Association [AHA], 2003). The information required to make informed decisions must be relevant, current, and clearly presented. As a nurse you often clarify information given by physicians and other health care providers and are the primary source for information when helping clients adjust to health problems.

Education often becomes the priority of nursing care when clients transition from an acute care setting back into the home. Discharge planning is an organized, coordinated, interdisciplinary

BOX 38-1 Topics for Health Education

Health Promotion and Illness Prevention
- Avoidance of risks (e.g., smoking, alcohol)
- Relaxation
- Growth and development
- Immunizations
- Prenatal care
- Childbirth education
- Nutrition
- Exercise
- Safety
- Screening (e.g., blood pressure, vision, cholesterol)

Coping with Impaired Function
- Long-term care
- Rehabilitation
- Environmental modifications
- Physical therapy
- Occupational therapy
- Speech therapy
- Prevention of complications
- Implications of noncompliance with therapy

Restoration of Health Related to Disease Process
- Body system affected
- Cause of disease
- Origin of symptoms
- Diagnostic tests
- Prognosis
- Limitation of function
- Treatment plan
- Dietary modifications
- Medication
- Surgical intervention (if appropriate)
- Client participation in care
- Adaptations in activities of daily living (e.g., bathing, toileting, eating)
- Activity modifications
- Self-help devices
- Home care

process that provides a plan of care for the client leaving the health care setting. The teaching and services provided should promote healthy behaviors, support recovery, and facilitate an effective return to normal function. Your role in discharge planning follows the nursing process. When initiating discharge planning, assess clients and their learning needs. After analyzing assessment data, determine clients' discharge needs and identify appropriate nursing diagnoses.

It is important to partner with the client in the planning phase to identify goals and expected outcomes. Because of shortened length of stays and complexity of client needs, nurses need to collaborate with other members of the health care team to prepare the client for discharge. Interdisciplinary team members usually include nurses; physicians; social workers; and respiratory, physical, and occupa-

tional therapists. Clear, concise, accurate documentation of the client's needs and abilities on the discharge plan improves the continuity of care. Therefore document the client's and family's understanding of and ability to follow through with discharge instructions.

Teaching more likely leads to learning when clients become actively involved in the learning process. The best way to evaluate a client's understanding of self-care behaviors is to have the client or family verbalize knowledge and demonstrate skills they need to perform to meet ongoing health care needs. Client education needs to include safe and effective use of medication and medical equipment, diet and nutrition, rehabilitation, educational resources in the community, and follow-up care (JCAHO, 2004). Confirm the discharge plan with the client and family after discharge. Telephone follow-up several days after discharge provides an opportunity to answer questions or refer the client to a home health agency if needed.

EVIDENCE IN PRACTICE

Wilson FL and others: Literacy, readability and cultural barriers: critical factors to consider when educating older African Americans about anticoagulation therapy, *J Clin Nurs* 12(2):275, 2003.

A group of researchers studied the readability and cultural sensitivity of written information given to older African-Americans attending an anticoagulation management clinic. They evaluated the clients' reading abilities to determine if there was a discrepancy between the clients' reading skills and the demands of the educational materials. Finally the researchers evaluated the clients' knowledge about the anticoagulant, warfarin (Coumadin). More than half of the clients were unable to read the written information given to them. As the age of the clients increased, their reading skills and knowledge about warfarin decreased. Furthermore, clients had only a moderate level of understanding about warfarin, and the majority did not understand the side effects or the food-drug interactions associated with warfarin. It is important for nurses to evaluate written materials given to clients. Written information needs to match clients' educational level, language, beliefs, cultural values, and experiences.

NURSING DIAGNOSES

Health-seeking behaviors is appropriate when a client or family is in stable health and is actively seeking to alter personal habits to achieve better health. **Ineffective health maintenance** applies when a client or family needs help to identify, manage, or seek resources to maintain or improve health. When the client has a complex treatment regimen, has little or no previous experience with the plan of care, or does not perceive susceptibility to complications, **ineffective management of therapeutic regimen** is relevant.

Impaired home maintenance applies when the client or family has difficulties maintaining the home. Inadequate support systems, decreased knowledge of available resources, and impaired cognitive or emotional functioning are contributing factors. **Caregiver role strain** applies when family members provide extensive or continuous complex care to clients, resulting in disruption of the family routines and roles.

Deficient knowledge is appropriate when the client is learning about a new procedure or does not remember or misinterprets information. **Anxiety** results when clients' concerns about illness interfere with the learning process. When clients have **altered sensory perception**, it becomes necessary to adapt teaching methods for successful learning and to make modifications in the home for client safety.

SKILL 38.1 Home Safety Assessment and Accident Prevention

This skill focuses on preparing the client to go home to a safe environment. Discharge from an agency is often stressful. Before discharge, you need to teach your client and family about any physical restrictions and the implications of new cognitive problems. Adequate discharge planning prepares the family to care for the client in the home and decreases the chance of readmission to the health care system. In some cases referral to a physical or occupational therapist is helpful. A home visit before discharge helps identify the need for any modifications for accident prevention.

Unintentional injuries and injuries related to violence are a major health problem and occur regardless of the client's age or developmental level (Hendrickson, 2005; King and others, 2005; Tideiksaar, 2003). Many of these injuries result from hazards that are easily overlooked and fixed. Therefore injury and prevention of violence is one of the leading health indicators identified by *Healthy People 2010* (Centers for Disease Control and Prevention [CDC], 2005). Knowledge of specific motor and cognitive developmental needs helps you to assess the potential for injury for each client. After you identify areas of risk, design interventions to eliminate or reduce threats to the client's safety.

ASSESSMENT

1 Determine client's actual or potential limitations resulting from sensory, motor, cognitive, or physical changes. *Rationale: These factors increase client's risk of injury.*

2 Assess client's physical and mental status before discharge and determine type of adaptations necessary in the home. *Rationale: The nature of physical and cognitive limitations determines the type of adjustments to be made in the home.*

3 Assess client's attitudes toward returning home and following health care provider recommendations. Determine the client's perceived benefit of action, perceived barrier to action, interpersonal influences such as family and peers, and commitment to a plan of action. *Rationale: These variables are major sources of motivation for changing behavior, and nursing interventions are targeted toward these variables (Pender and others, 2006).*

4 Consult other health care team members (e.g., physical, occupational, or respiratory therapist; dietitian; social worker; home care nurse) about needs after discharge. Make appropriate referrals. *Rationale: Members of all health care disciplines collaborate to determine client's needs and functional abilities.*

5 Assess developmental stage of client. *Rationale: Safety needs of clients vary based on their developmental age. For example, toddlers between ages 1 and 2 years are at a great risk for accidental poisoning, whereas young adult men are more frequently involved in firearm-related violence (Edelman and Mandle, 2006).*

6 Assess client's history of falls in the past. If client has fallen at home, use the mnemonic, SPLATT, to assess the client.
Symptoms at time of fall
Previous fall
Location of fall
Activity at time of fall
Time of fall
Trauma postfall (Meiner and Lueckenotte, 2006)

PLANNING

Expected Outcomes focus on identification of risk factors and provision of a safe environment in the home.
1 Client/family identify safety risks in the home.
2 Client/family identify community resources available and how to initiate contact.
3 Client/family do not experience injury in the home.

Delegation Considerations

The skill of risk assessment and accident prevention may not be delegated. However, you may need to consult with a physical or an occupational therapist to conduct a thorough home safety assessment and to determine appropriate adaptations needed based on client's physical and/or cognitive limitations.

Equipment

• Home safety checklist

IMPLEMENTATION *for Home Safety Assessment and Accident Prevention*

STEPS	RATIONALE
1 See Standard Protocol (inside front cover).	
2 Before discharge involve client and family as active participants in a home safety assessment using a checklist (Table 38-1). Validate the assessment later if necessary with client in the home. Use data gathered during assessment to determine learning priorities.	Active participation enhances learning and empowers client to be an active participant in making decisions about care (Bastable, 2003).
3 General safety in the home	
a. With client and family identify ways to make home environment safe; post emergency numbers (e.g., hospital, police, poison control center) near all telephones. Explore benefits and challenges of all recommendations.	A safe environment helps maintain or improve client's level of independence and function.

> **COMMUNICATION TIP** Because safety modifications affect all people living in a home, be sure to include client and caregivers in discussion. Be prepared to discuss concerns about the number of modifications required, the costs of modifications, and the change in home decor. Allowing the client and the caregiver to collaborate with you in making these decisions is needed to achieve a safer physical environment (Hurley and others, 2004).

STEPS	RATIONALE
b. If client is an older adult and is alone frequently, suggest use of personal emergency response system (PERS) and set a schedule for client to "check in" with family, neighbors, or friends.	Clients who use PERS wear a transmitter on the wrist or on a cord around the neck. The client pushes the button when help is needed. PERS often helps clients feel safer when home alone (Porter, 2005). Checking in with others at regular times communicates that client is safe at home (Meiner and Lueckenotte, 2006).
c. Reduce the number of different pain medications the client uses if possible.	Prevents oversedation and enhances ability of client to make safe decisions.
d. Offer client and family appropriate information about community health care resources, including homemakers, home health care agencies, transportation services, Meals on Wheels, retirement communities, home care, day care for children and/or adults, respite care, rehabilitation, and long-term care.	The emphasis is to keep client in the home for as long as it is safe and desirable to do so. During decision-making period regarding need for care outside the home, the role of the nurse is to support client and family and to provide information about options available (Hockenberry and others, 2005; Meiner and Lueckenotte, 2006).
4 Electrical safety	
a. Verify that major electrical appliances are grounded and that there are no overloaded plugs or sockets. Also ensure that no cords run under carpets.	Reduces risk of electrical shock and fire (Nemours Foundation, 2005).
b. If small children are in the house, cover unused outlets with safety plugs.	Prevents child from electrical shock (Nemours Foundation, 2005).
5 Prevention of burns	
a. Instruct client to keep thermostat on hot water heater below 120° F (49° C).	Prevents scalding burns (Meiner and Lueckenotte, 2006; Nemours Foundation, 2005).
b. Encourage client not to smoke. If client smokes, educate client not to smoke while tired or while in bed.	Smoking and secondhand smoke are both health hazards; falling asleep while smoking is associated with preventable deaths and injuries (Meiner and Lueckenotte, 2006).
c. Instruct clients, especially those with small children in the home, about stove safety (e.g., turn pot handles inward; install stove knob protectors and a stove lock).	Safe stove use helps prevent burns (Nemours Foundation, 2005).
6 Fall prevention	
a. Schedule diuretics early in the day and space antihypertensives and antiarrhythmics at different times to minimize side effects.	Appropriate diuretic schedule minimizes interruption in sleep and trips to the bathroom at night. Antihypertensives and antiarrhythmics often cause hypotension and dizziness, increasing risk of falls.

TABLE 38-1 Home Safety Checklist

CRITERIA	YES	NO
1. Walkways and steps are smooth and well lighted. Sturdy handrail is on both sides of stairs to entrance.	___	___
2. Nonskid strips/safety treads or bright paint is used on outdoor steps. All steps have the same depth and rise.	___	___
3. A shelf or bench is kept by front/back doors to place grocery bags or packages if needed.	___	___
Kitchen		
1. Client wears clothes with short or close-fitting sleeves when cooking.	___	___
2. Stove control dials are easy to see and use, and stovetop and oven are clean and grease free.	___	___
3. Items in kitchen cabinets and shelves are easy to reach.	___	___
4. Lighting over sink, stove, and work areas is bright.	___	___
Floors		
1. All carpeting and mats are secure. Skid backing is present under area rugs, or throw rugs are removed.	___	___
2. Walkways are free of clutter.	___	___
Bathrooms		
1. Door lock can be unlocked from both sides.	___	___
2. Tub or shower has nonskid mats or abrasive strips.	___	___
3. Tub or shower has at least one grab bar kept free of towels or other items.	___	___
4. Shower has a stable stool or chair and handheld sprayer.	___	___
5. Cold and hot water faucets are clearly marked, and temperature on water heater is 120° F or less.	___	___
6. A night-light is available.	___	___
Bedroom		
1. Client can turn on light without having to get out of bed in the dark.	___	___
2. Furniture is arranged to provide clear path from bed to bathroom.	___	___
3. Phone with emergency numbers is within easy reach of bed.	___	___
4. Alarm systems are available. There are listening devices for invalid clients.	___	___
Living Room/Family Room		
1. Light can be turned on without having to walk into dark room.	___	___
2. Lamp, extension, or phone cords are kept out of traffic ways.	___	___
3. Furniture is arranged so that it can be walked around easily.	___	___
Fire Safety		
1. Sufficient numbers of working smoke detectors are in appropriate locations.	___	___
2. Emergency exit plans are in place in case of fire.	___	___
3. Family has determined a meeting place outside the house.	___	___
4. Portable space heaters are used and kept 3 ft away from flammable items.	___	___
5. Furnace area is free of things that can catch on fire.	___	___
6. Furnace and chimney are checked annually by a qualified professional.	___	___
7. Emergency numbers for police, fire, and poison control are posted near phone.	___	___
8. Fire extinguisher is available and easy to handle and use.	___	___
Electrical Safety		
1. Electrical cords are in good condition and are not frayed, spliced, or cracked.	___	___
2. Electrical cords are kept away from water.	___	___
3. Extension cord/outlet extenders have built-in circuit breaker or fuse.	___	___
4. Wall outlets and switches have cover plates.	___	___
5. Light bulbs are of correct wattage for each fixture.	___	___
6. Fuse box is easily accessible and clearly labeled.	___	___
7. Lamp switches are easy to turn on to avoid burns from hot light bulbs.	___	___
Carbon Monoxide Prevention		
1. Furnace flues are checked regularly for patency	___	___
2. Carbon monoxide detector is in home.	___	___

Modified from Meiner SE, Lueckenotte AG: *Gerontologic nursing,* ed 3, St Louis, 2006, Mosby.

STEPS	RATIONALE
b. Consider changing the physical environment to reduce predisposition to falls, such as removing trip hazards on floor and stairs, using shower chairs, and installing safety grab bars in the bathroom.	Modifying the home environment to decrease fall risks and enhance safety is effective in preventing falls (Meiner and Lueckenotte, 2006; Tideiksaar, 2003).
c. Inspect client's shoes. Teach client to wear shoes with thin, firm soles and moderate traction, especially if client has a shuffling gait.	Better stability and proprioception is provided by shoes that have a thin, firm sole with moderate traction. Footwear with thicker soles (e.g., sneakers) can result in tripping if the client has a shuffling gait (Tideiksaar, 2003).
d. Refer client to physical therapist for rehabilitative and/or therapeutic exercise if indicated.	Tailored exercise programs help decrease the risk of falls (Tideiksaar, 2003).
e. Educate client and family about risks for falling, implications of illness, and plan for reducing falls in the home.	Fear of falling is a risk factor for falling. Clients who are educated about their fall risk and understand their illnesses are less fearful of falling (Tideiksaar, 2003).
f. Have client keep a fall diary if client falls or almost falls at home (Box 38-2). Instruct client to share diary with physicians, nurses, and other health care providers.	Information in diary provides helpful information about what happened before and after the fall. This information can be used by health care providers to develop fall prevention strategies with the client (Meiner and Lueckenotte, 2006).
g. Have a list of emergency phone numbers at each phone.	Increases emergency response.
7 Firearm safety	
a. Instruct client about dangers associated with keeping guns in the home.	The incidence of accidental injury in all age-groups as well as suicide in adolescents and adults is higher when there are guns in the household (Hockenberry and others, 2005; Shenassa and others, 2004).
b. If guns are in the home, instruct client to install trigger locks on all guns and store all guns unloaded and in a locked cabinet. Instruct client to store ammunition in a secured area separate from the guns. Store keys in a place unaccessible by children.	Following gun safety standards decreases the risk of injury and death related to gun use (Hockenberry and others, 2005; Shenassa and others, 2004).
8 Ask client to verbalize information taught.	Indicates learning (Bastable, 2003).
9 See Completion Protocol (inside front cover).	

BOX 38-2   Fall/Near Fall Diary

1 Keep a notebook with 8½ × 11-inch paper. Across longest edge of paper, write the headings: Date, Time of Fall, Activity at Time of Fall, Symptoms and Injury.

2 As soon as possible after the fall, client completes information under each heading.

3 If a family member witnessed the fall, the family member records what happened on a separate piece of paper.

4 List emergency contact numbers in the diary for client to call in case a fall results in serious injury.

5 Instruct client to bring diary to health care provider's office at the next scheduled visit or share information with home health nurse on next home visit.

Modified from Meiner SE, Lueckenotte AG: *Gerontologic nursing*, ed 3, St Louis, 2006, Mosby.

EVALUATION

1 Ask client to identify safety risks present in the home.
2 Have client describe plan that minimizes risk for injury and leads to safe health behavior choices.
3 Ask client and family to identify resources available for a particular problem and how to initiate contact with that resource.
4 Ask client and family if anyone has experienced an injury in the home.

Unexpected Outcomes and Related Interventions

1 Client is unable to identify safety risks.
a. Reevaluate home environment with client and family members.
b. Reinforce information about preventing and removing potential hazards from home environment with client.
2 Client and family do not follow through with plan to reduce risks in home.
a. Assess client's concerns or views about making changes.
b. Assess client's finances.
c. Establish a plan that includes changes client will accept.
3 Client and family are unaware of community resources.
a. Reinforce information about available resources.
b. Provide informational brochures and contact information for resources.
4 Client/family reports an injury has occurred in the home.
a. Determine cause and extent of injury.
b. Suggest further modifications that can be made in the home to prevent future injuries.

Recording and Reporting

- Retain copy of the home safety assessment in client's home health record.
- Record assessment of client's cognitive and mental status, recommended interventions, and client's and caregiver's response.
- Record any instruction provided, client's response, and changes made to environment.

Sample Documentation

0900 Safety checklist completed before discharge; family members present. Spouse states will remove throw rugs and have handrails installed in bathroom. Home health care agency referral made after discussion with client, family members, and advanced practice nurse.

Special Considerations
Pediatric Considerations

- Ensuring the safety of children in the home is based on child's developmental level. Instruct families to use safety devices (e.g., safety gates on staircases and cabinet locks) as applicable (Nemours Foundation, 2005).
- Suggest that parents or other caregivers get down on the floor to look at the environment from child's view to identify dangers present in the home to young children (Hockenberry and others, 2005).
- Children imitate and copy what they see and hear. Instruct parents that practicing safety teaches safety. Saying one thing and doing another confuses children (Hockenberry and others, 2005).
- Teach families car safety based on child's age, developmental level, and size. Children are placed in appropriate restraint system, and, if the car has airbags, children under 12 years of age need to ride in the back seat.

Geriatric Considerations

- Physiological and mental status changes that accompany aging, such as a slower reaction time, reduced pain and temperature perception, and reduced visual acuity, place older adults at risk for injury in the home environment.
- Older adults are usually more aware of potential dangers when they are in a familiar setting.
- Frail older adults should not ride in the passenger side of the car if the car has airbags. Teach them to sit in the back seat or sit at least 10 inches away from the airbag.

Home Care and Long-Term Care Considerations

- Make changes in client's home environment to keep client as independent as possible.
- Before making any revisions to a client's home, know client's financial resources and let client be the final decision maker in the types of changes to be made to the home whenever possible. Also consider client's physical strengths and remaining functional abilities, not just the disabilities.
- Teach caregivers the importance of preserving client autonomy.

Clients with different kinds of cognitive impairments and their families need assistance in making adaptations to preserve their ability to function safely within the home. To be safe, a person needs to be able to perform routine activities of daily living (ADLs) and to make sound decisions. This includes the use of the telephone, cleaning, shopping, money management, meal preparation, and taking medications. When there are cognitive limitations, a person's independence is clearly threatened. Family members often do not understand changes in cognition and function and need help to determine whether a client is competent to remain at home safely.

It is a myth that all older adults experience cognitive dysfunction. However, older adults are more likely to develop cognitive dysfunctions. Accurate assessment includes mental health, physical health, social and economic status, functional status, and the environment (Ebersole and others, 2004). A person may have certain mental processes intact (e.g., orientation to name, time, and place), while at the same time other processes are compromised (e.g., short-term memory of life events).

In addition to mental status and cognitive changes, it is important to recognize that many older adults suffer from depression, which also may result in cognitive impairment (Meiner and Lueckenotte, 2006). Depression occurs alone or in combination with cognitive disorders such as dementia. Depression often results from social isolation (e.g., the older adult is homebound and has few visitors).

ASSESSMENT

1 Assess client over a short period of time and be ready to adapt your assessment if the client has sensory disabilities. *Rationale: Improves likelihood of gathering relevant data (Ebersole and others, 2004).*

2 Listen carefully to the client in a quiet, well-lit space, and avoid interruptions or distractions. Speak slowly, clearly, and in a normal tone of voice. *Rationale: Providing an optimal environment ensures accurate assessment of client's cognitive and mental status.*

3 Ask client to describe own level of health and ability to provide self-care skills, including bathing, dressing, eating, and toileting. Ask family members to confirm description. Also assess for risky behaviors (e.g., unsupervised use of stove, handling of weapons). *Rationale: Question requires client to describe abilities and health challenges. Family members are able to provide helpful insight especially about risky behaviors. Minimizing risky behaviors is essential in making the environment safe (Hurley and others, 2004).*

4 Ask how the client is doing with home management responsibilities and with managing medical care. For example, ask the client, "Do you have problems following your diet?" or "Tell me what medications you take and when you take them." *Rationale: Data gathered allows you to assess short-term memory, judgment, and problem solving.*

5 If you suspect that your client is wandering or at risk for wandering, observe and assess for the following characteristics and behaviors or ask caregivers if these behaviors or characteristics exist:
Higher level of cognitive impairment
Difficulties sleeping
Active lifestyle before becoming cognitively impaired
Use of psychotropic medications
Pacing or walking that cannot be redirected easily
Getting lost in familiar places
Client explains he or she is searching for "missing" people or places
Rationale: Clients who exhibit these behaviors or have these characteristics are more prone to wandering (Futrell and Melillo, 2002; Lai and Arthur, 2003).

6 Determine if client has a family member or friend who helps with self-care or home management responsibilities. *Rationale: Determines availability of potential resources for client.*

7 Assess competency of caregiver (e.g., knowledge, skills and physical ability to provide care), as well as caregiver's perception of ability to care for client safely in the home. *Rationale: Caring for the caregiver and ensuring that the caregiver can care for the client competently is essential in providing a safe environment for the client (Hurley and others, 2004).*

PLANNING

Expected Outcomes focus on adaptation of the home environment and promoting the client's ability to perform ADLs.

1 Client is able to complete as many home management responsibilities as possible within existing limitations.

2 Family caregiver(s) use adaptations in the home that help client perform home management activities as needed.

Delegation Considerations

The skill of adapting the home setting for clients with cognitive deficits may not be delegated. The nurse directs personnel by:

- Reviewing to observe for and report back any changes in client mood, memory, and ability to maintain the home.

Equipment
- Mini-Mental State Examination (see Chapter 12)
- Calendar
- Paper for making lists
- Bulletin board or poster board (optional)
- Motion detector (optional)

IMPLEMENTATION *for Adapting the Home Setting for Clients with Cognitive Deficits*

STEPS	RATIONALE
1 See Standard Protocol (inside front cover).	
2 If client has difficulty remembering when to perform self-care routines, create a list or post reminder notes written in large print in a noticeable place. Suggest use of a wristwatch with an alarm to signal time of scheduled activity and use of a medication organization container to help with medication administration. Post a large calendar for appointments or special events.	Memory function in older adults tends to be preserved for relevant, well-known material (Meiner and Lueckenotte, 2006). Lists and other reminders will help client remember and complete required tasks. Large print is helpful when client has limited eyesight.
3 Schedule medications likely to cause confusion or drowsiness at bedtime.	Maintains mental status during the day at the maximum level possible.
4 Instruct caregiver to focus on client's abilities rather than disabilities.	Retains client's autonomy and sense of self-worth.
5 When client has difficulty completing tasks with multiple steps, reduce number of steps or simplify task.	Prevents frustration and/or forgetting one or more steps that lead to task being unfinished.
6 Help client and family develop a schedule for routine daily activities such as eating, bathing, and exercise.	Consistency creates a sense of security and helps keep client oriented to daily activities.
7 Have caregiver(s) set up activities so that client can complete them (e.g., lay out clothes to wear for the day, place food for meals out on the counter).	Helps client complete tasks even though unable to plan and perform all the steps.
8 Encourage caregivers to use simple and direct communication using calm and relaxed approach. Use eye contact and touch. Speak in simple words and short sentences. Use nonverbal gestures that complement verbal messages.	Facilitates effective communication and reduces anxiety.
9 Keep clocks, calendars, and personal items (pictures, scrapbooks, personal gifts from loved ones) throughout rooms where easily seen.	Reinforces reality orientation. Increasing visual appeal of environment helps to reduce wandering (Futrell and Melillo, 2002).
10 If client wanders, consider the following interventions:	
a. Provide a safe place (e.g., large room in den free of obstacles) for client to wander.	Reduces risk of client leaving residence.
b. Provide clues (e.g., pictures or signs) to guide client to a desired location.	Reduces aimless wandering (Futrell and Melillo, 2002).
c. Suggest that family members install multiple and different kinds of locks, as well as motion detectors with portable alarms at exit sites of the home.	Reduces ability of client to leave the home (Futrell and Melillo, 2002).
d. Address the cause of wandering (e.g., provide food if hungry) and eliminate stressors (e.g., changes in daily routine).	Reduces causes of wandering (Futrell and Melillo, 2002).
11 Routinely remind client of who caregiver is and what the next step is to be.	Improves client's responses to activities and environment (Meiner and Lueckenotte, 2006).
12 Facilitate regular naps or rest periods.	Fatigue adds to mental status changes.
13 Encourage and support frequent visits by family and friends. Encourage use of humor and reminiscing of favorite stories.	Prevents boredom and reduces restlessness.
14 See Completion Protocol (inside front cover).	

EVALUATION

1 Ask client to review the home management activities completed that day and the previous day.
2 Ask caregiver to describe approaches used to help client maintain independence.

Unexpected Outcomes and Related Interventions

1 Client is unable to complete daily activities as planned.
a. Review what occurred and identify barriers.
b. Identify strategies for maintaining adequate support and overcoming barriers.

2 Caregiver is unable to carry out techniques that improve orientation and ability of client to complete activities.

a. Offer reinstruction for caregiver.

b. Reassess caregiver's ability to provide necessary support. Consider other living arrangements or support services if indicated.

Recording and Reporting

- Record cognitive abilities and mental status, recommended interventions, and client's and caregiver's responses.
- Report significant decline in cognitive or mental status to physician or health care provider.

Sample Documentation

2100 Oriented to person and place but not to time. States is waiting for breakfast. Reoriented by having client look outside to see it is dark and telling her it will soon be bedtime. Sister reports client has wandered less since offering more frequent meals and planning naps.

Special Considerations
Pediatric Considerations

- Children with cognitive impairments are often not aware of dangers normally present during play and daily activities. Adult supervision is critical.

Geriatric Considerations

- Many clients experience progressive loss of function, requiring continuous adaptations and adjustments. If client becomes unable to complete any ADLs or experiences major behavioral changes (e.g., excessive wandering), you may need to help family member determine need for a skilled nursing facility (Aud, 2004).
- Caregiver stress may be reduced by educating caregiver about problematic behaviors and how to manage them (Meiner and Lueckenotte, 2006).

SKILL 38.3 Medication and Medical Device Safety

The safe use of medications and medical devices is a nursing priority. Researchers estimate that over half of clients who take prescribed medications at home fail to take them correctly (Haynes and others, 2002). This often happens for several reasons: clients stop taking medications once symptoms subside, regimens involving multiple drugs are confusing, the consequences of not taking medications are not understood, prescriptions are costly, and many clients fear addiction. If clients were educated about their medications, approximately 120,000 lives and $45.6 billion per year could be saved in the United States (Schommer and others, 2002).

The use of different medical devices in the home further complicates the ability of clients to care for themselves. Medical devices used in the home include syringes, blood glucose monitoring equipment, dressings, and intravenous devices. To use medications and medical devices safely in the home, clients need to understand medication administration, storage of medical devices and medications, proper waste disposal, and prevention of infection.

Clients who have special needs include those with acute sensory or neurological impairment, chronic illnesses such as diabetes or arthritis, and physical limitations that make manipulation of medical devices and handling medications difficult. In some cases a family member or other caregiver must learn to provide this care (Figure 38-1).

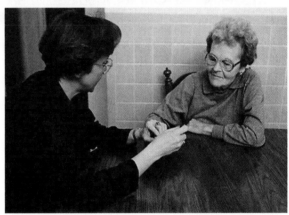

FIGURE 38-1 A family member or other caregiver often needs to learn about prescribed medications.

ASSESSMENT

1 Assess client's and caregiver's visual, cognitive, musculo-skeletal, and neurological function; level of consciousness or sedation; vision; hearing; literacy; and willing-ness to learn (see Chapter 12). *Rationale: Helps to identify approaches to use in instruction and appropriate assistive devices needed.*

2 Assess client's knowledge of medication regimen and compare with actual regimen. Also assess length of time client has been receiving each drug. *Rationale: Determines complexity of medication regimen and client's familiarity with each drug.*

3 Identify where medications are stored in the home and the type of storage containers used. *Rationale: Determines safe use of medications.*

4 Assess resources (e.g., transportation and financial) for obtaining medications when needed. *Rationale: Lack of resources interferes with self-medication at home.*

PLANNING

Expected Outcomes focus on the client's ability to manage medications and medical devices safely.

1 Client will state purpose of each medication, common side effects, and when to notify physician or health care provider about problems.
2 Client is able to read each label and explain when each drug is to be taken.
3 Client/caregiver will be able to prepare and administer prescribed medications independently.
4 Client/caregiver will store medications and medical devices properly and dispose of medical wastes safely.

Delegation Considerations

The skill of medication and medical device safety may not be delegated. The nurse directs personnel by:
- Reviewing to observe for and report unsafe behaviors, improper disposal of sharps and contaminated supplies, and use of infection control practices.

Equipment

- Written instructions or charts
- Medications
- Container for daily or weekly medication preparation
- Measuring devices (e.g., medicine cup, teaspoon, syringe) if needed
- Colored marking pens
- Labels
- Assistive device (e.g., syringe magnifier) or medical device (e.g., blood glucose monitor)
- Puncture-resistant sharps container or other hard plastic bottle (e.g., fabric softener bottle) with cap

IMPLEMENTATION *for Medication and Medical Device Safety*

STEPS	RATIONALE
1 See Standard Protocol (inside front cover).	
2 Instruct client and caregiver about prescribed medications and over-the-counter medications that are scheduled and taken prn, including:	Education about all medications enhances compliance with medication therapy and reduces errors in medication administration.
a. Purpose of medications and their expected effects.	
b. How medications work.	
c. Dosage schedules and rationale.	
d. Common side effects, what to do to relieve side effects.	
e. What to do if dose is missed.	
f. When to call the physician or health care provider.	
3 Suggest use of appropriate devices to help client take medications as scheduled:	Helps client decrease medication administration errors.
a. Make calendars for each week with plastic bags of medications to take at specific times.	
b. Divide egg cartons into color-coded sections with medications for the day, using color-coding for drug types (e.g., blue for sedative, red for pain pill).	
c. Use pillboxes that are set up daily or weekly to separate pills into slots for each day of the week and appropriate time of day (see illustration).	
4 Instruct client and caregiver in principles of safe medication administration and recommend modifications for safe administration.	Medication prescriptions specify frequency, dosage, and special instructions (e.g., take before meals).
a. Medicine prescribed must only be used as prescribed and by person for whom it was prescribed.	It is unsafe for members of the household to take medications prescribed for another person.
b. Do not take expired medications.	Medication may be toxic or no longer effective.
c. Keep medications in the container in which they came and make sure label is clearly legible. Have pharmacy provide large print or Braille labels if needed.	Putting several different kinds of medications in the same container is unsafe because client can mix up dosages or schedules of administration. Large print makes label reading easier.

STEPS	RATIONALE
d. Finish prescribed medications and, if ordered, get refills before container is empty.	Clients may be tempted to keep some medication when symptoms are gone, planning to use it later. This is an unsafe practice. It is essential to order refills so that there is no interruption in medication routine.
e. Have pharmacist put medications in a container client can open easily if manual dexterity is limited.	Most pharmacies dispense medications in childproof containers, which may be difficult to open if client has limited mobility of fingers/hands.

> **NURSE ALERT** If there are small children in the home or children who frequently visit, help identify a safe place for storage of medication to reduce risk of accidental ingestion.

STEPS	RATIONALE
f. Use a color-coding system when many medications are prescribed by marking tops of medication containers with the same color when they are taken at the same time.	Often helps clients take medications at right time.
5 Teach safe use and disposal of medical devices and supplies.	Prevents injuries from contaminated supplies.
a. Teach client or caregiver how to use medical device, using diagrams, written information, other resources (e.g., Internet, Intranet), and return demonstration when possible.	Clear written information, diagrams, and other resources enhance client learning and allow reinforcement of information (Bastable, 2003; Sorrentino and others, 2002).
b. Instruct client or caregiver on proper storage and care of medical device.	Ensures device will continue to work safely and accurately.
c. Instruct client to place needles, syringes, lancets, or other sharp objects in hard plastic or metal container such as a soda bottle or laundry detergent container with screw-on or tightly secured lid.	Reduces transmission of microorganisms and prevents exposure to body fluids (OSHA, 2001).
d. Instruct client to put soiled bandages, disposable sheets, and medical gloves in securely fastened plastic bag before being placed in garbage can.	Ensures safe disposal of medical supplies (OSHA, 2001).
6 See Completion Protocol (inside front cover).	

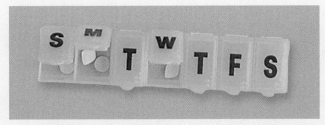

STEP 3c. Pill organizer for each day of the week.

EVALUATION

1 Ask client to state purpose of each medication, common side effects, and when to notify physician or health care provider about problems associated with medications.

2 Ask client to explain when each medication is to be taken.

3 Observe client/caregiver preparing and administering medications and using medical devices independently.

4 Complete a pill count at specific intervals.

5 Ask to see where client/caregiver stores items and observe disposal of medical supplies, including sharps and contaminated supplies.

Unexpected Outcomes and Related Interventions

1 Client makes errors in preparing medications or is unable to recall information.

a. Provide written instructions at client's/caregiver's level of understanding. Often pictures are very helpful (Wilson and others, 2003).

b. Repeat and reinforce important information. Give positive feedback for accurate recall of information.

c. Provide repeated supervised practice until client is able to self-administer medications safely.

2 Self-medication is not possible due to client's self-care deficits.

a. Develop alternate plan, which may require family, friends, or home health agency.

b. Consider need for alternative living arrangements.

3 Excess or insufficient pills are found in pill container during pill count.

a. Reevaluate use of dosage reminders.

b. Establish additional monitoring system until client is able to self-medicate accurately.

4 Medications and medical devices/supplies are not stored and/or disposed of in a secure or appropriate location.

a. Identify barriers and appropriate alternatives.

b. Explain risks posed when supplies/devices are not handled safely.

Recording and Reporting

- Document all instructions given, including details of medication administration, use of medical devices, and client's response to instruction.
- Describe system planned to ensure safe medication administration and use of medical devices.

Sample Documentation

Instructed on self-administration of digoxin and Lasix. States purpose of each medication, common side effects, and when to notify physician about medication-related concerns. Able to read each label and state when each drug is to be taken. Demonstrated how to take pulse correctly. Demonstrated use of pill dispenser.

Special Considerations
Pediatric Considerations

- All medications, medical supplies, and equipment must be kept safely out of reach of children.
- Tell caregivers not to compare medications to treats because this could add to risk of child overdosing by mistaking medicine for candy.

Geriatric Considerations

- Capacity for learning new information remains as adults age (in the absence of dementia). However, additional time is needed to accomplish learning. Allow adequate time and number of teaching sessions to support successful learning.
- A home health nurse is often needed to fill weekly pillbox if client/family cannot reliably complete this task.

PROCEDURAL GUIDELINE 38-1
Teaching Clients Self-Injections

Delegation Considerations
The skill of teaching clients self-injections may not be delegated.

Equipment
- Instruction booklet or chart with pictures, vial of medication, appropriate-size syringe and needle, antiseptic/alcohol swab, small gauze pad (optional), site rotation chart (optional), bottle of sterile saline, container for disposal of sharps

Procedural Steps
1. See Standard Protocol (inside front cover).
2. Explain importance of hand hygiene and ask client to perform hand hygiene.
3. Have client hold and manipulate syringe and medication vial. If client cannot manipulate syringe, develop another plan (e.g., involve family or significant other). Explain which parts of syringe need to remain sterile (free of germs) and which can be touched.
4. Discuss medication dosage and show client how much medication to draw into syringe. Show client where to find the name and concentration of the medication on the label.
5. Have client look for color change or clumping in medication vial. If appropriate, mix medication by gently rolling bottle. If medication has been refrigerated, allow it to warm to room temperature to minimize discomfort and regulate absorption.
6. Teach client how to prepare medication in syringe (see Tables 17-1 and 17-2 and Procedural Guideline 18.2). Instruct client to replace cap or sheath on needle without touching it after medication is prepared in syringe.
7. Teach client about appropriate injection sites and injection site rotation (see Skills 17.1 and/or 17-2). Help client choose appropriate injection site and wipe it with alcohol. Explain importance of wiping injection site with alcohol. Allow alcohol to dry.

PROCEDURAL GUIDELINE 38-1—cont'd

8   If subcutaneous (Sub-Q) injection is given, have client grasp or pinch injection site between thumb and forefingers of free hand (see illustration). To give Sub-Q injections in posterior upper arm, have client press back of arm against a wall or back of a chair and "roll" arm down to push up skin. If intramuscular (IM) injection is given, tell client to spread skin and hold skin taut.

a.   Instruct client on self-inspection technique.

b.   Teach client to insert needle quickly into prepared site all the way to hub. Most injections are given at a 90-dgree angle; a 45-degree angle is used with children or thin adults receiving Sub-Q injections.

> **COMMUNICATION TIP**   Tell client to inject on the count of 3; then count slowly and rhythmically and say "Go." Some clients may need you to gently push on their hand at first.

c.   Once needle is inserted, instruct client to slowly let go of skin and transfer free hand to barrel of syringe.

d.   If client is giving intramuscular injection, explain need to aspirate before injecting medication, show how to aspirate, and explain need to stop injection and start over if blood is aspirated. If client is giving Sub-Q injection, there is no need to aspirate.

e.   Have client push plunger all the way in at a slow and steady rate to administer the medication. Have client count to 5 before removing needle to ensure all medication is administered.

f.   Have client quickly remove needle at same angle at which it was inserted and exert gentle pressure on the site with a small gauze pad or cotton ball if desired.

9   Teach client appropriate disposal of uncapped needle or needle enclosed in safety shield in a sharps container or a hard plastic bottle (e.g., detergent or fabric softener bottle).

10   If client needs to reuse needles for economic reasons, explain safe reuse of needles. If client has adequate immune system and does

not contaminate or bend the needle during the injection process, the needle may be recapped and used for the next injection. Teach to dispose of syringes and needles when the needle becomes dull or if the syringe or needle become contaminated (American Diabetes Association [ADA], 2004).

11   Have client record on a chart where injection was given.

12   Encourage client to ask questions and provide client with written and visual instructions. Give client a bottle of sterile saline to avoid wasting medication while practicing medication preparation.

13   Discuss where medication and syringes will be stored at home so that children will not have access to them.

14   **See Completion Protocol (inside front cover).**

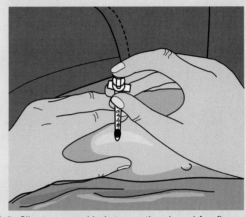

STEP 8   Client grasps skin between thumb and forefinger of free hand when giving self a Sub-Q injection and inserts needle to the hub.

SKILL 38.4 Using Home Oxygen Therapy

Clients with alterations in oxygenation often require continuous oxygen therapy. Oxygen therapy often lasts several weeks or months or for the rest of the client's life if the client has a chronic condition. Oxygen is a drug and is administered and monitored with the same care as any other medication.

Home oxygen equipment is classified as durable medical equipment (DME) and is often paid for by government or private insurance as long as it is prescribed by a physician or advanced practice nurse. A certificate of medical necessity is needed for clients who receive Medicare (Findeisen, 2001). Medicare has specific guidelines for reimbursement of oxygen therapy in the home (e.g., serious reduction in oxygenation during sleep or following exercise) (Positive Air, Inc., 2006). For example, indications for home oxygen therapy include specific PaO_2 (e.g., 55 mm Hg or less) or SaO_2 (88% or less) on room air, at rest, or with exercise (AARC, 1992).

Home oxygen therapy is usually administered using nasal cannula or different types of masks, depending on the needs

of the client (Table 38-2). Oxygen-conserving devices (OCDs) reduce the amount of oxygen the client uses; however, they are not usually covered by Medicare or private insurance. Three types of OCDs are available: reservoir nasal cannulas, demand oxygen delivery systems, and transtracheal oxygen catheters (Findeisen, 2001).

Three types of oxygen delivery systems are available for home use: compressed oxygen, oxygen concentrators (Figure 38-2), and liquid oxygen (Figure 38-3, A and B). Some oxygen tanks are large and stationary, while smaller tanks are considered portable or ambulatory. Portable tanks are easily moved but are not designed to be carried. Ambulatory tanks are light weight (less than 10 pounds) and can be carried (Findeisen, 2001). The type of oxygen delivery system ordered is based on a thorough assessment of the client's needs. Criteria for determining the right oxygen delivery system for the client include the client's activity level, the amount of oxygen prescribed for the client, the client's

TABLE 38-2 Oxygen Flow and Appropriate Uses for Oxygen Delivery Devices

DEVICE	FLOW (L/MIN)	Fio_2 RANGE (%)	USES
Nasal cannula	¼-8	22-45	Long-term oxygen therapy
Transtracheal catheter	¼-4	22-45	High oxygen flow through tracheostomy
Simple oxygen mask	6-12	35-50	Short-term oxygen therapy with moderate Fio_2 needs
Reservoir mask	6-10	35-60	Acute respiratory distress with moderate Fio_2 needs
Nonrebreather mask	10-15	80-100	Acute respiratory failure or emergency situations

Data from Petty TL: *Guide to prescribing home oxygen: home oxygen options,* available at http://www.nlhep.org/resources/Prescrb-Hm-Oxygen/home-oxygen-options-4.html. National Lung Health Education Program, 2004, accessed November 18, 2006.

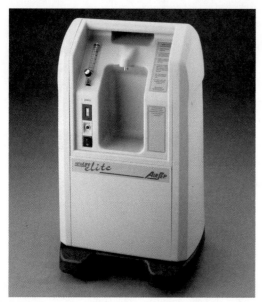

FIGURE 38-2 Oxygen concentrator. (Courtesy AirSep Corporation.)

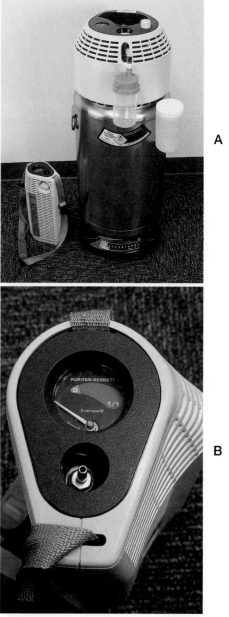

FIGURE 38-3 A, Liquid oxygen containers. Smaller container is ambulatory unit, and larger container is stationary reservoir. **B,** Control panel.

physical ability, the ability to get help for activities such as refilling a liquid tank and where the client lives. A client who is very mobile and active benefits from a liquid oxygen system because it allows the client to easily continue activities. A client who is homebound is best served with an oxygen concentrator and a smaller cylinder for infrequent trips outside the home.

Compressed oxygen requires a regulator and a flowmeter. The client receives delivery of several large oxygen tanks to the home. Table 38-3 shows how long compressed oxygen tanks last, depending on the prescribed flow rate. Liquid oxygen systems take up less space because oxygen is stored in a liquid state, at or below $-297°$ F. The client fills smaller portable units from a larger stationary unit in the home. Table 38-4 lists the length of time a liquid oxygen system will last, depending on the liter flow. Oxygen concentrators are moderate-size units that extract oxygen from the room air, concentrate it, and deliver the prescribed liter flow to the client. Because they deliver a lower percentage of oxygen to the flowmeter, you frequently need to adjust the flow rate when switching a client to a concentrator. A client who uses a concentrator needs to have a backup system such as a portable oxygen tank in case of power failure (Findeisen, 2001).

TABLE 38-3 Oxygen Cylinder Timetable*

| L/MIN | LARGE (H-K) TANK | | SMALL (E) TANK | |
	12,000 LB FULL	1,000 LB ½ FULL	625 LB FULL	284 LB ½ FULL
1	115 hr	52 hr	10 hr	5 hr
2	56 hr	26 hr	5 hr	2 hr
3	37 hr	17 hr	3 hr	1 hr
4	28 hr	13 hr	3 hr	1 hr
5	22 hr	10 hr	2 hr	54 min
6	18 hr	8 hr	<2 hr	417 min

Use the following formulas to determine the length of time a tank will last:
For E Cylinders: Pressure on cylinder gauge (psi) − 500 psi (safety factor) × 0.3 (E cylinder factor) ÷ L/min = minutes
For H Cylinders: Pressure on cylinder gauge (psi) − 500 psi (safety factor) × 3.1 (H cylinder factor) ÷ L/min = minutes
Example: if E cylinder reads 1500 psi and liter flow rate is 4L/min, time left = 1500 − 500 × 0.3 ÷ 4 = 75 minutes (1 hour, 15 minutes)
Note: Keep oxygen cylinder pressure above 500 psi to prevent running out of oxygen

*All times are approximate.

TABLE 38-4 Liquid Oxygen Timetable

| L/MIN | STATIONARY RESERVOIRS | | PORTABLE UNITS | |
	41 L (HR)	31L (HR)	½ L (HR)	1 L (HR)
0.25	1400	1060	28	44
0.5	1125	850	18	27
1	560	425	9	15½
1.5	375	283½	6	11½
2	281	213	4½	8½
3	187	142	3	6

Nasal cannulas are replaced weekly or cleaned with mild soap and water. Face masks, T tubes, and tracheostomy collars are cleaned daily with mild soap and water and allowed to air dry. Clients need to have more than one delivery device so they can clean and dry one while using the other.

ASSESSMENT

1 Assess client's and family's ability to apply and manipulate oxygen equipment while in hospital or home. *Rationale: Physical or mental impairment indicates need for assistance in home.*

2 Assess client's and family's knowledge of oxygen therapy and ability to determine signs and symptoms of hypoxia. *Rationale: Knowledge of oxygen therapy is needed for safe home therapy. Hypoxia can be caused by worsening of client's physical problem or an underlying change in respiratory status and needs to be reported to client's physician or health care provider immediately.*

3 Assess availability of community resources for home oxygen therapy. *Rationale: Ensures readily available assistance for home oxygen system.*

4 Assess home environment for adequate electrical service if concentrator is used. *Rationale: Adequate electrical source is required for oxygen concentrators to work (Findeisen, 2001).*

5 If compressor or concentrator is used, determine appropriate backup system in case of power failure (e.g., notify local emergency medical service [EMS]). Have spare oxygen tank available for emergency use. *Rationale: Many municipalities require that clients who have home oxygen equipment notify EMS before bringing equipment home. In case of power outage, EMS will call the home, and in some cases, the home is on priority list for restoration of power.*

PLANNING

Expected Outcomes focus on correct and safe use of home oxygen equipment.

1 Client's symptoms are minimized while receiving oxygen at prescribed rate.

2 Client and family verbalize the purpose and correct use of home oxygen by discharge.

3 Client and family demonstrate how to set up the oxygen system.

4 Client and family verbalize safety guidelines for oxygen use and troubleshoot problems (i.e., broken tubing, tubing disconnected, or not in nostrils correctly).

5 Client and family develop and verbalize emergency plan of care.

Delegation
The skill of home oxygen therapy may not be delegated. The nurse directs personnel by:
- Reviewing to observe for and report any changes in client's breathing, level of consciousness, and unsafe behaviors (e.g., smoking in the home).

Equipment
- Nasal cannula, oxygen mask, OCD, or other prescribed delivery device
- Oxygen tubing
- Home oxygen delivery system (compressed oxygen, oxygen concentrator, or liquid oxygen) with all required equipment (varies with supplier and system used)

IMPLEMENTATION *for Using Home Oxygen Therapy*

STEPS	RATIONALE
1 See Standard Protocol (inside front cover).	
2 Place oxygen system in clutter-free environment that is well ventilated, away from walls, drapes, bedding, and at least 8 feet from heat sources.	Keeps device balanced and prevents injury.
3 Demonstrate steps for preparation and delivery of oxygen therapy.	Demonstration is reliable technique for teaching psychomotor skill and allows client to ask questions (Falvo, 2004).
a. Compressed oxygen system	
(1) Turn cylinder valve counterclockwise two or three turns with wrench.	Turns on oxygen.
(2) Check cylinders by reading amount on pressure gauge.	Verifies adequate oxygen supply for client.
(3) Store wrench with oxygen tank or in other safe place.	Ensures wrench is available when needed.
b. Oxygen concentrator system	
(1) Plug concentrator into appropriate outlet.	Provides power safely to concentrator.
(2) Turn on power switch.	Starts concentrator motor.
(3) Alarm will sound for a few seconds.	Alarm turns off when desired pressure inside concentrator is reached.
c. Liquid oxygen system	
(1) Check system by pressing button at lower right corner and reading the dial on the stationary oxygen reservoir or the ambulatory tank (see Figure 38-3, *B*).	Verifies adequate oxygen supply for client use.
(2) Collaborate with DME provider to instruct on refilling ambulatory tank.	Ambulatory tanks of liquid oxygen need to be filled when empty.

> **NURSE ALERT** Only fill ambulatory tanks when they are empty. If cold oxygen stored in liquid reservoir mixes with warmer oxygen left in ambulatory tank, the ambulatory tank can malfunction.

(3) To refill liquid oxygen tank:	
(a) Wipe both filling connectors with a clean, dry, lint-free cloth.	Removes dust and moisture from system.
(b) Turn off flow selector of ambulatory unit.	Prevents oxygen from leaking.
(c) Attach ambulatory unit to stationary reservoir by inserting female adapter from ambulatory tank into male adapter of stationary reservoir.	Secures connection between oxygen reservoir and ambulatory tank.
(d) Open fill valve on ambulatory tank and apply firm pressure to top of stationary reservoir (see illustration). Stay with unit while it is filling. You will hear a loud hissing noise. Tank fills in about 2 minutes.	Prevents leakage of oxygen during filling process. If oxygen leaks during filling process, connection between ambulatory tank and reservoir can ice up and stick together.
(e) Disengage ambulatory unit from stationary reservoir when hissing noise changes and vapor cloud begins to form from stationary unit.	Overfilling can cause ambulatory tank to malfunction due to high pressure in tank.

> **NURSE ALERT** If ambulatory unit does not separate easily, valves from reservoir and ambulatory unit may be frozen together. Wait until valves warm to disengage (about 5 to 10 minutes). To prevent frostbite, do not touch any frosted areas.

(f) Wipe both filling connectors with clean, dry, lint-free cloth.	Ice can form during filling process; removes moisture from oxygen system.

STEPS

4 Connect oxygen delivery device (e.g., nasal cannula) to oxygen system.

5 Determine and set correct liter flow rate.
6 Place oxygen delivery device on client.
7 Instruct client about safe home oxygen use (Box 38-3).

8 Instruct client not to change oxygen flow rate.
9 Have client or family member perform each step with guidance if needed. Provide written material for reinforcement and review.
10 Discuss emergency plans for power loss, natural disaster, and acute respiratory distress.
11 **See Completion Protocol (inside front cover).**

RATIONALE

Connects oxygen source to delivery method.

Ensures delivery of prescribed amount of oxygen.
Delivers oxygen to client.
Safe use of oxygen in home is essential to prevent client injury.
Provides prescribed amount of oxygen.
Allows you to correct errors in technique and ensure safe oxygen use in home.

Ensures appropriate response to emergency situations.

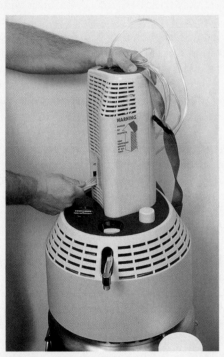

STEP 3c.(3)(d) Open fill valve on ambulatory tank while applying firm pressure to top of stationary reservoir.

BOX 38-3 Oxygen Safety Guidelines

Fire Safety
- Oxygen is not flammable; however, it supports combustion, therefore:
  - Use and store oxygen in a well-ventilated area.
  - Do not use petroleum-based ointments (e.g., Vaseline) around the nose to avoid burns.
  - Keep oxygen delivery systems at least 8 feet from open flames (e.g., stoves, fireplace).
  - Do not allow smoking in the house.
  - Avoid use of electrical appliances that produce sparks (e.g., electric razors).
  - Install smoke detectors and have a fire extinguisher in the home.
  - Help client and family plan a fire evacuation route.

Oxygen Storage and Handling
- Store cylinders upright in carts or stands to prevent from tipping or place tanks flat on floor when not in use.
- Never store oxygen tanks in a car.
- When oxygen tanks are transported in a car, secure them in the passenger area and keep the windows open 2-3 inches to allow for ventilation.

Concentrator Safety
- Plug concentrator into properly grounded outlets.
- Do not use extension cords, power strips, or multiple outlet adapters with concentrators.
- Ensure that power supply or electrical circuit meets or exceeds the electrical requirements of the concentrator.

Liquid Oxygen Safety
- Avoid direct contact with liquid oxygen; it can cause frostbite.
- Do not touch frosted or icy connectors.
- Keep ambulatory tanks upright; do not lay them down or place them on their sides.

Adapted from Findeisen M: Long-term oxygen therapy in the home, *Home Healthc Nurse* 19(11):692, 2001; Robb BW and others: Home oxygen therapy: adjunct or risk factor? *J Burn Care Rehabil* 24(6):403, 2003.

EVALUATION

1 Observe client's respiratory pattern and ask client if feeling short of breath to determine if oxygen therapy is effective as prescribed. Verify oxygen is being delivered at correct rate.

2 Ask client and family to describe reasons for home oxygen use.

3 Watch client and family set up equipment and use home oxygen system.

4 Ask client and family to describe safety guidelines for home oxygen use.

5 Ask client and family to verbalize plan in case of emergency.

Unexpected Outcomes and Related Interventions

1 Client develops signs and symptoms associated with hypoxemia (e.g., agitations, restlessness, dyspnea, confusion, delirium, or loss of consciousness).

a. Determine if oxygen delivery device and source are delivering oxygen properly and if flow rate is set correctly.

b. Assess client for change in respiratory status such as airway plugging, respiratory infection, or bronchospasm.

c. Notify client's physician or health care provider.

2 Client does not use oxygen therapy safely (e.g., uses oxygen near fire, smokes cigarettes).

a. Discuss risks created by unsafe behavior with client.

b. Attempt to identify reason client is unable to use oxygen correctly (e.g., health beliefs, incorrect information).

Recording and Reporting

• Record teaching plan for instructing client and family to use home oxygen and validation of learning on progress notes.

• Communicate client's or family's learning progress to other health care providers involved.

Sample Documentation

1600 Education about liquid oxygen system provided. Client and family gave return demonstration on appropriate use of system, including safety guidelines. Correctly stated signs and symptoms of hypoxemia.

Special Considerations
Pediatric Considerations

• Keep equipment out of reach of children.

• Children who receive home oxygen therapy have better long-term outcomes when they are followed by home oxygen programs run by advanced practice nurses (Kotecha and Allen, 2002).

Geriatric Considerations

• Older adults have less efficient respiratory systems and less surface area for gas exchange; thus their response to decreased oxygen often causes cerebral anoxia and leads to confusion. They may be unable to recognize respiratory problems or problems with the delivery system; therefore they must have frequent contact with a designated caregiver.

• Older adults are prone to skin breakdown. Assess the area behind the ears frequently. It is important to keep skin dry under the mask and wash with mild soap and water. Cotton balls or foam pads provided by vendor can be used to prevent skin breakdown from the cannula on the ears.

Home Care and Long-Term Care Considerations

• Oxygen desaturation and decreased oxygen delivery to the brain can impair the client's ability to remember previous learning; provide written or pictorial instructions for the home setting.

• Clients who receive long-term oxygen therapy often report poorer quality of life and have symptoms of depression. Provide emotional support and screen for depression as you visit clients in their homes (Ferreira and others, 2003; Lacasse and others, 2001).

• Some clients are able to manage portable oxygen system but are unable to fill portable system. If this happens, help client identify a family member or friend who can help fill tanks.

• Post oxygen provider's contact information, including phone numbers, in a place where it can be easily found.

NCLEX® Style Questions

1 When performing a home safety check in a home with a new infant, the nurse assesses that the hot water in the home is 145° F when it comes out of the faucet. What is the immediate nursing intervention?

1. Tell the mother to call her plumber immediately to fix the hot water heater.
2. Tell the mother that the hot water heater is set appropriately.
3. Show the mother how to adjust the hot water heater to make the temperature of the hot water 120° F or less.
4. Show the mother how to adjust the hot water heater to make the temperature of the hot water higher than 145° F.

2 A family with three school-age children asks the nurse to help them complete a home safety check. Which of the following findings require an immediate action? (Mark all that apply.)

1. The handle of a pot of boiling water is hanging over the edge of the stove.
2. Prescription medications are in a locked box in the parents' bathroom.
3. The stairs to the basement do not have a railing.
4. The father's guns are locked in a cabinet in the basement.
5. Fertilizer is stored in a bag on the floor of the garage.

3 The nurse is caring for a client who has Alzheimer's disease and who lives in her daughter's home. Which of the following statements, made by daughter, shows that she needs further education on adapting her home for her mother?

1. "I have put clocks and calendars in all the rooms of my house so my mom knows what day and time it is."
2. "My mom picks out clothes that do not match. The other day, she refused to put on a sweater, even though it was a cold day."

3. "I have found that, if I break my mom's favorite recipes down into simple steps, she is still able to cook, and she feels better because she is helping me."
4. "I have my mom's good friends come over for lunch once a week."

4 The nurse is visiting a client at home who has recently been discharged from the hospital. The client was discharged on eight medications. Which of the following assessment findings indicate the client is able to administer his own medications safely?

1. A list of medications from before the hospital stay is attached to the refrigerator.
2. Medications are correctly placed in a pill organizer.
3. There is one extra pill in the bottle of antibiotics when counted.
4. The client has poured all his medications into one container.

5 The nurse needs to teach a client how to administer an insulin injection subcutaneoulsy. The following steps must be completed when teaching the client. Put the steps in the correct order:

1. Encourage client to pinch injection site and then insert needle quickly at a 90-degree angle into the site all the way to the hub.
2. Have client manipulate the syringe and explain which parts of the syringe the client can touch.
3. Teach client how to properly dispose of the needle.
4. Have client push in on the plunger to administer the medication.
5. Explain choice and rotation of injection sites and help client select and prepare an appropriate site for injection.
6. Have client remove the syringe at a 90-degree angle.
7. Teach client how to prepare the medication in the syringe.

References for all chapters appear in Appendix D.

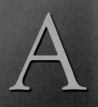

NCLEX® Answer Key

Chapter 1
1. 2
2. 4
3. 1
4. 4
5. 2,3

Chapter 2
1. 4
2. 1
3. 4
4. 2
5. 3

Chapter 3
1. 1, 4
2. 2
3. 2, 5, 7, 9, 4, 1, 8, 3, 6
4. 1, 3, 4, 5

Chapter 4
1. 2
2. 3, 4, 2, 6, 5, 1, 7
3. 2, 4, 5
4. 4
5. 1

Chapter 5
1. 1.S, 2.S, 3.M, 4.M, 5.S, 6.M
2. 1
3. 2
4. 3, 4

Chapter 6
1. 4
2. 4
3. 2, 3
4. 2, 4
5. 2

Chapter 7
1. 4
2. 6, 1, 5, 3, 4, 2
3. 2
4. 2
5. 4

Chapter 8
1. 3
2. 3
3. 1
4. 4
5. 2
6. 4

Chapter 9
1. 3
2. 3
3. 1
4. 2
5. In 1810, Out 1220

Chapter 10
1. 4
2. 2
3. 1
4. 2
5. 1
6. 1

Chapter 11
1. 2
2. 1
3. 4
4. 3
5. 3

Chapter 12
1. 1, 5, 6, 7
2. 3
3. 4
4. 2
5. 2, 3, 1
6. 3
7. 2

Chapter 13
1. 1
2. 1
3. 2
4. 4
5. 4
6. 7, 1, 3, 6, 4, 5, 2

Chapter 14
1. 2
2. 4
3. 1
4. 3, 4, 1, 2
5. 1

Chapter 15
1. 4
2. 3
3. medication, dose, client, route, time, and documentation
4. 0.5 or ½ tablet
5. 5 ml

Chapter 16
1. 4
2. 2
3. 3
4. 1
5. 3, 6, 4, 5, 1, 2

Chapter 17
1. 2
2. 2
3. 2
4. 1
5. 1.b, 2.c, 3.a

Chapter 18
1. 1
2. 3
3. 2
4. 3
5. 3, 1, 4, 2, 5

Chapter 19
1. 3
2. 4
3. 1
4. 3, 5, 7, 2, 4, 1, 6

Chapter 20
1. 4
2. 2
3. 1
4. 2
5. 3

Chapter 21
1. 3
2. 3
3. 2
4. 2

Chapter 22
1. 3
2. 2
3. 3
4. 1
5. 3

Chapter 23
1. 1
2. 3
3. 2, 4, 1, 5, 10, 9, 6, 7, 8, 3
4. 1
5. 3

Chapter 24
1. 1
2. 3
3. 2
4. 1
5. 2

Chapter 25
1. 4
2. 2
3. 2
4. 4
5. 2

Chapter 26
1. 1
2. 2
3. 2
4. 2
5. 2, 5

Chapter 27
1. 4
2. 2, 5
3. 3
4. 3
5. 3
6. 4

Chapter 28
1. 2, 4
2. 3
3. 4
4. 1
5. 1

Chapter 29
1. 3
2. 4
3. 1, 2, 3
4. 2
5. 2
6. 2, 3, 4

Chapter 30
1. 3
2. 2
3. 1
4. 4
5. 2

Chapter 31
1. 1
2. 3
3. 2
4. 4
5. 2

Chapter 32
1. 3
2. 3
3. 2
4. 1

Chapter 33
1. 3
2. 4
3. 3
4. 2
5. 1
6. 2, 5, 1, 3, 6, 4

Chapter 34
1. 1
2. 2
3. 2
4. 2
5. 3

Chapter 35
1. 1, 3, 2, 4, 6, 5
2. 2
3. 1
4. 2
5. 4

Chapter 36
1. 6, 3, 2, 4, 8, 1, 7, 5, 9
2. 4, 6, 1, 3, 7, 2, 5, 8, 9
3. 3
4. 2

Chapter 37
1. 3
2. 4, 3, 6
3. 4
4. 5, 3, 4, 1, 2
5. 1

Chapter 38
1. 3
2. 1, 3, 5
3. 2
4. 2
5. 2, 7, 5, 1, 4, 6, 3

B

Abbreviations and Equivalents

ABBREVIATIONS FOR CONVERSION USING HOUSEHOLD MEASURES

1 drop (gtt) = 1 minim
1 teaspoon (1 tsp) = 5 ml
3 tsp = 1 tablespoon (tbsp)
1 cup = 8 oz
16 oz = 1 pound (lb)

STANDARD EQUIVALENTS, ABBREVIATIONS, AND CONVERSIONS

1000 mg = 1 g
1000 ml = 1 liter (L)
2.2 lb = 1 kilogram (kg) = 1000 g
1 tsp = 5 ml
1 dr = 4 ml
mEq: milliequivalent
mcg (μg): microgram

SYMBOLS

/	Per
≤	Equal to or less than
≥	Equal to or more than
≅	Approximately equal to
+/−,‴±	Plus or minus
♂	Male
♀	Female
1°	Primary; first degree
2°	Secondary; second degree
3°	Tertiary; third degree
↑	Up; increase
↓	Down; decrease
μ	Micron

ABBREVIATIONS

ā: before
abd: abdomen
ABGs: arterial blood gases
ac: before meals
ad lib: as desired
ADH: antidiuretic hormone
ADLs: activities of daily living
AFB: acid-fast bacillus (related to tuberculosis)
AIDS: acquired immunodeficiency syndrome
ALL: acute lymphoblastic leukemia
AMB: ambulatory
AP (and lateral chest): anterior and posterior
ASA: aspirin
ASHD: arteriosclerotic heart disease
ax: axillary
BE: barium enema
bid: twice a day
BM: bowel movement
BP: blood pressure
BPH: benign prostatic hypertrophy
BR: bed rest
BRP: bathroom privileges
BSE: breast self-examination
BSI: body substance isolation
BUN: blood urea nitrogen
bx: biopsy
c̄: with
C&S: culture and sensitivity
CA: cancer
CABG: coronary artery bypass graft
CAD: coronary artery disease
cap: capsule
CBC: complete blood count
CBI: continuous bladder irrigation
CBR: complete bed rest
CC: chief complaint
CDC: Centers for Disease Control and Prevention
CHF: congestive heart failure
Cl: chloride
CN: cranial nerve
CNS: central nervous system

c/o: complains of
CO_2: carbon dioxide
COPD: chronic obstructive pulmonary disease
CPM: continuous passive motion
CPR: cardiopulmonary resuscitation
CSF: cerebrospinal fluid
CT: computed tomography
CVA: cerebrovascular accident (stroke)
CVP: central venous pressure
D5NS, D_5NS: 5% dextrose in 0.9% (normal) saline
D5 ½ NS, D_5½ NS: 5% dextrose in 0.45% saline
D5W, D_5W: 5% dextrose and water
DAT: diet as tolerated
D/C: discontinue
DM: diabetes mellitus
DNR: do not resuscitate
DSD: dry sterile dressing
DTR: deep tendon reflex
DVT: deep venous thrombosis
dx: diagnosis
EC: enteric coated
ECG, EKG: electrocardiogram
elix: elixir
ER: extended release
ESR: erythrocyte sedimentation rate
ESRD: end-stage renal disease
ET: enterostomal therapist
FUO: fever of unknown origin
fx: fracture
g: gram
GI: gastrointestinal
gtt: drops
GU: genitourinary
Hb, Hgb: hemoglobin
HBV: hepatitis B virus
HCO_3^-: bicarbonate
Hct: hematocrit
HCV: hepatitis C virus
HEPA: high-efficiency particulate air
HIV: human immunodeficiency virus
h/o: history of
HOB: head of bed
HR: heart rate
hs: at bedtime
HTN: hypertension
I&O: intake and output
ICP: intracranial pressure
ICU: intensive care unit
IDDM: insulin-dependent diabetes mellitus
IM: intramuscular
IPPB: intermittent positive-pressure breathing
IV: intravenous
JVD: jugular vein distention
K: potassium
KUB: kidney, ureter, bladder
KVO: keep vein open (run IV very slowly)

LLQ: left lower quadrant
LMP: last menstrual period
LOC: level of consciousness
LR: lactated Ringer's solution
lytes: electrolytes
MAP: mean arterial pressure
MCHC: mean corpuscular hemoglobin concentration
MCV: mean corpuscular volume
MI: myocardial infarction
MRI: magnetic resonance imaging
N: nitrogen
Na: sodium
NaCl: sodium chloride
neg: negative
NG: nasogastric
NPO: nothing by mouth
NS: normal saline
NSAIDs: nonsteroidal antiinflammatory drugs
O_2: oxygen
O.D.: right eye
OOB: out of bed
OR: operating room
O.S.: left eye
OT: occupational therapy
OTC: over the counter (medicine without prescription)
O.U.: both eyes
P: pulse
PACU: postanesthesia care unit
pc: after meals
PCA: patient-controlled analgesia
PE: pulmonary embolism
PID: pelvic inflammatory disease
PMH: past medical history
PMI: point of maximal impulse
PO: by mouth
postop: after surgery
preop: before surgery
prep: preparation
prn: as needed
pt: patient
PT: physical therapy
PT: prothrombin time
PTT: partial thromboplastin time
PVD: peripheral vascular disease
q: each
q__h (fill in number of hours), e.g., q3h: every 3 hours
qid: four times a day
qod: every other day
qs: sufficient quantity
R: respirations
RA: rheumatoid arthritis
RBC: red blood cell
R/O: rule out (eliminate possibility of a condition)
ROM: range of motion
ROS: review of systems
r/t: related to

RUQ: right upper quadrant
Rx: treatment
s̄: without
SC (SQ): subcutaneous
sl (SL): sublingual
SOB: shortness of breath
sp gr: specific gravity
SR: sustained release
STAT: immediately
STD: sexually transmitted disease
supp: suppository
susp: suspension
sx: symptoms, signs
T: temperature
T&C: type and crossmatch
tab: tablet
TB: tuberculosis

TCDB: turn, cough, deep breathe
tid: three times a day
TPN: total parenteral nutrition
TPR: temperature, pulse, respirations
TURP: transurethral resection of prostate
UA: urinalysis
up ad lib: up as desired
URI: upper respiratory infection
US: ultrasound
UTI: urinary tract infection
VS: vital signs
VTBI: volume to be infused
WBC: white blood cell
WC: wheelchair
WNL: within normal limits
wt: weight

Official "Do Not Use" List* 2006

DO NOT USE	POTENTIAL PROBLEM	USE INSTEAD
U (unit)	Mistaken for "O" (zero), the number "4" (four), or "cc"	Write "unit"
IU (International Unit)	Mistaken for IV (intravenous) or the number 10 (ten)	Write "International Unit"
Q.D., QD, q.d., qd (daily) Q.O.D, QOD, q.o.d., qod (every other day)	Mistake for each other Period after the Q mistaken for "I" and the "O" mistaken for "I"	Write "daily" Write "every other day"
Trailing zero (X.0 mg)†	Decimal point is missing	Write X mg
Lack of leading zero (.X mg)		Write 0.X mg
MS	Can mean morphine sulphate or magnesium sulphate	Write "morphine sulphate"
MSO4 and MgSO4	Confused for one another	Write "magnesium sulphate"

*Applies to all orders and all medication-related documentation that is handwritten (including free-text computer entry) or on preprinted forms.
†**Exception:** A "trailing zero" may be used only where required to demonstrate the level of precision of the value being reported, such as for laboratory results, imaging studies that report size of lesions, or catheter/tube sizes. It may not be used in medication orders or other medical-related documentation.
Official "Do Not Use" List, Joint Commission on Accreditation of Heathcare Organizations (April 19, 2006), www.jointcommission.org, accessed September 15, 2006.

Additional Abbreviations, Acronyms, and Symbols *(for possible future inclusion in the Official "Do Not Use" List)*

DO NOT USE	POTENTIAL PROBLEM	USE INSTEAD
> (greater than)	Misinterpreted as the number "&" (seven) or the letter "L"	Write "greater than"
< (less than)	Confused for one another	Write "less than"
Abbreviations for drug names	Misinterpreted due to similar abbreviations for multiple drugs	Write drug names in full
Apothecary units	Unfamiliar to many practitioners Confused with metric units	Write drug names in full
@	Mistaken for the number "2" (two)	Write "at"
cc	Mistaken for U (units) when written poorly	Write "ml" or "milliliters"
μg	Mistaken for mg (milligrams) resulting in one thousand-fold overdose	Write "mcg" or "micrograms"

Official "Do Not Use" List, Joint Commission on Accreditation of Heathcare Organizations (April 19, 2006), www.jointcommission.org, accessed September 15, 2006.
NANDA International APPROVED NURSING DIAGNOSES 2005-2006.

Activity intolerance
Activity intolerance, risk for
Adjustment, impaired
Airway clearance, ineffective
Allergy response, latex
Allergy response, latex, risk for
Anxiety
Anxiety, death
Aspiration, risk for
Attachment, impaired parent/infant/child, risk for
Autonomic dysreflexia
Autonomic dysreflexia, risk for
Body image, disturbed
Body temperature, imbalanced, risk for
Bowel incontinence
Breastfeeding, effective
Breastfeeding, ineffective
Breastfeeding, interrupted
Breathing pattern, ineffective
Cardiac output, decreased
Caregiver role strain
Caregiver role strain, risk for
Comfort, impaired
Communication, verbal, impaired
Communication, readiness for enhanced
Conflict, decisional (specify)
Conflict, parental role
Confusion, acute
Confusion, chronic
Constipation
Constipation, perceived
Constipation, risk for
Coping, ineffective
Coping, readiness for enhanced
Coping, community, ineffective
Coping, community, readiness for enhanced
Coping, defensive
Coping, family, compromised
Coping, family, disabled
Coping, family, readiness for enhanced

Death syndrome, sudden infant, risk for
Denial, ineffective
Dentition, impaired
Development, delayed, risk for
Diarrhea
Disuse syndrome, risk for
Diversional activity, deficient
Energy field, disturbed†
Environmental intrpretation syndrome, impaired
Failure to thrive, adult
Falls, risk for
Family processes: alcoholism, dysfunctional
Family processes, interrupted
Family processes, readiness for enhanced
Fatigue
Fear
Fluid balance, readiness for enhanced
Fluid volume, deficient
Fluid volume, excess
Fluid volume, deficient, risk for
Fluid volume, imbalanced, risk for
Gas exchange, impaired
Grieving
Grieving, anticipatory
Grieving, dysfunctional†
Grieving, risk for dysfunctional*
Growth and development, delayed
Growth disproportionate, risk for
Health maintenance, ineffective
Health-seeking behaviors
Home maintenance, impaired
Hopelessness
Hyperthermia
Hypothermia
Identity, personal, disturbed
Incontinence, urinary, functional
Incontinence, urinary, reflex
Incontinence, urinary, stress
Incontinence, urinary, total
Incontinence, urinary, urge
Incontinence, urinary, urge, risk for
Infant behavior, disorganized

*New diagnosis for 2005-2006.
†Revised diagnosis for 2005-2006.

Infant behavior, disorganized, risk for
Infant behavior, organized, readiness for enhanced
Feeding pattern, infant, ineffective
Infection, risk for
Injury, risk for
Injury, perioperative positioning, risk for
Intracranial adaptive capacity, decreased
Knowledge, deficient
Knowledge of (Specify), readiness for enhanced
Lifestyle, sedentary*
Loneliness, risk for
Memory, impaired
Mobility, bed, impaired
Mobility, physical, impaired
Mobility, wheelchair, impaired
Nausea
Neglect, unilateral
Noncompliance
Nutrition, readiness for enhanced
Nutrition: less than body requirements, imbalanced
Nutrition: more than body requirements, imbalanced
Nutrition: more than body requirements, risk for imbalanced
Oral mucous membrane, impaired
Pain, acute
Pain, chronic
Parenting, readiness for enhanced
Parenting, impaired
Parenting, impaired, risk for
Peripheral neurovascular dysfunction, risk for
Poisoning, risk for
Post-trauma syndrome
Post-trauma syndrome, risk for
Powerlessness
Powerlessness, risk for
Protection, ineffective
Rape-trauma syndrome
Rape-trauma syndrome: compound reaction
Rape-trauma syndrome: silent reaction
Religiosity, impaired
Religiosity, readiness for enhanced*
Religiosity, risk for impaired*
Relocation stress syndrome*
Relocation stress syndrome, risk for
Role performance, ineffective
Self-care deficit, bathing/hygiene
Self-care deficit, dressing/grooming
Self-care deficit, feeding

Self-care deficit, toileting
Self-concept, readiness for enhanced
Self-esteem, chronic low
Self-esteem, situational low
Self-esteem, situational low, risk for
Self-mutilation
Self-mutilation, risk for
Sensory perception, disturbed
Sexual dysfunction
Sexuality patterns, ineffective
Skin integrity, impaired
Skin integrity, impaired, risk for
Sleep deprivation
Sleep patterns, disturbed
Sleep, readiness for enhanced
Social interaction, impaired
Social isolation
Sorrow, chronic
Spiritual distress
Spiritual distress, risk for†
Spiritual well-being, readiness for enhanced
Suffocation, risk for
Suicide, risk for
Surgical recovery, delayed
Swallowing, impaired
Therapeutic regimen management, community, ineffective
Therapeutic regimen management, effective
Therapeutic regimen management, family, ineffective
Therapeutic regimen management, ineffective
Therapeutic regimen management, readiness for enhanced
Thermoregulation, ineffective
Thought processes, disturbed
Tissue integrity, impaired
Tissue perfusion, ineffective
Transfer ability, impaired
Trauma, risk for
Urinary elimination, readiness for enhanced
Urinary elimination, impaired
Urinary retention
Ventilation, spontaneous, impaired
Ventilatory weaning response, dysfunctional
Violence, other-directed, risk for
Violence, self-directed, risk for
Walking, impaired
Wandering

NANDA International: *NANDA International nursing diagnoses: definitions and classifications 2005-2006*, Philadelphia, 2005, NANDA-I.
*New diagnosis for 2005-2006.
†Revised diagnosis for 2005-2006.

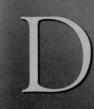

References

Chapter 1
Professional Nursing Practice

American Hospital Association: *The patient care partnership: understanding expectations, rights, and responsibilities*, Chicago, 2003, AHA.

American Nurses Association: ANA news, *Am J Nurs* 55:1474, 1955.

American Nurses Association: *Nursing: scope and standards of practice*, Washington, DC, 2004, ANA.

American Nurses Association: *Nursing's social policy statement*, ed 2, Washington, DC, 2003, ANA.

American Nurses Association: *Principles for delegation*, www.nursingworld.org, accessed October 22, 2006.

Cambridge Research Institute: *Trends affecting the US health care system*, 262, Health Planning Information Series, Human Resources Administration, Public Health Service, Department of Health, Education, and Welfare, Washington, DC, 1976, revised and updated 1992, US Government Printing Office.

Carpenito-Moyet LJ: *Nursing diagnosis application to clinical practice*, ed 11, Philadelphia, 2005, Lippincott Williams & Wilkins.

Christensen B, Kockrow E: *Foundations of nursing*, ed 5, St Louis, 2005, Mosby.

Dochterman JM, Bulechek GM: *Nursing interventions classification (NIC)*, ed 4, St Louis, 2004, Mosby.

Dudley A: Journey toward family-centered care, *Adv Nurse* 1(6):10, 2001.

Edelman CL, Mandle CL: *Health promotion throughout the lifespan*, ed 6, St Louis, 2005, Mosby.

Joint Commission on Accreditation of Healthcare Organizations: *Comprehensive accreditation manual for hospitals (CAMH)*, Chicago, 2005, JCAHO.

Joint Commission on Accreditation of Healthcare Organizations: *National patient safety goals: 2006 critical access hospital and hospital national patient safety goals*, http://www.jointcommission.org/PatientSafety/NationalPatientSafetyGoals, accessed May 15, 2006.

Kataoka-Yahiro M, Saylor C: A critical thinking model for nursing judgment, *J Nurs Educ* 33(8):351, 1994.

Keeling B and others: Appropriate delegation, *Am J Nurs* 100(12):24, 2000.

Leavell H, Clark AE: *Preventive medicine for doctors in the community*, ed 3, New York, 1965, McGraw-Hill.

Melnyk BM, Fineout-Overholt E: *Evidence-based practice in nursing & healthcare: a guide to best practice*, Philadelphia, 2005, Lippincott Williams & Wilkins.

Mikos C: Legal checkpoints, *Nurs Manage* 35(9):20, 2004.

NANDA: *NANDA nursing diagnoses: definitions and classifications 2005-2006*, Philadelphia, 2005, NANDA.

National Council of State Boards of Nursing: *Delegation: concepts and decision-making process*, Chicago, 1995, The Council.

National Council of State Boards of Nursing: *The Five Rights of Delegation*, http://www.ncsbn.org, accessed May 2006.

Paul R: The art of redesigning instruction. In Willsen J, Blinker AJA, editors: *Critical thinking: how to prepare students for a rapidly changing world*, Santa Rosa, Calif, 1993, Foundation for Critical Thinking.

US Department of Health and Human Services: *Healthy people 2010: national health promotion and disease prevention objectives*, Washington, DC, 2000, US Government Printing Office.

US Department of Health and Human Services: Standards for Privacy of Individually Identifiable Health Information, Health Insurance Portability and Accountability Act of 1996, *Fed Regist* 64:60053, 1999, www.hhs.gov/ocr/hippa, revised 2003, accessed August 2003.

Chapter 2
Facilitating Communication

Akamatsu C, Mayer C, Farelly S: An investigation of two-way text messaging use with deaf students at the secondary level, *J Deaf Stud Deaf Educ* 11(1):120-131, 2005.

Beck H and others: Computer skills in patients with movement disorders, *Parkinsonism Relat Disord* 11(7):421-426, 2005.

Dysart-Gale D: Communication models, professionalism, and the work of medical interpreters, *J Health Commun* 17(1):91-103, 2005.

Flores G: The impact of medical interpreter services on the quality of health care: a systematic review, *Med Care Res Rev* 62(3):255-299, 2005.

Fortinash K, Holoday-Worret P: *Psychiatric-mental health nursing*, ed 3, St Louis, 2004, Mosby.

Giger J, Davidhizar R: *Transcultural nursing: assessment and intervention*, ed 4, St Louis, 2004, Mosby.

Hagerty B, Patusky K: Reconceptualizing the nursing-patient relationship, *J Nurs Scholarsh* 35(2):145, 2003.

Hockenberry MJ : *Wong's essentials of pediatric nursing*, ed 7, St Louis, 2005, Mosby.

Houts P and others: The role of pictures in improving health communication: a review of the research on attention, comprehension, recall, and adherence, *Patient Educ Couns* 61(2):173-190, 2005.

Keltner N, Schwecke L, Bostrom C: *Psychiatric nursing: a psychotherapeutic management approach*, ed 4, St Louis, 2003, Mosby.

Lopez A and others: Use of American Sign Language in telepsychiatry consultation, *Telemed J E Health* 10(3):389-391, 2004.

Martin M and others: Enhancing patient-physician communication: a community and culturally based approach, *J Cancer Educ* 20(3):150-154, 2005.

Purnell L, Paulanka B: *Transcultural health care: a culturally competent approach*, ed 2, Philadelphia, 2003, FA Davis.

Sundin K, Jansson L: 'Understanding and being understood' as a creative caring phenomenon-in care of patients with stroke and aphasia, *J Clin Nurs* 12(1):107-116, 2003.

Chapter 3
Promoting a Safe Environment

Algase DL and others: The Algase wandering scale: initial psychometrics of a new caregiver reporting tool, *Am J Alzheimers Dis Other Demen* 16(3):141-152, 2001.

Brians LK and others: Development of the RISK tool for fall prevention, *Rehabil Nurs* 16(2):67, 1991.

Capezuti E and others: Side rail use and bed-related fall outcomes among nursing home residents, *J Am Geriatr Soc* 50(1):90-96, 2002.

Centers for Disease Control and Prevention, National Center for Injury Prevention and Control: *A tool kit to prevent senior falls*, http://www.cdc.gov/ncipc/pub-res/toolkit/toolkit.htm, accessed April 24, 2006.

Centers for Disease Control and Prevention, National Center for Injury Prevention and Control: *Web-based Injury Statistics Query and Reporting System (WISQARS)*, http://www.cdc.gov/ncipc/wisqars, accessed November 24, 2003.

Centers for Medicare & Medicaid Services: *Conditions of participation: interpretive guidelines*, Baltimore, Md, 2004, CMS.

Centers for Medicare & Medicaid Services: *Hospital conditions of participation: patients' rights (section 482.13): interpretive guidelines and survey procedures*, Baltimore, Md, 2000, CMS.

Cwikel G and others: Validation of a fall-risk screening test, the elderly fall screening test (EFST) for community-dwelling elderly, *Disabil Rehabil* 20:161-167, 2001.

Ebersole P, Hess P: *Geriatric nursing and healthy aging*, St Louis, 2001, Mosby.

Ebersole P and others: *Toward healthy aging: human needs and nursing response*, ed 6, St Louis, 2004, Mosby.

Elsaris Z and others: Medications and falls in the elderly: a review of the evidence and practical considerations, *P&T* 28(11):724-733, 2003.

Futrell M, Melillo KD, Titler MG: *Evidence-based protocol: wandering*, Iowa City, 2002, University of Iowa Gerontological Nursing Interventions Research Center, Research Dissemination Core.

Gallinagh R and others: Side rails as physical restraints in the care of older people: a management issue, *J Nurs Manag* 10(5):299-301, 2002.

Hockenberry MJ, Wilson D: *Wong's nursing care of infants and children*, ed 8, St Louis, 2007, Mosby.

Ignatavicius DD, Workman ML: *Medical-surgical nursing: critical thinking for collaborative care*, ed 4, Philadelphia, 2006, Saunders.

Joanna Briggs Institute: *Falls in hospitals*, http://www.joannabriggs.edu.au/best_practice/bp4.php, accessed July 2006.

Joint Commission on Accreditation of Healthcare Organizations: *Comprehensive accreditation manual for hospitals*, Chicago, 2005a, JCAHO.

Joint Commission on Accreditation of Healthcare Organizations: *Sentinel events*, http://www.jointcommission.org/SentinelEvents, accessed April 26, 2006.

Joint Commission on Accreditation of Healthcare Organizations: *2006 National patient safety goals: ambulatory care and office-based surgery*, Chicago, 2005b, JCAHO, http://www.jointcommission.org/Patient/Safety/NationalPatientSafetyGoals/, accessed September 24, 2006.

Lannon S: Epilepsy in the elderly, *Clin Nurs Pract Epilepsy* 2(2):5, 1995.

Ledford L, Mentes J: *Research-based protocol: restraints*, Iowa City, 1997, University of Iowa Gerontological Nursing Interventions Research Center, Research Dissemination Core.

Meiner SE, Lueckenotte AG: *Gerontologic nursing*, ed 3, St Louis, 2006, Mosby.

National Institute of Neurological Disorders and Stroke: *Seizures and epilepsy: hope through research*, Bethesda, Md, 2007, National Institutes of Health.

North American Nursing Diagnosis Association: *Nursing diagnoses: definitions and classification 2005-2006*, Philadelphia, 2005, NANDA.

Powell-Cope G and others: Modification of bed systems and use of accessories to reduce the risk of hospital-bed entrapment, *Rehabil Nurs* 30(1):9-17, 2005.

Registered Nurses' Association of Ontario: *Nursing best practice guideline: prevention of falls and fall injuries in the older adult*, Toronto, Ontario, January 2002, RNAO.

Riefkohl E and others: Medications and falls in the elderly: a review of the evidence and practical considerations, *P&T* 28(11):724, 2003.

Rogers P, Bocchino N: Restraint free care: is it possible? *Am J Nurs* 99(10):26, 1999.

Sorrentino SA: *Assisting with patient care*, St Louis, 1999, Mosby.

Sorrentino SA: *Mosby's textbook for nursing assistants*, ed 6, St Louis, 2000, Mosby.

Strumpf NE, Evans LK: Physical restraint of the hospitalized elderly: perceptions of clients and nurses, *Nurs Res* 37(3):132, 1988.

Strumpf N and others: *Restraint free care: individualized approaches for frail elders*, New York, 1998, Springer.

Tideiksaar R: Home safe home: practical tips for fall-proofing, *Geriatr Nurs* 11(6):284, 1989.

Tinetti ME: Preventing falls in elderly persons, *N Engl J Med* 348(1):42, 2003.

Chapter 4
Medical Aseptic Techniques

Arnold F, McDonald LC: Antimicrobials and resistance. In Carrico R, editor: APIC *text of infection control and epidemiology*, Washington, DC, 2005, Association for Professionals in Infection Control and Epidemiology.

Bobo L: The microbiologic environment. In Soule B, Larson E, Preson G, editors: *Infection and nursing practice: prevention and control*, St Louis, 1994, Mosby.

Boyce JM, Pittet D: *HICPAC/SHEA/APIC/IDSA Hand Hygiene Task Force and the CDC Healthcare Infection Control Practices Advisory Committee draft guideline for hand hygiene in health-care settings*, 2001.

Centers for Disease Control and Prevention: Controlling tuberculosis in the United States: recommendations from the American Thoracic Society, CDC, and the Infectious Disease Society of America, *MMWR Recomm Rep* 54(RR12):1-81, 2005a.

Centers for Disease Control and Prevention: Guidelines for preventing the transmission of *Mycobacterium tuberculosis* in health-care facilities, *MMWR Recomm Rep* 43(RR-13):1-132, 1994.

Centers for Disease Control and Prevention: *Healthcare-associated infections (HAIs)*, http://www.cdc.gov/ncidod/dhqp/healthdis.html, accessed April 17, 2006a.

Centers for Disease Control and Prevention: Perspectives in disease prevention and health promotion update: universal precautions for prevention of transmission of human immunodeficiency virus, hepatitis B virus, and other bloodborne pathogens in healthcare settings, *MMWR Morb Mortal Wkly Rep* 37(24):377, 1988.

Centers for Disease Control and Prevention, Division of Tuberculosis Elimination: *Fact sheets: QuantiFERON-TB Gold Test*, http://www.cdc.gov/nchstp/tb/pubs/tbfactsheets/250103.htm, accessed April 9, 2006b.

Centers for Disease Control and Prevention, Healthcare Infection Control Practices Advisory Committee and the HICPAC/SHEA/APIC/IDSA Hand Hygiene Task Force: Guideline for hand hygiene in health-care settings, *MMWR Recomm Rep* 51(RR16):1-44, 2002.

Centers for Disease Control and Prevention, U.S. Department of Health & Human Services: *Guidance for the selection and use of personal protective equipment (PPE) in the health care setting*, http:www.cdc.gov/ncidod/dhqp/pdf/ppe/PPEslides6-29-04.ppt, accessed December 2, 2005b.

DeCastro M: Aseptic technique. In Carrico R, editor: APIC *text of infection control and epidemiology*, Washington, DC, 2002, Association for Professionals in Infection Control and Epidemiology.

Garner JS: Guidelines for isolation precautions in hospitals, *Am J Infect Control* 24:24, 1996.

Girou E and others: Efficacy of handrubbing with alcohol based solution versus standard handwashing with antiseptic soap: randomized clinical trial, *BMJ* 325(7360):362, 2002.

Griffith CJ and others: Environmental surface cleanliness and the potential for contamination during handwashing, *Am J Infect Control* 31(2):93-96, 2003.

Guinto CH and others: Evaluation of dedicated stethoscopes as a potential source of nosocomial pathogens, *Am J Infect Control* 30(8):499, 2002.

Harrison and others: Bacterial transfer and cross-contamination potential associated with paper-towel dispensing, *Am J Infect Control* 31(7):387-391, 2003.

Hilburn J and others: Use of alcohol hand sanitizer as an infection control strategy in an acute care facility, *Am J Infect Control* 31(2):109-116, 2003.

Hospital Infection Control Practices Advisory Committee: Guidelines for isolation precautions in hospitals, *Am J Infect Control* 24:24, 1996.

Kim PW and others: Rates of hand disinfection associated with glove use, patient isolation, and changes between exposure to various body sites, *Am J Infect Control* 31(2):97, 2003.

Larson E: Antiseptic. In Olmsted R, editor: APIC *infection control and applied epidemiology: principles and practice*, St Louis, 2000, Mosby.

Larson E: APIC guideline for the use of topical antimicrobial agents, *Am J Infect Control* 16(6):253, 1996.

Mashaba G: South African culturally based health-illness patterns and humanistic care practices. In Leininger M, McFarland MR: *Transcultural nursing: theories, research, and practice*, New York, 2002, McGraw-Hill.

McCoy KD and others: Monitoring adherence to standard precautions, *Am J Infect Control* 29:24, 2001.

Occupational Safety and Health Administration: *Enforcement policies on procedures for occupational exposure to tuberculosis*, Washington, DC, 1993, OSHA.

Occupational Safety and Health Administration: Occupational exposure to bloodborne pathogens; needlesticks and other sharps injuries; final rule, *Fed Regist* 66:5318, 2001.

Occupational Safety and Health Administration: Respiratory protection, *Fed Regist* 59(219):58884, 1994.

Potter P and others: Evaluation of chemical dot thermometers for measuring body temperature of orally intubated patients, *Am J Crit Care* 12(5):403, 2003.

Rutala W: Disinfection and sterilization of patient-care items, *Infect Control Hosp Epidemiol* 17(6):377, 1996.

Sattar SA and others: Preventing the spread of hepatitis B and C viruses: where are germicides relevant? *Am J Infect Control* 29:187, 2001.

Siegel J: Isolation systems. In Carrico R, editor: *APIC text of infection control and epidemiology*, Washington, DC, 2005, Association for Professionals in Infection Control and Epidemiology.

Stricof RL: Endoscopy. In Carrico R, editor: *APIC text of infection control and epidemiology*, Washington, DC, 2005, Association for Professionals in Infection Control and Epidemiology.

Chapter 5
Basic Sterile Techniques

Association of Operating Room Nurses: *Standards, recommended practices, and guidelines*, Denver, 2005, AORN.

Burt S: What you need to know about latex allergy, *Nursing* 28(10):33, 1998.

Centers for Disease Control and Prevention, Healthcare Infection Control Practices Advisory Committee: Guideline for isolation precautions in hospitals, *Am J Infect Control* 24:24, 1996.

DeCastro M: Aseptic technique. In *APIC text of infection control and epidemiology*, Washington, DC, 2002, Association for Professionals in Infection Control and Epidemiology.

Fleischman CA, Olmstead RM: Ask APIC: a comprehensive reference anthology. In *APIC text of infection control and epidemiology*, Washington, DC, 2000, Association for Professionals in Infection Control and Epidemiology.

Gritter M: The latex threat, *Am J Nurs* 98(9):26, 1998.

Kim KT and others: Implementation recommendations for making health care facilities latex safe, *AORN J* 67(3):615, 1998.

Osborne S: Influences on compliance with standard precautions among operating room nurses, *Am J Infect Control* 31(7):415-423, 2003.

Chapter 6
Promoting Activity and Mobility

American Nurses Association: *Position statement on elimination of manual patient handling to prevent work-related musculoskeletal disorders*, http://www.nursingworld.org.readroom/position/workplac/pathand.htm, accessed August 2006.

Babis G and others: Poor outcomes of isolated tibial insert exchange and arthrolysis for the management of stiffness following total knee arthroplasty, *J Bone Joint Surg Am* 83(10):1534, 2001.

Branson J, Goldstein W: Sequential bilateral total knee arthroplasty, *AORN J* 73(3):608, 2001.

DeWit SC: *Fundamental concepts and skills for nursing*, ed 2, Philadelphia, 2005, Saunders.

Dingle M: Role of dangling when moving from supine to standing position, *Br J Nurs* 12(6):346, 2003.

Frederiks C and others: Evaluation of skills and knowledge on orthostatic blood pressure measurements in elderly patients, *Age Ageing* 31(3):211, 2003.

Groeneveld A, McKenzie ML, Williams D: Logrolling: establishing consistent practice, *Orthop Nurs* 20(2):45, 2001.

Hammesfahr R, Serafino M: Early motion gets the worm: continuous passive motion following total hip arthroplasty can aid in alleviating pain, edema, stiffness, deep vein thrombosis, and dislocation, and in controlling cost, *Rehab Manag* 15(2):20, 2002.

Hignett S: Systematic review of patient handling activities starting in lying, sitting and standing positions, *J Adv Nurs* 41(6):545, 2003.

Hockenberry MJ, Wilson D: *Wong's nursing care of infants and children*, ed 8, St Louis, 2007, Mosby.

Hoeman SP: *Rehabilitation nursing: process and application*, ed 3, St Louis, 2002, Mosby.

Huddleston JS: Exercise. In Edelman C, Mandle C, editors: *Health promotion throughout the lifespan*, ed 5, St Louis, 2002, Mosby.

Huether S, McCance K: *Understanding pathophysiology*, ed 3, St Louis, 2004, Mosby.

Ignatavicius D, Workman L: *Medical surgical nursing: critical thinking for collaborative care*, ed 5, St Louis, 2006, Mosby.

Jitramontree N: Evidence-based protocol: exercise promotion, *J Gerontol Nurs* 27(10):7, 2001.

Kenny R: Advances in the treatment of orthostatic hypotension, *Clin Geriatr* 8(suppl 7):S1, 2000.

Konradi DB, Anglin LT: Moderate-intensity exercise: for our patients, for ourselves, *Orthop Nurs* 20(1):47, 2001.

Lavender S and others: Postural analysis of paramedics simulating frequently performed strenuous work tasks, *Appl Ergon* 31:45, 2000.

Marion BS: A turn for the better: prone positioning of patients with ARDS, *Am J Nurs* 101(5):26, 2001.

Meiner SE, Lueckenotte AG: *Gerontologic nursing*, ed 3, St Louis, 2006, Mosby.

Nelson A and others: Preventing nursing back injuries: redesigning patient handling tasks, *AAOHN J* 51(3):126-134, 2003.

Neslon A, Baptiste AS: Evidence-based practices for safe patient handling and movement, *Online 2 Issues-Nurs* 9(3), manuscript 3, 2004.

Netea R and others: Body position and blood pressure measurement in patients with diabetes mellitus, *J Intern Med* 251:393, 2002.

Occupational Safety and Health Administration: *Guidelines for nursing homes: ergonomics for the prevention of musculoskeletal disorders*, Washington, DC, 2003, OSHA.

Owens B: Preventing injuries using an ergonomic approach, *AORN J* 72(6):1031, 2000.

Owens B, Welden N, Kane J: What are we teaching about lifting and transferring patients? *Res Nurs Health* 22:3, 1999.

Phipps W and others: *Medical-surgical nursing: concepts and clinical practice,* ed 8, St Louis, 2007, Mosby.

Tinkoff A and others: Musculoskeletal problems of the neck, shoulder, and back and functional consequences in nurses, *Am J Ind Med* 41(3):170, 2002.

Chapter 7
Promoting Hygiene

Agency for Health Care Policy and Research: *Pressure ulcers in adults: prediction and prevention,* Clinical practice guideline, Rockville, Md, 1992, US Department of Health and Human Services, Public Health Service, AHCPR.

American Diabetes Association: *Foot complications,* http://www.diabetes.org/type-1-diabetes/foot-complications.jsp, accessed August 2006.

American Diabetes Association: Preventive foot care in people with diabetes, *Diabetes Care* 21(suppl 1):S56, 2001.

American Society of Health-Systems Pharmacists: Clinical practice guidelines for sustained neuromuscular blockade in the adult critically ill patient, *Am J Health Syst Pharm* 59(2):179, 2002.

Bauroth K and others: The efficacy of an essential oil antiseptic mouthwash vs dental flossing in controlling interproximal gingivitis: a comparative study, *J Am Dent Assoc* 144(3):359, 2003.

Crute S, editor: *Health and healing for African-Americans,* Emmaus, Pa, 1997, Rodale Press.

Galanti G: *Caring for patients from different cultures,* ed 3, Philadelphia, 2004, University of Pennsylvania Press.

Grap MT and others: Oral care interventions in critical care: frequency and documentation, *Am J Crit Care* 12(2):114, 2003.

Greenberger NJ, Hinthorn DR: *History taking and physical examination: essentials and clinical correlates,* St Louis, 1993, Mosby.

Habif TP: *Clinical dermatology: a color guide to diagnosis and therapy,* ed 2, St Louis, 1990, Mosby.

Hockenberry MJ, Wilson D: *Wong's nursing care of infants and children,* ed 8, St Louis, 2007, Mosby.

Lecours AD: Understanding common oral lesions associated with HIV, *Clin Rev* 11(6):96, 2001.

Meiner SE, Lueckenotte AG: *Gerontologic nursing,* ed 3, St Louis, 2006, Mosby.

Sheppard CM, Brenner PS: The effects of bathing and skin care practices on skin quality and satisfaction with an innovative product, *J Gerontol Nurs* 26(10):36, 2000.

Strauss MB, Hart JD, Winant DM: Diabetic foot problems: keys to effective, aggressive prevention, *Consultant* 41(14):1693, 2001.

Weston WL, Lane AT: *Color textbook of pediatric dermatology,* ed 3, St Louis, 2002, Mosby.

Zitelli BJ, Davis HW: *Atlas of pediatric physical diagnosis,* ed 3, St Louis, 1997, Mosby.

Chapter 8
Promoting Nutrition

American Dietetic Association: Identifying patients at risk: ADA's definitions for nutrition screening and nutrition assessment. Council on Practice (COP) Quality Management Committee, *J Am Diet Assoc* 94(8):838-839, 1994.

American Heart Association: *Fiber,* http://www.americanheart.org/presenter.jhtml?identifier=4574, accessed August 2006.

American Society of Parenteral and Enteral Nutrition (ASPEN) Board of Directors and Clinical Guidelines Taskforce: Guidelines for the use of parenteral and enteral nutrition in adult and pediatric patients, *JPEN J Parenter Enteral Nutr* 26(1):1SA-138SA, 2002.

Bastian RW: Contemporary diagnosis of the dysphagic patient, *Otolaryngol Clin North Am* 31(3):489-506, 1998.

Bickford GR and others: Nutrition assessment outcomes: a strategy to improve health care, *Clin Lab Manage Rev* 13(6):357-364, 1999.

Cunningham RS: The anorexia-cachexia syndrome. In Yarbro C, Frogge MH, Goodman M: *Cancer symptom management,* Sudbury, Mass, 2003, Jones and Bartlett.

Dorner B: Tough to swallow, *Today's Dietitian,* August: 28-31, 2002.

Franz MJ and others: Nutrition principles and recommendations in diabetes, *Diabetes Care* 27(suppl 1):S36-S46, 2004.

Grodner M, Lon S, DeYoung S: *Foundations and clinical applications of nutrition,* ed 3, St Louis, 2004, Mosby.

Groher M: *Dysphagia: diagnosis and management,* Boston, Mass, 1997, Butterworth-Heinemann.

Goulding R, Bakheit AM: Evaluation of the benefits of monitoring fluid thickness in the dietary management of dysphagic stroke patients, *Clin Rehabil* 14(2):119, 2000.

Hammond K: Dietary and clinical assessment. In Mahan L, Escott-Stump S: *Krause's food nutrition and diet therapy,* Philadelphia, 2003, Saunders.

Hockenberry MJ, Wilson D: *Wong's nursing care of infants and children,* ed 8, St Louis, 2007, Mosby.

Joint Commission on Accreditation of Healthcare Organizations: *Comprehensive accreditation manual for hospitals: the official handbook,* Oakbrook Terrace, Ill, 2006, JCAHO; http://www.jcrinc.com, accessed May 2006.

Meals on Wheels Association of America: *FAQ,* http://www.mowaa.org/index.asp, accessed January 2006.

Meiner SE, Lueckenotte AG: *Gerontologic nursing,* ed 3, St Louis, 2006, Mosby.

National Dysphagia Diet Task Force (NDDTF): *National dysphagia diet: standardization for optimal care,* Chicago, 2002, American Dietetic Association.

Niedert KC: Position of the American Dietetic Association: liberalization of the diet prescription improves quality of life for older adults in long-term care, *J Am Diet Assoc* 105(12):1955-1965, 2005.

Perry L, Love C: Screening for dysphagia and aspiration in acute stroke: a systematic review, *Dysphagia* 16:7-18, 2001.

Perry L, McLaren S: Eating difficulties after stroke, *J Adv Nurs* 43(4):360, 2003.

Shanley C, O'Loughlin G: Dysphagia among nursing home residents: an assessment and management protocol, *J Gerontol Nurs* 26(8):35-48, 2000.

Shopbell J and others: Nutrition screening and assessment. In Gottschlich M: *The science and practice of nutrition support*, Dubuque, Iowa, 2001, American Society for Parenteral and Enteral Nutrition.

US Department of Agriculture: *USDA's food guide pyramid*, Washington, DC, 2005, US Government Printing Office; available at http://www.mypyramid.gov.

US Department of Health and Human Services: *Healthy people 2010: what are its goals?* Washington, DC, 2005, USDHHS; available at http://www.healthypeople.gov/About/goals.htm.

US Department of Health and Human Services, National Institutes of Health: *Calculate your BMI*, http://nhlbisupport.com/bmi, accessed January 2006.

US Department of Health and Human Services and US Department of Agriculture: *Dietary guidelines for Americans 2005*, ed 6, Washington, DC, 2005, US Government Printing Office.

Vanek V: The use of serum albumin as a prognostic or nutritional marker, *Nutr Clin Pract* 13:110-112, 1998.

Westergren A: Detection of eating difficulties after stroke: a systematic review, *Int Nurs Rev* 53(2):143-149, 2006.

Wong DL: *Whaley & Wong's nursing care of infants and children*, ed 6, St Louis, 1999, Mosby.

Chapter 9
Assisting with Elimination

Cravens D, Zweig S: Urinary catheter management, *Am Fam Physician* 61(2):369, 2000.

Ebersole P, Hess P: *Toward healthy aging: human needs and nursing response*, ed 6, St Louis, 2004, Mosby.

Hockenberry MJ, Wilson D: *Wong's nursing care of infants and children*, ed 8, St Louis, 2007, Mosby.

Lekan-Rutledge D and others: Promoting social continence: products and devices in the management of urinary incontinence, *Urol Nurs* 26(6):416, 2003.

Lewis S, Heitkemper M, Dirkson S: *Medical surgical nursing: assessment and management of clinical problems*, ed 6, St Louis, 2003, Mosby.

Marklew A: Urinary catheter care in the intensive care unit, *Nurs Crit Care* 9(1):21, 2004.

Meiner SE, Lueckenotte AG: *Gerontologic nursing*, ed 3, St Louis, 2006, Mosby.

Pomfret I: Catheter care in the community, *Nurs Stand* 14(27):46, 2000.

Sorrentino SA: *Assisting with patient care*, St Louis, 2000, Mosby.

Webster J and others: Water or antiseptic for periurethral cleaning before urinary catheterization: a randomized controlled trial, *Am J Infect Control* 29(6):389, 2001.

Chapter 10
Promoting Comfort and Pain Control

Agency for Health Care Policy and Research, Acute Pain Management Guideline Panel: *Acute pain management in infants, children and adolescents: operative or medical procedures and trauma*, Clinical practice guideline, AHCPR Pub No 92-0032, Rockville, Md, 1992a, Agency for Health Care Policy and Research, Public Health Service, US Department of Health and Human Services.

Agency for Health Care Policy and Research, *Acute Pain Management Guideline Panel:* Acute pain management: operative or medical procedures and trauma, *Clinical practice guideline*, AHCPR Pub No 92-0032, Rockville, Md, 1992b, Agency for Health Care Policy and Research, Public Health Service, US Department of Health and Human Services.

American Geriatrics Society: Clinical practice guidelines, *J Am Geriatr Soc* 60:S204, 2002.

American Medical Directors Association: *Chronic pain management in the long-term care setting: clinical practice guidelines*, New York, 1999, the Association.

American Nurses Association: *Code of ethics for nurses with interpretative statements*, Kansas City, 2001, ANA.

American Pain Society: *Analgesic use in the treatment of acute pain and cancer pain*, ed 6, Glenview, Ill, 2003, APS.

Antall GF, Kresevic D: The use of guided imagery to manage pain in an elderly orthopaedic population, *Orthop Nurs* 23(5):335-340, 2004.

Astin J and others: Complementary and alternative medicine use among elderly persons: one-year analysis of a Blue Shield Medicare supplement, *J Gerontol Med Sci* 55a(1):M4-M9, 2000.

Berry PH and others: *Pain: current understanding of assessment, management, and treatments*, Chicago, 2001, National Pharmaceutical Council, Inc. and Joint Commission on Accreditation of Healthcare Organizations.

Beyer J and others: The creation, validation, and continuing development of the Oucher; a measure of pain intensity in children, *J Pediatr Nurs* 7(5):335, 1992.

Bird A, Wallis M: Nursing knowledge and assessment skills in the management of patients receiving analgesia via epidural infusion, *J Adv Nurs* 40(5):522-531, 2002.

Block BM and others: Efficacy of postoperative epidural analgesia: a meta-analysis, *JAMA* 290(18):2455-2463, 2003.

Buffum M, Buffum J: Nonsteroidal anti-inflammatory drugs in elderly, *Pain Manag Nurs* 1(2):40, 2000.

Chumbley G and others: Patient-controlled analgesia: what information does the patient want? *J Adv Nurs* 39(5):459-471, 2002.

Cosentino B: Epidural pain management, *Nurs Spectr* 12A(4):NJ1, 2000.

Cox F: Clinical care of patients with epidural infusions, *Prof Nurs* 16(10):1429, 2001.

Feldt K: The checklist of nonverbal pain indicators (CNPI), *Pain Manag Nurs* 1(1):35, 2000.

Gerdner L: *Evidence-based protocol, individualized music,* Iowa City, 2001, University of Iowa Gerontological Nursing Interventions Research Center, Research Dissemination Core.

Good M and others: Relaxation and music reduce pain after gynecologic surgery, *Pain Manag Nurs* 3(2):61-70, 2002.

Gordon D: Nonopioid and adjuvant analgesics in chronic pain management: strategies for effective use, *Nurs Clin North Am* 38(3):447, 2003.

Gunnarsdottir S and others: Interventions to overcome clinician- and patient-related barriers to pain management, *Nurs Clin North Am* 38(3):419, 2003.

Herr K: Chronic pain in the older patient: management strategies, *J Gerontol Nurs* 28(2):28, 2002.

Hockenberry MJ, Wilson D: *Wong's nursing care of infants and children,* ed 8, St Louis, 2007, Mosby.

Joint Commission on Accreditation of Healthcare Organizations: *Sentinel event alert: patient controlled analgesia by proxy,* December 20, 2004; available at http://www.jointcommission.org/SentinelEvents/SentinelEventAlert/sea_33.htm.

Joint Commission on Accreditation of Healthcare Organizations: *2007 National patient safety goals;* available at http://www.jointcommission.org/PatientSafety/NationalPatientSafety, accessed January 4, 2007.

Kwekkeboom K and others: A pilot study to predict success with guided imagery for cancer pain, *Pain Manag Nurse* 4(3):112, 2003.

Lehr V, BeVier P: Patient-controlled analgesia for the pediatric patient, *Orthop Nurs* 22(4):298, 2003.

McCaffery M, Pasero C: *Pain: clinical manual,* ed 2, St Louis, 1999, Mosby.

Meiner SE, Lueckenotte AG: *Gerontologic nursing,* ed 3, St Louis, 2006, Mosby.

Mok E, Woo P: The effects of slow-stroke back massage on anxiety and shoulder pain in elderly stroke patients, *Complement Ther Nurs Midwifery* 10(4):209, 2004.

Pasero C: Continuous local anesthetics, *Am J Nurs* 100(8):22, 2000.

Pasero C: *Epidural analgesia for acute pain management: self-directed learning module,* Pensacola, Fla, 1999, American Society for Pain Management Nursing.

Pasero C: Epidural analgesia for postoperative pain, *Am J Nurs* 102(10):62, 2003a.

Pasero C: *Intravenous patient-controlled analgesia for acute pain management: self-directed learning module,* Pensacola, Fla, 2003b, American Society for Pain Management Nursing.

Pasero C and others: Using continuous infusion with PCA, *Am J Nurs* 99(2):22, 1999.

Pasero C, McCaffery M: Authorized and unauthorized use of PCA pumps: clarifying the use of patient-controlled analgesia, in light of recent alerts, *Am J Nurs* 105(7):30-32: 2005.

Pasero C, McCaffery M: Reversing respiratory depression with naloxone, *Am J Nurs* 100(2):26, 2000.

Perin M: Problems with propoxyphene, *Am J Nurs* 100(6):22, 2000.

Rakel B, Barr J: Physical modalities in chronic pain management, *Nurs Clin North Am* 38(3):477, 2003.

Horlocker TT and others: Regional anesthesia in the anticoagulated patient: defining the risks, *Reg Anesth Pain Med* 28:172-197, 2003; available at http://www.asra.com/Consensus_Conferences/Consensus_Statements.shtml.

Riordan S and others: Introducing patient-controlled oral analgesia, *Nursing 2005* 34(9):20-23, 2004.

Sinatra S: Spinal opioid analgesia: an overview. In Sinatra RS and others, editors: *Acute pain management,* St Louis, 1992, Mosby.

Tarzian A, Hoffmann DE: Barriers to managing pain in the nursing home: findings from a statewide survey, *J Am Med Dir Assoc* 5(2):82-88, 2004.

Waitman J: Meperidine—a liability, *Am J Nurs* 101(1):57, 2001.

Wentz J: Assessing pain in the cognitively impaired adult, *Nursing* 31(7):26, 2001.

Wheeler M and others: Adverse events associated with postoperative opioid analgesia: a systematic review, *J Pain* 3(3):159, 2002.

Wong DL, Baker CM: Pain in children: comparison of assessment scales, *Pediatr Nurs* 14(1):9, 1988.

Young-McCaughan S, Miaskowski C: Measurement of opiod-induced sedation, *Pain Manage Nurs* 2(4):132, 2001.

Chapter 11
Vital Signs

Armstrong RS: Nurses' knowledge of error in blood pressure measurement technique, *Int J Nurs Pract* 8:118, 2002.

Barkauskas VH and others: *Health and physical assessment,* ed 3, St Louis, 2002, Mosby.

Grap MJ: Pulse oximetry, *Crit Care Nurs* 22(3):69, 2002.

Holtzclaw BJ: Use of thermoregulatory principles in patient care: fever management, *Online J Clin Innov* 5(5):1-64, 2002.

Joint National Committee: The seventh report of the Joint National Committee on prevention, detection, evaluation, and treatment of high blood pressure, *JAMA* 289:2560, 2003.

Jones DW and others: Measuring blood pressure accurately, *JAMA* 289(8):1027, 2003.

Maxton FJ, Justin L, Gilles D: Estimating core temperature in infants and children after cardiac surgery: a comparison of six methods, *J Adv Nurs* 45(2):214-222, 2004.

Netea RT and others: Both body and arm position significantly influence blood pressure measurement, *J Hum Hypertens* 17(7):459, 2003.

Pickering TG and others: Recommendations for blood pressure measurement in humans and experimental animals, part I: blood pressure measurement in humans, *Hypertension* 45(1):142, 2005.

Potter P and others: Evaluation of chemical dot thermometers for measuring body temperature of orally intubated patients, *Am J Crit Care* 12(5):403, 2003.

Sorrentino S, Gorek B: *Basic skills for nursing assistants in long-term care*, St Louis, 2005, Mosby.

Stanley M, Blair K, Beare P: *Gerontological nursing: promoting successful aging with older adults*, Philadelphia, 2005, FA Davis.

Sund-Levander and others: Normal oral, rectal, tympanic and axillary body temperature in adult men and women: a systematic literature review, *Scand J Caring Sci* 16:112, 2002.

Thomas SA and others: A review of nursing research on blood pressure, *J Nurs Scholarsh* 34(4):313, 2002.

Chapter 12
Health Assessment

American Academy of Pediatrics Committee on Practice and Ambulatory Medicine and Section on Ophthalmology: Eye examination in infants, children, and young adults by pediatricians, *Pediatrics* 111(4):907, 2003.

American Cancer Society: *Cancer facts and figures 2004*, Atlanta, 2004, ACS.

Ball JW, Bindler RC: *Child health nursing: partnering with children and families*, Upper Saddle River, NJ, 2006, Pearson Prentice Hall.

Barkauskas VH and others: *Health and physical assessment*, ed 3, St Louis, 2002, Mosby.

Bartley MK: Preventing venous thromboembolism in medical/surgical patients, *Nurs Manage* 36:16-18, 2005.

Burke MM, Laramie JA: *Primary care of the older adult: a multidisciplinary approach*, St Louis, 2004, Mosby.

Cannobio MM: *Cardiovascular disorders*, St Louis, 1990, Mosby.

Day MW: Recognizing and managing DVT, *Nursing* 33(5):36, 2003.

Ebersole P, Hess P, Luggen A: *Toward healthy aging: human needs and nursing response*, ed 6, St Louis, 2004, Mosby.

Eggimann P and others: Overview of catheter-related infections with special emphasis on prevention based on educational programs, *Clin Microbiol Infect* 8(5):305, 2002.

Gareth E: The aged foot, *Cambridge University Press* 12:175, 2002.

Glover AL: How to detect and defend against DVI, *Nursing* 35(10):32, 2005.

Gray-Vickery P: Protecting the older adult, *Nurs Manage* 32(10):36, 2001.

Green B, Taplin S: Breast cancer screening controversies, *J Am Board Fam Pract* 16:233, 2002.

Hockenberry M, Wilson D: *Wong's nursing care of infants and children*, ed 8, St Louis, 2007, Mosby.

Joint Commission on Accreditation of Healthcare Organizations: *2007 National patient safety goals FAQs*, Oakbrook Terrace, Ill, 2006, JCAHO; available at http://www.jointcommission.org/GeneralPublic/NPSG/04_gp_npsg.htm.

Ladwig G, Ackley J: *Mosby's guide to nursing diagnosis*, St Louis, 2006, Mosby.

Martin CT and others: Factors contributing to low weight in community-living older adults, *J Am Acad Nurse Pract* 17(10):7, 2005.

Meiner SE, Lueckenotte AG: *Gerontologic nursing*, ed 3, St Louis, 2006, Mosby.

Moore MC: *Pocket guide to nutritional care*, ed 4, St Louis, 2001, Mosby.

Pachucki-Hyde L: Assessment of risk factors for oestoporosis and fracture, *Nurs Clin North Am* 36(3):401, 2001.

Phipps WJ and others: *Medical-surgical nursing: health and illness perspectives*, ed 7, St Louis, 2003, Mosby.

Reuben DB and others: *2005 Geriatrics at your fingertips*, ed 7, Williston, Vt, 2005, Blackwell.

Rosenblum RK and others: A guide to children with acute and chronic headaches, *J Pediatr Health Care* 15(5):229-235, 2001.

Seidel HM and others: *Mosby's guide to physical examination*, ed 5, St Louis, 2003, Mosby.

Seidel HM and others: *Mosby's guide to physical examination*, ed 6, St Louis, 2006, Mosby.

Tabloski PA: *Gerontological nursing*, Upper Saddle River, NJ, 2006, Pearson Prentice Hall.

Thompson JM and others: *Mosby's manual of clinical nursing*, ed 5, St Louis, 2001, Mosby.

Tryniszewski C: *Expert 10 minute physical examinations*, ed 2, St Louis, 2005, Mosby.

Urbano FL: Homans' sign in the diagnosis of deep venous thrombosis, *Hosp Physician* 37(3):22, 2001.

US Preventive Services Task Force: Screening for osteoporosis in postmenopausal women: recommendations and rationale, *Am J Nurs* 103(1):73, 2003.

Vahabi M: Breast cancer screening methods: a review of the evidence, *Health Care Women Int* 24(9):790, 2003.

Zitelli B, Davis H: *Atlas of pediatric physical diagnosis*, ed 4, St Louis, 2002, Mosby.

Zuguo M and others: Shifts in percentiles of growth during early childhood: analysis of longitudinal data from the California child health and development study, *Pediatrics* 113(6):e617, 2004.

Chapter 13
Laboratory Tests

American Association of Diabetes Educators: *A core curriculum for diabetes education*, ed 6, Chicago, 2006, AADE.

American Association of Diabetes Educators: *A core curriculum for diabetes education*, ed 5, Chicago, 2003, AADE.

American Diabetes Association: *2006 Clinical practice recommendations*, 2006a; available at http://www.diabetes.org.

American Diabetes Association: 2006 Resource guide, *Diabetes Forecast (supplement)* January, 2006b.

Cunningham MA: Glucose monitoring in type 2 diabetes, *Nurs Clin North Am* 36(2):361, 2001.

Grimes D: *Infectious diseases*, Mosby's clinical nursing series, St Louis, 1991, Mosby.

Hockenberry MJ, Wilson D: *Wong's nursing care of infants and children*, ed 8, St Louis, 2007, Mosby.

Joint Commission on Accreditation of Healthcare Organizations: *Manual of hospital accreditation: 2006 standards*, Chicago, 2006, JCAHO.

Joint Commission on Accreditation of Healthcare Organizations: *2007 Laboratory services national patient safety goals*, Chicago, 2007, JCAHO; available at http://www.jointcommission.org/PatientSafety/NationalPatientSafetyGoals/07_lab_npsgs.htm.

Lawrence P, Rozmus C: Culturally sensitive care of the Muslim patient, *J Transcult Nurs* 12(3):228, 2001.

Malarkey LM, McMorrow ME: *Saunders guide to laboratory and diagnostic tests*, Saunders, 2005, Philadelphia.

Mason NJ and others: *Murray and Nadel's textbook of respiratory medicine*, ed 4, Saunders, 2005, Philadelphia.

Mermel LA and others: Guidelines for the management of intravascular catheter-related infections, *Clin Infect Dis* 32:1249-1272, 2001.

National Committee for Clinical Laboratory Standards (NCCLS): *Urinalysis and collection, transportation, and preservation of urine specimens*, ed 2, Vol 18, No 7, 2001.

Occupational Safety and Health Administration (OSHA): Occupational exposure to bloodborne pathogens: final rule, *Fed Regist* 66(12):5318, January 18, 2001.

Pagana KD, Pagana TJ: *Mosby's diagnostic and laboratory tests reference*, ed 7, St Louis, 2005, Mosby.

Parini S: Combating infection: how to collect specimens, *Nursing* 30(5):66, 2000.

Roark DC, Miguel K: RFID: bar coding's replacement, *Nurs Manage* 37(2):28, 2006.

US Department of Health and Human Services (USDHHS): Standards for privacy of individuals. Health insurance portability and accountability act of 1996, 64 *Fed Regist* 60053 (1999). Identifiable health information, August 2003.

Chapter 14
Diagnostic Procedures

American Academy of Pediatrics: Guidelines for monitoring and management of pediatric patients during and after sedation for diagnostic and therapeutic procedures: addendum, *Pediatrics* 110(4):836-838, 2002.

American Society of Anesthesiologists: *Continuum of depth of sedation definition of general anesthesia and levels of sedation/analgesia* (approved October 13, 1999; amended October 27, 2004), Park Ridge, Ill, 2004a, ASA; available at http://www.asahq.org/publicationsAndServices/standards/20.pdf.

American Society of Anesthesiologists: *Relative value guide*, Park Ridge, Ill, 2004b, ASA.

Beare P, Myers J: *Adult health nursing*, ed 3, St Louis, 1998, Mosby.

Calabrese A and others: Evaluation of prescribing practices: risk of lactic acidosis with metformin therapy, *Arch Intern Med* 162:4, 2002.

Chernecky CC, Berger BJ: *Laboratory tests & diagnostic procedures*, ed 4, Philadelphia, 2004, Saunders.

Dougherty DB, Jackson DB: *Gastrointestinal disorders*, Mosby's clinical nursing series, St Louis, 1993, Mosby.

Evans RW and others: Assessment: prevention of post-lumbar puncture headaches: report of the Therapeutics and Technology Assessment Subcommittee of the American Academy of Neurology, *Neurology* 55(7):909-914, 2000.

Haiat H, Bar-Mor G, Shochat M: The world of the child: a world of play even in the hospital, *J Pediatr Nurs* 18(3):209-214, 2003.

Hoffman GM and others: Risk reduction in pediatric procedural sedation by application of an American Academy of Pediatrics/American Society of Anesthesiologists process model, *Pediatrics* 109(2):236-243, 2002.

Ignatavicius DD, Workman ML: *Medical-surgical nursing: critical thinking for collaborative care*, ed 4, Philadelphia, 2002, Saunders.

Joint Commission on Accreditation of Healthcare Organizations: *Implementation expectations for the universal protocol for preventing wrong site, wrong procedure and wrong person surgery*, Oakbrook Terrace, Ill, 2003, JCAHO; available at http://www.jointcommission.org/NR/rdonlyres/DEC4A816-ED52-4C04-AF8C-FEBA74A732EA/0/up_guidelines.pdf.

Joint Commission on Accreditation of Healthcare Organizations: *2006 National patient safety goals*, Oakbrook Terrace, Ill, 2006, JCAHO; available at http://www.jointcommission.org/PatientSafety/NationalPatientSafetyGoals/06_npsgs.htm.

Nagelhout JJ, Zaglaniczny KL: *Handbook of nurse anesthesia*, ed 3, St Louis, 2005, Elsevier.

Negishi C and others: Resistive-heating and forced-air warming are comparably effective, *Anesth Analg* 96(6):1683-1687, 2003.

Pagana KD, Pagana TJ: *Mosby's manual of diagnostic and laboratory tests*, ed 2, St Louis, 2002, Mosby.

Pagana KD, Pagana TJ: *Mosby's manual of diagnostic and laboratory tests*, ed 3, St Louis, 2005, Mosby.

Phipps WJ and others: *Medical-surgical nursing: health and illness perspectives*, ed 7, St Louis, 2003, Mosby.

Potter PA, Perry AG: *Basic nursing: a critical thinking approach*, ed 4, St Louis, 1999, Mosby.

Ramsay MA and others: Controlled sedation with alphaxalone-alphadolone, *Br Med J* 2(920):656-659, 1974.

van Crevel H, Hijdra A, de Gans J: Lumbar puncture and the risk of herniation: when should we first perform CT? *J Neurol* 249:129-137, 2002.

Wellens HJJ, Conover MB: *The ECG in emergency decision making*, ed 2, Philadelphia, 2006, Saunders.

Wong DL and others: *Whaley and Wong's nursing care of infants and children*, ed 7, St Louis, 2003, Mosby.

Yucel A and others: Intravenous administration of caffeine sodium benzoate for postdural puncture headache, *Reg Anesth Pain Med* 24(1):51, 1999.

Chapter 15
Preparation for Medication Administration

Benner P: Creating a culture of safety and improvement: a key to reducing medical error, *Am J Crit Care* 10(4):281, 2001.

Brager R, Sloan E: The spectrum of polypharmacy, *Nurse Pract* 30(6):44, 2005.

Clayton BD, Stock YN: *Basic pharmacology for nurses*, ed 13, St Louis, 2004, Mosby.

Hockenberry M: *Wong's clinical manual of pediatric nursing*, ed 6, St Louis, 2004, Mosby.

Joint Commission on Accreditation of Healthcare Organizations: *2005 Hospital national patient safety goals*, Oakbrook Terrace, Ill, 2005, JCAHO; available at http://www.jointcommission.org/PatientSafety/NationalPatientSafetyGoals/05_hap_npsgs.htm.

Joint Commission on Accreditation of Healthcare Organizations: *2006 Critical access hospital and hospital national patient safety goals*, Oakbrook Terrace, Ill, 2006, JCAHO; available at http://www.jointcommission.org/PatientSafety/NationalPatientSafetyGoals/06_npsg_cah.htm.

Kohn L, Corrigan J, Donaldson M, editors: *To err is human: building a safer health system*, Washington, DC, 1999, National Academy Press.

Meiner SE, Lueckenotte AG: *Gerontologic nursing*, ed 3, St Louis, 2006, Mosby.

McCaffery M, Robinson E: Your patient is in pain, *Nursing* 32(10):36, 2002.

Rich DS: Ask the Joint Commission, *Hosp Pharm* 37(6):1, 2002.

Skidmore-Roth L: *Mosby's drug guide for nurses*, ed 3, St Louis, 2006, Mosby.

Smetzer J: Take 10 giant steps to medication safety, *Nursing* 31(11):49, 2001.

Sullivan C and others: Medication reconciliation in the acute care setting, *J Nurs Care Qual* 20(2):95, 2005.

Chapter 16
Administration of Nonparenteral Medications

Capriotti T: Changes in inhaler devices for asthma and COPD, *Medsurg Nurs* 14(3):185-194, 2005.

Ebersole P, Hess P: *Toward healthy aging*, ed 6, St Louis, 2004, Mosby.

Galvan TJ: Dysphagia: going down and staying down, *Am J Nurs* 101(1):37-43, 2001.

Hockenberry MJ, Wilson D: *Wong's nursing care of infants and children*, ed 8, St Louis, 2007, Mosby.

Ignatavicius DD, Workman ML: *Medical-surgical nursing: critical thinking for collaborative care*, ed 5, Philadelphia, 2006, Saunders.

Institution for Safe Medication Practices (ISMP): Hazard alert: asphyxiation possible with syringe tip caps, *ISMP Medication Safety Alert Acute Care Edition Newsletter* August 22, 2001; available at http://www.ismp.org/hazardalerts/Hypodermic.asp.

Institution for Safe Medication Practices (ISMP): Suppository stories, *Medication Safety Alert* 2006; available at http://www.ismp.org/consumers/Suppository.asp.

Joint Commission on Accreditation of Healthcare Organizations: *2006 Disease-specific care national patient safety goals*, Oakbrook Terrace, Ill, 2006, JCAHO; available at http://www.jointcommission.org/PatientSafety/NationalPatientSafetyGoals/06_npsg_dsc.htm.

Lewis SM, Heitkemper MM, Dirksen SR: *Medical-surgical nursing, assessment and management of clinical problems*, ed 6, St Louis, 2004, Mosby.

Lilley LL, Harrington S, Snyder JS: *Pharmacology and the nursing process*, ed 4, St Louis, 2004, Mosby.

Mahan LK, Escott-Stump S: *Krause's food, nutrition, and diet therapy*, ed 11, Philadelphia, 2004, Saunders.

McConnell EA: Clinical do's and don'ts: applying nitroglycerin ointment, *Nursing* 31(6):17, 2001.

McKenry L, Tessier E, Hogan MA: *Mosby's pharmacology in nursing*, ed 22, St Louis, 2006, Mosby.

Metheny NA and others: Verification of inefficiency of the glucose method in detecting aspiration associated with tube feedings, *Medsurg Nurs* 14(2):112-121, 2005.

Miller D, Miller H: To crush or not to crush, *Nursing* 30(2):51, 2000.

Rubin DK, Durotoye L: How do clients determine that their metered dose inhaler is empty? *Chest* 126(4):1134-1137, 2005.

Schulmeister L: Transdermal drug patches: medicine with muscle, *Nursing* 35(1):48-53, 2005.

Terrado M, Russell C, Bowman JB: Dysphagia: an overview, *Medsurg Nurs* 10(5):233-247, 2001.

Togger DA, Brenner PS: Metered dose inhalers, *Am J Nurs* 101(10):26-32, 2001.

Chapter 17
Administration of Injections

American Diabetes Association: Continuous subcutaneous insulin infusion, *Diabetes Care* 27(suppl 1):S110, 2004a.

American Diabetes Association: Insulin administration: position statement, *Diabetes Care* 27(suppl 1):S106, 2004b.

American Diabetes Association: Insulin delivery, *Diabetes Forecast* 58(1):RG16, 2005.

American Nurses Association: *American Nurses Association's needlestick prevention guide: safe needles save lives*, Washington, DC, 2002, ANA; available at http://www.needlestick.org/needlestick/needleguide.pdf.

Aventis: *Lovenox (enoxaparin sodium injection)*, http://www.lovenox.com, accessed September 2006.

Beyea SC, Nicoll LH: Administration of medications via the intramuscular route: an integrative review of the literature and research-based protocol for the procedure, *Appl Nurs Res* 8(1):23, 1995.

Bick RL and others: Unfractionated heparin, LMW heparin, and pentasaccharide: basic mechanisms of action, pharmacology, and clinical use, *Hematol Oncol Clin North Am* 19(1):1-51, 2005.

Caffrey RM: Are all syringes created equal? *Am J Nurs* 103(6):46, 2003.

Centers for Disease Control and Prevention (CDC): *Mantoux tuberculin skin test facilitator guide*, http://www.cdc.gov/nchstp/tb/pubs/Mantoux/images/Mantoux.pdf, accessed September 2006.

Dawkins L and others: A randomized trial of winged Vialon cannulae and metal butterfly needles, *Int J Palliat Nurs* 6(3):110, 2000.

Environmental Protection Agency (EPA): *New information about disposing of medical sharps*, http://www.epa.gov/epaoswer/other/medical/errata.pdf, accessed September 2006.

Foley M: Update on needlestick and sharps injuries: the needle stick safety and prevention act of 2000, *Am J Nurs* 104:96, 2004.

Gilsenan I: A practical guide to giving injections, *Nurs Times* 96(33):43, 2000.

Hockenberry MJ, Wilson D: *Wong's nursing care of infants and children*, ed 8, St Louis, 2007, Mosby.

Hockenberry MJ and others: *Wong's essentials of pediatric nursing*, ed 7, St Louis, 2005, Mosby.

Joint Commission on Accreditation of Healthcare Organizations: *2006 Critical access hospital and hospital national patient safety goals*, Oakbrook Terrace, Ill, 2006, JCAHO; available at http://www.jointcommission.org/AccreditationPrograms/Hospitals/NPSG/06_npsg_cah.htm.

Katsma DL, Katsma R: The myth of the 90°-angle intramuscular injection, *Nurs Educ* 25(1):34, 2000.

Kuzu N, Ucar H: The effect of cold on the occurrence of bruising, haematoma and pain at the injection site in subcutaneous low molecular weight heparin, *Int J Nurs Stud* 38(1):51, 2001.

Lenhard MJ, Reeves GD: Continuous subcutaneous insulin infusion: a comprehensive review of insulin pump therapy, *Arch Intern Med* 161(19):2293, 2001.

Lilley LL, Harrington S, Snyder JS: *Pharmacology and the nursing process*, ed 4, St Louis, 2004, Mosby.

Litton J and others: Insulin pump therapy in toddlers and preschool children with type I diabetes mellitus, *J Pediatr* 141(4):490, 2002.

McConnell EA: Administering subcutaneous heparin, *Nursing* 36(6):17, 2000.

McKenry LM and others: *Mosby's pharmacology in nursing*, ed 22, St Louis, 2006, Mosby.

McKenry LM, Salerno E: *Pharmacology in nursing*, ed 21, St Louis, 2003, Mosby.

Medtronic MiniMed: *MiniMed Paradigm REAL-Time Insulin Pump and Continuous Glucose Monitoring System*, http://www.minimed.com/products/insulinpumps, accessed September 2006.

Nicoll LH, Hesby A: Intramuscular injection: an integrative research review and guideline for evidence-based practice, *Appl Nurs Res* 16(2):149, 2002.

Occupational Safety and Health Administration (OSHA): Occupational exposure to bloodborne pathogens; needlestick and other sharps injuries; final rule, *Fed Regist* 66:5317, January 18, 2001; available at http://needlestick.org.

Pasero C: Subcutaneous opioid infusion, *Am J Nurs* 102(7):61, 2002.

Perry J, Parker G, Jagger J: Nurses and needlesticks, then and now, *Nursing* 33(4):22, 2003.

Pope BA: How to administer subcutaneous and intramuscular injections, *Nursing* 32(1):50, 2002.

Rodger MA, King L: Drawing up and administering intramuscular injections: a review of the literature, *J Adv Nurs* 31(3):574, 2000.

Sparks L: Taking the "ouch" out of injections for children, *MCN Am J Matern Child Nurs* 26(2):72, 2001.

Stephens M: Subcutaneous injections, *Nurs Times* 99(36):29, 2003.

Strowig S: Insulin therapy, *RN* 64(9):38, 2001.

Torre MC: Subcutaneous infusion: non-metal cannulae vs. metal butterfly needles, *Br J Community Nurs* 7(7):365, 2002.

Weissberg-Benchell J and others: Insulin pump therapy: a meta analysis, *Diabetes Care* 26(4):1079, 2003.

Wilburn SQ: Needlestick and sharps injury prevention, *Online J Issues Nurs* 9(3):4, 2004; available at http://nursingworld.org/ojin/topic25/tpc25_4.htm.

Chapter 18
Preparing the Client for Surgery

American Society of Anesthesiologists: American Society of Anesthesiologists Task Force on Perioperative Fast: practice guidelines for preoperative fasting and the use of pharmacologic agents to reduce the risk of pulmonary aspiration, *Anesthesiology* 90(3):896, 1999.

Association of Operating Room Nurses: *Standards and recommended practices for perioperative nursing: perioperative care of patients with do-not-resuscitate (DNR) orders*, Denver, 2005, AORN.

Bartley MK: Preventing venous thromboembolism in medical/surgical patients, *Med/Surg Insider* 35(9):16, 2005.

Bernier JB and others: Preoperative teaching received and valued in a day surgery setting, *AORN J* 77(3):563, 2003.

Centers for Disease Control and Prevention: *National surgical infection prevention: Medicare quality improvement project-evidence base for duration of antimicrobial prophylaxis,* Atlanta, 2003, CDC.

Crowther M, McCourt K: Get the edge on deep vein thrombosis: head off progression of this deadly condition by knowing when to assess and what to look for during patient screening, *Nurs Manage* 35(1):21, 2004.

Day MW: Recognizing and managing deep vein thrombosis, *Nursing* 33(5):37, 2003.

Eliopoulos C: *Gerontological nursing,* ed 6, Philadelphia, 2005, Lippincott Williams & Wilkins.

Heizenroth PA: Positioning the patient for surgery. In Rothrock JC, editor: *Alexander's care of the patient in surgery,* ed 12, St Louis, 2003, Mosby.

Hockenberry MJ: *Wong's essentials of pediatric nursing,* ed 7, St Louis, 2005, Mosby.

Iowa Intervention Project: *Nursing interventions classification,* ed 3, St Louis, 2000, Mosby.

Joint Commission on Accreditation of Healthcare Organizations: *2006 Critical access hospital and hospital national patient safety goals,* Oakbrook Terrace, Ill, 2006, JCAHO; available at http://www.jointcommission.org/GeneralPublic/NPSG/06_npsg_cah.htm.

Lewis SM and others: *Medical-surgical nursing: assessment and management of clinical problems,* ed 6, St Louis, 2004, Mosby.

Oetker-Black SL and others: Preoperative teaching and hysterectomy outcomes, *AORN J* 77(6):1215, 2003.

Spry C: *Essentials of perioperative nursing,* ed 2, Gaithersburg, Md, 2003, Aspen.

Weiss BD: *Health literacy: a manual for clinicians,* Chicago, 2003, AMA Foundation.

Chapter 19
Intraoperative Techniques

Association of periOperative Registered Nurses: AORN official statement on RN first assistants. In *AORN standards and recommended practices for perioperative nursing,* Denver, 2005a, AORN.

Association of periOperative Registered Nurses: Position statement on unlicensed assistive personnel. In *AORN standards and recommended practices for perioperative nursing,* Denver, 2005b, AORN.

Association of periOperative Registered Nurses: Recommended practices for selection and use of surgical gowns and drapes. In *AORN standards and recommended practices for perioperative nursing,* Denver, 2005c, AORN.

Association of periOperative Registered Nurses: Recommended practices for surgical hand antisepsis/hand scrubs. In *AORN standards and recommended practices for perioperative nursing,* Denver, 2005d, AORN.

Boyce JM, Pittet D: Guidelines for hand hygiene in health care settings, *Am J Infect Control* 30(8):S1-S46, 2002.

Centers for Disease Control and Prevention: Guidelines for hand hygiene in health-care settings: recommendations and reports, *MMWR Morb Mortal Wkly Rep* 51:RR-16, 2002.

Connor R: Clinical issues: fire blankets; alcohol-based hand scrubs; peel pouch indicators; aseptic technique definitions; shaving, *AORN J* 78(3):484, 2003.

Gruendemann BJ, Bjerke NB: Is it time for brushless scrubbing with an alcohol-based agent? *AORN J* 74(6):859, 2001.

Joint Commission on Accreditation of Healthcare Organizations: *Universal protocol for preventing wrong site, wrong procedure, wrong person surgery,* Oakbrook Terrace, Ill, 2003, JCAHO.

Parienti JJ and others: Hand-rubbing with an aqueous alcoholic solution vs. traditional surgical hand-scrubbing and 30-day surgical site infection rates: a randomized equivalence study, *JAMA* 288(6):722-727, 2002.

Phillips N: *Berry and Kohn's operating room technique,* ed 10, St Louis, 2004, Mosby.

Chapter 20
Caring for the Postoperative Client

Aldrete JA: Modifications to the postanesthesia score for use in ambulatory surgery, *J Perianesth Nurs* 13(3):148, 1998.

American Society of PeriAnesthesia Nurses: *Clinical guideline for the prevention of unplanned perioperative hypothermia,* Cherry Hill, NJ, 1998, ASPAN; available at http://www.aspan.org/Hypothermia.htm.

American Society of PeriAnesthesia Nurses: *Standards of perianesthesia nursing practice,* Cherry Hill, NJ, 2004, ASPAN.

Hockenberry MJ, Wilson D: *Wong's nursing care of infants and children,* ed 8, St Louis, 2007, Mosby.

Kiekkas P and others: Effects of hypothermia and shivering on standard PACU monitoring of patients, *AANA J* 73(1):47, 2005.

Krenzischek DA and others: A survey of current perianesthesia nursing practice for pain and comfort management, *J Perianesth Nurs* 19(3):138, 2004.

Lewis SM and others: *Medical-surgical nursing: assessment and management of clinical problems,* ed 6, St Louis, 2004, Mosby.

Maldonado SS, LeBoeuf B: Pediatric surgery. In Rothrock JC, editor: *Alexander's care of the patient in surgery,* ed 12, St Louis, 2003, Mosby.

McKenry LM, Salerno E: *Mosby's pharmacology in nursing,* ed 21, St Louis, 2003, Mosby.

Ringdal M and others: A survey on incidence and factors that may influence first postoperative urination, *Urol Nurs* 23(5):341, 2003.

Rothrock JC: *Alexander's care of the patient in surgery,* ed 12, St Louis, 2003, Mosby.

Chapter 21
Surgical Wound Care

Colwell JC, Fichera A: Care of the obese patient with an ostomy, *J Wound Ostomy Continence Nurs* 32(6):378-383, 2005.

Hockenberry MJ, Wilson D: *Wong's nursing care of infants and children*, ed 8, St Louis, 2007, Mosby.

Kabon B and others: Obesity decreases perioperative tissue oxygenation, *Anesthesiology* 100(2):274, 2004.

Lewis SM and others: *Medical-surgical nursing: assessment and management of clinical problems*, ed 6, St Louis, 2004, Mosby.

Posthauer ME, Thomas DR: Nutrition and wound care. In Baranoski S, Ayello EA: *Wound care essentials*, Philadelphia, Pa, 2004, Lippincott Williams & Wilkins.

Sussman C: Wound healing biology and chronic wound healing. In Sussman C, Bates-Jensen BM: *Wound care*, ed 2, Gaithersburg, Md, 2001, Aspen.

Stotts NA, Hopf HW: Facilitating positive outcomes in older adults with wounds, *Nurs Clin North Am* 40(2):267-279, 2005.

Chapter 22
Pressure Ulcers

Ayello EA and others: Pressure ulcers. In Baranoski S, Ayello EA, editors: *Wound care essentials: practice principles*, Philadelphia, 2004, Lippincott Williams & Wilkins.

Baranoski S, Ayello EA: Wound assessment. In Baranoski S, Ayello EA, editors: *Wound care essentials: practice principles*, Philadelphia, 2004, Lippincott Williams & Wilkins.

Bates-Jensen BM: Pressure ulcers: pathophysiology and prevention. In Sussman C, Bates-Jenson BM: *Wound care*, Gaithersburg, Md, 1998, Aspen.

Bennett MA: Report of the task force on the implications for darkly pigmented intact skin in the prediction and prevention of pressure ulcers, *Adv Wound Care* 8(6):34, 1995.

Bergstrom N and others: The National Pressure Ulcer Long-Term Care Study: outcomes of pressure ulcer treatments in long-term care, *J Am Geriatr Soc* 53(10):1721-1729, 2005.

Bergstrom N and others: Predicting pressure ulcer risk: a multisite study of the predictive validity of the Braden scale, *Nurs Res* 47(5):261, 1998.

Bergstrom N and others: *Pressure ulcers in adults: prediction and prevention*, Clinical Practice Guideline No 3, AHCPR Pub No 92-0047, Rockville, Md, May 1992, Agency for Health Care Policy and Research, Public Health Service, US Department of Health and Human Services.

Bergstrom N and others: *Treatment of pressure ulcers*, Clinical Practice Guideline No 15, AHCPR Pub No 95-0652, Rockville, Md, December 1994, Agency for Health Care Policy and Research, Public Health Service, US Department of Health and Human Services.

Braden BJ, Bergstrom N: Clinical utility of the Braden scale for predicting pressure sore risk, *Decubitus* 2(3):441, 1989.

Braden BJ, Maklebust J: Preventing pressure ulcers with the Braden scale: an update on this easy-to-use tool that assesses a patient's risk, *Am J Nurs* 105(8):16, 2005.

Colburn L: Prevention of chronic wounds. In Krasner DL, Rodheaver GT, Sibald RG, editors: *Chronic wound care: a clinical source book for healthcare professionals*, ed 3, Wayne, Pa, 2001, HMP Communications.

Doughty D: Dressings and more: guidelines for topical wound management, *Nurs Clin North Am* 40(2):217-231, 2005.

Jones V, Bale S, Harding K: Acute and chronic wound healing. In Baranoski S, Ayello EA, editors: *Wound care essentials: practice principles*, Philadelphia, 2004, Lippincott Williams & Wilkins.

Maklebust J, Sieggreen M: *Pressure ulcers: guidelines for prevention and nursing management*, ed 2, Springhouse, Pa, 1996, Springhouse.

Mechanick J: Practical aspects of nutritional support for wound-healing patients, *Am J Surg* 188(suppl 1A):52-56, 2004.

National Pressure Ulcer Advisory Panel: Pressure ulcers prevalence, cost and risk assessment: consensus development conference statement, *Decubitus* 2(2):24-28, 1989.

National Pressure Ulcer Advisory Panel: Pressure Ulcer Stages revised by NPUAP, February 2007.

National Pressure Ulcer Advisory Panel: *Stage I assessment in darkly pigmented skin*, Washington, DC, 1998, NPUAP; available at http://www.NPUAP.org/positn4.html.

Posthauer ME, Thomas DR: Nutrition and wound care. In Baranoski S, Ayello EA, editors: *Wound care essentials: practice principles*, Philadelphia, 2004, Lippincott Williams & Wilkins.

Stotts NA, Wipke-Tevis DD: Co-factors in impaired wound healing. In Krasner DL, Rodheaver GT, Sibbald RG, editors: *Chronic wound care: a clinical source book for healthcare professionals*, ed 3, Wayne, Pa, 2001, HMP Communications.

Trott AT: *Wounds and lacerations*, ed 2, St Louis, 1997, Mosby.

Wound, Ostomy and Continence Nurses Society: *Guideline for prevention and management of pressure ulcers*, WOCN Clinical Practice Guidelines Series, Glenview, Ill, 2003, WOCN.

Chapter 23
Dressings

Agency for Health Care Policy and Research: *Treatment of pressure ulcers*, Clinical Practice Guideline No 15, Rockville, Md, 1994, Agency for Health Care Policy and Research, Public Health Service, US Department of Health and Human Services.

Beshara M, Jameson G, Barr B: Practice development in acute and long-term care settings. In Bryant RA, editor: *Acute and chronic wounds: nursing management*, ed 2, St Louis, 2000, Mosby.

Broussard CL, Mendez-Eastman S, Frantz R: Adjuvant wound therapies. In Bryant RA, editor: *Acute and chronic wounds: nursing management*, ed 2, St Louis, 2000, Mosby.

Chua PC and others: Vacuum-assisted wound closure, *Am J Nurs* 100(12):45, 2000.

Cuzzell J: Wound assessment and evaluation wound dressings: confusion or choice? *Dermatol Nurs* 14(3):187, 2002.

Doughty D, Gray M: Clean versus sterile technique when changing wound dressings, *J Wound Ostomy Continence Nurs* 28(3):125, 2001.

Evans L, Land L: Topical negative pressure for treating chronic wounds: a systematic review, *Br J Plast Surg* 54(3):238, 2001.

Hall P, Schumann L: Wound care: meeting the challenge, *J Am Acad Nurse Pract* 13(6):258-266, 2001.

Harvey C: Wound healing, *Orthop Nurs* 23(2):143, 2005.

Hess C: Quick tips: dressings for autolytic debridement, *Adv Skin Wound Care* 17(5):222, 2004.

Hockenberry MJ: *Wong's essentials of pediatric nursing*, ed 7, St Louis, 2005, Mosby.

Hockenberry MJ, Wilson D: *Wong's nursing care of infants and children*, ed 8, St Louis, 2007, Mosby.

Kaufman M, Pahl D: Vacuum assisted closure therapy: wound care and nursing implications, *Dermatol Nurs* 15(4):317, 2003.

Kinetic Concepts Inc (KCI): *The V.A.C. Vacuum Assisted Closure: V.A.C. Therapy clinical guidelines: a reference source for clinicians*, product information, San Antonio, Tex, 2004, KCI.

Meiner SE, Lueckenotte AG: *Gerontologic nursing*, ed 3, St Louis, 2006, Mosby.

Mendez-Eastman S: Using negative-pressure wound therapy for positive results, *Nursing 2005* 35(5):48, 2005.

Milne C, Houle T: Current trends in wound care management, *Orthop Nurs* 21(6):11, 2002.

Nelson D, Dilloway MA: Principles, products, and practical aspects of wound care, *Crit Care Nurs Q* 25(1):33, 2002.

Rolstad BS, Ovington LG, Harris A: Principles of wound management. In Bryant RA, editor: *Acute and chronic wounds: nursing management*, ed 2, St Louis, 2000a, Mosby.

Rolstad BS, Ovington LG, Harris A: Wound care product formulary. In Bryant RA, editor: *Acute and chronic wounds: nursing management*, ed 2, St Louis, 2000b, Mosby.

Stotts NA and others: Sterile versus clean technique in post-operative wound care of patients with open surgical wounds: a pilot study, *J Wound Ostomy Continence Nurs* 24:10, 1997.

Wooten M and others: *WOCN position statement: clean versus sterile: management of chronic wounds*, Glenview, Ill, 2005, Wound, Ostomy and Continence Nurses Society.

Worley C: So, what do I put on this wound? Making sense of the wound dressing puzzle: part I, *Dermatol Nurs* 17(2):143, 2005a.

Worley C: So, what do I put on this wound? Making sense of the wound dressing puzzle: part II, *Dermatol Nurs* 17(3):204, 2005b.

Wright K, McNichol LL: Home environment: implications for wound care practice development. In Bryant RA, editor: *Acute and chronic wounds: nursing management*, ed 2, St Louis, 2000, Mosby.

Chapter 24
Therapeutic Use of Heat and Cold

Airaksinen O and others: Efficacy of cold gel for soft tissue injuries, *Am J Sports Med* 31(5):680, 2003.

Hockenberry MJ, Wilson D: *Wong's nursing care of infants and children*, ed 8, St Louis, 2007, Mosby.

Mauer K and others: National practice patterns for the care of the patient with total joint replacement, *Orthop Nurs* 21(3):37, 2002.

Meiner SE, Lueckenotte AG: *Gerontologic nursing*, ed 3, St Louis, 2006, Mosby.

Nicoll L: Heat in motion: evaluating and managing temperature, *Nursing* 32(5):S1, 2002.

Poddar S: Heat or ice for acute ankle sprain, *J Fam Pract* 52(8):642, 2003.

Stitik T, Nadler S: Sports injuries: when and how to apply heat, *Consultant* 39(1):144, 1999.

Stitik T, Nadler S: Sports injuries: when- and how- to use cold most effectively, *Consultant* 38(12):2881, 1998.

Wilke B, Weiner RD: Postoperative cryotherapy; risks versus benefits of continuous-flow cryotherapy units, *Clin Podiatr Med Surg* 20(2):307, 2003.

Chapter 25
Special Mattresses and Beds

Agency for Health Care Policy and Research, Panel for the Treatment of Pressure Ulcers: *Treatment of pressure ulcers*, Clinical Practice Guideline No 15, AHCPR Pub No 95-0652, Rockville, Md, 1994, US Department of Health and Human Services.

Bergstrom N and others: Predicting pressure ulcer risk: a multisite study of the predictive validity of the Braden scale, *Nurs Res* 47(5):261, 1998.

Braden B, Maklebust J: Preventing pressure ulcers with the Braden scale: an update on this easy-to-use tool that assesses a patient's risk, *Am J Nurs* 105(6):70, 2005.

Brienza D, Geyer MJ: Using support surfaces to manage tissue integrity, *Adv Skin Wound Care* 18(3):152, 2005.

Bryant RA: *Acute and chronic wounds: nursing management*, ed 3, St Louis, 2007, Mosby.

Collins F: A practical guide to the provision of mattresses and cushions to relieve pressure, *Int J Ther Rehabil* 11(7):335, 2004.

Cullum N and others: Support surfaces for pressure ulcer prevention, *Cochrane Database of Systematic Reviews*, Hoboken, NJ, 2006, John Wiley & Sons.

Hockenberry MJ, Wilson D: *Wong's nursing care of infants and children*, ed 8, St Louis, 2007, Mosby.

Jiricka MC and others: Pressure ulcer risk factors in an ICU population, *Am J Crit Care* 4(5):361, 1995.

Lyder CH and others: Validating the Braden scale for the prediction of pressure ulcer risk in Black and Latino/Hispanic elders: a pilot study, *Ostomy Wound Manage* 44 (suppl A):42S, 1998.

Mackey D: Support surfaces: beds, mattresses, overlays-oh my! *Nurs Clin North Am* 40(2):21, 2005.

Maklebust J: Choosing the right support surface, *Adv Skin Wound Care* 18(3):158, 2005.

Meiner SE, Lueckenotte AG: *Gerontologic nursing*, ed 3, St Louis, 2006, Mosby.

Merk K: F314 and pressure relief, *Nurs Home Long Term Care Manage* 55(4):44, 2006.

Morrison MJ: *The prevention and treatment of pressure ulcers*, St Louis, 2001, Mosby.

Pieper B: Mechanical forces: pressure, shear, and friction. In Bryant RA: *Acute and chronic wounds: nursing management*, ed 2, St Louis, 2000, Mosby.

Tomaselli N, Goldberg E, Wind S: Pressure-reducing devices: lateral rotation therapy. In Lynn-McHale DJ, Carlson KK, editors: *AACN procedural manual for critical care*, ed 4, Philadelphia, 2001, Saunders.

Whittemore R: Pressure-reduction support surfaces: a review of the literature, *J Wound Ostomy Continence Nurs* 25(1):6, 1998.

Wound, Ostomy and Continence Nurses Society: *Guideline for prevention and management of pressure ulcers*, Glenview, Ill, 2003, WOCN.

Young T, Clark M: Re-positioning for pressure ulcer prevention, *Cochrane Database of Systematic Reviews* 3:1, 2006.

Chapter 26
Traction, Cast Care, and Immobilization Devices

Bakker JPJ and others: The effects of knee-ankle-foot orthoses in the treatment of Duchenne muscular dystrophy: review of the literature, *Clin Rehabil* 14(4):343, 2000.

Ball JW, Bindler RC: *Pediatric nursing: caring for children*, ed 3, Upper Saddle River, NJ, 2003, Prentice Hall.

Hockenberry MJ, Wilson D: *Wong's nursing care of infants and children*, ed 8, St Louis, 2007, Mosby.

Holmes SB, Brown SJ: Skeletal pin site care: National Association of Orthopaedic Nurses guidelines for orthopaedic nursing, *Orthop Nurs* 24(2):99-107, 2005.

Maher AB and others: *Orthopedic nursing*, ed 3, Philadelphia, 2002, Saunders.

Schoen DC: *Adult orthopaedic nursing*, Philadelphia, 2000, Lippincott.

Stanley M, Blaire KA, Beare PG: *Gerontological nursing: promoting successful aging with older adults*, ed 3, Philadelphia, 2005, FA Davis.

Yip E, Roman M: Latex protein allergy and your choice of gloves: a balanced consideration, *Medsurg Nurs* 12(1):20, 2003.

Chapter 27
Intravenous Therapy

American Association of Blood Banks: *Technical manual*, ed 15, Bethesda, Md, 2005, The Association.

Burke KG: Executive Summary: the state of the science on safe medication administration symposium, *J Infus Nurs* 28(2):87-92, 2005.

Centers for Disease Control and Prevention: Guidelines for the prevention of intravascular catheter-related infections, *MMWR* 52:No RR-10, 2002.

Cox JA and others: Home infusion therapy. Essential characteristics of a successful education process: a grounded theory study, *J Infus Nurs* 28(2):99-107, 2005.

Crosby CT, Mares AK: Skin antiseptic: past, present, and future, *J Vasc Access Devices* 6(2):26, 2001.

Curchoe RM: Weekly dressing changes linked to increased bacteremia rates, *Infect Control Hosp Epidemiol* 23(12):730-732, 2002.

Deacon VL: The safe medical device act and its impact on clinical practice, *J Infus Nurs* 27 (1):31-36, 2004.

Gillies D: Timing of intravenous administration set changes: a systemic review, *Infect Control Hosp Epidemiol* 25(3):240-250, 2004.

Hadaway LC: IV rounds. Skin flora: unwanted dead or alive, *Nursing* 35(7):20, 2005a.

Hadaway LC: Reopen the pipeline for IV therapy, *Nursing* 35(8):54-63, 2005b.

Hadaway LC: Technology of flushing vascular access devices, *J Infus Nurs* 29(3):137-145, 2006.

Hankins J and others: *Infusion therapy in clinical practice*, ed 2, Philadelphia, 2004, Saunders.

Hodgson B, Kizor RJ: *Saunders nursing drug handbook 2006*, St. Louis, 2006, Elsevier.

Infusion Nurses Society: *Back to basics: flushing 101*, INS Newsline 27(6):10, 2005, The Society.

Infusion Nurses Society: *Standards of practice* 29:(1S), 2006, The Society.

Joint Commission on Accreditation of Healthcare Organizations (JCAHO): 2007 Hospital/Critical Access Hospital National Patient Safety Goals, http://www.jointcommission.org/PatientSafety/NationalPatientSafetyGoals/07, accessed July 24, 2006.

Jones A: Dressings for the management of catheter sites: a review, *J Vasc Access Devices* 9(1):26-33, 2004.

Ketchum K and others: Medication reconciliation, *Am J Nurs* 105(11):78-85, 2005.

Macklin D, Chernecky C: Equipment and infusion regulation devices. In Macklin D, Chernecky C, editors: *Real world survival guide: IV therapy*, St Louis, 2004, Saunders.

Masoorli S: Consult stat. Can you really leave this dressing on all week? *RN* 68(7):58-60, 2005a.

Masoorli S: Consult stat. Help for nurses who flush too much, *RN* 68(5):72, 2005b.

McInally W: Whose line is it anyway? Management of central venous catheters in children, *Pediatr Nurs* 17(5):14-18, 2005.

McKnight S: Clinical practice. Nurse's guide to understanding and treating thrombotic occlusion of central venous devices, *Medsurg Nurs* 13(6):377-382, 2004.

Nakazawa N: Pharmacological management of vascular access devices, *Pharm Manage Vasc Devices* 11(1):1-7, 2005.

Occupational Safety and Health Administration: *Revision to OSHA's bloodborne pathogen standard*, April 2001, http://www.osha-sic.gov/needlesticks/needlefact.html.

Oncology Nursing Society: *Access device guidelines: recommendations for nursing practice and education*, ed 2, Pittsburgh, 2004, The Society.

Otto SE: *Pocket guide to infusion therapy*, ed 5, St Louis, 2005, Elsevier-Mosby.

Rickard CM: Routine changing of intravenous administration sets does not reduce colonization or infection in central venous catheters, *Infect Control Hosp Epidemiol* 25(8):650-655, 2004.

Rosenthal K: Guarding against vascular infection, *Nurs Manage* Suppl:4-10, November 2004.

Scarlet C: Anaphylaxis, *J Infus Nurs* 29(1):39-44, 2006.

Chapter 28
Fluid, Electrolyte, and Acid-Base Balance

Ebersole P and others: *Gerontological nursing & healthy aging*, ed 2, St Louis, 2005, Elsevier.

Hockenberry MJ, Wilson D: *Wong's nursing care of infants and children*, ed 8, St Louis, 2007, Mosby.

Lewis SM and others: *Medical-surgical nursing: assessment and management of clinical problems*, ed 6, St Louis, 2004, Mosby.

Meiner SE, Lueckenotte AG: *Gerontologic nursing*, ed 3, St Louis, 2006, Mosby.

Metheny N: *Fluid and electrolyte balance*, ed 4, Philadelphia, 2000, Lippincott.

Pullen RL: Performing a modified Allen test, *Nursing* 35(10):26, 2005.

Stotts NA, Hopf HW: The link between tissue oxygenation and hydration in nursing home residents with pressure ulcers: Preliminary data, *J Wound Ostomy Continence Nurs* 30:184-190, 2003.

Van Wissen K, Breton C: Perioperative influences on fluid distribution, *Medsurg Nurs* 13(5):304-311, 2004.

Chapter 29
Promoting Oxygenation

Allibone L: Nursing management of chest drains, *Nurs Stand* 17(22):45, 2003.

American Association of Respiratory Care: AARC clinical practice guideline, nasotracheal suction—2004 revision and update, *Resp Care* 49:1080, 2004.

American Association of Respiratory Care: AARC clinical practice guideline, suctioning of the patient in the home, *Resp Care* 44:99, 1999. http://www.rcjournal.com/online_resources/cpgs/pdtcpg.html, accessed November 2006.

Beers M and others, editors: *The Merk Manual of Geriatrics*, 2005, Merk and Co.

Carroll P: Improve your suctioning technique, *RN Web Magazine* 66(30), 2003, http://rnweb.com/rnweb/content/printContentPopup.jsp?id=107341, accessed November 15, 2005.

Carroll P: Providing age-appropriate pediatric respiratory care, *J Respir Care Pract*, vol 1, 2005, http://www.rtmagazine.com/articles.asp:articleid=r0501f02, accessed November 15, 2005.

Cigna J, Turner-Cigna L: Rehabilitation for the home care client with COPD, *Home Health Care Nurs* 23(9):578-584, 2005.

Finder JD: Airway clearance in the ICU: a critical need for improvement, *J Resp Care Pract* 18(3):28, 20005.

Fretag ML and others: Prolonged application of closed in-line suction catheters increase microbial colonization of lower respiratory tract bacterial growth on catheter surface, *Infection* 31(1):31, 2003.

Garp MJ and others: Oral care interventions in critical care: frequency and documentation, *Am J Crit Care* 12(2):114, 2005.

Garvey C: *Secretion clearance devices: coverage policies/cost*, 2005, ATS: American Thoracic Society Website Practice Tips.

Hockenberry MJ, Wilson D: *Wong's nursing care of infants and children*, ed 8, St Louis, 2007, Mosby.

Hockenberry MJ and others: *Wong's essentials of pediatric nursing*, ed 7, St Louis, 2005, Mosby.

Joanna Briggs Institute: *Best practice: tracheal suctioning of adults with an artificial airway*, vol 4, no 4, 2000, ISSN 1329-1874.

Lazzara D: 2002 Eliminate the air of mystery from chest tubes, *Nursing* 32(6):36-43, 2002, http://nursingcenter.com/prodev/cearticleprint.asp?CE_ID=272440, accessed November 15, 2005.

Lewis SL and others: *Medical surgical nursing, assessment and management of clinical problems*, ed 6, St Louis, 2004, Mosby.

Moore T: Suctioning techniques for the removal of respiratory secretions, *Nurs Stand* 18(9):47, 2003.

Pruitt WC, Jacobs M: Breathing lessons of oxygen therapy, *Nursing 2003* 13(10):43, 2003.

US Environmental Protection Agency: *Help your child gain control over asthma*, November 2004, http://www.epa.gov/asthma/pdfs/ll_asthma_brochure.pdf.

Zoidis JD: Peak flow monitoring for asthma, December 2005, *J Respir Care Pract*, Currant Communications, December 2005, http://www.rtmagazine.com/articles.asp:articleid=r0412f02, accessed November 15, 2005.

Chapter 30
Gastric Intubation

Colagiovanni L: Preventing and clearing blocked feeding tubes, *Nurs Times* 96(17 suppl):3-4, 2000.

Cottrell DB, Asturi E: Gastric intubation: assessment and intervention, *Crit Care Nurs Clin North Am* 16(4):489-493, 2004.

Ellett LMC and others: Gastric tube placement in young children, *Clin Nurs Res* 14(3):238-252, 2005.

Hockenberry MJ, Wilson D: *Wong's nursing care of infants and children*, ed 8, St Louis, 2007, Mosby.

Metheny and others: pH, color, and feeding tubes, *RN* 61(1):25, 1998a.

Metheny NA and others: Testing feeding tube placement auscultation vs. pH method, *Am J Nurs* 98(5):37, 1998b.

Metheny NA, Titler MG: Assessing placement of feeding tubes, *Am J Nurs* 101(5):36, 2001.

Chapter 31
Enteral Nutrition

American Association of Critical Care Nurses: Practice alert, Verification of Feeding Tube Placement, Aliso Viejo, Calif, 2005, The Association, http://www.aacn.org/AACN/aacnhome.nsf/vwdoc/ClinicalPractice, accessed December 2005.

ASPEN: American Society for Parenteral and Enteral Nutrition: Guidelines for the use of parenteral and enteral nutrition in adult and pediatric patients, *JPEN: J Parenter Enteral Nutr* 26:1SA-137SA, 2002.

Baskin WD: Acute complications associated with placement of feeding tube, *Nutr Clin Pract* 21(1):40, 2006.

Chen MY, Ott DJ, Gelfand DW: Nonfluoroscopic, postpyloric feeding tube placement: Number and cost of plain films for determining position, *Nutr Clin Pract* 14:40-44, 2000.

Gharpure V, Meert KL, Sarnaik AP, Metheny NA: Indicators of postpyloric feeding tube placement in children, *Crit Care Med* 28:2962-2966, 2000.

Hanson RL: Predictive criteria for length of nasogastric tube insertion for tube feeding, *JPEN: J Parenter Enteral Nutr* 3:160-163, 1979.

Hockenberry MJ, Wilson D: *Wong's nursing care of infants and children*, ed 8, St Louis, 2007, Mosby.

Lord LM and others: Comparison of weighted vs. unweighted enteral feeding tubes for efficacy of transpyloric intubation, *JPEN: J Parenter Enteral Nutr* 17:271-273, 1993.

Kittinger JW, Sandler RS, Heizer WD: Efficacy of metoclopramide as an adjunct to duodenal placement of small-bore feeding tubes: a randomized, placebo-controlled, double-blind study, *JPEN: J Parenter Enteral Nutr* 11:33-37, 1987.

Lebak KJ and others: What's new on defining diarrhea in tube-feeding studies? *Clin Nurs Res* 12:174, 2003.

McClave SA and others: Use of residual volume as a marker for enteral feeding intolerance: prospective blinded comparison with physical examination and radiographic findings, *JPEN J Parenter Enteral Nutr* 16(2):99, 1992.

Metheny N and others: Effectiveness of pH measurements in predicting feeding tube placement: an update, *Nurs Res* 42(6):323, 1993.

Metheny NA and others: pH testing of feeding-tube aspirates to determine placement, *Nutr Clin Pract* 9:185-190, 1994.

Metheny N and others: Detection of improperly positioned feeding tubes, *J Healthc Risk Manage* 18(3):37, 1998a.

Metheny N and others: pH, color, and feeding tubes, *RN* 61(1):25, 1998b.

Metheny N and others: Testing feeding tube placement: auscultation vs. pH method, *Am J Nurs* 98(5):37, 1998c.

Metheny NA: Inadvertent intracranial nasogastric tube placement, *Am J Nurs* 102:25, 2001, 2002.

Metheny NA, Titler MG: Assessing placement of feeding tubes, *Am J Nurs* 101:36-45, 2001.

Metheny NA, Stewart BJ: Testing feeding tube placement during continuous tube feedings, *Appl Nurs Res* 15:254-258, 2002.

Metheny NA, Schallom ML, and Edwards SJ: Effect of GI motility and feeding tube site on aspiration risk in critically ill patients: a review, *Heart Lung* 33:131, 2004.

Metheny NA and others: pH and concentration of bilirubin in feeding tube aspirates as predictors of tube placement, *Nurs Res* 48:189-197, 1999.

Metheny NA and others: Effect of feeding-tube properties on residual volume measurements in tube-fed patients, *JPEN: J Parenteral Enter Nutr* 29:192, 2005.

Padula CA and others: Enteral feedings: What the evidence says, *Am J Nurs* 104:62-70, 2004.

Pearce CB, Duncan HD: Enteral feeding. Nasogastric, nasojejunal, percutaneous endoscopic gastrostomy, or jejunostomy: Its indications and limitations, *Postgrad Med J* 78:198-204, 2002.

Silva CCR, Saconarto H, Atallah, AN: Metoclopramide for migration of naso-enteral tube, *Cochrane Database System Rev* 2002(4):CD003353, accessed August 10, 2006.

Welch SK: Certification of staff nurses to insert enteral feeding tubes using a research-based procedure, *Nutr Clin Pract* 11(1):21, 1996

Welch SJ and others: Comparison of four bedside indicators used to predict duodenal feeding tube placement with radiography, *JPEN: J Parenter Enteral Nutr* 18:525-530, 1994.

Chapter 32
Altered Bowel Elimination

Ball EM: Ostomy guide. II. A teaching guide for continent ileostomy, *RN* 63(12):35, 2000.

Black P: Practical stoma care, *Nurs Stand* 14(41):47, 2000.

Bliss DZ, Fischer LR, Savik K: Managing fecal incontinence-self care practices of older adults, *J Gerontol Nurs* 31(7):35, 2005.

Coggrave M and others: Management of faecal incontinence and constipation in adults with central neurological diseases (review), *Cochrane Database Systematic Rev*, The Cochrane Collaboration Volume (4), 2005.

Collwell JC, Goldberg MT, Carmel JE: *Fecal and urinary diversions, management principles*, St Louis, 2004, Mosby.

Collwell JC and others: The state of the standard diversion, *J Wound Ostomy Continence Nurse* 28(1):6, 2001.

Dosh SA: Evaluation and treatment of constipation, *J Fam Pract* 51(6):555, 2002.

Eberhardie C: Constipation: identifying the problem, *Nursing Older People* 15(9):22, 2003.

Ebersole P and others: *Toward a healthy aging: human needs and nursing response*, ed 6, St Louis, 2004, Mosby.

Erwin-Toth P: The effect of ostomy surgery between the ages of 6 and 12 years on psychosocial development during childhood, adolescence, and young adulthood, *J Wound Ostomy Continence Nurse* 16(2):77, 1999.

Erwin-Toth P: Ostomies and fistulas: prevention and management of peristomal skin complications, *Adv Skin Wound Care* 13(4):175, 2000.

Erwin-Toth P: Caring for a stoma is more than skin deep, *Nursing 2001* 31(5):36, 2001.

Erwin-Toth P: Ostomy pearls, *Adv Skin Wound Care* 16(3):146, 2003.

Hampton BG, Bryant RA: *Ostomies and continent diversions: nursing management*, St Louis, 1992, Mosby.

Hockenberry MJ, Wilson D: *Wong's nursing care of infants and children*, ed 8, St Louis, 2007, Mosby.

Jeffries C, MacKay AT: Improving stoma management in the low-vision patient, *J Wound Ostomy Continence Nurse* 24(6):302, 1997.

Lembo A, Camilleri M: Current concepts: chronic constipation, *N Engl J Med* 349(14):1360, 2003.

Meiner SE, Leuckenotte AG: *Gerontologic Nursing*, ed 3, St Louis, 2006, Mosby.

O'Shea HS: Teaching the adult ostomy patient, *J Wound Ostomy Continence Nurse* 28(1):47, 2001.

Prather C: Subtypes of constipation: sorting out the confusion, *Rev Gastroenterol Disorders* 4(suppl 2):S11-S16, 2004.

Rogers VE: Ostomy care: managing preemie stomas—more than just the pouch, *J Wound Ostomy Continence Nurse* 30(2):100, 2003.

Schiff L: Ostomy products, *RN* 63(11):71, 2000.

Thomason SS: Promoting outcomes for patients with spinal cord impairments and ostomies, *Medsurg Nurs* 9(2):77, 2000.

Thompson J: A practical ostomy guide, part I, *RN* 63(11):61, 2000.

Wound, Ostomy, and Continence Nurses Society (WOCN): *Peristomal skin complications: best practice for clinicians*, Glenview, Illinois, 2004a, WOCN Society.

Wound, Ostomy, and Continence Nurses Society (WOCN): *Basic ostomy skin care: a guide for patients and healthcare providers*, Glenview, Illinois, 2004b, WOCN Society.

Wound, Ostomy, and Continence Nurses Society (WOCN): *Stoma complications: best practice for clinicians*, Glenview, Illinois, 2005, WOCN Society.

Chapter 33
Altered Urinary Elimination

Brosnahan JE. Short-term indwelling catheters (a systematic review): evidence for a primary nursing decision, *Worldview Evidence-Based Nurs* 1(4):228, 2004.

Centers for Medicare & Medicaid Services: *Revised long-term care resident assessment instrument user's manual Version 2.0*, Miamisburg, Ohio, 2003, Heaton Resources Med-Pass.

Colwell JC, Goldberg, MT, Carmel, JE: *Fecal and urinary diversions: management principles*, Mosby, 2004, St Louis.

Daneshgari F and others: Evidence-based multidisciplinary practice: improving the safety and standards of male bladder catheterization, *MedSurg Nurs* 11(5):236, 2002.

Dixon L, Wasson D, JohnsonV: Urinary diversions: a review of nursing care, *Urologic Nurs* 21(5):337-346. 2001.

Emr K, Ryan R: Best practice for indwelling catheter in the home setting, *Home Health Nurs* 22(12):820-830, 2004.

Fallis WM: Indwelling Foley catheters. Is the current design a source of erroneous measurement of urine output? *Crit Care Nurs* 25(2):44-50, 2005.

Fernandez RS, Griffiths RD: Clamping short-term indwelling catheters: a systematic review of the evidence, *J Wound Ostomy Continence Nurse* 32(5):329-336, 2005.

Getliffe K: Managing recurrent urinary catheter blockage: problems, promises, and practicalities, *J Wound Ostomy Continence Nurse* 30(3):146-151, 2003.

Gray M: Expert review: best practices in managing the indwelling catheter, *Perspectives* 25(1):1-12, 2006.

Gray M: What nursing interventions reduce risk of symptomatic urinary tract infection in the patient with an indwelling catheter, *J Wound Ostomy Continence Nurse* 31(1):3-13, 2004.

Guidelines for preventing infections associated with insertion and maintenance of short-term indwelling urethral catheters, available at http://www.doh.gov.uk/HAI, accessed January 4, 2004.

Hanchett M: Techniques for stabilizing urinary catheters, *Am J Nurs* 102(3):44-48, 2002.

Hockenberry MJ, Wilson D: *Wong's nursing care of infants and children*, ed 8, St Louis, 2007, Mosby.

Horn SD and others: The national pressure ulcer long-term care study: pressure ulcer development in long-term care residents, *J Am Geriatric Soc* 52(3):359-367, 2004.

Joint Commission on the Accreditation of Healthcare Organization: *2005 national patient safety goals, 2005 critical access hospitals national patient safety goals*, www.jcaho.org/accredited+organization/patientsafety/npsg.htm, accessed July 2004.

Marklew A: Urinary catheter care in the intensive care unit, *Nurs Crit Care* 9(1):21-27, 2004.

Newman DK: Incontinence products and devices for the elderly, *Urol Nurs* 24(4):316-333, 2004.

Ryder MA: Catheter-related infections: it's all about biofilm, *Topics Adv Pract Nurs eJournal* 5(3), 2005, Medscape http://www.medscape.com/viewarticle/508109, accessed October 23, 2005.

Smith JM: Indwelling catheter management: from habit-based to evidence-based practice, *Ostomy Wound Manage* 49(12):34-45, 2003a.

Smith L: Which catheter? Criteria for selection of urinary catheters for children, *Pediatr Nurs* 15(2):14-18, 2003b.

Sparks A and others: The clinical benefits of the bladder scanner: a research synthesis, *J Nurs Care Quality* 19(3):188-192, 2004.

Stevens E: Bladder ultrasound: avoiding unnecessary catheterizations, *MedSurg Nurs* 14(4):249-253, 2005.

Teng D and others: Application of portable ultrasound scanners in the measurement of post-void residual urine, *J Nur Res* 13(3):216-224, 2005.

Toughill E: Indwelling urinary catheters, *Am J Nurs* 105(5):35-37, 2005.

Trautner BW, Hull R, Daroviche RO: Prevention of catheter-associated urinary tract infection, *Curr Opinion Infect Dis* 18(1):37-41, 2005.

Wilde MH: Urinary catheter management for the older adult patient, *Clin Geriatrics* 12(4):26-32, 2004.

Chapter 34
Altered Sensory Perception

Boyd-Monk H: Bringing common eye emergencies into focus, *Nursing 2005* 35(12):46-51, 2005.

Ebersole P, Hess P, Luggen A: *Toward healthy aging,* ed 6, St Louis, 2004, Mosby.

Hockenberry MJ, Wilson D: *Wong's nursing care of infants and children,* ed 8, St Louis, 2007, Mosby.

Kolberg Ocular Prosthetics: *Artificial eye information and patient support page,* available at http://www.artificialeye.net/index.html, last updated November 22, 2005.

McKenry LM and others: *Mosby's pharmacology in nursing,* ed 22, St Louis, 2006, Mosby.

National Institute on Deafness and Other Communication Disorders: *Health information: hearing aids,* available at http://www. nided.nih.gov/health/hearing/thebasics_hearingaid.asp, last updated June 28, 2004.

National Institute on Deafness and Other Communication Disorders: *Health information: hearing loss and older adults,* http://www. nided.nih.gov/health/hearing/older.asp, last updated February 25, 2005.

Occupational Safety & Health Administration: *Eye protection for the workplace,* 2005, US Department of Labor: available at http://www.osha.gov, last updated November 27, 2005.

Phipps W and others: *Medical-surgical nursing: health and illness perspectives,* ed 7, St Louis, 2003, Mosby.

Slaven A: Communication and the hearing impaired patient, *Nurs Standard* 18(12):39-41,2003.

Sommer S, Sommer N: When your patient is hearing impaired, *RN* 65(12):28-32, 2002.

Chapter 35
Emergency Measures for Life Support in the Hospital Setting

Aufderheide T and others: Community lay rescuer automated external defibrillation programs, *Circulation* 113(9):260-270, 2006.

American Heart Association: 2005 American Heart Association guidelines for cardiopulmonary resuscitation and emergency cardiovascular care, *Circulation* 112(Suppl I): IV1-IV5, 2005a.

American Heart Association: Part 3: Overview of CPR, *Circulation* 112(Suppl I):IV12-IV17, 2005b.

American Heart Association: Part 7.2: Management of cardiac arrest, *Circulation* 112(Suppl I):IV-58, 2005c.

Craig KJ, Hopkins-Pepe L: Understanding the new AHA guidelines, Part II, *Nursing 2006* 36(5):52, 2006.

Ditto PH and others: Advance directives as acts of communication: a randomized control trial, *Arch Intern Med* 161(3):421, 2001.

Hockenberry MJ, Wilson D: *Wong's nursing care of infants and children,* ed 8, St Louis, 2007, Mosby.

Chapter 36
Care of the Client with Special Needs

AACN: *Ventilator-associated pneumonia practice alert,* 2004, available at www.aacn.org.

Ahrens T, Sona C: Capnography application in acute and critical care, *AACN Clin Issues* 14(2):123, 2003.

American College of Emergency Physicians: Verification of endotracheal tube placement (Policy 400307 approved 2001), American College of Emergency Physicians, www.acep.org/Webportal/PracticeResources, accessed November 27, 2006.

Carey HB and others: Continuous peritoneal dialysis and the extended care facility, *Am J Kidney Dis* 37(3):580, 2001.

Centers for Disease Control and Prevention (CDC): *Guidelines for preventing health-care associated pneumonia,* MMWR 2003/53RR03;1, May, 2004.

Ely EW and others: Mechanical ventilator weaning protocols driven by non physician health care professionals: evidenced-based clinical practice guidelines, *Chest* 120(6 suppl):4545, 2001.

Garp MJ and others: Oral care interventions in critical care: frequency and documentation, *Am J Crit Care,* 12(2):114, 2003.

Ignatavicius DD, Workman ML: *Medical-surgical nursing: critical thinking for collaborative care,* ed 4, Philadelphia, 2002, Saunders.

Infusion Nurses Society: Infusion Nursing Standards of Practice, *J Infusion Nurs* 29S:1, 2006.

Joint Commission on the Accreditation of Health Care Organizations: *2006 Critical access hospital and hospital national patient safety goals,* Joint Commission International Center for Patient Safety, 2006, The Commission, available at http://www.jcipatientsafety.org, accessed May 12, 2006.

Mermel LA and others: Guidelines for the management of intravascular catheter-related infections, *Clin Infect Dis* 32:1249, 2001.

Robinson MK and others: Improved care and reduced costs for patients requiring peripherally inserted central catheters: the role of bedside ultrasound and a dedicated team, *JPEN: J Parenter Enteral Nutr* 29:374, 2005.

Chapter 37
Palliative Care

Briggs L, Colvin E: The nurse's role in end-of-life decision making for patients and families, *Geriatr Nurs* 23(6):302-310, 2002.

Buckley J, Herth K: Fostering hope in terminally ill patients, *Nurs Standard* 19(10):33-41, 2004.

Derby S, O'Mahony S: Elderly patients. In Ferrell B, Coyle N, editors: *Textbook of palliative nursing*, New York, 2006, Oxford Press, pp 635-659.

Douglass A, Maxwell T, Whitecar P: Principles of palliative care medicine, Part I, Patient assessment, *Adv Studies Med* 4(1):15-20, 2004.

Ersek M: Artificial nutrition and hydration: clinical issues, *J Hospice Palliative Nurs* 5(4):231-233, 2003.

Ferrell B, Coyle N: *Textbook of palliative nursing*, ed 2, New York, 2006, Oxford University Press.

Harstäde C, Andershed B: Good palliative care: How and where? The patient's opinions, *J Hospice Palliative Nurs* 6(1):27-35, 2004.

Hellsten M, Kane J: Symptom management in pediatric palliative care. In Ferrell B, Coyle N, editors: *Textbook of palliative nursing*, New York, 2006, Oxford Press, pp 895-908.

Kemp C, Bhungalia S: Culture and the end of life: a review of major world religions, *J Hospice Palliative Nurs* 4(4):235-242, 2002.

Kolcaba K and others: Efficacy of hand massage for enhancing the comfort of hospice patients, *J Hospice Palliative Nurs* 6(2):91-101, 2004.

Koenig H: *Spirituality in patient care: why, how, when and what*, Radnor, Penn, 2002, Templeton Press.

Kübler-Ross E: *On death and dying*, New York, 1969, Macmillan.

Matzo M, Sherman D: *Palliative care nursing: quality care to the end of life*, New York, 2006, Springer.

Mauk KL, Schmidt NK: *Spiritual care in nursing practice*, Philadelphia, 2004, Lippincott Williams & Wilkins.

Paice J, Fine P: Pain at the end of life. In Ferrell B, Coyle N, editors: *Textbook of palliative nursing*, New York, 2006, Oxford Press, pp 131-153.

Panke J: Difficulties in managing pain at the end of life, *J Hospice Palliative Nurs* 5(2):83-90, 2003.

Pitorak E: Care at the time of death, *Am J Nurs* 103(7):42-52, 2003.

Sherman D: Nurses' stress and burnout, *Am J Nurs* 104(5):48-56, 2004.

Stanley K: The healing power of presence: a respite from the fear of abandonment, *Oncol Nurs Forum* 29(6):935-940, 2002.

Valente S: End of life and ethnicity, *J Nurses Staff Dev* 20(6):285-293, 2004.

Vandecreek L, Lucas A, editors: *The discipline for pastoral caregiving: foundations for outcome oriented chaplaincy*, Binghamton, NY, 2001, Haworth Press.

Wakefield A: Nurses' response to death and dying: a need for relentless self-care, *Int J Palliative Nurs* 6(5):245-258, 2000.

Wentz DJ: Controlling pain: assessing pain at the end of life, *Nursing 2003* 33(8):22, 2003.

Whitecar P, Maxwell T, Douglass A: 2004 Principles of palliative care medicine, Part 2, Pain and symptom management, *Adv Studies Med* 4(2):88-99, 2004.

Chapter 38
Discharge Teaching and Home Health Management

American Association of Respiratory Care: AARC clinical practice guideline: oxygen therapy in the home of extended care facility, *Resp Care* 37:918, 1992.

American Diabetes Association: Insulin administration, *Diabetes Care* 27(S1):S106, 2004.

American Hospital Association: *Patient care partnership: understanding expectations, rights, and responsibilities*, Chicago, 2003, The Association.

Aud MA: Residents with dementia in assisted-living facilities: the role of behavior in discharge decisions, *J Gerontol Nurs* 30(6):6, 2004.

Bastable S: *Nurse as educator: principles of teaching and learning for nursing practice*, Sudbury, Mass, 2003, Jones & Bartlett Publishers.

Centers for Disease Control and Prevention (CDC): *Healthy people 2010*, 2005, available at http://www.cdc.gov/nchs/hphome.htm#Healthy%20People%202010.

Ebersole P and others: *Toward healthy aging: human needs and nursing response*, ed 6, St Louis, 2004, Mosby.

Edelman CL, Mandle CL: *Health promotion throughout the lifespan*, ed 6, St Louis, 2006, Mosby.

Falvo DR: *Effective patient education: a guide to increased compliance*, ed 3, Boston, 2004, Jones & Bartlett Publishers.

Ferreira CAS and others: Evaluation of health-related quality of life in low-income patients with COPD receiving long-term oxygen therapy, *Chest* 123(1):136, 2003.

Findeisen M: Long-term oxygen therapy in the home, *Home Healthc Nurse* 19(11):692, 2001.

Futrell M, Melillo KD: *Evidence-based protocol: wandering*, The University of Iowa Gerontological Nursing Interventions Research Center, Research Dissemination Core, Iowa City, Iowa, 2002, University of Iowa.

Haynes RB and others: Helping patients follow prescribed treatment: clinical applications, *JAMA* 288(22):2280, 2002.

Hendrickson SG: Reaching an underserved population with a randomly assigned home safety intervention, *Injury Prev* 11(5):313, 2005.

Hockenberry MJ and others: *Wong's essentials of pediatric nursing*, ed 7, St Louis, 2005, Mosby.

Hurley AC and others: Promoting safer home environments for persons with Alzheimer's disease: the home safety/injury model, *J Gerontol Nurs* 30(6):43, 2004.

Joint Commission on Accreditation of Healthcare Organizations: *Comprehensive accreditation manual for hospital standard: the official handbook*, Oak Brook, Ill, 2004, The Commission.

King WJ and others: Long-term effects of a home visit to prevent childhood injury: three year follow up of a randomized trial, *Injury Prev* 11(2):106, 2005.

Kotecha S, Allen J: Oxygen therapy for infants with chronic lung disease, *Arch Dis Child Fetal Neonatal Ed* 87(1):F11, 2002.

Lacasse Y: Prevalence of depressive symptoms and depression in patients with severe oxygen-dependent chronic obstructive pulmonary disease, *J Cardiopulmonary Rehabil* 21(2):80, 2001.

Lai CKY, Arthur DG: Wandering behaviour in people with dementia, *J Adv Nurs* 44(2):173, 2003.

Meiner SE, Lueckenotte AG: *Gerontologic nursing*, ed 3, St Louis, 2006, Mosby.

Nemours Foundation: Household safety checklists, 2005, available at http://www.kidshealth.org/parent/firstaid_safe/home/household_checklist.html.

Occupational Safety and Health Administration (OSHA): Occupational exposure to bloodborne pathogens; needlestick and other sharp injuries: final rule, *Fed Reg* CFR 29, part 1910(66:5317-5325), January 18, 2001, available at http://www.osha.gov/pls/oshaweb/owadisp.show_document?p_table=STANDARDS&p_id=10051.

Pender NJ and others: *Health promotion in nursing practice*, ed 5, Upper Saddle River, 2006, Prentice Hall.

Petty TL: *Guide to prescribing home oxygen: home oxygen options*, available at http://www.nlhep.org/resources/Prescb-Hm-Oxygen/home-oxygen-options-4.html, National Lung Health Education Program, 2004, accessed November 18, 2006.

Porter EJ: Wearing and using personal emergency response system buttons: older frail widows' intentions, *J Gerontol Nurs* 31(10):26, 2005.

Positive Air, Inc: *Medicare requirements for the home use of oxygen*, (see §60-9; Intermediary Manual, Part 3, §3113ff; and Medicare Carriers Manual, Part 3, §2100ff.), available at http://www.positiveair.com/medicare_home_use_of_oxygen.htm, accessed July 27, 2006.

Redman B: *The practice of patient education*, ed 9, St Louis, 2001, Mosby.

Schommer JC and others: Interdisciplinary medication education in a church environment, *Am J Health Syst Pharm* 59(5):423, 2002.

Shenassa, E and others: Safer storage of firearms at home and risk of suicide: a study of protective factors in a nationally representative sample, *J Epidemiol Commun Health* 58(10):841, 2004.

Sorrentino C and others: Using the Internet to deliver patient-education materials, *Clin J Oncol Nurs* 6(6):354, 2002.

Tideiksaar R: Best practice approach to fall prevention in community-living elders, *Geriatr Rehabil* 19(3):199, 2003.

Wilson FL and others: Literacy, readability and cultural barriers: critical factors to consider when educating older African-Americans about anticoagulation therapy, *J Clin Nurs* 12(2):275, 2003.

Index

*f indicates figure; t indicates table; b indicates box.